LANCHESTER LIBRARY
3 8001 00543 4570

KT-519-442

FOURTH EDITION

Handbook of VITAMINS

FOURTH
EDITION

Handbook of VITAMINS

Edited by

Janos Zempleni
Robert B. Rucker
Donald B. McCormick
John W. Suttie

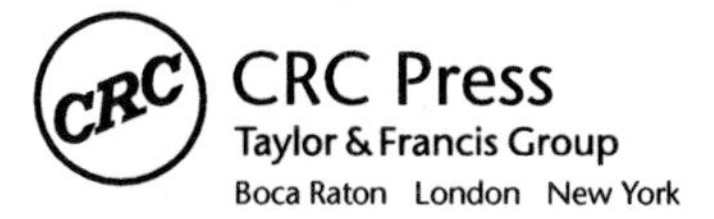

CRC Press is an imprint of the
Taylor & Francis Group, an **informa** business

CRC Press
Taylor & Francis Group
6000 Broken Sound Parkway NW, Suite 300
Boca Raton, FL 33487-2742

Printed in the United States of America on acid-free paper
10 9 8 7 6 5 4 3 2 1

International Standard Book Number-10: 0-8493-4022-5 (Hardcover)
International Standard Book Number-13: 978-0-8493-4022-2 (Hardcover)

Library of Congress Cataloging-in-Publication Data

Handbook of vitamins / editors, Robert B. Rucker ... [et al.]. -- 4th ed.
p. ; cm.
Includes bibliographical references and index.
ISBN-13: 978-0-8493-4022-2 (hardcover : alk. paper)
ISBN-10: 0-8493-4022-5 (hardcover : alk. paper)
1. Vitamins. 2. Vitamins in human nutrition. I. Rucker, Robert B.
[DNLM: 1. Nutrition Physiology--Handbooks. 2. Vitamins--Handbooks. QU 39 H361 2007]

QP771. H35 2007
612.3'99--dc22 2006100138

Visit the Taylor & Francis Web site at
http://www.taylorandfrancis.com

and the CRC Press Web site at
http://www.crcpress.com

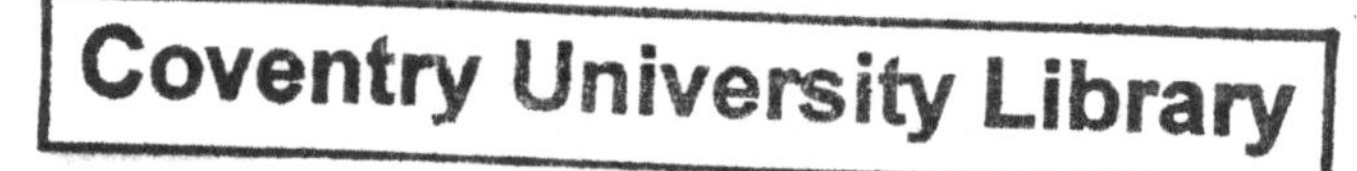

Table of Contents

Preface

In keeping with the tradition of previous editions, the fourth edition of the *Handbook of Vitamins* was assembled to update and provide contemporary perspectives on dietary accessory factors commonly classified as vitamins. One of the challenges in assembling this volume was to maintain the clinical focus of previous editions, while addressing important concepts that have evolved in recent years owing to the advances in molecular and cellular biology as well as those in analytical chemistry and nanotechnology. The reader will find comprehensive summaries that focus on chemical, physiological, and nutritional relationships and highlights of newly described and identified functions for all the recognized vitamins. Our goal was to assemble the best currently available reference text on vitamins for an audience ranging from basic scientists to clinicians to advanced students and educators with a commitment to better understanding vitamin function.

As examples, apparent vitamin-dependent modifications that are important to epigenetic events and genomic stability are described, as well as new information on the role and importance of maintaining optimal vitamin status for antioxidant and anti-inflammatory defense. Important analytical advances in vitamin analysis and assessment are discussed in a chapter dealing with accelerated mass spectrometry (AMS) applications. Recent AMS applications have provided the basis for studies of vitamin metabolism and turnover in humans at levels corresponding to physiological concentrations and fluxes. It is also important to underscore that much of the interest in vitamins stems from an appreciation that there remains regrettably sizable populations at risk for vitamin deficiencies. In this regard, classic examples are included along with examples of vitamin-related polymorphisms and genetic factors that influence the relative needs for given vitamins.

This volume is written by a group of authors who have made major contributions to our understanding of vitamins. Over half of the authors are new to this series; each chapter is written by individuals who have made clearly important contributions in their respective areas of research as judged by the scientific impact of their work. In addition, Dr. Janos Zempleni joins the group of editors who assembled the third edition. Dr. Zempleni adds a molecular biology perspective to complement the biochemical and physiological expertise of the other editors. We also wish to note that we miss the input of Dr. Lawrence Machlin, a renowned researcher on vitamin E, who was sole editor of the first two editions in this series and who died shortly after the release of the third edition. We know that he would be pleased with the progress and advances in vitamin research summarized in the fourth edition.

This volume comes at an important time and represents a new treatment of this topic. With the possible exception of the earlier days of vitamin discovery, this period of vitamin research is particularly exciting because of the newly identified roles of vitamins in cellular and organismal regulation and their obvious and continuing importance in health and disease.

Janos Zempleni
Robert B. Rucker
Donald B. McCormick
John W. Suttie

Editors

Janos Zempleni received his undergraduate and graduate training in nutrition at the University of Giessen in Germany. He received postdoctoral training in nutrition, biochemistry, and molecular biology at the University of Innsbruck (Austria), Emory University, and Arkansas Children's Hospital Research Institute. Janos Zempleni is currently an assistant professor of molecular nutrition at the University of Nebraska at Lincoln. He has published more than 100 manuscripts and books and is the recipient of the 2006 Mead Johnson Award by the American Society for Nutrition. Zempleni's research focuses on roles of the vitamin biotin in chromatin structure.

Robert B. Rucker received his PhD in biochemistry from Purdue University in 1968 and worked for two years as a postdoctoral fellow at the University of Missouri, before joining the faculty of nutrition at the University of California (UC), Davis, in 1970. He currently holds the title of distinguished professor. He serves as vice chair of the department of nutrition in the College of Agriculture and Environmental Sciences and holds an appointment in endocrinology, nutrition, and vascular medicine, department of internal medicine, UC Davis, School of Medicine.

Dr. Rucker's research focuses on cofactor function. His current research addresses problems associated with extracellular matrix assembly, the role of copper in early growth and development, and the physiological roles of quinone cofactors derived from tyrosine, such as pyrroloquinoline quinone.

Honors and activities include serving as a past president, American Society for Nutrition; appointment as a fellow in the American Association for the Advancement of Science and the American Society for Nutrition; service as chair or cochairperson for FASEB Summer and Gordon Conferences; service on Program and Executive Committees for American Society for Nutrition and FASEB, as well as service on committees of the Society for Experimental Biology and Medicine. He also currently serves as senior associate editor, *American Journal of Clinical Nutrition* and is a past editorial board member of the *Journal of Nutrition, Experimental Biology and Medicine, Nutrition Research*, and the *Annual Review of Nutrition.* He is a past recipient of UC Davis and the American Society for Nutrition Research awards.

Donald B. McCormick earned his bachelor's degree (chemistry and math, 1953) and doctorate (biochemistry, 1958) at Vanderbilt University in Nashville, Tennessee. His dissertation was on pentose and pentitol metabolism. He was then an NIH postdoctoral fellow (1958–1960) at the University of California-Berkeley, where his research was on enzymes that convert vitamin B_6 to the coenzyme pyridoxal phosphate. He has had sabbatics in the chemistry departments in Basel University (Switzerland) and in the University of Arizona, and in the biochemistry department in Wageningen (Netherlands).

Dr. McCormick's academic appointments have been at Cornell University (1960–1978) in Ithaca, New York, where he became the Liberty Hyde Bailey Professor of nutritional biochemistry and at Emory University (1979–present) in Atlanta, Georgia, where he served as the Fuller E. Callaway professor and chairman of the department of biochemistry and the executive associate dean for basic sciences in the school of medicine. His research has been on cofactors with emphases on chemistry, biochemistry, and nutrition of vitamins (especially B_6, riboflavin, biotin, and lipoate), coenzymes, and metal ions.

Dr. McCormick has been a consultant and served on numerous committees that include service for NIH, NCI, FASEB, IOM/NAS, NASA, FAO/WHO, and several organizing groups for international symposia on cofactors. He has been on the editorial boards of several journals of biochemistry and nutrition, and he has served as editor of volumes on vitamins and coenzymes in the *Methods in Enzymology* series, *Vitamins and Hormones*, the *Handbook of Vitamins*, and the *Annual Review of Nutrition.*

Dr. McCormick is a member of numerous scientific societies, including those in biochemistry and nutrition and has received such honors as a Westinghouse Science Scholarship, Guggenheim Fellowship, Wellcome Visiting Professorships (University of Florida, Medical College of Pennsylvania), and named visiting professorships (University of California-Davis, University of Missouri). He has received awards from the American Institute of Nutrition (Mead Johnson, Osborne and Mendel) and Bristol-Myers Squibb/Mead Johnson Award for Distinguished Achievement in Nutrition Research. He is a fellow of AAAS and a fellow of the American Society of Nutritional Sciences.

John W. Suttie is the Katherine Berns Van Donk Steenbock professor emeritus in the department of biochemistry and former chair of the department of nutritional sciences at the University of Wisconsin-Madison. He has broad expertise in biochemistry and human nutrition. Dr. Suttie received his BS, MS, and PhD degrees from the University of Wisconsin-Madison. He was an NIH postdoctoral fellow at the National Institute for Medical Research, Mill Hill, England, before joining the University of Wisconsin faculty. His research activities are directed toward the metabolism, mechanism of action, and nutritional significance of vitamin K. Dr. Suttie has served as president of the American Society for Nutritional Sciences (ASNS) and recently resigned his position as editor-in-chief of *The Journal of Nutrition.* He has received the Mead Johnson Award, the Osborne and Mendel Award, and the Conrad Elvehjem Award of the ASNS, the ARS Atwater Lectureship, and the Bristol Myers-Squibb Award for Distinguished Achievement in Nutrition Research. In 1996 Dr. Suttie was elected to the National Academy of Sciences. He has served as chairman of the Board of Experimental Biology, as president of the Federation of American Societies for Experimental Biology (FASEB), and as a member of the NRC's Board on Agriculture and Natural Resources, the FDA Blood Products Advisory Committee, and the American Heart Association Nutrition Committee. He presently serves on the Public Policy Committees of the ASNS and the American Society for Biochemistry and Molecular Biology (ASBMB), the USDA/NAREEE Advisory Board, the ILSI Food, Nutrition and Safety Committee, and the Food and Nutrition Board of the Institute of Medicine.

Contributors

Lynn B. Bailey
Department of Food Science and Human Nutrition
University of Florida
Gainesville, Florida

Susan I. Barr
Department of Food, Nutrition, and Health
University of British Columbia
Vancouver, British Columbia, Canada

Chris J. Bates
MRC Human Nutrition Research
Elsie Widdowson Laboratory
Cambridge, United Kingdom

Kathryn Bauerly
Department of Nutrition
University of California
Davis, California

Linda K. Buckles
Department of Biochemistry and Molecular Biology
University of Nebraska Medical Center
Omaha, Nebraska

Betty Jane Burri
Department of Nutrition
University of California
Davis, California

Judith K. Christman
Department of Biochemistry and Molecular Biology and UNMC/Eppley Cancer Center
University of Nebraska Medical Center
Omaha, Nebraska

Andrew J. Clifford
Department of Nutrition
University of California
Davis, California

Krishnamurti Dakshinamurti
Department of Biochemistry and Medical Genetics
University of Manitoba
Winnipeg, Manitoba, Canada

Shyamala Dakshinamurti
Department of Pediatrics and Physiology
University of Manitoba
Winnipeg, Manitoba, Canada

Timothy A. Garrow
Department of Food Science and Human Nutrition
University of Illinois at Urbana-Champaign
Urbana, Illinois

Ralph Green
Department of Pathology and Laboratory Medicine
University of California
Davis, California

Earl H. Harrison
Department of Human Nutrition
The Ohio State University
Columbus, Ohio

Helen L. Henry
Department of Biochemistry
University of California
Riverside, California

Carol S. Johnston
Department of Nutrition
Arizona State University
Mesa, Arizona

James B. Kirkland
Department of Human Health and Nutritional Sciences
University of Guelph
Guelph, Ontario, Canada

Donald B. McCormick
Department of Biochemistry
Emory University
Atlanta, Georgia

Joshua W. Miller
Department of Pathology and Laboratory Medicine
University of California
Davis, California

Donald M. Mock
Department of Biochemistry and Molecular Biology
University of Arkansas for Medical Sciences
Little Rock, Arkansas

Fabiana Fonseca de Moura
Department of Nutrition
University of California
Davis, California

Suzanne P. Murphy
Cancer Research Center of Hawaii
University of Hawaii
Honolulu, Hawaii

Anthony W. Norman
Department of Biochemistry
University of California
Riverside, California

Richard S. Rivlin
Department of Medicine
Weill Medical College of Cornell University
New York, New York

A. Catharine Ross
Department of Nutritional Sciences
Pennsylvania State University
University Park, Pennsylvania

Robert B. Rucker
Department of Nutrition
University of California
Davis, California

Francene M. Steinberg
Department of Nutrition
University of California
Davis, California

John W. Suttie
Department of Biochemistry
University of Wisconsin
Madison, Wisconsin

Maret G. Traber
Department of Nutrition and Exercise Sciences, Linus Pauling Institute
Oregon State University
Corvallis, Oregon

Janos Zempleni
Department of Nutrition and Health Sciences
University of Nebraska
Lincoln, Nebraska

1 Vitamin A: Nutritional Aspects of Retinoids and Carotenoids

A. Catharine Ross and Earl H. Harrison

CONTENTS

INTRODUCTION

Vitamin A (retinol) is an essential micronutrient for all vertebrates. It is required for normal vision, reproduction, embryonic development, cell and tissue differentiation, and immune function. Many aspects of the transport and metabolism of vitamin A, as well as its functions, are well conserved among species. Dietary vitamin A is ingested in two main forms—preformed vitamin A (retinyl esters and retinol) and provitamin A carotenoids (β-carotene, α-carotene, and β-cryptoxanthin)—although the proportion of vitamin A obtained from each of these form varies considerably among animal species and among individual human diets. These precursors serve as substrates for the biosynthesis of two essential metabolites of vitamin A: 11-*cis*-retinal, required for vision, and all-*trans*-retinoic acid, required for cell differentiation and the regulation of gene transcription in nearly all tissues.

Research on vitamin A now spans nine decades. Over 34,000 citations to vitamin A, 7,000 to β-carotene, and 20,000 to retinoic acid can be found in the National Library of Medicine's PubMed database [1], covering topics related to nutrition, biochemistry, molecular and cell biology, physiology, toxicology, public health, and medical therapy. Besides the naturally occurring forms of vitamin A indicated earlier, numerous structural analogs have been synthesized. Some retinoids have become widely used as therapeutic agents, particularly in the treatment of dermatological diseases and certain cancers.

In this chapter, we focus first on vitamin A from a nutritional perspective, addressing its chemical forms and properties, the nutritional equivalency of compounds that provide vitamin A activity, and current dietary recommendations. We then cover the metabolism of carotenoids and vitamin A. Finally, we provide a brief discussion of the key uses of vitamin A and retinoids in public health and medicine, referring to their benefits as well as some of the adverse effects caused by ingesting excessive amounts of this highly potent group of compounds.

NUTRITIONAL ASPECTS OF VITAMIN A AND CAROTENOIDS

Historical

Vitamin A was discovered in the early 1900s by McCollum and colleagues at the University of Wisconsin and independently by Osborne and Mendel at Yale. Both groups were studying the effects of diets made from purified protein and carbohydrate sources, such as casein and rice flour, on the growth and survival of young rats. They observed that growth ceased and the animals died unless the diet was supplemented with butter, fish oils, or a quantitatively minor ether-soluble fraction extracted from these substances, from milk, or from meats. The unknown substance was then called "fat-soluble A." Not long thereafter, it was recognized that the yellow carotenes present in plant extracts had similar nutritional properties, and it was postulated that this carotenoid fraction could give rise through metabolism to the bioactive form of fat-soluble A, now called vitamin A, in animal tissues. This was shown to be correct after β-carotene and retinol were isolated and characterized, and it was shown that dietary β-carotene gives rise to retinol in animal tissues. Within the first few decades of vitamin A research, vitamin A deficiency was shown to cause several specific disease conditions, including xerophthalmia; squamous metaplasia of epithelial and mucosal tissues; increased susceptibility to infections; and abnormalities of reproduction. Each of these seminal discoveries paved the way for many subsequent investigations that have greatly expanded our knowledge about vitamin A. Although the discoveries made in the early 1900s may now seem long ago, it is interesting to note, as reviewed by Wolf [2], that physicians in ancient Egypt, around 1500 BC, were already using the liver of ox, a very rich source of vitamin A, to cure what is now referred to as night blindness.

Definitions of Vitamin A, Retinoids, and Carotenoids

Vitamin A is a generic term that refers to compounds with the biological activity of retinol. These include the provitamin A carotenoids, principally β-carotene, α-carotene, and β-cryptoxanthin, which are provided in the diet by green and yellow or orange vegetables and some fruits and preformed vitamin A, namely retinyl esters and retinol itself, present in foods of animal origin, mainly in organ meats such as liver, other meats, eggs, and dairy products.

The term retinoid was coined to describe synthetically produced structural analogs of the naturally occurring vitamin A family, but the term is now used for natural as well as synthetic compounds [3]. Retinoids and carotenoids are defined based on molecular structure. According to the Joint Commission on Biochemical Nomenclature of the International Union of Pure and Applied Chemistry and International Union of Biochemistry and Molecular Biology (IUPAC–IUB), retinoids are "a class of compounds consisting of four isoprenoid units joined in a head-to-tail manner" [4]. All-*trans*-retinol is the parent molecule of this family. The retinoid molecule can be divided into three parts: a trimethylated cyclohexene ring, a conjugated tetraene side chain, and a polar carbon–oxygen functional group. Additional examples of key retinoids and structural subgroups, a history of the naming of these compounds, and current nomenclature of retinoids are available online [4].

The IUPAC–IUB defines carotenoids [5] as "a class of hydrocarbons (carotenes) and their oxygenated derivatives (xanthophylls) consisting of eight isoprenoid units joined in such a manner that the arrangement of isoprenoid units is reversed at the center of the molecule." All carotenoids may be formally derived from the acyclic $C_{40}H_{56}$ structure that has a long central chain of conjugated double bonds, by (i) hydrogenation, (ii) dehydrogenation, (iii) cyclization, or (iv) oxidation, or any combination of these processes.

Properties, Nutritional Equivalency, and Recommended Intakes

Properties of Nutritionally Important Retinoids

Nutritionally important retinoids and some of their metabolites are illustrated in Figure 1.1. The conventional numbering of carbon atoms in the retinoid molecule is shown in the structure of all-*trans*-retinol in Figure 1.1a. Due to the conjugated double-bond structure of retinoids and carotenoids, these molecules possess very characteristic UV or visible light absorption spectra that are useful in their identification and quantification [6,7].

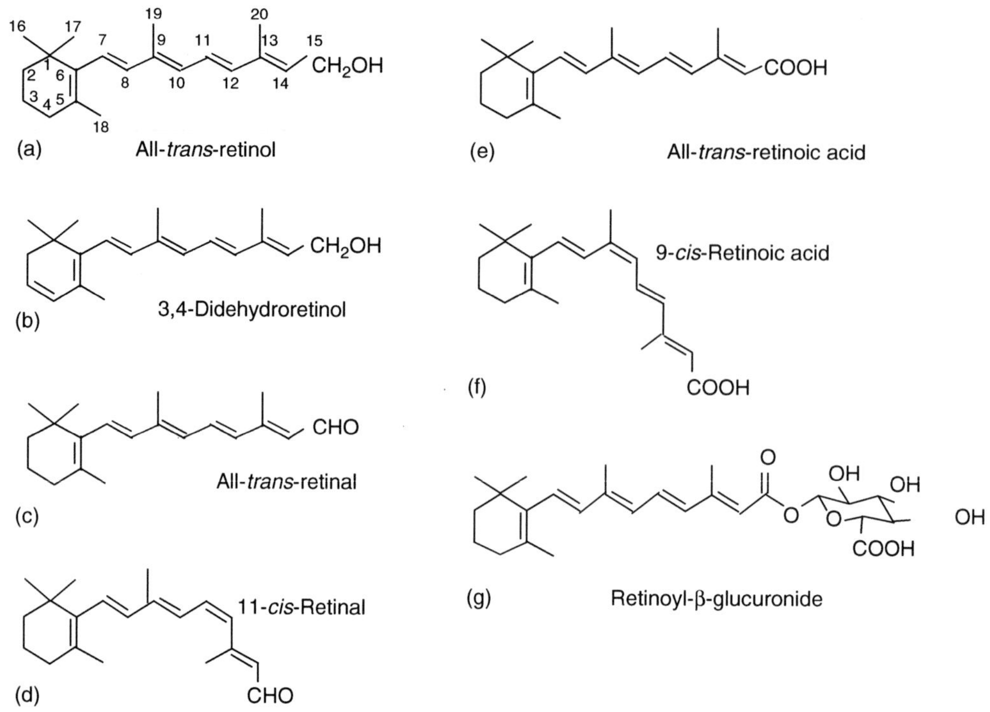

FIGURE 1.1 Nutritionally important retinoids and major metabolites. The conventional numbering system for retinoids is shown for all-*trans*-retinol, the parent molecule of the retinoid family.

Furr and colleagues have summarized the light absorption properties of over 50 retinoids [8] and nutritionally active carotenoids [9]. Some of the properties of several retinoids related to dietary vitamin A are summarized in Table 1.1.

Retinoids tend to be most stable in the all-*trans* configuration. Retinol is most often present in tissues in esterified form, where the fatty acyl group is usually palmitate with lesser amounts of stearate and oleate esters. Esterification protects the hydroxyl group from oxidation and significantly alters the molecule's physical properties (Table 1.1). Retinyl esters in tissues are usually admixed with triglycerides and other neutral lipids, including the antioxidant α-tocopherol. Retinyl esters are the major form of vitamin A in the body as a whole and the predominant form (often more than 95%) in chylomicrons, cellular lipid droplets, and milk fat globules. Thus, they are also the major form in foods of animal origin. Retinol contained in nutritional supplements and fortified foods is usually produced synthetically and is stabilized by formation of the acetate, propionate, or palmitate ester. Minor forms of vitamin A may be present in the diet, such as vitamin A_2 (3,4-didehydroretinol) (Figure 1.1b), which is present in the oils of fresh-water fish and serves as a visual pigment in these species [10].

Several retinoids that are crucial for function are either absent or insignificant in the diet, but are generated metabolically from dietary precursors. Due to the potential for the double bonds of the molecules in the vitamin A family to exist in either the *trans*- or *cis*-isomeric form, a large number of retinoid isomers are possible. The terminal functional group can be in one of several oxidation states, varying from hydrocarbon, as in anhydroretinol, to alcohol, aldehyde, and carboxylic acid. Many of these forms may be further modified through the addition of substituents to the ring, side chain, or end group. These changes in molecular structure significantly alter the physical properties of the molecules in the vitamin A family and may markedly affect their biological activity. While dozens of natural retinoids

TABLE 1.1
Properties of Vitamin A Compounds and Their Metabolites

Compound	Formula and Molecular Mass	Solvents in Which Soluble	Physical State	Wavelength of Maximum Absorption, λ_{max}	Molar Extinction Coefficient, ε, in Indicated Solvent
All-*trans*-retinol (vitamin A_1)	$C_{20}H_{30}O$ 286.44	Absolute alcohol, methanol, chloroform, petroleum ether, fats, and oils	Crystalline solid	324–325	52,770 in ethanol 51,770 in hexane
3,4-Didehydroretinol (vitamin A_2)	$C_{20}H_{28}O$ 284.44	Alcohols, ether	Crystalline solid	350	41,320 in ethanol
Retinyl palmitate	$C_{36}H_{60}O_2$ 528	Hexane, ether, dimethylsulfoxide	Viscous oil	325	49,260 in ethanol
All-*trans*-retinal	$C_{20}H_{28}O$; 284.44	Ethanol, chloroform, cyclohexane, petroleum ether, oils	Crystalline solid	383 368	42,880 in ethanol 48,000 in hexane
11-*cis*-Retinal	$C_{20}H_{28}O$; 284.44	Ethanol, chloroform, cyclohexane, petroleum ether, oils	Crystalline solid	380 365	24,935 in ethanol 26,360 in hexane
All-*trans*-retinoic acid	$C_{20}H_{28}O_2$; 300.4	Ethanol, methanol, isopropanol, dimethyl sulfoxide	Crystalline solid	350	45,300 in ethanol
9-*cis*-Retinoic acid	$C_{20}H_{28}O_2$; 300.4	Ethanol, methanol, isopropanol, dimethyl sulfoxide	Crystalline solid	345	36,900 in ethanol
13-*cis*-Retinoic acid	$C_{20}H_{28}O_2$; 300.4	Ethanol, methanol, isopropanol, dimethyl sulfoxide	Crystalline solid	354	39,750 in ethanol
Retinoyl-β-glucuronide	$C_{26}H_{36}O_8$ 476.1	Aqueous methanol	Crystalline solid	360	50,700 in methanol
4-Oxo-all-*trans*-retinoic acid	$C_{20}H_{26}O_3$; 314.4	Ethanol, methanol, dimethyl sulfoxide	Crystalline solid	360	58,220 in ethanol

Note: For additional absorption spectrum data, see Furr et al. [8,9].

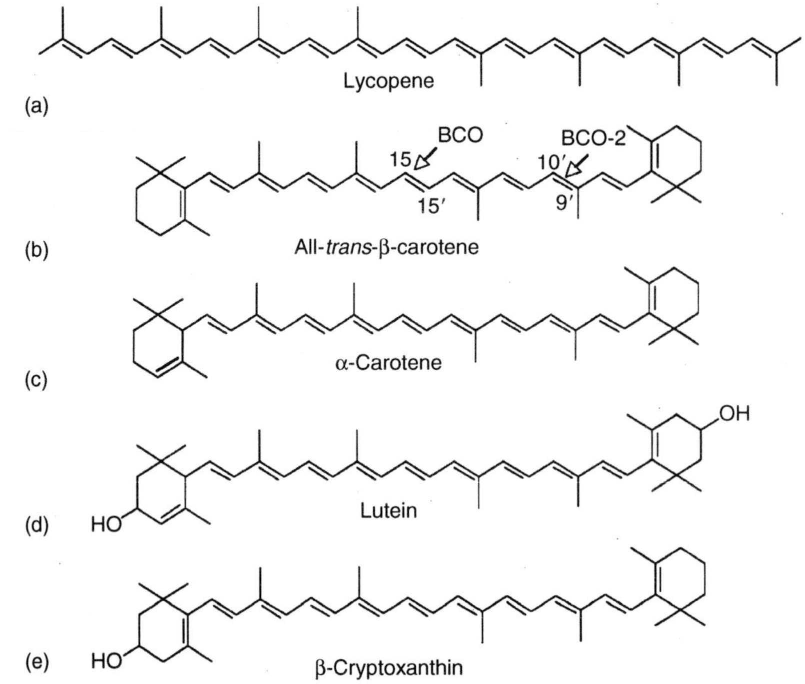

FIGURE 1.2 Nutritionally important carotenoids. (a) Lycopene, a nonprovitamin A carotene; (b) all-*trans*-ββ′-carotene; arrows indicate sites of cleavage by β-carotene monooxygenase, BCO, and BCO-2; (c) all-*trans* (α,β′) carotene; (d) lutein, a nonprovitamin A xanthophyll; (e) β-cryptoxanthin.

have been isolated, the molecules illustrated in Figure 1.1 and Figure 1.2 are the principal retinoids and carotenoids, respectively, of nutritional importance, and thus are the main focus of this chapter. Nevertheless, it is important to recognize that numerous minor metabolites can be formed at several branch points as retinol and the provitamin A carotenoids are metabolized.

All-*trans*-retinal (Figure 1.1c) is the immediate product of the central cleavage of β-carotene as well as an intermediate in the oxidative metabolism of retinol to all-*trans*-retinoic acid. The 11-*cis* isomer of retinal (Figure 1.1d) is formed in the retina and most of it is covalently bound to one of the visual pigments, rhodopsin in rods or iodopsin in cones. The aldehyde functional group of 11-*cis*-retinal combines with specific lysine residues in these proteins as a Schiff's base.

All-*trans*-retinoic acid (Figure 1.1e) is the most bioactive form of vitamin A. When fed to vitamin A-deficient animals, retinoic acid restores growth and tissue differentiation and prevents mortality, indicating that this form alone, or metabolites made from it, is able to support nearly all of the functions attributed to vitamin A. A notable exception is vision, which is not restored by retinoic acid because retinoic acid cannot be reduced to retinal in vivo. Retinoic acid is also the most potent natural ligand of the retinoid receptors, RAR and RXR (described later), as demonstrated in transactivation assays. Several *cis* isomers of retinoic acid have been studied rather extensively, but they are still somewhat enigmatic as to origin and function. 9-*cis*-Retinoic acid (Figure 1.1f) is capable of binding to the nuclear receptors and may be a principal ligand of the RXR. 13-*cis*-Retinoic acid is present in plasma, often at a concentration similar to all-*trans*-retinoic acid, and its therapeutic effects are well demonstrated (see the section Dermatology), but it is not known to be a high-affinity ligand for the nuclear retinoid receptors. It is possible that 13-*cis*-retinoic acid acts as a relatively stable precursor or prodrug that can be metabolized to all-*trans*-retinoic acid or perhaps another bioactive metabolite. Di-*cis* isomers of retinoic acid also have been detected in plasma, further illustrating the complex mix of retinoids in biological systems.

Retinoids that are more polar than retinol or retinoic acid are formed through oxidative metabolism of the ionone ring and side chain. These include 4-hydroxy, 4-oxo, 18-hydroxy, and 5,6-epoxy derivatives of retinoic acid, and similar modifications of other retinoids. Conjugation of the lipophilic retinoids with very polar molecules such as glucuronic acid renders them water-soluble. As an example, retinoyl-β-glucuronide (Figure 1.1g) is present as a significant metabolite in the plasma and bile. Although some of these polar retinoids are active in some assays, most of the more polar and water-soluble retinoids appear to result from phase I and phase II metabolic or detoxification reactions. They may, however, be deconjugated to some extent and recycled as the free compound.

Many retinoids have been chemically synthesized. A large number of structural analogs have been synthesized and tested for their potential as drugs that may be able to induce cell differentiation. In the field of dermatology, 13-*cis*-retinoic acid (isotretinoin) and the 1,2,4-trimethyl-3-methoxyphenyl analog of retinoic acid (acetretin) are prominent differentiation-promoting and keratinolytic compounds. Other retinoids have been developed as agents able to selectively bind to and activate only a subset of retinoid receptors. Some synthetic retinoids show none of the biological activities of vitamin A, but still are related in terms of structure. Retinoids that show selectivity in binding to the RXR receptors rather than RAR, sometimes referred to as rexinoids, also have been synthesized [11,12].

As analytical methods have improved, additional retinoids have been discovered. Retinol metabolites have been identified in which the terminal group is dehydrated (anhydroretinol); the 13,14 position is saturated or hydroxylated; or the double bonds of the retinoid side chain are flipped back into a form known as a retro retinoid [4]. These retinoids tend to be quantitatively minor or limited in their distribution, and their significance is still uncertain.

Properties of Nutritionally Important Carotenoids

Carotenoids are synthesized by photosynthetic plants and some algae and bacteria, but not by animal tissues. The initial stage of biosynthesis results in the formation of the basic poly-isoprenoid structure of the hydrocarbon lycopene (Figure 1.2a), a 40-carbon linear structure with an extended system of 13 conjugated double bonds. Further biosynthetic reactions result in the cyclization of the ends of this linear molecule to form either α- or β-ionone rings. The carotene group of carotenoids comprises hydrocarbon carotenoids in which the ionone rings bear no other substituents. The addition of oxygen to the carotene structure results in the formation of the xanthophyll group of carotenoids. The double bonds in most carotenoids are present in the more stable all-*trans* configuration, although *cis* isomers can exist. Carotenoids are widespread in nature and are responsible for the yellow, orange, red, and purple colors of many fruits, flowers, birds, insects, and marine animals. In photosynthetic plants, carotenoids improve the efficiency of photosynthesis, while they are important to insects, birds, animals, and humans for their colorful and attractive sensory properties.

Although some 600 carotenoids have been isolated from natural sources, only about one-tenth of them are present in human diets [13], and only about 20 have been detected in blood and tissues. β-carotene (Figure 1.2b), α-carotene (Figure 1.2c), lycopene, lutein (Figure 1.2d), and β-cryptoxanthin (Figure 1.2e) are the five most prominent carotenoids in the human body. However, only β-carotene, α-carotene, and β-cryptoxanthin possess significant vitamin A activity. To be active as vitamin A, a carotenoid must have an unsubstituted β-ionone ring and an unsaturated hydrocarbon chain. The bioactivity of all-*trans*-β-carotene, with two symmetrical halves, is about twice that of an equal amount of α-carotene and β-cryptoxanthin, in which only one unsubstituted β-ionone ring is present. Even though lycopene, lutein, and zeaxanthin can be relatively abundant in the diet and humans can absorb them across the intestine into plasma, they lack vitamin A activity because of the absence of a closed unsubstituted ring. In plants, provitamin A carotenoids are embedded in complex cellular structures such as the cellulose-containing matrix of chloroplasts or pigment-containing chromoplasts. Their association with these matrices of plants is a significant factor affecting the efficiency of their digestion, release, and bioavailability [14,15].

Nutritional Equivalency

Units of Activity

Different forms of vitamin A differ in their biological activity per unit of mass. For this reason, the bioactivity of vitamin A in the diet is expressed in equivalents (with respect to all-*trans*-retinol) rather than in mass units. Several different units have been adopted over time and most of them are still used in some capacity. In 1967, the World Health Organization (WHO)/FAO recommended replacing the international unit (IU), a bioactivity unit, with the retinol equivalent (RE); 1 RE was defined as 1 μg of all-*trans*-retinol or 6 μg of β-carotene in foods [16]. In 2001, the U.S. Institute of Medicine recommended replacing the RE with the retinol activity equivalent (RAE) and redefining the average equivalency values for carotenoids in foods in comparison with retinol [15]. These sequential changes in units were in large part a response to better knowledge of the efficiency of utilization of carotenoids [15,16]; 1 μg RAE is defined as 1 μg of all-*trans*-retinol, and therefore is the same as 1 μg RE. Both are equal to 3.3 IU of retinol. The equivalency of provitamin A carotenoids and retinol in the RAE system is illustrated in Figure 1.3. These currently adopted conversion factors are necessarily approximations. Because the RAE terminology is not yet fully used, the vitamin A values in some food tables, food labels, and supplements are still expressed in RE or IU.

Another term, daily value (% DV), is used in food labeling. It is not a true unit of activity, but provides an indication of the percentage of the recommended dietary allowance (RDA)* present in one serving of a given food.

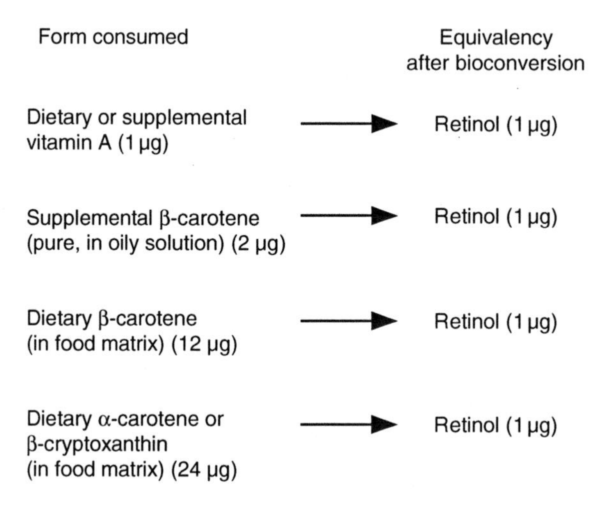

FIGURE 1.3 Approximate nutritional equivalency of dietary provitamin A carotenoids and retinol, as revised in 2001. The values shown are used to convert the contents of carotenoids in supplements and foods to equivalent amounts of dietary retinol. (From Institute of Medicine, *Dietary Reference Intakes for Vitamin A, Vitamin K, Arsenic, Boron, Chromium, Copper, Iodine, Iron, Manganese, Molybdenum, Nickel, Silicon, Vanadium, and Zinc,* National Academy Press, Washington, 2002, pp. 8–9.)

* Based on the percentage of the RDA of a nutrient, for a person consuming a 2000 kcal diet.

TABLE 1.2
Recommended Dietary Allowances (RDA) and Upper Level (UL) Values for Vitamin A by Life Stage Group

Life Stage Group	RDA (μg/day)[a]	UL (μg/day)[b]
Infants		
0–12 months	400[c]	600
Children		
1–3 years	300	600
4–8 years	400	900
Adolescent and adult males		
9–13 years	600	1700
14–18 years	900	2800
19 to ≥70 years	900	3000
Adolescent and adult females		
9–13 years	600	1700
14–18 years	700	2800
19 to ≥70 years	700	3000
Pregnancy		
<18 years	750	2800
19–50 years	770	3000
Lactation		
<18 years	1200	2800
19–50 years	1300	3000

Source: From Institute of Medicine in *Dietary Reference Intakes for Vitamin A, Vitamin K, Arsenic, Boron, Chromium, Copper, Iodine, Iron, Manganese, Molybdenum, Nickel, Silicon, Vanadium, and Zinc*, National Academy Press, Washington, 2002, pp. 8–9.

[a] As retinol activity equivalents (RAEs).
[b] As μg preformed vitamin A (retinol).
[c] Adequate intake (RAEs).

Recommended Intakes

The conceptual framework and values for dietary reference intakes (DRI) are discussed by Murphy and Barr in Chapter 18. DRI values for vitamin A, established in 2001 [15], are summarized in Table 1.2. A tolerable upper intake level (UL, see Chapter 18) for vitamin A was defined at this time [15]; similarly, a safe upper level for vitamin A and β-carotene has been defined in the United Kingdom [17]. It is important to note that the UL applies only to chronic intakes of preformed vitamin A (not carotenoids, which do not cause adverse effects). For several life stage groups, the UL values are less than three times higher than the RDA.

Dietary Sources

Detailed tables of the vitamin A contents of foods can be found in several reference sources and online resources. A database for carotenoids in foods is available online [18]. It should be noted that nutrient databases provide only approximate values. The contents of vitamin A and carotenoids in foods can vary substantially with crop variety or cultivar, the environment in which it is grown, and with processing and storage conditions [19,20].

Foods in the U.S. diet with the highest concentrations of preformed vitamin A are liver (4–20 mg retinol/100 g) and fortified foods such as powdered breakfast drinks (3–6 mg/100 g), ready-to-eat cereals (0.7–1.5 mg/100 g), and margarines (~0.8 mg/100 g) [18]. The highest levels of provitamin A carotenoids are found in carrots, sweet potatoes, pumpkin, kale, spinach, collards, and squash (roughly 5–10 mg RAE/100 g) [18].

Data from NHANES 2001–2002 for food consumption in the United States showed that the major contributors to the intake of preformed vitamin A are milk, margarine, eggs, beef liver, and ready-to-eat cereals, whereas the major sources of provitamin A carotenoids are carrots, cantaloupes, sweet potatoes, and spinach [21]. These data, compiled for both genders and all age groups, showed that the mean intake of vitamin A is ~600 μg RAE/day from food and that 70%–75% of this is as preformed vitamin A (retinol). The provitamin A carotenoids β-carotene, α-carotene, and β-cryptoxanthin were ingested in amounts of ~1750, 350, and 150 μg/day, respectively. By comparison, the intakes of the nonprovitamin A carotene lycopene and the xanthophylls (zeaxanthin and lutein) were ~6000 and 1300 μg/day, respectively. The Institute of Medicine's Micronutrients Report [15] includes sample menus to illustrate that an adequate intake of vitamin A can be obtained even if a vegetarian diet containing only provitamin A carotenoids is consumed.

TRANSPORT AND METABOLISM

Taken as a whole, the processes of vitamin A metabolism can be viewed as supporting two main biological functions: providing appropriate retinoids to tissues throughout the body for the local production of retinoic acid, which is required to maintain normal gene expression and tissue differentiation, and providing retinol to the retina for adequate production of 11-*cis*-retinal. Major interconversions and metabolic reactions are diagrammed in Figure 1.4.

TRANSPORT AND BINDING PROTEINS

Carotenoids and retinyl esters are transported by lipoproteins and stored within the fat fraction of tissues, whereas retinol, retinal, and retinoic acid are mostly found in plasma and cells in association with specific retinoid-binding proteins. The associations of carotenoids and retinoids with proteins greatly influence their distribution, metabolism, and physiological functions. Amphiphilic retinoids—principally retinol, retinal, and retinoic acid—bind to retinoid-binding proteins, which confer aqueous solubility on these otherwise insoluble molecules. The concentration of free retinoid is very low. Binding proteins thus reduce the potential for retinoids to cause membrane damage [22]. Different retinoid-binding proteins function in plasma, interstitial fluid, and the cytosolic compartment of cells as chaperones that direct the bound retinoids to enzymes that then carry out their metabolism. Table 1.3 summarizes

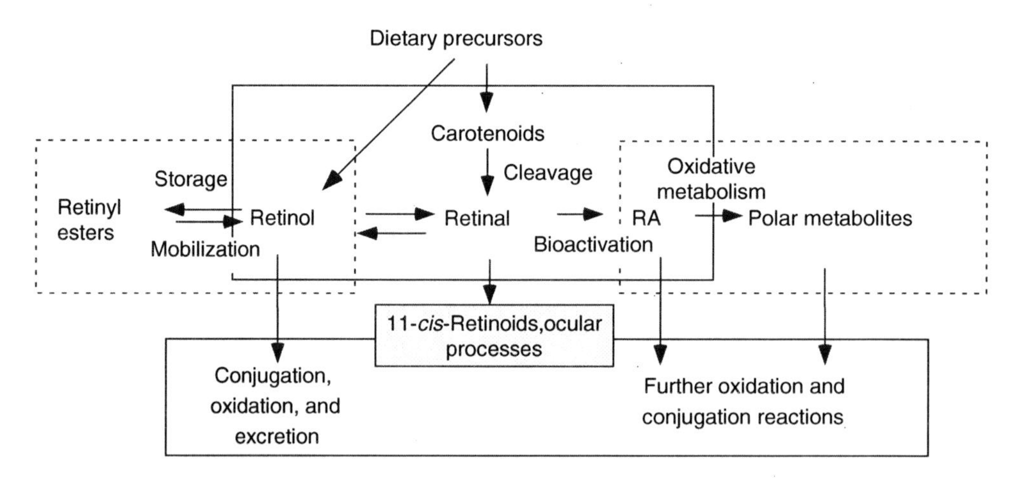

FIGURE 1.4 Principal metabolic reactions of vitamin A. RA, retinoic acid.

TABLE 1.3
Major Extracellular and Intracellular Retinoid-Binding Proteins

Protein	Gene Family/Type	Size	Ligand (All-*trans* Isomer Unless Indicated)	Function
Retinol-binding protein, RBP	Lipocalin	21 kDa	Retinol	Transport of retinol between liver and extrahepatic tissues
Cellular retinol-binding proteins, CRBP-I, CRBP-II, CRBP-III, CRBP-IV	Fatty acid-binding protein/cellular retinoid-binding protein	~14.6 kDa	CRBP-I: retinol CRBP-II: retinol and retinal CRBP-III: *trans*- and *cis*-retinol CRBP-IV: retinol	Binding of retinol and chaperone function to enzymes of metabolism
Cellular retinoic acid-binding proteins, CRABP-I, CRABP-II	Fatty acid-binding protein/cellular retinoid-binding protein	~14.8 kDa	CRABP-I: retinoic acid CRABP-II: retinoic acid	Binding of retinoic acid and chaperone function to enzymes of metabolism; possible coreceptor function for CRABP-II
Cellular retinal-binding protein, CRALBP	CRAL/TRIO	~36 kDa	All-*trans*-retinol and 11-*cis*-retinol; 11-*cis*-retinal	Binding of retinol, retinal; chaperone function to enzymes of retinoid cycle that regenerate visual pigments in the retina
Interstitial retinoid-binding protein, IRBP	Partial homology to enoyl-CoA isomerase/hydratases	136 kDa	All-*trans* and 11-*cis*-retinal; other lipophilic substances	Improving the efficiency of translocation of retinoids between the RPE and photoreceptor cells
Transthyretin, TTR	Transthyretin	55 kDa	Thyroxin homotetramer	Cotransport protein for holo-RBP; prevents rapid loss by renal filtration
Albumin	Albumin	67 kDa	Retinoic acid; other acidic retinoids; fatty acids	General carrier for acidic lipids

some of the characteristics of the retinoid-binding proteins involved in these absorptive, transport, and metabolic processes.

Retinol-Binding Protein

Plasma retinol is transported by a retinol-binding protein (RBP) [23]. One molecule of retinol is bound noncovalently within the beta-barrel pocket of the RBP protein. Although most RBP is produced in liver parenchymal cells, the kidney, adipose tissue, lacrimal gland, and some other extrahepatic organs also contain RBP mRNA, generally at levels less than 10% of that in hepatocytes, and may synthesize RBP [24]. The maintenance of a normal rate of RBP synthesis depends on an adequate intake of protein, calories, and some micronutrients (Table 1.4); conversely, a deficiency of any of these can reduce the plasma concentrations of retinol–RBP. RBP is synthesized in the endoplasmic reticulum of hepatocytes, transported through the Golgi apparatus where apo-RBP combines with a molecule of retinol to form holo-RBP [25], and then released into plasma. Nearly all circulating holo-RBP is bound noncovalently to another hepatically synthesized protein, transthyretin (TTR), which also binds thyroxine [26,27]. RBP protects retinol from oxidation, while TTR stabilizes the retinol–RBP interaction [28]. Although retinol is the natural ligand of RBP, other retinoids such as 4-hydroxyphenylretinamide (4HPR) can compete for binding to RBP in vitro [29], destabilize the RBP–TTR complex [30], and result in reduced levels of plasma retinol [31].

TABLE 1.4
Causes of a Low Level of Plasma Retinol

Etiology	Mechanisms
Nutritional	
Inadequate vitamin A in liver	Reduced secretion of holo-RBP
Inadequate protein or energy	
Inadequate micronutrients (zinc, iron)	Reduced RBP synthesis, release
Disease-related	
Infection or inflammation	Reduced production and section of RBP, and TTR (retinol not limiting)
Liver diseases	Reduced synthesis of hepatic proteins, including RBP, TTR
Renal diseases	Reduced reabsorption
Treatment-related	
Retinoid treatment (4HPR, RA)	Displacement of retinol from RBP; possibly altered synthesis is RBP
Genetic	
Hereditary disorders	Rare natural mutations that affect the production or the stability of RBP and TTR proteins
Toxicologic	
Alcohol-related	Impaired vitamin A storage; generally poor nutritional or health status
Environmental toxin-related	Altered retinol kinetics (e.g., dioxin or TCDD exposure)

Note: 4HPR, 4-hydroxphenylretinamide; RA, retinoic acid; RBP, retinol-binding protein; TCDD, 2,3,7,8-tetrachlorodibenzo-p-dioxin; TTR, transthyretin.

Albumin

Retinoic acid circulates in plasma bound to albumin [32], and it is likely that other retinoids with a carboxylic acid function also bind to albumin.

Lipoproteins

Retinyl esters, when present in plasma, are bound to lipoproteins. Retinyl esters are a normal constituent of chylomicrons and chylomicron remnants in the postprandial phase, but they are not present in appreciable amounts in the fasting state in humans, except in the pathophysiological state of hypervitaminosis A [33]. Plasma retinyl esters may also indicate delayed metabolism of retinyl ester-containing chylomicrons or remnants [34]. As noted later, some species (carnivores) carry most vitamin A as lipoprotein-bound retinyl esters.

Humans and a few other species absorb a fraction of intestinally absorbed carotenoids without cleaving them; thus, carotenoids are present transiently in chylomicrons and remnants, as well as low-density (LDL) and high-density lipoproteins (HDL) [35], which also carry carotenoids in the fasting state. The nonpolar carotenes and lycopene are associated mostly with LDL whereas the relatively more polar xanthophylls are equally distributed between LDL and HDL [36].

Intracellular Retinoid-Binding Proteins

CRBP Family

Cellular retinoid-binding proteins belonging to the fatty acid-binding or cellular retinoid-binding protein gene family are present in the cytoplasm of many types of cells [37]. The structural motif of this family has been described as a beta clam in which a single molecule of ligand fits into the binding pocket with the functional group (hydroxyl group of retinol) oriented inward. Various cellular retinoid-binding proteins bind ligands selectively (see Table 1.3). Four cellular RBPs (CRBP-I, CRBP-II, CRBP-III, and CRBP-IV) and two cellular retinoic acid-binding proteins (CRABP-I and CRABP-II), which may have arisen through gene duplication, are expressed at different levels in cell type-specific and tissue-specific patterns (reviewed by O'Bryne and Blaner [38] and Ross [39]). These proteins confer aqueous solubility on otherwise insoluble retinoids; protect them from degradation; protect membranes from accumulating retinoids; and escort retinoids to enzymes that metabolize them [39,40].

CRBP-I is widely distributed in retinol-metabolizing tissues. In liver, its principal endogenous ligand, all-*trans*-retinol, is a substrate for lecithin:retinol acyltransferase (LRAT) [41] and a retinol dehydrogenase [42]. It may also function in the uptake of retinol by effectively removing retinol from solution and providing a driving force for its continued uptake [43]. In the small intestine, CRBP-II is abundant and CRBP-II-bound retinol is the substrate for LRAT [44]. Apo-CRBP, when present, increases retinyl ester hydrolysis [42]. Mice lacking these proteins do not exhibit a significant phenotype so long as they are fed a diet high in vitamin A [45,46]. However, retinol is rapidly lost when the diet is low in vitamin A. Therefore, the CRBPs apparently serve as efficiency factors that help to conserve vitamin A, and therefore they may be of significant advantage when dietary vitamin A is scarce.

The sequences of CRBP-III and CRBP-IV are ~50%–60% homologous to CRBP-I and CRBP-II. CRBP-III is distributed mainly in liver, kidney, mammary tissue, and heart and binds, in addition to all-*trans*-retinol, several other retinoids as well as fatty acids [47,48]. Another member of the CRBP family, CRBP-IV, is more similar to CRBP-II than CRBP-I and CRBP-III [30]. CRBP-IV has a higher affinity for retinol and exhibits a somewhat different absorption spectrum, suggesting it binds retinol somewhat differently as compared with the binding of retinol by the other CRBPs. The mRNA for CRBP-IV is most abundant in kidney, heart, and colon, but is relatively widely expressed.

CRABP-I and CRABP-II bind all-*trans*-retinoic acid. CRABP-I is expressed, albeit at low concentrations, in numerous tissues whereas CRABP-II has a more limited distribution range but is inducible by retinoic acid [49]. These proteins have been studied most extensively for their roles in embryonic development and tissue differentiation [50–52]. CRABP-I has been implicated in the oxidation of retinoic acid [42], whereas CRABP-II may aid in the distribution of retinoic acid within cells and as a cotranscription factor in the nucleus [53,54]. Nevertheless, mice lacking either CRABP-I or CRABP-II, and even double-mutant mice lacking both proteins, appear essentially normal [55].

Specialized Intracellular and Extracellular Retinoid-Binding Proteins

Two proteins unrelated to CRBP and CRABP are highly expressed in the retina: an intracellular retinal-binding protein, CRALBP belonging to the CRAL-TRIO family [56], and interstitial retinoid-binding protein, IRBP, a large multiligand-binding protein that is abundant in the extracellular space of the retina, known as the interphotoreceptor matrix [57]. CRALBP binds 11-*cis*-retinoids, retinol, and retinal and functions in the retinal pigment epithelium (RPE) in the visual cycle. Disruption of this gene resulted in reduced dark adaptation after exposure to light [58]. IRBP is implicated in the transport, distribution, and protection of retinol and 11-*cis*-retinal between the RPE and photoreceptor cells [57]. Another protein, RPE65, which is also highly expressed in the retina, can bind retinyl esters and may facilitate the storage of vitamin A in the RPE [59].

Nuclear Retinoid Receptors

Nuclear retinoid receptor proteins may be considered a subset of retinoid-binding proteins, as ligand binding is crucial for their function. The nuclear retinoid receptors, RAR and RXR, are transcription factors that bind as dimers to specific DNA sequences present in retinoid responsive genes (RAREs and RXREs, respectively) and thereby induce or repress gene transcription. The retinoid receptor gene family, a subset of the superfamily of steroid hormone receptors [60], is composed of six genes, encoding RAR α, β, and γ, and RXR α, β, and γ. Each protein contains several domains that are similarly organized and well conserved within the RAR and RXR subfamilies, including a ligand-binding domain (LBD) that binds the preferred retinoid ligand with high affinity and a DNA-binding domain (DBD) that binds to the retinoic acid receptor response elements (RAREs). These are usually located within the promoter region upstream of the transcription start site of target genes [61]. All-*trans*-retinoic acid binds with high affinity to the RAR, while 9-*cis*-retinoic acid binds with high affinity to RXR and RAR proteins in vitro, but is believed to mainly activate members of the RXR family in vivo [62]. Each nuclear receptor protein also includes a dimerization domain and a transactivation domain through which the RAR–RXR heterodimer interacts with coreceptor molecules [63]. In the absence of ligand, RAR–RXR heterodimers associate with a multiprotein complex containing transcriptional repressor proteins (e.g., N-CoR and SMRT), which induce histone deacetylation, chromatin condensation, maintaining transcription in a repressed state. Crystallographic studies have shown that the binding of all-*trans*-retinoic acid to the RAR causes a change in receptor conformation [61], which induces the receptors to dissociate from their corepressors and associate with coactivators that have histone acetyltransferase activity and induce the local opening up of the condensed chromosome. In turn, these changes allow the binding of the RNA polymerase II complex, thus enabling the activation of the target gene and the transcription of DNA to RNA [63,64].

There are still many open questions about ligand-activated transcription involving the RAR and RXR receptors, including the significance of subtle differences between the three RARs, α, β, and γ [61,65]; the specificity of RARE to which these receptors bind; and how receptor levels are regulated. Regarding RARE, certain canonical elements are well defined, such as the direct repeat (DR)-2 and DR-5 nucleotide sequences of Pu/GGTCA-N(2 or 5)-Pu/GGTCA to which the RAR–RXR heterodimer binds well, but widely spaced or noncanonical response elements have also been discovered [66]. Regarding receptor levels, the expression RAR-β is regulated at least in part by retinoids through a DR-5 RARE in its promoter [67]. This receptor is frequently downregulated in cancers, possibly related to increased methylation of its gene or other changes in chromatin structure [68,69]. Other important but unresolved questions concern the role of posttranscriptional or posttranslational modifications in modulating retinoid receptor activity [64] and the ways in which coactivator and corepressor proteins are recruited and, in turn, regulate the outcome of gene expression by retinoids [63,70]. The ligand specificity of the RXR in vivo is still a subject of speculation. Although 9-*cis*-retinoic acid can bind to the RXR in vitro and is an excellent RXR ligand in transfection and gene promoter assays, it has been suggested that other ligands such as phytanic acid [71] and docosahexaenoic acid [72] might also be RXR ligands. Overall, the nature and the production of the endogenous ligands for the RXR are less clear than those for the RAR.

Besides forming heterodimers with RAR, the RXR also bind with several other ligand-activated nuclear receptors: the vitamin D receptor (VDR), thyroid hormone receptor (TR), and the PPAR, LXR, FXR, and CAR proteins.

It is interesting that mice do well in the absence of one and sometimes more of these binding proteins and nuclear receptors. However, mice do not survive a nutritional deficiency of vitamin A, which effectively knocks out all of these ligand-dependent functions.

Intestinal Metabolism

Conversion of Provitamin A Carotenoids to Retinoids

Humans are apparently relatively unusual in their ability to absorb an appreciable proportion of dietary β-carotene across the intestine in intact form. In contrast, most species cleave nearly all of the absorbed β-carotene during digestion and absorption [73]. Most of what is known about human carotenoid absorption has been derived directly from metabolic studies in humans and in vitro cell culture models. Ferrets, preruminant calves, and gerbils [74–76] have been used as models although none of these completely represents human carotenoid metabolism [77].

In human studies, the intestinal absorption of carotenoids has been estimated through the intake–excretion balance approach, and by assessing the total plasma carotenoid response to carotenoid ingestion, which provides only a rough estimate of intestinal absorption. The bioavailability of a single dose of purified oil-dissolved β-carotene appears to be relatively low: 9%–17% using the lymph-cannulation approach [78], 11% using the carotenoid and retinyl ester response in the triglyceride-rich lipoprotein plasma fraction [79], and 3%–22% using isotopic tracer approaches [80,81]. Even though quantitative data are few and numerous aspects of the absorption process require further study, the framework for the intestinal absorption of carotenoids is reasonably well known. The process can be divided into several steps: (1) release of carotenoids from the food matrix, (2) solubilization of carotenoids into mixed lipid micelles in the lumen, (3) cellular uptake of carotenoids by intestinal mucosal cells, (4) intracellular metabolism, and (5) incorporation of carotenoids into chylomicrons and their secretion into lymph.

Release of Carotenoids

The type of carotenoid and its physical form affect the efficiency of carotene absorption. Pure β-carotene in an oily solution or supplements is absorbed more efficiently than an equivalent amount of β-carotene in foods. Carotenoids in foods are often bound within plant matrices of indigestible polysaccharides, fibers, and phenolic compounds, which reduces the bioavailability of these carotenoids. Although the absorption of provitamin A carotenoids from fruits is generally more efficient than that from fibrous vegetables, it is still low as compared with β-carotene in oil (see the section Units of Activity).

Solubilization of Carotenoids and Retinoids

Almost no detailed information exists on the physical forms or phases of carotenoids or retinoids in the intestinal lumen. Nonetheless, both human and animal studies have shown that the coingestion of dietary fat is necessary for and markedly enhances the absorption of carotenoids and vitamin A [82,83]. In the lumen, fat stimulates the secretion of pancreatic enzymes and bile salts, and facilitates the formation of micelles that are required for absorption of preformed vitamin A and provitamin A. Within the enterocytes, fat promotes vitamin A and carotenoid absorption by providing the lipid components for intestinal chylomicron assembly. Diets critically low in fat (less than 5–10 g/day) [84] or disease conditions that cause steatorrhea reduce the absorption of retinoids and carotenoids.

Cellular Uptake

Only a few studies have addressed the kinetics of carotenoid absorption. Although earlier studies in rats [85,86] indicated that the uptake of carotenoids was by passive diffusion, determined by the concentration gradient of the carotenoid across the intestinal membrane, studies with Caco-2 (human intestinal cell) monolayers have shown cellular uptake and secretion in chylomicrons to be curvilinear, time-dependent, saturable, and concentration-dependent (apparent K_m of 7–10 μM) processes [87], more consistent with the participation of a specific epithelial transporter than with passive diffusion. The extent of absorption of all-*trans*-β-carotene through Caco-2 cell monolayers was 11%, a value similar to that reported from different human studies. Of the total β-carotene secreted by Caco-2 cells, 80% was associated with chylomicrons, 10% with very LDPs, and 10% with the nonlipoprotein fraction [87], pointing to the importance of chylomicron assembly for β-carotene secretion into the lymph in vivo.

Human studies [88–92] have consistently reported a preferential accumulation of all-*trans*-β-carotene, compared with its 9-*cis* isomer, in total plasma and in the postprandial lipoprotein fraction, suggesting either a selective intestinal transport of all-*trans*-β-carotene versus its 9-*cis* isomer or an intestinal *cis–trans* isomerization of 9-*cis*-β-carotene to all-*trans*-β-carotene. Indeed, a significant accumulation of [^{13}C]-all-*trans*-β-carotene was observed in plasma of subjects who ingested only [^{13}C]-9-*cis*-β-carotene [92]. In Caco-2 cells incubated with an initial concentration (1 μM) of the three geometrical isomers of β-carotene applied separately, both 9-*cis*- and 13-*cis*-β-carotenes were taken up but their absorption through the cell monolayer was less than 3.5%, compared with 11% for all-*trans*-β-carotene [87].

Intracellular Metabolism

Within the intestinal absorptive cells, carotenoids undergo cleavage to form vitamin A, or they may pass unmetabolized across the intestine. An intestinal β-carotene cleavage activity was described in the 1960s as a cytosolic, NADP+, and oxygen-requiring enzyme, called β-carotene 15,15′-dioxygenase. This activity was capable of cleaving β-carotene centrally (between the 15 and 15′ carbons, see Figure 1.2b), forming two molecules of retinal [73]. Later, excentric cleavage also was demonstrated, but its importance as compared to central cleavage has been uncertain. Recently, molecular and biochemical studies have clarified that the central cleavage reaction, which is mediated by a cytosolic enzyme now referred to as β-carotene 15,15′-dioxygenase (BCO) [93,94] generates 2 moles of retinal, and is the predominant pathway for β-carotene cleavage. The BCO cDNA codes for a 550 amino acids (~65 kDa) protein. The cloned sequence is well conserved among *Drosophila*, chicken, mouse, and human, and it is also highly homologous with RPE65, a protein thought to be important in vitamin A metabolism in the retina [95].

The eccentric or assymetrical cleavage pathway has also been demonstrated through cloning of a second cleavage enzyme, BCO-2, which cleaves specifically at the 9′,10′-double bond of β-carotene (see Figure 1.2b) to produce β-apo-10′-carotenal and β-ionone [93,94,96]. In this pathway, the polyene chain of β-carotene is cleaved at double bonds other than the central 15,15′-double bond and the products formed are β-apo-carotenals with different chain lengths. Trace amounts of apo-carotenals have been detected in vivo in animals fed β-carotene [97].

BCO activity has been reported to be increased in vitamin A deficiency [98], possibly due to the presence of an RAR–RXR responsive RARE in the promoter of the mouse *BCO* gene [99] and by dietary polyunsaturated fats [100], possibly through a PPAR–RXR mechanism [101].

Postintestinal Conversion

The conversion of β-carotene in humans takes place in the intestine during absorption, but the liver is also important in this process. The conversion of β-carotene can continue for days or longer after intestinal absorption [102]. It was estimated that adult human small intestine and liver together metabolize ~12 mg β-carotene/day [100]. Thus, the capacity for β-carotene metabolism exceeds its average daily intake in the United States (1.5 mg β-carotene/day) or even the higher daily intake of 6 mg β-carotene/day that may be needed to meet the dietary goal of consuming 90% of vitamin A from β-carotene [103].

Intestinal Absorption of Vitamin A

Digestion of Retinyl Esters

Retinyl esters must be hydrolyzed before the uptake of retinol. Based on earlier studies, it has been thought that pancreatic carboxylester lipase (CEL), which hydrolyzes cholesteryl esters, triglycerides, and lysophospholipids in the intestinal lumen, also hydrolyzes retinyl esters. However, studies showed that CEL knockout mice [104,105], in which cholesterol absorption from cholesteryl ester was reduced to half that of wild-type mice, absorbed a normal amount of retinol fed as retinyl ester. These data suggested that retinyl ester hydrolysis is required, but CEL is not the responsible enzyme, at least under the dietary conditions used in this study. Subsequent studies have provided evidence that the observed retinyl ester hydrolase (REH) activity is due to pancreatic triglyceride lipase (PTL) [106]. However, more than one enzyme, including pancreatic lipase-related proteins 2 and 1, may be involved in the lumenal hydrolysis of retinyl esters. Besides the REH activities secreted by the pancreas, a brush border-associated REH activity was demonstrated in the small intestines of rat and human [107,108]. This enzyme activity was suggested to be due to an intestinal phospholipase B (PLB) [109]. Further studies of retinyl ester absorption in appropriate knockout models are needed to clarify the involvement, and functional redundancy, of these several enzymes.

Cellular Uptake and Efflux of Vitamin A

The uptake of retinol by human CaCo-2 cells has been shown to occur rapidly (with a half-life of minutes [110]), by a saturable, carrier-mediated process when retinol is added at physiological concentrations and by a nonsaturable, diffusion-dependent process at pharmacological concentrations [111]. Uptake was not affected by the presence of high concentrations of free fatty acids, although retinol was rapidly esterified, mainly with palmitic and oleic acids, when these were present [111,112]. The basolateral lipid transporter ABCA1 may be involved in the efflux of retinol [113]. One interpretation of these data is that unesterified retinol, at physiological concentrations, enters from the luminal side by simple diffusion, while the secretion of retinol across the basolateral membrane requires facilitated transport.

Chylomicrons transport most retinol as retinyl esters from the intestine (for review [114]); however, the portal transport of retinol may also contribute to its uptake and could be especially important when chylomicron formation is impaired. In various physiological studies, between 20% and 60% of ingested retinol has been recovered in lymph [78,114,116]. In CaCo-2 cells, free retinol or its metabolized products were transported both in the presence and the absence of lipoprotein secretion [110]. In patients with abetalipoproteinemia, who do not form chylomicrons, oral treatment with vitamin A has ameliorated their vitamin A deficiency [114]. It is therefore likely that the portal transport of free retinol is physiologically significant in pathologic conditions that restrict the secretion of chylomicrons.

Recently, the uptake of retinol into cells has been ascribed to a newly defined gene, *Stra6* [115]. The Stra6 gene encodes a transmembrane protein that, when expressed by transfection in COS-1 cells, significantly increased the uptake of retinol from RBP and the RBP-TTR complex. Stra6 protein was also identified by immunohistochemistry in tissues including the retinal pigment epithelium and placenta, which are thought to obtain most of their vitamin A as retinol from RBP.

Reesterification, Incorporation into Chylomicrons, and Lymphatic Secretion

A large fraction of newly absorbed retinol is reesterified within enterocytes with long-chain fatty acids, packaged in the endoplasmic reticulum into the lipid core of nascent chylomicrons, and secreted into the lymphatic vessels (lacteals). Retinoid-binding proteins and microsomal enzymes are integral to this process. Retinol bound to CRBP-II is available for esterification by LRAT [117–119]. The K_m of LRAT for CRBP-II-bound retinol is in the low micromolar range, consistent with physiological concentrations, and its capacity is great enough for processing physiological amounts of vitamin A. Retinol in chylomicrons is almost entirely esterified and the fatty acyl group is limited to palmitic, stearic, and oleic acids, even if the fat absorbed at the time contains other fatty acids [116], consistent with the substrate specificity of LRAT for the sn-1 fatty acid of membrane-associated lecithin, which is predominantly acylated with palmitate, stearate, and oleate. Although CRBP-II-bound retinol is a substrate of LRAT, it is not used effectively by second microsomal retinol-esterifying activity, acyl-CoA:retinol acyltransferase (ARAT). Mice lacking LRAT had no detectable retinyl esters in their tissues [120]. ARAT activity was reduced in mice lacking the gene for acyl-CoA:diglyceride acyltransferase-1, DGAT1, and recombinant DGAT1 was able to esterify retinol [121], suggesting DGAT1 as possibly responsible for ARAT activity.

Newly formed retinyl esters are secreted in chylomicrons. Thus, plasma retinyl esters rise transiently after meals, proportionate to vitamin A intake. Usually less than 5% of total plasma retinol is esterified in fasting plasma [122]. The turnover of chylomicrons and chylomicron remnants is rapid, normally on the order of minutes, due to the rapid hydrolysis of triglycerides and the nearly immediate uptake of newly formed chylomicron remnants into the liver or extrahepatic tissues [123].

In pathophysiological conditions such as hypervitaminosis A (discussed later), retinyl esters are present even in the fasting state, bound to plasma lipoproteins, and they may exceed the concentration of unesterified retinol bound to RBP [33,124,125]. In some species, especially carnivores [126], retinyl esters are the predominant form of plasma vitamin A. Domestic dogs were shown to transport most of their plasma vitamin A as lipoprotein-associated retinyl esters, even in the fasting state, even after they were deprived of dietary vitamin A for several weeks [127].

Hepatic Uptake, Storage, and Release of Vitamin A

Hepatic Uptake

Because the majority of chylomicron remnants are cleared into the liver within a few minutes of their formation [128], newly absorbed retinyl esters circulate in plasma for only a short time. Other tissues active in metabolizing chylomicron triglyceride (adipose tissue, the mammary gland during lactation) may also acquire newly absorbed vitamin A during lipolysis [104,128]. Retinyl esters are rapidly hydrolyzed in the liver [129], most likely by the enzyme carboxylesterase ES10 in either endosomes or the endoplasmic reticulum [130].

Most of the released retinol makes its way by uncertain means to hepatic stellate cells, located in the perisinusoidal region but close to hepatocytes. Stellate cells, also known as Ito cells, vitamin A-storing cells, or fat-storing cells [131], are specialized for the storage of retinyl esters, which are contained in multiple large lipid droplets. CRBP-I and LRAT are implicated in forming stellate cell retinyl esters [132]. Cells with the same appearance as liver stellate cells, although fewer in number, have been described in extrahepatic tissues, implying that a system of vitamin A-storing cells exists throughout the body [133]. The capacity of liver stellate cells for retinyl esters is high and their concentration can increase rapidly—within a few hours—after a large dose of vitamin A is consumed (see the section Release).

Extrahepatic Uptake

Extrahepatic tissues clear relatively less chylomicron vitamin A than does the liver. The lactating mammary gland [128] and macrophage-like cells in bone marrow can take up chylomicron vitamin A [134]. As discussed in the section Plasma Retinol, most tissues are apparently able to obtain a sufficient amount of vitamin A from chylomicrons when delivery by RBP is absent (as in mice lacking RBP), or defective as in rare human mutations of the *RBP* gene.

Storage

Under conditions of vitamin A adequacy, most mammals, including humans, store more than 90% of their total body vitamin A in liver stellate cells. When vitamin A intake is inadequate, nearly all of the vitamin A stored in liver can be mobilized and used by various tissues. The storage of vitamin A in human liver was shown to increase during the postnatal period, from a median of 4 μg/g liver in infants less than 1 month, to 83 μg/g in children 2–9 years of age [135], and increasing to 89 μg/g in adults, but with a wide range of 7.5–3200 μg/g [136]. Retinyl ester storage varies considerably among species. Mice retain liver vitamin A tenaciously, and it is therefore difficult to induce vitamin A deficiency [137]. Fish-eating animals accumulate very high levels of vitamin A in their livers. Some other carnivores store very little vitamin A in liver, but have high concentrations in their kidneys [126].

Retinyl ester formation in the liver, similar to that in the small intestine, is catalyzed mainly by LRAT. This enzyme is present at higher levels in hepatic stellate cells than in parenchymal cells [132]. LRAT is encoded by a single gene [138,139] and its 230–231 amino acid protein is expressed in tissue-specific patterns. LRAT is most abundant in the liver, small intestine, testis and eyes [138,140].

LRAT activity and mRNA expression in the liver are highly regulated by vitamin A status. LRAT activity was almost undetectable in the liver of vitamin A-deficient rats [141]. However, LRAT activity was induced rapidly after treatment with retinol, as well as with retinoic acid or RAR-selective retinoids [141–143]. Hepatic LRAT activity was low in rats fed a diet marginal in vitamin A [144]. The ability of the liver to down-regulate LRAT mRNA and enzyme activity when retinoids are scarce could be an adaptive mechanism to conserve retinol for secretion into plasma, rather than converting it into retinyl esters for storage. However, LRAT in the small intestine and the testis was not reduced during vitamin A deficiency [140]. Thus, the small intestine is capable of esterifying retinol immediately after vitamin A is delivered, even if the animal has become vitamin A deficient. This result from animal studies is consistent with clinical reports that vitamin A deficient individuals recover very quickly when vitamin A is provided [145–147]. Apparently the mechanisms for retinol absorption and storage remain intact even when the diet is deficient in vitamin A.

CRBP delivers retinol to LRAT for esterification, and mice lacking CRBP [45] were able to store only about half the amount of retinyl esters as compared to wild-type controls. When switched from an adequate diet to a vitamin A-deficient diet, CRBP-deficient mice quickly lost stored retinol from their liver [45]. Plasma retinol fell and the visual response was slower [148]. Therefore, CRBP therefore can improve the efficiency of retinol storage, even though CRBP is not actually essential.

Olson [149] has shown that the relationship between liver vitamin A storage and plasma retinol concentrations is not linear. He showed that plasma retinol stays in a normal range, with little variation, so long as the liver total retinol concentration is between ~20 and 300 μg/g tissue (Figure 1.5a). However, as liver vitamin A falls below 20 μg retinol/g, plasma retinol concentration declines progressively [149a]. At such low concentrations of liver retinol, the release of holo-RBP is compromised. Conversely, when liver vitamin A concentration is elevated to above ~300–500 μg retinol/g of liver plasma unesterified retinol does not increase; rather, retinyl esters (not normally present) are then found in plasma lipoproteins [33]. Thus, total retinol (unesterified plus esterified retinol) increases. An increase in plasma retinyl esters is one of the signs of hypervitaminosis A, as discussed later.

Release

As retinol is required by peripheral tissues, retinyl esters within stellate cells are hydrolyzed by one or more yet-to-be-defined REHs, and retinol is transferred back to hepatocytes. Precisely what signals this process is uncertain, but apo-RBP and retinoic acid levels have been suggested as signals [150,151]. In vitamin A deficiency, as the retinol available for combination with apo-RBP falls below some critical level, apo-RBP mRNA and protein continue to be synthesized but RBP accumulates in the endoplasmic reticulum and thus the concentration of apo-RBP in liver rises [24,152]. When retinol is made available, by oral administration or direct administration into the portal vein, holo-RBP is released very rapidly and plasma retinol rises [145,152], as illustrated in Figure 1.5b. Even a small dose of vitamin A too low to increase liver stores was able to restore normal plasma retinol concentrations (Figure 1.5b and Figure 1.5c). The ability of retinol to stimulate the release of RBP from the vitamin A-inadequate liver has been applied as a clinical test, referred to as relative dose–response (RDR) test. In the RDR test, which in practice has several variations, plasma retinol is measured before and a few hours after the administration of a small test dose of vitamin A [153]. An increase above baseline that reaches a certain criterion level is taken as evidence that apo-RBP had accumulated in the liver, and it is inferred that vitamin A reserves are inadequate. In the vitamin A-adequate state, no increase in plasma retinol occurs or it is below the criterion level.

β-Carotene is stored at relatively low concentrations in liver and fatty tissues. Therefore, yellow color of adipose tissue can indicate that a species absorbs some of its ingested carotene intact. A prolonged slow rate of postabsorptive conversion to retinol has been observed in volunteers in isotope kinetic studies [102].

Plasma Transport

Plasma Retinol

In the fasting state, greater than 95% of plasma vitamin A is present as retinol bound to RBP. The term plasma vitamin A usually implies total retinol (determined after saponification of retinyl esters) whereas plasma retinol indicates unesterified retinol specifically. Plasma or

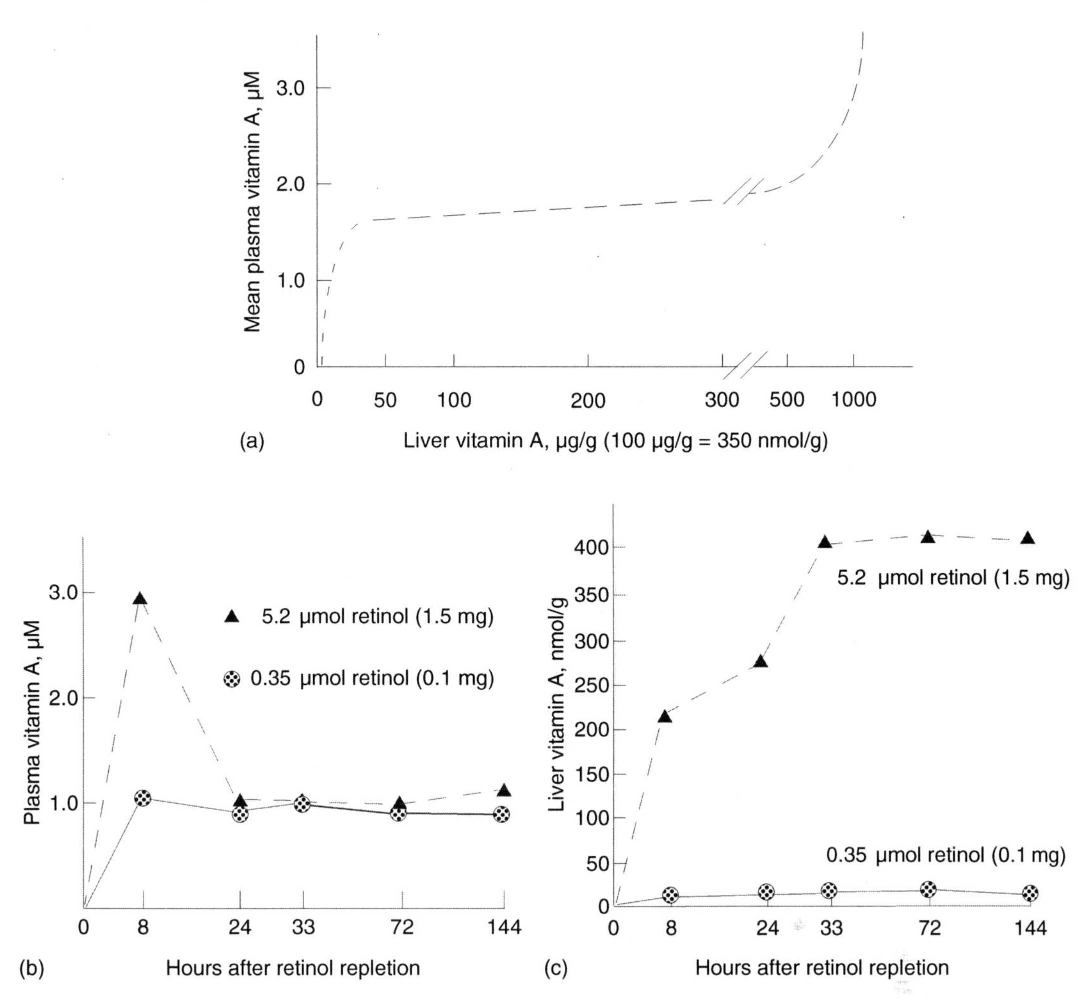

FIGURE 1.5 Relationships of plasma and liver vitamin A storage. (a) Relationship of plasma retinol concentration to liver retinol concentration. Three portions of the curve represent the following: left, inadequate liver vitamin A to maintain a normal level of plasma retinol; middle, homeostatic regulation of plasma retinol over a range of liver retinol concentrations from ~20 to ~300 μg/g liver; right, increasing plasma total retinol at liver concentrations greater than ~300 μg/g, due to presence in plasma of lipoprotein-associated retinyl esters. (From Olson, J.A., *J. Natl. Canc. Inst.*, 73, 1439, 1984. With permission.) (b) Plasma retinol response of vitamin A-deficient rats to oral repletion with a small (0.35 μmol) or large (5.2 μmol) dose of vitamin A. Initial spike of plasma retinol in rats that received the large dose is due to transient presence of retinyl esters. (c) Liver response to the same doses as in b; the 5.2 μmol dose was adequate to replete liver vitamin A stores, whereas the 0.35 μmol dose was not, although both increased plasma retinol to normal levels. (From Pasatiempo, A.M.G., Abaza, M., Taylor, C.E., and Ross, A.C., *Am. J. Clin. Nutr.*, 55, 443, 1992. With permission.)

serum retinol levels are normally very stable, with low inter- and intra-individual variations [122], averaging ~2–2.2 μM for adult men and women in NHANES III. Although lower in children and adolescents, concentrations increased progressively with age. All but a small portion of retinol is RBP-bound, and nearly all RBP is bound to TTR, but plasma contains additional TTR that is not associated with holo-RBP. Both RBP and TTR have high rates of turnover, with half-lives of ~0.5 and 2–3 days, respectively [154], and therefore must be constantly resynthesized. The plasma concentrations of RBP and TTR are sometimes used as an indicator of adequate visceral protein synthesis.

In healthy vitamin A-adequate individuals, the concentration of plasma retinol is tightly regulated. Plasma retinol falls only when vitamin A status is becoming precarious (marginal), and continues to decline as overt vitamin A deficiency develops. Vitamin A status has sometimes been categorized as sufficient, marginal, or deficient, based on somewhat arbitrary cut-off values, even though it is understood that vitamin A status actually represents a continuum of states. In general, plasma retinol values above 1.05 μM (30 μg/dL) are accepted as indicating vitamin A adequacy, values between 0.7 and 1.05 μM (20–30 μg/dL plasma) as indicating marginal vitamin A status, and less than 0.7 μM retinol as indicating vitamin A deficiency [122,155]. In experimental models of vitamin A deficiency, such as rats fed a vitamin A-free diet, plasma retinol has usually fallen to less than 0.10 μM before weight loss or external signs of deficiency are evident.

Conditions in Which Plasma Retinol May Be Low

Although low plasma retinol is a presumptive indicator that vitamin A status is inadequate, it can also result from impaired mobilization and transport of retinol [24]. Several conditions resulting in low plasma retinol are listed in Table 1.4. Nutritional deficiencies of protein, calories, or micronutrients limit the synthesis of RBP and release of holo-RBP, and plasma retinol may be low even if hepatic vitamin A is not limiting. Excessive alcohol intake depletes vitamin A stores and reduces retinol transport. Various liver diseases affect the synthesis of RBP and TTR [24,154]. Retinol also may be low due to renal diseases that impair the recovery of retinol after filtration of the holo-RBP complex. Mice lacking the multiligand protein receptor megalin, which has been implicated in the reuptake of RBP and TTR in renal tubules, were shown to lose retinol in their urine [156–158]. Retinol may be reduced in states of infection or inflammation because, during the acute-phase response, the synthesis of RBP and TTR is reduced [159].

Low plasma retinol also may be due to perturbations in the protein transport complex induced by retinoids used experimentally or therapeutically, such as 4HPR which binds to RBP, displacing retinol and destabilizing the association of RBP with TTR [28]. The concentrations of plasma retinol and RBP are also significantly reduced by supraphysiologic doses of retinoic acid [160].

Rare cases of hyporetinolemia of genetic origin have been described. In two teenage female siblings who presented with night blindness [161], plasma retinol and RBP were very low, even though vitamin A intake was apparently adequate. Molecular analysis revealed the presence of two single-point mutations in the *RBP* gene that were predicted to alter two amino acids in RBP protein [161]. Although the girls' plasma retinol levels were very low, less than 0.2 μM, their growth and development was normal, and their retinoic acid levels were similar to controls. Mice lacking the *RBP* gene showed a similar phenotype [162]. These results suggest that other retinoids (such as chylomicron retinyl esters) can compensate for RBP-bound retinol and, since vision was most affected, that the retina is more dependent than other tissues on the delivery of retinol by holo-RBP.

Because multiple nutritional and metabolic disturbances can lead to similar decreases in plasma retinol, RBP, and TTR, laboratory values must be interpreted cautiously. It can be unclear whether a reduction is the result of a nutritional deficiency of vitamin A or due to other factors, such as inflammation. Retinol dose–response tests and isotopic dilution methods [163,164] have been used to test whether hepatic vitamin A stores are sufficient for a normal rate of secretion of holo-RBP. Measuring acute-phase proteins along with retinol may help to determine whether low plasma retinol concentrations could be due to inflammation [155,165,166].

Other Retinoids in Plasma

Several acidic and more polar retinoids have been measured in human and animal plasma, but quantitative data are quite limited. In general, these retinoids are present in the nanomolar range, much lower than retinol, for which 1–3 μM is normal. In a study that measured several forms of retinoic acid at once, all-*trans*-retinoic acid, 13-*cis*-retinoic acid, and 13-*cis*-4-oxo-retinoic acid averaged 5.6–7 nM, compared with 2.2 μM for retinol [167]. The half-life of acidic retinoids is short, making metabolic studies at physiological concentrations difficult. In pharmacokinetic studies using high doses of all-*trans*-RA and 9-*cis*-RA in rhesus monkeys, plasma half-times were in the range of 15–30 min [168,169]. Rats that received a tracer amount of isotopically labeled retinoic acid complexed to albumin cleared more than 90% of retinoic acid from plasma in 3–5 min [170].

Plasma Carotenoids

Carotenoids circulate in plasma in association with LDLs and HDLs. The level of β-carotene reflects its recent intake, but is also increased when plasma lipoprotein levels are elevated.

Plasma Retinol Kinetics and Recycling

Computer-based compartmental modeling has been used to analyze the kinetics of plasma retinol turnover. Each molecule of retinol recirculates from liver to other tissues through the plasma compartment several times before it leaves the system and is irreversibly disposed [171]. In one young man who consumed 105 μmol of retinyl palmitate in a test meal, 50 μmol of retinol passed through his plasma per day, while only 4 μmol/day was degraded. Plasma retinol concentration itself was a significant predictor of the rate of retinol utilization [172]. Unlike retinol, RBP apparently is not recycled. Therefore, it appears that new RBP must be synthesized in extrahepatic tissues to release retinol back into plasma. As noted earlier, some extrahepatic tissues, such as kidney and adipose, contain RBP mRNA [24]. Holo-RBP can bind to renal epithelial cells and cross the epithelium by transcytosis, suggesting a mechanism for the recovery of retinol lost by filtration [173]. Megalin, a large protein implicated in the reuptake of several small nutrient-binding proteins in the kidney, has been shown to bind RBP and TTR [156,157], and its synthesis appears to be regulated by retinoic acid [174]. Retinoic acid also alters the plasma kinetics and tissue distribution of retinol [175].

Intracellular Retinoid Metabolism

Most tissues contain retinyl esters, at concentrations lower than those in liver, which appear to provide the substrate for the local generation of bioactive retinoids, as illustrated schematically in Figure 1.4.

Hydrolysis

The hydrolysis of retinyl esters is catalyzed by a variety of both secreted and intracellular enzymes of the lipase and carboxylesterase families. However, as most of the enzymes studied in detail to date were from pancreas, intestine, or liver, there is little detailed information on the exact nature of the enzymes responsible for the hydrolysis of retinyl esters in most peripheral tissues (see Harrison and Hussain [176] for review). It is likely, however, that one or more of the four major carboxylesterases, ES 2, ES 3, ES 4, or ES 10, are involved [130].

Oxidation–Reduction and Irreversible Oxidation Reactions

The oxidation of retinol to retinal, and reduction of retinal to retinol, can be catalyzed by several different enzymes; some are members of the alcohol dehydrogenase gene family and others of the short-chain dehydrogenase or reductase gene family [177]. All these can also metabolize other substrates, often steroids, as well as retinoids. The preferred substrates of these enzymes, their distribution and biological significance, and how they may respond to changes in vitamin A status are not well clarified. Some retinol dehydrogenases are capable of oxidizing CBP-bound retinol and are colocalized with CRBP in various tissues [178]. Therefore, they would appear most likely to be involved in retinol oxidation in vivo, but other enzymes cannot be ruled out. Vitamin A-sensitive tissues were shown to contain a cassette of CRBP-I, an epithelial retinol dehydrogenase, retinal dehydrogenase 2 (RALDH2), and CRABP-II, all implicated in the conversion of retinol to retinoic acid. However, because some epithelial cells possessed only some of these elements, it was proposed that the complete conversion of retinol to retinoic acid may involve cooperation between epithelial cells and neighboring mesenchymal cells [179].

The oxidation of the C-15 terminal group of retinal is a physiologically irreversible process that produces retinoic acid, the main hormonal metabolite of vitamin A. Many tissues contain retinoic acid, at nanomolar concentrations in tissues that have been analyzed, and several isomers are usually detectable. Retinoic acid levels are thought to be regulated through both biogenesis and catabolism [177]. Some tissues, such as liver and brain, obtain most of their retinoic acid by uptake from plasma, while other tissues, including testis, kidney, and adipose tissues, produce most by oxidative metabolism [170]. The rapid turnover of retinoic acid, as indicated in the section Other Retinoids in Plasma, implies that new retinoic acid molecules must be produced continuously from precursors to maintain physiological levels. Several enzymes have been implicated in retinoic acid biosynthesis, including enzymes belonging to the aldehyde dehydrogenase family (ALDH) and a family of retinal dehydrogenases (RALDH1, RALDH2, RALDH3, and RALDH4) [42]; however, their individual roles are still unclear. All four of the *RALDH* genes were found to be expressed in mouse liver [180], whereas RALDH2 was present in mouse embryos early in development [181], and RALDH4 was expressed later. 9-*cis*-Retinoic acid was formed by expressed RALDH4 [180], suggesting a pathway for the formation of this isomer.

Formation of More Polar Retinoids

Retinol and retinoic acid are also subject to oxidation of the ring and side chain, as well as chain-shortening reactions that apparently prepare the molecules for excretion [182]. A number of enzymatic activities have been implicated in these reactions, but the activity of one cytochrome P450 gene family, CYP26, appears to play a prominent role and to be highly inducible by retinoic acid. The CYP26 family comprises at least three genes, A, B, and C, that encode monooxygenases capable of converting retinoic acid into 4-hydroxy, 4-oxo, and 18-hydroxy metabolites [183–185]. The various *CYP26* genes are expressed in patterns that are specific with respect to location and timing during embryonic development and are essential for establishing the body pattern of the embryo [186,187]. Mouse embryos lacking CYP26A1, and presumably unable to control retinoic acid levels, were not viable [186]. Both CYP26A1 and CYP26B1 enzymes are very selective for the all-*trans* isomer of retinoic acid, but CYP26C1 can also metabolize 9-*cis*-retinoic acid [188]. The proximal promoter region of the *CYP26A1* gene contains a RARE of the DR-5 type, whereas the second RARE is located 2 kb further upstream [189]. The expression of CYP26A1 in rat liver was dose-dependently regulated by dietary vitamin A [190]. CYP26A1 was also rapidly and dose-dependently upregulated in the liver, intestine, and other tissues by short-term treatment with retinoic acid and related retinoid analogs [190–192]. In general, the oxidation of retinoic acid and the formation of more polar retinoids is considered an inactivation reaction (phase I reaction) that is important in the normal metabolism of retinoic acid and to prevent toxicity. Oxidation of the C-4 position of retinoic acid is apparently linked to conjugation (phase II metabolism) and excretion. Nonetheless, some studies support the idea that oxidized forms of retinoic acid may possess biological activity [193]. Although the enzymes mentioned earlier are thought to have a major role in retinoid metabolism, several different enzymes may contribute to the activation and catabolism of retinoids.

Conjugation

Members of the UDP-glucuronyltransferase gene family have been implicated in the glucuronidation of 4-oxo-retinoic acid, mainly on the C-4 position, although glucuronidation of the carboxyl group at C-15 should also be possible [194,195]. Glucuronidation of retinoic acid, or retinol, converts these lipophilic molecules into water-soluble forms [196]. Glucuronides comprise a substantial fraction of the total retinoid excreted in bile and eliminated by the fecal route [197].

While retinoyl-β-glucuronide seems to be an inactivation product, it has also been shown to have biological activity in vivo and in vitro [198]. It is notable as it is relatively nontoxic, compared with retinoic acid, in tests of teratogenicity [199,200]. Retinoyl-β-glucuronide is not known to bind to nuclear retinoid receptors [201], so its biological activity may be related to its distribution properties and potential for slow hydrolysis to retinoic acid.

Isomerization

How *cis* retinoids are formed remains poorly understood. 13-*cis*- and 9-*cis*-retinoids are found in extracts of plasma. The formation of 11-*cis*-retinal in the RPE is well described (see the section Retina), although the enzymology is still controversial. An unusual isomerohydrolase has been implicated, which can concomitantly hydrolyze all-*trans*-retinyl esters and, apparently, use the released energy to convert retinol to the 11-*cis* isomer, which can then be oxidized to 11-*cis*-retinal. The retinal protein RPE65 has also been implicated as a possible mechanism [202]. *Cis* retinoids have been detected in other tissues but yet there is no compelling evidence for their enzymatic formation; and they might form spontaneously, as has been seen in vitro. In general, *cis* retinoids do not bind to the cellular retinoid-binding proteins that are present in most tissues. The preference of the cellular retinoid-binding proteins for retinoids in the *trans* conformation may explain why all-*trans*-retinoids are predominant in nearly all tissues. In contrast, the retina contains CRALBP and IRBP, which are capable of binding both *cis* and *trans* retinoids, and both *cis* and *trans* retinoids are abundant in the retina.

VITAMIN A AND PUBLIC HEALTH

Prevention of Xerophthalmia

Vitamin A deficiency is a primary cause of xerophthalmia, which is manifested as night blindness and corneal abnormalities—softening of the cornea (keratomalacia) and ulceration—leading to irreversible blindness. In the early 1990s, the WHO estimated that approximately 3 million children, most living in India, parts of Southeast Asia, and sub-Saharan Africa, had some form of xerophthalmia annually, and, on the basis of blood retinol levels, another 250 million were subclinically deficient [14]. The use of vitamin A to prevent or treat xerophthalmia represents an important success story in the nutritional sciences [203]. The WHO, together with the International Vitamin A Consultative Group (IVACG) and foundations such as Helen Keller International, has been instrumental in establishing vitamin A supplementation programs in areas where xerophthalmia was, or still is, a public health concern. Because vitamin A is readily absorbed, even by vitamin A-deficient individuals, and can be stored in tissues in amounts that provide retinol for 4–6 months or longer, it is possible to distribute high-dose vitamin A supplements (20,000 IU or 60 mg) of retinol to children over 1 year and to adults [204,205] at infrequent intervals, often 4–6 months apart. Enough vitamin A is absorbed and stored quickly, and released and used slowly, to prevent the development of xerophthalmia over an extended period.

Actions of Vitamin A in the Eye

The biological basis for the prevention of xerophthalmia is twofold: 11-*cis*-retinal is specifically required for the production of rhodopsin in rods and analogous proteins in cones [206], whereas retinoic acid is required for the maintenance and integrity of the corneal epithelium, a role similar to the one it plays in many other epithelial tissues.

Retina

Night blindness is often the first detectable sign of vitamin A deficiency. It is experienced as a loss of the ability to quickly readapt to the dark, after the retina is exposed to bright light. The absorption of light by rhodopsin in the photoreceptor cells results in the instantaneous isomerization of its 11-*cis*-retinal moiety to all-*trans*-retinal, and this photoisomerization event initiates a signal cascade to nearby retinal ganglion cells, which is propagated to the visual cortex of the brain. For normal vision to continue, the all-*trans*-retinal, just released from rhodopsin, must be converted back to 11-*cis*-retinal and recombined with opsin, a process known as dark adaptation. Dark adaptation occurs through an elegant series of reactions, known as the visual cycle or retinoid cycle [206], which involve both RPE and photoreceptor cells and the cycling of retinoids between them. However, the reactions of the visual cycle take place over minutes, as compared with milliseconds for photoisomerization [207], and thus dark adaptation would be slow were it not for the ability of the retina to very quickly generate new molecules of 11-*cis*-retinal using retinyl esters stored in the RPE as substrate. Retinyl esters previously formed by LRAT [120] are rapidly hydrolyzed and isomerized to 11-*cis*-retinol. It has been proposed that these steps take place in a single enzymatic reaction catalyzed by isomerohydrolase, a unique enzyme expressed in the RPE [208]. However, alternative mechanisms have also been suggested [209]. In a subsequent reaction facilitated by CRALBP, 11-*cis*-retinol is oxidized to 11-*cis*-retinal [207]. Then, in a transport step facilitated by IRBP the 11-*cis*-retinal molecule formed in the RPE is returned to the rod cell for combination with opsin, thereby taking the place of a molecule of rhodopsin that was bleached [207,210]. If the storage of vitamin A in the RPE is not adequate, the synthesis of rhodopsin is necessarily delayed as the visual cycle is completed, and night blindness occurs as the functional outcome of this delay. Ultimately, an adequate supply of retinoids in the eye depends on the resupply of retinol by holo-RBP to the RPE, to refill the retinyl ester pool.

Although the retinoid cycle is best understood for rod cells, a recently described cone retinoid cycle shares some of the same features [211]. However, Müller glial cells located near the cones apparently store retinyl esters in the cone retinoid cycle, analogous to the role of the RPE in the rod retinoid cycle [211].

Cornea and Conjunctiva

The epithelial cells of the cornea and conjunctiva require retinoids for their differentiation and integrity. RBP is expressed in the lacrimal glands and present in tears [212], and retinol bound to RBP is likely to be used for the biogenesis of retinoic acid by the cornea. Retinoid deficiency results in a loss of secretory goblet cells in the conjunctival membranes, observable cytologically [213,214], and sometimes includes visible Bitôt's spots (foamy, bacteria-laden deposits in the outer quadrants of the eye). These early changes typically progress gradually and can be reversed by vitamin A. However, when corneal lesions have advanced to the point of xerosis, further deterioration leading to corneal ulceration, loss of the lens, and scarring can occur rapidly. The need for vitamin A to avert irreversible blindness is urgent.

Morbidity and Mortality

The association of vitamin A deficiency and increased risk of mortality was not fully appreciated until late in the twentieth century. In the early 1980s, Sommer and colleagues reported results from studies in Indonesia in which young children with what was referred to as mild xerophthalmia—night blindness and Bitôt's spots—were found to have died at a higher rate than children with normal eyes [215]. Follow-up intervention studies by these and other investigators, conducted in preschool-aged children in poor regions of Southeast Asia, India, and Africa, showed conclusively that risk of mortality is reduced by preventing vitamin A deficiency (reviewed by Sommer [216]). Sommer [217] estimated that vitamin A administered at doses of 200,000 IU (60 mg retinol) every 6 months would reduce total mortality by 35% in preschool children, at a cost of a few cents per child per year, while a metaanalysis of eight epidemiological studies, including one in which vitamin A was administered weekly in amounts similar to the RDA, estimated a 23% reduction in mortality in children less than 6 years of age who received vitamin A [218]. Subsequent studies have shown a similar decrease in mortality in newborns [219] and pregnant women supplemented with vitamin A [220,221].

Subclinical Deficiency

Based on these observations, there is now increased interest in subclinical forms of vitamin A deficiency that, while not causing overt deficiency symptoms, may nonetheless increase the risk of developing respiratory and diarrheal infections, decrease growth rate, slow bone development, and decrease likelihood of survival from serious illness [222]. In children at risk of vitamin A deficiency, providing vitamin A supplements, given most often as prophylaxis and in some instances for therapy during illness, has significantly reduced the severity of infectious diseases. Vitamin A reduced measles-related morbidity and mortality [223]. Due to the protective role of vitamin A, WHO/UNICEF recommended in 1987 that in those countries where the measles fatality rate is 1% or greater, all the children diagnosed with measles should receive 30–60 mg of vitamin A immediately [205]. The American Academy of Pediatrics has also recommended vitamin A in the treatment of high-risk children with measles [224]. To facilitate the delivery of vitamin A supplements to young children, the WHO has recommended integrating vitamin A supplementation into the expanded program of immunization (EPI), using contacts at the time of measles and diphtheria–pertussis–tetanus vaccinations to deliver vitamin A to infants and children in countries where vitamin A deficiency is prevalent [225].

Immune System Changes

The ability of vitamin A to reduce mortality is widely thought to be due to effects on the immune system, which collectively may reduce the severity of disease and increase the likelihood of survival [226]. A number of animal models have been used to better understand the effects of vitamin A deficiency, and repletion, on the immune system [227]. In brief, vitamin A deficiency results in multiple abnormalities in innate and adaptive immunity involving cell differentiation, hematopoiesis and blood and lymphoid organ cell populations, and the organism's ability to respond to challenges with pathogens, antigens, and mitogens. Changes, either increases or decreases, in the numbers and functions of B-cells, T-cells, natural killer cells, antigen-presenting cells, and macrophages have all been reported. Responses are often imbalanced or dysregulated, evident as imbalances in the production of cytokines and type 1 or type 2 immune responses and alterations in cell proliferation and cell–cell interactions. Generally, these abnormalities are mostly or completely reversible by treatment with vitamin A or retinoic acid. In normal animals, retinoic acid has been shown to stimulate innate and adaptive immune responses [228–231].

Medical Uses of Retinoids

Retinoids have come into prominence as drugs in the treatment of dermatological diseases and certain leukemias, and they have shown promise in the prevention of some forms of cancer. These topics are mentioned here only briefly, with references to reviews of these specialized topics.

Dermatology

Essentially all epithelial tissues are sensitive to a lack, as well as an excess, of vitamin A [232]. In the skin, vitamin A deficiency appears as dryness (follicular hyperkeratosis associated with changes in the layers of the skin, sebaceous glands, and numerous keratins and other proteins). 13-*cis*-Retinoic acid (isotretinoin, Accutane*) has been used for more than two decades to treat severe cystic acne. Acetretin (Soritane†) is prescribed for severe psoriasis. In addition, numerous topical preparations of these and other retinoids are available for treating less severe dermatological conditions. Retinoids significantly reduce the production of sebum and induce keratinocytes to differentiate. The use of isotretinoin in dermatology has been reviewed by the American Academy of Dermatology [233].

The serious side effects of retinoic acid, especially its teratogenicity, threaten the continued use of retinoids in dermatology. Since the 1940s, it has been known that an excess or a deficiency of vitamin A causes birth defects or the death of the embryo, and later studies using acidic retinoids and their analogs showed them to be highly teratogenic [200]. Teratogenicity is often related to abnormal development of the neural crest, the head and sensory organs, nervous system, heart, limbs, and skeletomuscular system. Similar fetal abnormalities, often manifested as craniofacial defects, have affected the offspring of women who have consumed an excess of dietary vitamin A early in pregnancy, or have used prescription retinoids such as 13-*cis*-retinoic acid early in pregnancy. Because retinoids used therapeutically may persist in tissues for some time after their use has been discontinued, even assuring they have been discontinued before conception may not be enough to safeguard the fetus. Although the use of isotretinoin by women who could become pregnant has been contraindicated for years, and birth control has been required, cases of retinoid-related birth defects have persisted, suggesting inadequate compliance and monitoring. Therefore, in 2005, the FDA approved new strengthened regulations that include the registry of all patients to whom retinoids have been prescribed, the use of two forms of birth control, and the frequent reporting by both the patient and the prescribing physician. Other potential adverse effects, including depression and suicidal thoughts, were also reasons for the FDA's decision to raise the level of monitoring for prescription retinoids [234].

---

* A registered trademark of Hoffman-La Roche Inc. in the United States and other countries.

† A registered trademark of Hoffman-La Roche Inc. in the United States and other countries.

Acute Promyelocytic Leukemia

All-*trans*-retinoic has gained prominence for its ability to induce the differentiation of leukemic promyelocytes in patients with acute promyelocytic leukemia (APL) [235]. This form of leukemia is associated with chromosomal translocations involving the RAR-α nuclear receptor that result in several aberrant forms of receptor proteins and altered retinoid signaling. Remarkably, the majority of patients have achieved complete remission either with all-*trans*-retinoic acid alone or combined with chemotherapy [236].

Although all-*trans*-retinoic acid has generally been well tolerated by APL patients, some of them have developed a serious and sometimes fatal condition termed the retinoic acid syndrome, manifested by fever, respiratory distress, changes in hemostasis, and acute renal failure [237]. Protocols for the treatment of APL have been modified to reduce the length of treatment with retinoic acid to the minimum time necessary for differentiation of APL blasts and to introduce adjunctive therapies in place of prolonged treatment with retinoids [236].

Prevention of Hypervitaminosis A of Nutritional Origin

Hypervitaminosis A refers to high storage levels of vitamin A in the body that can lead to toxic symptoms. Signs of vitamin A toxicity include nausea and vomiting, headache, dizziness, blurred vision, lack of muscular coordination, abnormal liver functions, and pain in weight-bearing bones and joints. Most vitamin A toxicity results from the accidental or inappropriate use of supplements containing high levels of vitamin A [222]. Although rarely does hypervitaminosis A result from ingestion of food sources of vitamin A, a few case reports have described vitamin A toxicity due to excessive intakes of liver, and the frequent intake of high vitamin A foods still is a concern. In 2005, the Scientific Advisory Committee on Nutrition (SACN) of the Foods Standards Agency, in the United Kingdom, issued a report stating that, as a precaution, people who eat liver regularly, that is more than once a week, should not increase this amount and should avoid taking vitamin A supplements [238]. Symptoms resembling hypervitaminosis A have also been reported in some patients taking retinoids under medical supervision.

There is no treatment or antidote for hypervitaminosis A. Elevated tissue retinol levels fall only slowly after intake has stopped, as the tendency of the body is to conserve vitamin A. Thus, great care should be taken to prevent the development of hypervitaminosis A by limiting the consumption of foods, such as liver, and avoiding the use of supplements containing high levels of retinol (see ULs, Table 1.2).

Intakes of retinol that are higher than recommended levels but not overtly toxic may still have adverse consequences. Results from epidemiological and clinical studies have suggested that intakes of retinol not far above the RDA may reduce bone mineral density of the lumbar, femoral neck, and trochanter regions and increase the risk of osteoporotic disease [239,240]. The relative risk of hip fracture increased in a graded manner with increasing retinol intake, attributable primarily to retinol (either from diet or supplements), but not β-carotene intake [241].

Excessive Consumption of β-Carotene

β-Carotene and other carotenoids in foods, even when consumed at high levels, have not produced toxicity. For this reason, the UL for vitamin A does not include carotenoids. Excessive intakes of carotenoids often are the result of food faddism, such as vegetable juice diets, or use of supplements. When carotene accumulates in fatty tissues, yellow discoloration of the skin (carotenodermia) may result. However, Krinsky [242], in a review of the safety of β-carotene, has commented on the lack of carotenodermia in subjects ingesting very large amounts of carotenoids in foods for 6 weeks, but the appearance of carotenodermia after an intake of a 30 mg/day supplement of β-carotene for the same period [243]. The condition is not known to be harmful, and the yellow color slowly subsides after the excessive consumption of β-carotene ceases.

While the consumption of high amounts of β-carotene in foods and even in supplements is generally considered safe, the results of two large-scale placebo-controlled trials of the efficacy of β-carotene in the chemoprevention of lung cancer have called into question the safety of large doses of carotenoid supplements [244]. Thus, in both the α-Tocopherol β-Carotene Trial (ATBC) in Finland and the β-Carotene Retinol Efficacy Trial (CARET) in the United States, persons at high risk for lung cancer (i.e., smokers and asbestos workers) showed a significantly increased risk of lung cancer when supplemented with 20–30 mg of β-carotene/day for periods of 4–6 years. Although the mechanism of this effect is still not entirely clear, it is likely related to the induction of P450 enzymes by oxidative metabolites of β-carotene and perhaps from disruption of normal retinoid-signaling processes in cells [245]. Thus, this effect is apparently attributable to the pro-oxidant effects of β-carotene that have been observed under certain conditions in vitro and in vivo and not to the nutritional provitamin A activity of β-carotene.

REFERENCES

1. National Library of Medicine, *PubMed*, National Center for Biotechnology Information, 2005, http://www.ncbi.nlm.nih.gov/entrez/query.fcgi.
2. Wolf, G., A history of vitamin A and retinoids. *FASEB J.* 10, 1102, 1996.
3. Sporn, M.B. and Roberts, A.B., Introduction: What is a retinoid? in: *Retinoids, Differentiation, and Disease*, Pitman: London, 1985, p. 1.
4. International Union of Pure and Applied Chemists (IUPAC), Nomenclature of retinoids. Recommendations 1981, in: *IUPAC-IUBMB Joint Commission on Biochemical Nomenclature and Nomenclature Commission of IUBMB*, 2nd edition, Liébecq, C., editor, Portland Press, 1992, http://www.chem.qmul.ac.uk/iupac/misc/ret.html.
5. International Union of Pure and Applied Chemists, Nomenclature of Carotenoids, World Wide Web version prepared by G.P. Moss, 1974, http://www.chem.qmul.ac.uk/iupac/carot/.
6. Gundersen, T.E. and Blomhoff, R., Qualitative and quantitative liquid chromatographic determination of natural retinoids in biological samples. *J. Chromatogr. A* 935, 13, 2001.
7. Gellermann, W. et al., Raman detection of carotenoids in human tissue, in: *Carotenoids and Retinoids: Molecular Aspects and Health Issues*, Packer, L. et al., editors, AOCS Press: Champaign, IL, 2005, p. 86.
8. Furr, H.C., Barua, A.B., and Olson, J.A., Analytical methods, in: *The Retinoids: Biology, Chemistry and Medicine*, Sporn, M.B., Roberts, A.B. and Goodman, D.S., editors, Raven Press: NY, 1994, p. 179.
9. Furr, H.C., Analysis of retinoids and carotenoids: problems resolved and unsolved. *J. Nutr.* 134(Suppl.), 281S, 2004.
10. Tsin, A.T., Gentles, S.N., and Castillo, E.A., Selective utilization of serum vitamin A for visual pigment synthesis. *J. Exp. Biol.* 142, 207, 1989.
11. Dawson, M.I. and Zhang, X.K., Discovery and design of retinoic acid receptor and retinoid X receptor class- and subtype-selective synthetic analogs of all-*trans*-retinoic acid and 9-*cis*-retinoic acid. *Curr. Med. Chem.* 9, 623, 2002.
12. Nagpal, S. and Chandraratna, R.A., Recent developments in receptor-selective retinoids. *Curr. Pharm. Des.* 6, 919, 2000.
13. Mangels, A.R. et al., Carotenoid content of fruits and vegetables: an evaluation of analytic data. *J. Am. Diet. Assoc.* 93, 284, 1993.
14. FAO/WHO, Human vitamin and mineral requirements, in: *Report of a Joint FAO/WHO Expert Consultation. Vitamin A (Chapter 7)*, Bangkok, 2001, http://www.fao.org/documents/show_cdr.asp?url_file = /DOCREP/004/Y2809E/y2809e00.htm.

15. Institute of Medicine, *Dietary Reference Intakes for Vitamin A, Vitamin K, Arsenic, Boron, Chromium, Copper, Iodine, Iron, Manganese, Molybdenum, Nickel, Silicon, Vanadium, and Zinc*, National Academy Press: Washington, 2002, pp. 8–9.
16. Bieri, J.G. and McKenna, M.C., Expressing dietary values for fat-soluble vitamins: changes in concepts and terminology. *Am. J. Clin. Nutr.* 34, 289, 1981.
17. Expert Group on Vitamins and Minerals, *Safe Upper Levels for Vitamins and Minerals*, Food Standards Agency, UK, 2003 (see pdf).
18. USDA, *USDA Nutrient Database for Standard Reference*, Laboratory, Agricultural Research Service, 2004, http://www.nal.usda.gov/fnic/foodcomp/search/.
19. Surles, R.L. et al., Carotenoid profiles and consumer sensory evaluation of specialty carrots (*Daucus carota*, L.) of various colors. *J. Agric. Food Chem.* 52, 3417, 2004.
20. Rodriguez-Amaya, D.B., Food carotenoids: analysis, composition and alterations during storage and processing of foods. *Forum Nutr.* 56, 35, 2003.
21. USDA, *What We Eat in America*, 2004. Citation: U.S. Department of Agriculture, Agriculture Research Service. 2004. What We Eat in America, Nhanes 2001–2002: Documentation and Data Files. Available: http://www.ars.usda.gov/ba/bhnrc/fsrg.
22. Bangham, A.D., Dingle, J.T., and Lucy, J.A., Studies on the mode of action of excess of vitamin A. *Biochem. J.* 90, 133, 1964.
23. Newcomer, M.E. and Ong, D.E., Plasma retinol binding protein: structure and function of the prototypic lipocalin. *Biochim. Biophys. Acta* 1482, 57, 2000.
24. Soprano, D.R. and Blaner, W.S., Plasma retinol-binding protein, in: *The Retinoids: Biology, Chemistry and Medicine*, Sporn, M.B., Roberts, A.B., and Goodman, D.S., editors, Raven Press: NY, 1994, p. 257.
25. Smith, J.E., Muto, Y., and Goodman, D.S., Tissue distribution and subcellular localization of retinol-binding protein in normal and vitamin A-deficient rats. *J. Lipid Res.* 16, 318, 1975.
26. Raghu, P. and Sivakumar, B., Interactions amongst plasma retinol-binding protein, transthyretin and their ligands: implications in vitamin A homeostasis and transthyretin amyloidosis. *Biochim. Biophys. Acta* 1703, 1, 2004.
27. Eneqvist, T. et al., The transthyretin-related protein family. *Eur. J. Biochem.* 270, 518, 2003.
28. Malpeli, G., Folli, C., and Berni, R., Retinoid binding to retinol-binding protein and the interference with the interaction with transthyretin. *Biochim. Biophys. Acta* 1294, 48, 1996.
29. Berni, R. et al., Retinoids: in vitro interaction with retinol-binding protein and influence on plasma retinol. *FASEB J.* 7, 1179, 1993.
30. Folli, C. et al., Ligand binding and structural analysis of a human putative cellular retinol-binding protein. *J. Biol. Chem.* 277, 41970, 2002.
31. Formelli, F. et al., Plasma retinol level reduction by the synthetic retinoid fenretinide: a one year follow-up study of breast cancer patients. *Cancer Res.* 49, 6149, 1989.
32. Smith, J.E. et al., The plasma transport and metabolism of retinoic acid in the rat. *Biochem. J.* 132, 821, 1973.
33. Smith, F.R. and Goodman, D.S., Vitamin A transport in human vitamin A toxicity. *New Engl. J. Med.* 294, 805, 1976.
34. Cabezas, M.C. et al., Delayed chylomicron remnant clearance in subjects with heterozygous familial hypercholesterolaemia. *J. Intern. Med.* 244, 299, 1998.
35. Parker, R.S., Absorption, metabolism, and transport of carotenoids. *FASEB J.* 10, 542, 1996.
36. Romanchik, J.E., Morel, D.W., and Harrison, E.H., Distributions of carotenoids and alpha-tocopherol among lipoproteins do not change when human plasma is incubated in vitro. *J. Nutr.* 125, 2610, 1995.
37. Banaszak, L. et al., Lipid-binding proteins: a family of fatty acid and retinoid transport proteins. *Adv. Protein Chem.* 45, 89, 1994.
38. O'Bryne, S.M. and Blaner, W.S., Introduction to retinoids, in: *Carotenoids and Retinoids: Molecular Aspects and Health Issues*, Packer, L. et al., editors, AOCS Press: Champaign, IL, 2005, p. 1.
39. Ross, A.C., Cellular metabolism and activation of retinoids: roles of the cellular retinoid-binding proteins. *FASEB J.* 7, 317, 1993.
40. Noy, N., Retinoid-binding proteins: mediators of retinoid action. *Biochem. J.* 348 Pt 3, 481, 2000.

41. Ross, A.C., Zolfaghari, R., and Weisz, J., Vitamin A: recent advances in the biotransformation, transport, and metabolism of retinoids. *Curr. Opin. Gastroenterol.* 17, 184, 2001.
42. Napoli, J.L., Interactions of retinoid binding proteins and enzymes in retinoid metabolism. *Biochim. Biophys. Acta* 1440, 139, 1999.
43. Noy, N. and Blaner, W.S., Interactions of retinol with binding proteins: studies with rat cellular retinol-binding protein and with rat retinol-binding protein. *Biochemistry* 30, 6380, 1991.
44. Li, E., Structure and function of cytoplasmic retinoid binding proteins. *Mol. Cell. Biochem.* 192, 105, 1999.
45. Ghyselinck, N.B. et al., Cellular retinol-binding protein I is essential for vitamin A homeostasis. *EMBO J.* 18, 4903, 1999.
46. E, X.P. et al., Increased neonatal mortality in mice lacking cellular retinol-binding protein II. *J. Biol. Chem.* 277, 36617, 2002.
47. Folli, C. et al., Identification, retinoid binding, and x-ray analysis of a human retinol-binding protein. *Proc. Natl. Acad. Sci. USA* 98, 3710, 2001.
48. Vogel, S. et al., Characterization of a new member of the fatty acid-binding protein family that binds all-*trans*-retinol. *J. Biol. Chem.* 276, 1353, 2001.
49. Åström, A. et al., Retinoic acid induction of human cellular retinoic acid-binding protein-II gene transcription is mediated by retinoic acid receptor–retinoid X receptor heterodimers bound to one far upstream retinoic acid-responsive element with 5-base pair spacing. *J. Biol. Chem.* 269, 22334, 1994.
50. Siegenthaler, G. and Saurat, J.H., Retinoid binding proteins and human skin. *Pharmacol. Ther.* 40, 45, 1989.
51. Stahl, W. and Sies, H., Carotenoids and protection against solar UV radiation. *Skin Pharmacol. Appl. Skin Physiol.* 15, 291, 2002.
52. Zhang, L. et al., Analysis of human cellular retinol-binding protein II promoter during enterocyte differentiation. *Am. J. Physiol. Gastrointest. Liver Physiol.* 282, G1079, 2002.
53. Delva, L. et al., Physical and functional interactions between cellular retinoic acid binding protein II and the retinoic acid-dependent nuclear complex. *Mol. Cell. Biol.* 19, 7158, 1999.
54. Budhu, A.S. and Noy, N., Direct channeling of retinoic acid between cellular retinoic acid-binding protein II and retinoic acid receptor sensitizes mammary carcinoma cells to retinoic acid-induced growth arrest. *Mol. Cell. Biol.* 22, 2632, 2002.
55. Lampron, C. et al., Mice deficient in cellular retinoic acid binding protein II (CRABPII) or in both CRABPI and CRABPII are essentially normal. *Development* 121, 539, 1995.
56. Panagabko, C. et al., Ligand specificity in the CRAL-TRIO protein family. *Biochemistry* 42, 6467, 2003.
57. Gonzalez-Fernandez, F., Interphotoreceptor retinoid-binding protein—an old gene for new eyes. *Vis. Res.* 43, 3021, 2003.
58. Saari, J.C. et al., Visual cycle impairment in cellular retinaldehyde binding protein (CRALBP) knockout mice results in delayed dark adaptation. *Neuron* 29, 739, 2001.
59. Thompson, D.A. and Gal, A., Vitamin A metabolism in the retinal pigment epithelium: genes, mutations, and diseases. *Prog. Retin. Eye Res.* 22, 683, 2003.
60. Wei, L.N., Retinoid receptors and their coregulators. *Annu. Rev. Pharmacol. Toxicol.* 43, 47, 2003.
61. Chambon, P., A decade of molecular biology of retinoic acid receptors. *FASEB J.* 10, 940, 1996.
62. Mangelsdorf, D.J. et al., Nuclear receptor that identifies a novel retinoic acid response pathway. *Nature* 345, 224, 1990.
63. Privalsky, M.L., The role of corepressors in transcriptional regulation by nuclear hormone receptors. *Annu. Rev. Physiol.* 66, 315, 2004.
64. Srinivas, H. et al., c-Jun N-terminal kinase contributes to aberrant retinoid signaling in lung cancer cells by phosphorylating and inducing proteasomal degradation of retinoic acid receptor alpha. *Mol. Cell. Biol.* 25, 1054, 2005.
65. Zhang, Z.P. et al., Arginine of retinoic acid receptor beta which coordinates with the carboxyl group of retinoic acid functions independent of the amino acid residues responsible for retinoic acid receptor subtype ligand specificity. *Arch. Biochem. Biophys.* 409, 375, 2003.
66. Kato, S. et al., Widely spaced directly repeated PuGGTCA elements act as promiscuous enhancers for different classes of nuclear receptors. *Mol. Cell. Biol.* 15, 5858, 1996.

67. Hoffmann, B. et al., A retinoic acid receptor-specific element controls the retinoic acid receptor-β promoter. *Mol. Endocrinol.* 4, 1727, 1990.
68. Sun, S.Y. et al., Evidence that retinoic acid receptor beta induction by retinoids is important for tumor cell growth inhibition. *J. Biol. Chem.* 275, 17149, 2000.
69. Widschwendter, M. et al., Methylation and silencing of the retinoic acid receptor-b2 gene in breast cancer. *J. Natl. Canc. Inst.* 92, 826, 2000.
70. Perissi, V. et al., A corepressor/coactivator exchange complex required for transcriptional activation by nuclear receptors and other regulated transcription factors. *Cell* 116, 511, 2004.
71. Lemotte, P.K., Keidel, S., and Apfel, C.M., Phytanic acid is a retinoid X receptor ligand. *Eur. J. Biochem.* 236, 328, 1996.
72. Lengqvist, J. et al., Polyunsaturated fatty acids including docosahexaenoic and arachidonic acid bind to the retinoid X receptor alpha ligand-binding domain. *Mol. Cell Proteomics* 3, 692, 2004.
73. Olson, J.A., Carotenoids, in: *Modern Nutrition in Health and Disease*, Shils, M.E. et al., editors, Williams & Wilkins: Baltimore, 1999, p. 525.
74. Wang, X.-D. et al., Intestinal uptake and lymphatic absorption of β-carotene in ferrets: a model for human β-carotene metabolism. *Am. J. Physiol.* 263, G480, 1992.
75. Poor, C.L. et al., Evaluation of the preruminant calf as a model for the study of human carotenoid metabolism. *J. Nutr.* 122, 262, 1992.
76. Pollack, J. et al., Mongolian gerbils (*Meriones unguiculatus*) absorb beta-carotene intact from a test meal. *J. Nutr.* 124, 869, 1994.
77. Lee, C.M. et al., Review of animal models in carotenoid research. *J. Nutr.* 129, 2271, 1999.
78. Goodman, D.S. et al., The intestinal absorption and metabolism of vitamin A and β-carotene in man. *J. Clin. Invest.* 45, 1615, 1966.
79. van Vliet, T., Schreurs, W.H.P., and van den Berg, H., Intestinal β-carotene absorption and cleavage in men: response of β-carotene and retinyl esters in the triglyceride-rich lipoprotein fraction after a single oral dose of β-carotene. *Am. J. Clin. Nutr.* 62, 110, 1995.
80. Novotny, J.A. et al., Compartmental analysis of the dynamics of beta-carotene metabolism in an adult volunteer. *J. Lipid Res.* 36, 1825, 1995.
81. Lin, Y. et al., Variability of the conversion of beta-carotene to vitamin A in women measured by using a double-tracer study design. *Am. J. Clin. Nutr.* 71, 1545, 2000.
82. Noh, S.K. and Koo, S.I., Intraduodenal infusion of lysophosphatidylcholine restores the intestinal absorption of vitamins A and E in rats fed a low-zinc diet. *Exp. Biol. Med.* 226, 342, 2001.
83. Tso, P., Lee, T., and DeMichele, S.J., Randomized structured triglycerides increase lymphatic absorption of tocopherol and retinol compared with the equivalent physical mixture in a rat model of fat malabsorption. *J. Nutr.* 131, 2157, 2001.
84. Jayarajan, P., Reddy, V., and Mohanram, M., Effect of dietary fat on absorption of beta carotene from green leafy vegetables in children. *Indian J. Med. Res.* 71, 53, 1980.
85. El-Gorab, M.I., Underwood, B.A., and Loerch, J.D., The roles of bile salts in the uptake of β-carotene and retinol by rat everted gut sacs. *Biochim. Biophys. Acta* 401, 265, 1975.
86. Hollander, D. and Ruble, P.E., Jr., Beta-carotene intestinal absorption: bile, fatty acid, pH, and flow rate effects on transport. *Am. J. Physiol.* 235, E686, 1978.
87. During, A. et al., Carotenoid uptake and secretion by CaCo-2 cells: beta-carotene isomer selectivity and carotenoid interactions. *J. Lipid Res.* 43, 1086, 2002.
88. Jensen, C.D. et al., Observations on the effects of ingesting *cis*- and *trans*-β-carotene isomers on human serum concentrations. *Nutr. Rep. Int.* 35, 413, 1987.
89. Stahl, W. et al., All-*trans* beta-carotene preferentially accumulates in human chylomicrons and very low density lipoproteins compared with the 9-*cis* geometrical isomer. *J. Nutr.* 125, 2128, 1995.
90. Gaziano, J.M. et al., Discrimination in absorption or transport of beta-carotene isomers after oral supplemenatation with either all-*trans*- or 9-*cis*-beta-carotene. *Am. J. Clin. Nutr.* 61, 1248, 1995.
91. Johnson, E.J. et al., Beta-carotene isomers in human serum, breast milk and buccal mucosa cells after continuous oral doses of all-*trans* and 9-*cis* beta-carotene. *J. Nutr.* 1127, 1993, 1997.
92. You, C.S. et al., Evidence of *cis-trans* isomerization of 9-*cis*-beta-carotene during absorption in humans. *Am. J. Clin. Nutr.* 64, 177, 1996.
93. von Lintig, J. and Wyss, A., Molecular analysis of vitamin A formation: cloning and characterization of beta-carotene 15,15′-dioxygenases. *Arch. Biochem. Biophys.* 385, 47, 2001.

94. von Lintig, J. et al., Towards a better understanding of carotenoid metabolism in animals. *Biochim. Biophys. Acta* 1740, 122, 2005.
95. Gollapalli, D.R., Maiti, P., and Rando, R.R., RPE65 operates in the vertebrate visual cycle by stereospecifically binding all-*trans*-retinyl esters. *Biochemistry* 42, 11824, 2003.
96. Kiefer, C. et al., Identification and characterization of a mammalian enzyme catalyzing the asymmetric oxidative cleavage of provitamin A. *J. Biol. Chem.* 276, 14110, 2001.
97. Barua, A.B. and Olson, J.A., β-Carotene is converted primarily to retinoids in rats *in vivo*. *J. Nutr.* 130, 1996, 2000.
98. van Vliet, T. et al., β-Carotene absorption and cleavage in rats is affected by the vitamin A concentration of the diet. *J. Nutr.* 126, 499, 1996.
99. Bachmann, H. et al., Feedback regulation of beta, beta-carotene 15,15′-monooxygenase by retinoic acid in rats and chickens. *J. Nutr.* 132, 3616, 2002.
100. During, A. et al., Beta-carotene 15,15′-Dioxygenase activity in human tissues and cells: evidence of an iron dependency. *J. Nutr. Biochem.* 12, 640, 2001.
101. Boulanger, A. et al., Identification of beta-carotene 15,15′-monooxygenase as a peroxisome proliferator-activated receptor target gene. *FASEB J.* 17, 1304, 2003.
102. Tang, G. et al., Short-term (intestinal) and long-term (postintestinal) conversion of beta-carotene to retinol in adults as assessed by a stable-isotope reference method. *Am. J. Clin. Nutr.* 78, 259, 2003.
103. Lachance, P., Dietary intake of carotenes and the carotene gap. *Clin. Nutr.* 7, 118, 1988.
104. van Bennekum, A.M. et al., Lipoprotein lipase expression level influences tissue clearance of chylomicron retinyl ester. *J. Lipid Res.* 40, 565, 1999.
105. Weng, W. et al., Intestinal absorption of dietary cholesteryl ester is decreased but retinyl ester absorption is normal in carboxyl ester lipase knockout mice. *Biochemistry* 38, 4143, 1999.
106. van Bennekum, A.M. et al., Hydrolysis of retinyl esters by pancreatic triglyceride lipase. *Biochemistry* 39, 4900, 2000.
107. Rigtrup, K.M. et al., Retinyl ester hydrolytic activity associated with human intestinal brush border membranes. *Am. J. Clin. Nutr.* 60, 111, 1994.
108. Rigtrup, K.M. and Ong, D.E., A retinyl ester hydrolase activity intrinsic to the brush border membrane of rat small intestine. *Biochemistry* 31, 2920, 1992.
109. Rigtrup, K.M., Kakkad, B., and Ong, D.E., Purification and partial characterization of a retinyl ester hydrolase from the brush border of rat small intestine mucosa: probable identity with brush border phospholipase B. *Biochemistry* 33, 2661, 1994.
110. Nayak, N., Harrison, E.H., and Hussain, M.M., Retinyl ester secretion by intestinal cells: a specific and regulated process dependent on assembly and secretion of chylomicrons. *J. Lipid Res.* 42, 272, 2001.
111. Quick, T.C. and Ong, D.E., Vitamin A metabolism in the human intestinal Caco-2 cell line. *Biochemistry* 29, 11116, 1990.
112. Levin, M.S., Cellular retinol-binding proteins are determinants of retinol uptake and metabolism in stably transfected Caco-2 cells. *J. Biol. Chem.* 268, 8267, 1993.
113. During, A., Dawson, H.D., and Harrison, E.H., Carotenoid transport is decreased and expression of the lipid transporters SR-BI, NPC1L1 and ABCA1 is down-regulated in Caco-2 cells treated with Ezetimibe. *J. Nutr.* 135, 2305, 2005.
114. Blomhoff, R. et al., Vitamin A metabolism: new perspectives on absorption, transport and storage. *Physiol. Rev.* 71, 951, 1991.
115. Huang, H.S. and Goodman, D.S., Vitamin A and carotenoids. I. Intestinal absorption and metabolism of ^{14}C-labeled vitamin A alcohol and β-carotene in the rat. *J. Biol. Chem.* 240, 2839, 1965.
116. Kawaguchi, R. et al., A membrane receptor for retinol binding protein mediates cellular uptake of vitamin A. *Science*, in press, 2007.
117. MacDonald, P.N. and Ong, D.E., A lecithin:retinol acyltransferase activity in human and rat liver. *Biochem. Biophys. Res. Commun.* 156, 157, 1988.
118. MacDonald, P.N. and Ong, D.E., Evidence for a lecithin–retinol acyltransferase activity in the rat small intestine. *J. Biol. Chem.* 263, 12478, 1988.
119. Yost, R.W., Harrison, E.H., and Ross, A.C., Esterification by rat liver microsomes of retinol bound to cellular retinol-binding protein. *J. Biol. Chem.* 263, 18693, 1988.

120. Batten, M.L. et al., Lecithin–retinol acyltransferase is essential for accumulation of all-*trans*-retinyl esters in the eye and in the liver. *J. Biol. Chem.* 279, 10422, 2004.
121. Yen, C.L. et al., The triacylglycerol synthesis enzyme DGAT1 also catalyzes the synthesis of diacylglycerols, waxes, and retinyl esters. *J. Lipid Res.* 46, 1502, 2005.
122. Pilch, S.M., Analysis of vitamin A data from the health and nutrition examination surveys. *J. Nutr.* 117, 636, 1987.
123. Ross, A.C. and Zilversmit, D.B., Chylomicron remnant cholesteryl esters as the major constituent of very low density lipoproteins in plasma of cholesterol-fed rabbits. *J. Lipid Res.* 18, 169, 1977.
124. Mallia, A.K., Smith, J.E., and Goodman, D.S., Metabolism of retinol-binding protein and vitamin A during hypervitaminosis A in the rat. *J. Lipid Res.* 16, 180, 1975.
125. Dawson, H.D. et al., Regulation of hepatic vitamin A storage in a rat model of controlled vitamin A status during aging. *J. Nutr.* 130, 1280, 2000.
126. Raila, J. et al., The distribution of vitamin A and retinol-binding protein in the blood plasma, urine, liver and kidneys of carnivores. *Vet. Res.* 31, 541, 2000.
127. Wilson, D.E. et al., Novel aspects of vitamin A metabolism in the dog: distribution of lipoprotein retinyl esters in vitamin A-deprived and cholesterol-fed animals. *Biochim. Biophys. Acta* 922, 247, 1987.
128. Ross, A.C., Pasatiempo, A.M., and Green, M.H., Chylomicron margination, lipolysis, and vitamin A uptake in the lactating rat mammary gland: implications for milk retinoid content. *Exp. Biol. Med.* (*Maywood*) 229, 46, 2004.
129. Goodman, D.S., Huang, H.S., and Shiratori, T., Tissue distribution and metabolism of newly absorbed vitamin A in the rat. *J. Lipid Res.* 6, 390, 1965.
130. Linke, T., Dawson, H., and Harrison, E.H., Isolation and characterization of a microsomal acid retinyl ester hydrolase. *J. Biol. Chem.* 280, 23287, 2005.
131. Sato, M., Suzuki, S., and Senoo, H., Hepatic stellate cells: unique characteristics in cell biology and phenotype. *Cell Struct. Funct.* 28, 105, 2003.
132. Matsuura, T. et al., Lecthin:retinol acyltransferase and retinyl ester hydrolase activities are differentially regulated by retinoids and have distinct distributions between hepatocyte and nonparenchymal cell fractions of rat liver. *J. Nutr.* 127, 218, 1997.
133. Yamada, E. and Hirosawa, K., The possible existence of a vitamin A-storing cell system. *Cell Struct. Funct.* 1, 201, 1976.
134. Hussain, M.M. et al., Chylomicron metabolism. Chylomicron uptake by bone marrow in different animal species. *J. Biol. Chem.* 264, 17931, 1989.
135. Dahro, M., Gunning, D., and Olson, J.A., Variations in liver concentrations of iron and vitamin A as a function of age in young American children dying of the sudden infant death syndrome as well as of other causes. *Int. J. Vitam. Nutr. Res.* 53, 13, 1983.
136. Suthutvoravoot, S. and Olson, J.A., Plasma and liver concentrations of vitamin A in a normal population of urban Thai. *Am. J. Clin. Nutr.* 27, 883, 1974.
137. Smith, J.E., Preparation of vitamin A-deficient rats and mice. *Meth. Enzymol.* 190, 229, 1990.
138. Ruiz, A. et al., Genomic organization and mutation analysis of the gene encoding lecithin retinol acyltransferase in human retinal pigment epithelium. *Invest. Ophthalmol. Vis. Sci.* 42, 31, 2001.
139. Zolfaghari, R. and Ross, A.C., Cloning, gene organization and identification of an alternative splicing process in lecithin:retinol acyltransferase cDNA from human liver. *Gene* 341, 181, 2004.
140. Zolfaghari, R. and Ross, A.C., Lecithin:retinol acyltransferase from mouse and rat liver: cDNA cloning and liver-specific regulation by dietary vitamin A and retinoic acid. *J. Lipid Res.* 41, 2024, 2000.
141. Randolph, R.K. and Ross, A.C., Vitamin A status regulates hepatic lecithin:retinol acyltransferase activity in rats. *J. Biol. Chem.* 266, 16453, 1991.
142. Matsuura, T. and Ross, A.C., Regulation of hepatic lecithin:retinol acyltransferase activity by retinoic acid. *Arch. Biochem. Biophys.* 301, 221, 1993.
143. Shimada, T. et al., Regulation of hepatic lecithin:retinol acyltransferase activity by retinoic acid receptor-selective retinoids. *Arch. Biochem. Biophys.* 344, 220, 1997.
144. Dawson, H.D. et al., Regulation of hepatic vitamin A storage in a rat model of controlled vitamin A status during aging. *J. Nutr.* 130, 1280, 2000.
145. Pasatiempo, A.M.G. et al., Effects of timing and dose of vitamin A on tissue retinol concentrations and antibody production in the previously vitamin A-depleted rat. *Am. J. Clin. Nutr.* 55, 443, 1992.

146. Underwood, B.A., Effect of protein quantity and quality on plasma response to an oral dose of vitamin A as an indicator of hepatic vitamin A reserves in rats. *J. Nutr.* 110, 1635, 1980.
147. Levin, M.S., Intestinal absorption and metabolism of vitamin A, in: *Physiology of the Gastrointestinal Tract*, Johnson, L.R., editor, Raven Press: NY, 1994, p. 1957.
148. Saari, J.C. et al., Analysis of the visual cycle in cellular retinol-binding protein type I (CRBPI) knockout mice. *Invest. Ophthalmol. Vis. Sci.* 43, 1730, 2002.
149. Olson, J.A., Serum level of vitamin A and carotenoids as reflectors of nutritional status. *J. Natl. Canc. Inst.* 73, 1439, 1984.
149a. Harrison, E.H. et al., Subcellular localization of retinoids, retinoid-binding proteins, and acyl-CoA: retinol acyltransferase in rat liver. *J. Lipid Res.* 28, 973, 1987.
150. Gerlach, T.H. and Zile, M.H., Effect of retinoic acid and apo-RBP on serum retinol concentration in acute renal failure. *FASEB J.* 5, 86, 1991.
151. Ross, A.C. and Zolfaghari, R., Regulation of hepatic retinol metabolism: perspective from studies on vitamin A status. *J. Nutr.* 134, 269 (suppl.) 2004.
152. Muto, Y. et al., Regulation of retinol-binding protein metabolism by vitamin A status in the rat. *J. Biol. Chem.* 247, 2542, 1972.
153. Tanumihardjo, S.A. et al., Refinement of the modified-dose-response test as a method for assessing vitamin A status in a field setting: experience with Indonesian children. *Am. J. Clin. Nutr.* 64, 966, 1996.
154. Goodman, D.S., Plasma retinol-binding protein, in: *The Retinoids*, vol. 2, Sporn, M.B., Roberts, A.B., and Goodman, D.S., editors, Academic Press: Orlando, FL, 1984, p. 42.
155. Semba, R.D. et al., Assessment of vitamin A status of preschool children in Indonesia using plasma retinol-binding protein. *J. Trop. Pediatr.* 48, 84, 2002.
156. Christensen, E.I. et al., Evidence for an essential role of megalin in transepithelial transport of retinol. *J. Am. Soc. Nephrol.* 10, 685, 1999.
157. Sousa, M.M. et al., Evidence for the role of megalin in renal uptake of transthyretin. *J. Biol. Chem.* 275, 38176, 2000.
158. Leheste, J.R. et al., Megalin knockout mice as an animal model of low molecular weight proteinuria. *Am. J. Pathol.* 155, 1361, 1999.
159. Rosales, F.J. et al., Effects of acute inflammation on plasma retinol, retinol-binding protein, and its mRNA in the liver and kidneys of vitamin A-sufficient rats. *J. Lipid Res.* 37, 962, 1996.
160. Ritter, S.J. and Smith, J.E., Retinol-binding protein secretion from the liver of *N*-(4-hydroxyphenyl) retinamide-treated rats. *Biochim. Biophys. Acta* 1290, 157, 1996.
161. Biesalski, H.K. et al., Biochemical but not clinical vitamin A deficiency results from mutations in the gene for retinol binding protein. *Am. J. Clin. Nutr.* 69, 931, 1999.
162. Quadro, L. et al., Impaired retinal function and vitamin A availability in mice lacking retinol-binding protein. *EMBO J.* 18, 4633, 1999.
163. Olson, J.A., Isotope-dilution technique: a wave of the future in human nutrition. *Am. J. Clin. Nutr.* 66, 186, 1997.
164. Haskell, M.J. et al., Assessment of vitamin A status by the deuterated-retinol-dilution technique and comparison with hepatic vitamin A concentration in Bangladeshi surgical patients. *Am. J. Clin. Nutr.* 66, 67, 1997.
165. Rosales, F.J. et al., Relation of serum retinol to acute phase proteins and malarial morbidity in Papua New Guinea children. *Am. J. Clin. Nutr.* 71, 1582, 2000.
166. Stephensen, C.B. and Gildengorin, G., Serum retinol, the acute phase response, and the apparent misclassification of vitamin A status in the third National Health and Nutrition Examination Survey. *Am. J. Clin. Nutr.* 72, 1170, 2000.
167. Teerlink, T. et al., Simultaneous analysis of retinol, all-*trans*- and 13-*cis*-retinoic acid and 13-*cis*-4-oxoretinoic acid in plasma by liquid chromatography using on-column concentration after single-phase fluid extraction. *J. Chromatogr. B Biomed. Sci. Appl.* 694, 83, 1997.
168. Adamson, P.C. et al., Dose-dependent pharmacokinetics of all-*trans*-retinoic acid. *J. Natl. Canc. Inst.* 84, 1332, 1992.
169. Adamson, P.C. et al., Pharmacokinetics of 9-*cis*-retinoic acid in the Rhesus monkey. *Cancer Res.* 55, 482, 1995.
170. Kurlandsky, S.B. et al., Plasma delivery of retinoic acid to tissues in the rat. *J. Biol. Chem.* 270, 17850, 1995.

171. Green, M.H. and Green, J.B., Quantitative and conceptual contributions of mathematical modeling to current views on vitamin A metabolism, biochemistry, and nutrition. *Adv. Food Nutr. Res.* 40, 3, 1996.
172. Kelley, S.K. and Green, M.H., Plasma retinol is a major determinant of vitamin A utilization in rats. *J. Nutr.* 128, 1767, 1998.
173. Marino, M. et al., Transcytosis of retinol-binding protein across renal proximal tubule cells after megalin (gp 330)-mediated endocytosis. *J. Am. Soc. Nephrol.* 12, 637, 2001.
174. Liu, W. et al., Regulation of gp330/megalin expression by vitamins A and D. *Eur. J. Clin. Invest.* 28, 100, 1998.
175. Cifelli, C.J., Green, J.B., and Green, M.H., Dietary retinoic acid alters vitamin A kinetics in both the whole body and in specific organs of rats with low vitamin A status. *J. Nutr.* 135, 746, 2005.
176. Harrison, E.H. and Hussain, M.M., Mechanisms involved in the intestinal digestion and absorption of dietary vitamin A. *J. Nutr.* 131, 1405, 2001.
177. Napoli, J.L., Enzymology and biogenesis of retinoic acid, in: *Vitamin A and Retinoids: An Update of Biological Aspects and Clinical Applications*, Livrea, M.A., editor, Birkhèuser Verlag: Basel, 2000, p. 17.
178. Zhai, Y., Higgins, D., and Napoli, J.L., Coexpression of the mRNAs encoding retinol dehydrogenase isozymes and cellular retinol-binding protein. *J. Cell. Physiol.* 173, 36, 1997.
179. Everts, H.B., Sundberg, J.P., and Ong, D.E., Immunolocalization of retinoic acid biosynthesis systems in selected sites in rat. *Exp. Cell Res.* 308, 309, 2005.
180. Lin, M. et al., Mouse retinal dehydrogenase 4 (RALDH4), molecular cloning, cellular expression, and activity in 9-*cis*-retinoic acid biosynthesis in intact cells. *J. Biol. Chem.* 278, 9856, 2003.
181. Ulven, S.M. et al., Identification of endogenous retinoids, enzymes, binding proteins, and receptors during early postimplantation development in mouse: important role of retinal dehydrogenase type 2 in synthesis of all-*trans*-retinoic acid. *Dev. Biol.* 220, 379, 2000.
182. Roberts, A.B. and DeLuca, H.F., Pathways of retinol and retinoic acid metabolism in the rat. *Biochem. J.* 102, 600, 1967.
183. White, J.A. et al., Identification of the human cytochrome P450, P450RAI-2, which is predominantly expressed in the adult cerebellum and is responsible for all-*trans*-retinoic acid metabolism. *Proc. Natl. Acad. Sci. USA* 97, 6403, 2000.
184. Nelson, D.R., A second CYP26P450 in humans and zebrafish: CYP26B1. *Arch. Biochem. Biophys.* 371, 345, 1999.
185. MacLean, G. et al., Cloning of a novel retinoic-acid metabolizing cytochrome P450, *CYP26B1*, and comparative expression analysis with *CYP26A1* during early murine development. *Mech. Dev.* 107, 195, 2001.
186. Abu-Abed, S. et al., Developing with lethal RA levels: genetic ablation of Rarg can restore the viability of mice lacking CYP26A1. *Development* 130, 1449, 2003.
187. Kudoh, T., Wilson, S.W., and Dawid, I.B., Distinct roles for Fgf, Wnt and retinoic acid in posteriorizing the neural ectoderm. *Development* 129, 4335, 2002.
188. Taimi, M. et al., A novel human cytochrome P450, CYP26C1 involved in metabolism of 9-*cis* and all-*trans*, isomers of retinoic acid. *J. Biol. Chem.* 279, 77, 2004.
189. Loudig, O. et al., Transcriptional co-operativity between distant retinoic acid response elements in regulation of CYP26A1 inducibility. *Biochem. J.* 392, 241, 2005.
190. Yamamoto, Y., Zolfaghari, R., and Ross, A.C., Regulation of CYP26 (cytochrome P450RAI) mRNA expression and retinoic acid metabolism by retinoids and dietary vitamin A in liver of mice and rats. *FASEB J.* 14, 2119, 2000.
191. Wang, Y., Zolfaghari, R., and Ross, A.C., Cloning of rat cytochrome P450RAI (CYP26) cDNA and regulation of hepatic CYP26 gene expression by retinoic acid in vivo. *FASEB J.* 15, A602, 2001.
192. Lampen, A., Meyer, S., and Nau, H., Effects of receptor-selective retinoids on CYP26 gene expression and metabolism of all-*trans*-retinoic acid in intestinal cells. *Drug Metab. Dispos.* 29, 742, 2001.
193. Idres, N. et al., Activation of retinoic acid receptor-dependent transcription by all-*trans*-retinoic acid metabolites and isomers. *J. Biol. Chem.* 277, 31491, 2002.
194. Samokyszyn, V.M. et al., 4-Hydroxyretinoic acid, a novel substrate for human liver microsomal UDP-glucuronosyltransferase(s) and recombinant UGT2B7. *J. Biol. Chem.* 275, 6908, 2000.

195. Radominska, A. et al., Glucuronidation of retinoids by rat recombinant UDP: glucuronosyltransferase 1.1 (bilirubin UGT). *Drug Metab. Dispos.* 25, 889, 1997.
196. Olson, J.A. et al., Enhancement of biological activity by conjugation reactions. *J. Nutr.* 122, 615, 1992.
197. Hicks, V.A., Gunning, D.B., and Olson, J.A., Metabolism, plasma transport and biliary excretion of radioactive vitamin A and its metabolites as a function of liver reserves of vitamin A in the rat. *J. Nutr.* 114, 1327, 1984.
198. Romans, D.A., Barua, A.B., and Olson, J.A., Pharmacokinetics of all-*trans* retinoyl beta-glucuronide in rats following intraperitoneal and oral administration. *Int. J. Vit. Nutr. Res.* 73, 251, 2003.
199. Gunning, D.B., Barua, A.B., and Olson, J.A., Comparative teratogenicity and metabolism of all-*trans* retinoic acid, all-*trans* retinoyl β-glucose, and all-*trans* retinoyl β-glucuronide in pregnant Sprague-Dawley rats. *Teratology* 47, 29, 1993.
200. Soprano, D.R. and Soprano, K.J., Retinoids as teratogens. *Annu. Rev. Nutr.* 15, 111, 1995.
201. Sani, B.P. et al., Retinoyl beta-glucuronide: lack of binding to receptor proteins of retinoic acid as related to biological activity. *Biochem. Pharmacol.* 43, 919, 1992.
202. Redmond, T.M. et al., Mutation of key residues of RPE65 abolishes its enzymatic role as isomerohydrolase in the visual cycle. *Proc. Natl. Acad. Sci. USA* 102, 13658, 2005.
203. Buyckx, M., The FAO programme for the prevention and control of vitamin A deficiency. *Food Nutr. Agric.* 2/3, 16, 1991.
204. WHO, Prevention and control of vitamin A deficiency, xerophthalmia and nutritional blindness, in: *Proposal for a Ten-Year Programme of Support to Countries*, ed. Organization, Geneva: WHO, Doc. NUT/84.5 Rev 1, 1985, As cited at: http://www.unsystem.org/scn/archives/rwns01/ch10.htm.
205. WHO/UNICEF, Vitamin A for measles. *Lancet* 2, 1067, 1987.
206. McBee, J.K. et al., Confronting complexity: the interlink of phototransduction and retinoid metabolism in the vertebrate retina. *Prog. Retin. Eye Res.* 20, 469, 2001.
207. Saari, J.C., Biochemistry of visual pigment regeneration: the Friedenwald lecture. *Invest. Ophthalmol. Vis. Sci.* 41, 337, 2000.
208. Gollapalli, D.R. and Rando, R.R., All-*trans*-retinyl esters are the substrates for isomerization in the vertebrate visual cycle. *Biochemistry* 42, 5809, 2003.
209. Jin, M. et al., Rpe65 is the retinoid isomerase in bovine retinal pigment epithelium. *Cell* 122, 449, 2005.
210. Gonzalez-Fernandez, F., Interphotoreceptor retinoid-binding protein—an old gene for new eyes. *Vis. Res.* 43, 3021, 2003.
211. Mata, N.L. et al., Isomerization and oxidation of vitamin A in cone-dominant retinas: a novel pathway for visual-pigment regeneration in daylight. *Neuron* 36, 69, 2002.
212. Lee, S.-Y., Ubels, J.L., and Soprano, D.R., The lacrimal gland synthesizes retinol-binding protein. *Exp. Eye Res.* 55, 163, 1992.
213. Gadomski, A.M. et al., Conjunctival impression cytology (CIC) to detect subclinical vitamin A deficiency: comparison of CIC with biochemical assessments. *Am. J. Clin. Nutr.* 49, 495, 1989.
214. Stoltzfus, R.J. et al., Conjuctival impression cytology as an indicator of vitamin A status in lactating Indonesian women. *Am. J. Clin. Nutr.* 58, 167, 1993.
215. Sommer, A. et al., Increased mortality in children with mild vitamin A deficiency. *Lancet* 2(8350), 585, 1983.
216. Sommer, A., Vitamin A deficiency and the global response. *Forum Nutr.* 56, 33, 2003.
217. Sommer, A., Vitamin A, infectious disease, and childhood mortality: a $.02 solution? *J. Infect. Dis.* 167, 1003, 1993.
218. Beaton, G.H. et al., Vitamin A supplementation and child morbidity and mortality in developing countries. *Food Nutr. Bull.* 15, 282, 1994.
219. Rahmathullah, L. et al., Impact of supplementing newborn infants with vitamin A on early infant mortality: community based randomised trial in southern India. *Br. Med. J.* 327, 254, 2003.
220. West, K.P., Jr. et al., Double blind, cluster randomised trial of low dose supplementation with vitamin A or β carotene on mortality related to pregnancy in Nepal. *Br. Med. J.* 318, 570, 1999.
221. Radhika, M.S. et al., Effects of vitamin A deficiency during pregnancy on maternal and child health. *BJOG* 109, 689, 2002.

222. Office of Dietary Supplements, N.I.H., *Dietary Supplement Fact Sheet: Vitamin A*, NIH: Washington, 2005, ods.od.nih.gov/factsheets/cc/vita.html.
223. D'Souza, R.M. and D'Souza, R., Vitamin A for the treatment of children with measles—a systematic review. *J. Trop. Pediatr.* 48, 323, 2002.
224. Committee on Infectious Diseases, Vitamin A treatment of measles. *Pediatrics* 91, 1014, 1993.
225. WHO/UNICEF, Integration of vitamin A supplementation with immunization: policy and programme implication, in: *Report of a meeting, 12–13 January 1998, UNICEF, New York*, New York, 1998, pp. 1–7, http://www.who.int/vaccines-documents/DocsPDF/www9837.pdf.
226. Villamor, E. and Fawzi, W.W., Effects of vitamin A supplementation on immune responses and correlation with clinical outcomes. *Clin. Microbiol. Rev.* 18, 446, 2005.
227. Stephensen, C.B., Vitamin A, infection, and immune function. *Annu. Rev. Nutr.* 21, 167, 2001.
228. Iwata, M., Eshima, Y., and Kagechika, H., Retinoic acids exert direct effects on T cells to suppress T(h)1 development and enhance T(h)2 development via retinoic acid receptors. *Int. Immunol.* 15, 1017, 2003.
229. Iwata, M. et al., Retinoic acid imprints gut-homing specificity on T cells. *Immunity* 21, 527, 2004.
230. Ma, Y., Chen, Q., and Ross, A.C., Retinoic acid and polyriboinosinic:polyribocytidylic acid stimulate robust anti-tetanus antibody production while differentially regulating type 1/type 2 cytokines and lymphocyte populations. *J. Immunol.* 174, 7961, 13556, 2005.
231. Ma, Y. and Ross, A.C., The anti-tetanus immune response of neonatal mice is augmented by retinoic acid combined with polyriboinosinic:polyribocytidylic acid. *Proc. Natl. Acad. Sci. USA* 102, 13556, 2005.
232. De Luca, L.M., Kosa, K., and Andreola, F., The role of vitamin A in differentiation and skin carcinogenesis. *J. Nutr. Biochem.* 8, 426, 1997.
233. Goldsmith, L.A. et al., American Academy of Dermatology Consensus Conference on the safe and optimal use of isotretinoin: summary and recommendations. *J. Am. Acad. Dermatol.* 50, 900, 2004.
234. Food and Drug Administration, *FDA Announces Strengthened Risk Management Program to Enhance Safe Use of Isotretinoin (Accutane) for Treating Severe Acne*, 2005, http://www.fda.gov/cder/drug/infopage/accutane/default.htm.
235. Hansen, L.A. et al., Retinoids in chemoprevention and differentiation therapy. *Carcinogenesis* 21, 1271, 2000.
236. Avvisati, G. and Tallman, M.S., All-*trans* retinoic acid in acute promyelocytic leukaemia. *Best Pract. Res. Clin. Haematol.* 16, 419, 2003.
237. Larson, R.S. and Tallman, M.S., Retinoic acid syndrome: manifestations, pathogenesis, and treatment. *Best Pract. Res. Clin. Haematol.* 16, 453, 2003.
238. Food Safety Agency, *Review of Dietary Advice on Vitamin A*, 2005, http://www.food.gov.uk/news/newsarchive/2005/sep/newadvicevita.
239. Promislow, J.H. et al., Retinol intake and bone mineral density in the elderly: the Rancho Bernardo Study. *J. Bone Miner. Res.* 17, 1349, 2002.
240. Feskanich, D. et al., Vitamin A intake and hip fractures among postmenopausal women. *J. Am. Med. Assoc.* 287, 47, 2001.
241. Crandall, C., Vitamin A intake and osteoporosis: a clinical review. *J. Womens Health (Larchmt).* 13, 939, 2004.
242. Krinsky, N.I., The safety of β-carotene, in: *Carotenoids and Retinoids: Molecular Aspects and Health Issues*, Packer, L. et al., editors, AOCS Press: Champaign, 2005, p. 338.
243. Micozzi, M.S. et al., Carotenodermia in men with elevated carotenoid intake from foods and beta-carotene supplements. *Am. J. Clin. Nutr.* 48, 1061, 1988.
244. Forman, M.R. et al., Nutrition and cancer prevention: a multidisciplinary perspective on human trials. *Annu. Rev. Nutr.* 24, 223, 2004.
245. Wang, X.D. and Russell, R.M., Procarcinogenic and anti carcinogenic effects of beta-carotene. *Nutr. Rev.* 57, 263, 1999.

2 Vitamin D

Anthony W. Norman and Helen L. Henry

CONTENTS

INTRODUCTION

The generic term vitamin D designates a group of chemically related compounds that possess antirachitic activity. The two most prominent members of this group are vitamin D_2 (ergocalciferol) and vitamin D_3 (cholecalciferol). Vitamin D_2 is derived from a common plant steroid, ergosterol, and is the form that was employed for nutritional vitamin D fortification of foods from the 1940s to 1960s. Vitamin D_3 is the form of vitamin D obtained when radiant energy from the sun strikes the skin and converts the precursor 7-dehydrocholesterol. Since the body is capable of producing vitamin D_3, vitamin D does not meet the classical definition of a vitamin. A more accurate description of vitamin D is that it is a prohormone; thus, vitamin D is metabolized to a biologically active form that functions as a steroid hormone [1,2]. However, since vitamin D was first recognized as an essential nutrient, it has historically been classified among the lipid-soluble vitamins. Even today it is thought of by many as a

TABLE 2.1
Biological Calcium and Phosphorus[a]

Calcium	Phosphorus
Utilization	
Body content: 70 kg man has 1200 g Ca^{2+}	Body content: 70 kg man has 770 g P
Structural: bone has 95% of body Ca	Structural: Bone has 90% of body P_i
Plasma [Ca^{2+}] is 2.5 mM, 10 mg %	Plasma [P_i] is 2.3 mM, 2.5–4.3 mg %
Muscle contraction	Intermediary metabolism (phosphorylated intermediates)
Nerve pulse transmission	
Blood clotting	Genetic information (DNA and RNA)
Membrane structure	Phospholipids
Enzyme cofactors (amylase, trypsinogen, lipases, ATPases)	Enzyme or protein components (phosphohistidine, phosphoserine)
Eggshell (birds)	Membrane structure
Daily Requirements (70 kg man)	
Dietary intake: 700[a]	Dietary intake: 1200[a]
Fecal excretion: 300–600[a,b]	Fecal excretion: 350–370[a,b]
Urinary excretion: 100–400[a,b]	Urinary excretion: 200–600[a,b]

Note: For more details see Chapter 9 in Norman A.W. and Litwack G.L., *Hormones*, 2nd Academic Press, San Diego, CA, 1997, 2nd Edition.

[a] Values in mg/day.
[b] Based on the indicated level of dietary intake.

vitamin for public health reasons [3], although it is now known that there exists a vitamin D endocrine system that generates the steroid hormone 1α,25-dihydroxyvitamin D_3 [1α,25$(OH)_2D_3$] [4].

Vitamin D functions to maintain calcium homeostasis together with two peptide hormones, calcitonin and parathyroid hormone (PTH). Vitamin D is also important for phosphorus homeostasis [5–7]. Calcium and phosphorus are required for a wide variety of biological processes (see Table 2.1). Calcium is necessary for muscle contraction, nerve pulse transmission, blood clotting, and membrane structure. It also serves as a cofactor for such enzymes as lipases and ATPases and is needed for eggshell formation in birds. It is an important intracellular signaling molecule for signal transduction pathways such as those involving calmodulin and protein kinase C (PKC). Phosphorus is an important component of DNA, RNA, membrane lipids, and the intracellular energy-transferring ATP system. The phosphorylation of proteins is important for the regulation of many metabolic pathways. The maintenance of serum calcium and phosphorus levels within narrow limits is important for normal bone mineralization. Any perturbation in these levels results in bone calcium accretion or resorption. Disease states, such as rickets, can develop if the serum ion product is not maintained at a level consistent with that required for normal bone mineralization. Maintaining a homeostatic state for these two elements is of considerable importance to a living organism.

The active form of vitamin D_3, 1α,25$(OH)_2D_3$, has been shown to act on novel target tissues not related to calcium homeostasis. There have been reports characterizing receptors for the hormonal form of vitamin D and activities in such diverse tissues as brain, pancreas, pituitary, hair follicle, skin, muscle, immune cells, and parathyroid (Table 2.2). These studies suggest that vitamin D status is important for insulin and prolactin secretion, hair growth, muscle function, immune and stress response, and melanin synthesis and cellular differentiation

TABLE 2.2
Distribution of $1,25(OH)_2D_3$ Biological Actions[a]

Tissue Distribution of Nuclear $1,25(OH)_2D_3$ Receptor		
Adipose	Intestine	Pituitary
Adrenal	Kidney	Placenta
Bone	Liver (fetal)	Prostrate
Bone marrow	Lung	Retina
Brain	Muscle, cardiac	Skin
Breast	Muscle, embryonic	Stomach
Cancer cells	Muscle, smooth	Testis
Cartilage	Osteoblast	Thymus
Colon	Ovary	Thyroid
Eggshell gland	Pancreas β cell	Uterus
Epididymus	Parathyroid	Yolk sac (bird)
Hair follicle	Parotid	

Distribution of Nongenomic Responses	
Intestine	Transcaltachia[b]
Osteoblast	Ca^{2+} channel opening
Osteoclast	Ca^{2+} channel opening
Pancreas β cells	Insulin secretion
Muscle	A variety

[a] Summary of the tissue location of the nuclear receptor for $1\alpha,25(OH)_2D_3$ (VDR) (*top* panel) and tissues displaying rapid or membrane-initiated biological responses (*bottom* panel) [483].
[b] Transcaltachia is the rapid stimulation of intestinal calcium transport that can be initiated by $1\alpha,25(OH)_2D_3$ [484,485].

of skin and blood cells. A number of recent and comprehensive reviews [1,8–22] cover many aspects of vitamin D and its endocrinology.

HISTORY OF VITAMIN D

Rickets, a deficiency disease of vitamin D, appears to have been a problem in ancient times. There is evidence that rickets occurred in Neanderthal man about 50,000 BC [23]. The first scientific descriptions of rickets were written by Dr. Daniel Whistler [24] in 1645 and by Professor Francis Glisson [25] in 1650. Rickets became a health problem in northern Europe, England, and the United States during the Industrial Revolution when many people lived in urban areas with air pollution and little sunlight. Before the discovery of vitamin D, the theories on the causative factors of rickets ranged from heredity to syphilis [2].

Some of the important scientific discoveries leading to the understanding of rickets were dependent on the development of an appreciation of the complexity of bone. As reviewed by Hess [26], the first formal descriptions of bone were made by Marchand (1842), Bibard (1844), and Friedleben (1860). In 1885, Pommer wrote the first pathological description of the rachitic skeleton. In 1849, Trousseau and Lasque recognized that osteomalacia and rickets were different manifestations of the same disorder. In 1886 and 1890, Hirsch and Palm did a quantitative geographical study of the worldwide distribution of rickets and found that the incidence of rickets paralleled the lack of sunlight [26]. This was substantiated in 1919 when Huldschinsky demonstrated that ultraviolet (UV) rays were effective in healing rickets [27].

In the early 1900s, the concept of vitamins was developed and nutrition emerged as an experimental science, allowing for further advances in understanding rickets. In 1919, Sir Edward Mellanby [28,29] was able to experimentally produce rickets in puppies by feeding synthetic diets to over 400 dogs. He further showed that rickets could be prevented by the addition of cod-liver oil or butterfat to the feed. He postulated that the nutritional factor preventing rickets was vitamin A since butterfat and cod-liver oil were known to contain vitamin A [29]. Similar studies were conducted and conclusions drawn by McCollum et al. [30].

The distinction between the antixerophthalmic factor, vitamin A, and the antirachitic factor, vitamin D, was made in 1922 when McCollum's laboratory showed that the antirachitic factor in cod-liver oil could survive both aeration and heating to 100°C for 14 h whereas the activity of vitamin A was destroyed by this treatment. McCollum named the new substance vitamin D [31].

Although it was known that UV light and vitamin D were both equally effective in preventing and curing rickets, the close interdependence of these two factors was not immediately recognized. Then, in 1923, Goldblatt and Soames [32] discovered that UV-irradiated food fed to rats could cure rickets in cats, but nonirradiated food could not cure rickets. In 1925, Hess and Weinstock [33,34] demonstrated that a factor with antirachitic activity was produced in the skin on UV irradiation. Both groups demonstrated that the antirachitic agent was in the lipid fraction. The action of the light appeared to produce a permanent chemical change in some component of the diet and the skin. They postulated that a provitamin D existed that could be converted to vitamin D by UV light absorption and ultimately demonstrated that the antirachitic activity resulted from the irradiation of 7-dehydrocholesterol.

The isolation and characterization of vitamin D_2 and vitamin D_3 was now possible. In 1932, the structure of vitamin D_2 was determined simultaneously by Windaus et al. [35] in Germany, who named it vitamin D_2, and by Angus et al. [36] in England, who named it ergocalciferol. In 1936, Windaus et al. [37] identified the structure of vitamin D_3 found in cod-liver oil. Thus, the naturally occurring vitamin is vitamin D_3, or cholecalciferol. This conclusion is derived from the fact that 7-dehydrocholesterol (precursor of D_3), but not ergosterol (precursor of D_2), is present in the skin of all higher vertebrates. The structure of vitamin D was determined to be that of a steroid, or more correctly, a secosteroid. However, the relationship between its structure and mode of action was not realized for an additional 30 years.

Vitamin D (both D_3 and D_2) was believed for many years to be the active agent in preventing rickets. It was assumed that vitamin D was a cofactor for reactions that served to maintain calcium and phosphorus homeostasis. However, when radioisotopes became available, more precise measurements of metabolism could be made. Using radioactive $^{45}Ca^{2+}$, Carlsson and Lindquist [38] found that there was a lag period between the administration of vitamin D and the initiation of its biological response. Stimulation of intestinal calcium absorption (ICA) required 36–48 h for a maximal response. Other investigators found delays in bone calcium mobilization (BCM) and serum calcium level increases after treatment with vitamin D [39–43]. The rapidity of the response to vitamin D and its magnitude were proportional to the dose of vitamin D used [40].

One explanation for the time lag was that vitamin D had to be further metabolized before it was active. With the development of radioactively labeled vitamin D, it became possible to study the metabolism of vitamin D. Norman et al. [44] detected three metabolites that possessed antirachitic activity. One of these metabolites was subsequently identified as the 25-hydroxy derivative of vitamin D_3 [25(OH)D_3] [45]. 25(OH)D_3 had 1.5 times more activity than vitamin D in curing rickets in the rat, so it was first thought to be the biologically active form of vitamin D [46]. However, in 1968, the Norman laboratory reported a more polar metabolite, which was found in the nuclear fraction of the intestine from chicks given tritiated vitamin D_3 [47]. Biological studies demonstrated that this new metabolite was 13–15 times more effective than vitamin D_3 in stimulating ICA and 5–6 times more effective in elevating serum calcium levels [48]. The new metabolite was also as effective as vitamin D in increasing total body growth rate and bone ash [48]. In 1971, the structural identity of this metabolite was reported to be the 1α,25-dihydroxy derivative of vitamin D [$1\alpha,25(OH)_2D_3$] [49–51], the biologically active metabolite of vitamin D.

In 1970, the site of production of $1\alpha,25(OH)_2D_3$ was demonstrated to be the kidney [52]. This discovery, together with the finding that $1\alpha,25(OH)_2D_3$ is found in the nuclei and chromatin of intestinal cells and the demonstration of the presence of a nuclear receptor for $1\alpha,25(OH)_2D_3$ [53], suggested that vitamin D was functioning as a steroid hormone [47,53]. The cDNA for the $1\alpha,25(OH)_2D_3$ nuclear receptor as well as the estrogen (ER), progesterone (PR), androgen, glucocorticoid (GR), and mineralocorticoid steroid receptors and the retinoic acid receptors were all cloned in the interval of 1986–1990; somewhat surprisingly, these receptors have significant amino acid sequence homology [54]. It is now appreciated that all of these receptors, including the vitamin D receptor (VDR), belong to a superfamily of evolutionarily related proteins [55]. The discovery that the biological actions of vitamin D could be explained by the classical model of steroid hormone action marked the beginning of the modern era of vitamin D.

CHEMISTRY OF VITAMIN D STEROIDS

STRUCTURE

Vitamin D refers to a family of structurally related compounds that display antirachitic activity. Members of the D-family are derived from the cyclopentanoperhydrophenanthrene ring system, which is common to other steroids, such as cholesterol [56]. However, in comparison with cholesterol, vitamin D has only three intact rings; the B ring has undergone fission of the 9,10-carbon bond resulting in the conjugated triene system that is present in all the D vitamins. The structure of vitamin D_3 is shown in Figure 2.1. Naturally occurring members of the vitamin D family differ from each other only in the structure of their side chains; the side-chain structures of the various members of the vitamin D family are given in Table 2.3.

The Nobel laureate Dorothy Crowfoot–Hodgkin, using the then relatively new technique of X-ray crystallography, was the first to develop a three-dimensional model of vitamin D_3 in her Ph.D. dissertation [57,58]. Because vitamin D is a secosteroid, the A ring is not rigidly fused to the B ring (compare 7-dehydrocholesterol with provitamin D_3 in Figure 2.1). As a result, the A ring exists in one of the two possible chair conformations, designated either as chair conformer A or conformer B (see Figure 2.2). The rapid chair–chair interconversion of the A-ring conformers of the vitamin D secosteroids was confirmed by Okamura et al. [59] using nuclear magnetic resonance (NMR) spectroscopy (Figure 2.2). This A-ring conformational mobility is unique to vitamin D family of molecules and is not observed for other steroid hormones. It is a direct consequence of the breakage of the 9,10-carbon bond of the B ring, which serves to free the A ring. As a result of this mobility, substituents on the A ring (e.g., a 1-α hydroxyl, as in $1\alpha,25(OH)_2D_3$) are rapidly and continually alternating between the axial and equatorial positions. A second hallmark of the secosteroid is that the presence of the 6,7 single bond in the broken B ring, which allows for complete (360°) conformational rotation, thus generating the 6-s-*cis* or 6-s-*trans* conformations (see *top* panel of Figure 2.2).

NOMENCLATURE

Vitamin D is named according to the new revised rules of the International Union of Pure and Applied Chemists (IUPAC). Since vitamin D is derived from a steroid, the structure retains its numbering from the parent steroid compound, cholesterol. Vitamin D is designated *seco* because its B ring has undergone fission. Asymmetric centers are named using R,S notation and Cahn's rules of priority. The configuration of the double bonds is notated E, Z; E for

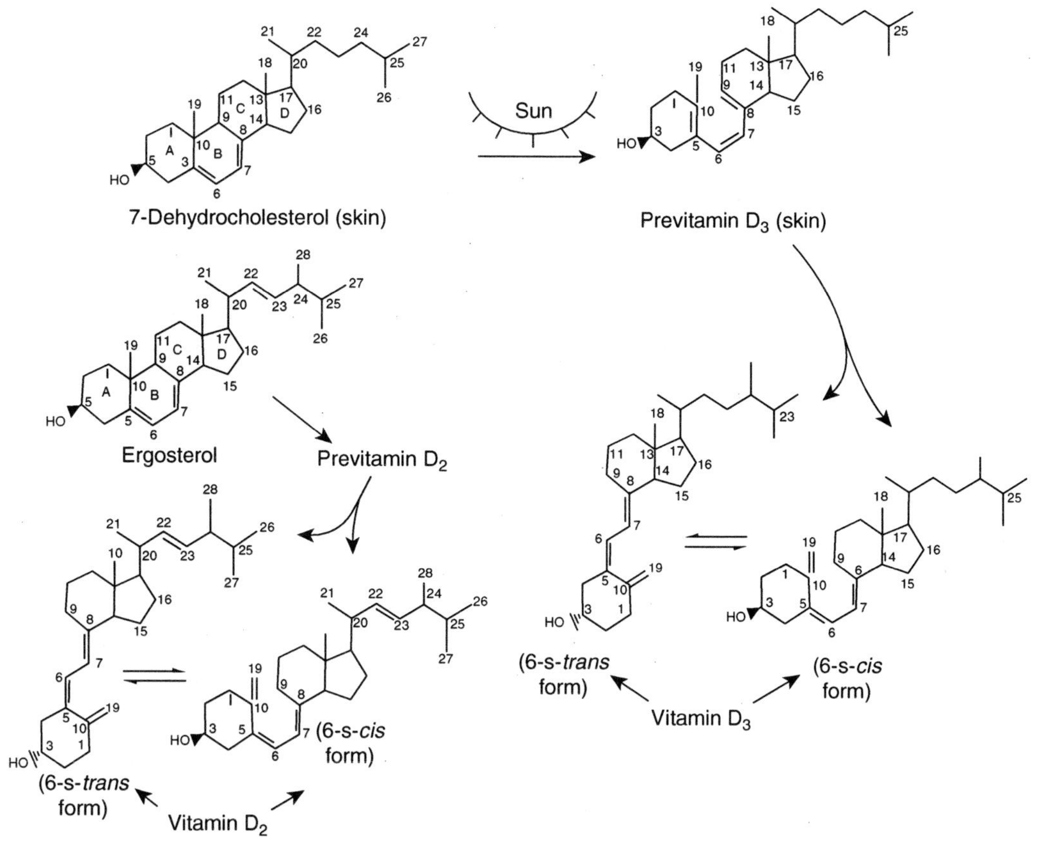

FIGURE 2.1 Chemistry and irradiation pathway for production of vitamin D_3 (a natural process) and vitamin D_2 (a commercial process). In each instance the provitamin, with a $\Delta 5,\Delta 7$ conjugated double-bond system in the B ring, is converted to the *seco*-B previtamin, with the 9,10 carbon–carbon bond broken. Then the previtamin D thermally isomerizes to the vitamin form, which contains a system of three conjugated double bonds. In solution, vitamin D is capable of assuming a large number of conformations because of the rotation about the 6,7 carbon–carbon bond of the B ring. The 6-s-*cis* conformer (the steroid-like shape) and the 6-s-*trans* conformer (the extended shape) are presented for both vitamin D_2 and vitamin D_3.

trans, Z for *cis*. The formal name for vitamin D_3 is 9,10-*seco*(5Z,7E)-5,7,10(19)-cholestatriene-3β-ol and for vitamin D_2 it is 9,10-*seco*(5Z,7E)-5,7,10(19),21-ergostatetraene-3β-ol.

Chemical Properties

Vitamin D_3 ($C_{27}H_{44}O$)

Three double bonds; melting point, 84°C–85°C; UV absorption maximum at 264–265 nm with a molar extinction coefficient of 18,300 in alcohol or hexane, $\alpha_D 20 + 84.8°$ in acetone; molecular weight, 384.65; insoluble in H_2O; soluble in benzene, chloroform, ethanol, and acetone; unstable in light; will undergo oxidation if exposed to air at 24°C for 72 h; best stored at 0°C.

Vitamin D_2 ($C_{28}H_{44}O$)

Four double bonds; melting point, 121°C; UV absorption maximum at 265 nm with a molar extinction coefficient of 19,400 in alcohol or hexane, $\alpha_D 20 + 106°$ in acetone; same solubility and stability properties as D_3.

TABLE 2.3
Side Chains of Provitamin D; It Includes Structures of the Side Chains of Vitamins $D_2 \gg D_7$

Provitamin Trivial Name	Vitamin D Produced upon Irradiation	Empirical Formula (Complete Steroid)	Side Chain Structure
Ergosterol	D_2	$C_{28}H_{44}O$	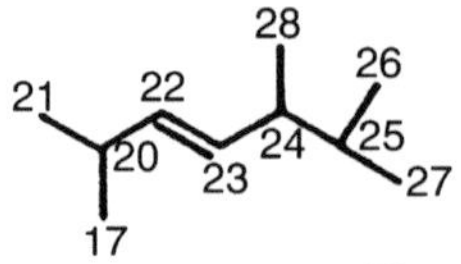
7-dehydrocholesterol	D_3	$C_{27}H_{44}O$	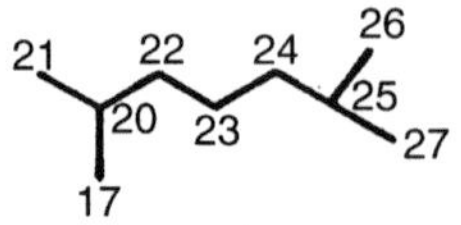
22,23-dihydroergosterol	D_4	$C_{28}H_{46}O$	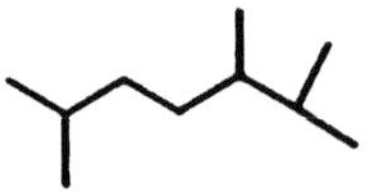
7-dehydrositosterol	D_5	$C_{29}H_{48}O$	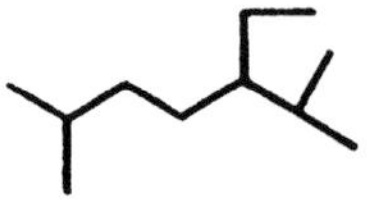
7-dehydrostigmasterol	D_6	$C_{29}H_{46}O$	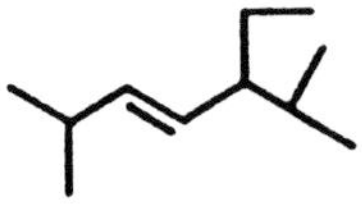
7-dehydrocampesterol	D_7	$C_{28}H_{46}O$	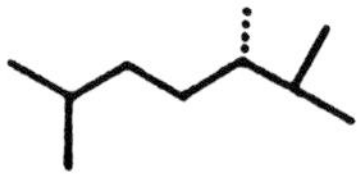

Isolation of Vitamin D Metabolites

Many of the studies that have led to our understanding of the mode of action of vitamin D have involved the tissue localization and identification of vitamin D and its 37 metabolites. Since vitamin D is a steroid, it is isolated from tissue by methods that extract total lipids. The technique most frequently used for this extraction is the method of Bligh and Dyer [60].

Over the years a wide variety of chromatographic techniques have been used to separate vitamin D and its metabolites. These include paper, thin-layer, column, and gas chromatographic methods. Paper and thin-layer chromatography usually require long development times, unsatisfactory resolutions, and have limited capacity. Column chromatography, using alumina, Floridin, celite, silica acid, and Sephadex LH-20 as supports, has been used to rapidly separate many closely related vitamin D compounds [2]. However, none of these methods is capable of resolving and distinguishing vitamin D_2 from vitamin D_3. Gas chromatography is able to separate these two compounds, but in the process vitamin D is thermally converted to pyrocalciferol and isopyrocalciferol, resulting in two peaks. High-pressure liquid chromatography (LC) has become the method of choice for the separation of vitamin D and its metabolites [61,62]. This powerful technique is rapid and gives good recovery with high resolution.

Synthesis of Vitamin D

Photochemical Production

In the 1920s, it was recognized that provitamins D were converted to vitamins D on treatment with UV radiation (see Figure 2.1). The primary structural requirement for a provitamin D is

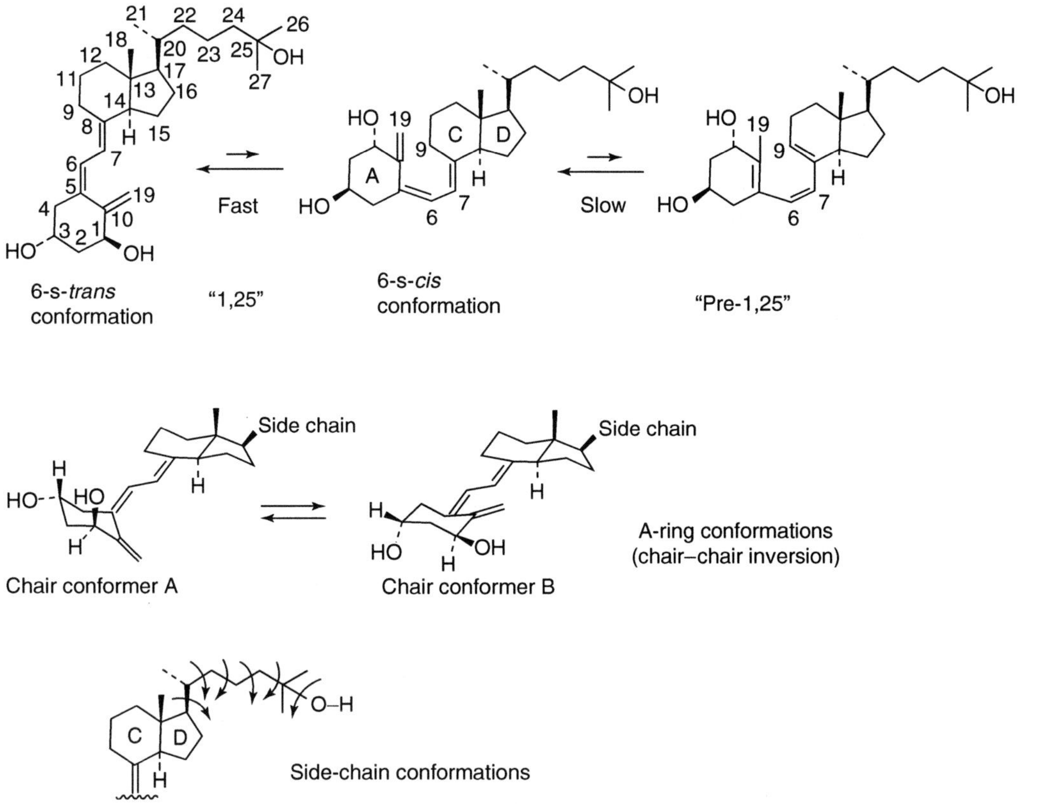

FIGURE 2.2 The dynamic behavior of $1\alpha,25(OH)_2D_3$. The topological features of the hormone $1\alpha,25(OH)_2D_3$ undergo significant changes as a consequence of rapid conformational changes (i.e., due to single-bond rotation) or, in one case, as a consequence of a hydrogen shift (resulting in the transformation of $1\alpha,25(OH)_2D_3$ to pre-$1\alpha,25(OH)_2D_3$). The *top* panel depicts the dynamic changes occurring within the *seco*-B conjugated triene framework of the hormone (C5, 6, 7, 8, 9, 10, 19). All the carbon atoms of the 6-s-*trans* conformer of $1\alpha,25(OH)_2D_3$ are numbered using standard steroid notation for the convenience of the reader. Selected carbon atoms of the 6-s-*cis* conformer are also numbered as are those of pre-$1\alpha,25(OH)_2D_3$. The *middle* panel depicts the rapid chair–chair inversion of the A ring of the secosteroid. The *lower* panel depicts the dynamic single-bond conformational rotation of the cholesterol-like side chain of the hormone. The C/D *trans*-hydrindane moiety is assumed to serve as a rigid anchor about which the A ring, *seco*-B triene, and side chain are in dynamic equilibrium.

a sterol with a C-5 to C-7 diene system in ring B. The conjugated double-bond system is a chromaphore, which on UV irradiation initiates a series of transformations resulting in the production of the vitamin D secosteroid structure. The two most abundant provitamins D are ergosterol (provitamin D_2) and 7-dehydrocholesterol (provitamin D_3).

Chemical Synthesis

There are two basic approaches to the synthesis of vitamin D. The first involves the chemical synthesis of a provitamin that can be converted to vitamin D by UV irradiation. The second is a total chemical synthesis.

Since vitamin D is derived from cholesterol, the first synthesis of vitamin D resulted from the first chemical synthesis of cholesterol. Cholesterol was first synthesized by Woodward and Robinson groups in the 1950s. The first method involves a 20-step conversion of

4-methoxy-2,5-toluquinone to a PR derivative, which is then converted in several more steps to PR, testosterone, cortisone, and cholesterol [63]. The other method used the starting material 1,6-dihydroxynaphthalene. This was converted to the B and C rings of the steroid. A further series of chemical transformations led to the attachment of the A ring and then the D ring. The final product of the synthesis was epiandrosterone, which could be converted to cholesterol [64]. The cholesterol was then converted to 7-dehydrocholesterol and UV irradiated to give vitamin D, with an overall yield of 10%–20%.

The first pure chemical synthesis of vitamin D, without any photochemical irradiation steps, was accomplished by the Lythgoe group in 1967 [65]. This continuing area of investigation allows for the production of many vitamin D metabolites and analogs, including radioactively labeled compounds, without the necessity of a photochemical step.

Figure 2.3 summarizes some of the currently used synthetic strategies [4]. Method A involves the photochemical ring opening of a 1-hydroxylated side-chain-modified derivative of 7-dehydrocholesterol 1 producing a provitamin that is thermolyzed to vitamin D [66,67]. Method B is useful in producing side chain and other analogs. In this method, the phosphine oxide 2 is coupled to a Grundmann's ketone derivative 3, producing the $1\alpha,25(OH)_2D_3$ skeleton [68,69]. In method C, dienynes like 4 are semihydrogenated to a previtamin structure that undergoes rearrangement to the vitamin D analog [70,71]. Method D involves the production of the vinylallene 6 from compound 5 and the subsequent rearrangement with

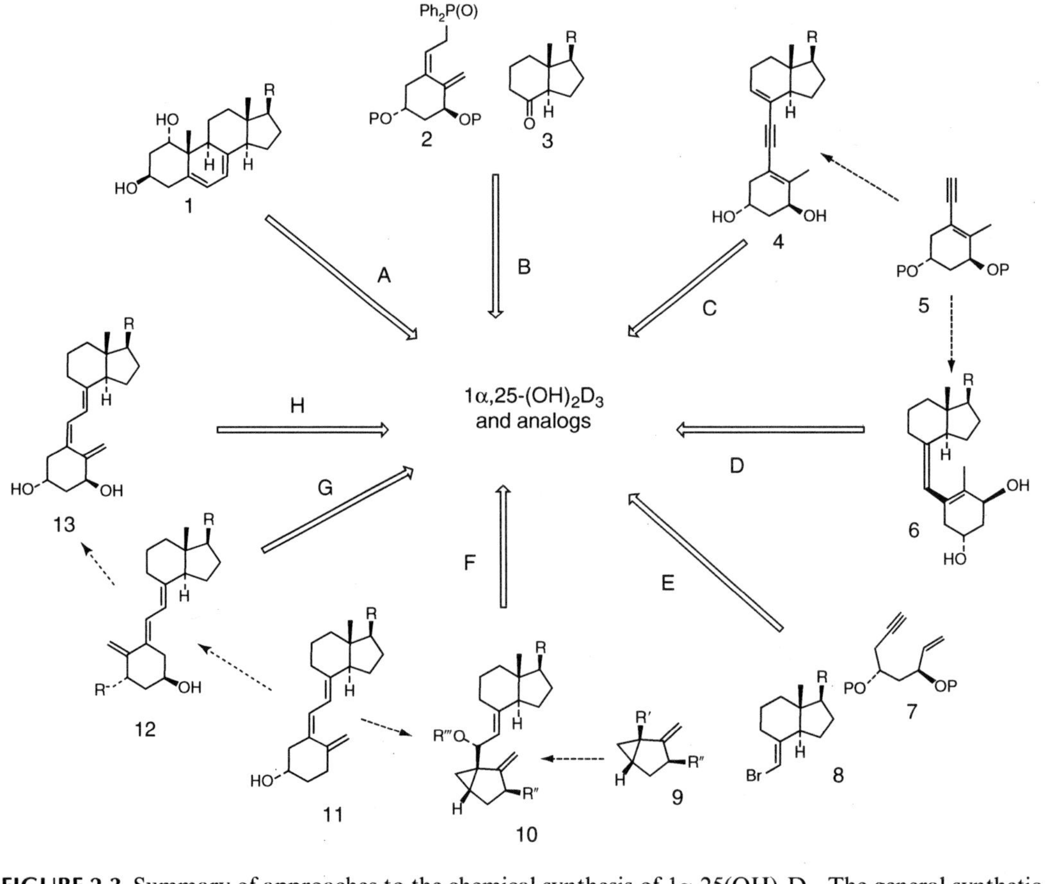

$1\alpha,25\text{-}(OH)_2D_3$ and analogs

FIGURE 2.3 Summary of approaches to the chemical synthesis of $1\alpha,25(OH)_2D_3$. The general synthetic approaches A–H, which are discussed in the text, represent some of the major synthetic approaches used in recent years to synthesize the hormone $1\alpha,25(OH)_2D_3$ and analogs of $1\alpha,25(OH)_2D_3$.

heat or metal-catalyzed isomerization followed by sensitized photoisomerization [72]. Method E starts with an acyclic A-ring precursor 7, which is intramolecularly cross-coupled to bromoenyne 8 resulting in the 1,25-skeleton [73,74]. Method F starts with the tosylate of 11, which is isomerized to the i-steroid 10. This structure can be modified at carbon-1 and then reisomerized under sovolytic conditions to $1\alpha,25(OH)_2D_3$ or analogs [75,76]. In method G, vitamin D derivatives 11 are converted to 1-oxygenated 5,6-*trans* vitamin D derivatives 12 [77]. Finally, method H involves the direct modification of $1\alpha,25(OH)_2D_3$ or an analog 13 through the use of protecting groups such as transition metal derivatives or by other direct chemical transformations on 13 [78]. These synthetic approaches have enabled the synthesis of over 1000 analogs of $1\alpha,25(OH)_2D_3$ [4].

PHYSIOLOGY OF VITAMIN D

INTRODUCTION

The elucidation of the metabolic pathway by which vitamin D is transformed into its biologically active form is one of the most important advances in our understanding of how vitamin D functions through its vitamin D endocrine system (see Figure 2.4). It is now known that vitamin D_3 must be sequentially hydroxylated at the C-25 position and then the C-1 position to generate the steroid hormone, $1\alpha,25(OH)_2D_3$, before it can produce any biological effects. The activation of vitamin D_2 occurs via the same metabolic pathway as that of vitamin D_3. Originally, it was believed that the biological activities of both vitamin D_2 and vitamin D_3 were approximately the same; however, it is now apparent that vitamin D_2 has significantly lower activity in birds [2] and the New World monkey [79]. Recent evidence indicates that in man, vitamin D_2 has only 25%–30% of the biological activity of vitamin D_3 [80].

ABSORPTION

Vitamin D can be obtained from the diet, in which case it is absorbed in the small intestine with the aid of bile salts [81,82]. In rats, baboons, and humans, the specific mode of vitamin D absorption is via the lymphatic system and its associated chylomicrons [83,84]. It has been reported that only about 50% of a dose of vitamin D is absorbed [83,84]. However, considering that sufficient amounts of vitamin D can be produced daily by exposure to sunlight, it is not surprising that the body has not evolved a more efficient mechanism for vitamin D absorption from the diet.

PHOTOCHEMICAL PRODUCTION OF VITAMIN D_3

Although the body can obtain vitamin D from the diet, the major source of this prohormone can be its production in the skin from 7-dehydrocholesterol. Skin consists of two primary layers: the inner dermis composed largely of connective tissue and the outer thinner epidermis. The epidermis contains five strata; from outer to inner they are the stratum corneum, lucidum, granulosum, spinosum, and basale. The highest concentrations of 7-dehydrocholesterol are found in the stratum basale and the stratum spinosum. Accordingly, of the five layers of the epidermis, these two have the greatest capability for production of previtamin D_3 and vitamin D_3.

Several types of cells characterize the epidermis. The most prevalent cell type is the keratinocytes that synthesize and excrete the insoluble keratin, which strengthens and waterproofs the outer surface of the skin. The second most abundant cells are the melanocytes that produce the pigment melanin, the amount of which determines the skin color characteristic of

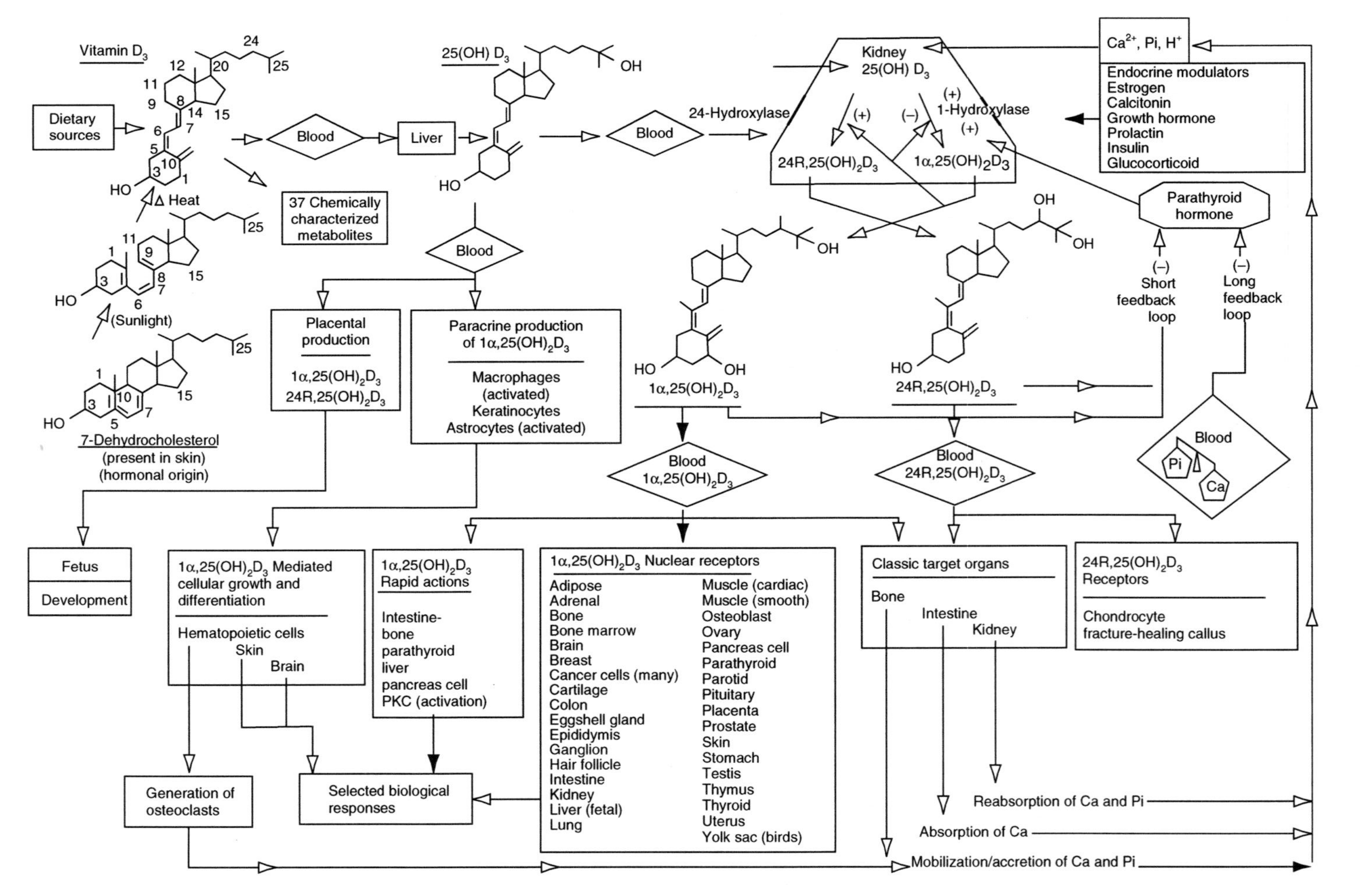

FIGURE 2.4 Overview of the vitamin D endocrine and paracrine system. Target organs and cells for $1\alpha,25(OH)_2D_3$ by definition contain receptors for the hormone. Biological effects are generated by both genomic and nongenomic signaling pathways.

racial groups [85]. Melanocytes are localized primarily in the innermost layer of the epidermis, the stratum basale. Here the enzyme tyrosinase synthesizes melanin from tyrosine. Importantly, the pigment granules that contain the melanin are transferred from the tips of long cytoplasmic processes of the melanocyte cells to other adjacent epidermal cells that are migrating upward toward the outer surface. Thus, melanin is present in all five strata of the epidermis and is the responsible agent that imparts a characteristic coloration to the skin. It normally takes 2 weeks for a cell present in the stratum basale to migrate up to the stratum corneum and another 2 weeks for the cell remnants to slough off.

There are four important variables that collectively determine the amount of vitamin D_3 that will be photochemically produced by an exposure of skin to sunlight. The two principal determinants are the quantity (intensity) and quality (appropriate wavelength) of the UV-B irradiation reaching the 7-dehydrocholesterol deep in the stratum basale and stratum spinosum. 7-Dehydrocholesterol absorbs UV light most efficiently over the wavelengths of 270–290 nm and thus only UV light in this wavelength range has the capability to produce vitamin D_3.

There have been many studies demonstrating the influence of season and latitude on the cutaneous photochemical synthesis of vitamin D_3 [86,87]; maximal vitamin D_3 production occurs in summer months, and depending on latitude little or no vitamin D_3 may be generated in winter months. [88,89]. The production of vitamin D_3 photochemically via exposure to sunlight is significantly higher at latitudes close to the equator and falls off significantly at higher latitudes. For example, at latitudes higher than 50° with clear atmospheric conditions no cutaneous production of vitamin D_3 occurs during some periods of the year, thus posing a serious vitamin D_3 nutritional problem for the citizens of Finland (e.g., Helsinki), Canada (e.g., Edmonton), or Alaska (e.g., Fairbanks). Clouds, aerosols, and thick ozone events can reduce the duration of vitamin D synthesis considerably, and can suppress vitamin D synthesis completely even at the equator [90].

The third potentially important variable governing the extent of vitamin D photosynthesis in the skin is the actual concentration of 7-dehydrocholesterol present in the strata spinosum and basale. However, under normal physiological circumstances in humans there are ample quantities of 7-dehydrocholesterol available in these two (of the order of 25–50 $\mu g/cm^2$ of skin).

The fourth determinant of vitamin D_3 production is the concentration of melanin present in the skin. Melanin, which absorbs UV-B in the 290–320 nm range, functions as a light filter and therefore determines the proportion of the incident UV-B that is actually able to penetrate the outer three strata and arrive at the strata basale and spinosum. Accordingly, skin pigmentation is, in fact, a dominant variable regulating the production of vitamin D_3 under circumstances of low levels of irradiation because the melanin absorbs UV photons in competition with the 7-dehydrocholesterol [91–93]. Appreciation of this fact allowed Loomis [94] to propose that the evolution of the world's racial distribution by latitude was due to regulation of vitamin D production. As people migrated to higher latitudes, their skin pigmentation was diminished to enable the adequate production of the vitamin by the skin [94].

Thus, there is a physiological connection between skin pigmentation (blacks versus whites), the seasons (with seasonally varying UV-B intensities), and the resulting conversion of 7-dehydrocholesterol into vitamin D_3 and then its subsequent metabolism by the vitamin D endocrine system to produce $25(OH)D_3$ and ultimately the steroid hormone, $1\alpha,25(OH)_2D_3$. Consistent with this are several reports showing that the circulating levels of $25(OH)D_3$ are substantially and significantly lower in black women than in white women in both the winter (February/March) and summer (June/July) months [92,95]. Once formed, the vitamin D_3 is preferentially removed from the skin into the circulatory system by the blood transport protein for vitamin D, the vitamin D-binding protein (DBP).

Transport by Vitamin D-Binding Protein

Vitamin DBP, also referred to as group-specific component of serum or Gc-globulin, was initially identified by its polymorphic migration pattern on serum electrophoresis. Although its function was quite unknown, its polymorphic properties allowed DBP (Gc) to play a significant role in human population genetics. In 1975 human Gc protein was found to specifically bind radioactive vitamin D_3 and 25(OH)-vitamin D_3, thus identifying one of its biological functions [96–98].

The vitamin DBP is the serum protein that serves as the transporter and reservoir for the principal vitamin D metabolites throughout the vitamin D endocrine system [99,100]. These include 25(OH)D_3, the major circulating metabolite ($K_D \sim 6 \times 10^{-9}$ M) [101,102], and the steroid hormone 1α,25$(OH)_2D_3$ ($K_D \sim 6 \times 10^{-8}$ M). DBP can be up to 5% glycosolated and is known to be one of the most polymorphic proteins, with 3 common allelic variants and over 124 rare variants known [102]. DBP's plasma concentration (4–8 μM) is approximately 20-fold higher than that of the total circulating vitamin D metabolites (~10^{-7} M). DBP binds 88% of the total serum 25(OH)D_3 and 85% of serum 1,25$(OH)_2D_3$, yet only 5% of the total circulating DBP actually carries vitamin D metabolites [103]. The concentration of the free hormone may be important in determining the biological activity of the 1α,25$(OH)_2D_3$ steroid hormone [104–106].

In addition to the vitamin D metabolite-binding properties of DBP, the protein has been shown to function as a high-affinity plasma actin-monomer scavenger functioning in concert with the protein gelsolin to prevent arterial congestion [107]. There are stoichiometric, 1:1, amounts of DBP and actin in their high-affinity heterodimer; the actin/DBP K_D ~10^{-9} M. The X-ray crystallographic structure of DBP–actin complexes has been recently determined [108,109]. This information is not considered in detail in this presentation.

DBP has been proposed to be involved in the transport of fatty acids [110]; the DBP K_D for binding fatty acids is ~10^{-6} M. In addition, DBP has also been implicated in playing a role in complement C5a-mediated chemotaxis [111] and has been found to be associated with immunoglobulin surface receptors on lymphocytes, monocytes, and neutrophils [112].

DBP (~53 kDa) is a member of the albumin multigene family of proteins, which also contains albumin (human serum albumin or HSA), α-fetoprotein (AFP), and afamin (AFM). AFP (~70 kDa) has an analogous function to albumin in the fetus and is measured clinically to diagnose or monitor fetal distress or fetal abnormalities, some liver disorders, and some cancers; however, AFP has no known function in adults. Albumin is the major protein component in human plasma and binds a number of relatively water-insoluble endogenous compounds, including fatty acids, bilirubin, and bile acids.

The known multifunctionality of DBP (both vitamin D metabolite and actin binding) separates it from other members of its family and other steroid transport proteins like retinal-binding protein (RBP) and thyroid-binding globulin (TBG). However, two proteins that bind and transport sterols, sex hormone-binding globulin (SHBG) and uteroglobulin (UG), have been implicated in physiological functions other than steroid transport. SHBG, which binds sex steroids in blood, triggers cAMP-dependent signaling through binding to specific cell surface receptors in prostate [113] and breast cancer cells [114].

The three-domain structure of DBP is shown in Figure 2.7A and is compared with the domain structure of the VDR. Domains I, II, and III have been postulated to have evolved from a progenitor that arose from the triple repeat of a 192 amino acid sequence [115]; however, domain III is significantly truncated at the C-terminus. The position of the vitamin D metabolite and actin-binding domains are specified in domain I and portions of domains I, II, and III, respectively.

The X-ray crystallographic structures of the human DBP with a bound ligand of 25(OH)-D_3 have been recently determined [116] (see Figure 2.7B and Figure 2.7C). The N-terminal region of DBP, helix 1–helix 6 of domain I, forms the ligand-binding domain (LBD), where $25(OH)D_3$ and other vitamin D metabolites bind. When bound to DBP, vitamin D sterols including $1\alpha,25(OH)_2D_3$ remain highly exposed to the external environment, which is not the case for internally sequestered ligands bound to the other plasma transport proteins (compare with the X-ray structure of the VDR in Figure 2.8), for example, SHBG, RBP, UG, and TBG. Virtually the whole α-face, top view, of the $25(OH)D_3$ molecule is exposed to the external environment when bound to the DBP, but the protein's affinity for $25(OH)D_3$ still remains high ($\sim 6 \times 10^{-9}$ M) presumably because of the relative strength of the protein–ligand interactions on the α-face of $25(OH)D_3$. A number of recent review articles on the DBP are available [12,106,117].

Storage of Vitamin D

Following intestinal absorption, vitamin D is rapidly taken up by the liver. Since it was known that the liver serves as a storage site for retinol, another fat-soluble vitamin, it was thought that the liver also functioned as a storage site for vitamin D. However, it has since been shown that blood has the highest concentration of vitamin D when compared with other tissues [118]. From studies in rats, it was concluded that no rat tissue can store vitamin D or its metabolites against a concentration gradient [83]. The persistence of vitamin D in rats during periods of vitamin D deprivation may be explained by the slow turnover rate of vitamin D in certain tissues, such as skin and adipose. Similarly, Mawer et al. [119] found that human adipose and muscle were found to be major storage sites for vitamin D and $25(OH)D_3$. It was also reported that in pigs, tissue concentrations of $1\alpha,25(OH)_2D_3$, especially in adipose tissue, are threefold to sevenfold higher than plasma levels [120].

In view of the current debate concerning what is a sufficient daily intake of vitamin D and suggestions by some that pharmacological amounts may have beneficial effects, our understanding of the storage of the parent vitamin is woefully inadequate and needs a great deal of research.

Metabolism of Vitamin D

The parent vitamin D is largely biologically inert; before vitamin D can exhibit any biological activity, it must first be metabolized to its active forms. $1\alpha,25(OH)_2D_3$ is the most active metabolite known, but there is evidence that $24,25(OH)_2D_3$ is required for some of the biological responses attributed to vitamin D [121–123]. Both these metabolites are produced in vivo following carbon-25 hydroxylation of the parent vitamin D molecule.

$25(OH)D_3$

In the liver, vitamin D undergoes its initial transformation with the addition of a hydroxyl group to the 25-carbon to form $25(OH)D_3$, the major circulating form of vitamin D. Although there is some evidence that other tissues, such as intestine and kidney, may have some 25-hydroxylase capacity, it is generally accepted that the formation of circulating $25(OH)D_3$ occurs predominantly in the liver.

The production of $25(OH)D_3$ is catalyzed by the cytochrome P450 enzyme, vitamin D_3 25-hydroxylase. The 25-hydroxylase activity is found in both liver microsomes and mitochondria [124–127]. It is a poorly regulated P450-dependent enzyme [128]. Therefore, circulating levels of $25(OH)D_3$ are a good index of vitamin D status, that is, they reflect the body content of the parent vitamin [129,130]. Cheng et al. [131,132] were the first to identify a microsomal CYP2R1 protein as a potential candidate for the liver vitamin D 25-hydroxylase based on the enzyme's biochemical properties, conservation, and expression pattern. In a breakthrough paper, this group provides molecular analysis of a patient with low circulating levels of $25(OH)D_3$ and classic symptoms of vitamin D deficiency. This individual was found to be homozygous for a transition mutation in exon 2 of the CYP2R1 gene on chromosome 11p15.2. The inherited mutation caused the substitution of a proline for an evolutionarily conserved leucine at amino acid 99 in the CYP2R1 protein and eliminated vitamin D 25-hydroxylase enzyme activity. These data identified CYP2R1 as a biologically essential vitamin D 25-hydroxylase and established the molecular basis of a new human genetic disease, namely, selective 25-hydroxyvitamin D deficiency.

$1\alpha,25(OH)_2D_3$

From the liver, $25(OH)D_3$ is returned to the circulatory system where it is transported via DBP to the kidney where a second hydroxyl group can be added at the C-1 position by the $25(OH)D_3$-1-α-hydroxylase [133]. The 1α-hydroxylase is a mitochondrial cytochrome P450-dependent mixed function oxidase. These enzymes consist of the two electron transport proteins, ferredoxin and ferredoxin reductase and cytochrome P450, which reduces molecular oxygen to one hydroxyl group to be incorporated into the substrate [$25(OH)D_3$] and to one molecule of water.

The most important point of regulation of the vitamin D endocrine system occurs through the stringent control of the activity of the renal-1α-hydroxylase [134]. In this way the production of the hormone $1\alpha,25(OH)_2D_3$ can be modulated according to the calcium needs of the organism. Although extrarenal production of $1\alpha,25(OH)_2D_3$ has been demonstrated in placenta [135,136], cultured pulmonary alveolar and bone macrophages [137–139], cultured embryonic calvarial cells [140], and cultured keratinocytes [141,142], which can provide the hormone to adjacent cells in a paracrine fashion, the kidney is considered the primary source of circulating $1\alpha,25(OH)_2D_3$. The major controls on the production of $1\alpha,25(OH)_2D_3$ are $1\alpha,25(OH)_2D_3$ itself, PTH, and the serum concentrations of calcium and phosphate [143].

Probably the most important determinant of 1α-hydroxylase activity in vivo is the vitamin D status of the animal. When circulating levels of $1\alpha,25(OH)_2D_3$ are low, the production of $1\alpha,25(OH)_2D_3$ in the kidney is high, and when circulating levels of $1\alpha,25(OH)_2D_3$ are high, synthesis of $1\alpha,25(OH)_2D_3$ is low [134]. The changes in enzyme activity induced by $1\alpha,25(OH)_2D_3$ can be inhibited by cycloheximide and actinomycin D [144], which suggests that $1\alpha,25(OH)_2D_3$ is acting, at least in part, at the level of transcription. PTH is secreted in response to low plasma calcium levels, and in the kidney it stimulates the activity of the 1α-hydroxylase. $1\alpha,25(OH)_2D_3$ operates in a feedback loop to modulate and reduce the secretion of PTH. In mammals, serum phosphate is also an important influence on the production of $1\alpha,25(OH)_2D_3$. Recently, substantial evidence has accumulated that the endocrine link mediating this regulatory effect of phosphate on the vitamin D endocrine system is fibroblast growth factor 23 (FGF23) [145–147].

$24,25(OH)_2D_3$

A second dihydroxylated metabolite of vitamin D produced in the kidney is $24R,25(OH)_2D_3$. In addition, virtually all other tissues that have receptors for $1\alpha,25(OH)_2D_3$ (VDR) can also produce $24R,25(OH)_2D_3$. There is some controversy concerning the possible unique biological actions of $24R,25(OH)_2D_3$. However, there is some evidence that $24,25(OH)_2D_3$ plays a role in the suppression of PTH secretion [148,149], in the mineralization of bone [150,151], and in fracture healing [152–155]. Other studies demonstrated that the combined presence of $24R,25(OH)_2D_3$ and $1\alpha,25(OH)_2D_3$ are required for normal egg hatchability in chickens [121] and quail [156]. From these studies, it is apparent that only combination doses of both metabolites are capable of eliciting the same response as the parent vitamin D. Thus, it appears that both 1α,25$(OH)_2D_3$ and 24R,25$(OH)_2D_3$ may be required for some of the known biological responses to vitamin D.

The enzyme responsible for the production of circulating 24R,25$(OH)_2D_3$ from 25$(OH)D_3$ in the kidney is the 25-hydroxyvitamin D_3-24R-hydroxylase, another mitochondrial cytochrome P450-dependent mixed function oxidase. The activity of the renal 24-hydroxylase is inversely proportional to circulating levels of 1α,25$(OH)_2D_3$. Under normal physiological circumstances, both 1α,25$(OH)_2D_3$ and 24R,25$(OH)_2D_3$ are secreted from the kidney and circulate in the plasma of all classes of vertebrates. The expression of the 24-hydroxylase is transcriptionally induced by 1α,25$(OH)_2D_3$ in virtually all target cells of the hormone where it undoubtedly contributes to the catabolism of the active hormone (see section Catabolism and Excretion).

In addition to these three metabolites of vitamin D_3, many others have been chemically characterized, and the existence of still others appears likely. The chemical structures of the 37 known metabolites are shown in Figure 2.5. Most of these appear to be intermediates in degradation pathways of 1α,25$(OH)_2D_3$ and none of these other metabolites have yet been shown to have biological activity except for the 1α,25$(OH)_2D_3$-26,23-lactone. The lactone is produced by the kidney when the plasma levels of 1α,25$(OH)_2D_3$ are very high. The metabolite appears to be antagonistic to 1α,25$(OH)_2D_3$, since it mediates a decrease in serum calcium levels in the rat. Other experiments suggest that the lactone inhibits bone resorption and blocks the resorptive action of 1α,25$(OH)_2D_3$ on the bone [157], perhaps functioning as a natural antagonist of 1α,25$(OH)_2D_3$ to prevent toxic effects from overproduction of 1α,25$(OH)_2D_3$. Interestingly structural analogs of the 1α,25$(OH)_2D_3$-26,23-lactone, namely (23S)-25-dehydro-1α-hydroxyvitamin-D_3-26,23-lactone, have been shown to function as antagonists of the nuclear VDR and can block the potent agonistic actions of 1α,25$(OH)_2D_3$ on gene transcription [158–160]. There is the possibility that a lactone analog may ultimately be used to treat the excessive bone resorption characteristic of Paget's disease by inhibiting the actions of osteoclasts (bone resorbing cells) [161].

Catabolism and Excretion

Several pathways exist in men and animals to further metabolize 1α,25$(OH)_2D_3$, all of which are depicted in Figure 2.5. These include: oxidative cleavage of the side chain following hydroxylation of C-24 to produce 1α,24,25$(OH)_3D_3$ and formation of 24-oxo-1α,25$(OH)_2D_3$, all catalyzed by the 24R-hydroxylase; formation of 1α,25$(OH)_2D_3$-26,23-lactone; and formation of 1α,25,26$(OH)_3D_3$. It is not clear which of these pathways predominate in the breakdown and clearance of 1α,25$(OH)_2D_3$ in man.

The catabolic pathway for vitamin D is obscure, but it is known that the excretion of vitamin D and its metabolites occurs primarily in the feces with the aid of bile salts. Very little appears in the urine. Studies in which radioactively labeled 1α,25$(OH)_2D_3$ was administered to humans have shown that 60%–70% of the 1α,25$(OH)_2D_3$ was eliminated in the feces as more polar metabolites, glucuronides, and sulfates of 1α,25$(OH)_2D_3$. The half-life of 1α,25$(OH)_2D_3$ in the plasma has two components. Within 5 min, only half of an administered dose of radioactive 1α,25$(OH)_2$D3 remains in the plasma. A slower component of elimination has a half-life of about 10 h. 1α,25$(OH)_2D_3$ is catabolized by a number of pathways that result in its rapid removal from the organism [162].

BIOCHEMICAL MODE OF ACTION

The major classical physiological effects of vitamin D are to increase the active absorption of Ca^{2+} from the proximal intestine and to increase the mineralization of bone. This is achieved

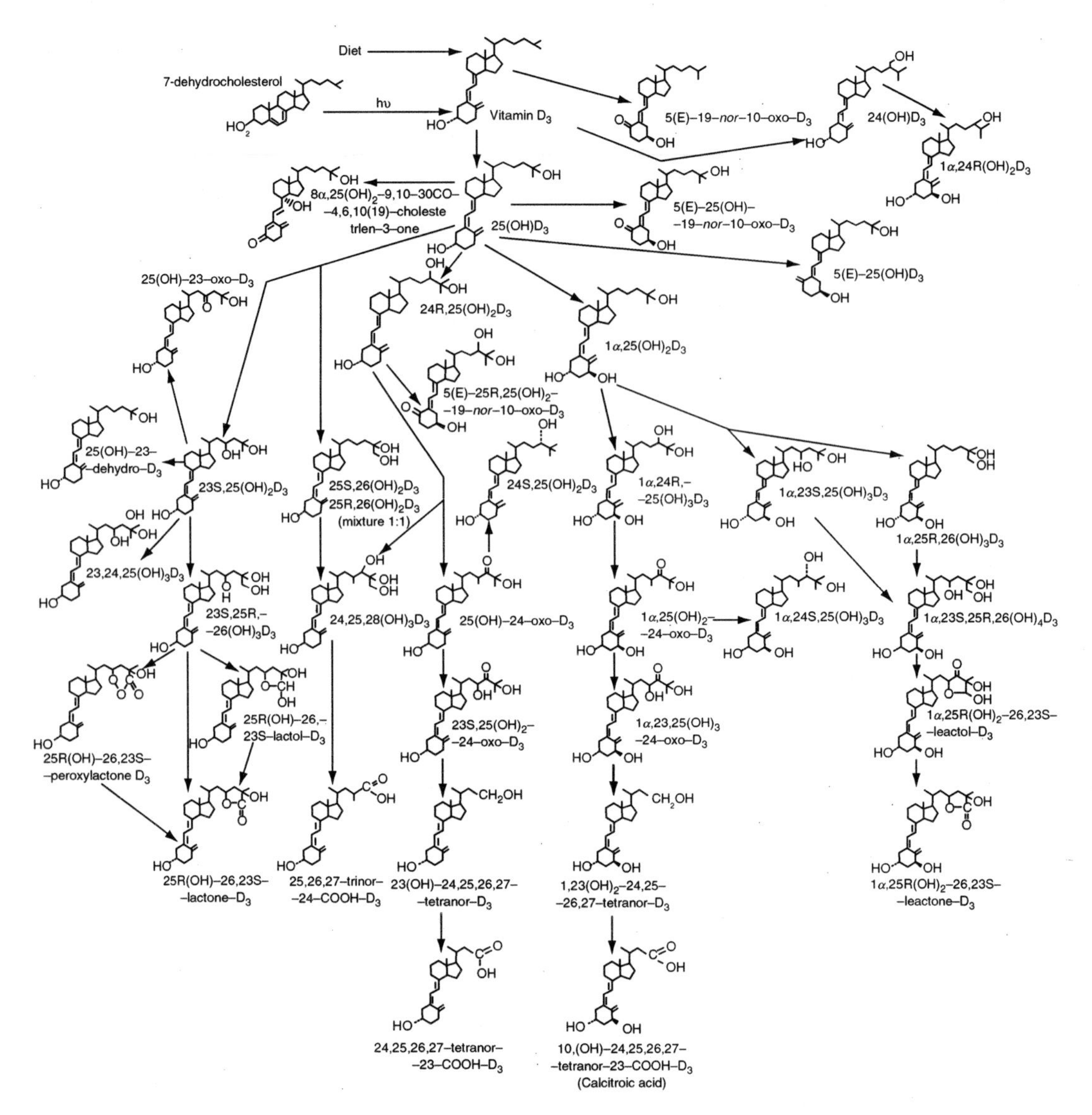

FIGURE 2.5 Summary of the metabolic transformations of vitamin D_3. Shown here are the structures of all known chemically characterized vitamin D_3 metabolites.

via two major signal transduction pathways, genomic and membrane-receptor-initiated rapid responses.

Genomic

Vitamin D, through its daughter metabolite, the steroid hormone $1\alpha,25(OH)_2D_3$, functions in a manner homologous to that of the classical steroid hormones. A model for steroid hormone action is shown in Figure 2.6. In the general model, a steroid hormone is produced in an endocrine gland in response to a physiological stimulus, then circulates in the blood, usually bound to a protein carrier, that is, DBP in the case of vitamin D, to target tissues where the hormone interacts with specific, high-affinity intracellular receptors. The receptor–hormone complex localizes in the nucleus, undergoes some type of activation perhaps involving phosphorylation [163–166], and binds to a hormone response element (HRE) on the DNA

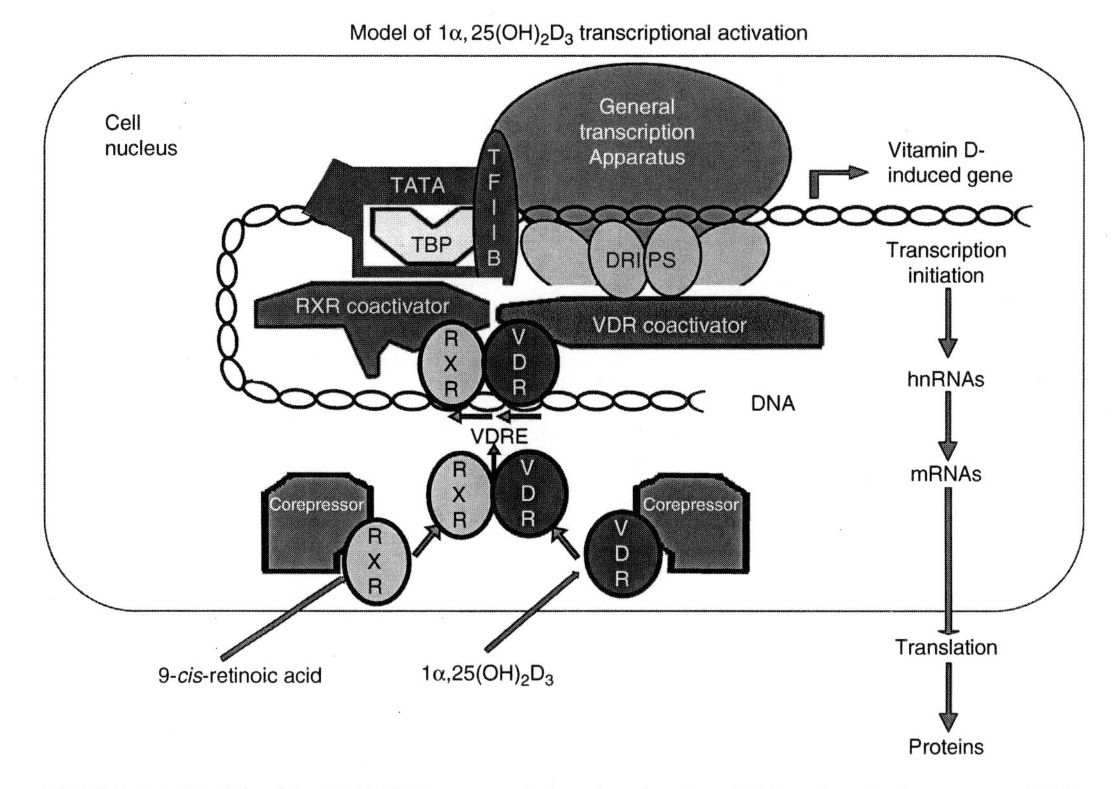

FIGURE 2.6 Model of $1\alpha,25(OH)_2D_3$ transcriptional activation. VDR, vitamin D receptor; RXR, retinoic acid X receptor; VDRE, vitamin D response element.

to modulate the expression of hormone-sensitive genes. The modulation of gene transcription results in either the induction or the repression of specific mRNAs, ultimately resulting in changes in protein expression needed to produce the required biological response. VDR has been identified in at least 30 target tissues [123,167,168] and with the advent of microarray analysis several hundred genes are known to be regulated by $1\alpha,25(OH)_2D_3$ [169–171]. A number of excellent recent reviews on the VDR regulation of gene transcription have appeared [9,10,16,172–176].

Nuclear Receptor

The $1\alpha,25(OH)_2D_3$ receptor was originally discovered in the intestine of vitamin D-deficient chicks [53,177]. It has been extensively characterized and the cDNA for the nuclear receptor has been cloned and sequenced [178,179]. The $1\alpha,25(OH)_2D_3$ receptor is a DNA-binding protein with a molecular weight of about 50,000 Da. It binds $1\alpha,25(OH)_2D_3$ with high affinity with a K_D in the range of $1–50 \times 10^{-10}$ M [180,181]. The ligand specificity of the nuclear $1\alpha,25(OH)_2D_3$ receptor is illustrated in Table 2.4. The $1\alpha,25(OH)_2D_3$ receptor protein belongs to the superfamily of homologous nuclear receptors [55,182]. To date only a single form of the receptor has been identified.

The protein superfamily to which the VDR belongs includes receptors for GR, PR, ER, aldosterone, androgens, thyroid hormone (T_3R), hormonal forms of vitamin A (RAR, RXR), the insect hormone, ecdysone, the peroxisome proliferator–activator receptor (PPAR), and several orphan receptors including the estrogen related receptor (ERR) and the cholic acid lipid sensing receptor, LXR [55,183]. To date biochemical evidence has been obtained for the

TABLE 2.4
Ligand Specificity of the Nuclear 1α,25(OH)$_2$D$_3$ Receptor

Ligand	Structural Modification	RCI[a] (%)
1α,25(OH)$_2$D$_3$		100
1α,25(OH)$_2$-24-*nor*-D$_3$	Shorten side chain by one carbon	67
1α,25(OH)$_2$-3-epi-D$_3$	Orientation of 3β-OH altered	24
1α,25(OH)$_2$-24a-dihomo-D$_3$	Lengthen side chain by two carbons	24
1β,25(OH)$_2$D$_3$	Orientation of 1α-OH changed	0.8
1α(OH)D$_3$	Lacks 25-OH	0.15
25(OH)D$_3$	Lacks 1α-OH	0.15
1α,25(OH)$_2$-7-dehydrocholesterol	Lacks a broken B ring; is not a secosteroid	0.10
Vitamin D$_3$	Lacks 1α and 25-OH	0.0001

Source: From Bouillon R., Okamura W.H., and Norman A.W., *Endocr. Rev.*, 16, 200, 1995.

[a] The relative competitive index (RCI) is a measure of the ability of a nonradioactive ligand to compete, under in vitro conditions, with radioactive 1α,25(OH)$_2$D$_3$ for binding to the nuclear 1α,25(OH)$_2$D$_3$ receptor (VDR).

existence of about 24 small molecules or steroid receptors and an equivalent number of orphan receptors for which a ligand has not yet been identified. Based on evaluation of the human genome database, it is believed that there are a total of 47 members of the steroid receptor superfamily [55].

VDR Domains

At the protein level, comparative studies of the VDR with all the steroid, retinoid, and thyroid receptors reveal that they have a common structural organization consisting of five domains [184] with significant amino acid sequence homologies (see Figure 2.8A). The different domains act as distinct modules that can function independently of each other [185].

The DNA-binding domain, C, is the most conserved domain throughout the family. About 70 amino acids fold into two zinc finger-like motifs in which conserved cysteines coordinate a zinc ion in a tetrahedral arrangement. The first finger, which contains four cysteines and several hydrophobic amino acids, determines the HRE specificity; an HRE is a specific nucleotide sequence located in the promoter region of the gene to be regulated by the receptor and cognate ligand [185–187]. The second zinc finger, which contains five cysteines and many basic amino acids, is also necessary for DNA binding and is involved in receptor dimerization [188,189]. The zinc fingers identify the receptor's cognate HRE and physically interact with the HRE to form a receptor + ligand + HRE–DNA complex.

The next most conserved region is the steroid-binding domain (region E). This region contains a hydrophobic pocket for ligand binding and also contains signals for several other functions including dimerization [190,191], nuclear translocation, and hormone-dependent transcriptional activation [192].

The A/B (transactivation) domain, which is quite small in the VDR (25 amino acids), is poorly conserved across the nuclear receptor superfamily and its function has not yet been clearly defined. An independent transcriptional activation function is located within the A/B region [188,192], which is constitutive in receptor constructs lacking the LBD (region E). The relative importance of the transcriptional activation by this domain depends on the receptor, the context of the target gene promoter, and the target cell type [192].

Domain D is the hinge region between the DNA-binding domain and the LBD. The hinge domain must be conformationally flexible because it allows the DNA-binding domains and

LBD some flexibility for their proper interactions with DNA and ligand, respectively. The VDR hinge region contains 65 amino acids and has immunogenic properties.

X-ray Structure of the VDR

The crystal structure of an engineered version of the LBD of the nuclear receptor for vitamin D, bound to $1\alpha,25(OH)_2D_3$, was determined in 2000 at a 1.8 Å resolution [193]. A follow-up X-ray crystallographic report compared the VDR LBD and bound ligand for $1\alpha,25(OH)_2D_3$ with that of four superagonist analogs of $1\alpha,25(OH)_2D_3$ [194]. Other X-ray structures of the VDR, which are all very similar to the original report, have appeared [195,196].

The structure of the LBD of the human VDR_{nuc} spans amino acid residues 143–427 (COOH-terminus) but without residues 165–215, which were in an undefined loop in the hinge region of domain D (see Figure 2.7A). The removal of the flexible insertion domain in the VDR LBD produced a more soluble protein, which was more amenable to crystallization. The VDR LBD protein structure is very similar to the LBD of the 5 other X-ray crystallographic nuclear receptor structures that had been determined before VDR in 2000 [192]. All nuclear steroid hormone receptors consist of a three-stranded β-sheet and 12 α-helices, which are arranged to create a three-layer sandwich that completely encompasses the ligand [$1\alpha,25(OH)_2D_3$ in the case of the VDR] in a hydrophobic core (see Figure 2.8). The X-ray structures of all six nuclear hormone receptors are so similar that their ribbon diagrams are virtually superimposable, indicating a remarkable spatial conservation of the secondary and tertiary structures [192]. In addition, the AF-2 domain of the C-terminal helix 12 (domain F; residues 404–427) contributes to the hormone-binding pocket.

Comparison of X-ray Structures VDR and DBP and Their Ligands

Table 2.5 summarizes the important similarities and differences in the structure of the two key proteins of the vitamin D endocrine system, the VDR LBD and DBP. Even though there is no

TABLE 2.5
Comparison of VDR and DBP Protein Crystal Structures

Property	VDR	DBP
Molecular weight (kDa)	51	58
Number of amino acid residues of intact protein	427	458
Number of residues in X-ray structure	158	458
Location of LBD on the protein	Interior pocket	Surface cleft
Ligand–protein contacts	Unique[a]	Unique[a]
Ligand A-ring conformation	β-chair	α-chair
3β-OH	Axial	Equatorial
C5–C6–C7–C8 torsion angle	+211°	+149°
General ligand shape	Bowl-shaped 6-s-*trans*	Twisted 6-s-*trans*
A-ring position	30° above C/D ring	31° below C/D ring
C17–C20–C22–C23 torsion angle	−156°	−70°
Side-chain orientation	Extended	Curled down
Distance from C-19 to oxygen on C-25	6.9 Å	3.8 Å
Overall ligand shape	Bowl	Hook

[a] The descriptor unique is used to indicate that the amino acid residues of the protein involved with the stabilizing hydrogen bond contact points with the respective ligands, $1\alpha,25(OH)_2D_3$ for VDR and $25(OH)D_3$ for DBP, are totally different.

amino acid or structural similarity between the two proteins, each has independently evolved to create a unique but highly effective LBD that can tightly bind its optimal vitamin D secosteroid ligand: for DBP, $25(OH)D_3$, $K_D \sim 6 \times 10^{-9}$ M; and for the VDR, $1\alpha,25(OH)_2D_3$, $K_Ds \sim 1 \times 10^{-9}$ M. However, the location of the two LBDs is vastly different for the two proteins. For the VDR, the ligand is sequestered inside the protein (see Figure 2.7C), whereas for DBP the ligand is held in a surface crevice (see Figure 2.7B) such that one face of the ligand is exposed to the solvent environment. Thus, there is a much greater freedom of ligand structure tolerated by the DBP ligand in comparison with the VDR; compare optimal DBP ligands with VDR ligand (Figure 2.8 and Table 2.2).

Calbindin-D

The first protein to be shown to be genomically regulated by $1\alpha,25(OH)_2D_3$ is a calcium-binding protein, named calbindin-D. In the mammalian kidney and brain and in all avian tissues, a larger form of the protein (calbindin-D_{28K}) is expressed, whereas in the mammalian intestine

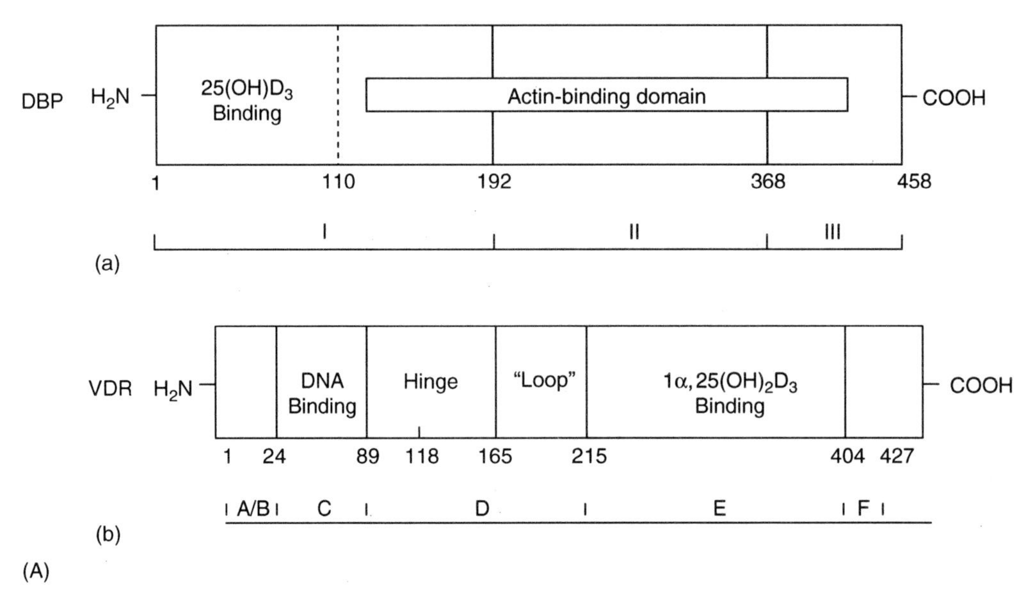

FIGURE 2.7 Three-dimensional structure of the vitamin D-binding protein (DBP). (A) Schematic models of the vitamin DBP (a) and the vitamin D receptor (b). (a) The DBP consists of 458 amino acid residues and is divided into three domains (I, II, and III). The numbers below the DBP indicate the amino acid residue boundaries for the various domains. The domains I, II, and III have been postulated to have evolved from a progenitor that arose from the triple repeat of a 192 amino acid sequence [115]. However, domain III is significantly truncated at the C-terminus. The $25(OH)D_3$-binding cleft is associated with the first six α-helices or residues 1–110 of domain I. The actin-binding property of DBP is associated with a portion of domains I and III, which clamp the actin while it rests on domain II. (b) The VDR comprises 427 amino acid residues that are divided into six domains (A–F). The numbers below the VDR indicate the amino acid residue boundaries for the various domains. The VDR belongs to a superfamily of nuclear receptors all of which have the same general A–F domain organization. The C domain, the most highly conserved, which contains the DNA-binding domain, defines the superfamily; it contains two zinc finger motifs. The E domain or ligand-binding domain (LBD) is less conserved and is responsible for binding $1\alpha,25(OH)_2D_3$ or its analogs and transcriptional activation. The A/B domain of the VDR is much smaller than other members of the superfamily. The portion of the intact VDR that was crystallized and subjected to X-ray crystallographic analysis included residues 118–427 but with deletion of the loop region of the hinge domain D, residues 165–215.

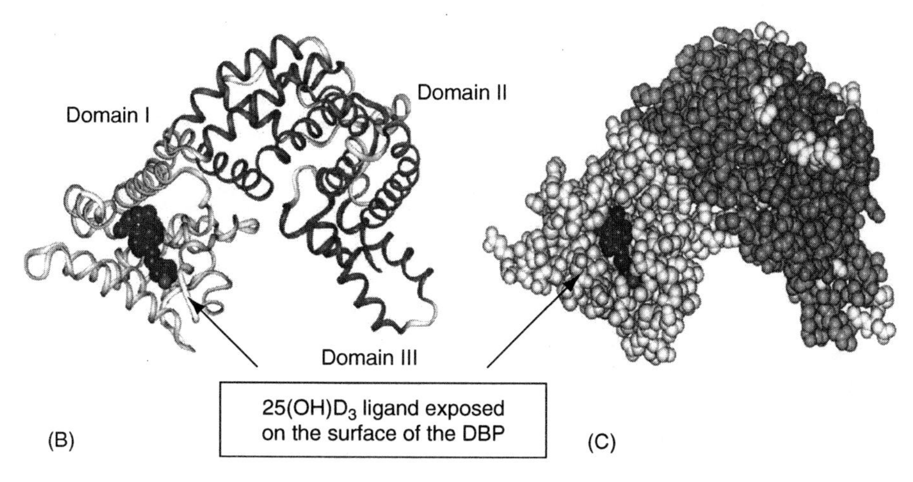

FIGURE 2.7 (continued) (B) Three-dimensional structure of DBP for residues 1–458 as determined via X-ray crystallography [116]. Illustration of the three domains (I, II, and III) of the DBP in a ribbon structure representation. The atoms of the ligand $25(OH)D_3$ are colored black. The X-ray structure of DBP was determined separately with two different ligands. These ligands were $25(OH)D_3$ and 22-(*m*-hydroxyphenyl)-23,24,25,26,27-pentanor vitamin D_3 (analog JY); both X-ray structures contained the same conformer shape of the bound ligands. The structure and the shape of $25(OH)D_3$ are presented in more detail in Figure 2.8C. (C) The LBD of the DBP is a crevice located on the surface of domain I. The figure illustrates the Corey–Pauling–Koltun (CPK) space-filling structure of DBP, with white regions indicating flexible regions of the molecule. Virtually the entire top face of the 25(OH) is exposed to the external environment.

and placenta a smaller form (calbindin-D_{9K}) is expressed [197]. The expression of calbindins in various tissues and species appears to be regulated to differing degrees by $1\alpha,25(OH)_2D_3$ [198]. The gene for calbindin-D_{28K} has now been cloned and sequenced [199], but there is still much to learn about the physiological importance of calbindins-D in its many tissues.

Nongenomic Actions of $1\alpha,25(OH)_2D_3$

The rapid or nongenomic responses mediated by $1\alpha,25(OH)_2D_3$ were originally postulated to be mediated through the interaction of $1\alpha,25(OH)_2D_3$ with a novel protein receptor located on the external membrane of the cell (see Figure 2.8) [200]. This membrane receptor has now been shown to be the classic VDR (heretofore largely found in the nucleus and cytosol) associated with caveolae present in the plasma membrane of a variety of cells [201]. Caveolae, also known as lipid rafts, are invaginations present in the plasma membrane of many cells; caveolae are believed to be docking platforms for protein components of many signal transduction systems [202–204]. Using VDR knockout (KO) and wild-type mice, rapid modulation of osteoblast ion channel responses by $1\alpha,25(OH)_2D_3$ was found to require the presence of a functional vitamin D nuclear or caveolae receptor [205].

Rapid responses stimulated by $1\alpha,25(OH)_2D_3$ or 6-s-*cis* locked analogs of $1\alpha,25(OH)_2D_3$ (see later) acting through the VDR_{mem} include the following: rapid stimulation by $1\alpha,25(OH)_2D_3$ of ICA (transcaltachia) (Figure 2.9) [206]; opening of voltage-gated Ca^{2+} and Cl^- [207] channels; store-operated Ca^{2+} influx in skeletal muscle cells as modulated by phospholipase C, PKC, and tyrosine kinases [208]; activation of PKC [209,210]; and inhibition of activation of apoptosis in osteoblasts mediated by rapid activation of Src, phosphatidyl inositol 3′-kinase, and JNK kinases [211].

Careful study using structural analogs of $1,25(OH)_2D_3$ has shown that the genomic and nongenomic responses to this conformationally flexible steroid hormone have different

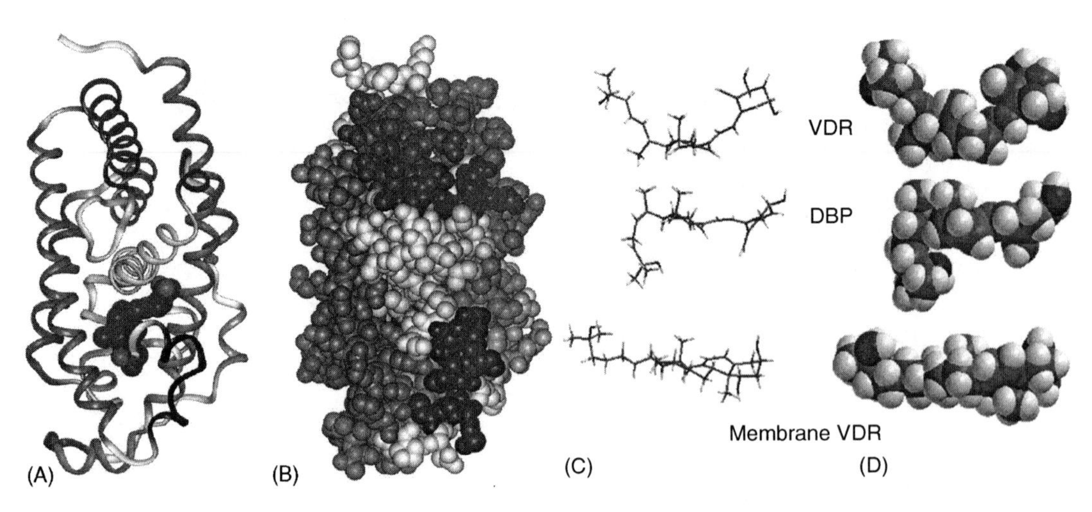

FIGURE 2.8 Three-dimensional structure of the vitamin D receptor (VDR) for the steroid hormone, 1α,25$(OH)_2D_3$. (A) Domains of the VDR. All steroid receptors, including the VDR, have a homologous domain structure. Domains A/B vary in size on the family of steroid receptors. The VDR domain A/B is small, by comparison, and is also referred to as the AF-1 domain or activation function-1 domain. Domain C is the site of two zinc fingers, which physically and very specifically interact with VDR HREs (specific sequences of deoxy nucleotides that are in the promoters of genes to be regulated by the VDR). Domain D is a linker region. Domain E comprises 12 helices (see B) and constitutes the ligand-binding domain (LBD) for 1α,25$(OH)_2D_3$. Domain F is also small and is the AF-2 domain. (B) Three-dimensional ribbon structure of the VDR LBD for residues 118–425 (Δ165–215) as determined via X-ray crystallography [193]; the helices are numbered H1–H12. In addition, the presence of the bound ligand 1α,25$(OH)_2D_3$ is shown; its structure and shape are presented in more detail in D. The white regions represent loops and other flexible regions of the molecule. The ligand 1α,25$(OH)_2D_3$ has its atoms indicated. (C) Illustration of the Corey–Pauling–Koltun (CPK) space-filling model of the VDR LBD. The position of helix-12 in the closed position effectively sequesters the ligand from the external environment of the protein, indicated by the absence of visible carbon and oxygen atoms from 1α,25$(OH)_2D_3$ in this view. (D) Conformation of the optimal ligands for the VDR and DBP as determined by X-ray crystallography. (*Top* structures) The shape of 1α,25$(OH)_2D_3$ as a ligand in the VDR LBD, in a stick (*left*) or CPK space-filling (*right*) rendition, is shown as a twisted or bowl-shaped 6-s-*trans* orientation. The A ring is in the β-chair conformation (see Figure 2.2) and the side chain is oriented northeasterly at 2 o'clock as defined by its global energy minimum [480, 481]. (*Middle* structures) The shape of the 25$(OH)D_3$ as a ligand for DBP is shown in a stick (*left*) and CPK space-filling (*right*) model. The side chain is organized as a hook. The A ring is in the α-chair conformation (see Figure 2.2) and the side chain is oriented behind and nearly perpendicular to the CD ring. The *bottom* structure is that of the optimal agonist for nongenomic or rapid responses 1α,25$(OH)_2$-lumisterol (analog JN). Both the stick and the space-filling presentations of JN are presented. It is apparent that the optimal ligand shapes for the VDR genomic responses, DBP, and VDR-mediated rapid responses are each unique [482].

requirements for ligand structure [9,212,213]. For example, a key consideration is the position of rotation about the 6,7 single carbon–carbon bond, which can either be in the 6-s-*cis* or 6-s-*trans* orientation (see Figure 2.1). The preferred shape of the ligand for VDR_{nuc}, determined from the X-ray crystal structure of the receptor occupied with ligand, is a 6-s-*trans*-shaped bowl with the A ring 30° above the plane of the C and D rings. In contrast, structure–function studies of rapid nongenomic actions of 1,25$(OH)_2D_3$ and its analogs show that the VDR_{mem} prefers its ligand to have a 6-s-*cis* shape.

Other steroid hormones, ER [214], PR [215–218], testosterone [219], GRs [220–222], and thyroid [223,224], have been shown to have similar membrane effects [225]. A model for the nongenomic signal transduction pathway is shown in Figure 2.8.

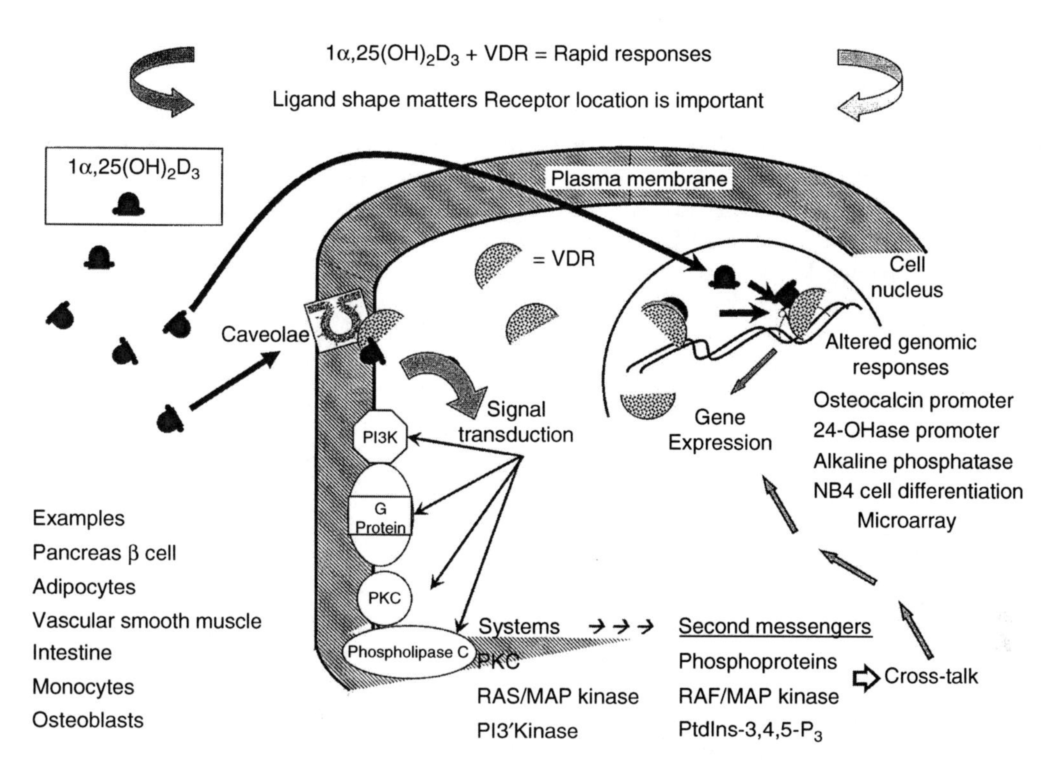

FIGURE 2.9 Schematic model describing how the conformationally flexible $1\alpha,25(OH)_2D_3$ can interact with a nuclear receptor to generate genomic responses or a plasma membrane receptor to generate rapid responses. Binding of $1\alpha,25(OH)_2D_3$ to the membrane surface receptor may result in the activation of one or more second messenger systems, including phospholipase C, protein kinase C, G protein coupled receptors, or phosphatidyl-inositol-3-kinase (PI3). There are a number of possible outcomes including opening of the voltage-gated calcium channel or generation of the indicated second messengers. Some of these second messengers, particularly RAF/MAP kinase, may engage in cross-talk with a nucleus to modulate gene expression. Evidence has been presented that rapid responses can modulate the list of specific genes tabulated in the figure.

SPECIFIC FUNCTIONS OF $1\alpha(OH)_2D_3$

$1\alpha,25(OH)_2D_3$ and Mineral Metabolism

The classical target tissues for $1\alpha,25(OH)_2D_3$ are those that are directly involved in the regulation of mineral homeostasis. In man, serum calcium and phosphorous levels are normally maintained between 9.5 and 10.5 mg/100 ml and between 2.5 and 4.3 mg/100 ml, respectively [2]. Together with PTH and calcitonin, $1\alpha,25(OH)_2D_3$ maintains serum calcium and phosphate levels by its actions on the intestine, kidney, bone, and parathyroid gland.

In the intestine, one of the best characterized effects of $1\alpha,25(OH)_2D_3$ is the stimulation of intestinal lumen-to-plasma flux of calcium and phosphate [41,226,227]. Although extensive evidence exists showing that $1\alpha,25(OH)_2D_3$, interacting with its receptor, upregulates calbindin-D in a genome-mediated fashion, the relationship between calbindin-D and calcium transport is not clear [228]. In the vitamin D-deficient state, both mammals and birds have severely decreased intestinal absorption of calcium with no detectable levels of calbindin. There is a linear correlation between the increased cellular levels of calbindin-D and calcium transport. When $1\alpha,25(OH)_2D_3$ is given to vitamin D-deficient chicks, the transport of calcium reaches maximal rates at 12–14 h whereas calbindin-D does not reach its maximal levels until 48 h [229].

In a study employing immunohistochemical techniques, it was demonstrated that the cellular location of calbindin-D_{28K} changed with the onset of calcium transport [230].

$1\alpha,25(OH)_2D_3$ treatment also alters the biochemical and morphological characteristics of the intestinal cells [231,232]. The size of the villus and the size of the microvilli increase on $1\alpha,25(OH)_2D_3$ treatment [233]. The brush border undergoes noticeable alterations in the structure and composition of cell surface proteins and lipids, occurring in a time frame corresponding to the increase in Ca^{2+} transport mediated by $1\alpha,25(OH)_2D_3$ [234]. However, despite extensive work, the exact mechanisms involved in the vitamin D-dependent intestinal absorption of calcium remain unknown [235–237].

The kidney is the major site of synthesis of $1\alpha,25(OH)_2D_3$ and of several other hydroxylated vitamin D derivatives. Probably the most important effect $1\alpha,25(OH)_2D_3$ has on the kidney is the inhibition of $25(OH)D_3$-1α-hydroxylase activity, which results in a decrease in the synthesis of $1\alpha,25(OH)_2D_3$ [238].

Simultaneously, the activity of the $25(OH)D_3$-24R-hydroxylase is stimulated. The actions of vitamin D on calcium and phosphorus metabolism in the kidney have been a controversial area and more research is needed to clearly define the actions of $1\alpha,25(OH)_2D_3$ on the kidney [239].

Recently, it has been found that $1\alpha,25(OH)_2D_3$ functions as a potent negative endocrine regulator of renin gene expression [240]. The renin–angiotensin system plays a central role in the regulation of blood pressure, volume, and electrolyte homeostasis. Epidemiological and clinical studies have long suggested an association of inadequate sunlight exposure or low serum $1\alpha,25(OH)_2D_3$ levels with high blood pressure and high plasma renin activity, but the mechanism is presently being elucidated [241–243].

Although vitamin D is a powerful antirachitic agent, its primary effect on bone is the stimulation of bone resorption leading to an increase in serum calcium and phosphorus levels [244]. With even slight decreases in serum calcium levels, PTH is synthesized, which then stimulates the synthesis of $1\alpha,25(OH)_2D_3$ in the kidney. Both of these hormones stimulate bone resorption. Maintaining constant levels of calcium in the blood is crucial, whether calcium is available in the diet or not. Therefore, the ability to release calcium from its largest body store, the bone, is vital. Bone is a dynamic tissue, which is constantly remodeled. Under normal physiological conditions, bone formation and bone resorption are tightly balanced [245]. The stimulation of bone growth and mineralization by $1\alpha,25(OH)_2D_3$ appears to be an indirect effect due to the provision of minerals for bone matrix incorporation through an increase in intestinal absorption of calcium and phosphorus. In bone, nuclear receptors for $1\alpha,25(OH)_2D_3$ have been detected in normal osteoblasts [246] and in osteoblast-like osteosarcoma cells, but not in mature osteoclasts. In addition, $1\alpha,25(OH)_2D_3$ can induce rapid changes in cytosolic Ca^{2+} levels in osteoblast and osteosarcoma cells by opening voltage-gated Ca^{2+} channels via a nongenomic signal transduction pathway [247,248].

Some of the actions of $1\alpha,25(OH)_2D_3$ in bone are related to changes in bone cell differentiation. For example, $1\alpha,25(OH)_2D_3$ decreases type-I collagen production [249], and increases alkaline phosphatase production and the proliferation of cultured osteoblasts [250]. $1\alpha,25(OH)_2D_3$ also increases the production of osteocalcin [251] and matrix Gla protein [252] and decreases the production of type-I collagen by fetal rat calvaria [253]. $1\alpha,25(OH)_2D_3$ also affects osteoclastogenesis from precursor cells through VDR-mediated effects on gene transcription and in this way can stimulate bone mineral resorption [254,255]. A particularly useful technique for studying the role of $1\alpha,25(OH)_2D_3$ in bone has been through the selective KO of either (or in combination) the genes encoding VDR, the 25(OH)D-1α-hydroxylase, or the 25(OH)D-24R-hydroxylase proteins. These studies have been reviewed in depth by Goltzman et al. and Panda et al. [15,256].

PTH is an important tropic stimulator of $1\alpha,25(OH)_2D_3$ synthesis by the kidney. High circulating levels of $1\alpha,25(OH)_2D_3$ have been shown to decrease the levels of PTH by an indirect mechanism involving increased serum calcium levels, which is an inhibitory signal for PTH production and a direct mechanism involving the direct suppression of the expression of the preprothyroid hormone gene by the $1\alpha,25(OH)_2D_3$–VDr complex. Collectively, $1\alpha,25(OH)_2D_3$ or analogs such as $1\alpha,25(OH)_2$-19-*nor*-D_2 (Zemplar; see Table 2.9) have been shown to be effective in reducing the secondary hyperparathyroidism commonly found in patients with renal failure [257–259].

During pregnancy and lactation, large amounts of calcium are needed for the developing fetus and for milk production. Hormonal adjustments in the vitamin D endocrine system are critical to prevent depletion of minerals leading to serious bone damage for the mother. Although receptors for $1\alpha,25(OH)_2D_3$ have been found in placental tissue [260] and in the mammary gland [261,262], the role vitamin D plays is not clear. In addition, there is an emerging view that there is a correlation between VDR polymorphism and the incidence of breast cancer [263,264].

VITAMIN D IN NONCLASSICAL SYSTEMS

In the 1970s and 1980s, nuclear receptors for $1\alpha,25(OH)_2D_3$ were discovered in a variety of tissues and cells not directly involved in calcium homeostasis (Table 2.2). Thus, the role of the vitamin D endocrine system has expanded to include a broader range of effects on cell regulation and differentiation [168,265]. Nuclear VDR is present in muscle, hematolymphopoietic, reproductive and nervous tissue as well as in other endocrine tissues, and skin. The expression of more than 100 proteins is known to be regulated by $1\alpha,25(OH)_2D_3$, including several oncogenes [266,267] by far extending the classical limits of vitamin D actions on calcium homeostasis. In many of these systems, the effect vitamin D has on the tissue or the details of its mechanism of action are not yet clear.

Skeletal muscle is a target organ for $1\alpha,25(OH)_2D_3$. Clinical studies have shown the presence of muscle weakness or myopathy during metabolic bone diseases related to vitamin D deficiency [25,268,269]. These abnormalities can be reversed with vitamin D therapy. Experimental evidence has shown that $1\alpha,25(OH)_2D_3$ has a direct effect on Ca^{2+} transport in cultured myoblasts and skeletal muscle tissue. Furthermore, there is evidence that the action of $1\alpha,25(OH)_2D_3$ on skeletal muscle may be important for the calcium homeostasis of the entire organism since the hormone induces a rapid release of calcium from muscle into the serum of hypocalcemic animals. $1\alpha,25(OH)_2D_3$ receptors have been detected in myoblast cultures and the changes in calcium uptake have been shown to be RNA- and protein synthesis-dependent, suggesting a genomic mechanism. $1\alpha,25(OH)_2D_3$ has also been shown to be important for cardiac muscle function [270–273].

The generation of VDR KO mice and the ability to maintain normal mineral ion homeostasis in these mice using a diet enriched in calcium and lactose have permitted investigations directed at identifying target tissues in which the actions of the VDR are critical for normal development, maturation, and homeostasis. These studies have demonstrated an important function in several nontraditional target tissues, including muscle [274–276].

In the skin, $1\alpha,25(OH)_2D_3$, acting through VDR, appears to exert effects on cellular growth and differentiation [277]. Receptors for $1\alpha,25(OH)_2D_3$ have been found in human [278] and mouse skin [279]. $1\alpha,25(OH)_2D_3$ inhibits the synthesis of DNA in mouse epidermal cells [279]. The hormone induces changes in cultured keratinocytes, which are consistent for terminal differentiation of nonadherent cornified squamous cells [280]. Additional experiments have shown that human neonatal foreskin keratinocytes produce $1\alpha,25(OH)_2D_3$ from $25(OH)D_3$ under in vitro conditions [281], suggesting that keratinocyte-derived $1\alpha,25(OH)_2D_3$ may affect epidermal differentiation locally. Psoriasis is a chronic hyperproliferative skin disease. Some forms of psoriasis have been shown to improve significantly when treated topically with calcipotriol, a nonhypercalcemic analog of

$1\alpha,25(OH)_2D_3$ [282–284]. In mouse skin carcinogenesis, $1\alpha,25(OH)_2D_3$ blocks the production of tumors induced by 12-*O*-tetradecanoyl-phorbol-12-acetate [285].

Recent work from the Demay laboratory emphasizes the critical role of the VDR functioning in the hair follicle; indeed a primary phenotype of the VDR KO mouse is that of alopecia [286]. Intriguingly, the presence of the VDR without any ligand [in the absence of $1\alpha,25(OH)_2D_3$ by genetic KO of the 25(OH)D-1α-hydroxylase] is essential for hair growth [287–289].

In the pancreas, $1\alpha,25(OH)_2D_3$ is essential for normal insulin secretion. Experiments with rats have shown the presence of the VDR in the pancreas [290] and that vitamin D and $1\alpha,25(OH)_2D_3$ increase insulin release from the isolated perfused pancreas, both in the presence and absence of normal serum calcium levels [291–295]. Human patients with vitamin D deficiency, even when serum calcium levels are normal, exhibit impaired insulin secretion but normal glucagon secretion, suggesting that $1\alpha,25(OH)_2D_3$ directly affects β-cell function [296]. More recent studies clearly indicate the role of $1\alpha,25(OH)_2D_3$ in preventing type-1 diabetes in mouse models [297,298]. It appears likely that in some circumstances type-1 diabetes is really an autoimmune disease that can be prevented by appropriate administration of vitamin D_3 or $1\alpha,25(OH)_2D_3$ or its analogs [298–301].

Receptors for $1\alpha,25(OH)_2D_3$ have been found in some sections of the brain. However, the role of $1\alpha,25(OH)_2D_3$ in the brain is not well understood. Both calbindins-D have been found in the brain but the expression of neither calbindin-D_{28K} nor calbindin-D_{9K} appears to be modulated directly by vitamin D [302,303]. In the rat, $1\alpha,25(OH)_2D_3$ appears to increase the activity of the choline acetyltransferase (CAT) in specific regions of the brain [302]. Other steroid hormones have also been shown to affect neurotransmitter metabolism in specific brain regions [304,305]. A recent report indicates that VDR KO mice exhibit both motor and behavioral changes that may be linked to disruption of normal brain activity [306,307]. Behavioral effects of vitamin D deficiency are currently under investigation in animal models and in humans [308].

Immunoregulatory Roles of $1\alpha,25(OH)_2D_3$

In the early 1980s, when the VDR was discovered in several neoplastic hematopoietic cell lines as well as in normal human peripheral blood mononuclear cells, monocytes, and activated lymphocytes [309,310], a role for $1\alpha,25(OH)_2D_3$ in immune function was suggested. Since then, $1\alpha,25(OH)_2D_3$ has been shown to affect cells of the immune system in a variety of ways. $1\alpha,25(OH)_2D_3$ reduces the proliferation of HL-60 cells and also induces their differentiation to monocytes and macrophages [311–313]. The actions of $1\alpha,25(OH)_2D_3$ on normal monocytes is controversial but it appears that it may enhance monocyte function. $1\alpha,25(OH)_2D_3$ appears to reduce levels of HLA-DR and CD4 + class II antigens on monocytes or macrophages with no effect on the expression of class I antigens [314]. The enhancement of class II antigen expression is a common feature of autoimmunity and often precedes the onset of autoimmune diseases.

$1\alpha,25(OH)_2D_3$ also promotes the differentiation of leukemic myeloid precursor cells toward cells with the characteristics of macrophages [309]. Subsequent experiments have shown that $1\alpha,25(OH)_2D_3$ does not alter the clonal growth of normal myeloid precursors but it does induce the formation of macrophage colonies preferentially over the formation of granulocyte colonies [312]. In addition, macrophages derived from different tissues are able to synthesize $1\alpha,25(OH)_2D_3$ when activated by γ-interferon [139]. In addition, $1\alpha,25(OH)_2D_3$ can suppress immunoglobulin production by activated B-lymphocytes [315] and inhibit DNA synthesis and proliferation of both activated B- and T-lymphocytes [316,317]. These findings suggest the existence of a vitamin D paracrine system involving activated macrophages and activated lymphocytes (Figure 2.4).

Current studies of 1α,25$(OH)_2D_3$ and the vitamin D endocrine system interactions with the immune system show many interesting new leads. A strain of mice (NOD) spontaneously develops a form of type-1 diabetes, which can be prevented by the administration of 1α,25$(OH)_2D_3$ [298,301,318]. 1α,25$(OH)_2D_3$ restores thymocyte apoptosis sensitivity in nonobese diabetic (NOD) mice through dendritic cells [319]. This has raised the possibility that analogs of 1α,25$(OH)_2D_3$ may be used to treat the autoimmune component of diabetes [320]. A similar approach has been proposed for autoimmune encephalomyelitis [321,322].

Still another immune system discovery has been the demonstration that tolerogenic dendritic cells induced by VDR ligands enhance the regulatory T-cells that inhibit allograft rejection and autoimmune diseases [323]. Similarly, Wang et al. [324] have found from microarray studies of gene expression a whole new category of 1α,25$(OH)_2D_3$-mediated responses. 1α,25$(OH)_2D_3$ is a direct regulator of antimicrobial innate immune responses. The promoters of the human cathelicidin antimicrobial peptide (camp) and defensin beta2 ($defB_2$) genes contain consensus vitamin D response elements that mediate 1,25$(OH)_2D_3$-dependent gene expression. Moreover, 1α,25$(OH)_2D_3$ induces corresponding increases in antimicrobial proteins and secretion of antimicrobial activity against pathogens including *Pseudomonas aeruginosa*. Thus, 1α,25$(OH)_2D_3$ directly regulates antimicrobial peptide gene expression, revealing the potential of its analogs in the treatment of opportunistic infections.

1α,25$(OH)_2D_3$ and cyclosporin, a potent immunosuppressive drug, appear to affect the immune system in a similar fashion. They affect T-lymphocytes during initial activation by antigen, select the generation of T-helper cells by inhibiting lymphokine production at a genomic level, and inhibit the generation of T-cytotoxic and NK cells. Both are involved in the enhancement of T-suppresser function, a key element in the efficacy of cyclosporin as a drug to reduce allograft tissue rejection [325]. 1α,25$(OH)_2D_3$ appears to work synergistically with cyclosporin when the two compounds are used in combination [326,327].

The use of nonhypercalcemic 1α,25$(OH)_2D_3$ analogs can result in enhanced immunosuppressive effects without the toxicity risks of 1α,25$(OH)_2D_3$. Because of the synergistic effects when 1α,25$(OH)_2D_3$ and cyclosporine are used in combination, synthetic 1α,25$(OH)_2D_3$ analogs may be used in the treatment of autoimmune diseases [328] or for transplantation [329] in combination with cyclosporin to reduce the toxicity of both compounds. The Koeffler lab has reported the consequences of administering separately to mice for 55 weeks 4 analogs of 1α,25$(OH)_2D_3$ that have potential as drugs for the immune system [330]. Thus, knowledge of long-term tolerability of vitamin D_3 analogs may be of interest in view of their potential clinical utility in the management of various pathologies such as malignancies, immunological disorders, and bone diseases.

Structures of Important Analogs

Studies using analogs of vitamin D have been used to address the question of the functional importance of the various structural features of the vitamin D and 1α,25$(OH)_2D_3$ molecules. Due to recent advances in new vitamin D syntheses described earlier and in Figure 2.3, analogs have been synthesized with modifications in all the key structural motifs of this secosteroid; these include the A ring, *seco*-B ring, C ring, C/D-ring junction, D ring, and side chain [4,331]. It is estimated that between 1973 and 2003 over 2000 analogs of 1α,25$(OH)_2D_3$ were synthesized by chemists in academia and pharmaceutical companies [172].

The importance of the configuration of the A ring has been studied by synthesizing 5,6-*trans* analogs. Because of the rotation of the A ring, these analogs cannot undergo 1α-hydroxylation and are only 1/1000 as biologically effective as 1α,25$(OH)_2D_3$. The relative significance of the 3β-hydroxyl group has been assessed by preparing analogs such as

3-deoxy-1α,25$(OH)_2D_3$. This analog has the interesting property that in vivo it preferentially stimulates ICA over BCM [332].

The length of the side chain also alters biological activity. 27-*Nor*-25$(OH)D_3$ and 26,27-bis-*nor*-25$(OH)D_3$ stimulate ICA and BCM in both normal and anephric rats, but are 10–100 times less active than 25$(OH)D_3$ [333]. 24-*Nor*-25$(OH)D_3$ was found to have no biological activity [334], although it was able to block the biological response to vitamin D, but not that of 25$(OH)D_3$ or 1α,25$(OH)_2D_3$. This suggests that it might have antivitamin D-metabolizing activity.

One of the most interesting side-chain analogs of 1α,25$(OH)_2D_3$ is 1$\alpha(OH)D_3$. This compound appears to have the same biological activity in chicks as 1α,25$(OH)_2D_3$ [335] and is approximately half as active in rats [336]. The 25-fluoro-1$\alpha(OH)D_3$ derivative, in which hydroxylation of the C-25 is inhibited, is only 1/50 as active as 1α,25$(OH)_2D_3$, suggesting that 1$\alpha(OH)D_3$ has some activity even without 25-hydroxylation [337].

From such studies, the particular attributes of the structure of 1α,25$(OH)_2D_3$ that enables it to elicit its biological responses are now defined. It is now known that the 3β-hydroxy group does not appear to be as important for biological activity as the 1α- or 25-hydroxyl groups; the *cis* configuration of the A ring is preferred over the *trans* configuration; and the length of the side chain appears critical, as apparently there is little tolerance for its shortened or lengthened state.

Analogs of 1α,25$(OH)_2D_3$ have also been used to study the in vivo metabolism and mode of action of vitamin D compounds. There is also widespread interest in developing 1α,25$(OH)_2D_3$ analogs to use as therapeutic agents in the treatment of osteoporosis, renal osteodystrophy, cancer, immunodeficiency syndromes, autoimmune diseases, and some skin disorders.

Of particular interest are analogs that separate the calcemic effects from the proliferation and differentiation effects of 1α,25$(OH)_2D_3$. Among these is a cyclopropyl derivative of 1α,25$(OH)_2D_3$, 1α,24*S*$(OH)_2$-22ene-26,27-dehydrovitamin D_3, designated calcipotriol; this analog has weak systemic effects on calcium metabolism but potent effects on cell proliferation and differentiation [338,339]. It is rapidly converted to inactive metabolites in vivo [340,341] and is 200-fold less potent than 1α,25$(OH)_2D_3$ in causing hypercalciuria and hypercalcemia in rats [338]. Calcipotriol is equally effective in binding to the nuclear receptor as 1α,25$(OH)_2D_3$ and has similar effects on the growth and differentiation of keratinocytes [340–343]. It is currently marketed as a topical treatment for psoriasis, a proliferative disorder of the skin [282,344–347].

Another analog that has potential as therapeutic agent is 22-oxa-1α,25$(OH)_2D_3$. This analog has been shown to suppress the secretion of PTH and may be useful in the treatment of secondary hyperparathyroidism [348]. It is 10 times more potent in suppressing proliferation and inducing differentiation than 1α,25$(OH)_2D_3$ with only 1/50 to 1/100 of the in vitro bone-resorbing activity of 1α,25$(OH)_2D_3$ [349].

Still another set of analogs of 1α,25$(OH)_2D_3$ with potential therapeutic applications are the compounds with a double bond at the 16-position and a triple bond at the 23-position. The best characterized of these compounds is 1α,25$(OH)_2$-16ene-23yne-D_3 [350,351], which is 300-fold less active than 1α,25$(OH)_2D_3$ in ICA and BCM and 10–15 times less active in inducing hypercalcemia in vivo in mice. In three leukemia models, therapy with this analog resulted in a significant increase in survival [351]. All of the 16-ene and or 23-yne analogs that have been tested are equivalent or more potent than 1α,25$(OH)_2D_3$ in the induction of HL-60 cell differentiation and inhibition of clonal proliferation [352] and 10-fold to 200-fold less active in intestinal calcium transport (ICT) and BCM [330,352].

Fluorinated analogs of 1α,25$(OH)_2D_3$ have been especially useful for studying the in vivo metabolism of 1α,25$(OH)_2D_3$. Fluorine groups have been substituted for the hydroxyls at positions C-25, C-1, and C-3 to study the importance of these hydroxylations for the biological activity of $1\alpha,25(OH)_2D_3$. In addition, fluorine groups have been substituted for hydrogens at positions C-23, C-24, and C-26 to study the catabolism of $1\alpha,25(OH)_2D_3$. The analog $1\alpha,25(OH)_2$-26,26,26,27,27,27-hexafluoro-D_3 has been shown to be 10 times more potent than $1\alpha,25(OH)_2D_3$ in calcium mobilization, with longer lasting effects due to its slower rate of catabolism and metabolic clearance [353]. This analog is also 10 times more potent than $1\alpha,25(OH)_2D_3$ in suppressing proliferation and inducing differentiation of HL-60 cells [312,354,355].

In the last decade, many other novel analogs have been chemically synthesized, which are capable of initiating biological responses in only one key target organ (e.g., intestine or bone) without affecting the many other potential target tissues (those which have the VDR; see Table 2.2). Thus, there are analogs that have been projected to be useful for renal osteodystrophy [356,357], leukemia [358,359], cardiovascular disease [360], prostate cancer [361], breast cancer [362], osteoporosis [363–365], secondary hyperparathyroidism [366], as well as in skin and immune disorders [367].

BIOLOGICAL ASSAYS FOR VITAMIN D ACTIVITY

With the exception of vitamin B_{12}, vitamin D is the most potent of the vitamins (as defined by the amount of vitamin required to elicit a biological response). Consequently, biological samples and animal tissues usually contain only very low concentrations of vitamin D. For example, the circulating plasma level of vitamin D_3 in humans is only 10–20 ng/ml or 2–5 $\times 10^{-8}$ M [368]. To be able to detect such low concentrations of vitamin D, assays that are specific for and sensitive to vitamin D and its biologically active metabolites are required.

RAT LINE TEST

From 1922 to 1958, the only official assay for the determination of the vitamin D content of pharmaceutical products or food was the rat line test. The term "official" indicates that the reproducibility and accuracy of the assay are high enough for the results of the test to be accepted legally. This assay, which is capable of detecting 1–12 IU (25–300 ng) of vitamin D, is still used by some agencies to authenticate the vitamin D content of many foods, particularly milk [369,370]. The rat line test for vitamin D employs recently weaned rachitic rats that are fed a rachitogenic diet for 19–25 days until severe rickets develops. The rats are then fed diets supplemented with either a graded series of known amounts of vitamin D_3 as standards or the unknown test sample. After 7 days on their respective diets, the animals are sacrificed and their radii and ulnae dissected out and stained with a silver nitrate solution. Silver is deposited in areas of bone where new calcium has been recently deposited. The regions turn dark when exposed to light; see Figure 2.10. Thus, the effects of the unknown sample on calcium deposition in the bone can be determined by visual comparison with the standards.

ASSOCIATION OF OFFICIAL ANALYTICAL CHEMISTS CHICK ASSAY

Since the rat line test is done in rats, it is unable to discriminate between vitamin D_2 and vitamin D_3. In the chick, vitamin D_3 is 10 times more potent than vitamin D_2, so it is important to accurately determine the amount of vitamin D_3 in poultry feeds. The AOAC (Association of Official Analytical Chemists) chick test was developed to specifically measure vitamin D_3 [371].

Groups of 20 newly hatched chicks are placed on D-deficient diets containing added levels of vitamin D_3 (1–10 IU) or the test substance. After 3 weeks on the diet, the birds are

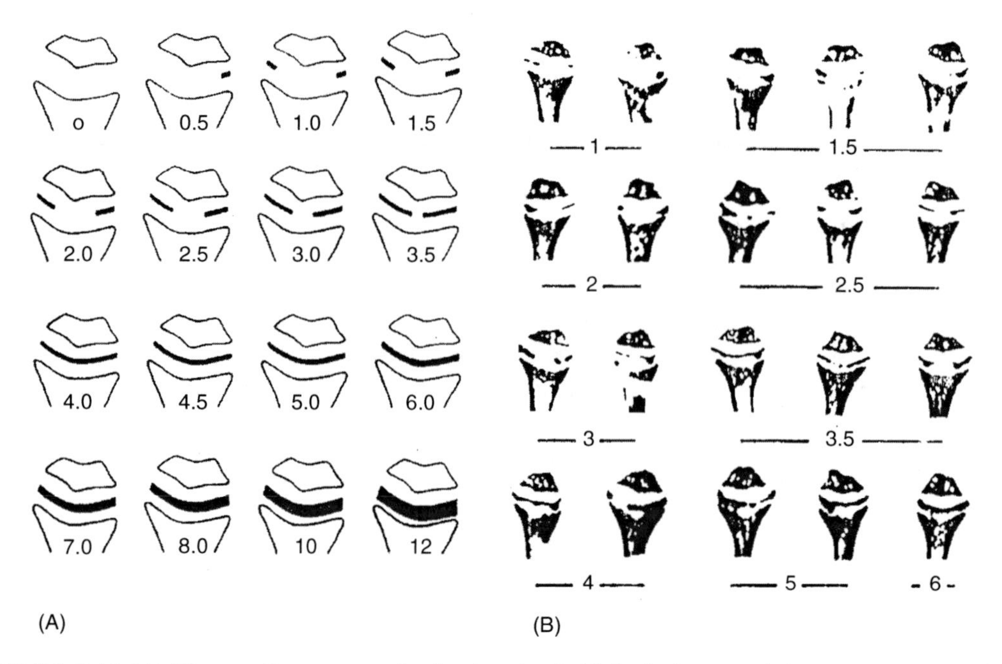

FIGURE 2.10 (A) The rat line test; a classic vitamin D biological assay. (B) Photographs of radii sections scored according to the line test chart.

sacrificed and the percentage of bone ash of their tibia is determined. A rachitic bird typically has 25%–27% bone ash whereas a vitamin D-supplemented bird has 40%–45% bone ash. This assay is not used frequently since it is time-consuming and somewhat expensive.

Intestinal Calcium Absorption

Biological assays have been developed that make use of the ability of vitamin D to stimulate the absorption of calcium across the small intestine. Two basic types of assays, in vivo [372] and in vitro [41,373], measure this process. Each assay is capable of detecting physiological quantities, that is, 2–50 IU (50–1250 ng: 0.13–3.2 nmol) of vitamin D.

In Vivo Technique

The in vivo technique for measuring ICA uses rachitic chicks that have been raised on a low-calcium (0.6%), rachitogenic diet for 3 weeks. The birds are then given one dose of the test compound orally, intraperitoneally, or intracardially. The chicks are anesthetized 12–48 h later, and 4.0 mg of $^{40}Ca^{2+}$ and approximately 6×10^6 dpm $^{45}Ca^{2+}$ are placed in the duodenal loop. The chicks are killed by decapitation 30 min later, and serum is collected. Aliquots of serum are measured for $^{45}Ca^{2+}$ in a liquid scintillation counter [372].

In Vitro Technique

The general design of this technique is the same as the in vivo technique since vitamin D activity is measured in terms of ICT. In these assays, a vitamin D standard or test compound is given orally or intraperitoneally 24–48 h before the assay. At the time of the assay, the animals are killed and a 10 cm length of duodenum is removed and turned inside out. A gut sac is formed by tying off the ends of the segment so that the mucosal surface is on the outside and the serosal surface on the inside. The everted intestinal loop is incubated with solutions of $^{45}Ca^{2+}$. The mucosal surface of the intestine actively transports the calcium through the tissue to the serosal side. The ratio of calcium concentration on the serosal versus the mucosal side of the intestine is a measure of the active transport of calcium [41,374,375]. In a vitamin D-deficient animal this ratio is 1–2.5, and in a vitamin D-dosed animal this ratio can be as high as 6–7. The chick in vivo assay is usually preferred because of the tedious nature of preparing the everted gut sacs. The in vitro technique is used primarily for studies with mammals rather than birds.

Bone Calcium Mobilization

Another assay for vitamin D activity often performed simultaneously with the chick in vivo ICA assay is the measurement of the vitamin D-mediated elevation of serum calcium levels. If 3 week old rachitic chicks are raised on a zero-calcium diet for at least 3 days before the assay and then are given a compound with vitamin D activity, their serum calcium levels will rise in a highly characteristic manner, proportional to the amount of steroid given [372]. Since there is no dietary calcium available, the only calcium source for elevation of serum calcium is bone. By carrying out this assay simultaneously with the ICA assay, it is possible to measure two different aspects of the animal's response to vitamin D simultaneously.

Growth Rate

The administration of vitamin D to animals raised on a vitamin D-deficient diet leads to an enhanced rate of whole body growth. An assay for vitamin D was developed in the chick using the growth-promoting properties of the steroid [48,376]. Chicks that are 1 day old are placed on a rachitogenic diet and given standard doses of vitamin D_3 or the test compound three times weekly. The birds are weighed periodically, and their weight is plotted versus age. In the absence of vitamin D, the rate of growth essentially plateaus by the fourth week, whereas 5–10 IU of vitamin D_3/day is sufficient to maintain a maximal growth rate in the chick. The disadvantage of this assay is the 3–4 week time period needed to accurately determine the growth rate.

Radioimmunoassay for Calbindin-D_{28K}

Additional biological assays use the presence of calbindin-D_{28K} protein as an indication of vitamin D activity. Calbindin-D_{28K} is not present in the intestine of vitamin D-deficient chicks and is only synthesized in response to the administration of vitamin D. Therefore, it is possible to use the presence of calbindin-D_{28K} to determine vitamin D activity. A radioimmunoassay (RIA) [377] and an enzyme-linked immunosorbent assay (ELISA) [378], both capable of detecting nanogram quantities of calbindin-D_{28K}, have been developed. A comparison of the sensitivity and working range of the biological assays for vitamin D are given in Table 2.6.

ANALYTICAL PROCEDURES FOR VITAMIN D-RELATED COMPOUNDS

Although considerable progress has been made in the development of chemical or physical means to measure vitamin D, these methods at present generally lack the sensitivity and selectivity of biological assays. Thus, they are not adequate for measuring samples that contain very low concentrations of vitamin D. However, these physical and chemical means of vitamin D determination have the advantage of not being as time-consuming as biological assays and so are frequently used on samples known to contain moderate levels of vitamin D.

TABLE 2.6
Comparison of Sensitivity and Working Range of Biological Assays for Vitamin D

Assay	Time Required for Assay	Minimal Level Detectable in Assay		Usual Working Range
		ng	nmol	
Rat line test	7 days	12	0.03	25–300 ng
AOAC chick	21 days	50	0.113	50–1250 ng
Intestinal Ca^{2+} absorption				
In vivo				
$^{45}Ca^{2+}$	1 day	125	0.33	0.125–25 g
$^{47}Ca^{2+}$	1 day	125	0.33	0.125–25 g
In vitro				
Everted sacs	1 day	250	0.65	250–1000 ng
Duodenal uptake of $^{45}Ca^{2+}$	1 day	250	0.65	250–1000 ng
Bone Ca^{2+} mobilization				
In vivo	24 h	125	0.32	0.125–25 g
Body growth	21–28 days	50	0.06	50–1250 ng
Immunoassays for calcium-binding protein	1 day	1	0.0025	1 ng

Source: From Bouillon R., Okamura W.H., and Norman A.W., *Endocr. Rev.*, 16, 200, 1995.

Ultraviolet Absorption

The first technique available for quantitation of vitamin D was based on the measurement of the UV absorption at 264 nm. The conjugated triene system of the vitamin D secosteroids produces a highly characteristic absorption spectrum (Figure 2.11). The absorption maximum for vitamin D occurs at 264 nm, and at this wavelength the molar extinction coefficient for both vitamins D_2 and D_3 is 18,300. Thus, the concentration of an unknown solution of vitamin D can be calculated once its absorption at 264 nm is known. Although this technique is both quick and straightforward, it suffers from the disadvantage that the sample must be scrupulously purified before assay to remove potential UV-absorbing contaminants.

Colorimetric Methods

Several colorimetric methods for the quantitation of vitamin D have been developed over the years. Among these is a method based on the isomerization of vitamin D to isotachysterol. This procedure, which employs antimony trichloride, can detect vitamin D in the range of 1–1000 μg. Because of its relative insensitivity, this assay is now used primarily to determine the vitamin D content of pharmaceutical preparations and has become the official United States Pharmacopeia (USP) colorimetric assay for vitamin D_3 [379].

Liquid Chromatography–Mass Spectrometry

One of the most powerful modern techniques available to steroid chemists for the analytical determination of samples containing mixtures of steroids is mass spectrometry [380] or mass spectrometry coupled with prior separation by LC [381,382]. The liquid chromatography–mass spectrometry (LC–MS) technique can be coupled to an online

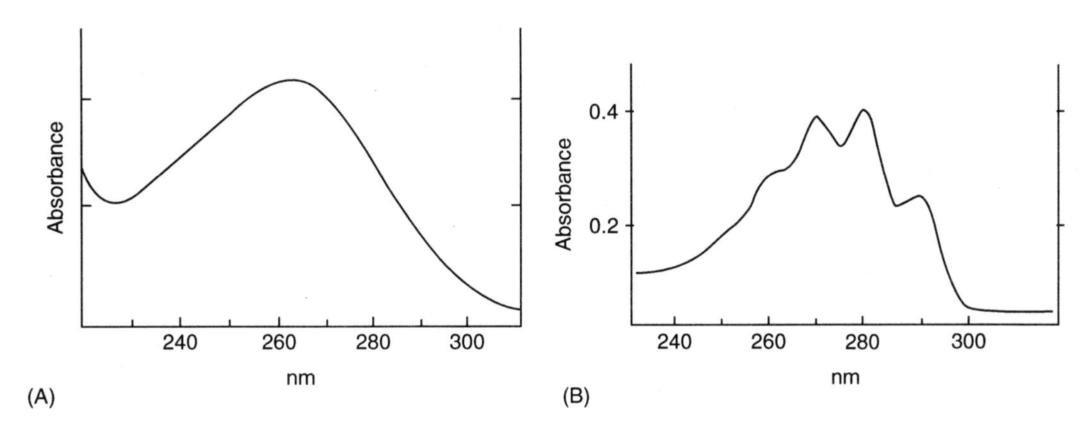

FIGURE 2.11 Ultraviolet (UV) spectrum of provitamin D and vitamin D. (A) Illustration of the characteristic UV absorption spectrum of provitamin D. The wavelengths of 7-dehydrocholesterol's several absorption maxima are 262, 271, 282, and 293 nm. The molar extinction coefficient at 282 nm is 11,500. (B) The characteristic UV spectrum of vitamin D. The molar extinction coefficient at the 264–265 nm absorption maxima is 18,300.

computer that collects information on the fragmentation patterns of steroids in the mass spectrometer. In this way, a sophisticated quantitative assay can be developed with a sensitivity and selectivity equaling that of RIAs. Thus, Higashi et al. [383] used LC–MS to characterize urinary metabolites of vitamin D_3 in man under physiological conditions.

Vogeser et al. [384] provided the first report of a candidate reference method for possible clinical assay of 25(OH)D_3 that employed LC–MS methodology. LC–MS methodology has also been employed to detect circulating concentrations of 22-oxacalcitriol, a drug candidate [381]. It is anticipated that the near future will bring many additional applications of LC–MS for the determination of vitamin D and its metabolites.

High-Performance Liquid Chromatography

The technique of high-performance liquid chromatography (HPLC) has become the separation procedure of choice for separating structurally related small organic molecules in many fields, including vitamin D metabolism and analytical determination of individual vitamin D metabolites. The HPLC separation process has an exceedingly high resolving capability because of the large number of theoretical plates present in a typical column. Of equal importance to this technique is the sensitivity of the detector used for observing the separated compounds. All the published procedures for the separation of vitamin D by HPLC have used an UV detector, and so their sensitivity is limited to approximately 5 ng. The chief advantages of using the HPLC are the reduced labor and time required to separate vitamin D and its metabolites.

A landmark paper in the vitamin D assay field that depended on the utilization of HPLC described the development of analytical assays for 25(OH)D_3, 1α,25$(OH)_2D_3$, 24R,25$(OH)_2D_3$, and 25,26$(OH)_2D_3$, as well as several metabolites of vitamin D_2 in small plasma samples. This was used to define the circulating concentrations of these metabolites in serum from five species of adult farm animals [385]. This assay or close variants have been widely used [386–392].

An older official USP method for the determination of vitamin D employed two prepurification steps, requiring up to 8 h, before the colorimetric analysis could be performed. However, with HPLC, reproducible separation of closely related compounds can be achieved in less than 1 h [393].

The technique of HPLC separation of vitamin D metabolites is now increasingly substituted for the classic rat line test biological assay (see earlier paragraphs) for the determination of the content of vitamin D_2 and vitamin D_3 in fortified milk samples [394,395] as well as in infant formula [396,397].

Competitive Binding Assays

Various competition assays that can specifically quantitate the levels of $25(OH)D_3$, $24,25(OH)_2D_3$, or $1\alpha,25(OH)_2D_3$ in a sample are now available. Such assays were developed as a consequence of the discovery of specific vitamin DBPs in the serum and tissues of mammals and birds; the availability of high specific activity tritiated $25(OH)D_3$ and $1\alpha,25(OH)_2D_3$; and HPLC separation procedures. The picogram sensitivity of these steroid competition assays allows them to be routinely used to measure vitamin D metabolite levels in plasma.

Two types of steroid competition assays have been developed for the detection of $1\alpha,25(OH)_2D_3$. The first employs incubation of intestinal mucosal cytosol and the nuclear chromatin fractions with standardized amounts of tritiated $1\alpha25(OH)_2D_3$ [398,399]. This technique requires a minimum of 10 ml plasma and involves a three-stage chromatographic procedure.

The second type of competition assay does not require any HPLC steps, uses calf thymus cytosol as the source of binding protein, and employs nonequilibrium assay conditions [400]. This procedure requires only 0.2–1.0 ml plasma and has a sensitivity of 0.7 pg. Similar assays using vitamin DBP have been developed for $25(OH)D_3$ and $24,25(OH)_2D_3$ [183,401,402].

Measurement of circulating 25-hydroxyvitamin D [25(OH)D] is important in the management of metabolic bone disease. Two companies have developed commercially available, Food and Drug Administration-approved, radioiodine ((125)I)-based RIA kits for the detection of $25(OH)D_3$ and $25(OH)D_2$ (DiaSorin, Stillwater, MN and IDS Ltd, Tyne and Wear, United Kingdom). These methods have been tested for general assay performance, including antibody specificity and were also compared with those of an HPLC-based direct UV detection method. Although both the within- and the between-run CVs were acceptable, both procedures quantitatively recovered $25(OH)D_3$ added to serum; only the DiaSorin kit quantitatively recovered $25(OH)D_2$ [403].

NUTRITIONAL REQUIREMENTS OF VITAMIN D

Humans

The vitamin D_3 requirement of healthy adults has never been precisely defined. Since vitamin D_3 is produced in the skin on exposure to sunlight and can be retained in vertebrate tissues, humans may not have a requirement for vitamin D when sufficient sunlight is available. However, vitamin D_3 does become an important nutritional factor in the absence of sunlight. In addition to geographical and seasonal factors, UV light from the sun may be blocked by factors such as air pollution, clothing, and sunscreens. In fact, as air pollution became prevalent during the industrial revolution, the incidence of rickets became widespread in industrial cities making it one of the first diseases attributable to air pollution. In addition to these man-made barriers to adequate sunlight exposure, there is insufficient sunlight at northerly latitudes to maintain adequate levels of vitamin D_3 in the skin. Under these conditions, vitamin D_3 becomes a true vitamin in that it must be supplied in the diet on a regular basis. The requirement for vitamin D_3 is also dependent on the concentration of calcium and phosphorus in the diet, the physiological stage of development, age, sex, degree of exposure to the sun, and the amount of pigmentation in the skin (see section Photochemical Production of Vitamin D_3).

RECOMMENDED DIETARY ALLOWANCE

The World Health Organization has defined the international unit (IU) of vitamin D_3 as "the vitamin D activity of 0.025 μg of the international standard preparation of crystalline vitamin D_3" [2]. Thus, 1.0 IU of vitamin D_3 is 0.025 μg, which is equivalent to 65.0 pmol. With the discovery of the metabolism of vitamin D_3 to other active secosteroids, particularly $1\alpha,25(OH)_2D_3$, it was recommended that 1.0 unit of $1\alpha,25(OH)_2D_3$ be set equivalent in molar terms to that of the parent vitamin D_3 [404]. Thus, 1.0 unit of $1\alpha,25(OH)_2D_3$ has been operationally defined to be equivalent to 65 pmol.

The current adequate intake allowance of vitamin D recommended in 1998 by the USA Food and Nutrition Board of the Institute of Medicine is 200 IU/day (5 μg/day) for infants, children, adult males, and females (including during pregnancy and lactation) up to age 51 [405]. For males and females ages 51–70 or more than 70, the adequate indicated level is set at 400 IU/day (10 μg/day) or 600 IU/day (15 μg/day), respectively.

It is known that a substantial proportion of the US population is exposed to suboptimal levels of sunlight; this is particularly true during winter months [87,406]. Under these conditions, vitamin D becomes a true vitamin, which indicates that it must be supplied in the diet on a regular basis. A recent work suggests that wintertime vitamin D insufficiency is common in young Canadian women and makes the observation that the levels of vitamin D in food did not prevent the deficiency [407]. This has led Vieth and others to ask the question whether the optimal requirement of vitamin D should be much higher than what is officially recommended [408]. In addition, a recent report documents the widespread deficiency of vitamin D in all regions of China, particularly in children [409].

It has been taught for the last seven decades that in humans, vitamin D_3 and vitamin D_2 (see Table 2.3 for the differences in their side-chain structures) are equally biologically efficacious. As a consequence, when vitamin D deficiency was encountered in the clinical setting (e.g., the older or sick individuals and newborn infants), the physician naturally desired to provide replacement or supplemental vitamin D; in the United States and Canada, this could be either in the form of vitamin D_3 or vitamin D_2. In Europe and Asia, the only form of vitamin D available for nutritional or clinical usage is vitamin D_3. However, with the realization that the serum $25(OH)D_3$ clinical assay provides the best assessment of vitamin D status [405], it became appropriate to determine whether vitamin D_2 was as effective in elevating serum 25(OH)D levels in humans as vitamin D_3. Earlier data suggesting that in humans vitamin D_3 is substantially more effective than vitamin D_2 [410] have been recently confirmed by Armas et al. [80], who found in a study in 20 healthy human volunteers that vitamin D_2 was less than one-third as vitamin D_3 in elevating serum 25(OH)D. Unfortunately, for patients who have a poor vitamin D status, there are currently no high-dose vitamin D_3 formulations approved by the USA FDA for clinical use; similarly there are no formulations of $25(OH)D_3$ approved in the United States.

ANIMALS

The task of assessing the minimum daily vitamin D requirement for animals is no easier than it is for humans. Factors such as the dietary calcium–phosphorus ratio, physiological stage of development, sex, the amount of fur or hair, color, and perhaps even breed affect the daily requirement of vitamin D in animals. In addition, some animals, such as chickens and turkeys, do not respond as well to vitamin D_2 as to vitamin D_3. As with humans, animals that are maintained in sunlight can normally produce their own vitamin D so that dietary supplementation is not really necessary. For animals that are kept indoors or that live in climates where the sunlight is not adequate for vitamin D production, the vitamin D content of food becomes important. Sun-cured hays are fairly good sources of vitamin D, but

TABLE 2.7
Vitamin D Requirements of Animals

Animal	Daily Requirements (IU)
Chickens, growing	90[a]
Dairy cattle	
Calves	660[b]
Pregnant, lactating	5000–6000[c]
Dogs	
Growing puppies	22[d]
Adult maintenance	11[d]
Ducks	100[d]
Monkey, growing rhesus	25[d]
Mouse, growing	167[d]
Sheep	
Lambs	300[e]
Adults	250[e]
Swine	
Breed sows	550[c]
Lactating sows	1210[c]
Young Boars	690[c]
Adult Boars	550[c]
Turkeys	400[a]

Source: Published information by the Committee of Animal Nutrition, Agricultural Board (National Research Council). Available at: http://dels.nas.edu/banr/nut_req.shtml

[a] IU required per pound of feed.
[b] IU required for 100 kg body weight.
[c] IU required per animal.
[d] IU required per kg body weight.
[e] IU required per 45 kg body weight.

dehydrated hays, green feeds, and seeds are poor sources. A brief list of the recommended daily allowances (RDAs) for animals is given in Table 2.7.

FOOD SOURCES OF VITAMIN D

In the United States, the FDA plays an active role in codifying the nutrition labeling of food [411]. The vitamin D_3 reference daily intake (RDI) values for males and females (nonpregnant) range from 200 IU at ages 1–50 years to 400 IU for ages 51–70 years and 600 IU for ages greater than 70 years. In contrast, the dietary reference intake (DRI), also known as the tolerable upper intakes or upper level (UL), is defined as the maximum level of a daily nutrient intake that is likely to pose no risk or adverse effects; for vitamin D, the DRI or UL is presently set at 2000 IU/day. The RDI and UL boundaries define the lower and upper daily intake values for vitamin D, which allow assessment of various food types to provide the desirable daily intake of vitamin D. Thus, the daily value (DV) or the amount of vitamin D to be provided per 2000 kcal each day is 400 IU.

TABLE 2.8
Selected Food Sources of Vitamin D in Unfortified Food

Food	International Units (IU) Per Serving	Percent DV[a]
Cod-liver oil, 1 tablespoon	1360	340
Salmon, cooked, 3½ ounces	360	90
Mackerel, cooked, 3½ ounces	345	90
Tuna fish, canned in oil, 3 ounces	200	50
Sardines, canned in oil, drained, 1¾ ounces	250	70
Milk, nonfat, reduced fat, and whole, vitamin D fortified, 1 cup	98	25
Margarine, fortified, 1 tablespoon	60	15
Pudding, prepared from mix and made with vitamin D fortified milk, ½ cup	50	10
Ready-to-eat cereals fortified with 10% of the DV for vitamin D, ¾ cup to 1 cup servings (servings vary according to the brand)	40	10
Egg, 1 whole (vitamin D is found in egg yolk)	20	6
Liver, beef, cooked, 3½ ounces	15	4
Cheese, Swiss, 1 ounce	12	4

Sources: From Pennington J.A.T. and Douglass J.S., in *Bowes and Church's Food Values of Portions Commonly Used*, Lippincott, Williams & Wilkins, Philadelphia, 2004, 18th Edition; US Department of Agriculture ARS., USDA Nutrient Database for Standard Reference, Release 16. http://www.nal.usda.gov/fnic/cgi-bin/nut_search.pl. 2003. Bethesda, MD, US Department of Agriculture.

Note: In addition, see the comprehensive tabulation of food values in Pennington and Douglass [486].
An assessment of human vitamin D requirements in 2005 is reviewed in Whiting and Calvo [420,488].

[a] DV, Daily value. DVs are reference numbers developed by the Food and Drug Administration (FDA) to help consumers determine if a food contains a high or a low amount of a specific nutrient. The DV for vitamin D is 400 IU (10 μg) for adults. Most food labels do not list vitamin D content unless a food has been fortified with this nutrient. The percent DV (%DV) listed on the table indicates the percent of the DV provided in one serving. A food providing 5% of the DV or less is a low source while a food that provides 10%–19% of the DV is a good source and a food that provides 20% or more of the DV is high in that nutrient. It is important to remember that foods that provide lower percentages of the DV also contribute to a healthy diet. For foods not listed in this table, please refer to the US Department of Agriculture's Nutrient Database Web site.

For the most part, vitamin D is present in unfortified foods in only very small and variable quantities (Table 2.8). The vitamin D that occurs naturally in unfortified foods is generally derived from animal products. Salt-water fish such as herring, salmon, and sardines contain substantial amounts of vitamin D, and fish-liver oils are extremely rich sources. However, eggs, veal, beef, unfortified milk, and butter supply only small quantities of the vitamin. Plants are extremely poor sources of vitamin D; fruits and nuts contain no vitamin D; and vegetable oils contain only negligible amounts of the provitamin. As a consequence, in the United States, dietary requirements for vitamin D can only be met by the fortification of suitable foods, including milk, both fresh and evaporated; margarine and butter; cereals; and chocolate mixes. Milk is usually fortified to supply 400 IU vitamin D/quart, and margarine usually contains 2000 IU or more per pound. A more complete listing of the vitamin D values of food is given by Booher et al. [412].

SIGNS OF VITAMIN D DEFICIENCY

HUMANS

A deficiency of vitamin D results in inadequate intestinal absorption and renal reabsorption of calcium and phosphate. As a consequence, serum calcium and phosphate levels fall and serum alkaline phosphatase activity increases. In response to these low serum calcium levels, hyperparathyroidism occurs [413]. Increased levels of PTH, along with whatever $1\alpha,25(OH)_2D_3$ is still present at the onset of the deficiency, result in the demineralization of bone. This ultimately leads to rickets in children and osteomalacia in adults. The classical skeletal symptoms associated with rickets, that is, bowlegs, knock-knees, curvature of the spine, and pelvic and thoracic deformities (Figure 2.12), result from the application of normal mechanical stress to demineralized bone. Enlargement of the bones, especially in the knees, wrists, and ankles, and changes in the costochondral junctions also occur. Since in children bone growth is still occurring, rickets can result in epiphyseal abnormalities not seen in adult osteomalacia. Rickets also results in inadequate mineralization of tooth enamel and dentin. If the disease occurs during the first 6 months of life, convulsions and tetany can occur. Few adults with osteomalacia develop tetany.

Low serum calcium levels in the range of 5–7 mg/100 ml and high serum alkaline phosphatase activity can be used to diagnose rickets and osteomalacia. In addition, a marked reduction in circulating $25(OH)D_3$ levels in individuals with osteomalacia or rickets has been reported [413]. As noted earlier in the section Nutritional Requirements for Vitamin D, a substantial proportion of the US population is exposed to suboptimal levels of sunlight; this is particularly true during winter months [87,406]. Under these conditions, vitamin D becomes a true vitamin, which indicates that it must be supplied in the diet on a regular basis. In the past 5 years, a substantial number of clinical reports

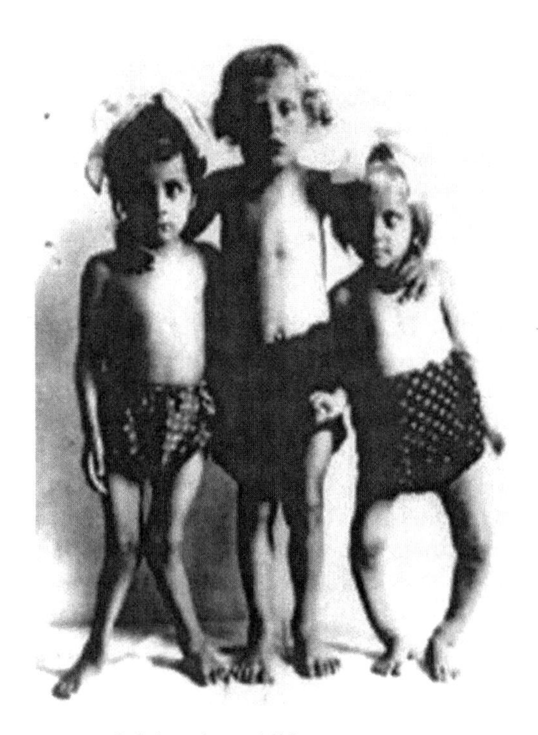

FIGURE 2.12 Classic appearance of rickets in a child.

from many countries and on many endpoints have indicated that there is likely a widespread vitamin D deficiency as defined by a serum level of $25(OH)D_3$ that is lower than 50 nmol/L (20 ng/ml). Low $25(OH)D_3$ levels in patients have been found to be associated with increased periodontal disease [414]. Secondary hyperparathyroidism linked with increased rates of hip fracture and osteoporosis in northern Europe [413] and the North American continent [415] and reduced bone mineral density (BMD) in persons with primary knee injury in association with osteoarthritis [416] and in both veiled and nonveiled Bangladeshi women [417].

Endemic hypovitaminosis D can lead to a variety of clinical problems. However, the problems of interlaboratory variation in the measurement of serum levels of $25(OH)D_3$ that has been reported also confound the diagnosis of vitamin D insufficiency or deficiency [387]. Further aggravating the validity of the $25(OH)D_3$ laboratory results is the problem of accurately determining both $25(OH)D_3$ and $25(OH)D_2$ in serum samples. In spite of these difficulties, in 2006 the view is emerging that there is a worldwide incidence of vitamin D malnutrition [408] and that current dietary recommendations of vitamin D_3 for children and adults are not sufficient to maintain circulating 25(OH)D levels at least 50 nmol/L [413,418–421].

Animals

The response to vitamin D deficiency in animals closely resembles that in humans. Among the first symptoms of the deficiency is a decline in the plasma concentration of calcium and phosphorus. This is followed by an abnormally low growth rate and the characteristic alteration of bones, including faulty calcification of the bone matrix. As the disease progresses, the forelegs bend sideways and the joints become swollen. In laying birds, egg production declines, the eggs are thin-shelled, and their hatchability is markedly reduced [121]; classic symptoms of rickets develop, followed by tetany and death. It is known that vitamin D_3 or $25(OH)D_3$ affects both the mineralization of avian bones and eggshell quality [422,423].

HYPERVITAMINOSIS D

Excessive amounts of vitamin D are not available from natural sources. However, vitamin D intoxication is a concern in those patients treated with vitamin D or vitamin D analogs for hypoparathyroidism, vitamin D-resistant rickets, renal osteodystrophy, osteoporosis, psoriasis, some cancers, or in those who are taking supplemental vitamins. Hypervitaminosis D is a serious problem as it can result in irreversible calcification of the heart, lungs, kidneys, and other soft tissues. Therefore, care should be taken to detect early signs of vitamin D intoxication in patients receiving pharmacological doses. Symptoms of intoxication include hypercalcemia, hypercalciuria, anorexia, nausea, vomiting, thirst, polyuria, muscular weakness, joint pains, diffuse demineralization of bones, and disorientation. If allowed to go unchecked, death will eventually occur.

One report of vitamin D intoxication occurred from drinking milk that had been fortified with inappropriately high (230,000 IU/quart) levels of vitamin D_3 [424]. A more recent report describes severe vitamin D intoxication of one family resulting from contamination of a household table sugar supply with extraordinary levels of vitamin D [425].

Vitamin D intoxication is thought to occur as a result of high 25(OH)D levels rather than high $1\alpha,25(OH)_2D$ levels [426,427]. Patients suffering from hypervitaminosis D have been shown to exhibit a 15-fold increase in plasma 25(OH)D concentration as compared with normal individuals. However, their $1\alpha,25(OH)_2D$ levels are not substantially altered [428]. Furthermore, anephric patients can still suffer from hypervitaminosis D even though they are, for the most part, incapable of producing circulating $1\alpha,25(OH)_2D_3$. It has also been shown that large concentrations of 25(OH)D can mimic the actions of 1α,25$(OH)_2$D at the level of the receptor [398,426,429,430]. Locally produced extrarenal 1α,25$(OH)_2D_3$ may also contribute to the symptoms of hypervitaminosis D.

The early effects of intoxication are usually reversible. Treatment consists of merely withdrawing vitamin D and perhaps reducing dietary calcium intake until serum calcium levels fall. In more severe cases, treatment with GRs, which are thought to antagonize some of the actions of vitamin D, may be required to facilitate the correction of hypercalcemia. Since calcitonin can bring about a decline in serum calcium levels, it may also be used in treatment.

FACTORS THAT INFLUENCE VITAMIN D STATUS

Disease

In view of the complexities of the vitamin D endocrine system, it is not surprising that many disease states are vitamin D-related. Figure 2.13 classifies some of the human disease states that are believed to be associated with vitamin D metabolism, according to the metabolic step in which the disorder occurs.

Intestinal Disorders

The intestine functions as the site of dietary vitamin D absorption and is also a primary target tissue for the hormonally active 1α,25$(OH)_2D_3$. Impairment of intestinal absorption of vitamin D can occur in intestinal disorders that result in the malabsorption of fat. Patients suffering from such disorders as tropical sprue, regional enteritis, and multiple jejunal diverticulosis often develop osteomalacia because of what appears to be a malabsorption of vitamin D from the diet [431]. Surgical conditions, such as gastric resection and jejunal–ileal bypass surgery for obesity, may also impair vitamin D absorption. In addition, patients receiving total parenteral nutrition in the treatment of the malnutrition caused by profound gastrointestinal disease often develop bone disease [432].

The intestinal response to vitamin D can be affected by certain disease states. Patients suffering from idiopathic hypercalciuria exhibit an increased intestinal absorption of calcium that may result from an enhanced intestinal sensitivity to 1α,25$(OH)_2D_3$ or from an overproduction of 1α,25$(OH)_2D_3$. Sarcoidosis is characterized by hypercalcemia and hypercalciuria in patients receiving only modest amounts of vitamin D. The enhanced sensitivity to the parent vitamin D is because of elevated levels of serum 1α,25$(OH)_2D_3$. The excess 1α,25$(OH)_2D_3$ is likely of extrarenal origin and therefore not regulated by circulating levels of PTH [433]. Other experiments have clearly shown that macrophages from patients with sarcoidosis can produce 1α,25$(OH)_2D_3$ [137,434].

Other disease states that can result in extrarenal production of 1α,25$(OH)_2D_3$ are tuberculosis [435,436], leprosy [437], and some lymphomas [438]. In one study of polymorphisms related to susceptibility to leprosy in more than 200 individuals from northern Malawi, it was found that individuals homozygous for a silent T→C change in codon 352 of the VDR gene appeared to be at high risk for this disease [439].

Liver Disorders

The liver plays an important role in the vitamin D endocrine system; not only it is the primary site for the production of 25(OH)D and the synthesis of plasma DBP, but it is also the source of the bile salts that aid in the intestinal absorption of vitamin D. Hence, malfunctions of the liver can interfere with the absorption, transport, and metabolism of vitamin D. Malabsorption of calcium and the appearance of bone disease have been reported in patients suffering

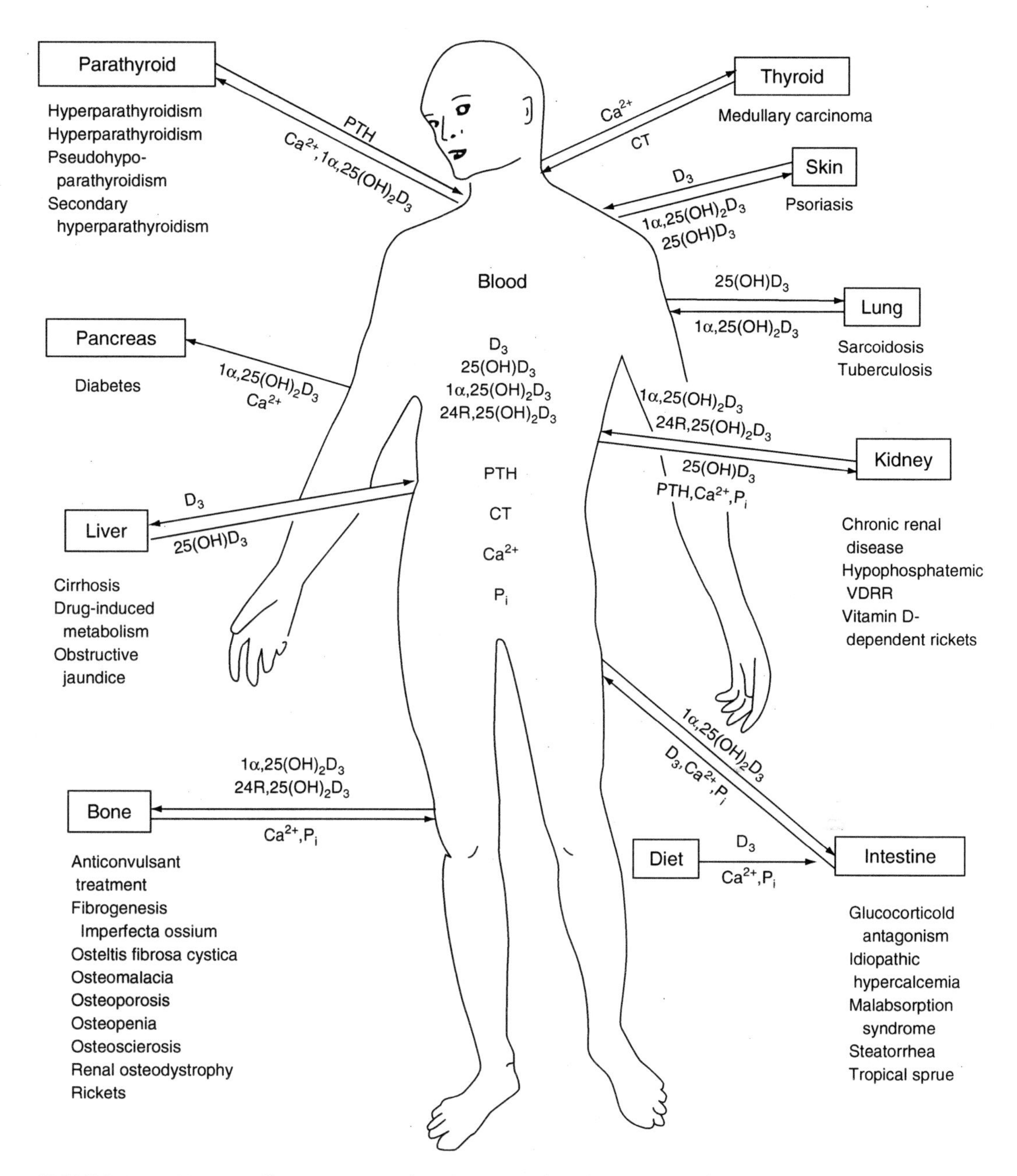

FIGURE 2.13 Human disease states related to the vitamin D endocrine system. Under the boxed headings (e.g., parathyroid, liver bone, etc.) are listed disease states occurring in man that have been shown or are believed to have some functional linkage between some aspect of the vitamin D endocrine system and that particular organ. The information associated with the arrows indicate the direction of flow of calcium phosphate, or the calcium-regulating hormone vitamin D_3, $25(OH)D_3$, $1\alpha,25(OH)_2D_3$, $24R,25(OH)_2D_3$, parathyroid hormone, and calcitonin (CT). A presentation on each of these disease states is given in Feldman, D., Pike, J.W., and Glorieux, F.H., eds., *Vitamin D*, Elsevier, San Diego, p. 1892, 2005. VDRR, vitamin D-resistant rickets; Pi, inorganic phosphate; Ca^{2+}, calcium.

from either primary biliary cirrhosis or from the prolonged obstructive jaundice. The disappearance of radioactive vitamin D from the plasma of these patients is much slower than that in normal subjects [440], and their plasma 25(OH)D levels are reduced [441]. Although these patients respond poorly to vitamin D treatment, they immediately respond if treated with 25(OH)D_3. Thus, it appears that the bone disease experienced by these patients results from their inability to produce 25(OH)D.

Renal Disorders

Since the kidney functions as the endocrine gland for 1α,25$(OH)_2D_3$, disease states that affect the kidney can alter the production of this calcium homeostatic hormone. It is well known that patients with renal failure often also suffer from skeletal abnormalities, termed renal osteodystrophy, a spectrum of disorders including growth retardation, osteitis fibrosa, osteomalacia, and osteosclerosis. Support for the idea that renal osteodystrophy is a result of the failure of the kidney to make 1α,25$(OH)_2D_3$ came from studies on the metabolism of radioactively labeled vitamin D in normal persons versus patients with chronic renal failure. In normal subjects, the circulating level of 1α,25$(OH)_2D_3$ is in the range of 30–35 pg/ml, whereas in chronic renal failure the levels have been reported as low as 3–6 pg/ml [442,443]. A successful renal transplant results in the return of 1α,25$(OH)_2D_3$ levels to the normal range. In addition, the administration of 1α,25$(OH)_2D_3$ to these patients results in the stimulation of ICA and an elevation of serum calcium levels [444,445].

Parathyroid Disorders

Since PTH stimulates the production of 1α,25$(OH)_2D_3$ in the kidney, any disease state that affects the secretion of PTH may, in turn, have an effect on the metabolism of vitamin D. Hyperactivity of the parathyroid glands, as in primary hyperparathyroidism, results in the appearance of bone disease resembling osteomalacia. Circulating 1α,25$(OH)_2D_3$ levels in these subjects have been reported to be significantly elevated [446], as is their ICT [447,448]. On the other hand, in hypoparathyroidism, hypocalcemia occurs. In these patients a slight reduction in circulating 1α,25$(OH)_2D_3$ levels has been reported [449]. When these patients are treated with 1α,25$(OH)_2D_3$, their serum levels of PTH and calcium return to normal. There are several review articles on the role of vitamin D in disease [1,3,265,450,451].

Genetics

Vitamin D-resistant rickets (hypophosphatemic rickets) appears to be an X-linked, dominant genetic disorder. Winters et al. [452] presented evidence that this disease is almost always inherited and is usually congenital. Males are usually more severely affected by this disease than females. Associated with the disease are skeletal abnormalities, such as rickets or osteomalacia, and a diminished renal tubular reabsorption of phosphate that results in hypophosphatemia. Individuals with this disease do not respond to physiological doses of vitamin D; treatment with 25(OH)D_3 and 1α,25$(OH)_2D_3$ is also ineffective, although an increase in ICA does occur [453]. Since these patients have been reported to have normal serum 1α,25$(OH)_2D_3$ levels, it appears that this disorder does not result from an alteration in the metabolism of vitamin D or from an impaired intestinal response to 1α,25$(OH)_2D_3$ but rather is a defect in phosphate reabsorption by the kidney, which is linked to the presence of an unknown humoral factor [454]. Very recent evidence suggests that this humoral factor is FGF23 secreted by osteoblasts. FGF23 lowers renal 25(OH)D_3-1α-hydroxylase activity and thereby lowers the circulating levels of 1α,25$(OH)_2D_3$ [145,455]. Thus, the physiologic role of FGF23 may be to act as a counterregulatory phosphaturic hormone to maintain phosphate homeostasis in response to vitamin D.

A genetic defect that interferes with vitamin D metabolism has also been suggested in vitamin D-dependent rickets type I. This ailment differs from rickets in that it appears in children who are receiving adequate amounts of vitamin D and it requires pharmacological doses of vitamin D or $25(OH)D_3$ to reverse the harmful effect this disease has on bone. However, the disease is responsive to physiological amounts of $1\alpha,25(OH)_2D_3$, suggesting that the defect occurs in the metabolism of $25(OH)D_3$ to $1\alpha,25(OH)_2D_3$. This disease state appears to be the result of an autosomal recessively inherited genetic defect [456]. It is not known how this defect affects the metabolism of $25(OH)D_3$ [457].

Vitamin D-dependent rickets type II also has a genetic basis [458]. This ailment is similar to type-I vitamin D-dependent rickets, except that children do not respond to large doses of vitamin D, $25(OH)D_3$ or $1\alpha,25(OH)_2D_3$. The combination of symptoms, that is, defective bone mineralization, decreased ICA, hypocalcemia, and increased serum levels of $1\alpha,25(OH)_2D_3$, suggests end-organ resistance to the action of $1\alpha,25(OH)_2D_3$, and in fact genetic analysis has shown that these children have single-point mutations in the nuclear receptor for $1\alpha,25(OH)_2D_3$ [459–462].

Drugs

Recent evidence suggests that the prolonged use of anticonvulsant drugs, such as diphenylhydantoin or phenobarbital, can result in an impaired response to vitamin D; this results in an alteration of calcium metabolism and the appearance of rickets or osteomalacia. Serum $25(OH)D_3$ levels in patients receiving these drugs have been reported to be markedly reduced [463], perhaps the result of drug-stimulated hepatic microsomal cytochrome P450 enzyme activity, which could lead to an increased catabolism of $25(OH)D_3$ [464]. On the other hand, circulating $1\alpha,25(OH)_2D_3$ levels are normal or even increased after drug treatment [465], suggesting that anticonvulsant osteomalacia may not be due to an effect of the drug on vitamin D metabolism. Studies on rat and chick duodena in organ culture indicate that anticonvulsant drugs directly affect the absorption of calcium by the gastrointestinal tract [466]. Anticonvulsant drugs have also been shown to inhibit calcium reabsorption in organ-culture mouse calvaria [467]. Further research is needed to determine the mechanism by which these anticonvulsant drugs affect calcium metabolism.

Alcohol

Persons suffering from chronic alcoholism exhibit a decrease in plasma $25(OH)D_3$ levels, ICA, and bone mineral content. This is observed in patients with and without cirrhosis of the liver. Current evidence indicates that the impairment of ICA is the result of low $25(OH)D_3$ levels [468,469]. However, how chronic alcoholism results in low $25(OH)D_3$ levels is at present not understood.

Age

The fact that changes in the metabolism of vitamin D may occur with aging has been suggested by the observation that the ability to absorb dietary calcium decreases with age [470]. In addition, loss of bone increases in the elderly along with age-related hypoplasia of bone cells. Further, $1\alpha,25(OH)_2D_3$ levels in the plasma and responsivity of the renal $25(OH)D_3$-1α-hydroxylase to PTH are both known to decrease with age [471].

Sex Differences

Gray et al. [472] demonstrated that men and women differ in their metabolism of vitamin D in response to various physiological stimuli. They observed that in women, but not in men,

TABLE 2.9
Drug Forms of Vitamin D Metabolites

Compound Name	Generic Name	Commercial Name	Pharmaceutical Company	Effective Daily Dose (μg)[a]	Approved Use
$1\alpha,25(OH)_2D_3$	Calcitriol	Rocaltrol	*X. HoffmannLa Roche*	0.5–1.0	RO, HP, O[b]
$1\alpha,25(OH)_2D_3$	Calcitriol	Calcijex	Abbott	0.5 (i.v.)	HC
$1\alpha,25(OH)_2$-19-*nor*-D_2	Paricalcitol	Zemplar	Abbott	2.8–7 (eod)	SHP
$1\alpha,24(OH)_2D_3$	Tacalcitol	Bonalfa	Teijin Ltd., Japan	40–80 (topical)	PP
$1\alpha,24S(OH)_2$-22-ene-24-cyclopropyl-D_3	Calcipotriene	Dovenex	Leo, Denmark	40–80 (topical)	PP
$1\alpha,24S(OH)_2$-22-ene-24-cyclopropyl-D_3	Calcipotriene	Dovenex	Westwood-Squibb	40–80 (topical)	PP
1α-OH-D_3	Alfacalcidol	One-Alfa	Leo, Denmark	1–2	RO, HP, O, VDRR
1α-OH-D_3	Alfacalcidol	Alpha-D_3	Teva, Israel	0.25–1.0	RO, O, HC, HP
1α-OH-D_3	Alfacalcidol	OneAlfa	Teijin Ltd., Japan	0.25–1.0	RO, O
1α-OH-D_3	Alfacalcidol	OneAlfa	Chugai, Japan	0.25–1.0	RO, O
1α-OH-D_2	Doxercalciferol	Hectorol	Bone Care	10 (4×/week, 15–30 μg/week)	SHP
$25(OH)D_3$	Calcifediol	Calderol	Organon,United States	50–500	RO
$25(OH)D_3$	Calcifediol	Dedrogyl	Roussel-UCLAF, France	50–500	RO
10,19-dihydrotachysterol$_3$	Dihydrotachysterol$_3$	XI. Hytakerol	Winthrop	200–1000	RO
$1\alpha,25(OH)_2$-22-oxa-D_3	Maxacalcitol	Oxarol	Chugai, Japan	5–10 (3×/week i.v.)	SHP
$1\alpha,25(OH)_2$-26,27-F_6-D_3	Falecalcitriol	Fulstan Tablets	Sumitomo Pharmaceuticals, Japan	0.15–0.35	HC, SHP, RO, O
$1\alpha,25(OH)_2$-26,27-F_6-D_3	Falecalcitriol	Hornel Tablets	Taisho Pharmaceuticals, Japan	0.15–0.35	HC, SHP, RO, O

Note: The key to the approved uses of the vitamin D analogs is as follows: RO, renal osteodystrophy, O, postmenopausal osteoporosis; PP, plaque psoriasis; HC, hypocalcemia (frequently present in patients with renal osteodystrophy who are subjected to hemodialysis); HP, hypoparathyroidism and associated hypocalcemia which may frequently be encountered in patients with hypoparathyroidism, pseudohypoparathyroidism or in circumstances of postsurgical hypoparathyroidism; SHP, secondary hyperparathyroidism associated with renal osteodystrophy; VDRR, vitamin D-resistant rickets.

[a] Oral dose unless otherwise indicated; eod, every other day.

[b] The use of Rocaltrol for postmenopausal osteoporosis is approved in Argentina, Australia, Austria, Czech Republic, Columbia, India, Ireland, Italy, Japan, Malaysia, Mexico, New Zealand, Peru, Philippines, South Korea, South Africa, Switzerland, Turkey, and the United Kingdom.

dietary phosphate deprivation resulted in decreased serum phosphorus levels with a concomitant increase in plasma $1\alpha,25(OH)_2D_3$ concentrations. The mechanism by which men and women respond to dietary phosphate deprivation seems to differ but the details of this difference are unknown.

EFFICACY OF PHARMACOLOGICAL DOSES

Several ailments are known to respond to massive doses of vitamin D. For example, the intestinal malabsorption of calcium that results from chronic renal failure and the subsequent development of rickets or osteomalacia can be overcome by administration of 100,000–300,000 IU vitamin D/day [471]. Patients suffering from hypoparathyroidism can usually be treated by giving 80,000–100,000 IU vitamin D/day [473]. Children afflicted with vitamin D-dependent rickets type I can be treated with 10,000–100,000 IU/day [2]. The therapeutic effect of such massive doses can be explained by the fact that 25(OH)D in sufficiently high concentrations will mimic the action of $1\alpha,25(OH)_2D_3$ at the receptor. However, as mentioned earlier, the administration of such pharmacological doses of vitamin D to patients over a prolonged period of time carries with it the danger of vitamin D toxicity.

Table 2.9 lists the drug forms of $1\alpha,25(OH)_2D_3$ that are currently available for treatment of several disease states including hypoparathyroidism, vitamin D-resistant rickets, renal osteodystrophy (calcitriol [474,475] and paricalcitol [476]), osteoporosis (calcitriol [477,478]), and psoriasis (calcipotriene [479]). The potential for vitamin D intoxication, that is, hypercalcemia and soft tissue calcification, is much higher when an individual has access to drug formulations of $1\alpha,25(OH)_2D_3$, since these medications bypass the stringent physiological control point of the vitamin D endocrine system, namely the $25(OH)D_3$-1-hydroxylase of the kidney.

CONCLUSIONS

Current evidence supports the concept that the classical biological actions of the nutritionally important fat-soluble vitamin D in mediating calcium homeostasis are part of a complex vitamin D endocrine system that coordinates the metabolism of vitamin D_3 into $1\alpha,25(OH)_2D_3$ and $24R,25(OH)_2D_3$. Further, it is clear that the vitamin D endocrine system embraces many more target tissues than simply the intestine, bone, and kidney. Notable additions to this list include the pancreas, pituitary, breast tissue, placenta, hematopoietic cells, hair follicle, skin, and cancer cells of various origins (see Table 2.2 and Figure 2.4). Key advances in understanding the mode of action of the steroid hormone, $1\alpha,25(OH)_2D_3$, have been made by a thorough study of the VDR as a classical nuclear receptor as well as the emerging studies describing the presence of VDR in the plasma membrane caveolae. Efforts are underway to define the signal transduction systems that are activated by the nuclear and membrane receptors for $1\alpha,25(OH)_2D_3$ and to obtain a thorough study of the tissue distribution and subcellular localization of the gene products induced by this steroid hormone. There are clinical applications for $1\alpha,25(OH)_2D_3$ and related analogs for treatment of the bone diseases of renal osteodystrophy and osteoporosis, psoriasis, and secondary hyperparathyroidism. Other clinical targets for $1\alpha,25(OH)_2D_3$ currently under investigation include its use in leukemia, breast, prostate, and colon cancer as well as use as an immunosuppressive agent. An emerging human nutritional issue is the question of whether the RDA for vitamin D_3 should be adjusted upward.

REFERENCES

1. Norman A.W. and Henry H.L., *Vitamin D*, Elsevier Academic Press, San Diego, 2005. 2nd Edition.
2. Norman A.W., *Vitamin D: The Calcium Homeostatic Steroid Hormone*, 1st Academic Press, NY, 1979, 1st Edition.
3. Heaney R.P., The vitamin D requirement in health and disease. *J. Steroid Biochem. Mol. Biol.*, 97, 13, 2005.
4. Bouillon R., Okamura W.H., and Norman A.W., Structure–function relationships in the vitamin D endocrine system. *Endocr. Rev.*, 16, 200, 1995.
5. Prie D., Beck L., Urena P., and Friedlander G., Recent findings in phosphate homeostasis. *Curr. Opin. Nephrol. Hypertens.*, 14, 318, 2005.
6. Radanovic T., Wagner C.A., Murer H., and Biber J., Regulation of intestinal phosphate transport. I. Segmental expression and adaptation to low-P(i) diet of the type IIb Na(+)-P(i) cotransporter in mouse small intestine. *Am. J. Physiol. Gastrointest. Liver Physiol.*, 288, G496–G500, 2005.
7. Marks J., Srai S.K., Biber J., Murer H., Unwin R.J., and Debnam E.S., Intestinal phosphate absorption and the effect of vitamin D: A comparison of rat with mouse. *Exp. Physiol.*, 3, 531–537, 2006.
8. Calvo M.S., Whiting S.J., and Barton C.N., Vitamin D intake: A global perspective of current status. *J. Nutr.*, 135, 310, 2005.
9. Norman A.W., 1α,25(OH)$_2$-vitamin D$_3$ mediated rapid and genomic responses are dependent upon critical structure–function relationships for both the ligand and receptor(s). In: *Vitamin D*, Eds. Feldman D., Pike J.W., and Glorieux F.H., p. 381. Elsevier Academic Press, San Diego, 2005.
10. Pike J.W. and Shevde N.K., The vitamin D receptor. In: *Vitamin D*, Eds. Feldman D., Pike J.W., and Glorieux F.H., p. 167. Elsevier Academic Press, San Diego, 2005.
11. Whitfield G.K., Jurutka P.W., Haussler C.A., Hsieh J.-C., Barthel T.K., Jacobs E.T., Encinas C., Thatcher M.L., and Haussler M.R., Nuclear vitamin D receptor: Structure–function, molecular control of gene transcription and novel bioactions. In: *Vitamin D*, Eds. Feldman D., Pike J.W., and Glorieux F.H., p. 219. Elsevier Academic Press, San Diego, 2005.
12. Laing C.J. and Cooke N.E., Vitamin D binding protein. In: *Vitamin D*, Eds. Feldman D., Glorieux F.H., and Pike J.W., p. 117. Elsevier Academic Press, San Diego, 2005.
13. Bikle D.D., Vitamin D and skin cancer. *J. Nutr.*, 134, 3472S, 2004.
14. Dietrich T., Joshipura K.J., Dawson-Hughes B., and Bischoff-Ferrari H.A., Association between serum concentrations of 25-hydroxyvitamin D$_3$ and periodontal disease in the US population. *Am. J. Clin. Nutr.*, 80, 108, 2004.
15. Goltzman D., Miao D., Panda D.K., and Hendy G.N., Effects of calcium and of the vitamin D system on skeletal and calcium homeostasis: Lessons from genetic models. *J. Steroid Biochem. Mol. Biol.*, 89–90, 485, 2004.
16. Kato S., Fujiki R., and Kitagawa H., Vitamin D receptor (VDR) promoter targeting through a novel chromatin remodeling complex. *J. Steroid Biochem. Mol. Biol.*, 89–90, 173, 2004.
17. Christakos S., Dhawan P., Liu Y., Peng X., and Porta A., New insights into the mechanisms of vitamin D action. *J. Cell. Biochem.*, 88, 695, 2003.
18. Mizwicki M.T. and Norman A.W., Two key proteins of the vitamin D endocrine system come into crystal clear focus: Comparison of the X-ray structures of the nuclear receptor for 1α,25(OH)$_2$-vitamin D$_3$, the plasma vitamin D binding protein, and their ligands. *J. Bone Miner. Res.*, 18, 795, 2003.
19. Adorini L., Immunomodulatory effects of vitamin D receptor ligands in autoimmune diseases. *Int. Immunopharmacol.*, 2, 1017, 2002.
20. Mathieu C. and Adorini L., The coming of age of 1,25-dihydroxyvitamin D$_3$ analogs as immunomodulatory agents. *Trends Mol. Med.*, 8, 174, 2002.
21. Omdahl J.L., Morris H.A., and May B.K., Hydroxylase enzymes of the vitamin D pathway: Expression, function, and regulation. *Annu. Rev. Nutr.*, 22, 139, 2002.
22. DeLuca H.F. and Cantorna M.T., Vitamin D: Its role and uses in immunology. *FASEB J.*, 15, 2579, 2001.
23. Soleki R.S., *Shanidar: The Humanity of Neanderthal Man*, Knopf, NY, 1971.
24. Whistler D., Morbo puerli Anglorum, quem patrio idiomate indigenae voacant or "Inaugural medical disputation on the disease of English children which is popularly termed the rickets." 1. 1645. University of Leiden, The Netherlands.

25. Glisson F., A treatise of the rickets being a disease common to children. 1. 1660. Cambridge University, England.
26. Hess A.F., *Rickets Including Osteomalacia and Tetany*, Lea & Febiger, Philadelphia, 1929.
27. Huldschinsky K., Heilung von rachitis durch kuenstliche hohensonne. *Dtsch. Med. Wschr.*, 45, 712, 1919.
28. Mellanby E. and Cantab M.D., Experimental investigation on rickets. *Lancet*, 196, 407, 1919.
29. Mellanby E., Experimental rickets. *Medical Research (G.B.), Special Report Series* SRS-61, 1. 1921. London, His Majesty's Stationery Office. Medical Research Council of Great Britain, Special Report Series.
30. McCollum E.V., Simmonds N., Parsons H.T., Shipley P.G., and Park E.A., Studies on experimental rickets. I. The production of rachitis and similar disease in the rat by deficient diets. *J. Biol. Chem.*, 45, 333, 1920.
31. McCollum E.V., Simmonds N., Becker J.E., and Shipley P.G., Studies on experimental rickets. XXI. An experimental demonstration of the existence of a vitamin which promotes calcium deposition. *J. Biol. Chem.*, 53, 293, 1922.
32. Goldblatt H. and Soames K.N., A study of rats on a normal diet irradiated daily by the mercury vapor quartz lamp or kept in darkness. *Biochem. J.*, 17, 294, 1923.
33. Hess A.F. and Weinstock M., The antirachitic value of irradiated cholesterol and phytosterol. II. Further evidence of change in biological activity. *Methods Enzymol.*, 64, 181, 1925.
34. Hess A.F. and Weinstock M., The antirachitic value of irradiated cholesterol and phytosterol. III. Evidence of chemical change as shown by absorption spectra. *Methods Enzymol.*, 64, 193, 1925.
35. Windaus A., Linsert O., Luttringhaus A., and Weidlinch G., Uber das krystallistierte vitamin D_2. *Justus. Liebigs. Ann. Chem.*, 492, 226, 1932.
36. Angus T.C., Askew F.A., Bourdillon R.B., Bruce H.M., Callow R., Fischmann C., Philpot L., and Webster T.A., A crystalline antirachitic substance. *Proc. R. Soc. Lond. B Biol. Sci.*, 108, 340, 1931.
37. Windaus A., Schenck Fr., and Werder V.F., Uber das antirachitisch wirksame bestrahlungsprodukt aus 7-dehydro-cholesterin. *H.-S. Zeit. Physiol. Chem.*, 241, 100, 1936.
38. Carlsson A. and Lindquist B., Comparison of intestinal and skeletal effects of vitamin D in relation to dosage. *Acta Physiol. Scand.*, 35, 53, 1955.
39. Migicovsky B.B., Influence of vitamin D on calcium resorption and accretion. *Can. J. Biochem. Phy.*, 35, 1267, 1957.
40. Norman A.W., Actinomycin D effect on lag in vitamin D-mediated calcium absorption in the chick. *Am. J. Physiol.*, 211, 829, 1966.
41. Schachter D., Kimberg D.V., and Schenker H., Active transport of calcium by intestine: Action and bio-assay of vitamin D. *Am. J. Physiol.*, 200, 1263, 1961.
42. Thompson V.W. and DeLuca H.F., Vitamin D and phospholipid metabolism. *J. Biol. Chem.*, 239, 984, 1964.
43. Zull J.E., Czarnowska-Misztal E., and DeLuca H.F., On the relationship between vitamin D action and actinomycin-sensitive processes. *Proc. Natl. Acad. Sci. USA*, 55, 177, 1966.
44. Norman A.W., Lund J., and DeLuca H.F., Biologically active forms of vitamin D_3 in kidney and intestine. *Arch. Biochem. Biophys.*, 108, 12, 1964.
45. Blunt J.W., DeLuca H.F., and Schnoes H.K., 25-Hydroxycholecalciferol: A biologically active metabolite of vitamin D_3. *Biochemistry*, 6, 3317, 1968.
46. DeLuca H.F., 25-Hydroxycholecalciferol. The probable metabolically active form of vitamin D_3: Its identification and subcellular site of action. *Arch. Intern. Med.*, 124, 442, 1969.
47. Haussler M.R., Myrtle J.F., and Norman A.W., The association of a metabolite of vitamin D_3 with intestinal mucosa chromatin, in vivo. *J. Biol. Chem.*, 243, 4055, 1968.
48. Norman A.W. and Wong R.G., The biological activity of the vitamin D metabolite 1,25-dihydroxycholecalciferol in chickens and rats. *J. Nutr.*, 102, 1709, 1972.
49. Norman A.W., Myrtle J.F., Midgett R.J., Nowicki H.G., Williams V., and Popjak G., 1,25-Dihydroxycholecalciferol: Identification of the proposed active form of vitamin D_3 in the intestine. *Science*, 173, 51, 1971.
50. Lawson D.E.M., Fraser D.R., Kodicek E., Morris H.R., and Williams D.H., Identification of 1,25-dihydroxycholecalciferol, a new kidney hormone controlling calcium metabolism. *Nature*, 230, 228, 1971.

51. Holick M.F., Schnoes H.K., DeLuca H.F., Suda T., and Cousins R.J., Isolation and identification of 1,25-dihydroxycholecalciferol. A metabolite of vitamin D active in intestine. *Biochemistry*, 10, 2799, 1971.
52. Fraser D.R. and Kodicek E., Unique biosynthesis by kidney of a biologically active vitamin D metabolite. *Nature*, 288, 764, 1970.
53. Haussler M.R. and Norman A.W., Chromosomal receptor for a vitamin D metabolite. *Proc. Natl. Acad. Sci. USA*, 62, 155, 1969.
54. Petkovich M., Brand N.J., Krust A., and Chambon P., A human retinoic acid receptor which belongs to the family of nuclear receptors. *Nature*, 330, 444, 1987.
55. Mangelsdorf D.J., Thummel C., Beato M., Herrlich P., Schütz G., Umesono K., Blumberg B., Kastner P., Mark M., Chambon P., and Evans R.M., The nuclear receptor superfamily: The second decade. *Cell*, 83, 835, 1995.
56. Norman A.W. and Litwack G.L., *Hormones*, 2nd Academic Press, San Diego, CA, 1997. 2nd Edition.
57. Crowfoot D. and Dunitz J.D., Structure of calciferol. *Nature*, 162, 608, 1948.
58. Hodgkin D.C., Rimmer B.M., Dunitz J.D., and Trueblood K.N., The crystal structure of a calciferol derivative. *J. Chem. Soc.*, 947, 4945, 1963.
59. Okamura W.H., Norman A.W., and Wing R.M., Vitamin D: Concerning the relationship between molecular topology and biological function. *Proc. Natl. Acad. Sci. USA*, 71, 4194, 1974.
60. Bligh E.G. and Dyer W.J., An extraction procedure for removing total lipids from tissue. *Can. J. Biochem.*, 37, 911, 1958.
61. Ikekawa N. and Koizumi N., Separation of vitamin D_3 metabolites and their analogs by high-pressure liquid chromatography. *J. Chromat.*, 119, 227, 1976.
62. Halloran B.P., Bikle D.D., and Whitney J.O., Separation of isotopically labeled vitamin-D metabolites by high-performance liquid-chromatography. *J. Chromat.*, 303, 229, 1984.
63. Woodward R.B., Sondheimer F., Taub D., Heusler K., and McLamore W.M., The total synthesis of steroids. *J. Am. Chem. Soc.*, 74, 4223, 1952.
64. Cardwell H.M.E., Cornforth J.W., Duff S.R., Holtermann H., and Robinson R., Experiments on the synthesis of substances related to the sterols. LI. Completion of the syntheses of androgenic hormones and of the cholesterol group of sterols. *Chem. Soc. Lond. J.*, 361, 1953.
65. Bruck P.R., Clark R.D., Davidson R.S., Gunther W.H., Littlewood P.S., and Lythgoe B., Calciferol and its relatives. VIII. Ring A intermediates for the synthesis of tachysterol. *J. Chem. Soc.*, 23, 2529, 1967.
66. Barton D.H.R., Hesse R.H., Pechet M.M., and Rizzardo E., A convenient synthesis of 1α-hydroxyvitamin D_3. *J. Am. Chem. Soc.*, 95, 2748, 1973.
67. Barton D.H.R., Hesse R.H., Pechet M.M., and Rizzardo E., Convenient synthesis of crystalline 1α,25-dihydroxyvitamin D_3. *J. Chem. Soc. Chem. Commun.*, 95, 203, 1974.
68. Baggiolini E.G., Iacobelli J.A., Hennessy B.M., Batcho A.D., Sereno J.F., and Uskokovic M.R., Stereocontrolled total synthesis of 1α,25-dihydroxycholecalciferol and 1α,25-dihydroxyergocalciferol. *J. Org. Chem.*, 51, 3098, 1986.
69. DeSchrijver J. and Declercq P.J., A novel synthesis of an A-ring precursor to 1α-hydroxyvitamin D. *Tetrahed. Lett.*, 34, 4369, 1993.
70. Barrack S.A., Gibbs R.A., and Okamura W.H., Potential inhibitors of vitamin D metabolism: An oxa analogue of vitamin D. *J. Org. Chem.*, 53, 1790, 1988.
71. Harrison R.G., Lythgoe B., and Wright P.W., Calciferol and its relatives; Part XVIII. Total synthesis of 1α-hydroxyvitamin D_3. *J. Chem. Soc. Perkin Trans. 1*, 1, 2654, 1974.
72. Okamura W.H., Aurrecoechea J.M., Gibbs R.A., and Norman A.W., Synthesis and biological activity of 9,11-dehydrovitamin D_3 analogues: Stereoselective preparation of 6β-vitamin D vinylallenes and a concise enynol synthesis for preparing the A-ring. *J. Org. Chem.*, 54, 4072, 1989.
73. Nagasawa K., Zako Y., Ishihara H., and Shimizu I., Stereoselective synthesis of 1α-hydroxyvitamin D_3 A-ring synthons by palladium-catalyzed cyclization. *Tetrahed. Lett.*, 32, 4937, 1991.
74. Trost B.M., Dumas J., and Villa M., New strategies for the synthesis of vitamin D metabolites via Pd-catalyzed reactions. *J. Am. Chem. Soc.*, 114, 9836, 1992.
75. Paaren H.E., DeLuca H.F., and Schnoes H.K., Direct C(1) hydroxylation of vitamin D_3 and related compounds. *J. Org. Chem.*, 45, 3253, 1980.

76. Sheves M. and Mazur Y., The vitamin D_3,5-cyclovitamin D rearrangement. *J. Am. Chem. Soc.*, 97, 6249, 1975.
77. Andrews D.R., Barton D.H.R., Cheng K.P., Finet J.P., Hesse R.H., Johnson G., and Pechet M.M., A direct, regioselective and stereoselective 1α-hydroxylation of (5E)-calciferol derivatives (Letter). *J. Org. Chem.*, 51, 1635, 1986.
78. Vanmaele L., Declercq P.J., and Vandewalle M., An efficient synthesis of 1α,25-dihydroxy vitamin D_3. *Tetrahedron*, 41, 141, 1985.
79. Hay A.W.M. and Watson G., Binding of 25-hydroxyvitamin D_2 to plasma protein in new world monkeys. *Nature*, 256, 150, 1975.
80. Armas L.A.G., Hollis B.W., and Heaney R.P., Vitamin D_2 is much less effective than vitamin D_3 in humans. *J. Clin. Endocrinol. Metab.*, 89, 5387, 2004.
81. Heymann W., Metabolism and mode of action of vitamin D. V. Intestinal excretion of vitamin D. *J. Biol. Chem.*, 122, 257, 1938.
82. Heymann W., Metabolism and mode of action of vitamin D. IV. Importance of bile in the absorption and excretion of vitamin D. *J. Biol. Chem.*, 12, 249, 1938.
83. Rosenstreich S.J., Rich C., and Volwiler W., Deposition in and release of vitamin D_3 from body fat: Evidence for a storage site in the rat. *J. Clin. Invest.*, 50, 679, 1971.
84. Schachter D., Finelstein J.D., and Kowarski S., Metabolism of vitamin D. I. Preparation of radioactive vitamin D and its intestinal absorption in the rat. *J. Clin. Invest.*, 43, 787, 1964.
85. Byard P.J., Quantitative genetics of human skin color. *Yearb. Phys. Anthropol.*, 24, 123, 1981.
86. Stamp T.C.B. and Round J.M., Seasonal changes in human plasma levels of 25-hydroxyvitamin D. *Nature*, 247, 563, 1974.
87. Webb A.R. and Holick M.F., The role of sunlight in the cutaneous production of vitamin D_3. *Ann. Rev. Nutr.*, 8, 375, 1988.
88. Holick M.F., Environmental factors that influence the cutaneous production of vitamin D. *Am. J. Clin. Nutr.*, 61, 638S, 1995.
89. Oliveri M.B., Mautalen C., Bustamante L., and Gomez G.V., Serum levels of 25-hydroxyvitamin D in a year of residence on the Antarctic continent. *Eur. J. Clin. Nutr.*, 48, 397, 1994.
90. Engelsen O., Brustad M., Aksnes L., and Lund E., Daily duration of vitamin D synthesis in human skin with relation to latitude, total ozone, altitude, ground cover, aerosols and cloud thickness. *Photochem. Photobiol.*, 81, 1287, 2005.
91. Clemens T.L., Adams J.S., Henderson S.L., and Holick M.F., Increased skin pigment reduces the capacity of skin to synthesize vitamin D_3. *Lancet*, 1, 74, 1982.
92. Matsuoka L.Y., Wortsman J., Haddad J.G., Kolm P., and Hollis B.W., Racial pigmentation and the cutaneous synthesis of vitamin D. *Arch. Dermatol.*, 127, 536, 1991.
93. Norman A.W., Sunlight, season, skin pigmentation, vitamin D, and 25-hydroxyvitamin D: Integral components of the vitamin D endocrine system. *Am. J. Clin. Nutr.*, 67, 1108, 1998.
94. Loomis W.F., Skin-pigment regulation of vitamin-D biosynthesis in man. Variation in solar ultraviolet at different latitudes may have caused racial differentiation in man. *Science*, 157, 501, 1967.
95. Harris S.S. and Dawson-Hughes B., Seasonal changes in plasma 25-hydroxyvitamin D concentrations of young American black and white women. *Am. J. Clin. Nutr.*, 67, 1232, 1998.
96. Daiger S.P., Schanfield M.S., and Cavalli-Sforza L.L., Group-specific component (Gc) proteins bind vitamin D and 25-hydroxyvitamin D. *Proc. Natl. Acad. Sci. USA*, 72, 2076, 1975.
97. Daiger S.P. and Cavalli-Sforza L.L., Detection of genetic variation with radioactive ligands. II. Genetic variants of vitamin D-labeled group-specific component (Gc) proteins. *Am. J. Hum. Genet.*, 29, 593, 1977.
98. Constans J., Cleve H., Dykes D., Fischer M., Kirk R.L., Papiha S.S., Scheffran W., Scherz R., Thymann M., and Weber W., The polymorphism of the vitamin D-binding protein (Gc); isoelectric focusing in 3M urea as additional method for identification of genetic variants. *Hum. Genet.*, 65, 176, 1983.
99. Bouillon R., Van Assche F.A., Van Baelen H., Heyns W., and DeMoor P., Influence of the vitamin D binding protein on the serum concentration of 1,25-dihydroxyvitamin D_3. *J. Clin. Invest.*, 67, 589, 1981.
100. Haddad J.G., Plasma vitamin D-binding protein (Gc-globulin): Multiple tasks. *J. Steroid Biochem. Mol. Biol.*, 53, 579, 1995.

101. Haddad J.G., Jr. and Walgate J., 25-Hydroxyvitamin D transport in human plasma. Isolation and partial characterization of calcifidiol-binding protein. *J. Biol. Chem.*, 251, 4803, 1976.
102. Song Y.H., Naumova A.K., Liebhaber S.A., and Cooke N.E., Physical and meiotic mapping of the region of human chromosome 4q11–q13 encompassing the vitamin D binding protein DBP/Gc-globulin and albumin multigene cluster. *Genome Res.*, 9, 581, 1999.
103. Bouillon R., Van Baelen H., and De Moor P., The measurement of the vitamin D-binding protein in human serum. *J. Clin. Endocrinol. Metab.*, 45, 225, 1977.
104. Bikle D.D., Siiteri P.K., Ryzen E., and Haddad J.G., Serum protein binding of 1,25-diyhydroxyvitamin D: A reevaluation by direct measurement of free metabolite levels. *J. Clin. Endocrinol. Metab.*, 61, 969, 1985.
105. Bouillon R. and Van Baelen H., Transport of vitamin D: Significance of free and total concentrations of the vitamin D metabolites. *Calcif. Tissue Int.*, 33, 451, 1981.
106. VanBaelen H., Allewaert K., and Bouillon R., New aspects of the plasma carrier protein for 25-hydroxycholecalciferol in vertebrates. *Ann. N.Y. Acad. Sci.*, 538, 60, 2001.
107. Haddad J.G., Harper K.D., Guoth M., Pietra G.G., and Sanger J.W., Angiopathic consequences of saturating the plasma scavenger system for actin. *Proc. Natl. Acad. Sci. USA*, 87, 1381, 1990.
108. Otterbein L.R., Cosio C., Graceffa P., and Dominguez R., Crystal structures of the vitamin D-binding protein and its complex with actin: Structural basis of the actin-scavenger system. *Proc. Natl. Acad. Sci. USA*, 99, 8003, 2002.
109. Swamy N., Head J.F., Weitz D., and Ray R., Biochemical and preliminary crystallographic characterization of the vitamin D sterol- and actin-binding by human vitamin D-binding protein. *Arch. Biochem. Biophys.*, 402, 14, 2002.
110. Bouillon R., Xiang D.-Z., Convents R., and Van Baelen H., Polyunsaturated fatty acids decrease the apparent affinity of vitamin D metabolites for human vitamin D-binding protein. *J. Steroid Biochem. Mol. Biol.*, 42, 855, 1992.
111. DiMartino S.J., Shah A.B., Trujillo G., and Kew R.R., Elastase controls the binding of the vitamin D-binding protein (Gc-globulin) to neutrophils: A potential role in the regulation of C5α co-chemotactic activity. *J. Immunol.*, 166, 2688, 2001.
112. DiMartino S.J. and Kew R.R., Initial characterization of the vitamin D-binding protein (Gc-globulin) binding site on the neutrophil plasma membrane: Evidence for a chondroitin sulfate proteoglycan. *J. Immunol.*, 163, 2135, 1999.
113. Nakhla A.M., Khan M.S., Romas N.P., and Rosner W., Estradiol causes the rapid accumulation of cAMP in human prostate. *Proc. Natl. Acad. Sci. USA*, 91, 5402, 1994.
114. Porto C.S., Lazari M.F., Abreu L.C., Bardin C.W., and Gunsalus G.L., Receptors for androgen-binding proteins: Internalization and intracellular signalling. *J. Steroid Biochem. Mol. Biol.*, 53, 561, 1995.
115. Gibbs P.E.M. and Dugaiczyk A., Origin of structural domains of the serum albumin gene family and a predicted structure of the gene for vitamin D binding protein. *Mol. Biol. Evol.*, 4, 364, 1987.
116. Verboven C., Rabijns A., De Maeyer M., Van Baelen H., Bouillon R., and De Ranter C., A structural basis for the unique binding features of the human vitamin D-binding protein. *Nat. Struct. Biol.*, 9, 131, 2002.
117. Gomme P.T. and Bertolini J., Therapeutic potential of vitamin D-binding protein. *Trends Biotechnol.*, 22, 340, 2004.
118. Compston J.E., Horton L.W.L., and Laker M.F., Vitamin D analogues and renal function. *Lancet*, 1, 386, 1979.
119. Mawer E.B., Backhouse J., Holman C.A., Lumb G.A., and Stanbury S.W., The distribution and storage of vitamin D and its metabolites in human tissues. *Clin. Sci.*, 43, 413, 1972.
120. Rungby J., Mortensen L., Jakobsen K., Brock A., and Mosekilde L., Distribution of hydroxylated vitamin D metabolites [250HD$_3$ and 1,25(OH)$_2$D$_3$] in domestic pigs: Evidence that 1,25(OH)$_2$D$_3$ is stored outside the blood circulation. *Comp. Biochem. Physiol.*, 104A, 483, 1993.
121. Henry H.L. and Norman A.W., Vitamin D: Two dihydroxylated metabolites are required for normal chicken egg hatchability. *Science*, 201, 835, 1978.
122. Norman A.W., Leathers V.L., and Bishop J.E., Studies on the mode of action of calciferol. XLVIII. Normal egg hatchability requires the simultaneous administration to the hen of 1α,25-dihydroxyvitamin D$_3$ and 24R,25-dihydroxyvitamin D$_3$. *J. Nutr.*, 113, 2505, 1983.

123. Norman A.W., Roth J., and Orci L., The vitamin D endocrine system: Steroid metabolism, hormone receptors and biological response (calcium binding proteins). *Endocr. Rev.*, 3, 331, 1982.
124. Axén E., Bergman T., and Wikvall K., Microsomal 25-hydroxylation of vitamin D_2 and vitamin D_3 in pig liver. *J. Steroid Biochem. Mol. Biol.*, 51, 97, 1994.
125. Bergman T. and Postlind H., Characterization of mitochondrial cytochromes P450 from pig kidney and liver catalysing 26-hydroxylation of 25-hydroxyvitamin D_3 and C_{27} steroids. *Biochem. J.*, 276, 427, 1991.
126. Bhattacharyya M.H. and DeLuca H.F., Subcellular location of rat liver calciferol-25-hydroxylase. *Arch. Biochem. Biophys.*, 160, 58, 1974.
127. Saarem K., Bergseth S., Oftebro H., and Pedersen J.I., Subcellular localization of vitamin D_3 25-hydroxylase in human liver. *J. Biol. Chem.*, 259, 10936, 1984.
128. Tucker G., Gagnon R.E., and Haussler M.R., Vitamin D_3-25-hydroxylase: Tissue occurrence and apparent lack of regulation. *Arch. Biochem. Biophys.*, 155, 47, 1973.
129. Mawer E.B., Clinical implication of measurements of circulating vitamin D metabolites. *Clin. Endocrinol. Metab.*, 9, 63, 1980.
130. Pettifor J.M., Ross F.P., and Wang J., Serum levels of 25-hydroxycholecalciferol as a diagnostic aid in vitamin D deficiency states. *S. Afr. Med. J.*, 51, 580, 1977.
131. Cheng J.B., Motola D.L., Mangelsdorf D.J., and Russell D.W., De-orphanization of cytochrome P450 2R1: A microsomal vitamin D 25-hydroxilase. *J. Biol. Chem.*, 278, 38084, 2003.
132. Cheng J.B., Levine M.A., Bell N.H., Mangelsdorf D.J., and Russell D.W., Genetic evidence that the human CYP2R1 enzyme is a key vitamin D 25-hydroxylase. *Proc. Natl. Acad. Sci. USA*, 101, 7711, 2004.
133. Henry H.L. and Norman A.W., Studies on calciferol metabolism. IX. Renal 25-hydroxyvitamin D_3-1-hydroxylase. Involvement of cytochrome P450 and other properties. *J. Biol. Chem.*, 249, 7529, 1974.
134. Henry H.L., Vitamin D hydroxylases. *J. Cell. Biochem.*, 49, 4, 1992.
135. Weisman Y., Harell A., Edelstein S., David M., Spirer Z., and Golander A., 1α,25-Dihydroxyvitamin D_3 and 24,25-dihydroxyvitamin D_3; in vitro synthesis by human decidua and placenta. *Nature*, 281, 317, 1979.
136. Tanaka Y., Halloran B.P., Schnoes H.K., and DeLuca H.F., In vitro production of 1,25-dihydroxyvitamin D_3 by rat placental tissue. *Proc. Natl. Acad. Sci. USA*, 76, 5033, 1979.
137. Adams J.S., Singer F.R., Gacad M.A., Sharma O.P., Hayes M.J., Vouros P., and Holick M.F., Isolation and structural identification of 1,25-dihydroxyvitamin D_3 produced by cultured alveolar macrophages in sarcoidosis. *J. Clin. Endocrinol. Metab.*, 60, 960, 1985.
138. Reichel H., Bishop J.E., Koeffler H.P., and Norman A.W., Evidence for 1,25-dihydroxyvitamin D_3 production by cultured porcine alveolar macrophages. *Mol. Cell. Endocrinol.*, 75, 163, 1991.
139. Reichel H., Koeffler H.P., and Norman A.W., Synthesis *in vitro* of 1,25-dihydroxyvitamin D_3 and 24,25-dihydroxyvitamin D_3 by interferon-gamma-stimulated normal human bone marrow and alveolar macrophages. *J. Biol. Chem.*, 262, 10931, 1987.
140. Puzas J.E., Turner R.T., Howard G.A., Brand J.S., and Baylink D.J., Synthesis of 1,25-dihydroxycholecalciferol and 24,25-dihydroxycholecalciferol by calvarial cells: Characterization of the enzyme systems. *Biochem. J.*, 245, 333, 1987.
141. Pillai S., Bikle D.D., and Elias P.M., 1,25-Dihydroxyvitamin D production and receptor binding in human keratinocytes varies with differentiation. *J. Biol. Chem.*, 263, 5390, 1988.
142. Matsumoto K., Azuma Y., Kiyoki M., Okumura H., Hashimoto K., and Yoshikawa K., Involvement of endogenously produced 1,25-dihydroxyvitamin D_3 in the growth and differentiation of human keratinocytes. *Biochim. Biophys. Acta*, 1092, 311, 1991.
143. Henry H.L., Dutta C., Cunningham N., Blanchard R., Penny R., Tang C., Marchetto G., and Chou S.-Y., The cellular and molecular regulation of 1,25$(OH)_2D_3$ production. *J. Steroid Biochem. Mol. Biol.*, 41, 401, 1992.
144. Colston K.W., Evans I.M., Spelsberg T.C., and Macintyre I., Feedback regulation of vitamin D metabolism by 1,25-dihydroxycholecalciferol. *Biochem. J.*, 164, 83, 1977.
145. Liu S., Tang W., Zhou J., Stubbs J.R., Luo Q., Pi M., and Quarles L.D., Fibroblast growth factor 23 is a counter-regulatory phosphaturic hormone for vitamin D. *J. Am. Soc. Nephrol.*, 17, 1305–1315, 2006.
146. Shimada T., Hasegawa H., Yamazaki Y., Muto T., Hino R., Takeuchi Y., Fujita T., Nakahara K., Fukumoto S., and Yamashita T., FGF-23 is a potent regulator of vitamin D metabolism and phosphate homeostasis. *J. Bone Miner. Res.*, 19, 429, 2004.

147. Ward L.M., Rauch F., White K.E., Filler G., Matzinger M.A., Letts M., Travers R., Econs M.J., and Glorieux F.H., Resolution of severe, adolescent-onset hypophosphatemic rickets following resection of an FGF-23-producing tumour of the distal ulna. *Bone*, 34, 905, 2004.
148. Henry H.L., Taylor A.N., and Norman A.W., Response of chick parathyroid glands to the vitamin D metabolites, 1,25-dihydroxycholecalciferol and 24,25-dihydroxycholecalciferol. *J. Nutr.*, 107, 1918, 1977.
149. Canterbury J.M., Gavellas G., Bourgoignie J.J., and Reise E., Metabolic consequences of oral administration of 24,25-dihydroxycholecalciferol to uremic dogs. *J. Clin. Invest.*, 65, 571, 1980.
150. Yamato H., Okazaki R., Ishii T., Ogata E., Sato T., Kumegawa M., Akaogi K., Taniguchi N., and Matsumoto T., Effect of 24R,25-dihydroxyvitamin D_3 on the formation and function of osteoclastic cells. *Calcif. Tissue Int.*, 52, 255, 1993.
151. Evans R.A., Hills E., Wong S.Y.P., Dunstan C.R., and Norman A.W., The use of 24,25-dihydroxycholecalciferol alone and in combination with 1,25-dihydroxycholecalciferol in chronic renal failure. In: *Vitamin D: Chemical, Biochemical and Clinical Endocrinology of Calcium Metabolism*, Eds. Norman A.W., Schaefer K., Grigoleit H.-G., and von Herrath D., p. 835. Walter de Gruyter and Company, Berlin, 1982.
152. Seo E.-G., Schwartz Z., Dean D.D., Norman A.W., and Boyan B.D., Preferential accumulation in vivo of 24R,25-dihydroxyvitamin D_3 in growth plate cartilage of rats. *Endocrine*, 5, 147, 1996.
153. Seo E.-G. and Norman A.W., Three-fold induction of renal 25-hydroxyvitamin D_3-24-hydroxylase activity and increased serum 24,25-dihydroxyvitamin D_3 levels are correlated with the healing process after chick tibial fracture. *J. Bone Miner. Res.*, 12, 598, 1997.
154. Seo E.-G., Einhorn T.A., and Norman A.W., 24R,25-dihydroxyvitamin D_3: An essential vitamin D_3 metabolite for both normal bone integrity and healing of tibial fracture in chicks. *Endocrinology*, 138, 3864, 1997.
155. Kato A., Seo E.-G., Einhorn T.A., Bishop J.E., and Norman A.W., Studies on 24R,25-dihydroxyvitamin D_3: Evidence for a non-nuclear membrane receptor in the chick tibial fracture-healing callus. *Bone*, 23, 141, 1998.
156. Norman A.W., Leathers V.L., Bishop J.E., Kadowaki S., and Miller B.E., 24R,25-dihydroxyvitamin D_3 has unique receptors (parathyroid gland) and biological responses (egg hatchability). In: *Vitamin D: Chemical, Biochemical, and Clinical Endocrinology of Calcium Metabolism*, Eds. Norman A.W., Schaefer K., Grigoleit H.-G., and von Herrath D., p. 147. Walter de Gruyter and Company, Berlin, 1982.
157. Ishizuka S., Ohba T., and Norman A.W., $1\alpha,25(OH)_2D_3$-26,23-lactone is a major metabolite of $1\alpha,25(OH)_2D_3$ under physiological conditions. In: *Vitamin D: Molecular, Cellular and Clinical Endocrinology*, Eds. Norman A.W., Schaefer K., Grigoleit H.G., and von Herrath D., p. 143. Walter de Gruyter, Berlin, 1988.
158. Saito N., Saito H., Anzai M., Yoshida A., Fujishima T., Takenouchi K., Miura D., Ishizuka S., Takayama H., and Kittaka A., Dramatic enhancement of antagonistic activity on vitamin D receptor: A double functionalization of 1α-hydroxyvitamin D_3-26,23-lactones. *Org. Lett.*, 5, 4859, 2003.
159. Ishizuka S., Miura D., Ozono K., Chokki M., Mimura H., and Norman A.W., Antagonistic actions in vivo of (23S)-25-dehydro-1α-hydroxyvitamin D_3-26,23-lactone on calcium metabolism induced by 1α,25-dihydroxyvitamin D_3. *Endocrinology*, 142, 59, 2001.
160. Bula C.M., Bishop J.E., Ishizuka S., and Norman A.W., 25-Dehydro-1α-hydroxyvitamin D_3-26-23S-lactone antagonizes the nuclear vitamin D receptor by mediating a unique noncovalent conformational change. *Mol. Endocrinol.*, 14, 1788, 2000.
161. Ishizuka S., Kurihara N., Miura D., Takenouchi K., Cornish J., Cundy T., Reddy S.V., and Roodman G.D., Vitamin D antagonist, TEI-9647, inhibits osteoclast formation induced by 1α,25-dihydroxyvitamin D_3 from pagetic bone marrow cells. *J. Steroid Biochem. Mol. Biol.*, 89–90, 331, 2004.
162. Kumar R., The metabolism and mechanism of action of 1,25-dihydroxyvitamin D_3. *Kidney Int.*, 30, 793, 1986.
163. Ortí E., Bodwell J.E., and Munck A., Phosphorylation of steroid hormone receptors. *Endocr. Rev.*, 13, 105, 1992.
164. Darwish H.M., Burmester J.K., Moss V.E., and DeLuca H.F., Phosphorylation is involved in transcriptional activation by the 1,25-dihydroxyvitamin D_3 receptor. *Biochim. Biophys. Acta*, 1167, 29, 1993.

165. Jurutka P.W., Hsieh J.-C., and Haussler M.R., Phosphorylation of the human 1,25-dihydroxyvitamin D_3 receptor by cAMP-dependent protein kinase, in vitro, and in transfected COS-7 cells. *Biochem. Biophys. Res. Commun.*, 191, 1089, 1993.
166. Hsieh J.-C., Jurutka P.W., Nakajima S., Galligan M.A., Haussler C.A., Shimizu Y., Shimizu N., Whitfield G.K., and Haussler M.R., Phosphorylation of the human vitamin D receptor by protein kinase C. Biochemical and functional evaluation of the serine 51 recognition site. *J. Biol. Chem.*, 268, 15118, 1993.
167. Lowe K.E., Maiyar A.C., and Norman A.W., Vitamin D-mediated gene expression. *Crit. Rev. Eukaryot. Gene Expr.*, 2, 65, 1992.
168. Walters M.R., Newly identified actions of the vitamin D endocrine system. *Endocr. Rev.*, 13, 719, 1992.
169. Norman A.W., Xu J., and Collins E.D., The vitamin D endocrine system: Metabolism, mode of action, and genetic evaluation. In: *Genetics in Endocrinology*, Ed. Baxter J.D., p. 445. Lippincott-Raven, Philadelphia, PA, 2002.
170. White J.H., Profiling 1,25-dihydroxyvitamin D_3-regulated gene expression by microarray analysis. *J. Steroid Biochem. Mol. Biol.*, 89–90, 239, 2004.
171. Eelen G., Verlinden L., Van Camp M., Mathieu C., Carmeliet G., Bouillon R., and Verstuyf A., Microarray analysis of 1α,25-dihydroxyvitamin D_3-treated MC3T3-E1 cells. *J. Steroid Biochem. Mol. Biol.*, 89–90, 405, 2004.
172. Bouillon R., Verstuyf A., Verlinden L., Eelen G., and Mathieu C., Prospects for vitamin D receptor modulators as candidate drugs for cancer and (auto)immune diseases. *Recent Results Cancer Res.*, 164, 353, 2003.
173. Lin R. and White J.H., The pleiotropic actions of vitamin D. *Bioessays*, 26, 21, 2004.
174. MacDonald P.N., Dowd D.R., Zhang C., and Gu C., Emerging insights into the coactivator role of NCoA62/SKIP in vitamin D-mediated transcription. *J. Steroid Biochem. Mol. Biol.*, 89–90, 179, 2004.
175. Sutton A.L. and MacDonald P.N., Vitamin D: More than a "bone-a-fide" hormone. *Mol. Endocrinol.*, 17, 777, 2003.
176. Rachez C. and Freedman L.P., Mechanisms of gene regulation by vitamin D_3 receptor: A network of coactivator interactions. *Gene*, 246, 9, 2000.
177. Tsai H.C. and Norman A.W., Studies on calciferol metabolism. VIII. Evidence for a cytoplasmic receptor for 1,25-dihydroxyvitamin D_3 in the intestinal mucosa. *J. Biol. Chem.*, 248, 5967, 1972.
178. Baker A.R., McDonnell D.P., Hughes M., Crisp T.M., Mangelsdorf D.J., Haussler M.R., Pike J.W., Shine J., and O'Malley B.W., Cloning and expression of full-length cDNA encoding human vitamin D receptor. *Proc. Natl. Acad. Sci. USA*, 85, 3294, 1988.
179. McDonnell D.P., Mangelsdorf D.J., Pike J.W., Haussler M.R., and O'Malley B.W., Molecular-cloning of complementary-DNA encoding the avian receptor for vitamin D. *Science*, 235, 1214, 1987.
180. Wecksler W.R., Ross F.P., Mason R.S., and Norman A.W., Studies on the mode of action of calciferol. XXI. Biochemical properties of the 1α,25-dihydroxyvitamin D_3 cytosol receptors from human and chicken intestinal mucosa. *J. Clin. Endocrinol. Metab.*, 50, 152, 1980.
181. Wecksler W.R., Ross F.P., Mason R.S., Posen S., and Norman A.W., Studies on the mode of action of calciferol. XXIV. Biochemical properties of the 1α,25-dihydroxyvitamin D_3 cytoplasmic receptors from human and chick parathyroid glands. *Arch. Biochem. Biophys.*, 201, 95, 1980.
182. Mangelsdorf D.J. and Evans R.M., The RXR heterodimers and orphan receptors. *Cell*, 83, 841, 1995.
183. Evans R.M., The steroid and thyroid hormone receptor superfamily. *Science*, 240, 889, 1988.
184. Brand N., Petkovich M., Krust A., Chambon P., de The H., Marchio A., Tiollais P., and Dejean A., Identification of a second human retinoic acid receptor. *Nature*, 332, 850, 1988.
185. Beato M., Gene regulation by steroid hormones. *Cell*, 56, 335, 1989.
186. McKenna N.J. and O'Malley B.W., Combinatorial control of gene expression by nuclear receptors and coregulators. *Cell*, 108, 465, 2002.
187. McKenna N.J. and O'Malley B.W., Minireview: Nuclear receptor coactivators—An update. *Endocrinology*, 143, 2461, 2002.
188. Green S. and Chambon P., Nuclear receptors enhance our understanding of transcription regulation. *Trends Genet.*, 4, 309, 1988.

189. Rastinejad F., Perlmann T., Evans R.M., and Sigler P.B., Structural determinants of nuclear receptor assembly on DNA direct repeats. *Nature*, 375, 203, 1995.
190. Bourguet W., Ruff M., Chambon P., Gronemeyer H., and Moras D., Crystal structure of the ligand-binding domain of the human nuclear receptor RXRα. *Nature*, 375, 377, 1995.
191. Renaud J.P., Rochel N., Ruff M., Vivat V., Chambon P., Gronemeyer H., and Moras D., Crystal structure of the RARγ ligand-binding domain bound to all-trans retinoic acid. *Nature*, 378, 681, 1995.
192. Weatherman R.V., Fletterick R.J., and Scanlon T.S., Nuclear receptor ligands and ligand-binding domains. *Annu. Rev. Biochem.*, 68, 559, 1999.
193. Rochel N., Wurtz J.M., Mitschler A., Klaholz B., and Moras D., The crystal structure of the nuclear receptor for vitamin D bound to its natural ligand. *Mol. Cell*, 5, 173, 2000.
194. Tocchini-Valentini G., Rochel N., Wurtz J.M., Mitschler A., and Moras D., Crystal structures of the vitamin D receptor complexed to superagonist 20-epi ligands. *Proc. Natl. Acad. Sci. USA*, 98, 5491, 2001.
195. Ciesielski F., Rochel N., Mitschler A., Kouzmenko A., and Moras D., Structural investigation of the ligand binding domain of the zebrafish VDR in complexes with $1\alpha,25(OH)_2D_3$ and Gemini: Purification, crystallization and preliminary X-ray diffraction analysis. *J. Steroid Biochem. Mol. Biol.*, 89–90, 55, 2004.
196. Tocchini-Valentini G., Rochel N., Wurtz J.M., and Moras D., Crystal structures of the vitamin D nuclear receptor liganded with the vitamin D side chain analogues calcipotriol and seocalcitol, receptor agonists of clinical importance. Insights into a structural basis for the switching of calcipotriol to a receptor antagonist by further side chain modification. *J. Med. Chem.*, 47, 1956, 2004.
197. Perret C., Desplan C., Brehier A., and Thomasset M., Characterization of rat 9-kDa cholecalcin (CaBP) messenger RNA using a complementary DNA: Absence of homology with 28-kDa cholecalcin mRNA. *Eur. J. Biochem.*, 148, 61, 1985.
198. Cancela L., Ishida H., Bishop J.E., and Norman A.W., Local chromatin changes accompany the expression of the calbindin-D_{28K} gene: Tissue specificity and effect of vitamin D activation. *Mol. Endocrinol.*, 6, 468, 1992.
199. Minghetti P.P., Cancela L., Fujisawa Y., Theofan G., and Norman A.W., Molecular structure of the chicken vitamin D-induced calbindin-D_{28K} gene reveals eleven exons, six Ca^{2+}-binding domains, and numerous promoter regulatory elements. *Mol. Endocrinol.*, 2, 355, 1988.
200. Nemere I., Dormanen M.C., Hammond M.W., Okamura W.H., and Norman A.W., Identification of a specific binding protein for 1α,25-dihydroxyvitamin D_3 in basal-lateral membranes of chick intestinal epithelium and relationship to transcaltachia. *J. Biol. Chem.*, 269, 23750, 1994.
201. Huhtakangas J.A., Olivera C.J., Bishop J.E., Zanello L.P., and Norman A.W., The vitamin D receptor is present in caveolae-enriched plasma membranes and binds $1\alpha,25(OH)_2$-vitamin D_3 in vivo and in vitro. *Mol. Endocrinol.*, 18, 2660, 2004.
202. Levin E.R., Integration of the extra-nuclear and nuclear actions of estrogen. *Mol. Endocrinol.*, 19, 1951, 2005.
203. Anderson R.G. and Jacobson K., A role for lipid shells in targeting proteins to caveolae, rafts, and other lipid domains. *Science*, 296, 1821, 2002.
204. Sowa G., Pypaert M., and Sessa W.C., Distinction between signaling mechanisms in lipid rafts vs. caveolae. *Proc. Natl. Acad. Sci. USA*, 98, 14072, 2001.
205. Zanello L.P. and Norman A.W., Rapid modulation of osteoblast ion channel responses by $1\alpha,25(OH)_2$-vitamin D_3 requires the presence of a functional vitamin D nuclear receptor. *Proc. Natl. Acad. Sci. USA*, 101, 1589, 2004.
206. Norman A.W., Okamura W.H., Farach-Carson M.C., Allewaert K., Branisteanu D., Nemere I., Muralidharan K.R., and Bouillon R., Structure–function studies of 1,25-dihydroxyvitamin D_3 and the vitamin D endocrine system. 1,25-dihydroxy-pentadeuterio-previtamin D_3 (as a 6-s-*cis* analog) stimulates nongenomic but not genomic biological responses. *J. Biol. Chem.*, 268, 13811, 1993.
207. Zanello L.P. and Norman A.W., Stimulation by $1\alpha,25(OH)_2$-vitamin D_3 of whole cell chloride currents in osteoblastic ROS 17/2.8 cells: A structure–function study. *J. Biol. Chem.*, 272, 22617, 1997.
208. Vazquez G., De Boland A.R., and Boland R.L., 1α,25-Dihydroxyvitamin D_3-induced store-operated Ca^{2+} influx in skeletal muscle cells—Modulation by phospholipase C, protein kinase C, and tyrosine kinases. *J. Biol. Chem.*, 273, 33954, 1998.

209. Schwartz Z., Ehland H., Sylvia V.L., Larsson D., Hardin R.R., Bingham V., Lopez D., Dean D.D., and Boyan B.D., 1α,25-Dihydroxyvitamin D_3 and 24R,25-dihydroxyvitamin D_3 modulate growth plate chondrocyte physiology via protein kinase C-dependent phosphorylation of extracellular signal-regulated kinase 1/2 mitogen-activated protein kinase. *Endocrinology*, 143, 2775, 2002.
210. Schwartz Z., Sylvia V.L., Larsson D., Nemere I., Casasola D., Dean D.D., and Boyan B.D., 1α,25$(OH)_2D_3$ regulates chondrocyte matrix vesicle protein kinase D (PKC) directly via G protein-dependent mechanisms and indirectly via incorporation of PKC during matrix vesicle biogenesis. *J. Biol. Chem.*, 277, 11828, 2002.
211. Vertino A.M., Bula C.M., Chen J.-R., Kousteni S., Han L., Bellido T., Norman A.W., and Manolagas S.C., Nongenotropic, anti-apoptotic signaling of 1α,25$(OH)_2$-vitamin D_3 and analogs through the ligand binding domain of the vitamin D receptor in osteoblasts and osteocytes. Mediation by Src, phosphatidylinositol 3-, and JNK kinases. *J. Biol. Chem.*, 280, 14130, 2005.
212. Norman A.W., Henry H.L., Bishop J.E., Song X., Bula C., and Okamura W.H., Different shapes of the steroid hormone 1α,25$(OH)_2$-vitamin D_3 act as agonists for two different receptors in the vitamin D endocrine system to mediate genomic and rapid responses. *Steroids*, 66, 147, 2001.
213. Mizwicki M.T., Keidel D., Bula C.M., Bishop J.E., Zanello L.P., Wurtz J.M., Moras D., and Norman A.W., Identification of an alternative ligand-binding pocket in the nuclear vitamin D receptor and its functional importance in 1α,25$(OH)_2$-vitamin D_3 signaling. *Proc. Natl. Acad. Sci. USA*, 101, 12876, 2004.
214. Morley P., Whitfield J.F., Vanderhyden B.C., Tsang B.K., and Schwartz J.L., A new, nongenomic estrogen action: The rapid release of intracellular calcium. *Endocrinology*, 131, 1305, 1992.
215. Mendoza C. and Tesarik J., A plasma-membrane progesterone receptor in human sperm is switched on by increasing intracellular free calcium. *FEBS Lett.*, 330, 57, 1993.
216. Aurell Wistrom C. and Meizel S., Evidence suggesting involvement of a unique human sperm steroid receptor/Cl^- channel complex in the progesterone-initiated acrosome reaction. *Dev. Biol.*, 159, 679, 1993.
217. Blackmore P.F., Beebe S.J., Danforth D.R., and Alexander N., Progesterone and 17α-progesterone: Novel stimulators of calcium influx in human sperm. *J. Biol. Chem.*, 265, 1376, 1990.
218. Majewska M.D. and Vaupel D.B., Steroid control of uterine motility via gamma-aminobutyric $acid_A$ receptors in the rabbit: A novel mechanism. *J. Endo.*, 131, 427, 1991.
219. Koenig H., Fan C.-C., Goldstone A.D., Lu C.Y., and Trout J.J., Polyamines mediate androgenic stimulation of calcium fluxes and membrane transport in rat myocytes. *Circ. Res.*, 64, 415, 1989.
220. Orchinik M., Murray T.F., and Moore F.L., A corticosteroid receptor in neuronal membranes. *Science*, 252, 1848, 1991.
221. Rehberger P., Rexin M., and Gehring U., Heterotetrameric structure of the human progesterone receptor. *Proc. Natl. Acad. Sci. USA*, 89, 8001, 1992.
222. Gametchu B., Watson C.S., and Wu S., Use of receptor antibodies to demonstrate membrane glucocorticoid receptor in cells from human leukemic patients. *FASEB J.*, 7, 1283, 1993.
223. Smith T.J., Davis F.B., and Davis P.J., Stereochemical requirements for the modulation by retinoic acid of thyroid hormone activation of Ca^{2+}-ATPase and binding at the human erythrocyte membrane. *Biochem. J.*, 284, 583, 1992.
224. Segal J., Thyroid hormone action at the level of the plasma membrane. *Thyroid*, 1, 83, 1990.
225. Nemere I., Zhou L.-X., and Norman A.W., Nontranscriptional effects of steroid hormones. *Receptor*, 3, 277, 1993.
226. Schachter D., Dowdle E.B., and Schenker H., Active transport of calcium by the small intestine of the rat. *Am. J. Physiol.*, 198, 263, 1960.
227. Harrison H.E. and Harrison H.C., Vitamin D and permeability of intestinal mucosa to calcium. *Am. J. Physiol.*, 208, 370, 1965.
228. Leathers V.L., Biophysical characterization and functional studies on calbindin-D-28K: A vitamin D-induced calcium binding protein. 1. 1989. University of California, Riverside.
229. Nemere I. and Norman A.W., Studies on the mode of action of calciferol. LII. Rapid action of 1,25-dihydroxyvitamin D_3 on calcium transport in perfused chick duodenum: Effect of inhibitors. *J. Bone Miner. Res.*, 2, 99, 1987.
230. Nemere I., Leathers V.L., Thompson B.S., Lüben R.A., and Norman A.W., Redistribution of calbindin-D_{28k} in chick intestine in response to calcium transport. *Endocrinology*, 129, 2972, 1991.

231. Putkey J.A., Spielvogel A.M., Sauerheber R.D., Dunlap C.S., and Norman A.W., Studies on the mode of action of calciferol. XXXIX. Vitamin D-mediated intestinal calcium transport: Effect of essential fatty acid deficiency and spin label studies of enterocyte membrane lipid fluidity. *Biochim. Biophys. Acta*, 688, 177, 1982.
232. Putkey J.A. and Norman A.W., Studies on the mode of action of calciferol (XLV) vitamin D: Its effect on the protein composition and core material structure of the chick intestinal brush border membrane. *J. Biol. Chem.*, 258, 8971, 1983.
233. Spielvogel A.M., Farley R.D., and Norman A.W., Studies on the mechanism of action of calciferol V. Turnover time of chick intestinal epithelial cells in relation to the intestinal action of vitamin D. *Exp. Cell Res.*, 74, 359, 1972.
234. McCarthy J.T., Barham S.S., and Kumar R., 1,25-Dihydroxyvitamin D_3 rapidly alters the morphology of the duodenal mucosa of rachitic chicks: Evidence for novel effects of 1,25-dihydroxyvitamin D_3. *J. Steroid Biochem. Mol. Biol.*, 21, 253, 1984.
235. Carmeliet G., Van Cromphaut S., Daci E., Maes C., and Bouillon R., Disorders of calcium homeostasis. *Best. Pract. Res. Clin. Endocrinol. Metab.*, 17, 529, 2003.
236. Gumbleton M., Abulrob A.G., and Campbell L., Caveolae: An alternative membrane transport compartment. *Pharmacol. Res.*, 17, 1035, 2000.
237. Hoenderop J.G., Willems P.H., and Bindels R.J., Toward a comprehensive molecular model of active calcium reabsorption. *Am. J. Physiol. Renal Physiol.*, 278, F352–F360, 2000.
238. Henry H.L. and Norman A.W., Vitamin D: Metabolism and biological action. *Ann. Rev. Nutr.*, 4, 493, 1984.
239. Anderson P.H., O'Loughlin P.D., May B.K., and Morris H.A., Determinants of circulating 1,25-dihydroxyvitamin D_3 levels: The role of renal synthesis and catabolism of vitamin D. *J. Steroid Biochem. Mol. Biol.*, 89–90, 111, 2004.
240. Li Y.C., Kong J., Wei M., Chen Z.F., Liu S.Q., and Cao L.P., 1,25-Dihydroxyvitamin D_3 is a negative endocrine regulator of the renin–angiotensin system. *J. Clin. Invest.*, 110, 229, 2002.
241. Li Y.C., Qiao G., Uskokovic M., Xiang W., Zheng W., and Kong J., Vitamin D: A negative endocrine regulator of the renin–angiotensin system and blood pressure. *J. Steroid Biochem. Mol. Biol.*, 89–90, 387, 2004.
242. Xiang W., Kong J., Chen S., Cao L.P., Qiao G., Zheng W., Liu W., Li X., Gardner D.G., and Li Y.C., Cardiac hypertrophy in vitamin D receptor knockout mice: Role of the systemic and cardiac renin–angiotensin systems. *Am. J. Physiol. Endocrinol. Metab.*, 288, 125–132, 2004.
243. Zheng W., Xie Y., Li G., Kong J., Feng J.Q., and Li Y.C., Critical role of calbindin-D_{28K} in calcium homeostasis revealed by mice lacking both vitamin D receptor and calbindin-D_{28K}. *J. Biol. Chem.*, 279, 52406–52413, 2004.
244. Underwood J.L. and DeLuca H.F., Vitamin D is not directly necessary for bone-growth and mineralization. *Am. J. Physiol.*, 246, E493–E498, 1984.
245. Norman A.W. and Hurwitz S., The role of the vitamin D endocrine system in avian bone biology. *J. Nutr.*, 123, 310, 1993.
246. Walters M.R., Rosen D.M., Norman A.W., and Luben R.A., 1,25-Dihydroxyvitamin D receptors in an established bone cell line: Correlation with biochemical responses. *J. Biol. Chem.*, 257, 7481, 1982.
247. Caffrey J.M. and Farach-Carson M.C., Vitamin D_3 metabolites modulate dihydropyridine-sensitive calcium currents in clonal rat osteosarcoma cells. *J. Biol. Chem.*, 264, 20265, 1989.
248. Lieberherr M., Effects of vitamin D_3 metabolites on cytosolic free calcium in confluent mouse osteoblasts. *J. Biol. Chem.*, 262, 13168, 1987.
249. Harrison J.R., Petersen D.N., Lichtler A.C., Mador A.T., Rowe D.W., and Kream B.E., 1,25-Dihydroxyvitamin D_3 inhibits transcription of type I collagen genes in the rat osteosarcoma cell line ROS 17/2.8. *Endocrinology*, 125, 327, 1989.
250. Kurihara N., Ikeda K., Hakeda Y., Tsunoi M., Maeda N., and Kumegawa M., Effect of 1,25-dihydroxyvitamin D_3 on alkaline phosphatase activity and collagen synthesis in osteoblastic cells, clone MC3T3-E1. *Biochem. Biophys. Res. Commun.*, 119, 767, 1984.
251. Pan L.C. and Price P.A., The effect of transcriptional inhibitors on the bone gamma-carboxyglutamic acid protein response to 1,25-dihydroxyvitamin D_3 in osteosarcoma cells. *J. Biol. Chem.*, 259, 5844, 1984.

252. Fraser J.D. and Price P.A., Induction of matrix Gla protein synthesis during prolonged 1,25-dihydroxyvitamin D_3 treatment of osteosarcoma cells. *Calcif. Tissue Int.*, 46, 270, 1990.
253. Rowe D.W. and Kream B.E., Regulation of collagen synthesis in fetal rat calvaria by 1,25-dihydroxyvitamin D_3. *J. Biol. Chem.*, 257, 8009, 1982.
254. Takasu H., Sugita A., Uchiyama Y., Katagiri N., Okazaki M., Ogata E., and Ikeda K., c-Fos protein as a target of anti-osteoclastogenic action of vitamin D, and synthesis of new analogs. *J. Clin. Invest*, 116, 528, 2006.
255. Kurihara N., Reddy S.V., Araki N., Ishizuka S., Ozono K., Cornish J., Cundy T., Singer F.R., and Roodman G.D., Role of TAFII-17, a VDR binding protein, in the increased osteoclast formation in Paget's disease. *J. Bone Miner. Res.*, 19, 1154, 2004.
256. Panda D.K., Miao D., Bolivar I., Li J., Huo R., Hendy G.N., and Goltzman D., Inactivation of the 25-hydroxyvitamin D 1α-hydroxylase and vitamin D receptor demonstrates independent and interdependent effects of calcium and vitamin D on skeletal and mineral homeostasis. *J. Biol. Chem.*, 279, 16754, 2004.
257. Dusso A., Cozzolino M., Lu Y., Sato T., and Slatopolsky E., 1,25-Dihydroxyvitamin D down-regulation of TGFα/EGFR expression and growth signaling: A mechanism for the antiproliferative actions of the sterol in parathyroid hyperplasia of renal failure. *J. Steroid Biochem. Mol. Biol.*, 89–90, 507, 2004.
258. Koshikawa S., Akizawa T., Kurokawa K., Marumo F., Sakai O., Arakawa M., Morii H., Seino Y., Ogata E., Ohashi Y., Akiba T., Tsukamoto Y., and Suzuki M., Clinical effect of intravenous calcitriol administration on secondary hyperparathyroidism. A double-blind study among 4 doses. *Nephron*, 90, 413, 2002.
259. Lippuner K., Perrelet R., Casez J.P., Popp A., Uskokovic M.R., and Jaeger P., 1,25-$(OH)_2$_16ene-23yne-D_3 reduces secondary hyperparathyroidism in uremic rats with little calcemic effect. *Horm. Res.*, 61, 7, 2004.
260. Pike J.W., Gooze L.L., and Haussler M.R., Biochemical evidence for 1,25-dihydroxyvitamin D_3 receptor macromolecules in parathyroid, pancreatic, pituitary, and placental tissues. *Life Sci.*, 26, 407, 1980.
261. Zinser G.M. and Welsh J., Vitamin D receptor status alters mammary gland morphology and tumorigenesis in MMTV-neu mice. *Carcinogenesis*, 2004.
262. Welsh J., Wietzke J.A., Zinser G.M., Byrne B., Smith K., and Narvaez C.J., Vitamin D_3 receptor as a target for breast cancer prevention. *J. Nutr.*, 133, 2425S, 2003.
263. Lowe L.C., Guy M., Mansi J.L., Peckitt C., Bliss J., Wilson R.G., and Colston K.W., Plasma 25-hydroxyvitamin D concentrations, vitamin D receptor genotype and breast cancer risk in a UK Caucasian population. *Eur. J. Cancer*, 41, 1164, 2005.
264. Guy M., Lowe L.C., Bretherton-Watt D., Mansi J.L., Peckitt C., Bliss J., Wilson R.G., Thomas V., and Colston K.W., Vitamin D receptor gene polymorphisms and breast cancer risk. *Clin. Cancer Res.*, 10, 5472, 2004.
265. Reichel H., Koeffler H.P., and Norman A.W., The role of the vitamin D endocrine system in health and disease. *New Engl. J. Med.*, 320, 980, 1989.
266. Minghetti P.P. and Norman A.W., 1,25$(OH)_2$-vitamin D_3 receptors: Gene regulation and genetic circuitry. *FASEB J.*, 2, 3043, 1988.
267. Norman A.W. and Collins E.D., Vitamin D and gene expression. In: *Nutrient–Gene Interactions in Health and Disease*, Eds. Moussa N.N. and Berdanier C., p. 348. CRC Press, Orlando, FL, 2001.
268. Peacock M. and Heyburn P.J., Effect of vitamin D metabolites on proximal muscle weakness. *Calcif. Tissue Int.*, 24, 78, 1977.
269. Boland R.L., Role of vitamin D in skeletal-muscle function. *Endocr. Rev.*, 7, 434, 1986.
270. Rabie A., Brehier A., Intrator S., Clavel M.C., Parkes C.O., Legrand C., and Thomasset M., Thyroid state and cholecalcin (calcium-binding protein) in cerebellum of the developing rat. *Dev. Brain Res.*, 29, 253, 1986.
271. Walters M.R., Wicker D.C., and Riggle P.C., 1,25-Dihydroxyvitamin D_3 receptors identified in the rat heart. *J. Mol. Cell. Cardiol.*, 18, 67, 1986.
272. Merke J., Hofmann W., Goldschm D., and Ritz E., Demonstration of 1,25$(OH)_2$ vitamin D_3 receptors and actions in vascular smooth-muscle cells in vitro. *Calcif. Tissue Int.*, 41, 112, 1987.

273. Boland R., Norman A.W., Ritz E., and Hasselbach W., Presence of a 1,25-dihydroxyvitamin D_3 receptor in chick skeletal muscle myoblasts. *Biochem. Biophys. Res. Commun.*, 128, 305, 1992.
274. Demay M., Muscle: A nontraditional 1,25-dihydroxyvitamin D target tissue exhibiting classic hormone-dependent vitamin D receptor actions. *Endocrinology*, 144, 5135, 2003.
275. Endo I., Inoue D., Mitsui T., Umaki Y., Akaike M., Yoshizawa T., Kato S., and Matsumoto T., Deletion of vitamin D receptor gene in mice results in abnormal skeletal muscle development with deregulated expression of myoregulatory transcription factors. *Endocrinology*, 144, 5138, 2003.
276. Buitrago C., Vazquez G., De Boland A.R., and Boland R., The vitamin D receptor mediates rapid changes in muscle protein tyrosine phosphorylation induced by $1,25(OH)_2D_3$. *Biochem. Biophys. Res. Commun.*, 289, 1150, 2001.
277. Chen C.H., Sakai Y., and Demay M.B., Targeting expression of the human vitamin D receptor to the keratinocytes of vitamin D receptor null mice prevents alopecia. *Endocrinology*, 142, 5386, 2001.
278. Stumpf W.E., Sar M., Reid F.A., Tanaka Y., and DeLuca H.F., Target cells for 1,25-dihydroxyvitamin D_3 in intestinal tract, stomach, kidney, skin, pituitary, and parathyroid. *Science*, 206, 1188, 1979.
279. Hosomi J., Hosoi J., Abe E., Suda T., and Kuroki T., Regulation of terminal differentiation of cultured mouse epidermal cells by 1α,25-dihydroxyvitamin D_3. *Endocrinology*, 113, 1950, 1983.
280. Regnier M. and Darmon M., 1,25-Dihydroxyvitamin D_3 stimulates specifically the last steps of epidermal differentiation of cultured human keratinocytes. *Differentiation*, 47, 173, 1991.
281. Bikle D.D., Nemanic M.K., Whitney J.O., and Elias P.W., Neonatal human foreskin keratinocytes produce 1,25-dihydroxyvitamin D_3. *Biochemistry*, 25, 1545, 1986.
282. Kragballe K., Beck H.I., and Sogaard H., Improvement of psoriasis by a topical vitamin D_3 analogue (MC 903) in a double-blind study. *Brit. J. Dermatol.*, 119, 223, 1988.
283. Kragballe K., Vitamin D analogues in the treatment of psoriasis. *J. Cell. Biochem.*, 49, 46, 1992.
284. Holick M.F., Will 1,25-dihydroxyvitamin D_3, MC 903, and their analogues herald a new pharmacologic era for the treatment of psoriasis? *Arch. Dermatol.*, 125, 1692, 1989.
285. Chida K., Hashiba H., Fukushim M., Suda T., and Kuroki T., Inhibition of tumor promotion in mouse skin by 1α,25-dihydroxyvitamin D_3. *Cancer Res.*, 45, 5426, 1985.
286. Li Y.C., Pirro A.E., Amling M., Delling G., Baroni R., Bronson R., and Demay M.B., Targeted ablation of the vitamin D receptor: An animal model of vitamin D-dependent rickets type II with alopecia. *Proc. Natl. Acad. Sci. USA*, 94, 9831, 1997.
287. Bergman R., Schein-Goldshmid R., Hochberg Z., Ben-Izhak O., and Sprecher E., The alopecias associated with vitamin D-dependent rickets type IIA and with hairless gene mutations: A comparative clinical, histologic, and immunohistochemical study. *Arch. Dermatol.*, 141, 343, 2005.
288. Hsieh J.C., Sisk J.M., Jurutka P.W., Haussler C.A., Slater S.A., Haussler M.R., and Thompson C.C., Physical and functional interaction between the vitamin D receptor and hairless corepressor, two proteins required for hair cycling. *J. Biol. Chem.*, 278, 38665, 2003.
289. Demay M.B., Mouse models of vitamin D receptor ablation. In: *Vitamin D*, Eds. Feldman D., Pike J.W., and Glorieux F.H., p. 341. Elsevier Academic Press, San Diego, 2005.
290. Ishida H. and Norman A.W., Demonstration of a high affinity receptor for 1,25-dihydroxyvitamin D_3 in rat pancreas. *Mol. Cell. Endocrinol.*, 60, 109, 1988.
291. Cade C. and Norman A.W., Vitamin D_3 improves impaired glucose-tolerance and insulin-secretion in the vitamin D-deficient rat in vivo. *Endocrinology*, 119, 84, 1986.
292. Kadowaki S. and Norman A.W., Studies on the mode of action of calciferol (XLIX). Dietary vitamin D is essential for normal insulin secretion from the perfused rat pancreas. *J. Clin. Invest.*, 73, 759, 1984.
293. Cade C. and Norman A.W., Rapid normalization/stimulation by $1,25(OH)_2$-vitamin D_3 of insulin secretion and glucose tolerance in the vitamin D-deficient rat. *Endocrinology*, 120, 1490, 1987.
294. Kadowaki S. and Norman A.W., Studies on the mode of action of calciferol (LIX). Time-course study of the insulin secretion after 1,25-dihydroxyvitamin D_3 administration. *Endocrinology*, 117, 1765, 1985.
295. Kadowaki S. and Norman A.W., Demonstration that the vitamin D metabolite $1,25(OH)_2$-vitamin D_3 and not $24R,25(OH)_2$-vitamin D_3 is essential for normal insulin secretion in the perfused rat pancreas. *Diabetes*, 34, 315, 1985.

296. Gedik O. and Akalin S., Effects of vitamin D deficiency and repletion on insulin and glucagon secretion in man. *Diabetologia*, 29, 142, 1986.
297. Mathieu C., Waer M., Casteels K., Laureys J., and Bouillon R., Prevention of type I diabetes in NOD mice by nonhypercalcemic doses of a new structural analog of 1,25-dihydroxyvitamin D_3, KH1060. *Endocrinology*, 136, 866, 1995.
298. Mathieu C., Waer M., Laureys J., Rutgeerts O., and Bouillon R., Prevention of autoimmune diabetes in NOD mice by 1,25-dihydroxyvitamin D_3. *Diabetologia*, 37, 552, 1994.
299. Gysemans C.A., Cardozo A.K., Callewaert H., Giulietti A., Hulshagen L., Bouillon R., Eizirik D.L., and Mathieu C., 1,25-Dihydroxyvitamin D_3 modulates expression of chemokines and cytokines in pancreatic islets: Implications for prevention of diabetes in nonobese diabetic mice. *Endocrinology*, 146, 1956, 2005.
300. Casteels K., Waer M., Laureys J., Valckx D., Depovere J., Bouillon R., and Mathieu C., Prevention of autoimmune destruction of syngeneic islet grafts in spontaneously diabetic nonobese diabetic mice by a combination of a vitamin D_3 analog and cyclosporine. *Transplantation*, 65, 1225, 1998.
301. Mathieu C., Casteels K., Waer M., Laureys J., Valckx D., and Bouillon R., Prevention of diabetes recurrence after syngeneic islet transplantation in NOD mice by analogues of $1,25(OH)_2D_3$ in combination with cyclosporin A: Mechanism of action involves an immune shift from TH1 to TH2. *Transplant Proc.*, 30, 541, 1998.
302. Sonnenberg J., Luine V.N., Krey L.C., and Christakos S., 1,25-Dihydroxyvitamin D_3 treatment results in increased choline acetyltransferase activity in specific brain nuclei. *Endocrinology*, 118 (4), 1433, 1986.
303. Thomasset M., Parkes C.O., and Cuisinier-Gleizes P., Rat calcium-binding proteins: Distribution, development, and vitamin D dependence. *Am. J. Physiol.*, 243, E483–E488, 1982.
304. Morrow A.L., Pace J.R., Purdy R.H., and Paul S.M., Characterization of steroid interactions with gamma-aminobutyric acid receptor-gated chloride ion channels: Evidence for multiple steroid recognition sites. *Mol. Pharmacol.*, 37, 263, 1990.
305. Bowers B.J. and Wehner J.M., Biochemical and behavioral effects of steroids on $GABA_A$ receptor function in long- and short-sleep mice. *Brain Res. Bull.*, 29, 57, 1992.
306. Burne T.H., McGrath J.J., Eyles D.W., and kay-Sim A., Behavioural characterization of vitamin D receptor knockout mice. *Behav. Brain Res.*, 157, 299, 2005.
307. Kalueff A.V., Lou Y.R., Laaksi I., and Tuohimaa P., Increased anxiety in mice lacking vitamin D receptor gene. *Neuroreport*, 15, 1271, 2004.
308. McGrath J., Feron F., and Eyles D., Vitamin D: The neglected neurosteroid? *Trends Neurosci.*, 24, 570, 2001.
309. Abe E., Miyaura C., Sakagami H., Takeda M., Konno K., Yamazaki T., Yoshiki S., and Suda T., Differentiation of mouse myeloid leukemia cells induced by 1α,25-dihydroxyvitamin D_3. *Proc. Natl. Acad. Sci. USA*, 78, 4990, 1981.
310. Provvedini D.M., Tsoukas C.D., Deftos L.J., and Manolagas S.C., 1,25-Dihydroxyvitamin D_3 receptors in human leukocytes. *Science*, 221, 1181, 1983.
311. McCarthy D.M., San Miguel J.F., Freake H.C., Green P.M., Zola H., Catovsky D., and Goldman J.M., 1,25-Dihydroxyvitamin D_3 inhibits proliferation of human promyelocytic leukaemia (HL60) cells and induces monocyte–macrophage differentiation in HL60 and normal human bone marrow cells. *Leuk. Res.*, 7, 51, 1983.
312. Koeffler H.P., Amatruda T., Ikekawa N., and Kobayashi Y., Induction of macrophage differentiation of human normal and leukemic myeloid stem-cells by 1,25-dihydroxyvitamin D_3 and its fluorinated analogs. *Cancer Res.*, 44, 5624, 1984.
313. Murao S., Gemmell M.A., Callaham M.F., Anderson N.L., and Huberman E., Control of macrophage cell differentiation in human promyelocytic HL-60 leukemia cells by 1,25-dihydroxyvitamin D_3 and phorbol-12-myristate-13-acetate. *Cancer Res.*, 43, 4989, 1983.
314. Rigby W.F.C., Waugh M., and Graziano R.F., Regulation of human monocyte HLA-DR and CD4 antigen expression, and antigen presentation by 1,25-dihydroxyvitamin D_3. *Blood*, 76, 189, 1990.
315. Iho S., Takahashi T., Kura F., Sugiyama H., and Hoshino T., The effect of 1,25-dihydroxyvitamin D_3 on in vitro immunoglobulin production in human β cells. *J. Immunol.*, 136, 4427, 1986.
316. Tsoukas C.D., Provvedini D.M., and Manolagas S.C., 1,25-Dihydroxyvitamin D_3: A novel immunoregulatory hormone. *Science*, 224, 1438, 1984.

317. Rigby W.F., Denome S., and Fanger M.W., Regulation of lymphokine production and human T lymphocyte activation by 1,25-dihydroxyvitamin D_3: Specific inhibition at the level of messenger RNA. *J. Clin. Invest.*, 79, 1659, 1987.
318. Mathieu C., Casteels K., Bouillon R., and Waer M., Protection against autoimmune diabetes in mixed bone marrow chimeras—Mechanisms involved. *J. Immunol.*, 158, 1453, 1997.
319. Decallonne B., van E.E., Overbergh L., Valckx D., Bouillon R., and Mathieu C., 1α,25-Dihydroxyvitamin D_3 restores thymocyte apoptosis sensitivity in non-obese diabetic (NOD) mice through dendritic cells. *J. Autoimmun.*, 24, 281, 2005.
320. Bouillon R., Garmyn M., Verstuyf A., Segaert S., Casteels K., and Mathieu C., Paracrine role for calcitriol in the immune system and skin creates new therapeutic possibilities for vitamin D analogs. *Eur. J. Endocrinol.*, 133, 7–16, 1995.
321. van Etten E., Branisteanu D.D., Overbergh L., Bouillon R., Verstuyf A., and Mathieu C., Combination of a 1,25-dihydroxyvitamin D_3 analog and a bisphosphonate prevents experimental autoimmune encephalomyelitis and preserves bone. *Bone*, 32, 397, 2003.
322. Spach K.M., Pedersen L.B., Nashold F.E., Kayo T., Yandell B.S., Prolla T.A., and Hayes C.E., Gene expression analysis suggests that 1,25-dihydroxyvitamin D3 reverses experimental autoimmune encephalomyelitis by stimulating inflammatory cell apoptosis. *Physiol. Genomics*, 18, 141, 2004.
323. Adorini L., Tolerogenic dendritic cells induced by vitamin D receptor ligands enhance regulatory T cells inhibiting allograft rejection and autoimmune diseases. *Kidney Int.*, 65, 1538, 2004.
324. Wang T.T., Nestel F.P., Bourdeau V., Nagai Y., Wang Q., Liao J., Tavera-Mendoza L., Lin R., Hanrahan J.H., Mader S., and White J.H., Cutting edge: 1,25-dihydroxyvitamin D_3 is a direct inducer of antimicrobial peptide gene expression. *J. Immunol.*, 173, 2909, 2004.
325. Hess A.D., Colobani P.M., and Esa A., *Kidney Transplantation. Diagnosis and Treatment*, Marcel Dekker Inc., NY, 1986.
326. Boissier M.-C., Chiocchia G., and Fournier C., Combination of cyclosporine A and calcitriol in the treatment of adjuvant arthritis. *J. Rheumatol.*, 19, 754, 1992.
327. Fournier C., Gepner P., Sadouk M., and Charreire J., In vivo beneficial effects of cyclosporin A and 1,25-dihydroxyvitamin D_3 on the induction of experimental autoimmune thyroiditis. *Clin. Immunol. Immunopathol.*, 54, 53, 1990.
328. Lillevang S.T., Rosenkvist J., Andersen C.B., Larsen S., Kemp E., and Kristensen T., Single and combined effects of the vitamin D analogue KH1060 and cyclosporin A on mercuric-chloride-induced autoimmune disease in the BN rat. *Clin. Exp. Immunol.*, 88, 301, 1992.
329. Lewin E. and Olgaard K., The in vivo effect of a new, in vitro, extremely potent vitamin D_3 analog KH1060 on the suppression of renal allograft rejection in the rat. *Calcif. Tissue Int.*, 54, 150, 1994.
330. Smith E.A., Frankenburg E.P., Goldstein S.A., Koshizuka K., Elstner E., Said J., Kubota T., Uskokovic M., and Koeffler H.P., Effects of long-term administration of vitamin D_3 analogs to mice. *J. Endocrinol*, 165, 163, 2000.
331. Gibbs R.A. and Okamura W.H., Studies on vitamin D (califerol) and its analogs 32: Synthesis of 3-deoxy-1α,25-dihydroxy-9,11-dehydroxyvitamin-D_3—Selective formation of 6-β-vitamin-D vinylallenes and their thermal -1,5*-sigmatropic hydrogen shift. *Tetrahed. Lett.*, 28, 6021, 1987.
332. Okamura W.H., Mitra M.N., Procsal D.A., and Norman A.W., Studies on vitamin D and its analogs. VIII. 3-Deoxy-1,25-dihydroxyvitamin D_3, a potent new analog of 1,25-$(OH)_2$-D_3. *Biochem. Biophys. Res. Commun.*, 65, 24, 1975.
333. Holick M.F., Garabedian M., Schnoes H.K., and DeLuca H.F., Relationship of 25-hydroxyvitamin D_3 side chain structure to biological activity. *J. Biol. Chem.*, 260, 226, 1975.
334. Johnson R.L., Okamura W.H., and Norman A.W., Studies on the mode of action of calciferol X: 24-*Nor*-25-hydroxyvitamin D_3, an analog of 25-hydroxyvitamin D_3 having "anti-vitamin" activity. *Biochem. Biophys. Res. Commun.*, 67, 797, 1975.
335. Haussler M.R., Zerwekh J.E., Hesse R.H., Rizzardo E., and Peche M.M., Biological activity of 1α hydroxycholecalciferol, a synthetic analog of the hormonal form of vitamin D_3. *Proc. Natl. Acad. Sci. USA*, 70, 2248, 1973.
336. Holick M.F., Kasten-Schraufrogel P., Tavela T., and DeLuca H.F., Biological activity of 1α-hydroxyvitamin D_3 in the rat. *Arch. Biochem. Biophys.*, 166, 63, 1975.
337. Napoli J.L., Fivizzani M.A., Schnoes H.K., and DeLuca H.F., 1α-Hydroxy-25-fluorovitamin D_3: A potent analogue of 1α,25-dihydroxyvitamin D_3. *Biochemistry*, 17, 2387, 1978.

338. Binderup L. and Bramm E., Effects of a novel vitamin D analogue MC-903 on cell proliferation and differentiation in vitro and on calcium metabolism in vivo. *Biochem. Pharmacol.*, 37, 889, 1988.
339. Bikle D.D., Gee E., and Pillai S., Regulation of keratinocyte growth, differentiation, and vitamin D metabolism by analogs of 1,25-dihydroxyvitamin D. *J. Invest. Dermatol.*, 101, 713, 1993.
340. Sorensen H., Binderup L., Calverley M.J., Hoffmeyer L., and Andersen N.R., In vitro metabolism of calcipotriol (MC 903), a vitamin D analogue. *Biochem. Pharmacol.*, 39, 391, 1990.
341. Masuda S., Strugnell S., Calverley M.J., Makin H.L.J., Kremer R., and Jones G., In vitro metabolism of the anti-psoriatic vitamin D analog, calcipotriol, in two cultured human keratinocyte models. *J. Biol. Chem.*, 269, 4794, 1994.
342. Pike J.W., Donaldson C.A., Marion S.L., and Haussler M.R., Development of hybridomas secreting monoclonal antibodies to the chicken intestinal 1α,25-dihydroxyvitamin D_3 receptor. *Proc. Natl. Acad. Sci. USA*, 79, 7719, 1982.
343. Itin P.H., Pittelkow M.R., and Kumar R., Effects of vitamin D metabolites on proliferation and differentiation of cultured human epidermal keratinocytes grown in serum-free or defined culture medium. *Endocrinology*, 135, 1793, 1994.
344. El-Azhary R.A., Peters M.S., Pittelkow M.R., Kao P.C., and Muller S.A., Efficacy of vitamin D_3 derivatives in the treatment of psoriasis vulgaris: A preliminary report. *Mayo Clin. Proc.*, 68, 835, 1993.
345. Nieboer C. and Verburgh C.A., Psoriasis treatment with vitamin D_3 analogue MC 903. *Brit. J. Dermatol.*, 126, 302, 1992.
346. Van de Kerkhof P.C.M. and De Jong E.M.G.J., Topical treatment with the vitamin D_3 analogue MC903 improves pityriasis *Rubra pilaris*: Clinical and immunohistochemical observations. *Brit. J. Dermatol.*, 125, 293, 1991.
347. Trydal T., Lillehaug J.R., Aksnes L., and Aarskog D., Regulation of cell growth, *c-myc* mRNA, and 1,25-$(OH)_2$ vitamin D_3 receptor in C3H/10T1/2 mouse embryo fibroblasts by calcipotriol and 1,25-$(OH)_2$ vitamin D_3. *Acta Endocrinol. (Copenh.)*, 126, 75, 1992.
348. Brown A.J., Ritter C.R., Finch J.L., Morrissey J., Martin K.J., Murayama E., Nishii Y., and Slatopolsky E., The noncalcemic analogue of vitamin D, 22-oxacalcitriol, suppresses parathyroid hormone synthesis and secretion. *J. Clin. Invest.*, 84, 728, 1989.
349. Abe J., Morikawa M., Miyamoto K., Kaiho S., Fukushima M., Miyaura C., Abe E., Suda T., and Nishii Y., Synthetic analogues of vitamin D_3 with an oxygen atom in the side chain skeleton. *FEBS Lett.*, 226, 58, 1987.
350. Jung S.J., Lee Y.Y., Pakkala S., De Vos S., Elstner E., Norman A.W., Green J., Uskokovic M.R., and Koeffler H.P., 1,25$(OH)_2$-16-ene-vitamin D_3 is a potent antileukemic agent with low potential to cause hypercalcemia. *Leuk. Res.*, 18, 453, 1994.
351. Zhou J.Y., Norman A.W., Chen D., Sun G., Uskokovic M.R., and Koeffler H.P., 1α,25-Dihydroxy-16-ene-23-yne-vitamin D_3 prolongs survival time of leukemic mice. *Proc. Natl. Acad. Sci. USA*, 87, 3929, 1990.
352. Zhou J.Y., Norman A.W., Lubbert M., Collins E.D., Uskokovic M.R., and Koeffler H.P., Novel vitamin D analogs that modulate leukemic cell growth and differentiation with little effect on either intestinal calcium absorption or bone calcium mobilization. *Blood*, 74, 82, 1989.
353. Tanaka Y., DeLuca H.F., Kobayashi Y., and Ikekawa N., 26,26,26,27,27,27-Hexafluoro 1,25-dihydroxyvitamin D_3: A highly potent, long-lasting analog of 1,25-dihydroxyvitamin D_3. *Arch. Biochem. Biophys.*, 229, 348, 1984.
354. Inaba M., Okuno S., Nishizawa Y., Yukioko K., Otani S., Matsui-Yuasa I., Morisawa S., DeLuca H.F., and Morii H., Biological activity of fluorinated vitamin D analogs at C-26 and C-27 on human promyelocytic leukemia cells, HL-60. *Arch. Biochem. Biophys.*, 258, 421, 1987.
355. Yukioka K., Otani S., Matsui-Yuasa I., Goto H., Morisawa S., Okuno S., Inaba M., Nishizawa Y., and Morii H., Biological activity of 26,26,26,27,27,27-hexafluorinated analogs of vitamin D_3 in inhibiting interleukin-2 production by peripheral blood mononuclear cells stimulated by phytohemagglutinin. *Arch. Biochem. Biophys.*, 260, 45, 1988.
356. Cunningham J., New vitamin D analogues for osteodystrophy in chronic kidney disease. *Pediatr. Nephrol.*, 19, 705, 2004.
357. Slatopolsky E., Dusso A., and Brown A.J., Control of uremic bone disease: Role of vitamin D analogs. *Kidney Int.*, 61 Suppl. 80, 143, 2002.

358. Elstner E., Lee Y.Y., Hashiya M., Pakkala S., Binderup L., Norman A.W., Okamura W.H., and Koeffler H.P., 1α,25-Dihydroxy-20-epi-vitamin D_3: An extraordinarily potent inhibitor of leukemic cell growth in vitro. *Blood*, 84, 1960, 1994.
359. Zhou J.Y., Norman A.W., Akashi M., Chen D.-L., Uskokovic M.R., Aurrecoechea J.M., Dauben W.G., Okamura W.H., and Koeffler H.P., Development of a novel 1,25$(OH)_2$-vitamin D_3 analog with potent ability to induce HL-60 cell differentiation without modulating calcium metabolism. *Blood*, 78, 75, 1991.
360. Reinhart G.A., Vitamin D analogs: Novel therapeutic agents for cardiovascular disease? *Curr. Opin. Investig. Drugs*, 5, 947, 2004.
361. Stewart L.V. and Weigel N.L., Vitamin D and prostate cancer. *Exp. Biol. Med. (Maywood.)*, 229, 277, 2004.
362. O'Kelly J. and Koeffler H.P., Vitamin D analogs and breast cancer. *Recent Results Cancer Res.*, 164, 333, 2003.
363. Nishii Y., Active vitamin D and its analogs as drugs for the treatment of osteoporosis: Advantages and problems. *J. Bone Miner. Metab.*, 20, 57, 2002.
364. Grzywacz P., Plum L.A., Sicinska W., Sicinski R.R., Prahl J.M., and DeLuca H.F., 2-Methylene analogs of 1α-hydroxy-19-norvitamin D_3: Synthesis, biological activities and docking to the ligand binding domain of the rat vitamin D receptor. *J. Steroid Biochem. Mol. Biol.*, 89–90, 13, 2004.
365. Plum L.A., Prahl J.M., Ma X., Sicinski R.R., Gowlugari S., Clagett-Dame M., and DeLuca H.F., Biologically active noncalcemic analogs of 1alpha,25-dihydroxyvitamin D with an abbreviated side chain containing no hydroxyl. *Proc. Natl. Acad. Sci. USA*, 101, 6900, 2004.
366. Slatopolsky E. and Brown A.J., Vitamin D analogs for the treatment of secondary hyperparathyroidism. *Blood Purif.*, 20, 109, 2002.
367. Verstuyf A., Segaert S., Verlinden L., Bouillon R., and Mathieu C., Recent developments in the use of vitamin D analogues. *Expert. Opin. Investig. Drugs*, 9, 443, 2000.
368. Belsey R., DeLuca H.F., and Potts J.T., Competitive binding assay for vitamin D and 25-OH vitamin D. *J. Clin. Endocrinol. Metab.*, 33, 554, 1971.
369. Committee of Revision, Vitamin D assay. In: *The United States Pharmacopeia*, p. 1756. United States Pharmacopeial Convention, Inc., Rockville, MD, 1995.
370. Vitamins and other nutrients: AOAC official method for determination of vitamin D in milk, vitamin preparations and feed concentrates via the rat bioassay. In: *Official Methods of Analysis of AOAC International*, Ed. Deutsch, M.J., p. 53. AOAC International, Arlington VA, 1995.
371. Vitamins and other nutrients: AOAC official method of determination of vitamin D_3 in poultry feed supplements via the chick bioassay. In: *Official Methods of Analysis of AOAC International*, p. 57. AOAC International, Arlington, VA, 1995.
372. Hibberd K.A. and Norman A.W., Comparative biological effects of vitamins D_2 and D_3 and dihydrotachysterol$_2$ and dihydrotachysterol$_3$ in the chick. *Biochem. Pharm.*, 18, 2347, 1969.
373. Olson E.B. and DeLuca H.F., 25-Hydroxycholecalciferol: Direct effect on calcium transport. *Science*, 165, 405, 1979.
374. Schachter D. and Rosen S.M., Active transport of Ca^{45} by the small intestine and its dependence on vitamin D. *Am. J. Physiol.*, 196, 357, 1959.
375. Kimberg D.V., Schachter D., and Schenker H., Active transport of calcium by intestine: Effects of dietary calcium. *Am. J. Physiol.*, 200, 1256, 1961.
376. Henry H.L., Norman A.W., Taylor A.N., Hartenbower D.L., and Coburn J.W., Biological activity of 24,25-dihydroxycholecalciferol in chicks and rats. *J. Nutr.*, 106, 724, 1976.
377. Christakos S. and Norman A.W., A radioimmunoassay for chick intestinal calcium binding protein. *Methods in Enzymology: Vitamins and Co-Enzymes*, 67, 500, 1980.
378. Miller B.E. and Norman A.W., Enzyme-linked immunoabsorbent assay (ELISA) and radioimmunoassay (RIA) for the viatmin D-dependent 28,000 dalton calcium-binding protein. In: *Methods in Enzymology: Hormone Action*, Eds. Means A.R. and O'Malley B.W., p. 291. Academic Press, NY, 1983.
379. Vitamins and other nutrients: AOAC official methods for vitamin D in vitamin preparations. In: *Official Methods of Analysis of the AOAC International*, Ed. Deutsch M.J., p. 19. AOAC International, Arlington, VA, 1995.

380. Wilson S.R., Tulchinsky M.L., and Wu Y., Electrospray ionization mass spectrometry of vitamin D derivatives. *Bioorg. Med. Chem. Lett.*, 3, 1805, 1993.
381. Ishigai M., Asoh Y., and Kumaki K., Determination of 22-oxacalcitriol, a new analog of 1α,25-dihydroxyvitamin D_3, in human serum by liquid chromatography mass spectrometry. *J. Chromatogr. B Biomed. Sci. Appl.*, 706, 261, 1998.
382. Yeung B., Vouros P., Siu-Caldera M.-L., and Satyanarayana Reddy G., Characterization of the metabolic pathway of 1,25-dihydroxy-16-ene vitamin D_3 in rat kidney by on-line high performance liquid chromatography-electrospray tandem mass spectrometry. *Biochem. Pharmacol.*, 49, 1099, 1995.
383. Higashi T., Homma S., Iwata H., and Shimada K., Characterization of urinary metabolites of vitamin D_3 in man under physiological conditions using liquid chromatography-tandem mass spectrometry. *J. Pharm. Biomed. Anal.*, 29, 947, 2002.
384. Vogeser M., Kyriatsoulis A., Huber E., and Kobold U., Candidate reference method for the quantification of circulating 25-hydroxyvitamin D_3 by liquid chromatography-tandem mass spectrometry. *Clin. Chem.*, 50, 1415, 2004.
385. Horst R.L., Littledike E.T., Riley J.L., and Napoli J.L., Quantitation of vitamin D and its metabolites and their plasma concentrations in five species of animals. *Anal. Biochem.*, 116, 189, 1981.
386. Glendenning P. and Fraser W.D., 25-OH-vitamin D assays. *J. Clin. Endocrinol. Metab.*, 90, 3129, 2005.
387. Binkley N., Krueger D., Cowgill C.S., Plum L., Lake E., Hansen K.E., DeLuca H.F., and Drezner M.K., Assay variation confounds the diagnosis of hypovitaminosis D: A call for standardization. *J. Clin. Endocrinol. Metab*, 89, 3152, 2004.
388. Shimada K., Mitamura K., Kitama N., and Kawasaki M., Determination of 25-hydroxyvitamin D_3 in human plasma by reversed-phase high-performance liquid chromatography with ultraviolet detection. *J. Chromatogr. B Biomed. Sci. Appl.*, 689, 409, 1997.
389. Frolich A., Storm T., and Thode J., Does the plasma concentration of 25-hydroxyvitamin D determine the level of 1,25-dihydroxyvitamin D in primary hyperparathyroidism? *Miner. Electrolyte Metab.*, 22, 203, 1996.
390. Mattila P.H., Piironen V.I., Uusi-Rauva E.J., and Koivistoinen P.E., New analytical aspects of vitamin D in foods. *Food Chem.*, 57, 95, 1996.
391. Mata-Granados J.M., Luque D.C., and Quesada J.M., Fully automated method for the determination of 24,25$(OH)_2$ and 25(OH) D3 hydroxyvitamins, and vitamins A and E in human serum by HPLC. *J. Pharm. Biomed. Anal.*, 35, 575, 2004.
392. Turpeinen U., Hohenthal U., and Stenman U.H., Determination of 25-hydroxyvitamin D in serum by HPLC and immunoassay. *Clin. Chem.*, 49, 1521, 2003.
393. Mulder F.J., De Vries E., and Borsje B., Analysis of fat-soluble vitamins. XXII. High performance liquid chromatographic determination of vitamin D in concentrates—A collaborative study. *J. Assoc. Off. Anal. Chem.*, 62, 1031, 1979.
394. Muniz J.F., Wehr C.T., and Wehr H.M., Reverse phase liquid chromatographic determination of vitamins D_2 and D_3 in milk. *J. Assoc. Off. Anal. Chem.*, 65, 791, 1982.
395. Faulkner H., Hussein A., Foran M., and Szijarto L., A survey of vitamin A and D contents of fortified fluid milk in Ontario. *J. Dairy Sci.*, 83, 1210, 2000.
396. Sertl D.C. and Molitor B.E., Liquid chromatographic determination of vitamin D in milk and infant formula. *J. Assoc. Off. Anal. Chem.*, 68, 177, 1985.
397. Agarwal V.K., Liquid chromatographic determination of vitamin D in infant formula. *J. Assoc. Off. Anal. Chem.*, 72, 1007, 1989.
398. Brumbaugh P.F. and Haussler M.R., 1α,25-Dihydroxyvitamin D_3 receptor: Competitive binding of vitamin D analogs. *Life Sci.*, 13, 1737, 1973.
399. Procsal D.A., Okamura W.H., and Norman A.W., Structural requirements for the interaction of 1α,25-$(OH)_2$-vitamin D_3 with its chick intestinal receptor system. *J. Biol. Chem.*, 250, 8382, 1975.
400. Reinhardt T.A., Horst R.L., Orf J.W., and Hollis B.W., A microassay for 1,25-dihydroxyvitamin D not requiring high performance liquid chromatography: Application to clinical studies. *J. Clin. Endocrinol. Metab.*, 58, 91, 1984.
401. Horiuchi N., Shinki T., Suda S., Takahashi N., Yamada S., Takayama H., and Suda T., A rapid and sensitive in vitro assay of 25-hydroxyvitamin D_3—1α-hydroxylase and 24-hydroxylase using rat kidney homogenates. *Biochem. Biophys. Res. Commun.*, 121(1), 174, 1984.

402. Reinhardt T.A. and Horst R.L., Simplified assays for the determination of 25(OH)D, $24,25(OH)_2D$ and $1,25(OH)_2D_3$. In: *Vitamin D: Molecular, Cellular and Clinical Endocrinology*, Eds. Norman A.W., Schaefer K., Grigoleit H.-G., and von Herrath D., p. 720. Walter de Gruyter, Berlin, 1988.
403. Hollis B.W., Comparison of commercially available (125)I-based RIA methods for the determination of circulating 25-hydroxyvitamin D. *Clin. Chem.*, 46, 1657, 2000.
404. Norman A.W., Problems relating to the definition of an international unit for vitamin D and its metabolites. *J. Nutr.*, 102, 1243, 1972.
405. Food and Nutrition Board, Dietary reference intakes for calcium, magnesium, phosphorus, vitamin D, and fluoride. Ed. Institue of Medicine. National Academy of Sciences, 1997.
406. Webb A.R., Pilbeam C., Hanafin N., and Holick M.F., An evaluation of the relative contributions of exposure to sunlight and of diet to the circulating concentrations of 25-hydroxyvitamin D in an elderly nursing home population in Boston. *Am. J. Clin. Nutr.*, 51(6), 1075, 1990.
407. Vieth R., Cole D.E., Hawker G.A., Trang H.M., and Rubin L.A., Wintertime vitamin D insufficiency is common in young Canadian women, and their vitamin D intake does not prevent it. *Eur. J. Clin. Nutr.*, 55, 1091, 2001.
408. Vieth R., Why the optimal requirement for vitamin D_3 is probably much higher than what is officially recommended for adults. *J. Steroid Biochem. Mol. Biol.*, 89–90, 575, 2004.
409. Fraser D.R., Vitamin D-deficiency in Asia. *J. Steroid Biochem. Mol. Biol.*, 89–90, 491, 2004.
410. Trang H., Cole D.E., Rubin L.A., Pierratos A., Siu S., and Vieth R., Evidence that vitamin D_3 increases serum 25-hydroxyvitamin D more efficiently that does vitamin D_2. *Am. J. Clin. Nutr.*, 68, 854, 1998.
411. Code of Federal Regulations FaD., Nutrition labeling of food. *Code of Federal Regulations, Food and Drugs* Title 21, Part 101.9. 2003. The Office of the Federal Register, National Archives and Records Administration. Washington DC. US Government Printing Office.
412. Booher L.E., Hartzler E.R., and Hewston E.M., A compilation of the vitamin values of foods in relation to processing and other variants. Circular 638. 1942. US Department of Agriculture.
413. Lips P., Which circulating level of 25-hydroxyvitamin D is appropriate? *J. Steroid Biochem. Mol. Biol.*, 89–90, 611, 2004.
414. Dietrich T., Joshipura K.J., wson-Hughes B., and Bischoff-Ferrari H.A., Association between serum concentrations of 25-hydroxyvitamin D_3 and periodontal disease in the US population. *Am. J. Clin. Nutr.*, 80, 108, 2004.
415. Hanley D.A. and Davison K.S., Vitamin D insufficiency in North America. *J. Nutr.*, 135, 332, 2005.
416. Bischoff-Ferrari H.A., Zhang Y., Kiel D.P., and Felson D.T., Positive association between serum 25-hydroxyvitamin D level and bone density in osteoarthritis. *Arthritis Rheum.*, 53, 821, 2005.
417. Islam M.Z., Akhtaruzzaman M., and Lamberg-Allardt C., Hypovitaminosis D is common in both veiled and nonveiled Bangladeshi women. *Asia Pac. J. Clin. Nutr.*, 15, 81, 2006.
418. Hollis B.W., Circulating 25-hydroxyvitamin D levels indicative of vitamin D sufficiency: Implications for establishing a new effective dietary intake recommendation for vitamin D. *J. Nutr.*, 135, 317, 2005.
419. Calvo M.S., Whiting S.J., and Barton C.N., Vitamin D intake: A global perspective of current status. *J. Nutr.*, 135, 310, 2005.
420. Whiting S.J. and Calvo M.S., Dietary recommendations for vitamin D: A critical need for functional end points to establish an estimated average requirement. *J. Nutr.*, 135, 304, 2005.
421. Dawson-Hughes B., Heaney R.P., Holick M.F., Lips P., Meunier P.J., and Vieth R., Estimates of optimal vitamin D status. *Osteoporos. Int.*, 16, 713, 2005.
422. Soares J.H., McLoughlin C.M., Swerdel M.R., and Bossard E., Effects of hydroxyl vitamin D metabolites on the mineralization of egg shells and bones. pp. 85–92, Proceedings of the Maryland Nutrition Conference. University of Maryland, College Park, MD, 1994.
423. Bar A., Striem S., Rosenberg J., and Hurwitz S., Egg shell quality and cholecalciferol metabolism in aged laying hens. *J. Nutr.*, 118, 1018, 1988.
424. Jacobus C.H., Holick M.F., Shao Q., Chen T.C., Holm I.A., Kolodny J.M., Fuleihan G.E., and Seely E.W., Hypervitaminosis D associated with drinking milk. *New Engl. J. Med.*, 326, 1173, 1992.

425. Vieth R., Pinto T.R., Reen B.S., and Wong M.M., Vitamin D poisoning by table sugar. *Lancet*, 359, 672, 2002.
426. Counts S.J., Baylink D.J., Shen F.-H., Sherrard D.J., and Hickman R.O., Vitamin D intoxication in an anephric child. *Ann. Intern. Med.*, 82, 196, 1975.
427. Pettifor J.M., Bikle D.D., Cavaleros M., Zachen D., Kamdar M.C., and Ross F.P., Serum levels of free 1,25-dihydroxyvitamin D in vitamin D toxicity. *Ann. Intern. Med.*, 122, 511, 1995.
428. Hughes M.R., Baylink D.J., Jones P.G., and Haussler M.R., Radioligand receptor assay for 25-hydroxyvitamin D_2/D_3 and 1α,25-dihydroxyvitamin D_2/D_3. *J. Clin. Invest.*, 58, 61, 1976.
429. Gertner J.M. and Domenech M., 25-Hydroxyvitamin D levels in patients treated with high-dosage ergo- and cholecalciferol. *Clin. Path.*, 30, 144, 1977.
430. Morrissey R.L., Cohn R.M., Empson R.N., Greene H.L., Taunton O.D., and Ziporin Z.Z., Relative toxicity and metabolic effects of cholecalciferol and 25-hydroxycholecalcifrol in chicks. *J. Nutr.*, 107, 1027, 1977.
431. Coburn J.W. and Brautbar N., Disease states in man related to vitamin D. In: *Vitamin D: Molecular Biology and Clinical Nutrition*, Ed. Norman A.W., p. 515. Marcel Dekker, NY, 1980.
432. Klein G.L., Targoff C.M., Ament M.E., Sherrard D.J., Bluestone R., Young J.H., Norman A.W., and Coburn J.W., Bone disease associated with total parenteral nutrition. *Lancet*, 15, 1041, 1980.
433. Maesaka J.K., Batuman V., Pablo N.C., and Shakamuri S., Elevated 1,25-dihydroxyvitamin D levels: Occurrence with sarcoidosis with end-stage renal disease. *Arch. Intern. Med.*, 142, 1206, 1982.
434. Reichel H., Koeffler H.P., Barbers R., and Norman A.W., Regulation of 1,25-dihydroxyvitamin D_3 production by cultured alveolar macrophages from normal human donors and from patients with pulmonary sarcoidosis. *J. Clin. Endocrinol. Metab.*, 65, 1201, 1987.
435. Epstein S., Stern P.H., Bell N.H., Dowdeswell I., and Turner R.T., Evidence for abnormal regulation of circulating 1α,25-dihydroxyvitamin D in patients with pulmonary tuberculosis and normal calcium metabolism. *Calcif. Tissue Int.*, 36, 541, 1984.
436. Liu P.T., Stenger S., Li H., Wenzel L., Tan B.H., Krutzik S.R., Ochoa M.T., Schauber J., Wu K., Meinken C., Kamen D.L., Wagner M., Bals R., Steinmeyer A., Zugel U., Gallo R.L., Eisenberg D., Hewison M., Hollis B.W., Adams J.S., Bloom B.R., and Modlin R.L., Toll-like receptor triggering of a vitamin D-mediated human antimicrobial response. *Science*, 311, 1770, 2006.
437. Hoffman V.N. and Korzenio O.M., Leprosy, hypercalcemia, and elevated serum calcitriol levels. *Ann. Intern. Med.*, 105, 890, 1986.
438. Mudde A.H., Van Den Berg H., Boshuis P.G., Breedveld F.C., Markusse H.M., Kluin P.M., Bijvoet O.L., and Papapoulos S.E., Ectopic production of 1,25-dihydroxyvitamin D by β-cell lymphoma as a cause of hypercalcemia. *Cancer*, 59, 1543, 1987.
439. Fitness J., Floyd S., Warndorff D.K., Sichali L., Mwaungulu L., Crampin A.C., Fine P.E., and Hill A.V., Large-scale candidate gene study of leprosy susceptibility in the Karonga district of northern Malawi. *Am. J. Trop. Med. Hyg.*, 71, 330, 2004.
440. Avioli L.V., Lee S.W., McDonald J.E., Lund J., and DeLuca H.F., Metabolism of vitamin D_3-^3H in human subjects: Distribution in blood, bile, feces, and urine. *J. Clin. Invest.*, 46, 983, 1967.
441. Haddad J.G. and Chyu K.J., Competitive protein-binding radioassay for 25-hydroxycholecalciferol. *J. Clin. Endocrinol. Metab.*, 33, 992, 1971.
442. Christiansen C., Christiansen M.S., Melsen F., Rodbro P., and DeLuca H.F., Mineral metabolism in chronic renal failure with special reference to serum concentrations of $1,25(OH)_2D$ and $24,25(OH)_2D$. *Clin. Nephr.*, 15, 18, 1981.
443. Mawer E.B., Taylor C.M., Backhouse J., Lumb G.A., and Stanbury S.W., Failure of formation of 1,25-dihydroxycholecalciferol in chronic renal insufficiency. *Lancet*, 1, 626, 1973.
444. Coburn J.W., Koppel M.H., Brickman A.S., and Massry S.G., Study of intestinal absorption of calcium in patients with renal failure. *Kidney Int.*, 3, 264, 1973.
445. Brickman A.S., Coburn J.W., Norman A.W., and Massry S.G., Short-term effects of 1,25-dihydroxycholecalciferol on disordered calcium metabolism of renal failure. *Am. J. Med.*, 57, 28, 1974.
446. Haussler M.R., Baylink D.J., Hughes M.R., Brumbaugh P.F., Wergedal J.E., Shen F.H., Nielsen R.L., Counts S.J., Bursac K.M., and McCain T.A., The assay of 1α,25-dihydroxyvitamin D_3: Physiologic and pathologic modulation of circulating hormone levels. *Clin. Endocrinology*, 5 Suppl., 151S, 1976.

447. Brickman A.S., Jowsey J., Sherrard D.J., Friedman G., Singer F.R., Baylink D.J., Maloney N., Massry S.G., Norman A.W., and Coburn J.W., Therapy with 1,25-dihydroxyvitamin D_3 in the management of renal osteodystrophy. In: *Vitamin D and Problems Related to Uremic Bone Disease*, Eds. Norman A.W., Schaefer K., Grigoleit H.G., von Herrath D., and Ritz E., p. 241. Walter de Gruyter, Berlin, 1975.
448. Akerstrom G. and Hellman P., Primary hyperparathyroidism. *Curr. Opin. Oncol.*, 16, 1, 2004.
449. Lund B., Sorensen O.H., Lund Bi., Bishop J.E., and Norman A.W., Vitamin D metabolism in hypoparathyroidism. *J. Clin. Endocrinol. Metab.*, 51, 606, 1980.
450. Reichel H. and Norman A.W., Systemic effects of vitamin D. *Ann. Rev. Med.*, 40, 71, 1989.
451. Nagpal S., Lu J., and Boehm M.F., Vitamin D analogs: Mechanism of action and therapeutic applications. *Curr. Med. Chem.*, 8, 1661, 2001.
452. Winters R.W., Graham J.B., Williams T.F., McFalls V.W., and Burnett C.H., A genetic study of familial hypophosphatemia and vitamin D resistant rickets with a review of the literature. *Medicine*, 37, 97, 1958.
453. Brickman A.S., Coburn J.W., Kurokawa K., Bethune J.E., Harrison H.E., and Norman A.W., Actions of 1,25-dihydroxycholecalciferol in patients with hypophosphatemic vitamin D-resistant rickets. *New Engl. J. Med.*, 289, 495, 1973.
454. Nesbitt T., Coffman T.M., Griffiths R., and Drezner M.K., Crosstransplantation of kidneys in normal and *Hyp* mice. Evidence that the *Hyp* mouse phenotype is unrelated to an intrinsic renal defect. *J. Clin. Invest.*, 89, 1453, 1992.
455. Strewler G.J., FGF23, hypophosphatemia, and rickets: Has phosphatonin been found? *Proc. Natl. Acad. Sci. USA*, 98, 5945, 2001.
456. Arnaud C.D., Maijer R., Reade T., Scriver C.R., and Whelan D.T., Vitamin D dependency: An inherited postnatal syndrome with secondary hyperparathyroidism. *Pediatrics*, 46, 871, 1970.
457. Malloy P.J., Xu R., Peng L., Peleg S., Al-Ashwal A., and Feldman D., Hereditary 1,25-dihydroxyvitamin D resistant rickets due to a mutation causing multiple defects in vitamin D receptor function. *Endocrinology*, 145, 5106, 2004.
458. Sultan A. and Vitale P., Vitamin D-dependent rickets Type II with alopecia: Two case reports and review of the literature. *Int. J. Dermatol.*, 42, 682, 2003.
459. Ritchie H.H., Hughes M.R., Thompson E.T., Malloy P.J., Hochberg Z., Feldman D., Pike J.W., and O'Malley B.W., An ochre mutation in the vitamin D receptor gene causes hereditary 1,25-dihydroxyvitamin D_3-resistant rickets in three families. *Proc. Natl. Acad. Sci. USA*, 86, 9783, 1989.
460. Sone T., Scott R.A., Hughes M.R., Malloy P.J., Feldman D., O'Malley B.W., and Pike J.W., Mutant vitamin D receptors which confer hereditary resistance to 1,25-dihydroxyvitamin D_3 in humans are transcriptionally inactive in vitro. *J. Biol. Chem.*, 264, 20230, 1989.
461. Rut A.R., Hewison M., Kristjansson K., Luisi B., Hughes M.R., and O'Riordan J.L.H., Two mutations causing vitamin D resistant rickets: Modelling on the basis of steroid hormone receptor DNA-binding domain crystal structures. *Clin. Endocrinol. (Oxf.)*, 41, 581, 1994.
462. Kristjansson K., Rut A.R., Hewison M., O'Riordan J.L.H., and Hughes M.R., Two mutations in the hormone binding domain of the vitamin D receptor cause tissue resistance to 1,25 dihydroxyvitamin D_3. *J. Clin. Invest.*, 92, 12, 1993.
463. Hahn T.J., Hendin B.A., Scharp C.R., and Haddad J.G., Effect of chronic anticonvulsant therapy on serum 25-hydroxycalciferol levels in adults. *New Engl. J. Med.*, 287, 900, 1972.
464. Norman A.W., Bayless J.D., and Tsai H.C., Biologic effects of short term phenobarbital treatment on the response to vitamin D and its metabolites in the chick. *Biochem. Pharm.*, 25, 163, 1976.
465. Jubiz W., Haussler M.R., McCain T.A., and Tolman K.G., Plasma 1,25-dihydroxyvitamin D levels in patients receiving anticonvulsant drugs. *J. Clin. Endocrinol. Metab.*, 44, 617, 1977.
466. Corradino R.A., Diphenylhydantoin: Direct inhibition of the vitamin D_3-mediated calcium absorptive mechanism in organ-cultured duodenum. *J. Clin. Invest.*, 74, 1451, 1976.
467. Jenkins M.V., Harris M., and Wills M.R., The effect of phenytoin on parathyroid extract and 25-hydroxycholecalciferol-induced bone resorption: Adenosine 3,5 cyclic monophosphate production. *Calcif. Tissue Int.*, 16, 163, 1974.
468. Mobarhan S.A., Russell R.M., Recker R.R., Posner D.B., Iber F.L., and Miller P., Metabolic bone-disease in alcoholic cirrhosis—A comparison of the effect of vitamin D_2, 25-hydroxyvitmain-D, or supportive treatment. *Hepathology*, 4, 266, 1984.

469. Barragry J.M., Long R.G., France M.W., Wills M.R., Boucher B.J., and Sherlock S., Intestinal absorption of cholecalciferol in alcoholic liver disease and primary biliary cirrhosis. *Gut*, 20, 559, 1979.
470. Bullamore J.R., Wilkinson R., Gallagher J.C., Nordin B.E., and Marshall D.H., Effect of age on calcium absorption. *Lancet*, 2, 535, 1970.
471. Lindeman R.D., Tobin J., and Shock N.W., Longitudinal studies on the rate of decline in renal function with age. *J. Am. Ger. So.*, 33, 278, 1985.
472. Gray R.W., Wilz D.R., Caldas A.E., and Lemann J., The importance of phosphate in regulating plasma 1,25-$(OH)_2$-vitamin D levels in humans: Studies in healthy subjects, in calcium-stone formers and in patients with primary hyperparathyroidism. *J. Clin. Endocrinol. Metab.*, 45, 299, 1977.
473. Ireland AW, Clubb J.S., Neale F.C., Posen S., and Reeve T.S., The calciferol requirements of patients with surgical hypoparathyroidism. *Ann. Intern. Med.* 69, 81, 1968.
474. Brickman A.S., Sherrard D.J., Jowsey J., Singer F.R., Baylink D.J., Maloney N., Massry S.G., Norman A.W., and Coburn J.W., 1,25-Dihydroxy-cholecalciferol: Effect on skeletal lesions and plasma parathyroid hormone levels in uremic osteodystrophy. *Ann. Intern. Med.*, 134, 883, 1974.
475. Henderson R.G., Ledingham J.G.G., Oliver D.O., Small D.G., Russell R.G.G., Smith R., Walton R.J., Preston C., Warner G.T., and Norman A.W., The effects of 1,25-dihydroxycholecalciferol on calcium absorption, muscle weakness and bone disease in chronic renal failure. *Lancet*, I, 379, 1974.
476. Martin K.J., González E.A., Gellens M., Hamm L.L., Abboud H., and Lindberg J., 19-*Nor*-1-α-25-dihydroxyvitamin D_2 (paricalcitol) safely and effectively reduces the levels of intact parathyroid hormone in patients on hemodialysis. *J. Am. Soc. Nephrol.*, 9, 1427, 1998.
477. Gallagher J.C., Metabolic effects of synthetic calcitriol (Rocaltrol) in the treatment of postmenopausal osteoporosis. *Metabolism*, 39 Suppl. 1, 27, 1990.
478. Tilyard M.W., Spears G.F.S., Thomson J., and Dovey S., Treatment of postmenopausal osteoporosis with calcitriol or calcium. *New Engl. J. Med.*, 326, 357, 1992.
479. Van de Kerkhof P.C., An update on vitamin D_3 analogues in the treatment of psoriasis. *Skin Pharmacol.*, 11, 2, 1998.
480. Midland M.M., Plumet J., and Okamura W.H., Effect of C20 stereochemistry on the conformational profile of the side chains of vitamin D analogs. *Bioorg. Med. Chem. Lett.*, 3, 1799, 1993.
481. Okamura W.H., Midland M.M., Hammond M.W., Rahman N.A., Dormanen M.C., Nemere I., and Norman A.W., Conformation and related topological features of vitamin D: Structure–function relationships. In: *Vitamin D, A Pluripotent Steriod Hormone: Structural Studies, Molecular Endocrinology and Clinical Applications*, Eds. Norman A.W., Bouillon R., and Thomasset M., p. 12. Walter de Gruyter, Berlin, 1994.
482. Norman A.W., Ishizuka I., and Okamura W.H., Ligands for the vitamin D endocrine system: Different shapes function as agonists and antagonists for genomic and rapid responses. *J. Steroid Biochem. Mol. Biol.*, 76, 49, 2001.
483. Norman A.W., Receptors for $1\alpha,25(OH)_2D_3$: Past, present, and future. *J. Bone Miner. Res.*, 13, 1360, 1998.
484. Nemere I., Yoshimoto Y., and Norman A.W., Calcium transport in perfused duodena from normal chicks: Enhancement within fourteen minutes of exposure to 1,25-dihydroxyvitamin D_3. *Endocrinology*, 115, 1476, 1984.
485. Nemere I. and Norman A.W., The rapid, hormonally stimulated transport of calcium (transcaltachia). *J. Bone Miner. Res.*, 2, 167, 1987.
486. Pennington J.A.T. and Douglass J.S., *Bowes and Church's Food Values of Portions Commonly Used*, Lippincott, Williams & Wilkins, Philadelphia, 2004. 18th Edition.
487. US Department of Agriculture ARS, USDA Nutrient Database for Standard Reference, Release 16. http://www.nal.usda.gov/fnic/cgi-bin/nut_search.pl. 2003. Bethesda, MD, US Department of Agriculture.
488. Whiting S.J. and Calvo M.S., Dietary recommendations to meet both endocrine and autocrine needs of Vitamin D. *J. Steroid Biochem. Mol. Biol.*, 97, 7, 2005.

3 Vitamin K

John W. Suttie

CONTENTS

HISTORY

The discovery of vitamin K was one of the outcomes of a series of experiments conducted by Henrik Dam who investigated the possible essential role of cholesterol in the diet of the chick. Dam [1] noted that chicks ingesting diets that had been extracted with nonpolar solvents to remove the sterols developed subdural or muscular hemorrhages and blood taken from these animals clotted slowly. Subsequently, McFarlane et al. [2] described a clotting defect seen when chicks were fed ether-extracted fish or meat meal, and Holst and Halbrook [3] observed scurvy-like symptoms including internal and external hemorrhages in chicks fed fish meal and yeast as a protein source. Studies in a number of laboratories soon demonstrated that this disease could not be cured by the administration of any of the known vitamins. Dam continued to study the distribution and lipid solubility of the active component in vegetable and animal sources and in 1935 proposed [4,5] that the antihemorrhagic vitamin of the chick was a new fat-soluble vitamin, which he called vitamin K. Not only was K the first letter of the alphabet that was not used to describe an existing or postulated vitamin activity at that time, but it was also the first letter of the German word *koagulation*. Dam's reported discovery of a new vitamin was closely followed by an independent report of Almquist and Stokstad [6,7] describing their success in curing the hemorrhagic disease with ether extracts of alfalfa and clearly pointing out that microbial action in fish meal and bran preparations could also lead to the development of antihemorrhagic activity.

A number of groups were involved in the attempts to isolate and characterize this new vitamin, and Dam's collaboration with Karrer of the University of Zurich resulted in the isolation of the vitamin from alfalfa as a yellow oil. Subsequent studies soon established that the active principle was a quinone and vitamin K_1 was characterized as 2-methyl-3-phytyl-1,4-naphthoquinone and synthesized by MacCorquodale et al. in St. Louis [8]. Their identification was confirmed by independent synthesis of this compound by Karrer et al. [9], Almquist and Klose [10], and Fieser [11]. The Doisy group also isolated a form of the vitamin from putrified fish meal, which in contrast to the oil isolated from alfalfa was a crystalline product. Subsequent studies demonstrated that this compound called vitamin K_2, contained an unsaturated side chain at the 3-position of the naphthoquinone ring. Early investigators recognized that sources of this form of the vitamin, such as putrified fish meal, contained a number of different vitamins of the K_2 series with differing chain length polyprenyl groups at the 3-position. The 1943 Nobel Prize in Physiology and Medicine was awarded to Dam and Doisy, and much of the early history of the discovery of vitamin K has been reviewed by them [12,13] and others [14,15].

CHEMISTRY

ISOLATION

Vitamin K can be isolated from biological material by standard methods used to obtain physiologically active lipids. The isolation is always complicated by the small amount of desired product in the initial extracts. Initial extractions are usually made with the use of some type of dehydrating conditions, such as chloroform–methanol, or by first grinding the wet tissue with anhydrous sodium sulfate and then extracting it with acetone followed by hexane or ether. Large samples (kilogram quantities) of tissues can be extracted with acetone alone, and this extract can be partitioned between water and hexane to obtain the crude vitamin. Small samples, such as in vitro incubation mixtures or buffered subcellular fractions, can be effectively extracted by shaking the aqueous suspension with a mixture of isopropanol and hexane. The phases can be separated by centrifugation and the upper layer analyzed directly.

Methods for the efficient extraction of vitamin K from various food matrices have been developed [16], and rather extensive databases of the vitamin K content of foods are now available.

Crude nonpolar solvent extracts of tissues contain large amounts of contaminating lipid in addition to the desired vitamin. Further purification and identification of vitamin K in this extract can be facilitated by a preliminary fractionation of the crude lipid extract on hydrated silicic acid [17]. A number of the forms of the vitamin can be separated from each other and from other lipids by reversed-phase partition chromatography, as described by Matschiner and Taggart [18]. These general procedures appear to extract the majority of vitamin K from tissues. Following separation of the total vitamin K fraction from much of the contaminated lipid, the various forms of the vitamin can be separated by the procedures described in the section Analytical Procedures and Vitamin K Content of Food.

Structure and Nomenclature

The nomenclature of compounds possessing vitamin K activity has been modified a number of times since the discovery of the vitamin. The nomenclature in general use at the present time is that of the most recently adopted IUPAC–IUB Subcommittee Report on Nomenclature of Quinones [19]. The term vitamin K is used as a generic descriptor of 2-methyl-1,4-naphthoquinone and all derivatives of this compound that exhibit an antihemorrhagic activity in animals fed a vitamin K-deficient diet. The compound 2-methyl-3-phytyl-1,4-naphthoquinone is produced in green plants and is generally called vitamin K_1, but is preferably called phylloquinone. The USP nomenclature for phylloquinone is phytonadione. The compound first isolated from putrified fish meal and called at that time, vitamin K_2 is one of a series of vitamin K compounds with unsaturated side chains called multiprenylmenaquinones that are synthesized by a number of facultative and obligate anaerobic bacteria [20]. The particular menaquinone shown in Figure 3.1 (2-methyl-3-farnesylgeranylgeranyl-1,4-naphthoquinone) has 7 isoprenoid units, or 35 carbons in the side chain and was once called vitamin K_2 but now is called menaquinone-7 (MK-7). Vitamins of the menaquinone series with up to 13 prenyl groups have been identified, as well as several partially saturated members of this series. The parent compound of the vitamin K series, 2-methyl-1,4-naphthoquinone, has often been called vitamin K_3 but is more commonly and correctly designated as menadione. MK-4 is a minor bacterial product but can be formed by animals by the alkylation of menadione or through the degradation of phylloquinone by a pathway not yet elucidated (see section Synthesis of Menaquinone-4).

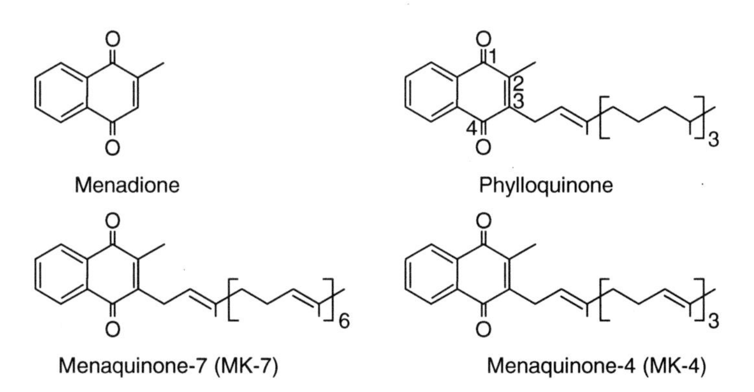

FIGURE 3.1 Structures of some compounds with vitamin K activity.

Structures of Important Analogs, Commercial Forms, and Antagonists

Analogs and Their Biological Activity

Following the discovery of vitamin K, a number of related compounds were synthesized in various laboratories and their biological activity compared with that of the isolated forms [21,22]. Structural features found to be essential for significant biological activity included: a naphthoquinone ring, a 2-Me group on the ring, an unsaturated isoprenoid unit adjacent to the ring, and *trans*-configuration of the polyisoprenoid side chain. The vitamin K analogs illustrated in Figure 3.2 have all been shown to have low or minimal activity relative to *trans* phylloquinone in whole-animal assays.

The activity of various structural analogs of vitamin K in whole-animal assay systems is, of course, a summation of the relative absorption, transport, metabolism, and effectiveness of this compound at the active site as compared with that of the reference compound. Much of the data on biological activity of various compounds were obtained by the use of an 18 h oral dose curative test using vitamin K-deficient chickens. It was found that when administered orally, isoprenalogs with 3–5 isoprenoid groups had maximum activity [22]. The lack of effectiveness of higher isoprenalogs in this type of assay may be due to the relatively poor absorption of these compounds. Matschiner and Taggart [23] have shown that when intracardial injection of vitamin K to deficient rats is used as a protocol, the very high molecular weight isoprenalogs of the menaquinone series are the most active; maximum activity was observed with MK-9. Structure–function relationships of vitamin K analogs have also been studied using in vitro assays of the vitamin K-dependent γ-glutamyl carboxylase, and these are discussed in the section Vitamin K-Dependent Carboxylase.

Commercial Form of Vitamin K

Only a few forms of vitamin K are commercially important. The major use of vitamin K in the animal industry is in poultry and swine diets. Chicks are very sensitive to vitamin K restriction, and antibiotics that decrease intestinal vitamin synthesis are often added to poultry diets. Phylloquinone is too expensive for this purpose, and different forms of menadione have been used. Menadione itself possesses high biological activity in a deficient chick, but its effectiveness depends on the presence of lipids in the diet to promote absorption. There are also problems of its stability in feed products, and because of this, water-soluble forms are used. Menadione forms a water-soluble sodium bisulfite addition product, menadione sodium bisulfite (MSB) (Figure 3.3), which has been used commercially but which is also somewhat

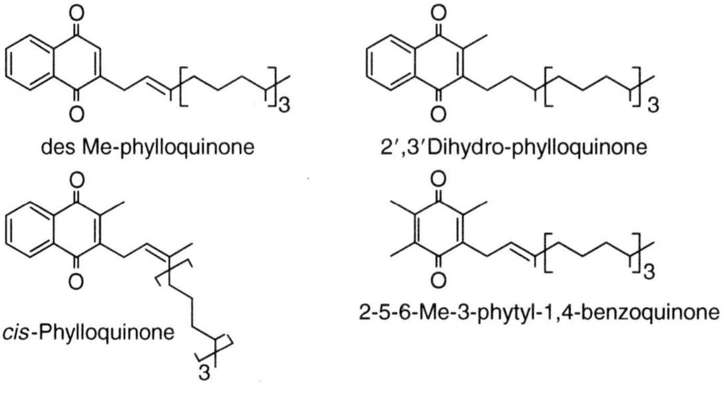

des Me-phylloquinone

2′,3′Dihydro-phylloquinone

cis-Phylloquinone

2-5-6-Me-3-phytyl-1,4-benzoquinone

FIGURE 3.2 Structures of vitamin K-related compounds lacking substantial biological activity.

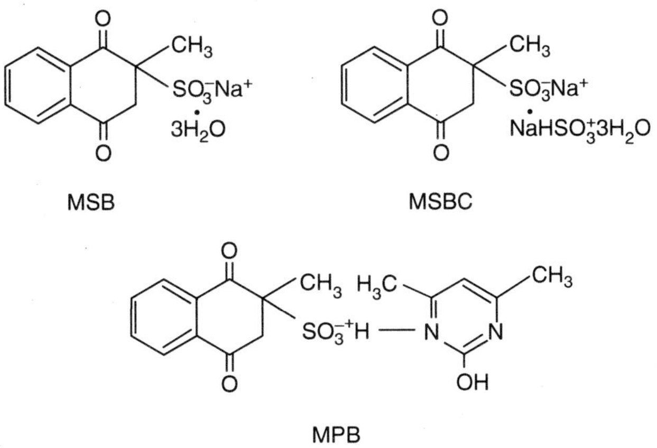

MSB

MSBC

MPB

FIGURE 3.3 Forms of vitamin K used in animal feeds.

unstable in mixed feeds. In the presence of excess sodium bisulfite, MSB crystallizes as a complex with an additional mole of sodium bisulfite; this complex, known as menadione sodium bisulfite complex (MSBC), has increased stability, and is widely used in the poultry industry. A third water-soluble compound is a salt formed by the addition of dimethylpyridinol to MSB; it is called menadione pyridinol bisulfite (MPB) [24]. Comparisons of the relative biopotency of these compounds have often been made on the basis of the weight of the salts rather than on the basis of menadione content, and this has caused some confusion in assessing their value in animal feeds.

The clinical use of vitamin K is largely limited to various preparations of phylloquinone. A water-soluble form of menadione, menadiol sodium diphosphate, which was sold as Kappadione or Synkayvite, was once used to prevent hemorrhagic disease of the newborn, but the danger of hyperbilirubinemia associated with menadione usage (see section Efficacy and Hazards of Pharmacological Doses of Vitamin K) has led to the use of phylloquinone as the desired form of the vitamin. Phylloquinone (USP phytonadione) is sold as AquaMEPHYTON, Konakion, Mephyton, and Mono-Kay. These preparations are detergent stabilized preparations of phylloquinone and are used as intramuscular injections to prevent hemorrhagic disease of the newborn. In some countries, oral prophylaxis of vitamin K has been promoted, and these preparations are not well absorbed. A lecithin and bile salt mixed micelle preparation, Konakion MM, is now available and has been shown [25] to be effective when administered orally. Although not currently used in the United States or Western Europe, pharmacological doses of MK-4, menatetrenone, are used as a treatment for osteoporosis in Japan and other Asian countries (see section Hemorrhagic Disease of the Newborn).

Antagonists of Vitamin Action

The history of the discovery of the first antagonists of vitamin K, the coumarin derivatives, has been documented and discussed by Link [26]. A hemorrhagic disease of cattle, traced to the consumption of improperly cured sweet clover hay, was described in Canada and the United States Midwest in the 1920s. The compound present in spoiled sweet clover that was responsible for this disease had been studied by a number of investigators but was finally isolated and characterized as 3′,3′-methylbis-(4-hydroxycoumarin) by Link's group during the period from 1933 to 1941 and was called dicumarol (Figure 3.4). Dicumarol was successfully used as a clinical agent for anticoagulant therapy in some early studies, and a large number of

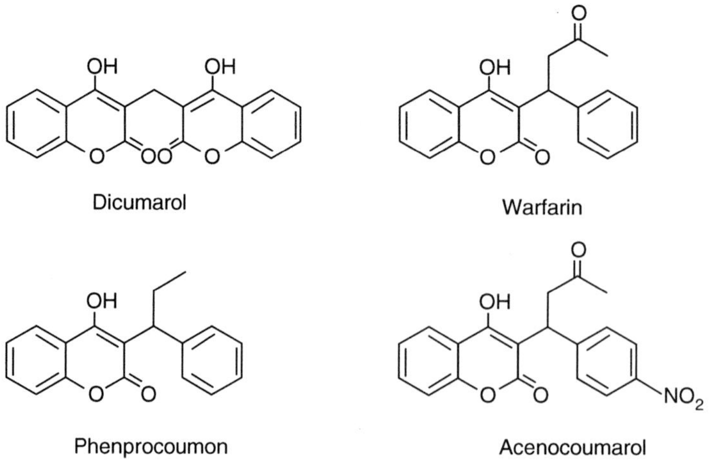

Dicumarol

Warfarin

Phenprocoumon

Acenocoumarol

FIGURE 3.4 Oral anticoagulants that antagonize vitamin K action.

substituted 4-hydroxycoumarins were synthesized both in Link's laboratory and elsewhere. The most successful of these, both clinically for long-term lowering of the vitamin K-dependent clotting factors and subsequently as a rodenticide, has been warfarin, 3-(α-acetonylbenzyl)-4-hydroxycoumarin. Although warfarin is the most extensively used drug worldwide for oral anticoagulant therapy, other coumarin derivatives with the same therapeutic mechanism such as its 4′-nitro analog, acenocoumarol, and phenprocoumon have been used. These drugs differ in the degree to which they are absorbed from the intestine, in their plasma half-life, and presumably in their effectiveness as a vitamin K antagonist at the active site. Because of this, their clinical use differs. Much of the information on the structure–activity relationships of the 4-hydroxycoumarins has been reviewed by Renk and Stoll [27]. The clinical use of these compounds and many of their pharmacodynamic interactions have been reviewed by O'Reilly [28].

Warfarin has been widely used as a rodenticide and, as might have been predicted, continual use led to development of anticoagulant-resistant populations [29,30]. More hydrophobic derivatives of 4-hydroxycoumarins are cleared from the body much more slowly and are effective rodenticides in warfarin-resistant rat strains. Compounds such as difenacoum and brodifacoum are now widely used for rodent control [31] but should be used with care as consumption of carcasses by birds or cats can lead to death.

A second class of compounds with anticoagulant activity that can be reversed by vitamin K administration [32] are the 2-substituted 1,3-indandiones such as 2-phenyl-1, 3-indandione (Figure 3.5). These compounds appear [33] to act by the same mechanism as the 4-hydroxycoumarins, and although they were administered as clinical anticoagulants and rodenticides at one time, they are currently seldom used. Some structural analogs of the vitamin have also been shown to antagonize its action. Early studies of the structural requirements for vitamin K activity [34] demonstrated that replacement of the 2-methyl group of phylloquinones by a chlorine atom to form 2-chloro-3-phytyl-1,4-naphthoquinone resulted in a compound that was a potent antagonist of vitamin K. In contrast to the coumarin and indandione derivatives, chloro-K acts like a true competitive inhibitor of the vitamin at its active site; and, as it is an effective anticoagulant in coumarin anticoagulant-resistant rats [35], it has been suggested as a possible rodenticide. Another structurally unrelated compound, 2,3,5,6-tetrachloro-4-pyridinol, has anticoagulant activity [36]; and, on the basis of its action in warfarin-resistant rats [33], it would appear that it is functioning as a direct antagonist of the vitamin. Subsequent studies have demonstrated [37] that other polychlorinated phenols are also effective

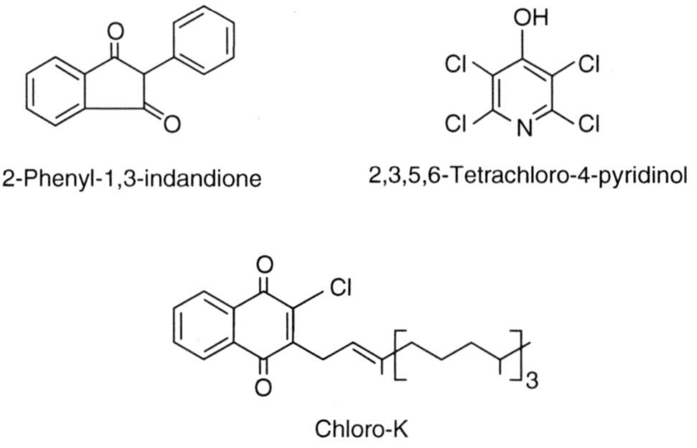

2-Phenyl-1,3-indandione

2,3,5,6-Tetrachloro-4-pyridinol

Chloro-K

FIGURE 3.5 Other vitamin K antagonists.

vitamin K antagonists. Studies of vitamin K antagonists have more recently been studied using in vitro assays and are discussed in the section Vitamin K-Dependent Carboxylase.

Synthesis of Vitamin K

The methods used in the synthesis of vitamin K by early investigators involved the condensation of phytol or its bromide with menadiol or its salt to form the reduced addition compound, which was then oxidized to the quinone. These reactions have been reviewed in considerable detail, as have methods to produce the specific menaquinones rather than phylloquinone [38,39]. The major side reactions in this general scheme are the formation of the *cis* rather than the *trans* isomer at the Δ^2 position and alkylation at the 2-position rather than the 3-position to form the 2-methyl-2-phytyl derivative. The use of monoesters of menadiol and newer acid catalysts for the condensation step [40] is the basis for the general method of industrial preparation used at the present time. Naruta [41] has described a new method for the synthesis of compounds of the vitamin K series based on the coupling of polyprenyltrimethyltins to menadione. This method is a regio- and stereocontrolled synthesis that gives a high yield of the desired product. Analytical methods based on high-performance liquid chromatography (HPLC)/MS or GC/MS have been reported, and methods for the high-yield synthesis of ^{18}O- or ^{2}H-labeled vitamin K homologs have been described [42–44].

Physical and Chemical Properties

Compounds with vitamin K activity are substituted 1,4-naphthoquinones and, therefore, have the general chemical properties expected of all quinones. The chemistry of quinoids has been reviewed in a book edited by Patai [45], and much of the data on the special and other physical characteristics of phylloquinone and the menaquinones have been summarized by Sommer and Kofler [46] and Dunphy and Brodie [47]. The oxidized form of the K vitamins exhibits an ultraviolet (UV) spectrum that is characteristic of the naphthoquinone nucleus, with four distinct peaks between 240 and 280 nm and a less sharp absorption at around 320–330 nm. The molar extinction value ε for both phylloquinone and the various menaquinones is about 19,000. The absorption spectrum changes drastically on reduction to the hydroquinone, with an enhancement of the 245 nm peak and disappearance of the 270 nm peak. Vitamin K-active compounds also exhibit characteristic infrared and nuclear magnetic resonance (NMR) absorption spectra that are largely those of the naphthoquinone ring. NMR analysis of phylloquinone has been used to firmly establish that natural phylloquinone is the *trans* isomer and can be used to establish the *cis–trans* ratio in synthetic mixtures of the vitamin. Mass spectroscopy has been useful in determining the length of the side chain and the degree of saturation of vitamins of the menaquinone series isolated from natural sources. Phylloquinone is an oil at room temperature; the various menaquiones can easily be crystallized from organic solvents and have melting points from 35°C to 60°C, depending on the length of the isoprenoid chain.

ANALYTICAL PROCEDURES AND VITAMIN K CONTENT OF FOOD

Chemical reactivity of vitamin K is a function of the naphthoquinone nucleus, and as other quinones also react with many of the colorimetric assays that have been developed [46,47], they are of little analytical value. The number of interfering substances present in crude extracts is also such that a significant amount of separation is required before UV absorption spectra can be used to quantitate the vitamin. These simple methods are therefore not practical in the determination of the small amount of vitamin present in natural sources. All oral bioassay procedures are complicated by the effects of different rates and extents of absorption of the desired nutrients from the various products assayed. They have been superseded by HPLC techniques and have little use at the present time.

Analytical methods suitable for the small amounts of vitamin K present in tissues and most food sources have been available only recently. The separation of the extensive mixtures of menaquiniones in bacteria and animal sources was first achieved with various thin-layer or paper chromatographic systems [38,46–48]. All separations involving concentrated extracts of vitamin K should be carried out in subdued light to minimize UV decomposition of the vitamin. Compounds with vitamin K activity are also sensitive to alkali, but they are relatively stable to an oxidizing atmosphere and to heat and can be vacuum-distilled with little decomposition. Interest in the quantitation of vitamin K in serum and animal tissues eventually led to the use of HPLC as an analytical tool to investigate vitamin K metabolism [49].

Satisfactory tables of the vitamin K content of various commonly consumed foods were not made available until the early 1990s. Many of the values previously quoted in various publications have apparently been recalculated in an unspecified way from data obtained by a chick bioassay that was not intended to be more than qualitative and should not be used to calculate intake. Tables of food vitamin K content in various older texts and reviews may also contain data from this source, as well as considerable amounts of unpublished data.

Current methodology uses HPLC analysis of lipid extracts, and has been reported [16] to have a within-sample coefficient of variation for different foods in the range of 7%–14% and a between-sample coefficient of variation of 9%–45%. Although green leafy vegetables have been known for some time to be the major source of vitamin K in the diet, it is now apparent that cooking oils, particularly soybean oil and rapeseed oil [50], are major contributors. Human milk contains about 1 ng/ml of phylloquinone [51–54], which is only 20%–30% of that found in cow's milk. Infant formulas are currently supplemented with vitamin K, providing a much higher intake than that provided by breast milk.

The data in Table 3.1 are taken from a survey of literature [55], which considered most of the reported HPLC-derived values for various food items and from analyses of the FDA total diet study. An extensive USDA database containing the vitamin K content of a large number of foods can be accessed at http://www.nal.usda.gov/fnic/foodcomp. In general, green and leafy vegetables are the best sources of the vitamin, and cooking oils are the next major sources. In addition to the data from the United States, there are databases published from a number of other countries [56–58] as well as reports of the vitamin K content of fast foods [59], mixed dishes [60], and baby food products [61]. The major source of vitamin K in foods, and the source usually reported, is phylloquinone. Significant amounts of MK-4 are

TABLE 3.1
Vitamin K Content of Ordinary Foods

μg Phylloquinone/100 g of Edible Portion									
Vegetables		Nuts, Oils, Seeds		Fruits		Grains		Meats and Dairy	
Kale	817	Soybean oil	193	Avocado	40	Bread	3	Ground beef	0.5
Parsley	540	Rapeseed oil	141	Grapes	3	Oat meal	3	Chicken	0.1
Spinach	400	Olive oil	49	Cantaloupe	1	White rice	1	Pork	<0.1
Endive	231	Walnut oil	15	Bananas	0.5	Wheat flour	0.6	Turkey	<0.1
Green onions	207	Safflower oil	11	Apples	0.1	Dry spaghetti	0.2	Tuna	<0.1
Broccoli	205	Sunflower oil	9	Oranges	0.1	Shredded wheat	0.7	Butter	7
Brussels sprouts	177	Corn oil	3			Corn flakes	<0.1	Cheddar cheese	3
Cabbage	147	Dry soybeans	47					3.5% Milk	0.3
Lettuce	122	Dry kidney beans	19					Yogurt	0.3
Green beans	47	Sesame seeds	8					Skim milk	<0.1
Peas	36	Dry navy beans	2					Mayonnaise	81
Cucumbers	19	Raw peanuts	0.2					Egg yolk	2
Tomatoes	6							Egg white	<0.1
Carrots	5								
Cauliflower	5								
Beets	3								
Onions	2								
Potatoes	0.8								
Sweet corn	0.5								
Mushrooms	<0.1								

Note: Values are taken from a provisional table [55] and are median values from a compilation of reported assays.

found in poultry meat and egg yolk as poultry rations are commonly supplemented with menadione, and some cheeses can have appreciable amounts of long-chain menaquinones [62] due to the bacterial action during aging. Using the available food composition data and food consumption data, it is possible to calculate average daily intakes of phylloquinone. Based on the Third National Health and Nutrition Examination Survey (NHANES III) data [63], the adult U.S. male and female intakes were about 115 and 100 μg/day, respectively. This is somewhat higher than some previous estimates [64,65]. Mean phylloquinone intakes in Ireland for adult men and women have been reported to be 84 and 74 μg/day [56], in Scotland 72 and 64 μg/day [66], in Britain 70 and 61 μg/day [67], and in The Netherlands 257 and 244 μg/day [58]. The high consumption of cheese in The Netherlands also provides an intake of about 20 μg/day of long-chain menaquinones. As different databases are used, variations in the assumed vitamin K content of those few foods that contribute the most vitamin to the diet can result in large differences. In a study where four metabolic ward diets were directly analyzed to contain about 100 μg/day, the amount calculated by two different databases ranged from 84 to 160 μg/day [68]. Use of the current database information has, however, made it possible to formulate nutritionally adequate diets that contain only 10 μg/day of phylloquinone [69].

The conversion of liquid oils to solid margarines by commercial hydrogenation results in the formation of substantial amounts of 2′,3′-dihydrophylloquinone, which in the case of some of the harder margarines can exceed the amount of unmodified phylloquinone [70,71]. Because of the large contribution of high phylloquinone vegetable oils to many diets, the amount of the hydrogenated form represents around 20% of the total vitamin K in American diets [72]. Although this form of the vitamin has some biological activity, the degree of this response has not been well established in either human subjects or experimental animals.

METABOLISM

Absorption and Transport of Vitamin K

The absorption of nonpolar lipids, such as vitamin K, into the lymphatic system requires incorporation into mixed micelles, and early studies [73] demonstrated that these phylloquinone-containing micellar structures required the presence of both bile and pancreatic juice. Using an in vitro recirculating perfused isolated rat intestine preparation [74], it was found that the absorption of radiolabeled phylloquinone was energy-dependent and saturable. Normal human subjects were found [75] to excrete less than 20% of a large (1 mg) dose of phylloquinone in the feces, but as much as 70%–80% of the ingested phylloquinone was excreted unaltered in the feces of patients with impaired fat absorption caused by obstructive jaundice, pancreatic insufficiency, or adult celiac disease.

The bioavailability of phylloquinone from different food sources has not been extensively studied, and the results reported are somewhat variable. Phylloquinone in spinach was found to be absorbed only about 15% as well as from a detergent-solubilized preparation (Konakion) when it was consumed with 25 g of butter [76], and less than 2% as well when butter was omitted. A second similar study [77] indicated that phylloquinone in broccoli, spinach, or romaine lettuce, consumed with a diet containing 30% fat, was only about 15%–20% as bioavailable as added phylloquinone. A comparison [78] of the absorption of about 300 μg/day of phylloquinone in the form of broccoli or 300 μg/day added to corn oil indicated that bioavailability from the food source was only about 50% that of phylloquinone in corn oil. Some cheeses and a fermented soybean product, natto, consumed mainly in the Japanese market, do contain substantial amounts of long-chain menaquinones, and there are indications [62] that these forms may be more bioavailable than phylloquinone from vegetable sources. The limited available data would suggest that bioavailability of vitamin K from food is rather low and variable and very dependent on both the individual food sources and total diet composition.

Substantial amounts of vitamin K are present in the human gut in the form of long-chain menaquinones. Relatively few of the bacteria that comprise the normal intestinal flora are major producers of menaquinones, but obligate anaerobes of the *Bacteroide fragilis*, *Eubacterium*, *Propionibacterium*, and *Arachnia* groups are, as are facultatively anaerobic organisms such as *Escherichia coli*. The amount of vitamin K in the gut can be quite large, and the amounts found in total intestinal tract contents from five colonoscopy patients have been reported [79] to range from 0.3 to 5.1 mg, with MK-9 and MK-10 as the major contributors. The total amount of long-chain menaquinones, mainly MK-6, MK-7, MK-10, and MK-11, present in human liver also greatly exceed the phylloquinone concentration, which represents only about 10% of the total [80]. There is some evidence [81] that the hepatic turnover of long-chain menaquinones is slower than that of phylloquinone, which would account for the increased concentration observed, but a major question remaining is how these very lipophylic compounds that are present as constituents of bacterial membranes are absorbed from the lower bowel. Absorption of menaquinones from rat colonic gut sacs has been reported [82], but in the absence of bile no uptake of MK-9 from the rat colon to lymph or blood occurred within 6 h [83]. In the presence of bile, MK-9 is absorbed via the lymphatic pathway from rat jejunum [83]. The oral administration of 1 mg mixed long-chain menaquinones to anticoagulated human subjects [84] effectively decreased the extent of the acquired hypoprothrombinemia, demonstrating that the human digestive tract can absorb these forms of the vitamin from the small intestine but does not address their absorption from the large bowel. However, a small but nutritionally significant portion of the intestinal content of the vitamin is located not in the large bowel but in a region where bile acid-mediated absorption could occur [79].

Menadione is widely used in poultry, swine, and laboratory animal diets as a source of vitamin K. It can be absorbed from both the small intestine and the colon by a passive process [85]. Menadione itself does not have biological activity, but after absorption it can be alkylated to MK-4, a biologically active form of the vitamin.

Absorption of phylloquinone from the intestine is via the lymphatic system [75] and is decreased in individuals with biliary insufficiency or various malabsorption syndromes. Phylloquinone in plasma is predominantly carried by the triglyceride-rich lipoprotein fraction containing very low density lipoproteins (VLDL) and chylomicrons, although significant amounts are located in the low-density lipoprotein (LDL) fraction [86,87]. In a study [88] comparing the transport of different forms of vitamin K, significant amounts of MK-4 were found in the high-density lipoprotein (HDL) fraction, and the half-life of MK-9 was found to be substantially greater than that of either phylloquinone or MK-4. As expected from lipoprotein transport, plasma phylloquinone concentrations are strongly correlated with plasma lipid levels [89,90]. The major route of entry of phylloquinone into tissues appears to be via clearance of chylomicron remnants by apolipoprotein E (apoE) receptors. The polymorphism of apoE has been found to influence the fasting plasma phylloquinone concentrations in patients undergoing hemodialysis therapy [89], and plasma phylloquinone concentrations have been shown to decrease according to apoE genotype: apoE2 > apoE3 > apoE4. This response is correlated to the hepatic clearance of chylomicron remnants from the circulation, with apoE2 that has the slowest rate of removal. Removal of circulating phylloquinone by osteoblasts has also been shown [91] to be modulated by the apoE genotype. Details of the secretion of phylloquinone from liver and the movement of the vitamin between organs are not available. The total human body pool of phylloquinone is very small, and early studies [75] using pharmacologic doses of radioactive phylloquinone indicated that the turnover is rapid. There are only limited available data assessing the disappearance of small amounts (<1 μg) of infused ^{3}H-phylloquinone from human subjects, and these [92] are consistent with a body pool turnover of about 1.5 days and a body pool size of about 100 μg. Other data, based on liver biopsies of patients fed diets very low in vitamin K before surgery [93], indicated that about two-thirds of hepatic phylloquinone was lost in 3 days. These findings are also consistent with a small pool size of phylloquinone that turns over very rapidly.

Plasma and Tissue Concentrations of Vitamin K

Measurements of endogenous plasma phylloquinone concentrations have been available only since the early 1980s. The early history of the development of HPLC techniques to quantitate plasma phylloquinone concentrations has been reviewed [49]. These methods require a preliminary semipreparative column to rid the sample of contaminating lipids followed by an analytical column. The chief alterations and improvement in methodology in recent years have been associated with the use of different methods of detection. Early methods used UV detectors, which lack sensitivity, and electrochemical detection or fluorescence detection of the vitamin following chemical or electrochemical reduction have replaced this methodology. Comprehensive reviews of the procedures used to determine plasma phylloquinone concentrations by both detection methodologies are available [94,95]. The most commonly used methodology at present involves fluorescence detection following zinc postcolumn reduction.

Continued modification of this technique [96] has greatly increased its sensitivity and reproducibility. Although earlier reports of plasma phylloquinone concentrations were somewhat higher, it now appears that normal fasting values are around 0.5 ng/ml (1.1 nmol/L). There is a strong positive correlation between plasma triglycerides and plasma phylloquinone [97], and the variation between samples measured at different days from the same subject is much higher than that for other fat-soluble vitamins [98]. Because of this, extreme caution should be used in attempts to determine vitamin K status of an individual from a single day's sample of plasma. Circulating phylloquinone concentrations do respond to daily changes in intake and fall rather rapidly when intake is restricted [93,99,100]. Although there are very few foods containing appreciable amounts of long-chain menaquinones, they are detectable in plasma, and in some cases have been reported to present at substantial levels [101–103].

Tissue Distribution and Storage of Vitamin K

The distribution of vitamin K in various body organs of the rat was first studied with radioactive forms of the vitamin, using both massive [104] and more physiological [105] amounts of phylloquinone. The liver was found to retain the majority of the vitamin at early time points, but as the half-life in the liver appears to be in the range of 10–15 h [105,106], it is rapidly lost. Studies using radioactive phylloquinone [107] indicated that more than 50% of the liver radioactivity was recovered in the microsomal fraction, and substantial amounts were found in the mitochondria and cellular debris fractions. The specific activity (picomoles of vitamin K/mg protein) of injected radioactive phylloquinone has been assessed [108], and only the mitochondrial and microsomal fractions had a specific activity that was enriched over that of the entire homogenate, with the highest activity in the microsomal fraction. A more detailed study [109] found the highest specific activity of radioactive phylloquinone to be in the Golgi and smooth microsomal membrane fractions. Only limited data on the distribution of menaquinones are available, and MK-9 has been reported [110] to be preferentially localized in a mitochondrial rather than a microsomal subcellular fraction. Factors influencing intracellular distribution of the vitamin are not well understood, and only preliminary evidence of an intracellular vitamin K-binding protein that might facilitate intraorganelle movement has been presented [111].

Because of the small amounts of vitamin K in animal tissues, it is difficult to determine which of the vitamers are present in tissue from different species. Only limited data are available, and they have been compiled and reviewed by Duello and Matschiner [112]. These data, obtained largely by thin-layer chromatography, indicate that phylloquinone is found in the liver of those species ingesting plant material and that, in addition to this, menaquinones containing 6–13 prenyl units in the alkyl chain are found in the liver of most species. More recently, analysis of a limited number of human liver specimens has shown that phylloquinone represents only about 10% of the total vitamin K pool and that a broad mixture (Table 3.2) of menaquinones is present. The predominant forms appear to be MK-7, MK-8, MK-10, and MK-11. Kayata et al. [113] have reported that the hepatic menaquinone content of five 24 month old infants was approximately sixfold higher than that of three infants less than 2 weeks of age, and another study [114] failed to find menaquinones in neonatal livers. Although the long-chain menaquinones are potential sources of vitamin K activity in liver, the extent to which they are used is not known. A study conducted in rats [110] has demonstrated that the utilization of MK-9 as a substrate for the vitamin K-dependent carboxylase is only about 20% as extensive as phylloquinone when the two compounds are present in the liver in equal concentrations. Recent data have suggested that MK-4 may play a role in satisfying a unique vitamin K requirement of some tissues. Most analyses of liver from various species have not detected significant amounts of MK-4. As commercially raised chickens are fed menadione as a source of vitamin K, chicken liver has been shown [112,115,116] to contain more MK-4 than

TABLE 3.2
Vitamin K Content of Human Liver

Vitamer	pmol/g Liver[a]		
	Study A	Study B	Study C
Phylloquinone	22 ± 5	18 ± 4	28 ± 4
MK-5	12 ± 18	NR	NR
MK-6	12 ± 13	NR	NR
MK-7	57 ± 59	122 ± 61	34 ± 12
MK-8	95 ± 157	11 ± 2	9 ± 2
MK-9	2 ± 4	4 ± 2	2 ± 1
MK-10	67 ± 71	96 ± 16	75 ± 10
MK-11	90 ± 15	94 ± 36	99 ± 15
MK-12	15 ± 13	21 ± 6	14 ± 2
MK-13	5 ± 6	8 ± 3	5 ± 1

[a] Values are means ± SEM for six or seven subjects in each study; study A [294], study B [295], and study C [93]. Values from studies A and B have been recalculated from data presented as ng/g liver. NR, not reported.

phylloquinone, and some nonhepatic tissues of the rat have also been shown [117] to contain much more MK-4 than phylloquinone.

Synthesis of Menaquinone-4

Long-chain menaquinones are synthesized by bacteria via pathways that have been well established [20]. It is now well established that MK-4 is not a major product of bacterial menaquinone biosynthesis, but that tissue MK-4 is formed by an alternate pathway. Menadione can be converted to MK-4 by in vitro incubation of rat or chick liver homogenates with geranylgeranyl pyrophosphate [118], and it has been demonstrated [119] that other isoprenoid pyrophosphates can serve as alkyl donors for menaquinone synthesis. Early animal studies [120] also suggested that both phylloquinone and other long-chain menaquiniones could be converted to MK-4. It was originally believed that the dealkylation and subsequent realkylation with a geranylgeranyl side chain occurred in the liver, but it was subsequently concluded that phylloquinone was not efficiently converted to MK-4 unless it was administered orally. This suggested that intestinal bacterial action was required for the dealkylation step. More recent studies [115–117,121] have demonstrated that the phylloquinone-to-MK-4 conversion is very extensive in tissues such as brain, pancreas, and salivary gland and that its concentrations in those tissues exceed that of phylloquinone. Similar distributions of MK-4 have been observed in human tissues [122], and it has been established that high tissue concentrations of MK-4 are more readily obtained in rats by phylloquinone supplementation than by administering MK-4 [123]. Gut bacteria are not needed for this conversion [124,125], and cultures of kidney cells are able to convert phylloquinone to MK-4 in a sterile incubation medium [124]. As both phylloquinone and MK-4 are effective substrates for the only known function of vitamin K, the vitamin K-dependent γ-glutamyl carboxylase, the metabolic significance of this conversion is not yet apparent.

Metabolic Degradation and Excretion

The conversion of phylloquinone or long-chain menaquiniones to MK-4 is a major metabolic pathway of vitamin K utilization in some tissues, but does not indicate ultimate excretion pathways. Evidence for metabolism of the naphthoquinone ring is lacking, and the phosphate, sulfate, and glucuronide of administered menadiol have been identified [126,127] in urine and bile. Studies with hepatectomized rats [128] have indicated that extrahepatic metabolism is also significant. Early studies of phylloquinone metabolism [104] demonstrated that the major route of excretion was in the feces and that very little unmetabolized phylloquinone was present. The side chains of phylloquinone and MK-4 are shortened by the rat to seven carbon atoms, yielding a terminal carboxylic acid group that cyclized to form a γ-lactone [129]. This lactone is excreted in the urine, presumably as a glucuronic acid conjugate. Studies [75] of the metabolism of radioactive phylloquinone in humans indicated that about 20% of an injected dose of either 1 or 45 mg of vitamin K was excreted in the urine in three days, and that 40%–50% was excreted in the feces via the bile. Two different aglycones of phylloquinone were tentatively identified as the 5- and 7-carbon side-chain carboxylic acid derivatives (Figure 3.6). These studies concluded that the γ-lactone previously identified was an artifact formed by the acidic extraction conditions used in previous studies.

The most abundant metabolite of phylloquinone is its 2,3-epoxide (Figure 3.6) formed as a product of the action of the vitamin K-dependent γ-glutamyl carboxylation. This metabolite was discovered by Matschiner et al. [130] who was investigating an observation [107] that warfarin treatment caused a buildup of radioactive vitamin K in the liver. This increase was shown to be due to the presence of a significant amount of a metabolite more polar than phylloquinone that was isolated and characterized as phylloquinone 2,3-epoxide. Further studies of this compound [131] revealed that about 10% of the vitamin K in the liver of a normal rat is present as the epoxide and that this can become the predominant form of the vitamin following treatment with coumarin anticoagulants. Warfarin administration also greatly increases urinary excretion and decreases fecal excretion of phylloquinone [132]. The distribution of the various urinary metabolites of phylloquinone is also substantially altered by warfarin administration. The 7-carbon and 5-carbon side-chain major urinary glucuronides (Figure 3.6) are decreased [133], and other uncharacterized metabolites, presumably arising from the epoxide, are increased. The major degradation products of vitamin K metabolism appear to have been identified and they are apparently formed from either phylloquinone or menaquinones, but there may be a number of urinary and biliary products not yet characterized. Methodology useful for the routine analysis of the two major urinary

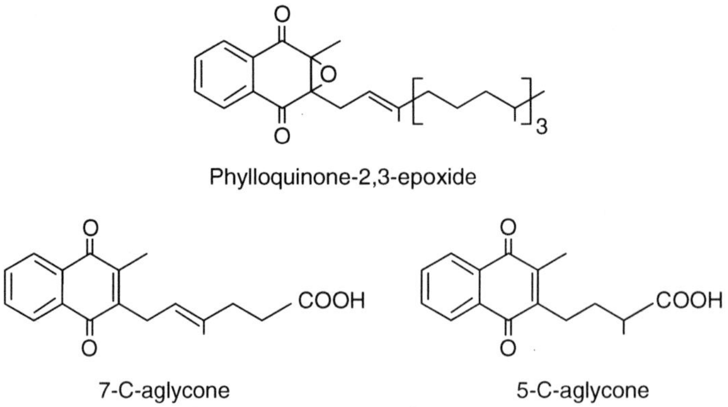

Phylloquinone-2,3-epoxide

7-C-aglycone

5-C-aglycone

FIGURE 3.6 Phylloquinone metabolites. The 7C-aglycone is 2-methyl-3-(5′-carboxy-3′-methyl-2′-pentenyl)-1,4-naphthoquinone and the 5C-aglycone is 2-methyl-3-(3′-carboxy-3′-methylpropyl) 1,4-naphthoquinone.

aglycones of vitamin K has been developed [134], and it has been suggested that quantitation of these metabolites might be a useful noninvasive marker of vitamin K status.

VITAMIN K-DEPENDENT PROTEINS

PLASMA-CLOTTING FACTORS

Soon after Dam's discovery of a hemorrhagic condition in chicks that could be cured by certain plant extracts, it was demonstrated that the plasma of these chicks contained a decreased concentration of prothrombin. This protein (also called clotting factor II) was the first plasma protein-clotting factor to be discovered. It is the most abundant of these proteins and was also the first protein demonstrated to contain γ-carboxyglutamic acid (Gla) residues. Plasma-clotting factor VII, factor IX, and factor X were all initially identified because their activity was decreased in the plasma of a patient with a hereditary bleeding disorder [135] and were subsequently shown to depend on vitamin K for their synthesis. Until the mid-1970s these four vitamin K-dependent clotting factors were the only proteins known to require this vitamin for their synthesis.

The process of blood coagulation is essential for hemostasis and, along with platelet activation, involves a complex series of events (Figure 3.7) which lead to the generation of thrombin by proteolytic activation of protease zymogens [136,137]. The vitamin K-dependent clotting factors are involved in these activation and propagation events through membrane-associated complexes with each other and with accessory proteins. These proteins are characterized by an amino terminal domain which contains a number of glutamic acid residues which have been posttranslationally converted to γ-carboxyglutamyl residues (see section Biochemical Role of Vitamin K). The Gla domain of the four vitamin K-dependent procoagulants is very homologous, and the 10–13 Gla residues in each are in essentially the same position as in prothrombin.

Following the discovery of Gla residues in vitamin K-dependent proteins, three more Gla containing plasma proteins with similar homology were discovered. Protein C [138,139] and protein S [140] are involved in a thrombin-initiated inactivation of factor V_a, a clotting factor which is not vitamin K-dependent, and therefore plays an anticoagulant rather than procoagulant role in normal hemostasis [141]. In addition to the approximately 40 residue Gla domain, the vitamin K-dependent proteins have other common features. The Gla domain of prothrombin is followed by two kringle domains, which are also found in plasminogen, and a serine protease domain. Factor VII, factor IX, factor X, and protein C contain two epidermal growth factor domains and a serine protease domain, whereas protein S contains four epidermal growth factor domains, but is not a serine protease. The function of protein Z [142], the seventh Gla-containing plasma protein which is also not a protease zymogen, was not known for some time, but has now been shown [143] to have an anticoagulant function under some conditions. As these proteins play a critical role in hemostasis, they have been extensively studied, the cDNA and genomic organization of each of them is well-documented [144], and a large number of genetic variants of these proteins have been identified as risk factors in coagulation disorders [145].

CALCIFIED TISSUE PROTEINS

The first vitamin K-dependent protein discovered that was not located in plasma was isolated from bone [146,147]. This 49 residue protein contained 3 Gla residues, was called osteocalcin (OC) or bone Gla protein (BGP), and had little structural homology to the vitamin K-dependent plasma proteins. Although it is the second most abundant protein in bone,

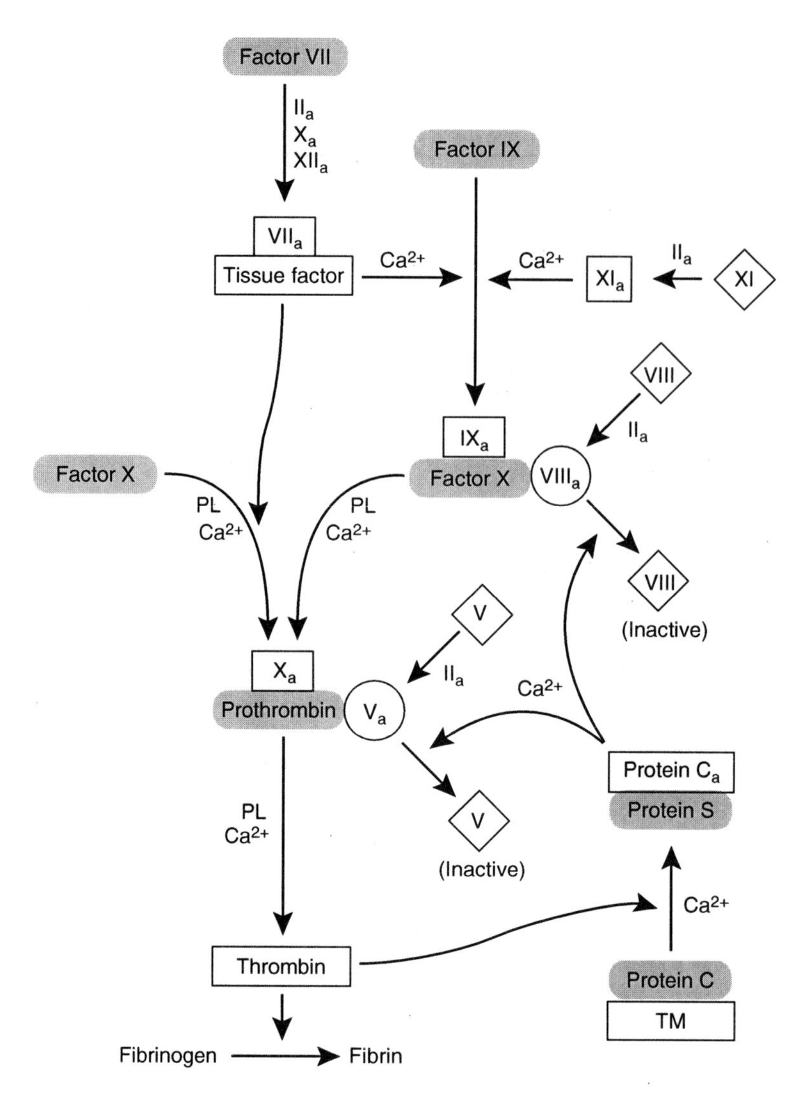

FIGURE 3.7 Vitamin K-dependent clotting factors. The vitamin K-dependent procoagulants (gray ovals) are zymogens of the serine proteases; prothrombin, factor VII, factor IX, and factor X. Coagulation is initiated when they are converted to their active (subscript a) forms. This process can be initiated by an extrinsic pathway when vascular injury exposes tissue factor to blood. The product of the activation of one factor can activate a second zymogen, and this cascade effect results in the rapid activation of prothrombin to thrombin and the subsequent conversion of soluble fibrinogen to the insoluble fibrin clot. A number of steps in this series of activations involve an active protease, a second vitamin K-dependent protein substrate, and an additional plasma protein cofactor (circles) to form a Ca^{2+}-mediated association with a phospholipid surface. The formation of activated factor X can also occur through an intrinsic pathway involving thrombin activation of factor XI and subsequently factor IX. Two other vitamin K-dependent proteins participate in hemostatic control as anticoagulants, not procoagulants. Protein C is activated by thrombin (II_a) in the presence of an endothelial cell protein called thrombomodulin (TM). Protein C is then able to function in a complex with protein S to inactivate V_a and VIII_a and to limit clot formation.

its function has been very difficult to define. Production of the biologically active Gla form of osteocalcin can be blocked when rats are fed a diet containing the anticoagulant warfarin and also given large amounts of vitamin K to maintain plasma vitamin K-dependent protein production. Using this protocol, no defects in bone were seen when bone osteocalcin was decreased to about 2% of normal after 2 months, and fusion of the proximal tibia growth plate was observed after 8 months [148,149]. These observations indicate that osteocalcin is involved in some manner in the control of tissue mineralization or skeletal turnover. However, osteocalcin gene knockout mice have been shown [150] to produce more dense bone rather than a defect in bone formation. Some of the osteocalcin produced in bone does appear in plasma at concentrations that are high in young children and approach adult levels at puberty.

A second low-molecular-weight (79 residue) protein with five Gla residues was also first isolated from bone [151] and called matrix Gla protein (MGP). This protein is structurally related to osteocalcin but is also present in other tissues and has been shown to be synthesized in cartilage and many other soft tissues [152]. MGP has been difficult to study because of its hydrophobic nature, relative insolubility, and tendency to aggregate. The details of this physiological role are unclear, but it has been shown that MGP knockout mice die from spontaneous calcification of arteries and cartilage [153], and arterial calcification has been demonstrated in a warfarin-treated rat model [154]. Although evidence to support a specific function in calcified tissues is lacking, the plasma protein, protein S, which is produced in the liver, is also synthesized by bone cells.

Other Vitamin K-Dependent Proteins

A relatively small number of other mammalian proteins have now been shown to contain Gla residues and are therefore dependent on vitamin K for their synthesis. The most extensively studied is Gas 6, a ligand for the tyrosine kinase Axl [155], which appears to be a growth factor for mesangial and epithelial cells. The physiological function of the protein is not clearly defined, but there are indications of its possible role in nervous system function [156], vascular cell function [157], and platelet activation [158]. Two proline-rich Gla proteins (PRGP-1, PRGP-2) were discovered [159] as integral membrane proteins with an extracellular amino terminal domain that is rich in Gla residues. Subsequently, two other members of this transmembrane Gla protein family (TMG-3 and TMG-4) have been cloned [160]. The specifics of the role of these cell-surface receptors are not yet known. Vitamin K deficiency has been reported to alter brain sphingolipid synthesis [121,161], but the mechanism of the response or the role that it plays in neural function has not been clearly identified [162]. There have also been reports of other peptide-bound Gla residues in mammalian tissues, but no specific proteins have been identified.

Vitamin K-dependent proteins are not confined to vertebrates, and a large number of the toxic venom peptides secreted by marine Conus snails are rich in Gla residues [163]. Vitamin K-dependent proteins have also been found in snake venom [164,165], and the carboxylase has been cloned from a number of vertebrates, the Conus snail, a tunicate, zebrafish, and drosophila [166–168], and has been identified in the genome of bacteria and archaea [169]. The strong sequence homology of the enzyme from these phyllogenetic systems suggests that this posttranslational modification of glutamic acid is of ancient evolutionary origin, and that numerous vitamin K-dependent proteins are yet to be discovered within the wide range of organisms capable of synthesizing this modified amino acid.

BIOCHEMICAL ROLE OF VITAMIN K

Discovery of γ-Carboxyglutamic Acid

A period of approximately 40 years elapsed between the discovery of vitamin K and the determination of its metabolic role. Beginning in the early 1960s, studies of prothrombin production in humans and experimental animals eventually led to an understanding of the metabolic role of vitamin K. Early theories that vitamin K controlled the production of specific proteins at a transcriptional level could not be proven, and alternate hypotheses were considered. Involvement of an intracellular precursor in the biosynthesis of prothrombin was first clearly stated by Hemker et al. [170] who postulated that an abnormal clotting time in anticoagulant-treated patients was due to a circulating inactive form of plasma prothrombin. It was subsequently demonstrated [171] that the plasma of patients treated with coumarin anticoagulants contained a protein that was antigenically similar to prothrombin but lacked biological activity. A circulating inactive form of prothrombin was first demonstrated in bovine plasma by Stenflo [172], but it appears [173] to be present in low concentrations or altogether absent in many other species. Other observations [174] were consistent with the presence of a hepatic precursor protein pool in the hypoprothrombinemic rat that was rapidly synthesized and that could be converted to prothrombin in a step that did not require protein synthesis.

Studies of the inactive abnormal prothrombin [175] demonstrated that it contained normal thrombin, had the same molecular weight and amino acid composition, but did not adsorb to insoluble barium salts as did normal prothrombin. This difference, and the altered calcium-dependent electrophoretic and immunochemical properties, suggested a difference in calcium-binding properties of these two proteins that was subsequently demonstrated by direct calcium-binding measurements. The critical difference in the two proteins was the inability of the abnormal protein to bind to calcium ions, which are needed for the phospholipid-stimulated activation of prothrombin by factor X_a [176]. Acidic, Ca^{2+}-binding, peptides could be isolated from a tryptic digest of the amino terminal domain of normal bovine prothrombin but could not be obtained when similar isolation procedures were applied to preparations of abnormal prothrombin. Stenflo et al. [177] succeeded in isolating an acidic tetrapeptide (residues 6–9 of prothrombin) and demonstrated that the glutamic acid residues of this peptide were modified so that they were present as γ-carboxyglutamic acid (3-amino-1,1,3-propanetricarboxylic acid) residues (Figure 3.8). Nelsestuen et al. [178] independently characterized γ-carboxyglutamic acid (Gla) from a dipeptide (residues 33 and 34 of prothrombin), and these characterizations of the modified glutamic acid residues in prothrombin were confirmed by Magnusson et al. [179], who demonstrated that all of the 10 Glu residues in the first 33 residues of prothrombin are modified in this fashion.

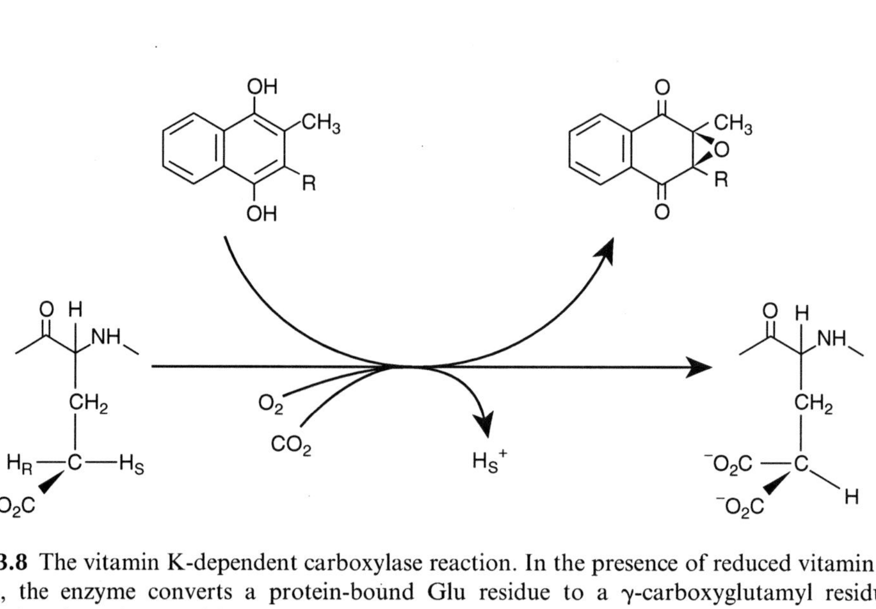

FIGURE 3.8 The vitamin K-dependent carboxylase reaction. In the presence of reduced vitamin K, O_2, and CO_2, the enzyme converts a protein-bound Glu residue to a γ-carboxyglutamyl residue and generates vitamin K-2,3-epoxide.

VITAMIN K-DEPENDENT CARBOXYLASE

The discovery of Gla residues in prothrombin led to the demonstration [180] that crude rat liver microsomal preparations contained an enzymatic activity (the vitamin K-dependent carboxylase) that promoted a vitamin K-dependent incorporation of $H^{14}CO_3^-$ into endogenous precursors of vitamin K-dependent proteins present in these preparations. The fixed $^{14}CO_2$ was present in Gla residues, and subsequent studies [181] established that detergent-solubilized microsomal preparations retained this carboxylase activity. The same microsomal preparations and incubation conditions that fixed CO_2 would convert vitamin K to its 2,3-epoxide [182] (Figure 3.8). In the solubilized preparation, small peptides containing adjacent Glu–Glu sequences such as Phe–Leu–Glu–Glu–Val were substrates for the enzyme [183], and they were used to study the properties of this unique carboxylase. The rough microsomal fraction of liver was found to be highly enriched in carboxylase activity, and lower but significant activity was found in smooth microsomes. These initial studies were consistent with the hypothesis that the carboxylation event occurs on the lumenal side of the rough endoplasmic reticulum [184].

A general understanding of the properties of the vitamin K-dependent carboxylase was gained from studies using this crude detergent-solubilized enzyme preparation, and these data have been adequately reviewed [185–189]. The vitamin K-dependent carboxylation reaction does not require ATP, and the energy to drive this carboxylation reaction is derived from the oxidation of the reduced, hydronaphthoquinone, form of vitamin K (vitamin KH_2) by O_2 to form vitamin K-2,3-epoxide (Figure 3.8). The lack of a requirement for biotin and studies of the CO_2 or HCO_3 requirement indicate that carbon dioxide rather than HCO_3^- is the active species in the carboxylation reaction. Studies of substrate specificity at the vitamin K-binding site of the enzyme have shown that active substrates are 2-methyl-1,4-naphthoquinones substituted at the 3-position with a rather hydrophobic group. Although some differences in carboxylase activity can be measured, phylloquinone, MK-4, and the predominant intestinal forms of the vitamin, MK-6 and MK-8, are all effective substrates. The 2-ethyl and des-methyl analogs of the vitamin have little activity, and methyl substitution of the benzenoid ring has little effect, or decreases substrate binding. The vitamin K antagonist, 2-chloro-3-phytyl-1,4-naphthoquinone, is an antagonist of the enzyme, and the reduced form has been shown to be a competitive inhibitor. Synthesis and assay of a large number of rather high K_m low-molecular-weight peptide substrates of the enzyme have failed to reveal any unique sequences surrounding the Glu residue that are needed as a signal for carboxylation.

Normal functioning of the vitamin K-dependent carboxylase poses an interesting question in terms of enzyme–substrate recognition. This microsomal enzyme recognizes a small fraction of the total hepatic secretory protein pool and then carboxylates 9–12 Glu sites in the first 45 residues of these proteins. Cloning of the vitamin K-dependent proteins has revealed that the primary gene products contain a very homologous propeptide between the amino terminus of the mature protein and the signal peptide [144]. This region appears to be a docking or recognition site for the enzyme [190] and has also been shown [191] to be a modulator of the activity of the enzyme by decreasing the apparent K_m of the Glu site substrate. Although the carboxylase-binding affinities of the propeptides for different proteins differ significantly [192], propeptides are required for efficient carboxylation, and glutamate-containing peptides with no homology to vitamin K-dependent proteins are substrates for the carboxylase if a propeptide is attached [193,194].

The role of vitamin K in the overall reaction catalyzed by the enzyme is to abstract the hydrogen on the γ-carbon of the glutamyl residue to allow attack of CO_2 at this position coupled to conversion of the vitamin to its 2,3-epoxide. A number of studies [195–197] that used substrates tritiated at the γ-carbon of each Glu residue have defined the action and the stoichiometry involved. The enzyme catalyzes a vitamin KH_2 and O_2-dependent, but

CO_2^--independent, release of tritium from the substrate and at saturating concentrations of CO_2 there is an apparent equivalent stoichiometry between vitamin K-2,3-epoxide formation and Gla formation. The mechanism by which epoxide formation is coupled to γ-hydrogen abstraction is key to a complete understanding of the role of vitamin K. The enzyme has been shown to catalyze a vitamin KH_2 and O_2-dependent exchange of ^3H from ^3H_2O into the γ-position of a Glu residue, and this exchange reaction is decreased as the concentration of HCO_3^- in the media is increased. The reaction efficiency defined as the ratio of Gla residues formed to γ–C–H bonds cleaved has been shown to be independent of Glu substrate concentrations, and to approach unity at high CO_2 concentrations [198].

Experiments designed to identify an intermediate chemical form of vitamin K, which is sufficiently basic to abstract the γ-hydrogen of the glutamyl residue, have been a challenge. The most likely hypothesis is that first proposed by Dowd et al. [199], who suggested that an initial attack of O_2 at the naphthoquinone carbonyl carbon adjacent to the methyl group results in the formation of a dioxetane ring that generates an alkoxide intermediate. This intermediate is hypothesized to be the strong base that abstracts the γ-methylene hydrogen and leaves a carbanion that can interact with CO_2. Although the general scheme [200] shown in Figure 3.9 is consistent with all of the available data, the mechanism remains a hypothesis at this time.

A general understanding of the mechanism of action of the vitamin K-dependent carboxylase was gained through studies of very impure preparations. Progress in purifying the enzyme was slow, but the enzyme was eventually purified to near homogeneity and cloned [201].

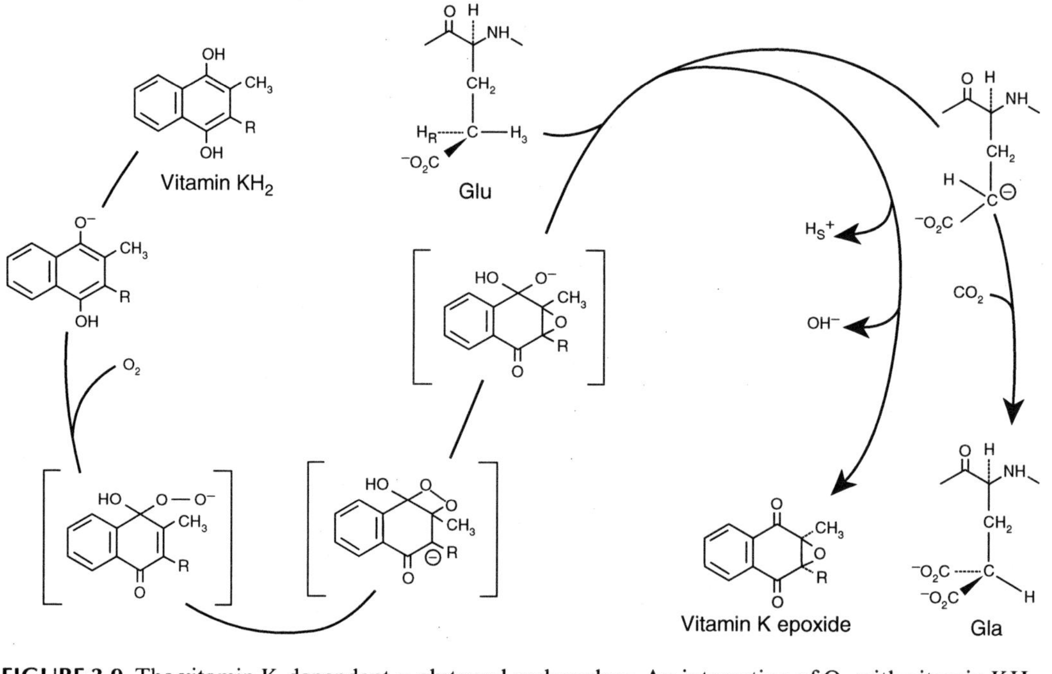

FIGURE 3.9 The vitamin K-dependent γ-glutamyl carboxylase. An interaction of O_2 with vitamin KH_2, the reduced (hydronaphthoquinone) form of vitamin K, generates intermediates eventually leading to an oxygenated metabolite that is sufficiently basic to abstract the γ-hydrogen of the glutamyl residue. The products of this reaction are vitamin K-2,3-epoxide and a glutamyl carbanion. Attack of CO_2 on the carbanion leads to the formation of a γ-carboxyglutamyl residue (Gla). The bracketed peroxy, dioxetane, and alkoxide intermediates have not been identified in the enzyme-catalyzed reaction but are postulated based on model organic reactions. The available data are consistent with their presence.

The carboxylase is a unique 758 amino acid residue protein with a sequence suggestive of an integral membrane protein with a number of membrane-spanning domains in the N-terminus, and a C-terminal domain located in the lumen of the endoplasmic reticulum. It has been demonstrated that the multiple Glu sites on the substrate for this enzyme are carboxylated processively as they are bound to the enzyme via their propeptide [202,203], while the Gla domain undergoes intramolecular movement to reposition each Glu for catalysis, and that release of the carboxylated substrate is the rate-limiting step in the reaction [204].

The membrane topology of the carboxylase has not yet been firmly established. The amino acid sequence of the carboxylase indicates seven hydrophobic regions in the protein [205], and it has been proposed that the enzyme has five transmembrane regions spanning the endoplasmic reticulum [206]. Alternative models of the topology [207] are also possible, and additional data are needed. To generate the strong vitamin K base needed to generate a carbanion on the γ-carbon of the Glu residue would require deprotonation of the reduced form of the vitamin so that it could react with O_2. For some time, the available data suggested that specific active-site Cys residues performed this function, but more recent data indicate that an activated His residue carries out this function during catalysis [208]. Further details of progress in an understanding of the details of the action of this unique fat-soluble vitamin-dependent reaction are available in recent reviews [207,209,210].

Vitamin K-Epoxide Reductase

The degradation of vitamin K-dependent proteins generates Gla residues which are not metabolized but are excreted in the urine [211]. Human adult Gla excretion is in the range of 50 μmol/day, indicating that a similar amount is formed each day. The average dietary intake of vitamin K is only about 0.2 μmol/day, and a mole of vitamin is oxidized for each mole of Gla formed. It is clear that the vitamin K 2,3-epoxide generated by the carboxylase must be actively recycled, and the hepatic ratio of the epoxide relative to that of the vitamin is increased in animals administered the 4-hydroxycoumarin anticoagulant warfarin [212]. This suggested that warfarin inhibition of vitamin K action was indirect through an inhibition of the enzyme called the vitamin K-epoxide reductase [213]. Blocking of the reductase prevents the reduction of the epoxide to the quinone form of the vitamin and eventually to the carboxylase substrate, vitamin KH_2. Widespread use of warfarin as an anticoagulant rodenticide led to the appearance of strains of warfarin-resistant rats [214], and the study of the activity of the epoxide redutcase in livers of these animals was key to an understanding [215, 216] of the details of what is now referred to as the "vitamin K cycle" (Figure 3.10). Three forms of vitamin K (the quinone (K), the hydronaphthoquinone (KH_2), and the 2,3-epoxide (KO)) can feed into this liver vitamin K cycle. In normal liver, the ratio of vitamin K-2,3-epoxide to the less oxidized forms of the vitamin is about 1:10 but can increase to a majority of epoxide in an anticoagulated animal. The quinone and hydronaphthoquinone forms of the vitamin can also be interconverted by a number of NAD(P)H-linked reductases including one that appears to be a microsomal-bound form of the extensively studied liver DT-diaphorase activity. The epoxide reductase uses a sulfhydryl compound as a reductant in vitro, but the physiological reductant has not been identified. Efforts to purify and characterize the protein or proteins responsible for this enzyme activity from liver have not been successful, and a clear understanding of the enzymatic mechanism of the reduction is not available. Recent identification of the human and rat genes for the vitamin K epoxide reductase [217,218] will aid in efforts to more completely understand this enzyme. It is not yet established if the small, 18 kDa protein expressed by this gene is completely responsible for the observed activity, or if other as-of-yet-unidentified proteins of the endoplasmic reticulum are needed to form an active complex [219]. The presence of the identified gene in *Drosophila* and other insects [220] suggests that this activity may be as widespread as the carboxylase. The importance

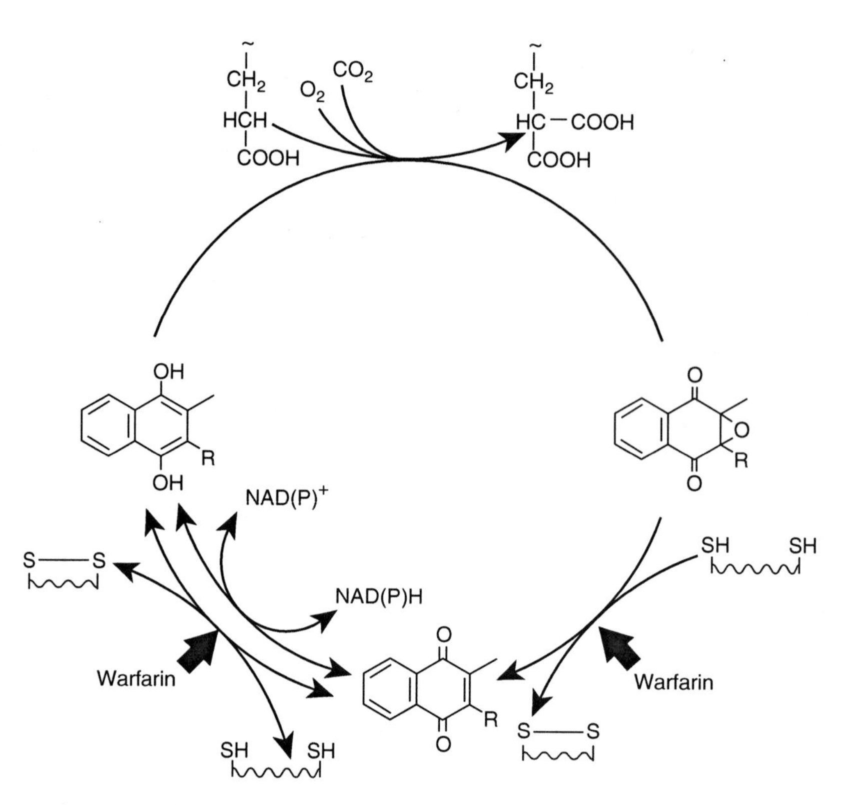

FIGURE 3.10 Tissue recycling of vitamin K. Vitamin K epoxide formed in the carboxylation reaction is reduced to the quinone form of the vitamin by a warfarin-sensitive enzyme, the vitamin K epoxide reductase. This reaction is driven by a reduced dithiol. The naphthoquinone form of the vitamin can be reduced to the hydronaphthoquinone form either by the same warfarin-sensitive dithiol-driven reductase or by one or more of the hepatic NADH- or NADPH-linked quinone reductases that are less sensitive to warfarin.

of the epoxide reductase for the synthesis of vitamin K-dependent proteins is illustrated by observations [204,221] that the production of reduced vitamin K by this enzyme rather than the activity of the carboxylase is the rate-limiting step in the production of these important proteins.

HEALTH IMPACTS OF ALTERED VITAMIN K STATUS

METHODOLOGY

The classical method used to define an inadequate intake of vitamin K was to measure the plasma concentration of one of the vitamin K-dependent clotting factors: prothrombin (factor II), factor VII, factor IX, or factor X. The various tests of clotting function used in clinical practice, which are based on the activity of these factors, have been summarized [222]. Standard tests currently in use measure the time it takes recalcified citrated or oxalated plasma to form a fibrin clot. The standard prothrombin time or PT (historically called a quick prothrombin time) assay measures clotting times in plasma after the addition of calcium and a lung or brain extract (thromboplastin) preparation to furnish phospholipids and tissue factors. Variations of this assay have been developed, and commercial reagent kits are available. The assay responds to the levels of prothrombin and factor VII and factor X, and as factor VII has the shortest half-life, it is likely that these one-stage prothrombin assays often measure the level of factor VII rather than prothrombin. Specific assays for factor VII and factor X are also available but are seldom used in studies of vitamin K sufficiency. A number of snake venom preparations liberate thrombin from prothrombin and have been used [173,223] to develop one-stage clotting assays more specific for prothrombin. The enzymes in these preparations do not require that prothrombin be present in a calcium-dependent phospholipid complex for activation, and they will therefore activate the descarboxyprothrombin formed in vitamin K-deficient animals. For this reason, they cannot be used to monitor a vitamin K deficiency. As the vitamin K-dependent clotting factors are serine proteases, chromogenic substrates can also be used to assay their activity. These assays, when used to assay prothrombin activity, actually measure the concentration of thrombin that has been generated from prothrombin by various methods [223]. Because of their relative lack of sensitivity, these historical clotting factor assays have had little value in determining vitamin K status.

Human vitamin K deficiency results in the secretion into the plasma of partially carboxylated species of vitamin K-dependent proteins. Because they lack the full complement of γ-carboxyglutamic acid residues, their calcium-binding affinity is altered, and they can be separated from normal prothrombin by alterations in their ability to bind to barium salts or by electrophoresis. Antibodies that are specific for these abnormal prothrombins have been developed and can also be used to detect vitamin K deficiency. These assays or similar methods used to detect the concentration of under-γ-carboxylated osteocalcin (ucOC) have greatly increased the sensitivity with which a vitamin K deficiency can be detected [102]. Vitamin K status is also reflected in alterations of circulating levels of the vitamin, but these values are subject to day-to-day variation based on recent intake of the vitamin. The extremely low concentration of vitamin K in plasma made these measurements very difficult at one time, but satisfactory HPLC methods for the determination of plasma or serum phylloquinone have now been developed (see section Plasma and Tissue Concentrations of Vitamin K). The amount of vitamin K found in normal plasma appears to be about 0.5 ng/ml, and limited information on the response of circulating vitamin K to changes in dietary vitamin K is currently available.

Adult Human Deficiencies

The human population normally consumes a diet containing an amount of vitamin K in excess of that needed to maintain normal hemostasis, but a vitamin K-responsive human hypoprothrombinemia can sometimes be a clinically significant response. O'Reilly [28] has reviewed the potential problem areas and has pointed out the basic factors needed to prevent a vitamin K deficiency: (a) a normal diet containing the vitamin, (b) the presence of bile in the intestine, (c) a normal absorptive surface in the small intestine, and (d) a normal liver. Cases of an acquired vitamin K deficiency do, therefore, occur in the adult population and, though relatively rare, present a significant problem for some individuals. It has usually been assumed that a general deficiency in the population is not possible, but Hazell and Baloch [224] have observed that a relatively high percentage of an older adult hospital-admitted population has a hypoprothrombinemia that responds to administration of oral vitamin K. The basis for this apparent increase in vitamin K requirement was not determined and was probably multicausal. Vitamin K-responsive hemorrhagic events have frequently been reported in patients receiving antibiotics and have been extensively reviewed [225]. These episodes have usually been assumed to be due to decreased menaquinone availability from the gut, but it is possible that many cases may represent low dietary intake alone and that the presumed effect on gut bacteria was not related to the hypoprothrombinemia. Some second- and third-generation cephalosporins have been implicated in a large number of hypoprothrombinemic episodes

[226], and it is likely that they are exerting a weak vitamin K-dependent carboxylase inhibition [227] or a coumarin-like response [228,229] which might be more important than an influence on the gut bacterial population.

Experimentally induced vitamin K deficiencies that are sufficiently severe to reduce PT measurements have been rare. An often cited study [230] investigated the vitamin K requirement of starved intravenously fed debilitated patients given antibiotics to decrease intestinal vitamin K synthesis. A significant degree of vitamin K-responsive hypoprothrombinemia was clearly established in these subjects. More recently, a number of controlled studies using diets containing approximately 10 μg/day or less of phylloquinone [100,231,232] have demonstrated alterations using more sensitive markers of vitamin K status, but a clinically significant decrease in PTs was not seen.

Anticoagulant Therapy

A vitamin K deficiency acquired by treatment with oral anticoagulants is a common occurrence. Inhibition of the vitamin K epoxide reductase by warfarin results in the secretion to the plasma of vitamin K-dependent proteins lacking all or a portion of the normal number of Gla residues. The relationship between the concentration of various partially γ-carboxylated clotting factors and the response seen in the assays used to monitor warfarin therapy is not yet clear. The magnitude of the anticoagulant effect produced by a given dose of warfarin varies by as much as 20-fold between individuals and may vary substantially in an individual patient over time. Drug interactions have been found to be responsible for some of this variation, and drugs have been shown to: alter displacement of warfarin from its plasma albumin carrier; induce the hepatic P450 that metabolizes warfarin; interfere with warfarin clearance; or bind to warfarin in the gut. Alterations of vitamin K intake or absorption can also alter warfarin efficacy [233,234], and genetic variability is also undoubtedly important. Polymorphisms of the reductase gene itself [235,236] or of the P450 variant CYP2C9 [237] appear to be responsible for most of the variation in effective warfarin dose. In extreme cases, a genetic alteration of the warfarin sensitivity of the epoxide reductase has been shown to result in an enzyme that is very difficult to inhibit to a desired therapeutic level [238].

The anticoagulant effect of warfarin therapy is monitored by measurement of the PT, a measure of combined procoagulant status rather than a true measure of prothrombin activity. As thromboplastin reagents vary widely in their sensitivity to depressed levels of various clotting factors, plasma from a warfarin-treated patient may yield very different PTs when tested with different thromboplastins. To overcome this problem, the international normalized ratio (INR) is now used as a standardized method for reporting PT results. The INR allows interconversion of PT ratios (patient PT/mean normal PT) by use of an international sensitivity index (ISI) that corrects for differences in thromboplastin sensitivities. The goal of anticoagulant therapy is steady-state levels of vitamin K-dependent procoagulants in the range of 20%–30% of normal, which would be an INR of 2–3 [239]. The most common complication of anticoagulant therapy, bleeding, is directly related to the INR with few bleeds at a stable INR less than 4.0 and a relatively high incidence with INR greater than 7.0. Overanticoagulation can be brought back to the desired level by lowering the warfarin dose, or if severely out of range by s.c. or even slow i.v. infusion of phylloquinone.

Hemorrhagic Disease of the Newborn

Hemorrhagic disease of the newborn or early vitamin K deficiency bleeding (VKDB) occurring during the first week of life in healthy appearing neonates [240] is the classic example of a human vitamin K deficiency. The low vitamin K content of breast milk, low placental transfer of phylloquinone, low clotting factor levels, and a sterile gut all contribute to the disease. Although the incidence is low, the mortality rate from intracranial bleeding is high, and prevention by oral or intramuscular administration of vitamin K immediately following birth is the standard cure. Late VKDB is a syndrome occurring between 2 and 12 weeks of age predominantly in exclusively breastfed infants [52,241] or infants with severe intestinal malabsorption problems. Although oral administration of vitamin appears to be as effective as parenteral administration to prevent early VKDB, it may not be as effective for preventing late VKDB. A report in the early 1990s [242] suggested that intramuscular injection of vitamin K to infants was associated with an increased incidence of certain childhood cancers. This led to a switch to oral administration of vitamin K in some countries and an increase in the incidence of late VKDB. Subsequent studies have failed to show a correlation between the use of intramuscular vitamin K and the incidence of childhood leukemia or other cancers [243,244]. The current recommendations of the American Academy of Pediatrics [245] advise that "vitamin K (phylloquinone) should be given to all newborns as a single, intramuscular dose of 0.5 to 1 mg."

Possible Role in Skeletal and Vascular Health

Osteocalcin, MGP, and protein S are all known to be synthesized in bone. Because of its relatively high concentration in bone, attention has been directed toward osteocalcin as a possible factor in bone health. Small amounts of this protein circulate in plasma at concentrations that are fourfold to fivefold higher in young children than in adults, and reach the adult levels at puberty.

Some of the circulating osteocalcin in individuals within the normal population is not completely γ-carboxylated, and the extent of undercarboxylation can be influenced by vitamin K status [232,246,247]. An immunochemical assay for the des-γ-carboxylated form of osteocalcin is available, but most studies have defined ucOC as a fraction that does not adsorb to hydroxyapatite under standard conditions [248]. Depending on assay conditions and the specific epitopes detected by the assay kits used, the fraction of ucOC reported in normal healthy populations has ranged from 30%–40% to <10%. These data have established that the normal dietary intake of vitamin K is not sufficient to maximally γ-carboxylate osteocalcin, and it has been shown [249] that supplementation with 1 mg phylloquinone/day (~10 × the current RDI) is required to achieve maximal γ-carboxylation. Attempts to link this apparent marker of vitamin K insufficiency with bone health have included epidemiological observations that a low vitamin K intake is associated with increased hip fracture risk [250,251] and reports that ucOC is correlated with low bone mass [252]. These associations do not necessarily imply causation, and they might simply be surrogate markers of general nutrient deficiencies. Patients receiving oral anticoagulant therapy have very high circulating ucOC levels, but attempts to correlate this treatment with alterations in bone mineral density have not yielded consistent outcomes [253].

At present, there is no clear evidence to support a link between increased ucOC and decreased mineralization. When γ-carboxylation of osteocalcin is effectively blocked in a rat model [149], a mineralization disorder characterized by complete fusion of proximal tibia growth plate and cessation of longitudinal growth has been observed. These data suggest that a skeletal vitamin K-dependent protein, probably osteocalcin, is involved in regulating bone mineralization, but does not indicate that low vitamin K status would decrease mineralization. Studies using transgenic mice lacking the osteocalcin gene [150] have demonstrated that the phenotype is increased bone mineralization rather than a decrease of bone mass.

Although near-maximal carboxylation of osteocalcin does not appear to be needed for normal bone mineralization, supplementation with one form of the vitamin, MK-4, is a common therapy for osteoporosis in Japan and other Asian countries. The standard therapy is 45 mg of MK-4/day, a pharmacological rather than a nutritional approach. Positive responses in bone mineral density at specific sites or reduction in fracture rates of postmenopausal osteoporotic women have been reported [254,255], and MK-4 has been reported [256,257] to increase markers of bone formation or to increase bone mineral density in experimental animals or human subjects. The response to administration of a similar pharmacological dose of phylloquinone has not been studied, although supplementation of 1 mg phylloquinone/day to postmenopausal women between 50 and 60 years of age for 3 years has been reported [258] to marginally reduce ($P < 0.05$) the decrease in bone mineral density of the femoral neck. The decrease in mineral loss from the lumbar spine in this study was not altered by phylloquinone supplementation. MK-4 has effects on cultured bone cells that are not seen with phylloquinone [259] and has apoptotic effects on malignant cell lines [260] that are seen by other medium-chain-length menaquinones, but not by phylloquinone. MK-4 has also been identified as a ligand for the steroid xenobiotic receptor in bone cells [261], where it influences the expression of osteoblastic markers. Although most cells appear to obtain MK-4 by synthesis [124,262], it is possible that high doses do have an effect on bone cells that would explain the responses reported. Efforts to reproduce the ability of MK-4 to decrease bone loss have been studied in rat models, with success in some studies [263,264] but not in others [265]. Studies of the efficacy of 45 mg of MK-4 in maintaining the skeletal health of women in North America or Western Europe have not yet been reported, and it is likely that a clear understanding of the influence of vitamin K status on bone health will require substantially more study.

Studies of the MGP knockout mouse indicated that these animals died from massive calcifications of the large arteries within 8 weeks of birth [153], and a rapid calcification of the elastic lamellae of arteries and heart valves has been seen in a rat model in which MGP carboxylation was blocked [154]. Calcification of vascular smooth muscle cells appears to be associated with chondrocyte differentiation and cartilage formation [266], and it has been reported that the ability of γ-carboxylated MGP to prevent soft tissue calcification is mediated through an interaction with cellular growth factors [267,268]. It has been found [269] that mutations in the MGP are associated with the phenotype of the Keutel syndrome, a rare autosomal recessive condition characterized by abnormal cartilage calcification. The action of MGP requires the γ-carboxylated form, and studies of the relationship between aortic calcification and phylloquinone [270] or total vitamin K [271] intake have shown no relationship or slightly lower aortic calcification in subjects with a lower vitamin K intake. A much larger epidemiological study has shown, however, an inverse relationship between dietary menaquinone and aortic calcification, myocardial infarction, and sudden cardiovascular death [272]. There are, however, no data to link a low intake of menaquinone to under-γ-carboxylation. Whether or not individuals with low vitamin K status, or more specifically a low intake of menaquinones, are at risk for cardiovascular disease is not yet clear, and a great deal of additional data would be needed to classify low vitamin K status as a risk factor for cardiovascular disease.

Other Factors Influencing Vitamin K Status

Although it is easily demonstrated that the vitamin K requirement of the rat is greatly increased under germ-free conditions [273], the significance of the utilization of gut menaquinones by humans has been difficult to quantitate. Dietary butylated hydroxytoluene has been reported [274] to cause a hemorrhagic condition in rats that can be cured by vitamin K supplementation, but the mechanism of this response has not been clarified. Phenobarbital and diphenylhydantoin administration to pregnant women has been reported [275] to produce a vitamin K-responsive hemorrhage in the newborn.

Early studies of vitamin K requirements indicated that female rats had a lower vitamin K requirement, and nutritional deficiencies are much more readily produced in male rats.

Castration of both sexes unifies that vitamin K response, and in the castrated rat, prothrombin concentrations can be increased with estrogens and decreased with androgens [276]. The available evidence suggests that the influence of estrogens on rate of synthesis is reflected in a higher rate of synthesis and accumulation of prothrombin precursors in the microsomes [277,278]. Hypothyroidism in humans results in a decrease in both the rate of synthesis and the destruction of the vitamin K-dependent clotting factors [279], and it is likely that these hormonal effects are related to rates of synthesis of the proteins involved rather than to any effect on vitamin K metabolism.

Early studies of vitamin K function [280] established that the inclusion of mineral oil in diets prevented its absorption, and mineral oil has often been used in vitamin K-deficient diets. High dietary vitamin A has also been recognized for some time to adversely influence vitamin K action [281]. Whether this is a general effect on nonpolar lipid absorption or a specific vitamin K antagonism is not clear, but it can be observed at relatively low dietary levels of retinol acetate and retinoic acid. Administration of D-α-tocopherol hydroquinone has been shown to produce a vitamin K-responsive hemorrhagic syndrome in the pregnant rat [282], and the addition of vitamin E to the diet of a patient on coumarin anticoagulant therapy has been reported [283] to result in a hemorrhagic episode. This suggests that this interaction may be of clinical significance, and it is possible that high vitamin E intakes may exacerbate a borderline vitamin K deficiency. The vitamin K-dependent carboxylase is competitively inhibited by vitamin E, and there are indications that the α-tocopherol quinone, rather than α-tocopherol [284,285], may be the causative agent. More recent studies [286] using a rat model have indicated that vitamin E may adversely influence vitamin K absorption as well as inhibiting the carboxylase.

VITAMIN K REQUIREMENTS

ANIMALS

The establishment of a dietary vitamin K requirement for various species has been difficult because of the varying degrees to which they use the large amount of vitamin K synthesized by intestinal bacteria and the degree to which different species practice coprophagy. A spontaneous deficiency of vitamin K was first noted in chicks, and poultry are much more likely to develop symptoms of a dietary deficiency than any other species. This has usually been assumed to be due to the rapid transit rate of material through the relatively short intestinal tract of the chick or to limited synthesis of menaquinones in this species. A more recent study [287] suggests that limited recycling of vitamin K because of low epoxide reductase activity may be the cause of the increased requirement.

Ruminal microorganisms synthesize large amounts of vitamin K, and ruminants do not appear to need a source of vitamin in the diet. Deficiencies have, however, been produced in most monogastric species. Estimations of vitamin K requirements by different workers are difficult to compare. The majority of the data are old, different forms of the vitamin were used, and different methods were employed to establish the requirement. Phylloquinone has been used for most experimental nutrition studies, whereas other forms of vitamin K are usually used in practical rations. Menadione is usually considered to be from 20% to 40% as effective as phylloquinone on a molar basis, but this depends a great deal on the type of assay that is used. It is rather ineffective in a curative assay, where the rate of its alkylation to menaquinone-4 is probably the rate-limiting factor, but often shows activity nearly equal to phylloquinone in a long-term preventive assay. Commercial livestock rations usually use a water-soluble form of menadione, such as MSBC. This compound appears to be about as active on a molar basis as phylloquinone in poultry rations, and at least in this species, the activity of menadione, MSBC, and phylloquinone is roughly equal on a weight basis.

TABLE 3.3
Vitamin K Requirements of Various Species

Species	Daily Intake (μg/kg/day)	Dietary Concentration (μg/kg diet)
Dog	1.25	60
Pig	5	50
Rhesus monkey	2	60
Rat, male	11–16	100–150
Chicken	80–120	530
Turkey poult	180–270	1200

Note: Data have been summarized from a more extensive table [289] and are presented as the amount of vitamin needed to prevent the development of a deficiency. No correction for differences in potency of equal weights of different forms of the vitamin has been made.

Detailed discussions of the vitamin K requirements of various species are available [281,288,289]. The data indicate that the requirement for most species falls in a range of 2–200 μg vitamin K/kg body weight/day. The data in Table 3.3, which have been adopted from a table presented by Griminger [289], give an indication of the magnitude of the requirement for various species. It should be remembered that this requirement can be altered by age, sex, or strain, and that any condition influencing lipid absorption or conditions altering intestinal flora will have an influence of these values. A considerably higher level of dietary vitamin K has been recommended for most laboratory animals by the National Academy of Sciences [290]. Recommendations for most species are in the range of 3000 μg/kg of diet, but the rat requirement has been set at 50 μg/kg. Although this level is sufficient in most cases, it does not prevent all signs of deficiency [106], and the American Institute of Nutrition [291] has now recommended that purified diets for laboratory rodents should have 750 μg of phylloquinone added to each kilogram of diet.

Humans

The most recent values for vitamin K intake were established in 2001 as part of the comprehensive dietary reference intakes (DRI) project of the Food and Nutrition Board/Institute of Medicine and have been published by the National Academy of Sciences [63]. There are ample data to establish that very few, if any, individuals consume sufficient vitamin K to maximally γ-carboxylate their circulating osteocalcin and that supplementation with about 1 mg/day of phylloquinone is needed to achieve this response. As there appears to be no clinical significance of this apparent deficiency, this index of adequacy was not used to set a reference value.

The only indicator of vitamin K status with clinical significance is the PT, and alterations in the PT by changes in dietary intake alone are uncommon to nonexistent. As circulating phylloquinone concentration is very dependent on previous day intakes, it is also not a satisfactory indicator of an adequate intake (AI). Intakes of vitamin K that are in the range of 10% of normal have been demonstrated under controlled conditions to result in decreases in urinary Gla excretion and increases in under-γ-carboxylated prothrombin which can be measured by a commercially available immunoassay. However, no studies using a range of intakes that would allow the calculation of an estimated average requirement (EAR) based on these markers are available. Reports that might implicate bone or vascular health (see section Hemorrhagic Disease of the Newborn) to alterations in vitamin K status also

TABLE 3.4
Adequate Intakes of Vitamin K

Population	Vitamin K (μg/day)
0–6 Month old infants	2.0
7–12 Month old infants	2.5
1–3 Year old children	30
4–8 Year old children	55
9–13 Year old boys and girls	60
14–18 Year old boys and girls[a]	75
19 to >70 Year old men	120
19 to >70 Year old women[a]	90

Note: Food and Nutrition Board, IOM [63].

[a] No alteration of intake for pregnancy or lactation.

fail to provide the data needed to establish an EAR. If available data allow the determination of an EAR, the historical term used to indicate nutrient requirements, the recommended dietary allowance (RDA), can be calculated. As sufficient data to determine an EAR are not available, the RDI currently in use is the AI for different age groups shown in Table 3.4. The value is defined as "the recommended average daily intake level based on observed or experimentally determined approximations or estimates of nutrient intake by a group or groups of apparently healthy people that are assumed to be adequate." AIs of infants are based on the phylloquinone content of human milk and assume that infants also receive prophylactic vitamin K at birth. AIs for children, adolescents, and adults are based on the highest median intake for each age group reported by NHANES III. Based on those data, the intakes of pregnant or lactating women do not differ from those of the general population.

EFFICACY AND HAZARDS OF PHARMACOLOGICAL DOSES OF VITAMIN K

No hazards attributed to the long-term ingestion of elevated amounts of the natural forms of vitamin K have been reported [292,293]. For treatment of prolonged clotting times when hemorrhage is not a problem, vitamin K can be given orally or parenterally. If given orally to patients with impaired biliary function, bile salts should also be administered. Vitamin K_1 is available as the pure compound or as an aqueous colloidal solution that can be given intramuscularly or intravenously. Some adverse reactions have been noted following intravenous administration, and unless a severe hemorrhagic episode is present, intramuscular injection is the recommended route of therapy. Effective therapy requires synthesis of normal clotting factors, and a number of hours may be necessary before a substantial decrease in clotting times is apparent.

The relative safety of phylloquinone and, presumably, menaquinones does not hold for menadione or its water-soluble derivatives. These compounds can be safely used at low levels to prevent the development of a deficiency but should not be used as a pharmacological treatment for a hemorrhagic condition. Although once prescribed for treatment of the hemorrhagic disease of the newborn, these compounds are known to react with free sulfhydryl groups of various tissues and to cause hemolytic anemia, hyperbilirubinemia, and kernicterus. This marked increase in conjugated bilirubin is extremely toxic to the neonatal brain and has caused death in some instances [292].

REFERENCES

1. Dam, H., Cholesterinositoffwechsel in huhnereiern und huhnchen. *Biochem. Z.*, 1929. 215: pp. 475–492.
2. McFarlane, W.D., W.R. Graham, and F. Richardson, The fat-soluble vitamin requirements of the chick. I. The vitamin A and vitamin D content of fish meal and meat meal. *Biochem. J.*, 1931. 25: pp. 358–366.
3. Holst, W.F. and E.R. Halbrook, A "scurvy-like" disease in chicks. *Science*, 1933. 77: p. 354.
4. Dam, H., The antihaemorrhagic vitamin of the chick. *Biochem. J.*, 1935. 29: pp. 1273–1285.
5. Dam, H., The antihaemorrhagic vitamin of the chick. Occurrence and chemical nature. *Nature*, 1935. 135: pp. 652–653.
6. Almquist, H.J. and E.L.R. Stokstad, Dietary haemorrhagic disease in chicks. *Nature*, 1935. 136: p. 31.
7. Almquist, H.J. and E.L.R. Stokstad, Haemorrhagic chick disease of dietary origin. *J. Biol. Chem.*, 1935. 111: pp. 105–113.
8. MacCorquodale, D.W., L.C. Cheney, S.B. Binkley, W.F. Holcomb, R.W. McKee, S.A. Thayer, and E.A. Doisy, The constitution and synthesis of vitamin K_1. *J. Biol. Chem.*, 1939. 131: pp. 357–370.
9. Karrer, P., A. Geiger, R. Legler, A. Ruegger, and H. Salomon, Uber die isolierung des alpha-phyllochinones (vitamin K aus alfalfa) sowie uber dessen entdeckungsgeschechter. *Helv. Chim. Acta*, 1939. 22: pp. 1464–1470.
10. Almquist, H.J. and A.A. Klose, Synthetic and natural antihemorrhagic compounds. *J. Am. Chem. Soc.*, 1939. 61: pp. 2557–2558.
11. Fieser, L.F., Synthesis of 2-methyl-3-phytyl-1,4-naphthoquinone. *J. Am. Chem. Soc.*, 1939. 61: pp. 2559–2561.
12. Dam, H., Vitamin K, its chemistry and physiology. *Adv. Enzymol.*, 1942. 2: pp. 285–324.
13. Doisy, E.A., S.B. Binkley, and S.A. Thayer, Vitamin K. *Chem. Rev.*, 1941. 28: pp. 477–517.
14. Almquist, H.J., The early history of vitamin K. *Am. J. Clin. Nutr.*, 1975. 28: pp. 656–659.
15. Jukes, T.H., Vitamin K—a reminiscence. *TIBS*, 1980. 5: pp. 140–141.
16. Booth, S.L., K.W. Davidson, and J.A. Sadowski, Evaluation of an HPLC method for the determination of phylloquinone (vitamin K_1) in various food matrices. *J. Agric. Food Chem.*, 1994. 42: pp. 295–300.
17. Matschiner, J.T., W.V. Taggart, and J.M. Amelotti, The vitamin K content of beef liver, detection of a new form of vitamin K. *Biochemistry*, 1967. 6: pp. 1243–1248.
18. Matschiner, J.T. and W.V. Taggart, Separation of vitamin K and associated lipids by reversed-phase partition column chromatography. *Anal. Biochem.*, 1967. 18: pp. 88–93.
19. IUPAC–IUB Committee on Biochemistry Nomenclature, Nomenclature of quinones with isoprenoid side chains recommendations (1973). *Eur. J. Biochem.*, 1975. 53: pp. 15–18.
20. Bentley, R. and R. Meganathan, Biosynthesis of vitamin K (menaquinone) in bacteria. *Microbiol. Rev.*, 1982. 46: pp. 241–280.
21. Griminger, P., Biological activity of the various vitamin K forms. *Vitam. Horm.*, 1966. 24: pp. 605–618.
22. Weber, F. and O. Wiss, Vitamin K group: Active compounds and antagonists, *The Vitamins*, 2nd ed. 1971, New York: Academic Press. pp. 457–466.
23. Matschiner, J.T. and W.V. Taggart, Bioassay of vitamin K by intracardial injection in deficient adult male rats. *J. Nutr.*, 1968. 94: pp. 57–59.
24. Griminger, P., Relative vitamin K potency of two water-soluble menadione analogues. *Poult. Sci.*, 1965. 44: pp. 211–213.
25. Greer, F.R., S.P. Marshall, R.R. Severson, D.A. Smith, M.J. Shearer, D.G. Pace, and P.H. Jobe, A new mixed micellar preparation for oral vitamin K prophylaxis: Randomised controlled comparison with an intramuscular formulation in breast fed infants. *Arch. Dis. Child.*, 1998. 79: pp. 300–305.
26. Link, K.P., The discovery of dicumarol and its sequels. *Circulation*, 1959. 19: pp. 97–107.
27. Renk, E. and W.G. Stoll, Orale antikoagulantien. *Prog. Drug. Res.*, 1968. 11: pp. 226–355.
28. O'Reilly, R.A., Vitamin K and the oral anticoagulant drugs. *Annu. Rev. Med.*, 1976. 27: pp. 245–261.
29. Drummond, D., Rats resistant to warfarin. *New Sci.*, 1966. 30: pp. 771–772.
30. Greaves, J.H. and P. Ayres, Heritable resistance to warfarin in rats. *Nature*, 1967. 215: pp. 877–878.

31. Lund, M., Comparative effect of the three rodenticides warfarin, difenacoum and brodifacoum on eight rodent species in short feeding periods. *J. Hyg. Camb.*, 1981. 87: pp. 101–107.
32. Kabat, H., E.F. Stohlman, and M.I. Smith, Hypoprothrombinemia induced by administration of indandione derivatives. *J. Pharmacol. Exp. Ther.*, 1944. 80: pp. 160–170.
33. Ren, P., R.E. Laliberte, and R.G. Bell, Effects of warfarin, phenylindanedione, tetrachlorophyridinol, and chloro-vitamin K_1 on prothrombin synthesis and vitamin K metabolism in normal and warfarin-resistant rats. *Mol. Pharmacol.*, 1974. 10: pp. 373–380.
34. Lowenthal, J., J.A. MacFarlane, and K.M. McDonald, The inhibition of the antidotal activity of vitamin K_1 against coumarin anticoagulant drugs by its chloro analogue. *Experentia*, 1960. 16: pp. 428–429.
35. Suttie, J.W., Anticoagulant-resistant rats: Possible control by the use of the chloro analog of vitamin K. *Science*, 1973. 180: pp. 741–743.
36. Marshall, F.N., Potency and coagulation factor effects of 2,3,5,6-tetrachloro-pyridinol compared to warfarin and its antagonism by vitamin K. *Proc. Soc. Exp. Biol. Med.*, 1972. 139: pp. 806–810.
37. Grossman, C.P. and J.W. Suttie, Vitamin K-dependent carboxylase: Inhibitory action of polychlorinated phenols. *Biochem. Pharmacol.*, 1990. 40: pp. 1351–1355.
38. Mayer, H. and O. Isler, Vitamin K group—chemistry, *The Vitamins*, 2nd ed. 1971, New York: Academic Press. pp. 418–443.
39. Mayer, H. and O. Isler, Synthesis of vitamins K. *Meth. Enzymol.*, 1971. XVIII-C: pp. 491–547.
40. Mayer, H. and O. Isler, Vitamin K group—industrial, *The Vitamins.*, 2nd ed. 1971, New York: Academic Press. pp. 444–445.
41. Naruta, Y., Allylation of quinones with allyltin reagents. *J. Am. Chem. Soc.*, 1980. 102: pp. 3774–3783.
42. Suhara, Y., M. Kamao, N. Tsugawa, and T. Okano, Method for the determination of vitamin K homologues in human plasma using high-performance liquid chromatography-tandem mass spectrometry. *Anal. Chem.*, 2005. 77: pp. 757–763.
43. Fauler, G., H.J. Leis, J. Schalamon, W. Muntean, and H. Gleispach, Method for the determination of vitamin $K_1(20)$ in human plasma by stable isotope dilution/gas chromatography/mass spectrometry. *J. Mass. Spectrom.*, 1996. 31: pp. 655–660.
44. Payne, R.J., A.M. Daines, B.M. Clark, and A.D. Abell, Synthesis and protein conjugation studies of vitamin K analogues. *Bioorg. Med. Chem.*, 2004. 12: pp. 5785–5791.
45. Patai, S., *The Chemistry of the Quinonoid Compounds*, Parts 1 & 2. 1974, New York: John Wiley & Sons. p. 1274.
46. Sommer, P. and M. Kofler, Physicochemical properties and methods of analysis of phylloquinones, menaquinones, ubiquinones, phostoquinones, menadione, and related compounds. *Vitam. Horm.*, 1966. 24: pp. 349–399.
47. Dunphy, P.J. and A.F. Brodie, The structure and function of quinones in respiratory metabolism. *Meth. Enzymol.*, 1971. XVIII-C: pp. 407–461.
48. Matschiner, J.T. and J.M. Amelotti, Characterization of vitamin K from bovine liver. *J. Lipid. Res.*, 1968. 9: pp. 176–179.
49. Shearer, M.J., High-performance liquid chromatography of K vitamins and their antagonists. *Adv. Chromatogr.*, 1983. 21: pp. 243–301.
50. Ferland, G. and J.A. Sadowski, Vitamin K_1 (phylloquinone) content of edible oils: Effects of heating and light exposure. *J. Agric. Food Chem.*, 1992. 40: pp. 1869–1873.
51. Fomon, S.J. and J.W. Suttie, Vitamin K, *Nutrition of Normal Infants*. 1993, St. Louis, MO: Mosby. pp. 348–358.
52. Kries, R.V., M. Shearer, P.T. McCarthy, M. Haug, G. Harzer, and U. Gobel, Vitamin K_1 content of maternal milk: Influence of the stage of lactation, lipid composition, and vitamin K_1 supplements given to the mother. *Pediatr. Res.*, 1987. 22: pp. 513–517.
53. Indyk, H.E. and D.C. Woollard, Vitamin K in milk and infant formulas: Determination and distribution of phylloquinone and menaquinone-4. *Analyst*, 1997. 122: pp. 465–469.
54. Indyk, H.E. and D.C. Woollard, Determination of vitamin K in milk and infant formulas by liquid chromatography: Collaborative study. *J. AOAC. Int.*, 2000. 83: pp. 121–130.
55. Booth, S.L., J.A. Sadowski, J.L. Weihrauch, and G. Ferland, Vitamin K_1 (phylloquinone) content of foods: A provisional table. *J. Food Compost. Anal.*, 1993. 6: pp. 109–120.
56. Duggan, P., K.D. Cashman, A. Flynn, C. Bolton-Smith, and M. Kiely, Phylloquinone (vitamin K_1) intakes and food sources in 18–64-year-old Irish adults. *Br. J. Nutr.*, 2004. 92: pp. 151–158.

57. Bolton-Smith, C., R.J.G. Price, S.T. Fenton, D.J. Harrington, and M.J. Shearer, Compilation of a provisional UK database for the phylloquinone (vitamin K_1) content of foods. *Br. J. Nutr.*, 2000. 83: pp. 389–399.
58. Schurgers, L.J., J.M. Geleijnse, D.E. Grobbee, H.A.P. Pols, A. Hofman, J.C.M. Witteman, and C. Vermeer, Nutritional intake of vitamins K_1 (phylloquinone) and K_2 (menaquinone) in The Netherlands. *J. Nutr. Environ. Med.*, 1999. 9: pp. 115–122.
59. Weizmann, N., J.W. Peterson, D. Haytowitz, P.R. Pehrsson, V.P. de Jesus, and S.L. Booth, Vitamin K content of fast foods and snack foods in the US diet. *J. Food Compost. Anal.*, 2004. 17: pp. 379–384.
60. Dumont, J.F., J. Peterson, D. Haytowitz, and S.L. Booth, Phylloquinone and dihydrophylloquinone contents of mixed dishes, processed meats, soups and cheeses. *J. Food Compost. Anal.*, 2003. 16: pp. 595–603.
61. Majchrzak, D. and I. Elmadfa, Phylloquinone (vitamin K_1) content of commercially-available baby food products. *Food Chem.*, 2001. 74: pp. 275–280.
62. Schurgers, L.J. and C. Vermeer, Determination of phylloquinone and menaquinones in food. *Haemostasis*, 2000. 30: pp. 298–307.
63. Food and Nutrition Board and Institute of Medicine, eds. *Dietary Reference Intakes: Vitamin A, Vitamin K, Arsenic, Boron, Chromium, Copper, Iodine, Iron, Manganese, Molybdenum, Nickel, Silicon, Vanadium, and Zinc.* 2001, Washington, DC: National Academy Press.
64. Booth, S.L., D.R. Webb, and J.C. Peters, Assessment of phylloquinone and dihydrophylloquinone dietary intakes among a nationally representative sample of U.S. consumers using 14-day food diaries. *J. Am. Diet. Assoc.*, 1999. 99: pp. 1072–1076.
65. Booth, S.L., A.T. Pennington, and J.A. Sadowski, Food sources and dietary intakes of vitamin K_1 (phylloquinone) in the American Diet: Data from the FDA total diet study. *J. Am. Diet. Assoc.*, 1996. 96: pp. 149–154.
66. Price, R., S. Fenton, M.J. Shearer, and C. Bolton-Smith, Daily and seasonal variation in phylloquinone (vitamin K_1) intake in Scotland. *Proc. Nutr. Soc.*, 1996. 55: p. 266A.
67. Thane, C.W., A.A. Paul, C.J. Bates, C. Bolton-Smith, A. Prentice, and M.J. Shearer, Intake and sources of phylloquinone (vitamin K_1): Variation with socio-demographic and lifestyle factors in a national sample of British elderly people. *Br. J. Nutr.*, 2002. 87: pp. 605–613.
68. McKeown, N.M., H.M. Rasmussen, J.M. Charnley, R.J. Wood, and S.L. Booth, Accuracy of phylloquinone (vitamin K_1) data in 2 nutrient databases as determined by direct laboratory analysis of diets. *J. Am. Diet. Assoc.*, 2000. 100: pp. 1201–1204.
69. Ferland, G., D.L. MacDonald, and J.A. Sadowski, Development of a diet low in vitamin K_1 (phylloquinone). *J. Am. Diet. Assoc.*, 1992. 92: pp. 593–597.
70. Peterson, J.W., K.L. Muzzey, D. Haytowitz, J. Exler, L. Lemar, and S.L. Booth, Phylloquinone (vitamin K_1) and dihydrophylloquinone content of fats and oils. *JAOCS*, 2002. 79: pp. 641–646.
71. Cook, K.K., G.V. Mitchell, E. Grundel, and J.I. Rader, HPLC analysis for *trans*-vitamin K_1 and dihydro-vitamin K in margarines and margarine-like products using the C30 stationary phase. *Food Chem.*, 1999. 67: pp. 79–88.
72. Booth, S.L., J.A.T. Pennington, and J.A. Sadowski, Dihydro-vitamin K_1: Primary food sources and estimated dietary intakes in the American diet. *Lipids*, 1996. 31: pp. 715–720.
73. Hollander, D., Intestinal absorption of vitamins A, E, D, and K. *J. Lab. Clin. Med.*, 1981. 97: pp. 449–462.
74. Hollander, D. and E. Rim, Factors affecting the absorption of vitamin K_1 in vitro. *Gut*, 1976. 17: pp. 450–455.
75. Shearer, M.J., A. McBurney, and P. Barkhan, Studies on the absorption and metabolism of phylloquinone (vitamin K_1) in man. *Vitam. Horm.*, 1974. 32: pp. 513–542.
76. Gijsbers, B.L.M.G., K.-S.G. Jie, and C. Vermeer, Effect of food composition on vitamin K absorption in human volunteers. *Br. J. Nutr.*, 1996. 76: pp. 223–229.
77. Garber, A.K., N.C. Binkley, D.C. Krueger, and J.W. Suttie, Comparison of phylloquinone bioavailability from food sources or a supplement in human subjects. *J. Nutr.*, 1999. 129: pp. 1201–1203.
78. Booth, S.L., A.H. Lichtenstein, and G.E. Dallal, Phylloquinone absorption from phylloquinone-fortified oil is greater than from a vegetable in younger and older men and women. *J. Nutr.*, 2002. 132: pp. 2609–2612.

79. Conly, J.M. and K. Stein, Quantitative and qualitative measurements of K vitamins in human intestinal contents. *Am. J. Gastroenterol.*, 1992. 87: pp. 311–316.
80. Suttie, J.W., The importance of menaquinones in human nutrition. *Annu. Rev. Nutr.*, 1995. 15: pp. 399–417.
81. Will, B.H. and J.W. Suttie, Comparative metabolism of phylloquinone and menaquinone-9 in rat liver. *J. Nutr.*, 1992. 122: pp. 953–958.
82. Hollander, D., K.S. Muralidhara, and E. Rim, Colonic absorption of bacterially synthesized vitamin K_2 in the rat. *Am. J. Physiol.*, 1976. 230: pp. 251–255.
83. Ichihashi, T., Y. Takagishi, K. Uchida, and H. Yamada, Colonic absorption of menaquinone-4 and menaquinone-9 in rats. *J. Nutr.*, 1992. 122: pp. 506–512.
84. Conly, J.M. and K.E. Stein, The absorption and bioactivity of bacterially synthesized menaquinones. *Clin. Invest. Med.*, 1993. 16: pp. 45–57.
85. Hollander, D. and T.C. Truscott, Mechanism and site of vitamin K_3 small intestinal transport. *Am. J. Physiol.*, 1974. 226: pp. 1516–1522.
86. Kohlmeier, M., A. Salomon, J. Saupe, and M.J. Shearer, Transport of vitamin K to bone in humans. *J. Nutr.*, 1996. 126: pp. 1192S–1196S.
87. Lamon-Fava, S., J.A. Sadowski, K.W. Davidson, M.E. O'Brien, and J.R. McNamara, Plasma lipoproteins as carriers of phylloquinone (vitamin K_1) in humans. *Am. J. Clin. Nutr.*, 1998. 67: pp. 1226–1231.
88. Schurgers, L.J. and C. Vermeer, Differential lipoprotein transport pathways of K-vitamins in healthy subjects. *Biochim. Biophys. Acta*, 2002. 1570: pp. 27–32.
89. Kohlmeier, M., J. Saupe, H.J. Drossel, and M.J. Shearer, Variation of phylloquinone (vitamin K_1) concentrations in hemodialysis patients. *Thromb. Haemost.*, 1995. 74: pp. 1252–1254.
90. Saupe, J., M.J. Shearer, and M. Kohlmeier, Phylloquinone transport and its influence on gamma-carboxyglutamate residues of osteocalcin in patients on maintenance hemodialysis. *Am. J. Clin. Nutr.*, 1993. 58: pp. 204–208.
91. Newman, P., F. Bonello, A.S. Wierzbicki, P. Lumb, G.F. Savidge, and M.J. Shearer, The uptake of lipoprotein-borne phylloquinone (vitamin K_1) by osteoblasts and osteoblast-like cells: Role of heparan sulfate proteoglycans and apolipoprotein E. *J. Bone Miner. Res.*, 2002. 17: pp. 426–433.
92. Olson, R.E., J. Chao, D. Graham, M.W. Bates, and J.H. Lewis, Total body phylloquinone and its turnover in human subjects at two levels of vitamin K intake. *Br. J. Nutr.*, 2002. 88: pp. 543–553.
93. Usui, Y., H. Tanimura, N. Nishimura, N. Kobayashi, T. Okanoue, and K. Ozawa, Vitamin K concentrations in the plasma and liver of surgical patients. *Am. J. Clin. Nutr.*, 1990. 51: pp. 846–852.
94. Davidson, K.W. and J.A. Sadowski, Determination of vitamin K compounds in plasma or serum by high-performance liquid chromatography using postcolumn chemical reduction and fluorimetric detection. *Meth. Enzymol.*, 1997. 282: pp. 408–421.
95. McCarthy, P.T., D.J. Harrington, and M.J. Shearer, Assay of phylloquinone in plasma by high-performance liquid chromatography with electrochemical detection. *Meth. Enzymol.*, 1997. 282: pp. 421–433.
96. Wang, L.Y., C.J. Bates, L. Yan, D.J. Harrington, M.J. Shearer, and A. Prentice, Determination of phylloquinone (vitamin K_1) in plasma and serum by HPLC with fluorescence detection. *Clin. Chim. Acta*, 2004. 347: pp. 199–207.
97. Sadowski, J.A., S.J. Hood, G.E. Dallal, and P.J. Garry, Phylloquinone in plasma from elderly and young adults: Factors influencing its concentration. *Am. J. Clin. Nutr.*, 1989. 50: pp. 100–108.
98. Booth, S.L., K.L. Tucker, N.M. McKeown, K.W. Davidson, G.E. Dallal, and J.A. Sadowski, Relationships between dietary intakes and fasting plasma concentrations of fat-soluble vitamins in humans. *J. Nutr.*, 1997. 127: pp. 587–592.
99. Ferland, G., J.A. Sadowski, and M.E. O'Brien, Dietary induced subclinical vitamin K deficiency in normal human subjects. *J. Clin. Invest.*, 1993. 91: pp. 1761–1768.
100. Booth, S.L., M.E. O'Brien-Morse, G.E. Dallal, K.W. Davidson, and C.M. Gundberg, Response of vitamin K status to different intakes and sources of phylloquinone-rich foods: Comparison of younger and older adults. *Am. J. Clin. Nutr.*, 1999. 70: pp. 368–377.
101. Hodges, S.J., M.J. Pilkington, M.J. Shearer, L. Bitensky, and J. Chayen, Age-related changes in the circulating levels of congeners of vitamin K_2, menaquinone-7 and menaquinone-8. *Clin. Sci.*, 1990. 78: pp. 63–66.

102. Suttie, J.W., Vitamin K and human nutrition. *J. Am. Diet. Assoc.*, 1992. 92: pp. 585–590.
103. Hodges, S.J., K. Akesson, P. Vergnaud, K. Obrant, and P.D. Delmas, Circulating levels of vitamin K_1 and K_2 decreased in elderly women with hip fracture. *J. Bone Miner. Res.*, 1993. 8: pp. 1241–1245.
104. Taylor, J.D., G.J. Millar, L.B. Jaques, and J.W.T. Spinks, The distribution of administered vitamin K_1–^{14}C in rats. *Can. J. Biochem. Physiol.*, 1956. 34: pp. 1143–1152.
105. Thierry, M.J., M.A. Hermodson, and J.W. Suttie, Vitamin K and warfarin distribution and metabolism in the warfarin-resistant rat. *Am. J. Physiol.*, 1970. 219: pp. 854–859.
106. Kindberg, C.G. and J.W. Suttie, Effect of various intakes of phylloquinone on signs of vitamin K deficiency and serum and liver phylloquinone concentrations in the rat. *J. Nutr.*, 1989. 119: pp. 175–180.
107. Bell, R.G. and J.T. Matschiner, Intracellular distribution of vitamin K in the rat. *Biochim. Biophys. Acta*, 1969. 184: pp. 597–603.
108. Thierry, M.J. and J.W. Suttie, Effect of warfarin and the chloro analog of vitamin K on phylloquinone metabolism. *Arch. Biochem. Biophys.*, 1971. 147: pp. 430–435.
109. Nyquist, S.E., J.T. Matschiner, and D.J.J. Morre, Distribution of vitamin K among rat liver cell fractions. *Biochim. Biophys. Acta*, 1971. 244: pp. 645–649.
110. Reedstrom, C.K. and J.W. Suttie, Comparative distribution, metabolism, and utilization of phylloquinone and menaquinone-9 in rat liver. *Proc. Soc. Exp. Biol. Med.*, 1995. 209: pp. 403–409.
111. Kight, C.E., C.K. Reedstrom, and J.W. Suttie, Identification, isolation, and partial purification of a cytosolic binding protein for vitamin K from rat liver. *FASEB J.*, 1995. 9: pp. A725.
112. Duello, T.J. and J.T. Matschiner, Characterization of vitamin K from human liver. *J. Nutr.*, 1972. 102: pp. 331–335.
113. Kayata, S., C. Kindberg, F.R. Greer, and J.W. Suttie, Vitamin K_1 and K_2 in infant human liver. *J. Pediatr. Gastroenterol. Nutr.*, 1989. 8: pp. 304–307.
114. Shearer, M.J., P.T. McCarthy, O.E. Crampton, and M.B. Mattock, The assessment of human vitamin K status from tissue measurements, *Current Advances in Vitamin K Research*. 1988, New York: Elsevier. pp. 437–452.
115. Will, B.H., Y. Usui, and J.W. Suttie, Comparative metabolism and requirement of vitamin K in chicks and rats. *J. Nutr.*, 1992. 122: pp. 2354–2360.
116. Guillaumont, M., H. Weiser, L. Sann, B. Vignal, M. Leclerq, and A. Frederich, Hepatic concentration of vitamin K active compounds after application of phylloquinone to chickens on a vitamin K deficient or adequate diet. *Int. J. Vitam. Nutr. Res.*, 1992. 62: pp. 15–20.
117. Thijssen, H.H.W. and M.J. Drittij-Reijnders, Vitamin K distribution in rat tissues: Dietary phylloquinone is a source of tissue menaquinone-4. *Br. J. Nutr.*, 1994. 72: pp. 415–425.
118. Martius, C., The metabolic relationships between the different K vitamins and the synthesis of the ubiquinones. *Am. J. Clin. Nutr.*, 1961. 9: pp. 97–103.
119. Dialameh, G.H., K.G. Yekundi, and R.E. Olson, Enzymatic alkylation of menaquinone-o to menaquinones by microsomes from chick liver. *Biochim. Biophys. Acta*, 1970. 223: pp. 332–338.
120. Martius, C., Recent investigations on the chemistry and function of vitamin K, *Quinones in Electron Transport*. 1961, Boston: Little Brown. pp. 312–326.
121. Sundaram, K.S., J.A. Engelke, A.L. Foley, J.W. Suttie, and M. Lev, Vitamin K status influences brain sulfatide metabolism in young mice and rats. *J. Nutr.*, 1996. 126: pp. 2746–2751.
122. Thijssen, H.H.W. and M.J. Drittij-Reijnders, Vitamin K status in human tissues: Tissue-specific accumulation of phylloquinone and menaquinone-4. *Br. J. Nutr.*, 1996. 75: pp. 121–127.
123. Thijssen, H.H.W., M.J. Drittij-Reijnders, and M.A.J.G. Fischer, Phylloquinone and menaquinone-4 distribution in rats: Synthesis rather than uptake determines menaquinone-4 organ concentrations. *J. Nutr.*, 1996. 126: pp. 537–543.
124. Davidson, R.T., A.L. Foley, J.A. Engelke, and J.W. Suttie, Conversion of dietary phylloquinone to tissue menaquinone-4 in rats is not dependent on gut bacteria. *J. Nutr.*, 1998. 128: pp. 220–223.
125. Ronden, J.E., H.H.W. Thijssen, and C. Vermeer, Tissue distribution of K-vitamers under different nutritional regimens in the rat. *Biochim. Biophys. Acta*, 1998. 1379: pp. 16–22.
126. Hart, K.T., Study of hydrolysis of urinary metabolites of 2-methyl-1,4-naphthoquinone. *Proc. Soc. Exp. Biol. Med.*, 1958. 97: pp. 848–851.
127. Hoskin, F.C.G., J.W.T. Spinks, and L.B. Jaques, Urinary excretion products of menadione (vitamin K_3). *Can. J. Biochem. Physiol.*, 1954. 32: pp. 240–250.

128. Losito, R., C.A. Owen, and E.V. Flock, Metabolic studies of vitamin K_1–^{14}C and menadione–^{14}C in the normal and hepatectomized rats. *Thromb. Diath. Heamorrh.*, 1968. 19: pp. 383–388.
129. Wiss, O. and H. Gloor, Absorption, distribution, storage and metabolites of vitamin K and related quinones. *Vitam. Horm.*, 1966. 24: pp. 575–586.
130. Matschiner, J.T., R.G. Bell, J.M. Amelotti, and T.E. Knauer, Isolation and characterization of a new metabolite of phylloquinone in the rat. *Biochim. Biophys. Acta*, 1970. 201: pp. 309–315.
131. Bell, R.G., J.A. Sadowski, and J.T. Matschiner, Mechanism of action of warfarin. Warfarin and metabolism of vitamin K_1. *Biochemistry*, 1972. 11: pp. 1959–1961.
132. Shearer, M.J., A. McBurney, and P. Barkhan, Effect of warfarin anticoagulation on vitamin K_1 metabolism in man. *Br. J. Haematol.*, 1973. 24: pp. 471–479.
133. Shearer, M.J., A. McBurney, A.M. Breckenridge, and P. Barkhan, Effect of warfarin on the metabolism of phylloquinone (vitamin K_1): Dose–response relationships in man. *Clin. Sci. Mol. Med.*, 1977. 52: pp. 621–630.
134. Harrington, D.J., R. Soper, C. Edwards, G.E. Savidge, S.J. Hodges, and M.J. Shearer, Determination of the urinary aglycone metabolites of vitamin K by HPLC with redox-mode electrochemical detection. *J. Lipid. Res.*, 2005. 46: pp. 1053–1060.
135. Giangrande, P.L.F., Six characters in search of an author: The history of the nomenclature of coagulation factors. *Br. J. Haematol.*, 2003. 121: pp. 703–712.
136. Dahlback, B., Blood coagulation. *Lancet*, 2000. 355: pp. 1627–1632.
137. Mann, K.G., Thrombin formation. *Chest*, 2003. 124: pp. 4S–10S.
138. Stenflo, J., A new vitamin K-dependent protein. Purification from bovine plasma and preliminary characterization. J. Biol. Chem., 1976. 251: pp. 355–363.
139. Dahlback, B. and B.O. Villoutreix, The anticoagulant protein C pathway. *FEBS Lett.*, 2005. 579: pp. 3310–3316.
140. DiScipio, R.G. and E.W. Davie, Characterization of protein S, a gamma-carboxyglutamic acid containing protein from bovine and human plasma. *Biochemistry*, 1979. 18: pp. 899–904.
141. Esmon, C.T., The protein C pathway. *Chest*, 2003. 124: pp. 26S–32S.
142. Prowse, C.V. and M.P. Esnouf, The isolation of a new warfarin-sensitive protein from bovine plasma. *Biochem. Soc. Trans.*, 1977. 5: pp. 255–256.
143. Broze, G.J., Jr, Protein Z-dependent regulation of coagulation. Thromb Haemost, 2001. 86: pp. 8–13.
144. Ichinose, A. and E.W. Davie, The blood coagulation factors: Their cDNAs, genes, and expression, *Hemostasis and Thrombosis: Basic Principles and Clinical Practice*, 3rd ed. 1994, Philadelphia, PA: J.B. Lippincott. pp. 19–54.
145. Endler, G. and C. Mannhalter, Polymorphisms in coagulation factor genes and their impact on arterial and venous thrombosis. *Clin. Chim. Acta*, 2003. 330: pp. 31–55.
146. Hauschka, P.V., J.B. Lian, and P.M. Gallop, Direct identification of the calcium-binding amino acid gamma-carboxyglutamate, in mineralized tissue. *Proc. Natl. Acad. Sci. USA*, 1975. 72: pp. 3925–3929.
147. Price, P.A., A.S. Otsuka, J.W. Poser, J. Kristaponis, and N. Raman, Characterization of a gamma-carboxyglutamic acid-containing protein from bone. *Proc. Natl. Acad. Sci. USA*, 1976. 73: pp. 1447–1451.
148. Price, P.A. and M.K. Williamson, Effects of warfarin on bone. Studies on the vitamin K-dependent protein of rat bone. *J. Biol. Chem.*, 1981. 256: pp. 12754–12759.
149. Price, P.A., M.K. Williamson, T. Haba, R.B. Dell, and W.S.S. Jee, Excessive mineralization with growth plate closure in rats on chronic warfarin treatment. *Proc. Natl. Acad. Sci. USA*, 1982. 79: pp. 7734–7738.
150. Ducy, P., C. Desbois, B. Boyce, G. Pinero, B. Story, C. Dunstan, E. Smith, J. Bonadio, S. Goldstein, C. Gundberg, A. Bradley, and G. Karsenty, Increased bone formation in osteocalcin-deficient mice. *Nature*, 1996. 382: pp. 448–452.
151. Price, P.A. and M.K. Williamson, Primary structure of bovine matrix Gla protein, a new vitamin K-dependent bone protein. *J. Biol. Chem.*, 1985. 260: pp. 14971–14975.
152. Fraser, J.D. and P.A. Price, Lung, heart, and kidney express high levels of mRNA for the vitamin K-dependent matrix Gla protein. *J. Biol. Chem.*, 1988. 263: pp. 11033–11036.

153. Luo, G., P. Ducy, M.D. McKee, G.J. Pinero, E. Loyer, R.R. Behringer, and G. Karsenty, Spontaneous calcification of arteries and cartilage in mice lacking matrix Gla protein. *Nature*, 1997. 386: pp. 78–81.
154. Price, P.A., S.A. Faus, and M.K. Williamson, Warfarin causes rapid calcification of the elastic lamellae in rat arteries and heart valves. *Arterioscler. Thromb. Vasc. Biol.*, 1998. 18: pp. 1400–1407.
155. Manfioletti, G., C. Brancolini, G. Avanzi, and C. Schneider, The protein encoded by a growth arrest-specific gene (gas6) is a new member of the vitamin K-dependent proteins related to protein S, a negative coregulator in the blood coagulation cascade. *Mol. Cell. Biol.*, 1993. 13: pp. 4976–4985.
156. Prieto, A.L., J.L. Weber, S. Tracy, M.J. Heeb, and C. Lai, Gas6, a ligand for the receptor protein-tyrosine kinase tyro-3, is widely expressed in the central nervous system. *Brain Res.*, 1999. 816: pp. 646–661.
157. Melaragno, M.G., Y.-W.C. Fridell, and B.C. Berk, The Gas6/Axl system. A novel regulator of vascular cell function. *TCM*, 1999. 9: pp. 250–253.
158. Gould, W.R., S.M. Baxi, R. Schroeder, Y.W. Peng, R.J. Leadley, J.T. Peterson, and L.A. Perrin, Gas6 receptors AX1, Sky and Mer enhance platelet activation and regulate thrombotic responses. *J. Thromb. Haemost.*, 2005. 3: pp. 733–741.
159. Kulman, J.D., J.E. Harris, L. Xie, and E.W. Davie, Primary structure and tissue distribution of two novel proline-rich gamma-carboxyglutamic acid proteins. *Proc. Natl. Acad. Sci. USA*, 1997. 94: pp. 9058–9062.
160. Kulman, J.D., J.E. Harrais, L. Xie, and E.W. Davie, Identification of two novel transmembrane gamma-carboxyglutamic acid proteins expressed broadly in fetal and adult tissues. *Proc. Natl. Acad. Sci. USA*, 2001. 98: pp. 1370–1375.
161. Sundaram, K.S. and M. Lev, Regulation of sulfotransferase activity by vitamin K in mouse brain. *Arch. Biochem. Biophys.*, 1990. 277: pp. 109–113.
162. Denisova, N.A. and S.L. Booth, Vitamin K and sphingolipid metabolism: Evidence to date. *Nutr. Rev.*, 2005. 63: pp. 111–121.
163. McIntosh, J.M., B.M. Olivera, L.J. Cruz, and W.R. Gray, Gamma-carboxyglutamate in a neuroactive toxin. *J. Biol. Chem.*, 1984. 259: pp. 14343–14346.
164. Brown, M.A., B. Hambe, B. Furie, B.C. Furie, J. Stenflo, and L.M. Stenberg, Detection of vitamin K-dependent proteins in venoms with a monoclonal antibody specific for gamma-carboxyglutamic acid. *Toxicon*, 2002. 40: pp. 447–453.
165. Aguilar, M.B., E. Lopez-Vera, J.S. Imperial, A. Falcon, B.M. Olivera, and E.P. Heimer de la Cotera, Putative gamma-conotoxins in vermivorous cone snails: The case of Conus delessertii. *Peptides*, 2005. 26: pp. 23–27.
166. Bandhyopadhyay, P.K., J.E. Garrett, R.P. Shetty, T. Keate, C.S. Walker, and B.M. Olivera, Gamma-glutamyl carboxylation: An extracellular posttranslational modification that antedates the divergence of molluscs, arthropods, and chordates. *Proc. Natl. Acad. Sci. USA*, 2002. 99: pp. 1264–1269.
167. Li, T., LCl-T. Yang, D. Jin, and D.W. Stafford, Identification of a Drosophila vitamin K-dependent gamma-glutamyl carboxylase. *J. Biol. Chem.*, 2000. 275: pp. 18291–18296.
168. Hanumanthaiah, R., B. Thankavel, K. Day, M. Gregory, and P. Jagadeeswaran, Developmental expression of vitamin K-dependent gamma-carboxylase activity in Zebrafish embryos: Effect of warfarin. *Blood Cells Mol. Dis.*, 2001. 27: pp. 992–999.
169. Schultz, J., HTTM, a horizontally transferred transmembrane domain. *Trends Biochem. Sci.*, 2004. 29: pp. 4–7.
170. Hemker, H.C., J.J. Veltkamp, A. Hensen, and E.A. Loeliger, *Nature* of prothrombin biosynthesis: Preprothrombinaemia in vitamin K-deficiency. *Nature*, 1963. 200: pp. 589–590.
171. Ganrot, P.O. and J.E. Nilehn, Plasma prothrombin during treatment with dicumarol. II. Demonstration of an abnormal prothrombin fraction. *Scand. J. Clin. Lab. Invest.*, 1968. 22: pp. 23–28.
172. Stenflo, J., Dicoumarol-induced prothrombin in bovine plasma. *Acta Chem. Scand.*, 1970. 24: pp. 3762–3763.
173. Carlisle, T.L., D.V. Shah, R. Schlegel, and J.W. Suttie, Plasma abnormal prothrombin and microsomal prothrombin precursor in various species. *Proc. Soc. Exp. Biol. Med.*, 1975. 148: pp. 140–144.
174. Shah, D.V. and J.W. Suttie, Mechanism of action of vitamin K: Evidence for the conversion of a precursor protein to prothrombin in the rat. *Proc. Natl. Acad. Sci. USA*, 1971. 68: pp. 1653–1657.

175. Stenflo, J. and J.W. Suttie, Vitamin K-dependent formation of gamma-carboxyglutamic acid. *Annu. Rev. Biochem.*, 1977. 46: pp. 157–172.
176. Esmon, C.T., J.W. Suttie, and C.M. Jackson, The functional significance of vitamin K action. Difference in phospholipid binding between normal and abnormal prothrombin. *J. Biol. Chem.*, 1975. 250: pp. 4095–4099.
177. Stenflo, J., P. Fernlund, W. Egan, and P. Roepstorff, Vitamin K dependent modifications of glutamic acid residues in prothrombin. *Proc. Natl. Acad. Sci. USA*, 1974. 71: pp. 2730–2733.
178. Nelsestuen, G.L., T.H. Zytkovicz, and J.B. Howard, The mode of action of vitamin K. Identification of gamma-carboxyglutamic acid as a component of prothrombin. *J. Biol. Chem.*, 1974. 249: pp. 6347–6350.
179. Magnusson, S., L. Sotrup-Jensen, T.E. Petersen, H.R. Morris, and A. Dell, Primary structure of the vitamin K-dependent part of prothrombin. *FEBS Lett.*, 1974. 44: pp. 189–193.
180. Esmon, C.T., J.A. Sadowski, and J.W. Suttie, A new carboxylation reaction. The vitamin K-dependent incorporation of $H^{14}CO_3$ into prothrombin. *J. Biol. Chem.*, 1975. 250: pp. 4744–4748.
181. Esmon, C.T. and J.W. Suttie, Vitamin K-dependent carboxylase: Solubilization and properties. *J. Biol. Chem.*, 1976. 251: pp. 6238–6243.
182. Sadowski, J.A., H.K. Schnoes, and J.W. Suttie, Vitamin K epoxidase: Properties and relationship to prothrombin synthesis. *Biochemistry*, 1977. 16: pp. 3856–3863.
183. Suttie, J.W., J.M. Hageman, S.R. Lehrman, and D.H. Rich, Vitamin K-dependent carboxylase: Development of a peptide substrate. *J. Biol. Chem.*, 1976. 251: pp. 5827–5830.
184. Carlisle, T.L. and J.W. Suttie, Subcellular location of enzymes involved in vitamin K activity in rat liver. *Fed. Proc.*, 1978. 37: p. 708.
185. Olson, R.E., The function and metabolism of vitamin K. *Annu. Rev. Nutr.*, 1984. 4: pp. 281–337.
186. Suttie, J.W., Vitamin K-dependent carboxylase. *Annu. Rev. Biochem.*, 1985. 54: pp. 459–477.
187. Suttie, J.W., Synthesis of vitamin K-dependent proteins. *FASEB J.*, 1993. 7: pp. 445–452.
188. Vermeer, C. and M.A.G.d.B.-v.d. Berg, Vitamin K-dependent carboxylase. *Haematologia*, 1985. 18: pp. 71–97.
189. Vermeer, C., Gamma-carboxyglutamate-containing proteins and the vitamin K-dependent carboxylase. *Biochem. J.*, 1990. 266: pp. 625–636.
190. Furie, B. and B.C. Furie, Molecular and cellular biology of blood coagulation. *New. Eng. J. Med.*, 1992. 326: pp. 800–806.
191. Knobloch, J.E. and J.W. Suttie, Vitamin K-dependent carboxylase. Control of enzyme activity by the "propeptide" region of factor X. *J. Biol. Chem.*, 1987. 262: pp. 15334–15337.
192. Stanley, T.B., D-Y. Jin, P-J. Lin, and D.W. Stafford, The propeptides of the vitamin K-dependent proteins possess different affinities for the vitamin K-dependent carboxylase. *J. Biol. Chem.*, 1999. 274: pp. 16940–16944.
193. Furie, B.C., J.V. Ratcliffe, J. Tward, M.J. Jorgensen, L.S. Blaszkowsky, D. DiMichele, and B. Furie, The gamma-carboxylation recognition site is sufficient to direct vitamin K-dependent carboxylation on an adjacent glutamate-rich region of thrombin in a propeptide-thrombin chimera. *J. Biol. Chem.*, 1997. 272: pp. 28258–28262.
194. Stanley, T.B., S-M. Wu, R.J.T.J. Houben, V.P. Mutucumarana, and D.W. Stafford, Role of the propeptide and gamma-glutamic acid domain of factor IX for in vitro carboxylation by the vitamin K-dependent carboxylase. *Biochemistry*, 1998. 37: pp. 13262–13268.
195. Friedman, P.A., M.A. Shia, P.M. Gallop, and A.E. Griep, Vitamin K-dependent gamma-carbon-hydrogen bond cleavage and the non-mandatory concurrent carboxylation of peptide bound glutamic acid residues. *Proc. Natl. Acad. Sci. USA*, 1979. 76: pp. 3126–3129.
196. Larson, A.E., P.A. Friedman, and J.W. Suttie, Vitamin K-dependent carboxylase: Stoichiometry of carboxylation and vitamin K 2,3-epoxide formation. *J. Biol. Chem.*, 1981. 256: pp. 11032–11035.
197. McTigue, J.J. and J.W. Suttie, Vitamin K-dependent carboxylase: Demonstration of a vitamin K- and O_2-dependent exchange of ^3H from ^3H_2O into glutamic acid residues. *J. Biol. Chem.*, 1983. 258: pp. 12129–12131.
198. Wood, G.M., S. Funakawa, and J.W. Suttie, Stoichiometry of partial reactions of the vitamin K-dependent carboxylase system. *Fed. Proc.*, 1985. 44: p. 1155.
199. Dowd, P., S.W. Ham, and S.J. Geib, Mechanism of action of vitamin K. *J. Am. Chem. Soc.*, 1991. 113: pp. 7734–7743.

200. Dowd, P., S-W. Ham, S. Naganathan, and R. Hershline, The mechanism of action of vitamin K. *Annu. Rev. Nutr.*, 1995. 15: pp. 419–440.
201. Wu, S.M., W-F. Cheung, D. Frazier, and D. Stafford, Cloning and expression of the cDNA for human gamma-glutamyl carboxylase. *Science*, 1991. 254: pp. 1634–1636.
202. Morris, D.P., R.D. Stevens, D.J. Wright, and D.W. Stafford, Processive post-translational modification. Vitamin K-dependent carboxylation of a peptide substrate. *J. Biol. Chem.*, 1995. 270: pp. 30491–30498.
203. Stenina, O., B.N. Pudota, B.A. McNally, E.L. Hommema, and K.L. Berkner, Tethered processivity of the vitamin K-dependent carboxylase: Factor IX is efficiently modified in a mechanism which distinguishes Gla's from Glu's and which accounts for comprehensive carboxylation in vivo. *Biochemistry*, 2001. 40: pp. 10301–10309.
204. Hallgren, K.W., E.L. Hommema, B.A. McNally, and K.L. Berkner, Carboxylase overexpression effects full carboxylation but poor release and secretion of factor IX: Implications for the release of vitamin K-dependent proteins. *Biochemistry*, 2002. 41: pp. 15045–15055.
205. Tie, J-K., S.M. Wu, D. Jin, C.V. Nicchitta, and D.W. Stafford, A topological study of the human gamma-glutamyl carboxylase. *Blood*, 2000. 96: pp. 973–978.
206. Lin, P.-J., D.L. Straight, and D.W. Stafford, Binding of the factor IX gamma-carboxyglutamic acid domain to the vitamin K-dependent gamma-glutamyl carboxylase active site induces an allosteric effect that may ensure processive carboxylation and regulate the release of carboxylated product. *J. Biol. Chem.*, 2004. 279: pp. 6560–6566.
207. Berkner, K.L., The vitamin K-dependent carboxylase. *Annu. Rev. Nutr.*, 2005. 25: pp. 127–149.
208. Rishavy, M.A., B.N. Pudota, K.W. Hallgren, W. Qian, A.V. Yakubenko, J-H. Song, K.W. Runge, and K.L. Berkner, A new model for vitamin K-dependent carboxylation: The catalytic base that deprotonates vitamin K hydroquinone is not Cys but an activated amine. *Proc. Natl. Acad. Sci. USA*, 2004. 101: pp. 13732–13737.
209. Presnell, S.R. and D.W. Stafford, The vitamin K-dependent carboxylase. *Thromb. Haemost.*, 2002. 87: pp. 937–946.
210. Furie, B., B.A. Bouchard, and B.C. Furie, Vitamin K-dependent biosynthesis of gamma-carboxyglutamic acid. *Blood*, 1999. 93: pp. 798–1808.
211. Shah, D.V., J.K. Tews, A.E. Harper, and J.W. Suttie, Metabolism and transport of gamma-carboxyglutamic acid. *Biochim. Biophys. Acta.*, 1978. 539: pp. 209–217.
212. Bell, R.G. and J.T. Matschiner, Warfarin and the inhibition of vitamin K activity by an oxide metabolite. *Nature*, 1972. 237: pp. 32–33.
213. Sadowski, J.A. and J.W. Suttie, Mechanism of action of coumarins. Significance of vitamin K epoxide. *Biochemistry*, 1974. 13: pp. 3696–3699.
214. Lund, M., Resistance to warfarin in the common rat. *Nature*, 1964. 203: p. 778.
215. Fasco, M.J., P.C. Preusch, E. Hildebrandt, and J.W. Suttie, Formation of hydroxy vitamin K by vitamin K epoxide reductase of warfarin-resistant rats. *J. Biol. Chem.*, 1983. 258: pp. 4372–4380.
216. Hildebrandt, E.F. and J.W. Suttie, Mechanism of coumarin action: Sensitivity of vitamin K metabolizing enzymes of normal and warfarin-resistant rat liver. *Biochemistry*, 1982. 21: pp. 2406–2411.
217. Rost, S., A. Frogin, V. Ivaskeviciu, E. Conzelmann, K. Hortnagel, H-J. Pelz, K. Lappegard, E. Seifried, I. Scharrer, E.G.D. Tuddenham, C.R. Muller, T.M. Strom, and J. Oldenburg, Mutations in VKORC1 cause warfarin resistance and multiple coagulation factor deficiency type 2. *Nature*, 2004. 427: pp. 537–541.
218. Li, T., C-Y. Chang, D-Y. Jin, P-J. Lin, A. Khvorova, and D.W. Stafford, Identification of the gene for vitamin K epoxide reductase. *Nature*, 2004. 427: pp. 541–544.
219. Wallin, R. and S.M. Hutson, Warfarin and the vitamin K-dependent gamma-carboxylation system. *Trends Mol. Med.*, 2004. 10: pp. 299–302.
220. Robertson, H.M., Genes encoding vitamin-K epoxide reductase are present in drosophila and trypanosomatid protists. *Genetics*, 2004. 168: pp. 1077–1080.
221. Wajih, N., D.C. Sane, S.M. Hutson, and R. Wallin, Engineering of a recombinant vitamin K-dependent gamma-carboxylation system with enhanced gamma-carboxyglutamic acid forming capacity. Evidence for a functional CXXC redox center in the system. *J. Biol. Chem.*, 2005. 280: pp. 10540–10547.

222. Denson, K.W.E. and R. Biggs, Laboratory diagnosis, tests of clotting function and their standardization, *Human Blood Coagulation, Haemostasis and Thrombosis*. 1972, Oxford: Blackwell Scientific. pp. 278–332.
223. Kirchhof, B.R.J., C. Vermeer, and H.C. Hemker, The determination of prothrombin using synthetic chromogenic substrates; choice of a suitable activator. *Thromb. Res.*, 1978. 13: pp. 219–232.
224. Hazell, K. and K.H. Baloch, Vitamin K deficiency in the elderly. *Gerentol. Clin.*, 1970. 12: pp. 10–17.
225. Savage, D. and J. Lindenbaum, Clinical and experimental human vitamin K deficiency, *Nutrition in Hematology*. 1983, New York: Churchill Livingstone. pp. 271–320.
226. Weitekamp, M.R. and R.C. Aber, Prolonged bleeding times and bleeding diathesis associated with moxalactam administration. *JAMA*, 1983. 249: pp. 69–71.
227. Lipsky, J.J., Mechanism of the inhibition of the gamma-carboxylation of glutamic acid by N-methylthiotetrazole-containing antibiotics. *Proc. Natl. Acad. Sci. USA*, 1984. 81: pp. 2893–2897.
228. Suttie, J.W., J.A. Engelke, and J. McTigue, Effect of N-methyl-thiotetrazole on rat liver microsomal vitamin K-dependent carboxylation. *Biochem. Pharmacol.*, 1986. 35: pp. 2429–2433.
229. Creedon, K.A. and J.W. Suttie, Effect of N-methyl-thiotetrazole on vitamin K epoxide reductase. *Thromb. Res.*, 1986. 44: pp. 147–153.
230. Frick, P.G., G. Riedler, and H. Brogli, Dose response and minimal daily requirement for vitamin K in man. *J. Appl. Physiol.*, 1967. 23: pp. 387–389.
231. Allison, P.M., L.L. Mummah-Schendel, C.C. Kindberg, C.S. Harms, N.U. Bang, and J.W. Suttie, Effects of a vitamin K-deficient diet and antibiotics in normal human volunteers. *J. Lab. Clin. Med.*, 1987. 110: pp. 180–188.
232. Sokoll, L.J., S.L. Booth, M.E. O'Brien, K.W. Davidson, K.I. Tsaioun, and J.A. Sadowski, Changes in serum osteocalcin, plasma phylloquinone, and urinary gamma-carboxyglutamic acid in response to altered intakes of dietary phylloquinone in human subjects. *Am. J. Clin. Nutr.*, 1997. 65: pp. 779–784.
233. Schurgers, L.J., M.J. Shearer, K. Hamulyak, E. Stocklin, and C. Vermeer, Effect of vitamin K intake on the stability of oral anticoagulant treatment: Dose–response relationships in healthy subjects. *Blood*, 2004. 104: pp. 2682–2689.
234. Johnson, M.A., Influence of vitamin K on anticoagulant therapy depends on vitamin K status and the source and chemical forms of vitamin K. *Nutr. Rev.*, 2005. 63: pp. 91–97.
235. D'Andrea, G., R.L. D'Ambrosio, P. Di Perna, M. Chetta, R. Santacroce, V. Brancaccio, E. Grandone, and M. Margaglione, A polymorphism in the VKORC1 gene is associated with an interindividual variabilty in the dose-anticoagulant effect of warfarin. *Blood*, 2005. 105: pp. 645–649.
236. Rieder, M.J., A.P. Reiner, B.F. Gage, D.A. Nickerson, C.S. Eby, H.L. McLeod, D.K. Blough, K.E. Thummel, D.L. Veenstra, and A.E. Rettie, Effect of VKORC1 haplotypes on transcriptional regulation and warfarin dose. *New. Eng. J. Med.*, 2005. 352: pp. 2285–2293.
237. Takahashi, H. and H. Echizen, Pharmacogenetics of CYP2C9 and interindividual variability in anticoagulant response to warfarin. *Pharmacogenomics J.*, 2003. 3: pp. 202–214.
238. O'Reilly, R.A. and P.M. Aggeler, Coumarin anticoagulant drugs: Hereditary resistance in man. *Fed. Proc.*, 1965. 24: pp. 1266–1273.
239. Williams, E.C. and J.W. Suttie, Vitamin K antagonists, *Cardiovascular Thrombosis: Thrombocardiology and Thromboneurology*, M. Verstraete, V. Fuster, and E.J. Topol, eds. 1998, Lippincott-Raven Publishers: Philadelphia.
240. Lane, P.A. and W.E. Hathaway, Vitamin K in infancy. *J. Pediatrics.*, 1985. 106: pp. 351–359.
241. Greer, F.R., The importance of vitamin K as a nutrient during the first year of life. *Nutr. Res.*, 1995. 15: pp. 289–310.
242. Golding, J., R. Greenwood, K. Birmingham, and M. Mott, Childhood cancer, intramuscular vitamin K, and pethidine given during labour. *Br. Med. J.*, 1992. 305: pp. 341–346.
243. Roman, E., N.T. Fear, P. Ansell, D. Bull, G. Draper, P. McKinney, J. Michaelis, S.J. Passmore, and R. von Kries, Vitamin K and childhood cancer: Analysis of individual patient data from six case-control studies. *Br. J. Cancer*, 2002. 86: pp. 63–69.
244. Fear, N.T., E. Roman, P. Ansell, J. Simpson, N. Day, and O.B. Eden, Vitamin K and childhood cancer: A report from the United Kingdom childhood cancer study. *Br. J. Cancer*, 2003. 89: pp. 1228–1231.

245. American Academy of Pediatrics, Committee on Food and Nutrition, Policy statement: Controversies concerning vitamin K and the newborn. *Pediatrics*, 2003. 112: pp. 191–192.
246. Sokoll, L.J. and J.A. Sadowski, Comparison of biochemical indexes for assessing vitamin K nutritional status in a healthy adult population. *Am. J. Clin. Nutr.*, 1996. 63: pp. 566–573.
247. Binkley, N.C., D. Krueger, J. Engelke, T. Crenshaw, and J. Suttie, Vitamin K supplementation reduces serum concentrations of under-gamma-carboxylated osteocalcin in healthy young and elderly adults. *Am. J. Clin. Nutr.*, 2000. 72: pp. 1523–1528.
248. Gundberg, C.M., S.D. Nieman, S. Abrams, and H. Rosen, Vitamin K status and bone health: An analysis of methods for determination of undercarboxylated osteocalcin. *J. Clin. Endocrinol. Metab.*, 1998. 83: pp. 3258–3266.
249. Binkley, N.C., D.C. Krueger, T.N. Kawahara, J.A. Engelke, R.J. Chappell, and J.W. Suttie, A high phylloquinone intake is required to achieve maximal osteocalcin gamma-carboxylation. *Am. J. Clin. Nutr.*, 2002. 76: pp. 1055–1060.
250. Feskanich, D., P. Weber, W.C. Willett, H. Rockett, S.L. Booth, and G.A. Colditz, Vitamin K intake and hip fractures in women: A prospective study. *Am. J. Clin. Nutr.*, 1999. 69: pp. 74–79.
251. Booth, S.L., K.L. Tucker, H. Chen, M.T. Hannan, D.R. Gagnon, L.A. Cupples, P.W.F. Wilson, J. Ordovas, E.J. Schaefer, B. Dawson-Hughes, and D.P. Kiel, Dietary vitamin intakes are associated with hip fracture but not with bone mineral density in elderly men and women. *Am. J. Clin. Nutr.*, 2000. 71: pp. 1201–1208.
252. Vergnaud, P., P. Garnero, P.J. Meunier, G. Breart, K. Kamilhagi, and P.D. Delmas, Undercarboxylated osteocalcin measured with a specific immunoassay predicts hip fracture in elderly women: The EPIDOS study. *J. Clin. Endocrinol. Metab.*, 1997. 82: pp. 719–724.
253. Caraballo, P.J., S.E. Gabriel, M.R. Castro, E.J. Atkinson, and L.J. Melton, III, Changes in bone density after exposure to oral anticoagulants: A meta-analysis. *Osteoporos. Int.*, 1999. 9: pp. 441–448.
254. Orimo, H., M. Shiraki, A. Tomita, H. Morii, T. Fujita, and M. Ohata, Effects of menatetrenone on the bone and calcium metabolism in osteoporosis: A double-blind placebo-controlled study. *J. Bone Miner. Metab.*, 1998. 16: pp. 106–112.
255. Shiraki, M., Y. Shiraki, C. Aoki, and M. Miura, Vitamin K_2 (menatetrenone) effectively prevents fractures and sustains lumbar bone mineral density in osteoporosis. *J. Bone Miner. Res.*, 2000. 15: pp. 515–521.
256. Iwamoto, I., S. Kosha, T. Fujino, and Y. Nagata, Effects of vitamin K_2 on bone of ovariectomized rats and on a rat osteoblastic cell line. *Gynecol. Obstet. Invest.*, 2002. 53: pp. 144–148.
257. Ozuru, R., T. Sugimoto, T. Yamaguchi, and K. Chihara, Time-dependent effects of vitamin K_2 (menatetrenone) on bone metabolism in postmenopausal women. *Endocrine. J.*, 2002. 49: pp. 363–370.
258. Braam, L.A., M.H. Knapen, P. Geusens, F. Brouons, K. Hamulyak, M.J. Gerichhausen, and C. Vermeer, Vitamin K_1 supplementation retards bone loss in postmenopausal women between 50 and 60 years of age. *Calcif. Tissue Int.*, 2003. 73: pp. 21–26.
259. Binkley, N.C. and J.W. Suttie, Vitamin K nutrition and osteoporosis. *J. Nutr.*, 1995. 125: pp. 1812–1821.
260. Yoshida, T., K. Miyazawa, I. Kasuga, T. Yokoyama, K. Minemura, K. Ustumi, M. Aoshima, and K. Ohyashiki, Apoptosis induction of vitamin K_2 in lung carcinoma cell lines: The possibility of vitamin K_2 therapy for lung cancer. *Int. J. Oncol.*, 2003. 23: pp. 627–632.
261. Tabb, N.M., A. Sun, C. Zhou, F. Grun, J. Errandi, K. Romero, H. Pham, S. Inoue, S. Mallick, M. Lin, B.M. Forman, and B. Blumberg, Vitamin K_2 regulation of bone homeostasis is mediated by the steroid and xenobiotic receptor SXR. *J. Biol. Chem.*, 2003. 278: pp. 43919–43927.
262. Ronden, J.E., M-J. Drittij-Reijnders, C. Vermeer, and H.H.W. Thijssen, Intestinal flora is not an intermediate in the phylloquinone–menaquinone-4 conversion in the rat. *Biochim. Biophys. Acta*, 1998. 1379: pp. 69–75.
263. Akiyama, Y., K. Hara, M. Kobayashi, T. Tomiuga, and T. Nakamura, Inhibitory effect of vitamin K_2 (menatetrenone) on bone resorption in ovariectomized rats: A histomorphometric and dual energy x-ray absorptiometric study. *Jpn. J. Pharmacol.*, 1999. 80: pp. 67–74.
264. Hara, K., Y. Akiyama, I. Ohkawa, and T. Tajima, Effects of menatetrenone on prednisolone-induced bone loss in rats. *Bone*, 1993. 14: pp. 813–818.

265. Binkley, N., D. Krueger, J. Engelke, T. Crenshaw, and J. Suttie, Vitamin K supplementation does not affect ovariectomy-induced bone loss in rats. *Bone*, 2002. 30: pp. 897–900.
266. El-Maadawy, S., M.T. Kaartinen, T. Schinke, M. Murshed, G. Karsenty, and M.D. McKee, Cartilage formation and calcification in arteries of mice lacking matrix Gla protein. *Connect. Tissue Res.*, 2003. 44 (Suppl): pp. 272–278.
267. Zebboudj, A.F., M. Imura, and K. Bostrom, Matrix Gla protein, a regulatory protein for bone morphogenetic protein-2. *J. Biol. Chem.*, 2002. 277: pp. 4388–4394.
268. Bostrom, K., A.F. Zebboudj, Y. Yao, T.S. Lin, and A. Torres, Matrix Gla protein stimulates VEGF expression through increased transforming growth factor-beta1 activity in endothelial cells. *J. Biol. Chem.*, 2004. 279: pp. 52904–52913.
269. Hur, D.J., G.V. Raymond, S.G. Kahler, D.L. Riegert-Johnson, B.A. Cohen, and S.A. Boyadjiev, A novel MGP mutation in a consanguineous family: Review of the clinical and molecular characteristics of Keutel syndrome. *Am. J. Med. Genet.*, 2005. 135A: pp. 36–40.
270. Villines, T.C., C. Hatzigeorgiou, I.M. Feuerstein, P.G. O'Malley, and A.J. Taylor, Vitamin K_1 intake and coronary calcification. *Coron. Artery Dis.*, 2005. 16: pp. 199–203.
271. Jie, K.S., M.L. Bots, C. Vermeer, J.C. Witteman, and D.E. Grobbee, Vitamin K intake and osteocalcin levels in women with and without aortic atherosclerosis: A population-based study. *Atherosclerosis*, 1995. 116: pp. 117–123.
272. Geleijnse, J.M., C. Vermeer, D.E. Grobbee, L.J. Schurgers, M.H.J. Knapen, I.M. van der Meer, A. Hofman, and J.C.M. Witteman, Dietary intake of menaquinone is associated with a reduced risk of coronary heart disease: The Rotterdam study. *J. Nutr.*, 2004. 134: pp. 3100–3105.
273. Gustafsson, B.E., F.S. Daft, E.G. McDaniel, J.C. Smith, and R.J. FitzGerald, Effects of vitamin K-active compounds and intestinal microorganisms in vitamin K-deficient germfree rats. *J. Nutr.*, 1962. 78: pp. 461–468.
274. Takahashi, O. and K. Hiraga, Preventive effects of phylloquinone on hemorrhagic death induced by butylated hydroxytoluene in male rats. *J. Nutr.*, 1979. 109: pp. 453–457.
275. Mountain, K.R., A.S. Gallus, and J. Hirsh, Neonatal coagulation defect due to anticonvulsant drug treatment in pregnancy. *Lancet*, 1970. i: pp. 265–268.
276. Matschiner, J.T. and A.K. Willingham, Influence of sex hormones on vitamin K deficiency and epoxidation of vitamin K in the rat. *J. Nutr.*, 1974. 104: pp. 660–665.
277. Jolly, D.W., B.M. Kadis, and T.E. Nelson, Estrogen and prothrombin synthesis. The prothrombinogenic action of estrogen. *Biochem. Biophys. Res. Commun.*, 1977. 74: pp. 41–49.
278. Siegfried, C.M., G.R. Knauer, and J.T. Matschiner, Evidence for increased formation of preprothrombin and the noninvolvement of vitamin K-dependent reactions in sex-linked hyperprothrombinemia in the rat. *Arch. Biochem. Biophys.*, 1979. 194: pp. 486–495.
279. Oosterom, A.T.V., P. Kerkhoven, and J.J. Veltkamp, Metabolism of the coagulation factors of the prothrombin complex in hypothyroidism in man. *Thromb. Haemost.*, 1979. 41: pp. 273–285.
280. Elliott, M.V., B. Isaacs, and A.C. Ivy, Production of "prothrombin deficiency" and response to vitamins A, D and K. *Proc. Soc. Exp. Biol. Med.*, 1940. 43: pp. 240–245.
281. Doisy, E.A. and J.T. Matschiner, *Biochemistry* of vitamin K, *Fat-Soluble Vitamins*. 1970, Oxford: Pergamon Press. pp. 293–331.
282. Rao, G.H. and K.E. Mason, Antisterility and antivitamin K activity of d-alpha-tocopheryl hydroquinone in the vitamin E-deficient female rat. *J. Nutr.*, 1975. 105: pp. 495–498.
283. Corrigan, J.J. and L.L. Ulfers, Effect of vitamin E on prothrombin levels in warfarin-induced vitamin K deficiency. *J. Nutr.*, 1981. 34: pp. 1701–1705.
284. Olson, R.E. and J.P. Jones, The inhibition of vitamin K action by D-alpha-tocopherol and its derivatives. *Fed. Proc.*, 1979. 38: p. 710.
285. Uotila, L., Inhibition of vitamin K-dependent carboxylase by vitamin E and its derivatives, *Current Advances in Vitamin K Research*. 1988, New York: Elsevier. pp. 59–64.
286. Alexander, C.D. and J.W. Suttie, The effects of vitamin E on vitamin K activity. *FASEB J.*, 1999. 13: p. A535.
287. Will, B.H., Y. Usui, and J.W. Suttie, Comparative vitamin K metabolism in chick and rat liver. *FASEB J.*, 1992. 6: p. A1940.
288. Scott, M.L., Vitamin K in animal nutrition. *Vitam. Horm.*, 1966. 24: pp. 633–647.

289. Griminger, P., Nutritional requirements for vitamin K-animal studies, *Symposium Proceedings on the Biochemistry, Assay, and Nutritional Value of Vitamin K and Related Compounds*. 1971, Chicago: Asso. Vitamin Chemists. pp. 39–59.
290. National Academy of *Sciences*, *Nutrient Requirements of Laboratory Animals*, 3rd ed. 1978, Washington, DC: National Academy Press. p. 96.
291. Reeves, P.G., F.H. Nielsen, and G.C. Fahey Jr, AIN-93 purified diets for laboratory rodents: Final report of the American Institute of Nutrition ad hoc writing committee on the reformulation of the AIN-76A rodent diet. *J. Nutri.*, 1993. 123: pp. 1939–1951.
292. Owen, C.A., Vitamin K group XI pharmacology and toxicology, *The Vitamins*, 2nd ed. 1971, New York: Academic Press. pp. 492–509.
293. National Research Council, *Vitamin Tolerance of Animals*. 1987, Washington, DC: National Academy Press. p. 96.
294. Uchida, K. and T. Komeno, Relationships between dietary and intestinal vitamin K, clotting factor levels, plasma vitamin K and urinary Gla, *Current Advances in Vitamin K Research*. 1988, New York: Elsevier. pp. 477–492.
295. Usui, Y., N. Nishimura, N. Kobayashi, T. Okanoue, M. Kimoto, and K. Ozawa, Measurement of vitamin K in human liver by gradient elution high-performance liquid chromatography using platinum-black catalyst reduction and fluorimetric detection. *J. Chromatog.*, 1989. 489: pp. 291–301.

4 Vitamin E

Maret G. Traber

CONTENTS

INTRODUCTION

Vitamin E is unique because it remains a vitamin without a specific function. Other vitamins are cofactors, hormones, or have specific roles in metabolism. Vitamin E deficiency symptoms are varied because the major function of vitamin E is that of a lipid-soluble antioxidant. Therefore, vitamin E deficiency symptoms are dependent on α-tocopherol content, uptake and turnover, as well as susceptibility to and the degree of oxidative stress in a given tissue. Furthermore, vitamin E concentrations depend on the presence of other antioxidants to maintain α-tocopherol in its unoxidized state (1).

Importantly, vitamin E's antioxidant function cannot be fulfilled by just any antioxidant. Specifically, only α-tocopherol meets human vitamin E requirements (2). Plasma α-tocopherol is controlled by the hepatic α-tocopherol transfer protein (α-TTP) (3,4) and, in humans, a genetic defect in α-TTP results in severe vitamin E deficiency (5). α-TTP is necessary for the facilitated transfer of α-tocopherol from the liver to the plasma (6,7).

This chapter describes vitamin E structures, antioxidant function, lipoprotein transport, and delivery to tissues. Requirements, intake, human deficiency symptoms, and the role of vitamin E in the prevention of chronic disease are discussed.

HISTORY

Vitamin E deficiency in rats fed rancid fat was first described in 1922 by Evans and Bishop (8). In 1936, Evans et al. (9) isolated vitamin E from wheat germ and named this factor, "α-tocopherol;" a name derived from the Greek "tokos" (offspring) and "pherein" (to bear) with an "ol" to indicate that it was an alcohol. Subsequently, β-tocopherol and γ-tocopherol were isolated from vegetable oils (10), demonstrating that various forms of vitamin E exist, but that α-tocopherol is the most effective form in preventing vitamin E deficiency symptoms. Today, it seems likely that the minor α-tocopherol contaminant in these vitamin E preparations provided their vitamin E biologic activity.

Specific vitamin E deficiency symptoms (e.g., fetal resorption, muscular dystrophy, and encephalomalacia) were observed in experimental animals fed vitamin E-deficient diets (11). The most popular, though most tedious and time-consuming, assay for the biologic activity of vitamin E is the fetal resorption assay (11). Here, vitamin E-depleted virgin female rats are mated with normal males. After successful mating, various levels of single vitamin E forms are fed in several divided doses to the females, which are killed 20–21 days after mating. The number of living, dead, and resorbed fetuses are counted and the percentage of live young determined. Thus, the vitamin E biologic activity depends on the amount necessary to maintain the maximum number of live fetuses. The results of this assay remain in use today to define the international units (IUs) of vitamin E activity.

Horwitt (12,13) attempted to induce vitamin E deficiency in men by feeding a diet low in vitamin E (2–4 mg α-tocopherol) for six years to volunteers at the Elgin State Hospital in Illinois. After about two years, their serum vitamin E levels decreased into the deficient range. Although their erythrocytes were more sensitive to peroxide-induced hemolysis, overt anemia did not develop. The data from the Horwitt study was used in 2000 to set the recommended dietary allowance (RDA) for vitamin E (2). These latest RDAs are discussed later.

STRUCTURES AND ANTIOXIDANT CHEMISTRY

STRUCTURE

Vitamin E is the name for molecules with α-tocopherol antioxidant activity, including all tocol and tocotrienol derivatives (14). These antioxidants include four tocopherols and four

	R_1	R_2	R_3
α	CH_3	CH_3	CH_3
β	CH_3	H	CH_3
γ	H	CH_3	CH_3
δ	H	H	CH_3

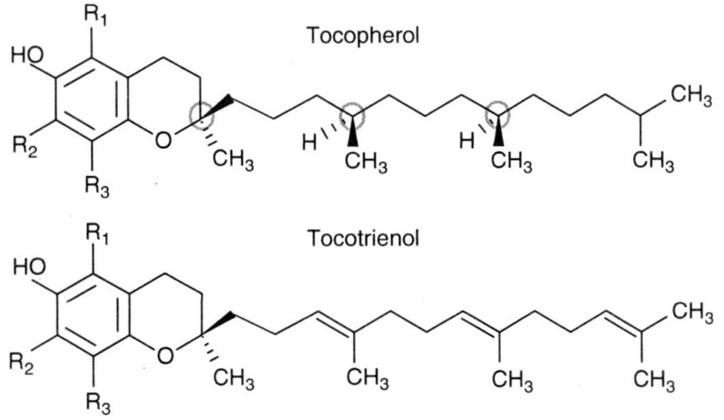

FIGURE 4.1 Vitamin E structures are shown. The methyl groups on the chromanol head determine whether the molecule is α-, β- or γ-, or δ-, while the tail determines whether the molecule is a tocopherol or a tocotrienol.

tocotrienols, which have similar chromanol structures: trimethyl (α-), dimethyl (β- or γ-), and monomethyl (δ-). Tocotrienols differ from tocopherols in that they have an unsaturated tail. However, in 2000, the Food and Nutrition Board (FNB) (2) defined α-tocopherol as the only form that meets human vitamin E requirements, because only α-tocopherol has been shown to reverse human vitamin E deficiency symptoms.

Unlike most other vitamins, chemically synthesized α-tocopherol is not identical to the naturally occurring form. α-Tocopherol synthesized by condensation of trimethyl hydroquinone with racemic isophytol (15) contains eight stereoisomers, arising from the three chiral centers (2,4′, and 8′, Figure 4.1), and is designated *all-rac*-α-tocopherol (incorrectly called D,L-α-tocopherol). The FNB (2) defined that only 2*R*-α-tocopherol forms meet human vitamin E requirements. Thus, only half of the stereoisomers in *all-rac*-α-tocopherol meet the vitamin E requirement.

Vitamin E supplements often contain α-tocopherol esters, including α-tocopheryl acetate, succinate, or nicotinate. The ester form is not an antioxidant and thus has a long shelf life. Vitamin E esters are readily hydrolyzed in the gut and are absorbed as α-tocopherol (16).

Nomenclature

The FNB (2) definition of vitamin E has led to confusion about vitamin E units. The vitamin E unit currently used on supplement labels was defined by the U.S. Pharmacopoeia (17). The IU of vitamin E equals 1 mg *all-rac*-α-tocopheryl acetate, 0.67 mg *RRR*-α-tocopherol, or 0.74 mg *RRR*-α-tocopheryl acetate. However, the FNB (Table 6.1 in (2)) defined the vitamin E requirement in milligrams of 2*R*-α-tocopherol and provided conversion factors, such that *all-rac* is equal to 1/2 *RRR*-α-tocopherol. To estimate the number of milligrams of 2*R*-α-tocopherol, IU *all-rac*-α-tocopherol (or its esters) must be multiplied by 0.45; whereas IU *RRR*-α-tocopherol (or its esters) is multiplied by 0.67.

Chemical Properties

All vitamin E forms act as lipid-soluble chain-breaking antioxidants (18). Vitamin E is a potent peroxyl radical scavenger and especially protects PUFA within phospholipids of biological membranes and in plasma lipoproteins. When lipid hydroperoxides are oxidized to peroxyl radicals (ROO•), these react 1,000 times faster with vitamin E (Vit E-OH) than with PUFA (RH) (19). The chromanol hydroxyl group reacts with a peroxyl radical to form a hydroperoxide and the chromanoxyl radical (Vit E-O•):

In the presence of vitamin E, ROO• + Vit E-OH → ROOH + Vit E-O•

In the absence of vitamin E, ROO• + RH → ROOH + R•

R• + O2 → ROO•

In this way, vitamin E acts as a chain-breaking antioxidant, preventing further autooxidation of lipids.

Antioxidant Network

Vitamin E interacts with other antioxidants to remain in the unoxidized form. The chromanoxyl radical Vit E-O• reacts with vitamin C (or other reductants serving as hydrogen donors, AH), oxidizing the other antioxidant and reducing vitamin E.

Vit E-O• + AH → Vit E-OH + A•

Biologically important antioxidants that regenerate chromanols from chromanoxyl radicals include ascorbate (vitamin C) and thiols, especially glutathione. Various metabolic processes can then reduce these other antioxidants. This phenomenon has led to the idea of vitamin E recycling, where vitamin E is restored by other antioxidants. Since the α-tocopheroxyl radical can readily be reduced to α-tocopherol, the amount of vitamin E that is recycled is likely much larger than the amount that is further oxidized.

Oxidized Vitamin E

The primary oxidation product of α-tocopherol is α-tocopheryl quinone, which can be conjugated to yield the glucuronide after reduction to the hydroquinone. The glucuronide can be excreted into bile or further degraded in the kidneys to α-tocopheronic acid, which is excreted in the urine (20). Other oxidation products, including dimers and trimers, as well as other adducts have also been described (18).

Specific vitamin E oxidation products have been generated in vitro (21,22). These include 4a,5-epoxy- and 7,8-epoxy-8a(hydroperoxy)tocopherones and their respective hydrolysis products, 2,3-epoxy-tocopherol quinone and 5,6-epoxy-α-tocopherol quinone. However, these products are formed during in vitro oxidation; their importance in vivo is unknown.

PHYSIOLOGIC RELATIONSHIPS

Absorption

The absorption of vitamin E from the intestinal lumen is dependent on processes necessary for fat digestion and uptake into enterocytes (23). Pancreatic esterases are required for release of free fatty acids from dietary triglycerides. Esterases are also required for the hydrolytic cleavage of tocopheryl esters, present in dietary supplements. Bile acids, monoglycerides, and free fatty acids are important components of mixed micelles. Bile acids are required for the formation of mixed micelles and are essential for vitamin E absorption. In the absence of both pancreatic and biliary secretions, only negligible amounts of vitamin E are absorbed. Thus, human vitamin E deficiency occurs as a result of fat malabsorption (24).

The bioavailability of vitamin E appears also to be dependent on the fat content of the meal. Hayes et al. (25) reported that plasma α-tocopherol concentrations doubled when α-tocopheryl acetate (100–200 mg/day) was provided as a microdispersion in milk, compared with providing the same dose in orange juice. Vitamin E absorption is relatively poor when it is consumed without fat, as was observed when vitamin E pills were consumed without food (26).

It is well known that increasing dietary fat increases absorption of vitamin E supplements (26,27). Roodenberg et al. (28) suggested that a 3% fat intake was sufficient for optimal vitamin E bioavailability. However, they measured bioavailability as increased plasma α-tocopherol concentrations following one week of supplementation with 50 mg α-tocopherol in either 50 g of a low- or high-fat spread, such that hot meals contained either less than 6.5 g fat or less than 45 g fat. Thus, dissolving the vitamin E in the spread may have allowed normal vitamin E absorption.

During fat absorption, enterocytes synthesize chylomicrons that contain triglycerides, free and esterified cholesterol, phospholipids, and apolipoproteins (especially apolipoprotein [apo] B48). In addition, fat-soluble vitamins, carotenoids, and other fat-soluble dietary components are incorporated into chylomicrons. Chylomicrons are then secreted into the lymph. The movement of vitamin E through the absorptive cells is not well understood; no intestinal TTPs have been described. Even in healthy individuals, the efficiency of vitamin E absorption is low (<50%). Recent findings in the cholesterol field suggest that lipid-soluble nutrient absorption may be modulated by adenosine triphosphate-binding cassette (ABC) transporters, nuclear receptors, and various intracellular trafficking proteins (29).

Often it is assumed that differences in plasma concentrations of various forms of vitamin E result from differences in the degree of intestinal absorption, but this is not the case. Discrimination between forms of vitamin E does not occur during their absorption by the intestine and their secretion in chylomicrons (30,31). Thus, all dietary forms of vitamin E are absorbed and secreted into chylomicrons.

Lipoprotein Transport

During chylomicron catabolism by lipoprotein lipase in the circulation, some of the newly absorbed vitamin E is transferred to high-density lipoproteins (HDL) and some remains with the chylomicron remnants. Because HDL readily transfer vitamin E to other lipoproteins, the newly absorbed vitamin E is distributed to all of the circulating lipoproteins. Although the process can occur spontaneously, the phospholipid transfer protein (PLTP) may also be involved. PLTP catalyzes vitamin E exchange between lipoproteins at a rate that represents transfer of approximately 10% of the plasma vitamin E/h (32).

Chylomicron remnants are taken up by the liver, delivering the newly absorbed vitamin E. The liver repackages dietary fats, secreting them into the plasma in very low density lipoproteins (VLDL). Unlike other fat-soluble vitamins, which have specific plasma transport proteins, vitamin E is transported nonspecifically in lipoproteins in the plasma. However, plasma vitamin E concentrations do depend on α-tocopherol secretion from the liver (33). Additionally, the newly absorbed vitamin E appears to be preferentially secreted into the plasma from the liver (34). Thus, the liver, not the intestine, discriminates between tocopherols.

Tissue Delivery

No plasma-specific vitamin E transport proteins have been described, but rather mechanisms of lipoprotein metabolism determine the delivery of vitamin E to tissues. There are at least three major routes by which tissues likely acquire vitamin E: (i) via lipoprotein lipase-mediated lipoprotein catabolism, (ii) via lipoprotein receptors, and (iii) mediated by membrane lipids transporters. In addition, vitamin E rapidly exchanges between lipoproteins, and between lipoproteins and membranes.

Delivery of vitamin E from both chylomicrons and VLDL is likely mediated by lipoprotein lipase. This mechanism may be particularly important for tissues that express lipoprotein lipase, such as adipose tissue, muscle, and brain. Sattler et al. (35) tested this hypothesis directly by overexpressing lipoprotein lipase in mouse muscle and found increased delivery of α-tocopherol to the muscle.

Another important mechanism for the delivery of tocopherols to tissues is via the LDL receptor (24). Other lipoprotein receptors are also involved in tissue uptake of tocopherols. The scavenger receptor-BI (SR-BI) mediates transfer of lipids from HDL, whereas the protein is released into the circulation (36). Apparently, SR-BI similarly delivers vitamin E from HDL to cells. HDL are major α-tocopherol transporters to lung (37–40), brain (41,42), and liver (43).

Vitamin E delivery by HDL to the liver appears analogous to reverse cholesterol transport (44), in that HDL via SR-BI deliver vitamin E for excretion into bile (45). Vitamin E-deficient rats increase liver SR-BI suggesting that SR-BI is regulated by α-tocopherol (43). Increased SR-BI would serve to increase vitamin E delivery to the liver.

ABCA1 is an ABC transporter that transfers cholesterol and phospholipids to HDL. ABCA1 is also responsible for the cellular secretion of α-tocopherol (46). Mice lacking ABCA1 have severe α-tocopherol deficiency (47). Clearly, ABCA1 is important in α-tocopherol trafficking, and its physiologic role appears to be involved in cellular tocopherol efflux; but further investigations into its role in regulating tissue vitamin E concentrations are warranted.

Storage Sites

No organ functions as an α-tocopherol storage site, releasing it on demand (24). More than 90% of the human body α-tocopherol is located in the adipose tissue. It has been estimated that more than two years are required to reach new steady state levels in response to changes in dietary intake (48). Thus, the analysis of adipose tissue α-tocopherol content is a useful estimate of long-term vitamin E intakes. El-Sohemy et al. (49) reported in nearly 500 Costa Rican subjects that adipose tissue γ-tocopherol concentrations were related to dietary γ-tocopherol intakes; whereas adipose tissue α-tocopherol concentrations were not related to intakes. Nonetheless, adipose tissue α-tocopherol concentrations were higher than γ-tocopherol concentrations. These findings suggest that the ability of α-TTP in its role of discriminating between tocopherols and maintaining plasma α-tocopherol concentrations is ultimately important for determining tissue, including adipose tissue concentrations.

VITAMIN E-SPECIFIC PROTEINS

α-Tocopherol Transfer Protein

α-TTP (calculated molecular weight 31,883 Da) has been detected in the liver of rats, humans, mice, dogs, chickens, and so on. The gene has been localized to the human 8q13.1–13.3 region of chromosome 8 (50,51). α-TTP mRNA has been detected in rat brain, spleen, lung, and kidney (52), as well as in human brain (53). α-TTP is also present in pregnant mouse uterus and human placenta (54–56), suggesting that it functions to ensure adequate α-tocopherol concentrations during pregnancy.

α-TTP preferentially transfers α-tocopherol, compared with other dietary vitamin E forms (57,58). Hypothetically, this ability to transfer tocopherol is necessary for the observed in vivo α-TTP action because nascent VLDL, secreted from the monkey liver, are preferentially enriched in *RRR*-α-tocopherol (59). However, when this hypothesis was tested in an α-TTP-expressing hepatic cell line (McARH7777 cells), α-TTP-mediated α-tocopherol secretion was not associated with VLDL secretion (60).

Although the mechanism by which α-TTP facilitates α-tocopherol secretion into plasma is unknown, some progress has been made in this area. α-TTP is a cytosolic protein in

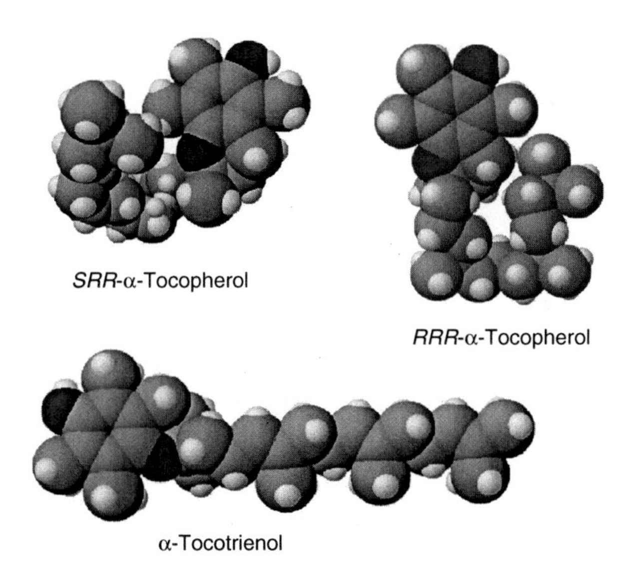

FIGURE 4.2 Space-filling structures of *RRR*-α-tocopherol and *SRR*-α-tocopherol and α-tocotrienol are shown to illustrate the conformation that *RRR*-α-tocopherol takes when it is bound to the α-tocopherol transfer protein. (Adapted from Min, K.C., Kovall, R.A., and Hendrickson, W.A., *Proc. Natl. Acad. Sci. USA*, 100, 14713, 2003.)

hepatocytes; however, following chloroquine treatment, α-TTP was associated with the cytosolic surface of late endosomes (61). Hypothetically, α-TTP translocates from the cytosol to late endosomes to acquire α-tocopherol and then α-TTP-α-tocopherol moves to the plasma membrane where α-TTP releases α-tocopherol to the membrane (61). Thus, chylomicron remnant-α-tocopherol could be released from the lipoprotein, enriching the inner leaflet of the endosomal membrane. Zha et al. (62) have reported that ABCA1 in the endosomal compartment also plays a role in endocytosis by acting as a flippase to translocate phosphatidyl serine to the outer membrane and potentiate membrane budding. Since ABCA1 can also transfer α-tocopherol (46), ABCA1 could enrich the outer membrane of the endocytic vesicles with both *RRR*- and *SRR*-α-tocopherols; α-TTP could then preferentially remove *RRR*-α-tocopherol from the outer leaflet of the endosomal membrane for transfer to the plasma membrane. It remains to be clarified as to whether ABCA1 participates in α-tocopherol transfer to α-TTP, as suggested by Horiguchi et al. (61), or if some other transporters or flippases are also involved in α-tocopherol trafficking.

α-TTP crystal structure has also been described (63,64). Importantly, the protein has a pocket that specifically binds α-tocopherol. The phytyl tail is bent to fit the pocket (Figure 4.2), thus the 2-position is critical for this conformation. Additionally, there are coordinating sites in the pocket that only allow α-tocopherol, and not other tocopherols, to bind. Clearly, the tocotrienols do not fit this binding pocket.

Other Tocopherol-Binding Proteins

α-TTP belongs to a family of hydrophobic ligand-binding proteins that have a *cis*-retinal binding motif sequence (CRAL_TRIO). This motif is also shared with the cellular retinaldehyde binding protein (CRALBP) and yeast phosphatidylinositol transfer protein (Sec14p). Panagabko et al. (65) showed that all of the CRAL_TRIO members bind α-tocopherol to some extent, but only α-TTP appears to have high enough affinity to serve as a physiological α-tocopherol mediator. The search for tissue α-tocopherol-regulating proteins led to the identification of the tocopherol-associated protein (TAP), a 46 kDa cytosolic, CRAL_TRIO protein in bovine liver (66). TAP is controversial because its sequence is identical to supernatant protein factor (SPF). SPF stimulates squalene conversion to lanosterol, and thus enhances cholesterol biosynthesis (67). The actual function of TAP/SPF remains under intense investigation. Both the liver and the heart contain an α-tocopherol-binding protein with a mass of 14.2 kDa (68).

PLASMA VITAMIN E KINETICS

Plasma vitamin E kinetics have been studied in humans using deuterium-labeled stereoisomers of α-tocopherol (*RRR*- and *SRR*-) (69). In normal subjects, the fractional disappearance rates of *RRR*-α-tocopherol (0.4 ± 0.1 pools/day) were significantly ($p < 0.01$) slower than those for *SRR*- (1.2 ± 0.6). In patients with a genetic defect in α-TTP, the fractional disappearance rates of both *RRR*- and *SRR*-α-tocopherols were fast and the same as for *SRR*-α-tocopherol in the control subjects.

The *RRR*-α-tocopherol half-life in normal subjects was approximately 48 h, consistent with the slow disappearance of *RRR*-α-tocopherol from the plasma (69). Because *RRR*-α-tocopherol is taken up by the liver and is returned to the plasma, its apparent turnover is slow. This hepatic recirculation of *RRR*-α-tocopherol results in the daily replacement of nearly all of the circulating *RRR*-α-tocopherol.

α-Tocopherol and γ-tocopherol E kinetics have also been evaluated in humans using differently deuterated α-tocopherol and γ-tocopherol (70). Like *SRR*-α-tocopherol, plasma γ-tocopherol fractional disappearance rates (1.4 ± 0.4 pools/day) were triple those of α-tocopherol (0.3 ± 0.1). In this study, γ-tocopherol half-lives were 13 ± 4 h compared with 57 ± 19 h for α-tocopherol. These data suggest that non-*RRR*-α-tocopherols are quickly removed from plasma.

Vitamin E kinetics in endurance exercisers suggests that a burst of oxidative stress can increase α-tocopherol depletion (71). Moreover, studies in cigarette smokers, a model of chronic oxidative stress and inflammation, not only demonstrate a faster α-tocopherol disappearance compared with nonsmokers, but faster disappearance in smokers with the lowest plasma ascorbate concentrations (72). These data demonstrate the in vivo antioxidant role of vitamin E in humans.

METABOLISM AND EXCRETION

Vitamin E is not accumulated in the liver (73), suggesting that excretion and metabolism are important. The vitamin E metabolites, α-CEHC (2,5,7,8-tetramethyl-2-(2′-carboxyethyl)-6-hydroxychroman) and γ-CEHC (2,7,8-trimethyl-2-(2′-carboxyethyl)-6-hydroxychroman), are derived from α-tocopherols and α-tocotrienols and from γ-tocopherols and γ-tocotrienols, respectively (74,75). Initially, the tail is hydroxylated, then β-oxidation takes place (75,76) (Figure 4.3).

Vitamins E appear to be metabolized similarly to xenobiotics, in that they are ω-oxidized by cytochrome P450s (CYPs), then conjugated and excreted in urine (77) or bile (78). Hepatic CYP 4F2 is involved in ω-oxidation of α-tocopherol and γ-tocopherol (76); but CYP 3A may also be involved (75,79–81). Similar to other xenobiotics, CEHCs are sulfated or glucuronidated (82–84). Xenobiotic transporters are likely candidates for mediating hepatic CEHC excretion because CEHCs are found in plasma, urine, and bile (85).

High α-tocopherol intakes, for example, most vitamin E supplements, lead to plasma increases of α-tocopherol, decreases of γ-tocopherol (86), and increases in excretion of both α-CEHC (87) and γ-CEHC (74,88). In cultured hepatocytes, γ-CEHC production is 100 times greater than that of α-CEHC from similar amounts of tocopherols added to the medium (75).

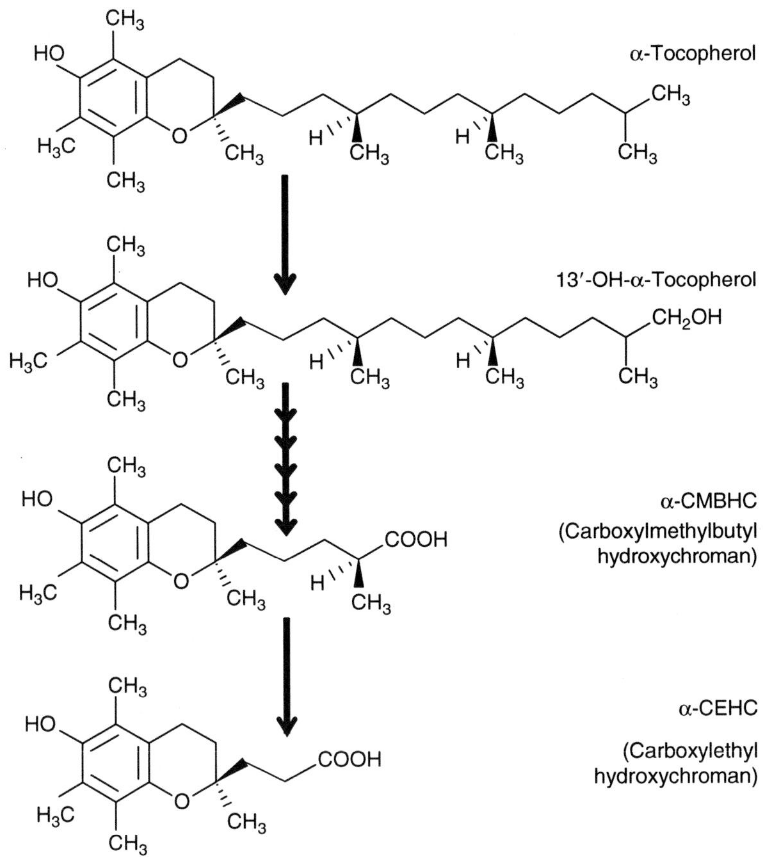

FIGURE 4.3 Proposed pathway for the metabolism of α-tocopherol to α-CEHC. (Adapted from Birringer, M., Pfluger, P., Kluth, D., Landes, N., and Brigelius-Flohé, R., *J. Nutr.*, 132, 3113, 2002.)

When humans were given equimolar amounts of labeled tocopherols (~50 mg each d_6-α-tocopheryl acetate and d_2-γ-tocopheryl acetate), plasma d_6-α-CEHC concentrations were below levels of detection, but γ-CEHC and γ-tocopherol rates of disappearance from plasma were similar (70). Thus, dietary γ-tocopherol is rapidly metabolized (within 9–12 h) by humans. Studies in mice suggest that γ-CEHC excretion increases because α-tocopherol upregulates hepatic xenobiotic metabolism (89). Additionally, studies in end-stage renal disease patients demonstrated that vitamin E supplementation was accompanied by a concomitant decrease (~1 μM) in circulating γ-tocopherol and about 1 μM increase in γ-CEHC (88). Thus, metabolism appears to be a regulator of plasma γ-tocopherol concentrations.

The mechanisms for the regulation of CEHC production are, however, unknown, but α-tocopherol appears to play an important role in the regulatory process (89). Studies thus far in isolated hepatocytes or liver cell lines (76) have not provided complete answers to the mystery of why α-tocopherol and γ-tocopherol, despite their very similar structures and antioxidant activities, are so differently handled by the liver. There is speculation, however, that the chemical properties of γ-tocopherol and other non-α-tocopherols make them toxic to cells (90).

The major route of excretion of ingested vitamin E is fecal elimination. Excretion of hepatic vitamin E into the bile has been demonstrated to be mediated by the ABC transporter, p-glycoprotein (MDR2) (91), a transporter that also facilitates biliary phospholipid excretion into bile.

CELLULAR AND BIOCHEMICAL FUNCTIONS

α-Tocopherol appears to modulate some cellular functions. For example, α-tocopherol inhibits protein kinase C (PKC) and thus inhibits smooth muscle cell proliferation (92), as well as platelet aggregation and adhesion (93,94). α-Tocopherol supplementation to humans (1200 IU or 900 mg/day) also decreases monocyte superoxide production via inhibition of PKC (95,96), decreases IL-1β release from monocytes by inhibiting 5-lipoxygenase (97), and decreases monocyte–endothelial cell adhesion in vitro, which correlated with decreases in message and cell surface expression of E-selectin in endothelial cells (98). Treatment of endothelial cells (HUVEC) with α-tocopherol significantly reduced the expression of the adhesion molecules, ICAM-1 and VCAM-1, on HUVEC induced by oxidized LDL (99). Enrichment of human aortic endothelial cells with α-tocopherol significantly inhibited LDL-induced adhesion of monocytes to endothelial cells in a dose-dependent manner with a concomitant reduction in levels of sICAM-1 (100). This decreased adhesion was mediated by decreased expression of CD11b and VLA-4, by inhibiting the activation of NFκB (96). Another key function that α-tocopherol regulates is vascular homeostasis through its action on PKC in endothelial cells; α-tocopherol has been shown to mediate NO production (101).

Singh et al. (102) have recently reviewed the data with respect to inflammation. α-Tocopherol decreased the release of proinflammatory cytokines and chemokines (IL-8 and plasminogen activator inhibitor-1 [PAI-1]). It decreased C-reactive protein level in patients with and those at risk for cardiovascular disease. The mechanisms proposed for these α-tocopherol actions include the inhibition of PKC, 5-lipoxygenase, tyrosine kinase, as well as cyclooxygenase-2 (102). Unfortunately, many of the studies described in this section were carried out in tissue culture or are a result of ex vivo treatments with α-tocopherol. Very few measurements have been carried out showing changes in humans, so the health benefits of these tissue culture observations are lacking.

NUTRITIONAL REQUIREMENT

The dietary reference intakes (DRIs) for Vitamin C, Vitamin E, Selenium, and Carotenoids were published in 2000 by the Panel on Dietary Antioxidants and Related Compounds, FNB, Institute of Medicine (2). The α-tocopherol health benefits described were primarily those related to the prevention of deficiency symptoms (2). The estimated average requirement (EAR) was based on the amount of 2*R*-α-tocopherol intake that reversed erythrocyte hemolysis in men who were vitamin E-deficient as a result of consuming a vitamin E-deficient diet for five years (2). The EAR of 12 mg 2*R*-α-tocopherol was chosen because intakes at this level prevented in vitro hydrogen peroxide-induced erythrocyte hemolysis. The 2000 RDA for adults (both men and women $\geq$19 years) defined as 2*R*-α-tocopherol is 15 mg/day (Table 4.1).

The tolerable upper intake level (UL) was set at 1000 mg/day for vitamin E (any form of supplemental α-tocopherol). This was one of the few UL that was set using data in rats, because sufficient and appropriate quantitative data assessing long-term adverse effects of vitamin E supplements in humans was not available.

There have been several reports carrying out mathematical analyses of adverse outcomes in clinical trials of vitamin E supplements. A meta-analysis that combined the results of 19 trials in normal subjects, as well as those with various diseases, including heart disease, end-stage renal failure, and Alzheimer's disease, suggested that adults who took supplements of 400 IU/day or more were 6% more likely to die from any cause than those who did not take vitamin E supplements (103). This report was highly criticized for using unorthodox methodology to reach their conclusions, given that simpler mathematical analyses did not find any statistical relationship between all-cause mortality and vitamin E supplement dose. Furthermore, three other meta analyses that combined the results of randomized controlled trials

TABLE 4.1
Criteria and Dietary Reference Intake Values for Vitamin E by Life Stage Group

		RDA[b]			UL[c]		
Life Stage Group	**Criterion**	**mg/day**	**IU *RRR***	**IU *all-rac***	**mg/day**	**IU *RRR***	**IU *all-rac***
Adult	Intakes sufficient to prevent hydrogen peroxide-induced hemolysis in vivo	15	23	34	1000	1500	1100
Pregnancy	Adult EAR[a]	15	23	34	1000	1500	1100
Lactation	Adult EAR plus average amount secreted in human milk	19	29	43	1000	1500	1100

Source: Adapted from Food and Nutrition Board, Institute of Medicine in *Dietary Reference Intakes for Vitamin C, Vitamin E, Selenium, and Carotenoids*, National Academy Press, Washington, 2000, pp. 186–283.

[a] EAR, Estimated Average Requirement. The intake that meets the estimated nutrient needs of half the individuals in a group.
[b] RDA, Recommended Dietary Allowance. The intake that meets the nutrient needs of almost all (97%–98%) of individuals in a group.
[c] UL, Tolerable Upper Intake Level. The highest level of daily nutrient intake that is likely to pose no risk of adverse health effects in almost all individuals.

designed to evaluate the efficacy of vitamin E supplementation for the prevention or treatment of cardiovascular disease found no evidence that vitamin E supplementation up to 800 IU/day significantly increased or decreased cardiovascular disease mortality or all-cause mortality (104–106). Moreover, an intervention trial in 40,000 women, half of whom took vitamin E supplements (600 IU every other day) for ten years found no increase in mortality with vitamin E (107). Thus, it appears that the Miller et al. (103) meta analysis overstated the risks of vitamin E supplements.

Adequacy of Vitamin E Intakes in Normal U.S. Populations

The amount of vitamin E consumed by most U.S. adults is sufficient to prevent overt symptoms of deficiency; however, the actual quantities consumed by U.S. adults, as assessed by various surveys (108–110), are closer to 8 mg than the required 15 mg. Estimates are that 92% of men and 98% of women did not meet the EAR for α-tocopherol (111). These low intakes may be real, or they may result from underreporting of fat intakes. Nevertheless, it is quite possible that many people do not consume a diet that contains 15 mg α-tocopherol; however, supplement intake is high (112).

Food Sources of Vitamin E

The richest dietary sources of vitamin E are edible vegetable oils (113), because only plants synthesize vitamin E (14). *RRR*-α-tocopherol is especially high in wheat germ, safflower, and sunflower oils. Soybean and corn oils contain predominantly γ-tocopherol, as well as some tocotrienols. Cottonseed oil, as well as palm oil, contain both α-tocopherol and γ-tocopherol in equal proportion. In addition, palm oil contains large amounts of α-tocotrienol and γ-tocotrienol (113). Vitamin E is found in relatively low concentrations in fruits and vegetables (Table 4.2).

TABLE 4.2
α-Tocopherol Contents of Selected Foods

Food	Measure	α-Tocopherol (mg)
Cereals, ready-to-eat, fortified	3/4 cup	13.50
Sunflower seeds, dry roasted	1/4 cup	8.35
Almonds	1 oz (24 nuts)	7.33
Oil, sunflower	1 tbsp	5.59
Tomato sauce	1 cup	5.10
Oil, safflower	1 tbsp	4.64
Turnip greens, cooked	1 cup	4.36
Hazelnuts	1 oz	4.26
Carrot juice	1 cup	2.74
Beet greens, cooked	1 cp	2.61
Potato chips	1 oz	2.58
Sweet potato, canned	1 cup	2.55
Broccoli, chopped, cooked	1 cup	2.43
Oil, canola	1 tbsp	2.39
Peppers, sweet, red, raw	1 cup	2.35

The major source of vitamin E in the American diet is desserts (108). Thus, it is not surprising that decreasing fat intake decreases vitamin E intake. Decreasing intake of saturated fats and increasing intake of PUFA-containing fats, usually corn oil or soybean oil, which contain high γ-tocopherol and lesser α-tocopherol amounts, decreases vitamin E intake (14).

Probably, the most important source of vitamin E in the American diet is the supplement pill (112). Pills containing vitamin E with natural stereochemistry (*RRR*-α-tocopherol) are labeled D-α-tocopherol, while those containing synthetic (*all-rac*-α-tocopherol) are labeled DL. Each IU contains either 0.91 mg *all-rac*-α-tocopherol or 0.67 mg *RRR*-α-tocopherol. The FNB (2) defined that the equivalence of natural and synthetic is such that 2 mg *all-rac*-α-tocopherol is needed to provide 1 mg 2*R*-α-tocopherol. Thus, a 400 IU pill of D-α-tocopherol contains 268 mg 2*R*-α-tocopherol (400 IU times 0.67 mg/IU), whereas a 400 IU pill of DL-α-tocopherol contains 180 mg 2*R*-α-tocopherol (400 IU times 0.91 mg/IU divided by 2).

DEFICIENCY SIGNS AND METHODS OF NUTRITIONAL ASSESSMENT

Overt vitamin E deficiency occurs only rarely in humans and virtually never as a result of dietary deficiencies. Vitamin E deficiency does occur as a result of genetic abnormalities in α-TTP and as a result of various fat malabsorption syndromes (Table 4.3).

VITAMIN E DEFICIENCY CAUSED BY GENETIC DEFECTS IN THE α-TOCOPHEROL TRANSFER PROTEIN

Genetic defects in α-TTP are associated with a characteristic syndrome, ataxia with vitamin E deficiency (AVED) (previously called familial isolated vitamin E [FIVE] deficiency). AVED patients have neurologic abnormalities characterized by a progressive peripheral neuropathy with a specific dying back of the large caliber axons of the sensory neurons, which results in ataxia.

These patients are responsive to oral α-tocopherol supplements. A dose of 800–1,200 mg/day is usually sufficient to prevent further deterioration of neurologic function and in some cases improvements have been noted, as reviewed by Sokol (114). Most of the patients

TABLE 4.3
Neurological Abnormalities of Vitamin E Deficiency

	Peripheral Neurology	Spinal Cord	Brain
Histology	Loss of large-caliber myelinated axons in peripheral sensory nerve	Axonal dystrophy in the posterior columns of the spinal cord and dorsal and ventral spinocerebellar tracts	Mild atrophy of the cerebellar hemispheres
Electrophysiology	Diminished amplitude of sensory nerve action potentials, delayed conduction velocity is unusual	Central delay in sensory nerve conduction	

described by Ouahchi et al. (115) have a truncation of the C-terminal portion of α-TTP that causes an inability to discriminate between *RRR*- and *SRR*-α-tocopherols (116).

Retinitis pigmentosa commonly accompanies vitamin E deficiency in humans (24). Importantly, α-tocopherol supplementation stops or slows the progression of retinitis pigmentosa caused by vitamin E deficiency (117). However, the results from a trial of vitamins E and A supplements in patients with many common forms of retinitis pigmentosa showed that there was a beneficial effect of 15,000 IU/day of vitamin A and a possible adverse effect of 400 IU vitamin E (118). Therefore, the plasma vitamin E concentrations should be measured in patients with retinitis pigmentosa to evaluate their vitamin E status before supplementation. Only those retinitis pigmentosa patients with vitamin E deficiency should be supplemented with α-tocopherol.

Vitamin E Deficiency Caused by Genetic Defects in Lipoprotein Synthesis

Studies of patients with hypobetalipoproteinemia or abetalipoproteinemia (low to nondetectable circulating chylomicrons, VLDL, or LDL) have demonstrated that lipoproteins containing apoB are necessary for effective absorption and plasma transport of vitamin E (24). Clinically, both groups become vitamin E-deficient and develop a progressive peripheral neuropathy if they are not given large vitamin E supplements. Daily doses of 100–200 mg/kg, or about 5–7 g of *RRR*-α-tocopherol are recommended (114). Although plasma concentrations of α-tocopherol concentrations never reach normal levels, adipose tissue α-tocopherol concentrations do reach normal levels (119).

Vitamin E Deficiency as a Result of Fat Malabsorption Syndromes

Vitamin E deficiency occurs secondary to fat malabsorption because vitamin E absorption requires biliary and pancreatic secretions (24). Vitamin E deficiency occurs in children with chronic cholestatic disease, who have impaired secretion of bile into the small intestine, resulting in severe fat malabsorption. Neurologic abnormalities, which appear as early as the second year of life, become irreversible if the vitamin E deficiency is uncorrected.

Children with cystic fibrosis can also become vitamin E deficient because the impaired secretion of pancreatic digestive enzymes causes steatorrhea and vitamin E malabsorption, even when pancreatic enzyme supplements are administered orally. More severe vitamin E deficiency occurs if bile secretion is impaired.

It should be emphasized that any disorder that causes fat malabsorption can lead to vitamin E deficiency. The development of neurologic symptoms of vitamin E deficiency in adults who acquire these disorders, however, takes decades (114). The prolonged time for onset of symptoms results from the earlier accumulation of vitamin E in most tissues and its relatively slow release from nervous tissues.

Vitamin E supplementation in patients with fat malabsorption syndromes is very difficult to achieve because they malabsorb vitamin E. Sokol (114) suggests treatment with *RRR*-α-tocopherol (not the ester) at 25–50 mg/kg/day, advancing by 50 mg/kg/day up to 150–200 mg/day if the ratio of serum α-tocopherol to total lipids does not normalize (>0.8 mg/g).

Pathology of Human Vitamin E Deficiency

The primary manifestations of human vitamin E deficiency include spinocerebellar ataxia, skeletal myopathy, and pigmented retinopathy (24). Hypo- or a-reflexia is the earliest symptom observed. By the end of the first decade of life, untreated patients with chronic cholestatic hepatobiliary disease have a combination of spinocerebellar ataxia, neuropathy, and opthalmoplegia. The progression of neurologic symptoms appears to be dependent on the level of oxidative stress accompanying the vitamin E deficiency.

The large-caliber, myelinated axons in peripheral sensory nerves are the predominant target in vitamin E deficiency in humans (120). In deficient humans, diminished amplitudes of sensory nerve action potential are common, whereas delayed conduction velocity, an indicator of demyelination, is unusual. Thus, axonal degeneration rather than demyelination is the primary sensory nerve abnormality. However, motor nerve demyelination has also been reported (121). Axonal dystrophy has been observed in the posterior columns of the spinal cord and the dorsal and ventral spinocerebellar tracts (120). Specifically, swollen, dystrophic axons (spheroids) have been observed in the gracille and cuneate nuclei of the brain stem. Lipofuscin accumulation has been observed in dorsal sensory neurons and peripheral Schwann cell cytoplasm. Electromyographic studies show denervation injury of muscles in patients with advanced vitamin E deficiency. Somatosensory-evoked potential testing has shown a central delay in sensory conduction, correlating with degeneration of the posterior columns of the spinal cord.

Assessment of Vitamin E Status

The FNB determined that a plasma concentration of less than 12 μmol α-tocopherol/L was associated with an increased tendency for hemolysis (2). The usual plasma α-tocopherol concentration in normal subjects is approximately 20 μmol/L. Although low serum or plasma α-tocopherol concentrations are indicative of vitamin E deficiency, measurement of plasma levels are insufficient for patients with various forms of lipid malabsorption. Calculation of effective plasma α-tocopherol concentrations needs to take into account plasma lipid levels when lipids are high or low. These are calculated by dividing the plasma α-tocopherol by the sum of plasma cholesterol and triglycerides (122). For example, Sokol et al. (123) showed that plasma vitamin E concentrations were in the normal range in patients with vitamin E deficiency resulting from cholestatic liver disease because they had extraordinarily high circulating lipid levels. Adipose tissue concentrations can also be used as an indicator of long-term vitamin E status (48,49,124).

Any patient presenting with peripheral neuropathies or retinitis pigmentosa with unknown causes should be evaluated to assess if they are vitamin E-deficient. The ataxia of Friedreich's ataxia is so remarkably similar to that of AVED patients that plasma concentrations of vitamin E in all patients with ataxia should definitely be measured or their genotypes defined (125).

EFFICACY OF PHARMACOLOGICAL DOSES OF VITAMIN E

Vitamin E has antioxidant benefits and is generally considered to be nontoxic even in relatively high doses (>1000 mg) (2). Moreover, several studies have reported that vitamin E is associated with decreased chronic disease risk. The Women's Health Study, a 10 year prevention trial in normal, healthy women, found that 600 IU vitamin E decreased cardiovascular mortality by 24% and in women over 65 by 49% (107). Antioxidant treatment with the combination of vitamins E and C slowed atherosclerotic progression in intimal thickness of coronary and carotid arteries in hypercholesterolemic (126) and in heart-transplant patients (127). Epidemiologic studies indicate a beneficial role of vitamin E supplements in decreasing risk of degenerative diseases, such as cardiovascular disease and atherosclerosis (128,129), cancer (130), and cataract formation (131). The Cache County Study reported that antioxidant use (vitamin E > 400 IU and vitamin C > 500 mg) was associated with reduced Alzheimer's disease prevalence and incidence in the elderly (132). Regular vitamin E supplement use for ten years or more was associated with a lower risk of dying of amyotrophic lateral sclerosis (ALS, Lou Gehrig's disease) (133). It is, therefore, not surprising that vitamin E supplements are taken daily by more than 35 million people in the United States (112).

Another important area of investigation is the maintenance of immune function. Meydani et al. (134–136) have demonstrated in a series of trials that immune function is compromised in the elderly, and that vitamin E supplements can improve immune responses.

No clinical trial in healthy people has shown that any supplemental dose of vitamin E causes adverse effects, with the exception of an increased tendency to bleed (137). However, an antioxidant intervention trial suggested adverse vitamin E effects in patients taking antihyperlipidemic drug therapy. The intervention study was a three year, double-blind trial of antioxidants (vitamins E and C, β-carotene, and selenium) or placebos in 160 subjects taking both simvastatin and niacin (138,139). Simvastatin is a 3-hydroxy-3-methylglutaryl coenzyme A (HMG-CoA) reductase inhibitor that is widely used in the treatment of hypercholesterolemia. The protective increase in HDL2 with simvastatin plus niacin was attenuated by concurrent therapy with antioxidants. The average stenosis progressed by 3.9% with placebos, 1.8% with antioxidants ($p = 0.16$ for the comparison with the placebo group), and 0.7% with simvastatin–niacin plus antioxidants ($p = 0.004$) and regressed by 0.4% with simvastatin–niacin alone ($p < 0.001$) (139). The other study reporting adverse vitamin E effects was the Women's Angiographic Vitamin and Estrogen (WAVE) Trial, a randomized, double-blind trial of 423 postmenopausal women with at least one coronary stenosis at baseline coronary angiography. In postmenopausal women on hormone replacement therapy, all-cause mortality was increased in women assigned to antioxidant vitamins compared with placebo (HR, 2.8; 95% CI, 1.1–7.2; $p = 0.047$) (140). Finally, the HopeToo trial suggested that patients at high risk for coronary heart disease taking vitamin E were at increased risk of left-ventricular dysfunction, but no specific mechanism was proposed (141).

One possibility for adverse vitamin E effects is vitamin E-dependent alterations in xenobiotic metabolism (142). Studies in mice showed that hepatic cytochrome P450 3a (analogous to CYP3A in humans) protein concentrations were correlated with hepatic α-tocopherol concentrations (89). CYP3A4 is responsible for the metabolism of more than 50% of prescription drugs, including statins (143). Both simvastatin (143) and estrogen (144) are metabolized by CYP3A4, lending support to the hypothesis that α-tocopherol in pharmacologic doses stimulates drug metabolism, potentially decreasing beneficial drug concentrations (145). These data suggest that α-tocopherol could stimulate xenobiotic metabolism, but clearly further studies are needed.

CONCLUSION

Vitamin E is clearly a lipid-soluble antioxidant. There remains huge enthusiasm for the concept that α-tocopherol has some specific molecular role of regulation of cellular functions, but efforts to document such a role along with its physiological significance have been limited. Numerous investigators have used gene chip technology to demonstrate specific vitamin E or α-tocopherol effects (146–152), but no consistent findings have emerged. Clinical trials to demonstrate that vitamin E supplements reverse chronic diseases have largely been disappointing. However, disease prevention shows more promise, but it is much more difficult to carry out the very long trials necessary to show benefit (107,153). Overall, it is important to recognize that vitamin E is a required nutrient, that its concentrations are regulated in vivo, that it has antioxidant benefits, and its role may be to prevent oxidative damage caused during lipid peroxidation. Thus, those people consuming diets that are low in α-tocopherol may be at risk for increased oxidative damage because they have insufficient protection from oxidative stress.

ACKNOWLEDGMENT

This work was supported in part by grants from NIH NIEHS (ES11536) and NIDDK (DK59576).

REFERENCES

1. Buettner, G.R., The pecking order of free radicals and antioxidants: lipid peroxidation, alpha-tocopherol, and ascorbate, *Arch. Biochem. Biophys.*, 300, 535, 1993.
2. Food and Nutrition Board and Institute of Medicine, *Dietary Reference Intakes for Vitamin C, Vitamin E, Selenium, and Carotenoids*, National Academy Press, Washington, 2000, pp. 186–283.
3. Hosomi, A. et al., Affinity for alpha-tocopherol transfer protein as a determinant of the biological activities of vitamin E analogs, *FEBS Lett.*, 409, 105, 1997.
4. Yokota, T. et al., Delayed-onset ataxia in mice lacking alpha-tocopherol transfer protein: model for neuronal degeneration caused by chronic oxidative stress, *Proc. Natl. Acad. Sci. USA*, 98, 15185, 2001.
5. Cavalier, L. et al., Ataxia with isolated vitamin E deficiency: heterogeneity of mutations and phenotypic variability in a large number of families, *Am. J. Hum. Genet.*, 62, 301, 1998.
6. Terasawa, Y. et al., Increased atherosclerosis in hyperlipidemic mice deficient in alpha-tocopherol transfer protein and vitamin E, *Proc. Natl. Acad. Sci. USA*, 97, 13830, 2000.
7. Leonard, S.W. et al., Incorporation of deuterated *RRR*- or *all rac* α-tocopherol into plasma and tissues of α-tocopherol transfer protein null mice, *Am. J. Clin. Nutr.*, 75, 555, 2002.
8. Evans, H.M. and Bishop, K.S., On the existence of a hitherto unrecognized dietary factor essential for reproduction, *Science*, 56, 650, 1922.
9. Evans, H.M., Emerson, O.H., and Emerson, G.A., The isolation from wheat germ oil of an alcohol, alpha-tocopherol, having the properties of vitamin E, *J. Biol. Chem.*, 113, 319, 1936.
10. Emerson, O.H. et al., The chemistry of vitamin E. Tocopherols from natural sources, *J. Biol. Chem.*, 22, 99, 1937.
11. Machlin, L.J., Vitamin E, in *Handbook of Vitamins*, 2nd ed., Hoffman-La Rouche, Inc., Nutley, New Jersey, 1991, p. 99.
12. Horwitt, M.K. et al., Effects of limited tocopherol intake in man with relationships to erythrocyte hemolysis and lipid oxidations, *Am. J. Clin. Nutr.*, 4, 408, 1956.
13. Horwitt, M.K., Vitamin E and lipid metabolism in man, *Am. J. Clin. Nutr.*, 8, 451, 1960.
14. Sheppard, A.J., Pennington, J.A.T., and Weihrauch, J.L., Analysis and distribution of vitamin E in vegetable oils and foods, in *Vitamin E in Health and Disease*, Packer, L. and Fuchs, J. (eds), Marcel Dekker, Inc., New York, 1993, p. 9.
15. Kasparek, S., Chemistry of tocopherols and tocotrienols, in *Vitamin E: A Comprehensive Treatise*, Machlin, L.J. (ed.), Marcel Dekker, New York, 1980, p. 7.

16. Cheeseman, K.H. et al., Biokinetics in humans of *RRR*-alpha-tocopherol: the free phenol, acetate ester, and succinate ester forms of vitamin E, *Free Radic. Biol. Med.*, 19, 591, 1995.
17. Anonymous, The United States Pharmacopeia. The National Formulary, *The United States Pharmacopeial Convention, Inc.* Rockville, 1979.
18. Kamal-Eldin, A. and Appelqvist, L.A., The chemistry and antioxidant properties of tocopherols and tocotrienols, *Lipids*, 31, 671, 1996.
19. Burton, G.W., Joyce, A., and Ingold, K.U., Is vitamin E the only lipid-soluble, chain-breaking antioxidant in human blood plasma and erythrocyte membranes? *Arch. Biochem. Biophys.*, 221, 281, 1983.
20. Drevon, C.A., Absorption, transport and metabolism of vitamin E, *Free Radic. Res. Commun.*, 14, 229, 1991.
21. Liebler, D.C. and Burr, J.A., Antioxidant stoichiometry and the oxidative fate of vitamin E in peroxyl radical scavenging reactions, *Lipids*, 30, 789, 1995.
22. Liebler, D.C. et al., Gas chromatography–mass spectrometry analysis of vitamin E and its oxidation products, *Anal. Biochem.*, 236, 27, 1996.
23. Traber, M.G. and Sies, H., Vitamin E in humans: demand and delivery, *Annu. Rev. Nutr.*, 16, 321, 1996.
24. Traber, M.G., Vitamin E, in *Modern Nutrition in Health and Disease*, Shils, M.E. et al. (eds), Williams & Wilkins, Baltimore, 1999, p. 347.
25. Hayes, K.C., Pronczuk, A., and Perlman, D., Vitamin E in fortified cow milk uniquely enriches human plasma lipoproteins, *Am. J. Clin. Nutr.*, 74, 211, 2001.
26. Leonard, S.W. et al., Vitamin E bioavailability from fortified breakfast cereal is greater than that from encapsulated supplements, *Am. J. Clin. Nutr.*, 79, 86, 2004.
27. Jeanes, Y.M. et al., The absorption of vitamin E is influenced by the amount of fat in a meal and the food matrix, *Br. J. Nutr.*, 92, 575, 2004.
28. Roodenburg, A.J. et al., Amount of fat in the diet affects bioavailability of lutein esters but not of alpha-carotene, beta-carotene, and vitamin E in humans, *Am. J. Clin. Nutr.*, 71, 1187, 2000.
29. Traber, M.G., The ABCs of vitamin E and beta-carotene absorption, *Am. J. Clin. Nutr.*, 80, 3, 2004.
30. Traber, M.G. et al., *RRR*- and *SRR*-alpha-tocopherols are secreted without discrimination in human chylomicrons, but *RRR*-alpha-tocopherol is preferentially secreted in very low density lipoproteins, *J. Lipid Res.*, 31, 675, 1990.
31. Traber, M.G. et al., Impaired ability of patients with familial isolated vitamin E deficiency to incorporate alpha-tocopherol into lipoproteins secreted by the liver, *J. Clin. Invest.*, 85, 397, 1990.
32. Kostner, G.M. et al., Human plasma phospholipid transfer protein accelerates exchange/transfer of alpha-tocopherol between lipoproteins and cells, *Biochem. J.*, 305, 659, 1995.
33. Kaempf-Rotzoli, D.E., Traber, M.G., and Arai, H., Vitamin E and transfer proteins, *Curr. Opin. Lipidol.*, 14, 249, 2003.
34. Traber, M.G. et al., Vitamin E dose response studies in humans using deuterated *RRR*-α-tocopherol, *Am. J. Clin. Nutr.*, 68, 847, 1998.
35. Sattler, W. et al., Muscle-specific overexpression of lipoprotein lipase in transgenic mice results in increased alpha-tocopherol levels in skeletal muscle, *Biochem. J.*, 318, 15, 1996.
36. Trigatti, B.L., Krieger, M., and Rigotti, A., Influence of the HDL receptor SR-BI on lipoprotein metabolism and atherosclerosis, *Arterioscler. Thromb. Vasc. Biol.*, 23, 1732, 2003.
37. Guthmann, F. et al., Interaction of lipoproteins with type II pneumocytes in vitro: morphological studies, uptake kinetics and secretion rate of cholesterol, *Eur. J. Cell Biol.*, 74, 197, 1997.
38. Kolleck, I. et al., HDL and vitamin E in plasma and the expression of SR-BI on lung cells during rat perinatal development, *Lung*, 178, 191, 2000.
39. Kolleck, I., Sinha, P., and Rustow, B., Vitamin E as an antioxidant of the lung: mechanisms of vitamin E delivery to alveolar type II cells, *Am. J. Respir. Crit. Care Med.*, 166, S62, 2002.
40. Rustow, B. et al., Type II pneumocytes secrete vitamin E together with surfactant lipids, *Am. J. Physiol.*, 265, L133, 1993.
41. Goti, D. et al., Scavenger receptor class B, type I is expressed in porcine brain capillary endothelial cells and contributes to selective uptake of HDL-associated vitamin E, *J. Neurochem.*, 76, 498, 2001.
42. Goti, D. et al., Uptake of lipoprotein-associated alpha-tocopherol by primary porcine brain capillary endothelial cells, *J. Neurochem.*, 74, 1374, 2000.

43. Witt, W. et al., Regulation by vitamin E of the scavenger receptor BI in rat liver and HepG2 cells, *J. Lipid Res.*, 41, 2009, 2000.
44. Oram, J.F. and Lawn, R.M., ABCA1. The gatekeeper for eliminating excess tissue cholesterol, *J. Lipid Res.*, 42, 1173, 2001.
45. Mardones, P. et al., Alpha-tocopherol metabolism is abnormal in scavenger receptor class B type I (SR-BI)-deficient mice, *J. Nutr.*, 132, 443, 2002.
46. Oram, J.F., Vaughan, A.M., and Stocker, R., ATP-binding cassette transporter A1 mediates cellular secretion of alpha-tocopherol, *J. Biol. Chem.*, 276, 39898, 2001.
47. Orso, E. et al., Transport of lipids from golgi to plasma membrane is defective in Tangier disease patients and Abc1-deficient mice, *Nat. Genet.*, 24, 192, 2000.
48. Handelman, G.J. et al., Human adipose alpha-tocopherol and gamma-tocopherol kinetics during and after 1 y of alpha-tocopherol supplementation, *Am. J. Clin. Nutr.*, 59, 1025, 1994.
49. El-Sohemy, A. et al., Population-based study of alpha- and gamma-tocopherol in plasma and adipose tissue as biomarkers of intake in Costa Rican adults, *Am. J. Clin. Nutr.*, 74, 356, 2001.
50. Arita, M. et al., Human alpha-tocopherol transfer protein: cDNA cloning, expression and chromosomal localization, *Biochem. J.*, 306, 437, 1995.
51. Doerflinger, N. et al., Ataxia with vitamin E deficiency: refinement of genetic localization and analysis of linkage disequilibrium by using new markers in 14 families, *Am. J. Hum. Genet.*, 56, 1116, 1995.
52. Hosomi, A. et al., Localization of alpha-tocopherol transfer protein in rat brain, *Neurosci. Lett.*, 256, 159, 1998.
53. Copp, R.P. et al., Localization of alpha-tocopherol transfer protein in the brains of patients with ataxia with vitamin E deficiency and other oxidative stress related neurodegenerative disorders, *Brain Res.*, 822, 80, 1999.
54. Kaempf-Rotzoll, D.E. et al., Human placental trophoblast cells express alpha-tocopherol transfer protein, *Placenta.*, 24, 439, 2003.
55. Kaempf-Rotzoll, D.E. et al., Alpha-tocopherol transfer protein is specifically localized at the implantation site of pregnant mouse uterus, *Biol. Reprod.*, 67, 599, 2002.
56. Muller-Schmehl, K. et al., Localization of alpha-tocopherol transfer protein in trophoblast, fetal capillaries' endothelium and amnion epithelium of human term placenta, *Free Radic. Res.*, 38, 413, 2004.
57. Sato, Y. et al., Purification and characterization of the alpha-tocopherol transfer protein from rat liver, *FEBS Lett.*, 288, 41, 1991.
58. Panagabko, C. et al., Expression and refolding of recombinant human alpha-tocopherol transfer protein capable of specific alpha-tocopherol binding, *Protein Expr. Purif.*, 24, 395, 2002.
59. Traber, M.G. et al., Nascent VLDL from liver perfusions of cynomolgus monkeys are preferentially enriched in *RRR*-compared with *SRR*-α tocopherol: studies using deuterated tocopherols, *J. Lipid Res.*, 31, 687, 1990.
60. Arita, M. et al., Alpha-tocopherol transfer protein stimulates the secretion of alpha-tocopherol from a cultured liver cell line through a brefeldin A-insensitive pathway, *Proc. Natl. Acad. Sci. USA*, 94, 12437, 1997.
61. Horiguchi, M. et al., pH-Dependent translocation of alpha-tocopherol transfer protein (alpha-TTP) between hepatic cytosol and late endosomes, *Genes Cells*, 8, 789, 2003.
62. Zha, X., Genest, J., Jr. and McPherson, R., Endocytosis is enhanced in Tangier fibroblasts: possible role of ATP-binding cassette protein A1 in endosomal vesicular transport, *J. Biol. Chem.*, 276, 39476, 2001.
63. Meier, R. et al., The molecular basis of vitamin E retention: structure of human alpha-tocopherol transfer protein, *J. Mol. Biol.*, 331, 725, 2003.
64. Min, K.C., Kovall, R.A., and Hendrickson, W.A., Crystal structure of human α-tocopherol transfer protein bound to its ligand: implications for ataxia with vitamin E deficiency, *Proc. Natl. Acad. Sci. USA*, 100, 14713, 2003.
65. Panagabko, C. et al., Ligand specificity in the CRAL-TRIO protein family, *Biochemistry*, 42, 6467, 2003.
66. Stocker, A. et al., Identification of a novel cytosolic tocopherol-binding protein: structure, specificity, and tissue distribution, *IUBMB Life*, 48, 49, 1999.

67. Shibata, N. et al., Supernatant protein factor, which stimulates the conversion of squalene to lanosterol, is a cytosolic squalene transfer protein and enhances cholesterol biosynthesis, *Proc. Natl. Acad. Sci. USA*, 98, 2244, 2001.
68. Dutta-Roy, A.K. et al., Identification of a low molecular mass (14.2 kDa) alpha-tocopherol-binding protein in the cytosol of rat liver and heart, *Biochem. Biophys. Res. Commun.*, 196, 1108, 1993.
69. Traber, M.G., Ramakrishnan, R., and Kayden, H.J., Human plasma vitamin E kinetics demonstrate rapid recycling of plasma *RRR*-α-tocopherol, *Proc. Natl. Acad. Sci. USA*, 91, 10005, 1994.
70. Leonard, S.W. et al., Studies in humans using deuterium-labeled α- and γ-tocopherol demonstrate faster plasma γ-tocopherol disappearance and greater γ-metabolite production, *Free Radic. Biol. Med.*, 38, 857, 2005.
71. Mastaloudis, A., Leonard, S.W., and Traber, M.G., Oxidative stress in athletes during extreme endurance exercise, *Free Radic. Biol. Med.*, 31, 911, 2001.
72. Bruno, R.S. et al., α-Tocopherol disappearance is faster in cigarette smokers and is inversely related to their ascorbic acid status, *Am. J. Clin. Nutr.*, 81, 95, 2005.
73. Leonard, S.W. et al., Quantitation of rat liver vitamin E metabolites by LC-MS during high-dose vitamin E administration, *J. Lipid Res.*, 46, 1068, 2005.
74. Lodge, J.K. et al., α- and γ-Tocotrienols are metabolized to carboxyethyl-hydroxychroman (CEHC) derivatives and excreted in human urine, *Lipids*, 36, 43, 2001.
75. Birringer, M. et al., Identities and differences in the metabolism of tocotrienols and tocopherols in HepG2 cells, *J. Nutr.*, 132, 3113, 2002.
76. Sontag, T.J. and Parker, R.S., Cytochrome P450 omega-hydroxylase pathway of tocopherol catabolism: novel mechanism of regulation of vitamin E status, *J. Biol. Chem.*, 277, 25290, 2002.
77. Brigelius-Flohé, R. and Traber, M.G., Vitamin E: function and metabolism, *FASEB J.*, 13, 1145, 1999.
78. Kiyose, C. et al., Alpha-tocopherol affects the urinary and biliary excretion of 2,7,8-trimethyl-2 (2′-carboxyethyl)-6-hydroxychroman, gamma-tocopherol metabolite, in rats, *Lipids*, 36, 467, 2001.
79. Birringer, M., Drogan, D., and Brigelius-Flohé, R., Tocopherols are metabolized in HepG2 cells by side chain omega-oxidation and consecutive beta-oxidation, *Free Radic. Biol. Med.*, 31, 226, 2001.
80. Parker, R.S., Sontag, T.J., and Swanson, J.E., Cytochrome P4503A-dependent metabolism of tocopherols and inhibition by sesamin, *Biochem. Biophys. Res. Commun.*, 277, 531, 2000.
81. Ikeda, S., Tohyama, T., and Yamashita, K., Dietary sesame seed and its lignans inhibit 2,7,8-trimethyl-2(2′-carboxyethyl)-6-hydroxychroman excretion into urine of rats fed gamma-tocopherol, *J. Nutr.*, 132, 961, 2002.
82. Swanson, J.E. et al., Urinary excretion of 2,7,8-trimethyl-2-(beta-carboxyethyl)-6-hydroxychroman is a major route of elimination of gamma-tocopherol in humans, *J. Lipid Res.*, 40, 665, 1999.
83. Stahl, W. et al., Quantification of the alpha- and gamma-tocopherol metabolites 2,5,7,8-tetramethyl-2-(2′-carboxyethyl)-6-hydroxychroman and 2,7,8-trimethyl-2-(2′-carboxyethyl)-6-hydroxychroman in human serum, *Anal. Biochem.*, 275, 254, 1999.
84. Pope, S.A. et al., Synthesis and analysis of conjugates of the major vitamin E metabolite, alpha-CEHC, *Free Radic. Biol. Med.*, 33, 807, 2002.
85. Hattori, A., Fukushima, T., and Imai, K., Occurrence and determination of a natriuretic hormone, 2,7,8-trimethyl-2-(beta-carboxyethyl)-6-hydroxy chroman, in rat plasma, urine, and bile, *Anal. Biochem.*, 281, 209, 2000.
86. Handelman, G.J. et al., Oral α-tocopherol supplements decrease plasma γ-tocopherol levels in humans, *J. Nutr.*, 115, 807, 1985.
87. Schultz, M. et al., alpha-Carboxyethyl-6-hydroxychroman as urinary metabolite of vitamin E, *Meth. Enzymol.*, 282, 297, 1997.
88. Smith, K.S. et al., Vitamin E supplementation increases circulating vitamin E metabolites tenfold in end-stage renal disease patients, *Lipids*, 38, 813, 2003.
89. Traber, M.G. et al., α-Tocopherol modulates CYA3A expression, increases γ-CEHC production and limits tissue γ-tocopherol accumulation in mice fed high γ-tocopherol diets, *Free Radic. Biol. Med.*, 38, 773, 2005.
90. Sachdeva, R. et al., Tocopherol metabolism using thermochemolysis: chemical and biological properties of gamma-tocopherol, gamma-carboxyethyl-hydroxychroman, and their quinones, *Chem. Res. Toxicol.*, 18, 1018, 2005.

91. Mustacich, D.J. et al., Biliary secretion of alpha-tocopherol and the role of the mdr2 P-glycoprotein in rats and mice, *Arch. Biochem. Biophys.*, 350, 183, 1998.
92. Azzi, A. et al., Vitamin E: a sensor and an information transducer of the cell oxidation state, *Am. J. Clin. Nutr.*, 62, 1337S, 1995.
93. Freedman, J.E. et al., Alpha-tocopherol inhibits aggregation of human platelets by a protein kinase C-dependent mechanism, *Circulation*, 94, 2434, 1996.
94. Steiner, M., Influence of vitamin E on platelet function in humans, *J. Am. Coll. Nutr.*, 10, 466, 1991.
95. Cachia, O. et al., Alpha-tocopherol inhibits the respiratory burst in human monocytes. Attenuation of p47(phox) membrane translocation and phosphorylation, *J. Biol. Chem.*, 273, 32801, 1998.
96. Islam, K.N., Devaraj, S., and Jialal, I., Alpha-tocopherol enrichment of monocytes decreases agonist-induced adhesion to human endothelial cells, *Circulation*, 98, 2255, 1998.
97. Devaraj, S. and Jialal, I., alpha-Tocopherol decreases interleukin-1beta release from activated human monocytes by inhibition of 5-lipoxygenase, *Arterioscler. Thromb. Vasc. Biol.*, 19, 1125, 1999.
98. Faruqi, R., de la Motte, C., and DiCorleto, P.E., Alpha-tocopherol inhibits agonist-induced monocytic cell adhesion to cultured human endothelial cells, *J. Clin. Invest.*, 94, 592, 1994.
99. Cominacini, L. et al., Antioxidants inhibit the expression of intercellular cell adhesion molecule-1 and vascular adhesion molecule-1 induced by oxidized LDL on human umbilical vein endothelial cells, *Free Rad. Biol. Med.*, 22, 117, 1997.
100. Martin, A. et al., Vitamin E inhibits low-density lipoprotein-induced adhesion of monocytes to human aortic endothelial cells in vitro, *Arterioscler. Thromb. Vasc. Biol.*, 17, 429, 1997.
101. Keaney, J.F., Jr., Simon, D.I., and Freedman, J.E., Vitamin E and vascular homeostasis: implications for atherosclerosis, *FASEB J.*, 13, 965, 1999.
102. Singh, U., Devaraj, S., and Jialal, I., Vitamin E, oxidative stress, and inflammation, *Annu. Rev. Nutr.*, 25, 151, 2005.
103. Miller, E.R., III et al., Meta-analysis: high-dosage vitamin E supplementation may increase all-cause mortality, *Ann. Intern. Med.*, 142, 37, 2005.
104. Eidelman, R.S. et al., Randomized trials of vitamin E in the treatment and prevention of cardiovascular disease, *Arch. Intern. Med.*, 164, 1552, 2004.
105. Shekelle, P.G. et al., Effect of supplemental vitamin E for the prevention and treatment of cardiovascular disease, *J. Gen. Intern. Med.*, 19, 380, 2004.
106. Vivekananthan, D.P. et al., Use of antioxidant vitamins for the prevention of cardiovascular disease: meta-analysis of randomised trials, *Lancet*, 361, 2017, 2003.
107. Lee, I.M. et al., Vitamin E in the primary prevention of cardiovascular disease and cancer: the Women's Health Study: a randomized controlled trial, *JAMA*, 294, 56, 2005.
108. Ma, J., Hampl, J.S., and Betts, N.M., Antioxidant intakes and smoking status: data from the continuing survey of food intakes by individuals 1994–1996, *Am. J. Clin. Nutr.*, 71, 774, 2000.
109. Ford, E.S. and Sowell, A., Serum alpha-tocopherol status in the United States population: findings from the Third National Health and Nutrition Examination Survey, *Am. J. Epidemiol.*, 150, 290, 1999.
110. Kushi, L.H. et al., Intake of vitamins A, C, and E and postmenopausal breast cancer. The Iowa Women's Health Study, *Am. J. Epidemiol.*, 144, 165, 1996.
111. Maras, J.E. et al., Intake of alpha-tocopherol is limited among US adults, *J. Am. Diet. Assoc.*, 104, 567, 2004.
112. Ford, E.S., Ajani, U.A., and Mokdad, A.H., Brief communication: the prevalence of high intake of vitamin E from the use of supplements among U.S. adults, *Ann. Intern. Med.*, 143, 116, 2005.
113. Eitenmiller, R. and Lee, J., *Vitamin E: Food Chemistry, Composition, and Analysis*, Marcel Dekker, Inc., New York, 2004.
114. Sokol, R.J., Vitamin E deficiency and neurological disorders, in *Vitamin E in Health and Disease*, Packer, L. and Fuchs, J. (eds), Marcel Dekker, Inc., New York, 1993, p. 815.
115. Ouahchi, K. et al., Ataxia with isolated vitamin E deficiency is caused by mutations in the alpha-tocopherol transfer protein, *Nat. Genet.*, 9, 141, 1995.
116. Traber, M.G. et al., Impaired discrimination between stereoisomers of α-tocopherol in patients with familial isolated vitamin E deficiency, *J. Lipid Res.*, 34, 201, 1993.
117. Yokota, T. et al., Postmortem study of ataxia with retinitis pigmentosa by mutation of the alpha-tocopherol transfer protein gene, *J. Neurol. Neurosurg. Psychiatry*, 68, 521, 2000.

118. Berson, E.L. et al., A randomized trial of vitamin A and vitamin E supplementation for retinitis pigmentosa, *Arch. Ophthalmol.*, 111, 761, 1993.
119. Traber, M.G. et al., Discrimination between *RRR*- and *all rac*-α-tocopherols labeled with deuterium by patients with abetalipoproteinemia, *Atherosclerosis*, 108, 27, 1994.
120. Sokol, R.J. et al., Isolated vitamin E deficiency in the absence of fat malabsorption—familial and sporadic cases: characterization and investigation of causes, *J. Lab. Clin. Med.*, 111, 548, 1988.
121. Puri, V. et al., Isolated vitamin E deficiency with demyelinating neuropathy, *Muscle Nerve*, 32, 230, 2005.
122. Traber, M.G. and Jialal, I., Measurement of lipid-soluble vitamins—further adjustment needed? *Lancet*, 355, 2013, 2000.
123. Sokol, R.J. et al., Vitamin E deficiency with normal serum vitamin E concentrations in children with chronic cholestasis, *N. Engl. J. Med.*, 310, 1209, 1984.
124. Andersen, L.F. et al., Evaluation of a food frequency questionnaire with weighed records, fatty acids, and alpha-tocopherol in adipose tissue and serum, *Am. J. Epidemiol.*, 150, 75, 1999.
125. Marzouki, N. et al., Vitamin E deficiency ataxia with (744 del A) mutation on alpha-TTP gene: genetic and clinical peculiarities in Moroccan patients, *Eur. J. Med. Genet.*, 48, 21, 2005.
126. Salonen, R.M. et al., Six-year effect of combined vitamin C and E supplementation on atherosclerotic progression: the Antioxidant Supplementation in Atherosclerosis Prevention (ASAP) Study, *Circulation*, 107, 947, 2003.
127. Fang, J.C. et al., Effect of vitamins C and E on progression of transplant-associated arteriosclerosis: a randomised trial, *Lancet*, 359, 1108, 2002.
128. Rimm, E.R. et al., Vitamin E consumption and the risk of coronary heart disease in men, *N. Engl. J. Med.*, 328, 1450, 1993.
129. Stampfer, M. et al., Vitamin E consumption and the risk of coronary disease in women, *N. Engl. J. Med.*, 328, 1444, 1993.
130. Blot, W.J. et al., Nutrition intervention trials in Linxian, China: supplementation with specific vitamin/mineral combinations, cancer incidence, and disease-specific mortality in the general population, *J. Natl. Cancer Inst.*, 85, 1483, 1993.
131. Trevithick, J.R., Robertson, J.M., and Mitton, K.P., Vitamin E and the eye, in *Vitamin E in Health and Disease*, Packer, L. and Fuchs, J. (eds), Marcel Dekker, Inc., New York, 1993, p. 873.
132. Zandi, P.P. et al., Reduced risk of Alzheimer disease in users of antioxidant vitamin supplements: the Cache County Study, *Arch. Neurol.*, 61, 82, 2004.
133. Ascherio, A. et al., Vitamin E intake and risk of amyotrophic lateral sclerosis, *Ann. Neurol.*, 57, 104, 2005.
134. Meydani, S.N. et al., Vitamin E supplementation enhances cell-mediated immunity in healthy elderly subjects, *Am. J. Clin. Nutr.*, 52, 557, 1990.
135. Meydani, S.N. et al., Vitamin E supplementation and in vivo immune response in healthy elderly subjects. A randomized controlled trial, *JAMA*, 277, 1380, 1997.
136. Meydani, S.N. et al., Vitamin E and respiratory tract infections in elderly nursing home residents: a randomized controlled trial, *JAMA*, 292, 828, 2004.
137. Hathcock, J.N. et al., Vitamins E and C are safe across a broad range of intakes, *Am. J. Clin. Nutr.*, 81, 736, 2005.
138. Cheung, M.C. et al., Antioxidant supplements block the response of HDL to simvastatin–niacin therapy in patients with coronary artery disease and low HDL, *Arterioscler. Thromb. Vasc. Biol.*, 21, 1320, 2001.
139. Brown, B.G. et al., Simvastatin and niacin, antioxidant vitamins, or the combination for the prevention of coronary disease, *N. Engl. J. Med.*, 345, 1583, 2001.
140. Waters, D.D. et al., Effects of hormone replacement therapy and antioxidant vitamin supplements on coronary atherosclerosis in postmenopausal women: a randomized controlled trial, *JAMA*, 288, 2432, 2002.
141. Lonn, E. et al., Effects of long-term vitamin E supplementation on cardiovascular events and cancer: a randomized controlled trial, *JAMA*, 293, 1338, 2005.
142. Brigelius-Flohé, R., Vitamin E and drug metabolism, *Biochem. Biophys. Res. Commun.* 305, 737, 2003.

143. Williams, D. and Feely, J., Pharmacokinetic-pharmacodynamic drug interactions with HMG-CoA reductase inhibitors, *Clin. Pharmacokinet.*, 41, 343, 2002.
144. Lee, A.J. et al., Characterization of the NADPH-dependent metabolism of 17beta-estradiol to multiple metabolites by human liver microsomes and selectively expressed human cytochrome P450 3A4 and 3A5, *J. Pharmacol. Exp. Ther.*, 298, 420, 2001.
145. Traber, M.G., Vitamin E, nuclear receptors and xenobiotic metabolism, *Arch. Biochem. Biophys.*, 423, 6, 2004.
146. Fischer, A. et al., Effect of selenium and vitamin E deficiency on differential gene expression in rat liver, *Biochem. Biophys. Res. Commun.*, 285, 470, 2001.
147. Gohil, K. et al., Gene expression profile of oxidant stress and neurodegeneration in transgenic mice deficient in α-tocopherol transfer protein, *Free Radic. Biol. Med.*, 35, 1343, 2003.
148. Gohil, K. et al., Alpha-tocopherol transfer protein deficiency in mice causes multi-organ deregulation of gene networks and behavioral deficits with age, *Ann. N.Y. Acad. Sci.*, 1031, 109, 2004.
149. Barella, L. et al., Identification of hepatic molecular mechanisms of action of alpha-tocopherol using global gene expression profile analysis in rats, *Biochim. Biophys. Acta*, 1689, 66, 2004.
150. Doring, F., Rimbach, G., and Lodge, J.K., In silico search for single nucleotide polymorphisms in genes important in vitamin E homeostasis, *IUBMB Life*, 56, 615, 2004.
151. Rota, C. et al., Dietary alpha-tocopherol affects differential gene expression in rat testes, *IUBMB Life*, 56, 277, 2004.
152. Azzi, A. et al., Regulation of gene expression by alpha-tocopherol, *Biol. Chem.*, 385, 585, 2004.
153. Age-Related Eye Disease Study Research Group, A randomized, placebo-controlled, clinical trial of high-dose supplementation with vitamins C and E, beta carotene, and zinc for age-related macular degeneration and vision loss: AREDS report no. 8, *Arch. Ophthalmol.*, 119, 1417, 2001.

5 Bioorganic Mechanisms Important to Coenzyme Functions

Donald B. McCormick

CONTENTS

INTRODUCTION

Definition

With the use (and misuse) of terms over significant periods of time, there is sufficient uncertainty regarding a specific word; it is best to avoid confusion by defining it. This is the case for the word coenzyme, which together with cofactor and prosthetic group has to some become ambiguous biochemical jargon [1]. As defined succinctly, a coenzyme is a natural, organic molecule that functions in a catalytic enzyme system [2]. Coenzymes bind specifically within protein apoenzymes to constitute catalytically competent holoenzymes. Hence, coenzymes are organic cofactors that augment the diversity of reactions that otherwise would be limited to chemical properties, principally simple acid–base catalysis of side-chain substituents from amino acid residues within enzymes. With tight binding, coenzymes may be referred to as prosthetic groups; with loose binding, they may be called cosubstrates.

The focus of this chapter is on the molecular means or mechanisms by which coenzymes participate as the loci of bond making and breaking steps in holoenzyme-catalyzed reactions. Most coenzymes are more complex metabolic derivatives of water-soluble vitamins. Since the subject of this volume is vitamins, as in the previous edition, coverage of coenzyme mechanisms will bear emphasis on those coenzymes derived from such vitamins covered in other regards in subsequent chapters; however, this edition also includes some information on quinone cofactors as well as some more recently identified functions of vitamin derivatives. References are sparsely used for typical or recent material that otherwise has largely become the domain of mechanistically inclined textbooks of biochemistry [3–5], especially when set for the more advanced student or professional [6].

Groupings

Attempts to place each coenzyme in a singular mechanistic group are sometimes fraught with difficulty because some can arguably fit into more than one category. For example, the lipoyl residues of transacylases undergo oxidation–reduction as well as participate in acyl transfers, but it is the latter that distinguishes the biological function. In at least a few instances, the tetrahydro forms of pterin coenzymes are oxidized to the dihydro level during operations of the enzymic systems, for example, 5,10-methylene tetrahydrofolate in thymidylate synthase and tetrahydrobiopterin in phenylalanine hydroxylase. More conventionally, folyl coenzymes are pulled together in a broad mechanistic view under one-carbon transfers.

The six groups that are subdivisions of this chapter reasonably imply the mechanistic and functional connections of principal coenzymes. These are oxidation–reduction reactions, generation of leaving group potential, acyl activation and transfer, carboxylations, one-carbon transfers, and rearrangements on vicinal carbons. These groupings follow a conventional pattern of biochemical recognition of what major purposes are served by vitamin-derived coenzymes.

OXIDATION–REDUCTION REACTIONS

Nicotinamide Coenzymes

Nicotinamide adenine dinucleotide (NAD) and its phosphate (NADP) are the two natural pyridine nucleotide coenzymes derived from niacin, as discussed in Chapter 6. Both contain an *N*(1)-substituted pyridine-3-carboxamide (nicotinamide) that is essential to function in redox reactions with a potential near −0.32 V. The nicotinamide coenzymes function in numerous oxidoreductase systems, usually of the dehydrogenase or reductase type, which include such diverse reactions as the conversion of alcohols (often sugars and polyols) to aldehydes or ketones, hemiacetals to lactones, aldehydes to acids, and certain amino acids to keto acids [7]. The general reaction stoichiometry is written as

$$\text{Substrate} + \text{NAD(P)}^+ \rightleftharpoons \text{Product} + \text{NAD(P)H} + \text{H}^+.$$

The common stereochemical mechanism of operation of nicotinamide coenzymes when associated with enzymes involves the stereospecific abstraction of a hydride ion (H^-) from the substrate, with para addition to one or the other side of C-4 in the pyridine ring of the coenzyme, as shown in Figure 5.1. The second hydrogen of the substrate group oxidized is concomitantly removed, typically from an electronegative atom (e.g., N, O, or S), as a proton (H^+) that ultimately exchanges as a hydronium ion. The sidedness of the pyridine ring is such that the para hydrogen up from the plane, when the carboxyamide function is near (or to the right) and the pyridine N is on the left (or at the bottom), is prochiral R because it is oriented

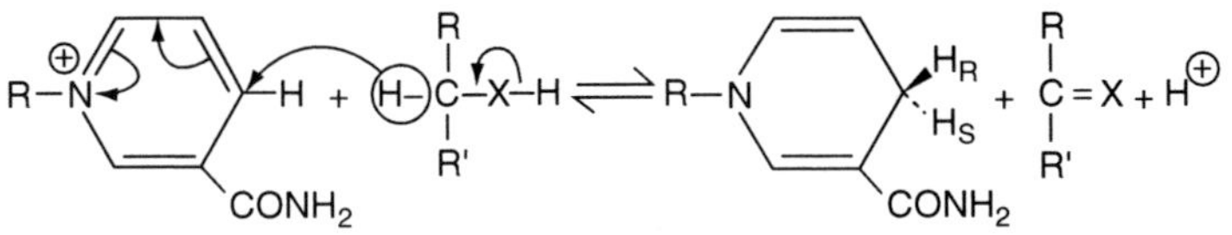

FIGURE 5.1 The stereospecific hydride ion transfer to and from nicotinamide coenzymes generating prochiral R and S forms.

toward the *re* face (A side). The hydrogen down from the plane of the ring is then prochiral S and oriented toward the *si* face (B side). There are numerous examples of nicotinamide coenzyme-dependent enzymes that are stereospecific as regards addition or removal of the hydride ion from the prochiral R (A) or S (B) position relative to the pyridine ring. These include, for A sidedness, NAD-dependent alcohol dehydrogenase and NADP-dependent cytoplasmic isocitrate dehydrogenase; for B sidedness, NAD-dependent D-glyceraldehyde-3-phosphate dehydrogenase and NADP-dependent D-glucose-6-phosphate dehydrogenase [8]. In general, A-side hydrogenases bind a conformation of the coenzyme in which the nicotinamide ring has an antiorientation with respect to the ribosyl ring, that is, the carboxamide groups points away; B-side dehydrogenases usually have syn conformation. This is probably due to stabilization of the dihydronicotinamide in the boat conformation attributable to orbital overlap between the lone *n* pair of electrons on the pyridine nitrogen and the antiboding σ orbital of the ribosyl C–O moiety, as depicted in Figure 5.2. The pseudoaxial hydrogens, either pro-R with anti or pro-S with syn orientation, are then more easily transferred because of orbital overlap in the transition state.

Nicotinamide coenzymes also participate in other (nonredox) biological reactions that involve ADP ribosylations; however, these are properly considered as substrate rather than coenzymic functions (see Chapter 6). The larger nucleotide-like structure of nicotinamide coenzymes is important with regard to coenzymic roles primarily to facilitate recognition and specific binding by the protein apoenzymes with which they interact.

Flavocoenzymes

Flavin mononucleotide (FMN), flavin adenine dinucleotide (FAD), and covalently linked flavocoenzymes (usually 8α-substituted FAD) are the natural coenzymes derived from riboflavin (vitamin B_2), which is discussed in Chapter 7. All contain an isoalloxazine ring system with a redox potential near -0.2 V when free in solution, but the potential is subject to considerable variation when bound within functional flavoproteins. This propensity for shifting potential gives flavoenzymes a wider operating range for oxidation–reduction reactions than is the case for enzymes dependent on nicotinamide coenzymes.

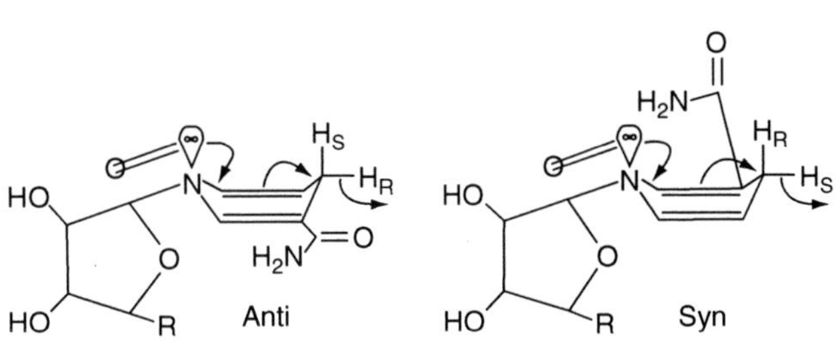

FIGURE 5.2 The syn and anti conformations of bound nicotinamide coenzymes that putatively transfer pro-S hydrogen and pro-R hydrogen, respectively.

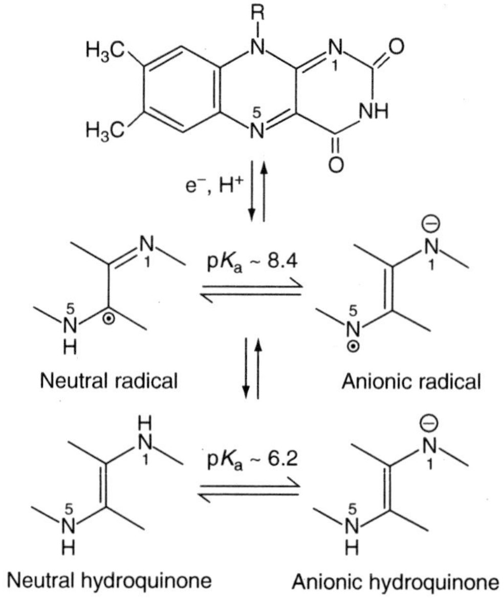

FIGURE 5.3 Biologically important redox states of flavocoenzymes with pK_a, values for interconversions of the free species.

Flavoproteins are variably able to catalyze both one- and two-electron redox reactions. The ring portion involving nitrogens 1 and 5 and carbon 4a reflects sequential addition or loss of electrons and hydrogen ions in one-electron processes and addition or loss of other transitory adducts with two-electron processes. There are nine chemically discernible redox forms, that is, three levels of oxidation–reduction and three species for acid, neutral, and base conditions. Of these only five have biological relevance because of pH considerations [2]. These biological forms are summarized in Figure 5.3. It should also be noted that free flavin semiquinones (radicals) are quite unstable, and the free flavia hydroquinones react very rapidly with molecular oxygen to become reoxidized. The latter is kinetically dissimilar to reduced nicotinamide coenzymes, which reoxidize more slowly with O_2. Binding to specific enzymes markedly affects the kinetic stability of the half-reduced and reduced forms of flavocoenzymes and again allows for diverse reactions under biological situations. An example of a flavoprotein undergoing a one-electron transfer is with the microsomal NADPH-cytochrome P450 reductase. This enzyme contains both FAD and FMN, and the latter cycles between a neutral semiquinone and fully reduced form [9]. The FAD in the electron-transferring flavoprotein, which mediates electron flow from fatty acyl coenzyme A (CoA) to the mitochondrial electron transport chain, cycles between oxidized quinone and anionic semiquinone. In addition, a single-step, two-electron transfer from substrate can occur in the nucleophilic reactions shown in Figure 5.4. Such cases as hydride ion transfer from reduced nicotinamide coenzymes or the carbanion generated by base abstraction of a substrate proton may lead to attack at the flavin N-5 positions; some nucleophiles, such as the hydrogen peroxide anion, are added on the C-4a position with its frontier orbital.

As regards stereochemistry, the transfer of hydrogen on and off N-5 can take place to or from one or the other face of the isoalloxazine ring system. When visualized with the benzenoid ring to the left and side chain at top (as in the top of Figure 5.3), orientation is to the *si* face with *re* on the opposite side. A fair number of flavoproteins have now been categorized on this steric basis [8]. Examples include the FAD-dependent glutathione reductase from human erythrocytes, which uses HADPH as substrate and is *re* side interacting, and

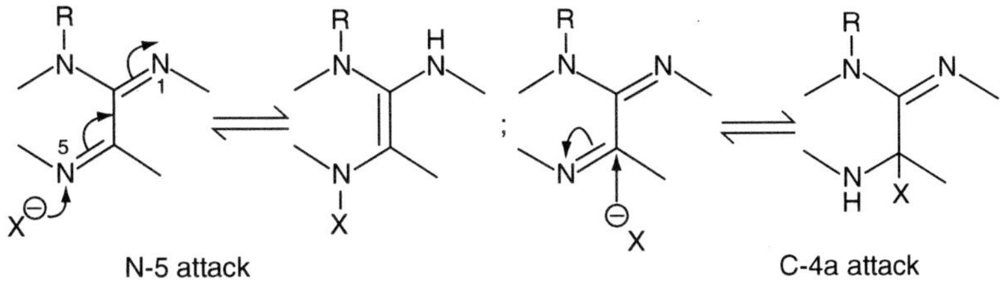

N-5 attack C-4a attack

FIGURE 5.4 Reaction types encountered with flavoquinone coenzymes and natural nucleophiles to generate N-5 and C-4a adducts as intermediates.

the FMN-dependent spinach glycolate oxidase, which is *si* side interacting. It should be noted that reduced flavins free in solution have bent or butterfly conformations, since the dihydroisoalloxazine has a 144° angle between benzenoid and phyrimidinoid portions. The orientations taken when bound to enzymes, however, may vary and can influence the redox potential.

There are flavoprotein-catalyzed dehydrogenations that are both nicotinamide coenzyme-dependent and -independent, reactions with sulfur-containing compounds, hydroxylations, oxidative decarboxylations, dioxygenations, and reduction of O_2 to hydrogen peroxide. The diversity of these systems is covered in periodic symposia on flavins and flavoproteins [10]. The intrinsic ability of flavins to be variably potentiated as redox carriers on differential binding to proteins, to participate in both one- and two-electron transfers, and in reduced (1,5-dihydro) form to react rapidly with oxygen permits wide scope in their operation. An interesting extension of the photoactivity of flavins is the vitamin B_2-based blue light photoreceptor (cryptochrome) found in the retinohypothalamic tract involved in setting the circadian clock in mammals [11].

Quinones and Quinoproteins

Among coenzymes that are not formed from vitamins because they can be biosynthesized by at least most of the organisms that require them are quinones that are both noncovalently and covalently bound within systems that operate generally in oxidation–reduction modes [12].

The ubiquinones (coenzyme Qs) are a group of ubiquitous substituted benzoquinones with variable-length terpenoid chains, as shown in Figure 5.5. In eukaryotes, they are found mainly in the mitochondrial inner membrane where they function to accept electrons from several different dehydrogenases and relay them to the cytochrome system. In this process, the quinone can be cyclically reduced and reoxidized with generation of intermediate radicals. Evidence has been found for a function of CoQ in plasma membrane electron transport, which influences mammalian cell growth.

More recently discovered redox cofactors [13] include pyrroloquinoline quinone (PQQ), originally called methoxatin, required in the pyridine nucleotide-independent primary alcohol dehydrogenase of methylotrophic bacteria. The structure of PQQ is illustrated in Figure 5.6. Though PQQ has been shown to function only in bacterial methanogens, its ubiquitous

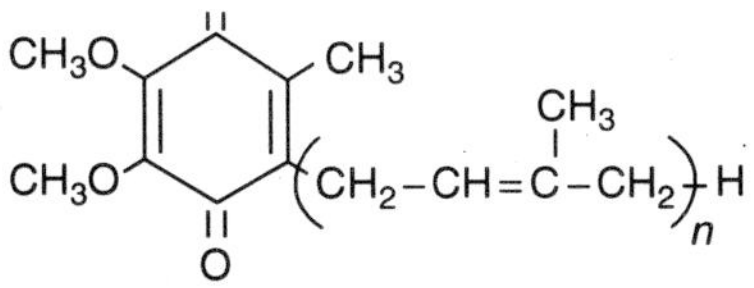

FIGURE 5.5 Ubiquinones (CoQ is ubiquinone-10).

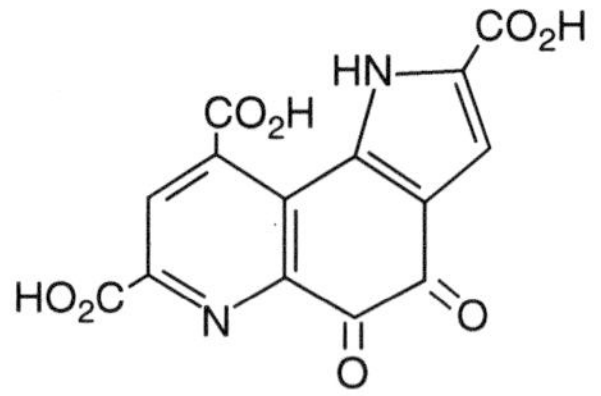

FIGURE 5.6 Pyrroloquinoline quinone (PQQ).

though trace occurrence in the environment and its ready accessibility in the human diet have raised questions concerning its role as a vitamin, or an essential or helpful nutrient. In particular, there are reported benefits for mice as regards growth, reproduction, and immunologic competence. However, as reviewed previously [13,14], there is a lingering question as to whether PQQ serves any unique role for humans and other mammals.

There are coenzymatically operating quinones that are within peptidic structures of a bacterial alkyl amine oxidase (trytophan tyrtophanal quinone, TTQ) and a fungal galactose oxidase (cysteinyl tyrosine cofactor, CT). At present, though, only a lysine tyrosyl quinone (LTQ) isolated from the Cu-containing lysyl oxidase from collagen and elastin and a tyrosyl quinone (TPQ) found in Cu-containing amine oxidase from almost every form of life are known to function in our bodies [13]. The structures of the later two topa quinones operating in the human are given in Figure 5.7. Such covalently bound coenzymes arise biosynthetically from the amino acid side chains of proenzymes and are released only by extensive proteolysis. The free quinones do not serve as vitamins.

GENERATION OF LEAVING GROUP POTENTIAL

THIAMINE PYROPHOSPHATE

Thiamine pyrophosphate (TPP) is the coenzyme derived from thiamine (vitamin B_1), which is discussed in Chapter 8. Though the substituted pyrimidyl portion shares a role in apoenzymic recognition and binding, the thiazole moiety not only is important in that regard but is involved with substrates to provide a transitory matrix that provides good leaving group potential [2,15]. Specifically, TPP as an Mg^{3+} ternary complex within enzymes can react as an ylid, resonance-stabilized carbanion that attacks carbonyl functions as illustrated in Figure 5.8.

In all cases, the bond to be labilized (from R′ to the C of the original carbonyl carbon) must be oriented for maximal σ–π orbital overlap with the periplanar system extending to the electron-deficient quaternary nitrogen of the thiazole ring. There are two general types of biological reactions in which TPP functions in so-called active aldehyde transfers. First, in decarboxylation of α-keto acids, the condensation of the thiazole moiety of TPP with the α-carbonyl carbon on the acid leads to loss of CO_2 and production of a resonance-stabilized carbanion. Protonation and release of aldehyde occur in fermentative organisms such as yeast, which have only the TPP-dependent decarboxylase, but reaction of the α-hydroxalkyl-TPP

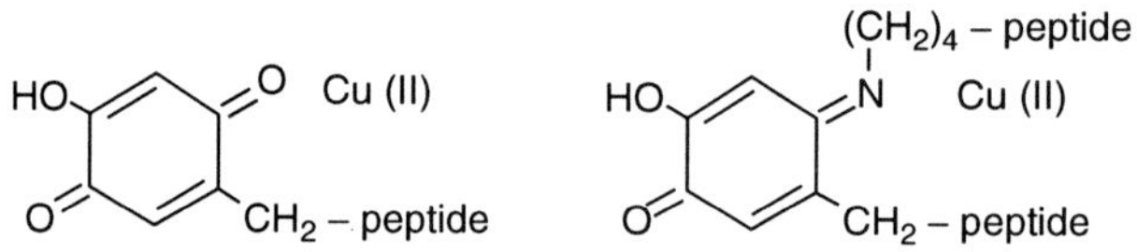

FIGURE 5.7 Topa quinone (TPQ) (left) and lysl topa quinone (LTQ) (right).

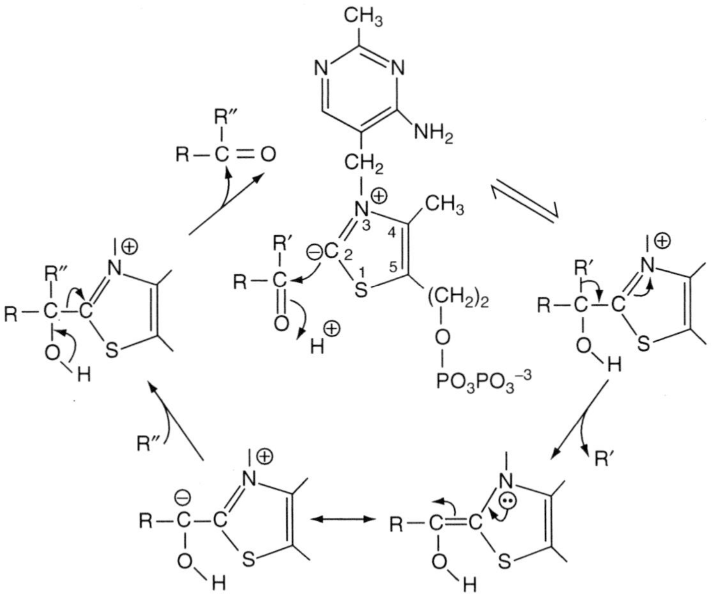

FIGURE 5.8 Function of the thiazole of the thiazole moiety of thiamine pyrophosphate. In α-keto acid decarboxylations, R′ is a carboxylate lost as CO_2 and R″ is a proton generating an aldehyde. In ketolations (both *trans*- and phospho-), R and R′ are part of a ketose phosphate generating a bound glycoaldehyde intermediate and R″ is an aldose phosphate or inorganic phosphate generating a different ketose phosphate or acetyl phosphate, respectively.

with lipoyl residues and ultimate conversion to acyl-CoA occurs in higher eukaryotes, including humans with multienzymic dehydrogenase complexes (see section Lipoic Acid). A lyase that is required to shorten 3-methyl-branched fatty acids, for example, phytanic acid, by α-oxidation also requires TPP. The other general reaction involving TPP is the transformation of α-ketols (ketose phosphates). Specialized phosphoketolases in certain bacteria and higher plants can split ketose phosphates, for example, D-glyceraldehyde-3-phosphate and acetyl phosphate. However, the reaction of importance to humans and most animals is a transketolation. Transketolase is a TPP-dependent enzyme found in the cytosol of many tissues, especially liver and blood cells, where principal carbohydrate pathways exist. This enzyme catalyzes the reversible transfer of a glycoaldehyde moiety (α,β-dihydroxyethyl-TPP) from the first two carbons of a donor ketose phosphate, that is, D-sylulose-5-phosphate, to the aldehyde carbon of an aldose phosphate, that is, D-ribose-5-phosphate, of the pentose phosphate pathway wherein D-sedoheptulose-7-phosphate and D-glyceraldehyde-3-phosphate participate as the other substrate–product pair.

Pyridoxal-5′-Phosphate

Two of the three natural forms of vitamin B_6, which are discussed in Chapter 10, can be phosphorylated to yield directly functional coenzymes, that is, pyridoxal-5′-phosphate (PLP) and pyridoxamine-5′-phosphate (PMP). PLP is the predominant and more diversely functional coenzymic form, although PMP interconverts as coenzyme during transaminations [2–6,16]. At physiological pH, the dianionic phosphates of these coenzymes exist as zwitterionic *meta*-phenolate phridinium compounds. Both natural and synthetic carbonyl reagents (e.g., hydrazines and hydroxylamines) form Schiff bases with the 4-formyl function of PLP, thereby removing the coenzyme and inhibiting PLP-dependent reactions.

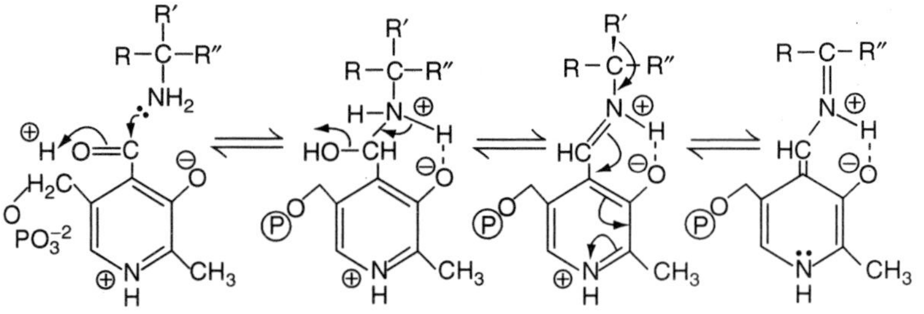

FIGURE 5.9 Operation of pyridoxal-5′-phosphate with a biological primary amine. Loss of R′ shown from the aldimine can be generalized for side-chain cleavages and eliminations, loss of CO_2 in decarboxylations, or loss of a proton in aminotransferations and racemizations.

PLP functions in numerous reactions that embrace the metabolism of proteins, carbohydrates, and lipids. Especially diverse are PLP-dependent enzymes that are involved in amino acid metabolism. By virtue of the ability of PLP to condense its 4-formyl substituent with an amine, usually the α-amino group of an amino acid, to form an azomethine (Schiff base) linkage, a conjugated double-bond system extending from the α carbon of the amine (amino acid) to the pyridinium nitrogen in PLP results in reduced electron density around the α carbon. This potentially weakens each of the bonds from the amine (amino acid) carbon to the adjoined functions (hydrogen, carboxyl, or side chain). A given apoenzyme then locks in a particular configuration of the coenzyme–substrate compound such that maximal overlap of the bond to be broken occurs with the resonant, coplanar, electron-withdrawing system of the coenzyme complex. These events are depicted in Figure 5.9.

Selection of the σ bond to be cleaved (R′–C) is achieved by stabilizing a conformation of the external aldimine in which the leaving group is orthogonal to the plane of the ring system, thus ensuring maximal orbital overlap with the π system in the transition state. The type of stereochemistry involved is characteristic of a given coenzyme system. Both *re* and *si* faces of the PLP complex can orient toward a reactive function, such as a base, contributed by enzyme protein. This is the case, for instance, with aspartate aminotransferase whereby a base function abstracts a proton from the α position and transfers it to the same side of the π system (syn transfer), adding it to the *si* face of the azomethine group in the ketimine. In this case, the hydrogen is incorporated in a pro-S position at carbon 4′ (the methylene of PMP).

Aminotransferases effect rupture of the α-hydrogen bond of an amino acid with ultimate formation of an α-keto acid and PMP; this reversible reaction proceeds by a double-displacement mechanism and provides an interface between amino acid metabolism and that for ketogenic and glucogenic reactions. Amino acid decarboxylases catalyze breakage of the α-carboxyl bond and lead to irreversible formation of amines, including several that are functional in nervous tissue (e.g., epinephrine, norepinephrine, serotonin, and γ-aminobutyrate). The biosynthesis of heme depends on the early formation of δ-aminolevulinate from PLP-dependent condensation of glycine and succinyl-CoA followed by decarboxylation. There are many examples of enzymes, such as cysteine desulfhydrase and serine hydroxymethyltransferase, that affect the loss or transfer of amino acid side chains. PLP is the essential coenzyme for phosphorylase that catalyzes phosphorolysis of the α-1,4 linkages of glycogen. An important role in lipid metabolism is the PLP-dependent condensation of L-serine with palmitoyl-CoA to form 3-dehydrosphinganine, a precursor of sphingolipids. The diversity of PLP functions is covered in periodic symposia that now include other carbonyl compounds as cofactors (pyruvyl enzymes, quinoproteins, etc.) [17,18]. A simpler but less-frequently encountered variation on the way in which PLP operates is provided by the pyruvoyl N-terminus of some enzymes [12,17]. In these electrophilic centers, the amino function of a substrate amino acid condenses to form a ketimine, which facilitates loss of a carboxyl group from the attached amino acid moiety. For example, S-adenosylmethionine decarboxylases from mammals as well as from *Escherichia coli* use such a subsystem to form spermidine from putrescine and methionine.

ACYL ACTIVATION AND TRANSFER

PHOSPHOPANTETHEINE COENZYMES

4′-Phosphopantetheine is a phosphorylated amide of β-mercaptoethylamine and the vitamin pantothenate, which is discussed in Chapter 9. The phosphopantetheinyl moiety serves as a functional component within the structure of CoA and as a prosthetic group covalently attached to a seryl residue of acyl carrier protein (ACP). Because of a thiol (sulfhydryl) terminus with a pK_a near 9, phosphopantetheine and its coenzymic forms are readily oxidized to the catalytically inactive disulfides.

Esterification of the thiol function to many carboxylic acids is the prelude to numerous acyl group transfers and enolizations [2–6]. In classic terminology, the thiol ester enhances both head and tail activations of acyl compounds, as illustrated in Figure 5.10. In head activation, the carbonyl function is attacked by a nucleophile and releases the original thiol. The carbonyl carbon of a thiol ester is more positively polarized than would be an oxy ester counterpart. Hence, the acyl moiety is relatively activated for transfer. The phosphopantetheine terminus of CoA and ACP both function in acyl transfer, the latter only within the fatty acid synthase complex. In tail activation, there is greater tendency for thio than oxy esters to undergo enolization by permitting removal of an α hydrogen as a proton. The enolate is stabilized by delocalization of its negative charge between the α carbon and the acyl oxygen, which makes it thermodynamically accessible as an intermediate. Since the developing charge is also stabilized in the transition state that precedes the enolate, it is also kinetically accessible. This process leads to facile condensation whereby nucleophilic addition of the carbanion-like carbon of the enolate to a neutral activated acyl group (another thiol ester) is a favored process. CoA is a good leaving group from the tetrahedral intermediate. From the above, it follows that thio esters are more like a ketone than an oxy ester. The degree of resonance electron delocalization from the overlap of sulfur p orbitals with the acyl π bond is less than that with oxygen in oxy esters.

The myriad acyl thio esters of CoA are central to the metabolism of numerous compounds, especially lipids and the penultimate catabolites of carbohydrates and ketogenic

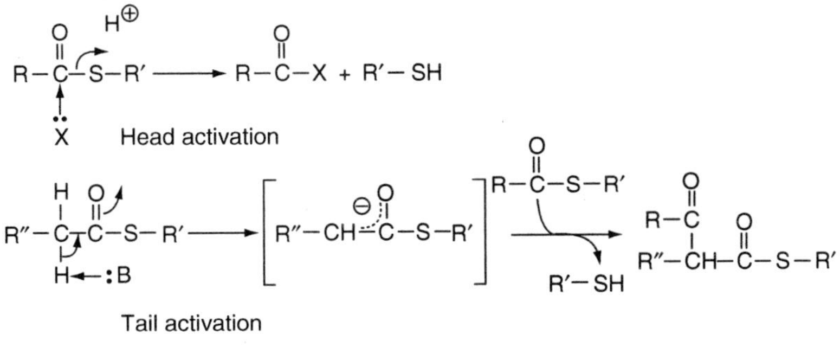

FIGURE 5.10 Activations of acyl moieties enhanced by formation of thio esters with phosphopantetheine coenzymes.

amino acids. For example, acetyl-CoA, which is formed during metabolism of carbohydrates, fats, and some amino acids, can acetylate compounds such as choline and hexosamines to produce essential biochemicals. It can also condense with other metabolites, such as oxalacetate, to supply citrate, and it can lead to formation of cholesterol. The reactive sulfhydryl termini of ACP provide exchange points for acetyl-CoA and malonyl-CoA. The ACP-*S*-malonyl thio ester can chain-elongate during fatty acid biosynthesis in a synthase complex.

Lipoic Acid

α-Lipoic (thioctic) acid is not a vitamin for humans and other animals because it can be biosynthesized from longer-chain, essential fatty acids. However, it is indispensable in its coenzymic role, which interfaces with some of the functions of TPP and CoA [2–5]. The natural D isomer of 6,8-dithiooctanoic (1,2-dithiolane-3-pentanoic) acid occurs in amide linkage to the ∈-amino group of lysyl residues within transacylases that are core protein subunits of α-keto acid dehydrogenase complexes of some prokaryotes and all eukaryotes. In such transacylases, the functional dithiolane ring is on an extended flexible arm. The lipoyl group mediates the transfer of the acyl group from an α-hydroxyalkyl-TPP to CoA in a cyclic system that transiently generates the dihydrolipoyl residue, as shown in Figure 5.11. Hence, the lipoyl/dihydrolipoyl pair in this cycle serves a dual role of electron transfer and acyl group vector by coupling the two processes.

The three α-keto acid dehydrogenase complexes of mammalian mitochondria are for pyruvate and α-ketoglutarate of the Krebs citric acid cycle and for the branched-chain α-keto acids from some amino acids. All involve participation of lipoyl moieties within core transacylase subunits surrounded by subunits of TPP-dependent α-keto acid decarboxylase, which generate α-hydroxyalkyl-TPP, and are further associated with subunits of FAD-dependent dihydrolipoyl (lipoamide) dehydrogenase. The number of subunits and their packing varies among cases. For instance, a single particle of *E. coli* pyruvate dehydrogenase consists of at least 24 chains of each decarboxylase and transacetylase plus 12 chains of the flavoprotein.

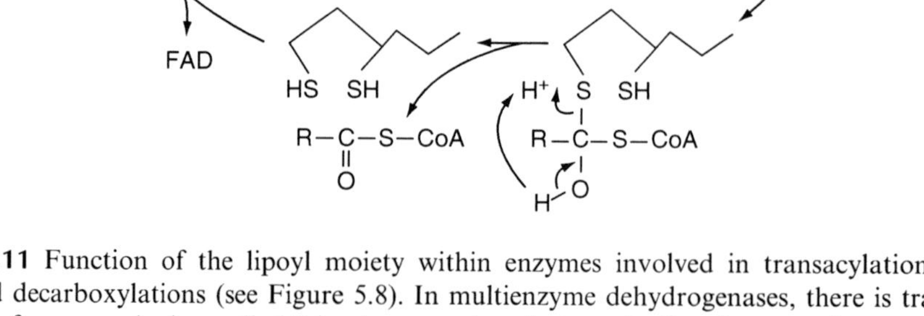

FIGURE 5.11 Function of the lipoyl moiety within enzymes involved in transacylations following α-keto acid decarboxylations (see Figure 5.8). In multienzyme dehydrogenases, there is transfer of an acyl moiety from an α-hydroxyalkyl thiamine pyrophosphate to the lipoyl group of a transacylase core and thence to CoA. This results in formation of the dihydrolipoyl group, which is cyclically reoxidized by the FAD-dependent dihydrolipoyl dehydrogenase.

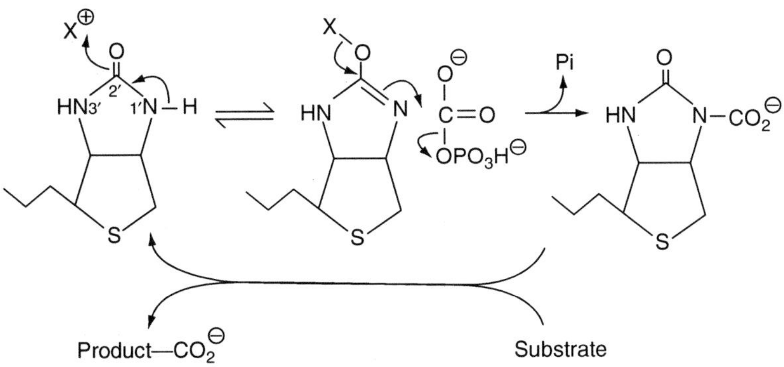

FIGURE 5.12 Function of the biotinyl moiety within enzymes involved in carboxylations with the intermediacy of the putative carbonyl phosphate.

CARBOXYLATIONS

BIOTIN

The characteristics of the vitamin biotin are discussed in Chapter 11. The coenzymic form of this vitamin occurs only as the vitamin with its valeric acid side chain amide linked to the ε-amino group of specific lysyl residues in carboxylase and transcarboxylase [2–6]. The length of this flexible arm (~14 Å) is similar to that encountered with the lipoyl attachments in transacylases. Biotin-dependent carboxylases operate by a common mechanism illustrated in Figure 5.12. This involves tautomerization of the ureido 1′-N to enhance its nucleophilicity. Though the two ureido nitrogens are essentially isoelectronic in the imidazoline portion of biotin, the steric crowding of the thiolane side chain near the 3′-N essentially prevents chemical additions to position 3′. Phosphorylation of bicarbonate by ATP to form carbonyl phosphate provides an electrophilic mixed-acid anhydride. The latter can then react at the nucleophilically enhanced 1′-N to generate reactive N(1′)-carboxylbiotinyl enzyme. This in turn can exchange the carboxylate function with a reactive center in a substrate, typically at a carbon with incipient carbanion character [19].

There are nine known biotin-dependent enzymes: six carboxylases, two decarboxylases, and a transcarboxylase. Of these, only four carboxylases have been found in tissues of humans and other mammals. Acetyl-CoA carboxylase is a cytosolic enzyme that catalyzes formation of malonyl-CoA for fatty acid biosynthesis. Pyruvate carboxylase is a mitochondrial enzyme that forms oxalacetate for citrate formation. Propionyl-CoA carboxylase forms the D isomer of methylmalonyl-CoA on a pathway toward succinyl-CoA in the Krebs cycle. Finally, β-methylcrotonyl-CoA carboxylase forms β-methylglutaconyl-CoA in the catabolic pathway from L-leucine.

ONE-CARBON TRANSFER: TETRAHYDROFOLYL COENZYMES

Among natural compounds with a pteridine nucleus, those most commonly encountered are derivatives of 2-amino-4-hydroxypteridines, which are trivially named pterins. Humans and other mammals normally require only folic acid as a vitamin of the pterion type. This is discussed in Chapter 12. Although a number of pterins when reduced to the 5,6,7,8-tetrahydro level function as coenzymes, the most generally used are poly-γ-glutamates of tetrahydrofolate (THF) [2,12,20,21]. Tetrahydropteroylglutamates and forms of its natural derivatives responsible for vectoring one-carbon units in different enzymic reactions are

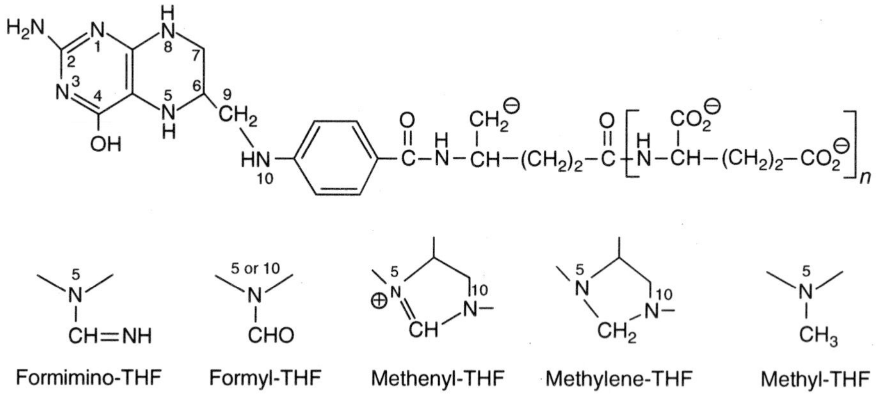

Formimino-THF Formyl-THF Methenyl-THF Methylene-THF Methyl-THF

FIGURE 5.13 Structures with numbering for tetrahydropteroyl-L-glutamates, including the biological derivatives for one-carbon transfers.

shown in Figure 5.13. All of these bear the substituent for transfer at nitrogen 5 or 10 or are bridged between these basic centers. The number of glutamate residues varies, usually from one to seven, but a few to several glutamyls optimize binding of tetrahydrofolyl coenzymes to most enzymes requiring their function. Less broadly functional, but essential for some coenzymic roles of pterins, is tetrahydrobiopterin, which cycles with its quinoid 7,8-dihydro form during O_2-dependent hydroxylation of such aromatic amino acids as in the conversion of phenylalanine to tyrosine. Tetrahydrobiopterin also serves as a one-electron donor in NO synthase catalysis. In addition, the recently elucidated molybdopterin functions in some Mo/Fe flavoproteins, such as xanthine dehydrogenase. Structures for tetrahydrobiopterin and molybdopterin are shown in Figure 5.14. Pterin coenzymes, most of them at the tetrahydro level, are sensitive to oxidation.

These interconversions of folate with the initial coenzymic relatives, the tetrahydrofolyl polyglutamates, involve dihydrofolate reductase, necessary for reducing the vitamin level compound through 7,8-dihydro to 5,6,7,8-tetrahydro levels. This enzyme is the target of such inhibitory drugs as aminopterin and amethopterin (methotrexate). A similar dihydropterin reductase catalyzes reduction of dihydrobiopterin to tetrahydrobiopterin. THF is trapped intracellularly and extended to polyglutamate forms that operate with THF-dependent systems. In some cases (e.g., thymidylate synthetase), there is a redox change in tetrahydro to dihydro coenzyme, which is rejected by the NADPH-dependent reductase.

There are different redox levels for the one-carbon fragment carried by THF systems. With formate, physphorylation by ATP leads to formyl phosphate, a reactive mixed-acid anhydride. This can react with nitrogens at either position 5 or 10 in THF to form the formyl compounds; on cyclization, the 5,10-methenyl-THF results. With formaldehyde, which becomes an electrophilic cation when protonated ($^+CH_2OH$), the reaction shown in Figure 5.15 ensues. This reaction is initiated at the most basic N-5 (pK_a ~ 4.8) of THF to generate an *N*-hydroxymethyl intermediate. The high electron charge (high basicity) and large free valence (high polarizability) confer a low

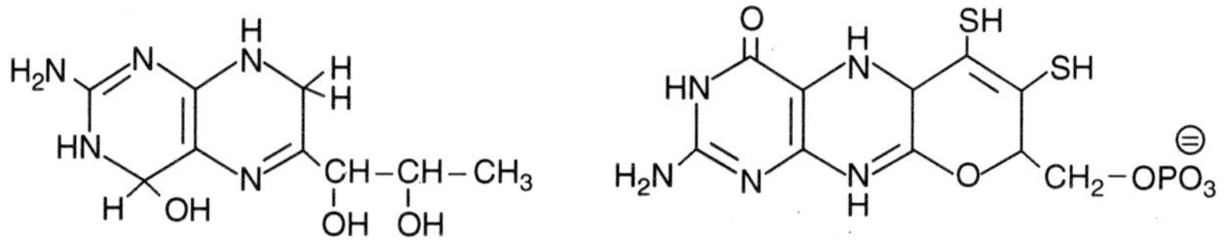

FIGURE 5.14 Tetrahydrobiopterin (left) and molybdopterin (right).

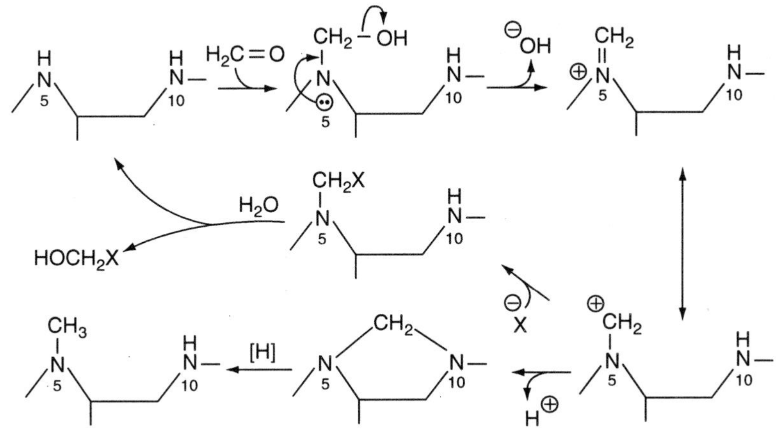

FIGURE 5.15 Reaction of formaldehyde with the basic N-5 of tetrahydrofolyl coenzyme to generate an N-hydroxymethyl intermediate that leads to a mesomeric carbocation. The latter can react intermolecularly in a Mannich-like reaction or intramolecularly to form 5,10-methylene tetrahydrofolate.

activation energy for electrophilic substitution at N-5. With loss of a hydroxyl and quaternization of this nitrogen, the one-carbon unit becomes canonically equivalent to a carbocation, which can react either inter- or intramolecularly. In the former instance, reaction with a nucleophile can lead to another hydroxymethyl compound; in the latter, 5,10-methylene-THF is formed. For the methyl level, reduction of the methylene-THF occurs.

An overview of some of the major interconnections among the one-carbon-bearing THF coenzymes and their metabolic origins and roles include a fair range of reaction types. As mentioned earlier, there is generation and utilization of formate. The important de novo biosynthesis of purine includes two steps wherein glycinamide ribonucleotide and 5-amino-4-imidazole carboxamide ribonucleotide are transformylated by 5,10-methenyl-THF and 10-formyl-THF, respectively. In pyrimidine nucleotide biosynthesis, deoxyuridylate and 5,10-methylene-THF form thymidylate and dihydrofolyl coenzyme in a mechanism whereby the tetrahydro coenzyme is oxidized to the dihydro level, as shown in Figure 5.16. There are

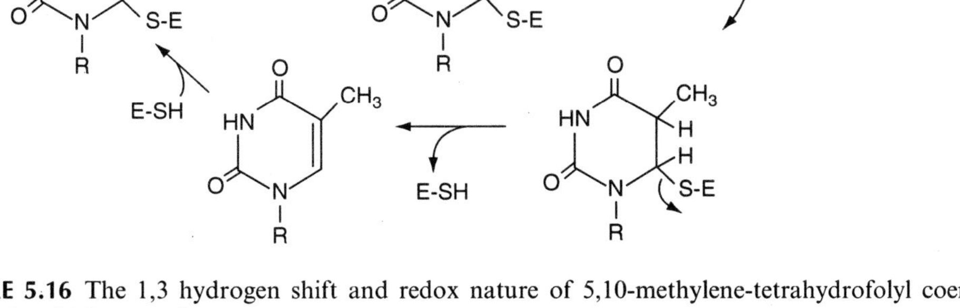

FIGURE 5.16 The 1,3 hydrogen shift and redox nature of 5,10-methylene-tetrahydrofolyl coenzyme within thymidylate synthase.

conversions of some amino acids, namely, *N*-formimino-L-glutamate (from histidine catabolism) with THF to L-glutamate and 5,10-methenyl-THF (via 5-formimino-THF), L-serine with THF to glycine and 5,10-methylene-THF, and L-homocysteine with 5-methyl-THF to L-methionine and regenerated THF.

REARRANGEMENTS ON VICINAL CARBONS: B_{12} COENZYMES

Though there are several biologically active forms derived from vitamin B_{12} discussed in Chapter 13, only a couple warrant attention as coenzymes in higher eukaryotes [2,22]. The coenzyme B_{12} (CoB_{12}) known to function in most organisms, including humans, is 5′-deoxyadenosylcobalamin. A second important coenzyme form is methylcobalamin (methyl-B_{12}), in which the methyl group replaces the deoxyadenosyl moiety of CoB_{12}. Some prokaryotes use other bases (e.g., adenine) in this position originally occupied by the cobalt-coordinated cyanide anion in cyanocobalamin, the initially isolated form of vitamin B_{12}.

The metabolic interconversion of vitamin B_{12} as the naturally occurring hydroxocobalamin (B_{12a}) with other vitamin and coenzyme level forms involves sequential reduction of B_{12a} to the paramagnetic or radical B_{12r} and further to the very reactive B_{12s}. The latter reacts in enzyme-catalyzed nucleophilic displacements of tripolyphosphate from ATP to generate CoB_{12} or of THF from 5-methyl-THF to generate methyl-B_{12}.

Seemingly all CoB_{12}-dependent reactions react through a radical mechanism, and all but one (*Lactobacillus leichmanii* ribonucleotide reductase) involve a rearrangement of a vicinal group (X) and a hydrogen atom. This general mechanism is illustrated in Figure 5.17. For the CoB_{12}-dependent mammalian enzyme, L-methylmalonyl-CoA mutase, X is the CoA-S-CO-group, which moves with retention of configuration from the carboxyl-bearing carbon of L(*R*)-methylmalonyl-CoA to the carbon β to the carboxyl group in succinyl-CoA. This reaction is essential for funneling propionate to the tricarboxylic acid cycle. Without CoB_{12} (from vitamin B_{12}), more methylmalonate is excreted, but also the CoA ester competes with malonyl-CoA in normal fatty acid elongation to form instead abnormal, branched-chain fatty acids. Methyl-B_{12} is necessary in the transmethylase-catalyzed formation of L-methionine and

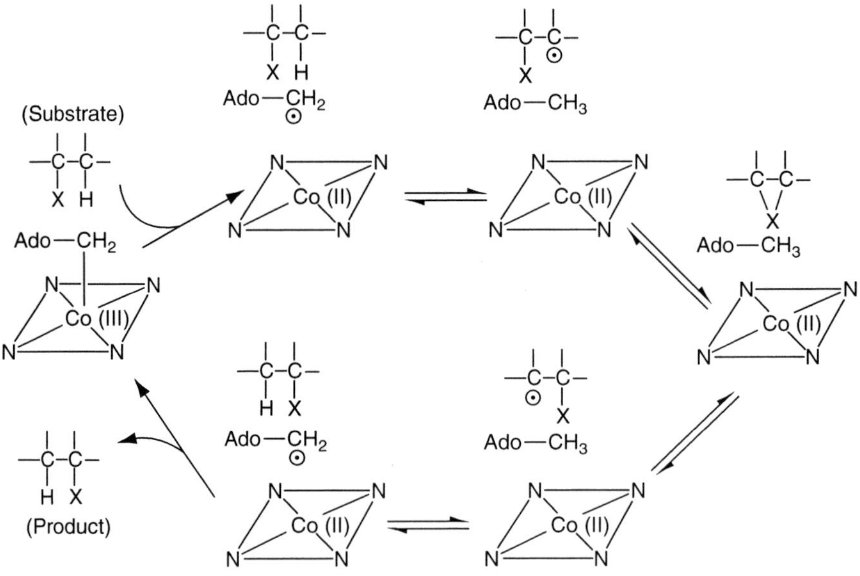

FIGURE 5.17 Radical intermediates in vicinal rearrangements catalyzed by enzymes using 5′-deoxyadenosyl-B_{12}.

regeneration of THF. Without this role, there would not only be no biosynthesis of the essential amino acid, but increased exogenous supply of folate would be necessary to replenish THF, which would not otherwise be recovered from its 5-methyl derivative.

REFERENCES

1. O.H. Hasim and N. Azila Adnan, Coenzyme, cofactor and prosthetic group—ambiguous biochemical jargon, *Biochem. Ed.* 22:93 (1994).
2. D.B. McCormick, Coenzymes, biochemistry, in *Encyclopedia of Human Biology*, Vol. 2 (R. Dulbecco, ed.-in-chief), Academic Press, San Diego, 1997, pp. 847–964.
3. D.E. Metzler, *Biochemistry: The Chemical Reactions of Living Cells*, 2nd ed., Vol. 1, Academic Press, San Diego, 2003.
4. D.E. Metzler, *Biochemistry: The Chemical Reactions of Living Cells*, 2nd ed., Vol. 2, Academic Press, San Diego, 2002.
5. P.A. Frey, Vitamins, coenzymes, and metal cofactors, in *Biochemistry* (G. Zubay, ed.), Wm. C. Brown, Dubuque, 1993, pp. 278–304.
6. C.T. Walsh, *Enzymatic Reaction Mechanisms*, Freeman, San Francisco, 1977.
7. D. Dolphin, R. Poulson, and O. Avamovic (eds.), *Pyridine Nucleotide Coenzymes*, Parts A and B, Wiley-Interscience, New York, 1987.
8. D.J. Creighton and N.S.R.K. Murthy, Stereochemistry of enzyme-catalyzed reactions at carbon, in *The Enzymes*, Vol. 19 (D.S. Sigmon and P.D. Boyer, eds.), Academic Press, San Diego, 1990, pp. 323–421.
9. A.H. Merrill, Jr., J.D. Lambeth, D.E. Edmondson, and D.B. McCormick, Formation and mode of action of flavoproteins, *Annu. Rev. Nutr.*, 1:281–317 (1981).
10. S. Chapman, R. Perman, and N. Scrutton (eds.), *Flavins and Flavoproteins*, 14th ed., Rudolf Weber Agency for Scientific Publ., Berlin, 2002.
11. Y. Miyamoto and A. Sancar, Vitamin B_2-based blue-light photoreceptors in the retinohypothalamic tract as the proactive pigments for setting the circadian clock in mammals, *Proc. Natl. Acad. Sci. USA*, 95:6097–6102 (1998).
12. D.B. McCormick, Organic cofactors as coenzymes, in *Encyclopedia of Molecular Cell Biology*, Wiley-VCH Verlag, Weinheim, Germany, 2004.
13. W.S. McIntire, Newly discovered redox cofactors: Possible nutritional, medical, and pharmacological relevance to higher animals, *Annu. Rev. Nutr.*, 18:145–177 (1998).
14. H.N. Christensen, Is PQQ a significant nutrient in addition to its role as a therapeutic agent in higher animals?, *Nutr. Rev.*, 52:24–25 (1994).
15. H.Z. Sable and C.J. Gubler (eds.), Thiamin. Twenty years of progress, *Ann. N.Y. Acad. Sci.*, 378 (1982).
16. D. Dolphin, R. Poulson, and O. Avamovic (eds.), *Pyridoxal Phosphate*, Parts A and B, Wiley-Interscience, New York, 1987.
17. T. Fukui, H. Kagamiyama, K. Soda, and H. Wada (eds.), *Enzymes Dependent on Pyridoxal Phosphate and Other Carbonyl Compounds as Cofactors*, Pergamon Press, Oxford, 1991.
18. A. Iriarte, H.M. Kagan, and M. Martinez-Carrion (eds.), *Biochemistry and Molecular Biology of Vitamin* B_6 *and PQQ-dependent Proteins*, Birkhäusen Verlag, Basel, 2000.
19. J.R. Knowles, The mechanism of biotin-dependent enzymes, *Annu. Rev. Biochem.*, 58:195 (1989).
20. R.L. Blakley and T.J. Benkovic, *Folate and Pterins*, Vol. 1, John Wiley and Sons, New York, 1986.
21. R.L. Blakley and V.M. Whitehead, *Folate and Pterins*, Vol. 3, John Wiley and Sons, New York, 1986.
22. D. Dolphin (ed.), B_{12}, Vols. 1 and 2, Wiley-Interscience, New York, 1982.

6 Niacin

James B. Kirkland

CONTENTS

HISTORICAL PERSPECTIVE

The identification of niacin as a vitamin resulted from an urgent need to cure pellagra, which ravaged low socioeconomic groups of the Southeastern United States in the early twentieth century and various European populations for the previous two centuries [1,2]. Corn had been introduced to Europe from the Americas and quickly became a staple food, as it could produce more calories per acre than wheat or rye. In 1735, the Spanish physician Casal became the first to describe the strange new disease, which he termed *mal de la rosa* (disease of the rose) and the characteristic rash around the neck of pellagrins is still referred to as "Casal's necklace." The disease spread geographically with the cultivation of corn, and became known as *pelle agra* (rough skin) in Italy.

Due to the widespread incidence of pellagra in eighteenth century Europe and the establishment of whole hospitals for victims of the disease, there was a painstaking documentation of its symptoms [1,2]. These include diarrhea and neurological disturbances (dementia) [3], as well as the sun-sensitive dermatitis, which, along with the eventual death of the patient, are often referred to as the 4 D's of pellagra. The disease was recognized in populations in Egypt, South Africa, and India in the late 1800s and early 1900s. The disease reached epidemic proportions in the United States in the first half of the 1900s, producing at least 250,000 cases and 7,000 deaths per year for several decades in the southern states alone [4]. Serious outbreaks continue to occur in some developing countries [5]. An improved standard of living and fortification of grain products have limited the disease in developed countries, but cases of pellagra still occur and they are likely underreported because of a lack of familiarity of modern physicians with this disease. Pellagra may be found in the homeless [6] and associated with alcohol abuse [7]. In these cases it may be complicated by deficiency of other nutrients, including thiamine, generating complex patterns of dementia [7]. Pellagra may occur in AIDS patients [8] and is associated with anorexia nervosa [9]. Low niacin status is also very common in cancer patients [10,11] and pellagra may be induced by chemotherapy [11,12]. Carcinoid cancers produce high levels of serotonin from tryptophan, and these patients will be at risk for deficiency if their intake of preformed niacin is low [13]. In all of these conditions, pellagra may be difficult to recognize if it does not present with the traditional outward signs of the disease [14]. For most of the cases given earlier, sun exposure is less of a factor compared with the historical pellagra outbreaks, and current patients may present with nondescript combinations of diarrhea and depression. Interestingly, if poorly diagnosed niacin-deficient patients are supplemented with micronutrients lacking sufficient niacin, they appear to move rapidly toward a full pellagrous dementia [14,15]. In addition to true pellagra, it is also likely that subclinical deficiencies of niacin exist in developed countries; 15% of women surveyed in Malmo, Sweden, had blood nucleotide pools which indicated a suboptimal niacin intake [16].

Until the first half of the twentieth century, the etiology of pellagra was unknown. Early theories suggested it was a type of leprosy; that it resulted from a toxin in moldy corn; or that it was an infectious disease communicated through an insect vector. Gradually, an association between pellagra and corn consumption became apparent, even in the absence of mold contamination. This was confirmed by Joseph Goldberger [17], who determined that a pellagra-preventative (P-P) factor, missing from corn, was necessary to prevent and cure pellagra in humans. In 1937, Elvehjem et al. [18] discovered that nicotinic acid could cure black tongue in dogs, an early animal model for pellagra. Paradoxically, chemical analysis of corn revealed that it was not especially low in nicotinic acid content. However, Krehl et al. [19] induced niacin deficiency in rats by feeding the animals a corn-based diet and the symptoms were alleviated with the addition of casein, a protein source rich in tryptophan. There had been suggestions that tryptophan deficiency caused pellagra and, in 1921, a pellagrous patient was treated successfully with tryptophan supplementation [20]. It was eventually realized that tryptophan can be used, with low efficiency, as a substrate for the synthesis of nicotinamide adenine dinucleotide (NAD) [21]. In 1951, Carpenter's group found that niacin in corn is biologically unavailable and can be released only following prolonged exposure to extremes in pH [22]. These findings eventually led to a better understanding of the contribution of a corn-based diet to the development of pellagra; corn-based diets are low in tryptophan and the preformed nicotinic acid is tightly bound, preventing its absorption. The release of niacin from this complex at elevated pH explained the good health of native Americans who used corn as a dietary staple: in most cases, these societies processed their corn with alkali before consumption. Corn was in use throughout North and South America for thousands of years as a domesticated crop, and methods of preparation ranged from treatment of corn with ashes from the fireplace, to the well-known use of limewater (water and calcium hydroxide) in the making of tortillas. In addition, niacin in immature corn is far more available, and the native practice of roasting and drying "green" corn provided another source of available niacin [23]. Had the explorers brought native American cooking techniques along with corn to sixteenth century Europe, pellagra epidemics might never have occurred.

Pellagra may be difficult to identify, as the symptoms of dermatitis, diarrhea, and dementia occur in an unpredictable order, and it is uncommon to find all three aspects until the disease is very advanced. The earliest sign of deficiency is often inflammation in the oral cavity, which progresses to include the esophagus and eventually the whole digestive tract, associated with a severe diarrhea [1]. Burning sensations often discourage food consumption, and the patient may progress toward a state of marasmus. The cause of death in many cases results from the effects of general malnutrition, poor disease resistance, and diarrhea [1]. Due to the sensitivity to sunlight, and possibly due to dietary variation, the incidence of pellagra is seasonal. The dermatitis can become severe rapidly, with exposed skin showing hyperpigmentation, bullous lesions, and desquamation (Figure 6.1a and Figure 6.1b). The skin may heal during fall and winter, leaving pink scars, only to revert to open sores the following summer. The other dramatic symptom of pellagra is dementia, which progresses beyond the type of depression associated with general malnutrition. Neurological changes in pellagra patients begin peripherally, with signs such as muscle weakness, twitching and burning feelings in the extremities, and altered gait [24]. Early psychological changes include depression and apprehension, but these progress to more severe changes, such as vertigo, loss of memory, deep depression, paranoia and delirium, hallucinations, and violent behavior [25]. This type of dementia is very similar to schizophrenia [26]. There are examples of the pellagrous insane committing murder, although it was more common for these patients to turn to suicide [1]. While there are pathological changes in the spinal cord in advanced pellagra, and some of the motor disturbances are permanent [1], there is a striking recovery of psychological function when insane pellagra patients are treated with nicotinic acid, with a disappearance of many symptoms in 1 to 2 days [25]. These observations suggest that a compound derived from niacin is involved in neural signaling pathways.

The first biochemical role established for niacin was its involvement in redox reactions and energy metabolism. For many years, however, the symptoms of pellagra remained mysterious when viewed from this perspective. Other nutrients involved in energy metabolism do not cause similar deficiency symptoms. Riboflavin-containing coenzymes are often coupled with nicotinamide-dependent reactions in the transfer of electrons, but riboflavin deficiency is not very similar to pellagra. Iron is intimately involved in electron transport and

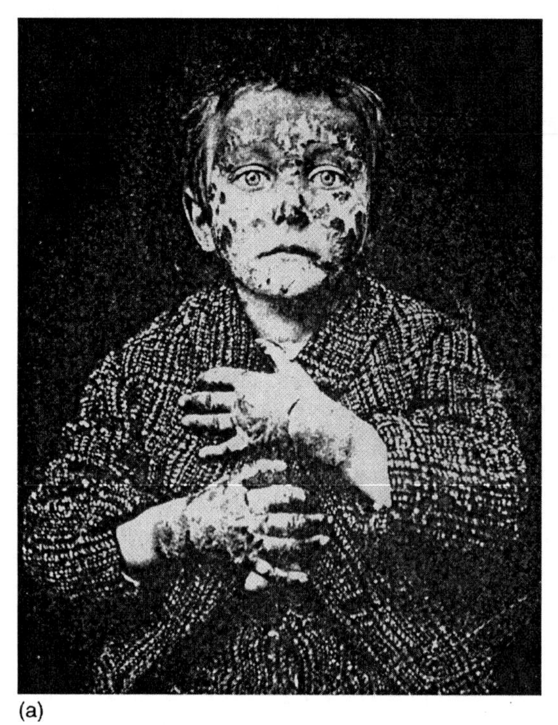
(a)

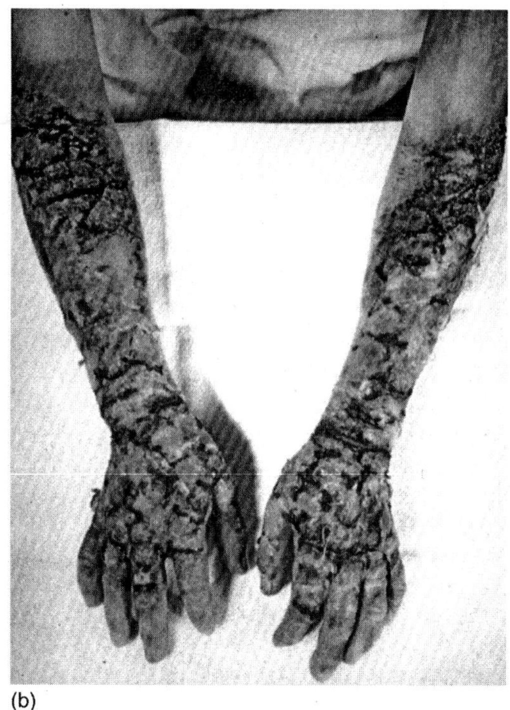
(b)

FIGURE 6.1 (a) An Austrian child with pellagra, showing dermatitis on the exposed skin of the face and hands. Note the unaffected skin on the wrists where the cuffs of the coat are turned up. (Reproduced from Roberts, S.R., *Pellagra: History, Distribution, Diagnosis, Prognosis, Treatment, Etiology*, C.V. Mosby, St. Louis, 1914. With permission.) (b) Severe pellagrous lesions on the arms of a 32 year old woman. They did not respond to riboflavin supplementation, but cleared up with the use of Valentine's whole liver extract, a good source of niacin. (Reproduced from Harris, S., *Clinical Pellagra*, C.V. Mosby, St. Louis, 1941. With permission.)

ATP production and it functions closely with nicotinamide cofactors in energy metabolism. Iron deficiency and pellagra both cause general weakness, which could be associated with disrupted energy metabolism, but the pellagra patient displays several unique and dramatic clinical characteristics. While other nutrient deficiencies cause dermatitis, only in niacin deficiency is this condition induced by exposure to sunlight. While thiamine deficiency also causes changes in energy metabolism and neural function, the behavioral effects reflect a severe depression (dry beriberi) rather than dementia.

Recently, insights into the function of nicotinamide coenzymes in metabolism have improved our appreciation of the biochemical changes that may underlie the 4 D's of pellagra. Table 6.1 lists the general categories of enzymes now known to require nicotinamide nucleotides as cofactors. In the end, the etiology of pellagra, and the impact of subclinical deficiencies of niacin, will be understood from a perspective of the relative disruption of these different areas of NADP-dependent metabolism.

In 1967, poly(ADP-ribosyl)ation was identified and recognized as a posttranslational modification of nuclear proteins. Poly(ADP-ribose) synthesis makes use of NAD^+ as substrate, rather than as an electron-transporting intermediate. Poly(ADP-ribose) formation has been shown to be important in DNA repair and genomic stability and provides an explanation for sensitivity to ultraviolet radiation observed in pellagra. Mono(ADP-ribosyl)ation was characterized, beginning in the mid-1960s, as a mechanism of action for many bacterial

TABLE 6.1
Summary of Reaction Types That Are Dependent on Nicotinamide Nucleotides

Category of Reaction	Enzymes	Main Products	Metabolic Roles
NAD^+/NADH redox exchanges	Numerous NAD-dependent enzymes throughout oxidative metabolism	NADH and oxidized metabolites, e.g., TCA cycle intermediates	Transfer of electrons from macronutrient substrates to the ETC, ATP production Numerous oxidative reactions are enabled by the high ratio of NAD^+:NADH
$NADP^+$/NADPH redox exchanges	Numerous NADP-dependent enzymes involved in reductive metabolism	$NADP^+$ and reduced metabolites, e.g., fatty acids	Biosynthetic metabolism, oxidant defense Numerous reductive reactions are enabled by the high ratio of NADPH:$NADP^+$, which is maintained by the pentose phosphate pathway
Poly(ADP-ribosyl)ation reactions	Up to 18 different PARP enzymes, mainly nuclear and DNA associated	Poly(ADP-ribose) covalently bound to proteins, free polymer resulting from catabolism	Diverse functions, but many related to DNA metabolism and genomic stability Polyanionic nature controls protein function High-affinity polymer binding by other proteins
Mono(ADP-ribosyl)ation reactions	Numerous poorly characterized transferases	Mono(ADP-ribose) covalently bound to proteins, many of which are G-proteins	Diverse and poorly characterized
Cyclic ADP-ribose and NAADP formation	ADP-ribosyl cyclases, which also have the potential to form NAADP	Cyclic ADP-ribose NAADP	Control of intracellular calcium levels, and thereby control of almost all cellular signaling events
SIR2/SIRT1 deacetylation reactions	SIR2 (rats) SIRT1 (humans)	Deacetylated proteins, including histones, p53 *O*-Acetyl-ADP-ribose	Control of p53 function and chromatin structure, central to life extension through caloric restriction

toxins. Mono(ADP-ribosyl)ation is now thought to be important in the endogenous regulation of many aspects of signal transduction and membrane trafficking in eukaryotic cells. In 1989, cyclic ADP-ribose was identified as another product of NAD metabolism and shown to have the ability to regulate cellular calcium homeostasis, a central process in neural transmission. Interestingly, the enzymes that make and degrade cyclic ADP-ribose and the proteins that bind this second messenger are present in the brain in relatively larger quantities than other tissues. The same enzymes that make cyclic ADP-ribose have now been found to produce nicotinic acid adenine dinucleotide phosphate (NAADP), using NADP as a substrate. NAADP also appears to have distinct functions in the regulation of intracellular calcium stores. The studies of mono-ADP-ribose, cyclic ADP-ribose, and NAADP function are in their early stages, but they may soon provide explanations for the dementia of the pellagra patient and the changes in intestinal cell function that lead to diarrhea.

CHEMISTRY

Nicotinic Acid and Nicotinamide

The term niacin is accepted as a broad descriptor of vitamers that have the biological activity associated with nicotinamide, including nicotinamide, nicotinic acid, and a variety of pyridine nucleotide structures. In the past, niacin has been used to specifically refer to nicotinic acid (pyridine-3-carboxylic acid, Figure 6.2a) but, for the purposes of this discussion, "niacin" is used in reference to all forms with vitamin activity whereas "nicotinic acid" refers to pyridine-3-carboxylic acid. Nicotinic acid is a white crystalline solid, stable in air at normal room temperature. It is moderately soluble in water and alcohol, but insoluble in ether. An aqueous solution has maximum ultraviolet absorbance at 263 nm.

Like nicotinic acid, nicotinamide (niacinamide; pyridine-3-carboxamide) (see structure, Figure 6.2b) is a white crystalline substance with a maximal ultraviolet absorbance at 263 nm. In contrast to nicotinic acid, nicotinamide is highly soluble in water, and is soluble in ether, characteristics that allow separation of the two vitamers.

Niacin Coenzymes

The biologically active forms of niacin compounds are the NAD and NADP coenzymes (Figure 6.2c and Figure 6.2d). The C-4 position on the pyridine ring of the nicotinamide moiety participates in oxidation and reduction reactions. Due to the electronegativity of the amide group and the nitrogen at position 1 on this ring, hydride ions can readily reduce the oxidized C-4 position. This is the basis for the enzymatic hydrogen-transfer reactions that are ubiquitous among organisms. In relation to the nonredox functions of NAD, the glycosidic linkage between nicotinamide and ribose is a high-energy bond and cleavage of this bond drives all types of ADP-ribose-transfer reactions in the forward direction.

The oxidized and reduced forms of the coenzymes are designated NAD^+ or $NADP^+$ and NADH or NADPH, respectively. The designations NAD and NADP are used to describe the total pools. This is often necessary if the method of quantification does not distinguish between oxidized and reduced forms or if a general statement about the nucleotide pool is made. The total pool of all four forms may be referred to as NAD(P). Both NAD and NADP are white powders, which are freely soluble in water and poorly soluble in ether. Both compounds have strong ultraviolet absorption at 340 nm in their reduced forms, with a weaker absorption at 260 nm when oxidized or reduced. The absorbance at 340 nm is often used to monitor the oxidation or reduction of these cofactors in enzyme assays.

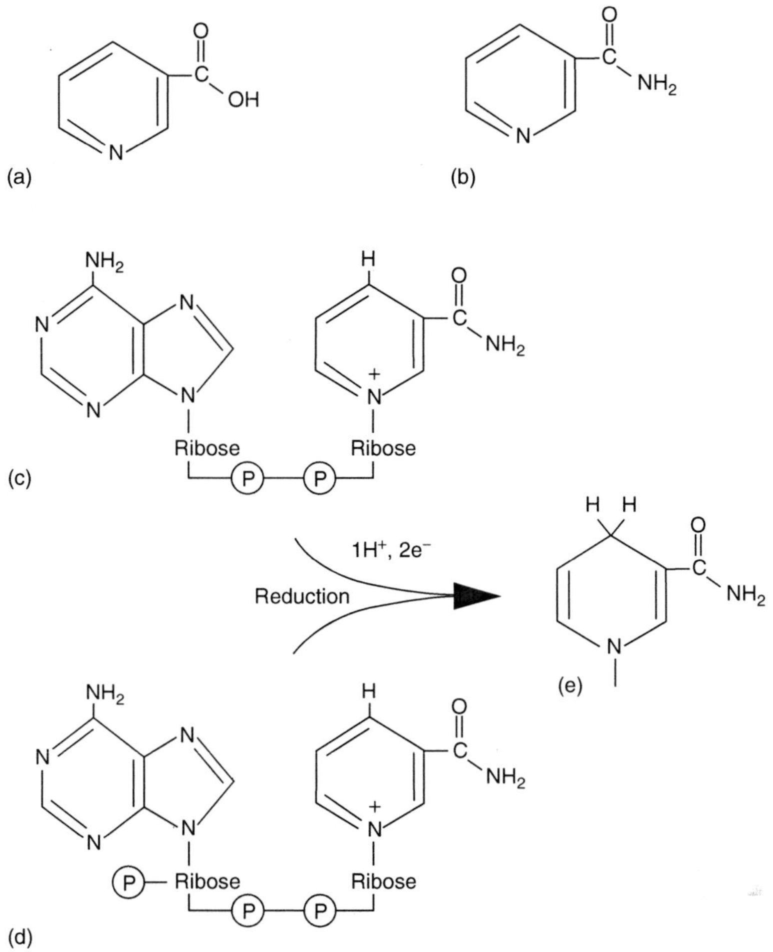

FIGURE 6.2 Chemical structures of niacin compounds. (a) Nicotinic acid, (b) nicotinamide, (c) NAD^+, (d) $NADP^+$, and (e) site of reduction.

FOOD CONTENT, DIETARY REQUIREMENTS, AND ASSESSMENT OF STATUS

QUANTIFICATION

The traditional analysis for nicotinic acid entails cleavage of the pyridine ring with cyanogen bromide (the Koenig reaction) and then reaction with an aromatic amine to yield a colored product that can be assayed spectrophotometrically [27]. Microbiological assay of nicotinic acid and nicotinamide is possible [28,29] and fluorometric measurement of nicotinamide is very sensitive [30]. These traditional methods for the analysis of nicotinic acid and nicotinamide are replaced by new techniques including gas chromatography and mass spectroscopy [31,32] or HPLC [33].

Measurement of pyridine nucleotides is easier than measurement of the vitamin precursors. Oxidized forms (NAD^+, $NADP^+$) are extracted by acid, usually 1 N perchlorate. This causes destruction of the reduced forms (NADH, NADPH). The reduced nucleotides are extracted by base, which causes destruction of the oxidized forms [34]. The extracted nucleotides are generally quantified by enzyme-cycling techniques, which recognize oxidized or reduced nucleotides, but are specific to either NAD or NADP [34]. The oxidized forms can also be measured by HPLC techniques, which provide additional data on ATP, ADP, and AMP levels [35].

Food Content

The niacin content of human foods is usually expressed as niacin equivalents (NE), which are equivalent to niacin content (mg) and 1/60 tryptophan content (mg). This relationship is not really constant across a range of niacin and tryptophan intake, as it may be less efficient with low tryptophan intakes [36,37] and more efficient with low niacin intake [2,36]. The efficiency of conversion may also be affected by other amino acids and dietary fat, as discussed in subsequent sections. Niacin in plant products is mainly in the form of nicotinic acid, although much of it exists in poorly understood bound forms. These bound forms have been studied in wheat bran, corn, and other grains and are heterogeneous mixtures of polysaccharides and glycopeptides to which nicotinic acid is esterified [38]. Niacin in immature corn is much more bioavailable [23]. Niacin in mature corn is about 35% available, even with cooking, but alkaline treatment frees the niacin for effective absorption [39]. Animal products initially contain mainly NAD and NADP coenzymes, although these tend to release nicotinamide during the aging and cooking of meats. Because plant products contain less tryptophan than animal products, and because the nicotinic acid may be largely bound in unavailable forms, some grain products such as breakfast cereals are supplemented with nicotinic acid. Diet fortification, together with the widespread occurrence of niacin and tryptophan in a mixed diet, has greatly diminished clinically obvious cases of pellagra in developed countries. Subclinical niacin deficiency may still be common in developed countries [16,31] and clinical pellagra still occurs in association with alcoholism [14]. Outbreaks of pellagra continue in some areas of the world where populations rely on corn as a staple [5]. The degree of nutrient deficiency in a population is always based on the current perception of optimal intake or function. As our understanding of niacin function evolves, we should be open to revising these end points and re-evaluating niacin status. Later sections in this chapter show that higher intakes of niacin may decrease the risk of various forms of cancer.

Dietary Requirements and Assessment of Status

Canada and the United States have harmonized dietary reference intakes (DRI) for essential nutrients, including niacin. There are recommended dietary allowances (RDA) and tolerable upper intake levels (UL) set out for niacin intake. The new RDA values for niacin range from 2 mg of preformed niacin per day for infants up to 18 NE/day during pregnancy [40]. Niacin status has traditionally been tested by measuring the urinary excretion of various niacin metabolites or the urinary ratio of *N*-methyl-2-pyridone-5-carboxamide to *N*-methylnicotinamide [41]. The 2-pyridone form decreases to a greater extent in response to a low dietary intake, and a ratio of less than 1.0 is indicative of niacin deficiency. More recently, it has been found that the NAD pool in red blood cells decreases rapidly during niacin deficiency in men whereas the NADP pool is quite stable [36]. This has led to the suggested use of (NAD/NAD + NADP) $\times$ 100, referred to as the niacin number, as an easily obtained index of niacin deficiency in humans [13,16,42]. Studies using animal models have also shown that blood NAD pools deplete more rapidly and to a greater extent than those of tissues such as the liver, heart, or kidney [43], suggesting that a portion of blood NAD may represent a labile storage pool.

The UL values for niacin apply only to supplements and fortified foods and range from 10 mg/day in young children to 35 mg/day in adults. The UL is based on the risk of skin flushing [40], which, alone, does not reflect serious health risks. Many vitamin B supplements contain 50–100 mg per tablet, and about half of all supplement users are found to exceed the

UL for niacin [44]. As Canada moves toward a more regulated natural product industry, these high-niacin supplements may not receive natural product numbers, and may not be available for purchase. On the other hand, future research may extend the results of animal studies and show that larger niacin supplements decrease cancer risk in human populations, and the recommendations for niacin supplementation may be increased. Very high levels of niacin intake can stress methyl donor status [45] and increase blood homocysteine levels [46]. (See Pharmacology and Toxicology in page 220.)

PHYSIOLOGY

Pathways of Synthesis

Although plants and most microorganisms can synthesize the pyridine ring of NAD de novo from aspartic acid and dihydroxyacetone phosphate [47], animals do not have this ability. Nicotinic acid, nicotinamide, pyridine nucleotides, and tryptophan represent the dietary sources for the pyridine ring structure in mammals. Animals may also practice coprophagy to take advantage of colonic synthesis of niacin by microflora. Ruminants receive an ample supply of niacin from foregut bacteria.

In 1958, Preiss and Handler [48] proposed a pathway for the conversion of nicotinic acid to NAD in yeast and erythrocytes (shown in reactions 9, 5, and 6 of Figure 6.3). Initially, it was believed that nicotinamide was also metabolized through the Preiss–Handler pathway, following the conversion of nicotinamide to nicotinic acid by nicotinamide deamidase (reaction 8, Figure 6.3). However, it was soon demonstrated by Dietrich et al. [49] that nicotinamide reacts first with phosphoribosyl pyrophosphate and then ATP to produce NAD directly (reactions 10 and 11, Figure 6.3). Interestingly, there is a common enzyme in the de novo and salvage routes of NAD synthesis. Nicotinamide mononucleotide (NMN) and nicotinic acid mononucleotide (NAMN) adenylyltransferase activities reside within a common protein; this enzyme catalyzes the last step in the conversion of nicotinamide and the second last step in the conversion of nicotinic acid to NAD. It was thought to exist only in the nucleus, but now three distinct forms of the enzyme have been characterized, including nuclear, mitochondrial, and Golgi isoforms [50].

Tryptophan catabolism plays an important role in niacin status. The majority of tryptophan is catabolized through kynurenine and 2-amino-3-carboxymuconic-6-semialdehyde (ACMS) to acetyl CoA. Quinolinic acid can react with phosphoribosyl pyrophosphate to produce NAMN. This reaction predominates in the kidney and in the liver in mammals because of the localization of quinolinate phosphoribosyltransferase in these tissues [51]. NAD is then synthesized from NAMN via the Preiss–Handler pathway. A number of reactions are required to convert tryptophan to quinolinic acid. ACMS, an intermediate in this pathway, is catabolized toward acetyl CoA and CO_2 (reaction 2, Figure 6.3) by 2-amino-3-carboxymuconic-6-semialdehyde decarboxylase (ACMSD, previously called picolinate carboxylase). If ACMS accumulates, some of it degrades spontaneously to quinolinic acid (reaction 3, Figure 6.3), allowing the formation of NAD. The formation of quinolinate and NAD is impaired if there is a high activity of ACMSD, and this appears to be a main source of variation between species in the efficiency of conversion of tryptophan to niacin [52]. The production of NAD from tryptophan is favored by a high activity of tryptophan or indoleamine 2,3-dioxygenase, a low activity of ACMSD, and a high activity of quinolinate phosphoribosyltransferase. These requirements restrict this pathway to the liver and kidney and lead to a wide range in the efficiency of tryptophan utilization among species and individuals. The following is a subjective observation, but the conversion of tryptophan to niacin seems like a poorly regulated pathway with respect to niacin status. NAD production is dependent on a nonenzymatic conversion, and the enzymes that are required to create

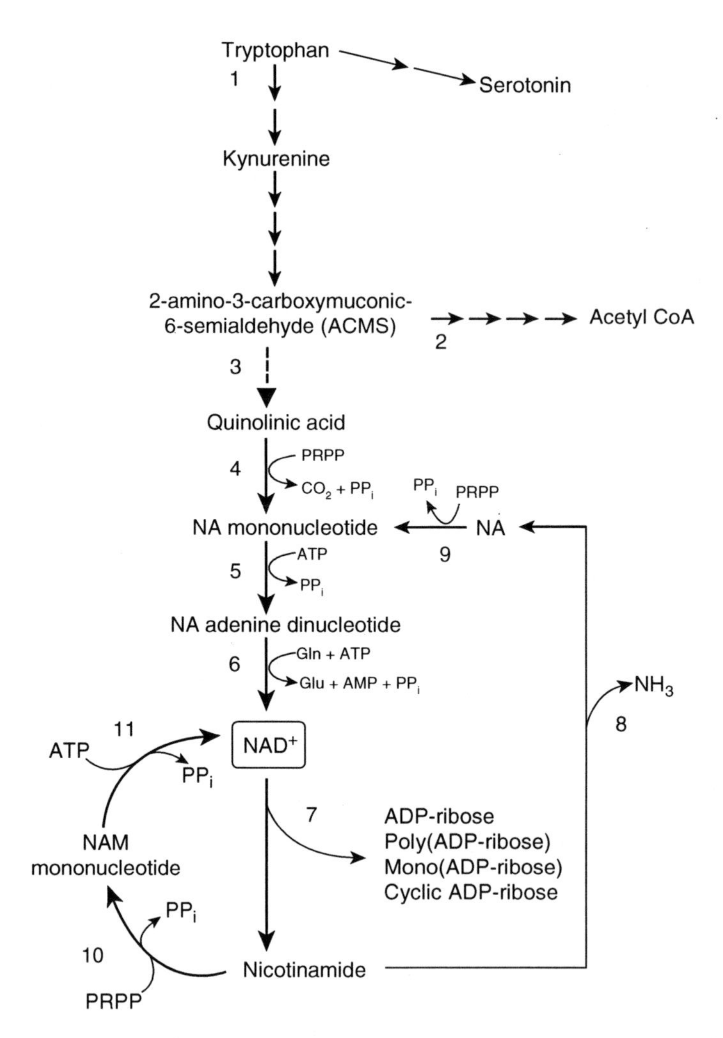

FIGURE 6.3 Pathways of NAD^+ synthesis in mammals. Reactions 5, 6, 8, and 9 comprise the Preiss–Handler pathway whereas reactions 10 and 11 form the Dietrich pathway. The following enzymes correspond to the numbered reactions: 1, tryptophan 2,3-dioxygenase (hepatic) or indoleamine 2,3-dioxygenase (extrahepatic), which start the five-step conversion to ACMS and nine-step catabolism of tryptophan to acetyl CoA; 2, ACMS decarboxylase (ACMSD); 3, spontaneous chemical reaction; 4, quinolinic acid phosphoribosyltransferase; 5, NAMN adenylyltransferase (enzymes 5 and 11 may be identical proteins); 6, NAD synthetase; 7, NAD glycohydrolases, various ADP-ribosylation reactions; 8, nicotinamide deamidase; 9, nicotinic acid phosphoribosyltransferase; 10, nicotinamide phosphoribosyltransferase; 11, NMN adenylyltransferase.

the required accumulation of ACMS are regulated by many factors unrelated to niacin status [53–55]. It appears that this pathway may be regulated, in part, to minimize quinolinate neurotoxicity during high protein intake [56], starvation, and ketosis [57].

In nutritionally replete humans, there is thought to be a 60:1 ratio between tryptophan supply and niacin formation, although individual variation is significant [58]. Because of this relationship, dietary niacin content is described in niacin equivalents (1 NE = mg niacin + 1/60 mg tryptophan). More recent work has suggested that humans may not utilize tryptophan for niacin synthesis when tryptophan levels are limited in the diet [36]. In these experiments, young men were placed on a diet containing 6 NE/day (RDA = 16 NE), and their blood NAD^+ levels decreased by 70% over 5 weeks, indicating a significant degree of niacin deficiency. Subsequent addition of 240 mg/day of tryptophan to this diet had no effect on blood NAD, although it prevented the decrease in plasma tryptophan that had been caused by the consumption of the unsupplemented diet. This tryptophan represented, in theory, an additional 4 NE/day, but it appears that protein turnover takes precedence over niacin synthesis when tryptophan levels are low. NE calculations for diets with marginal niacin status may be inaccurate because of this relationship. At the same time, tryptophan supplements have been reported to cure pellagra and a genetic defect in tryptophan absorption, known as Hartnup's disease, which also causes pellagra-like signs and symptoms. Carcinoid tumors, which catabolize tryptophan, are also seen to be associated with poor niacin status [13]. While the efficiency of conversion of tryptophan to NAD is thought to be increased by niacin deficiency [2], it is also apparent that at low tryptophan intakes, needs for protein metabolism dominate over conversion to NAD [36].

The conversion of tryptophan to NAD varies between individuals, because of genetic variation, disease states (e.g., carcinoid syndrome), and the effect of other dietary components. High-leucine diets [54] and high-fat diets [55] depress tryptophan to NAD conversion, apparently through a similar mechanism involving excess formation of ketone bodies. The impact of ketosis is supported by the finding that uncontrolled diabetes increases ACMSD expression [59], thereby depressing tryptophan to niacin conversion. This is interesting from the perspective that the diet of pellagrins in the southern United States has been described as a combination of corn bread and pork fat, which would create a ketotic environment that would discourage tryptophan conversion, in combination with a low-tryptophan diet and niacin in a form with low bioavailability.

Species vary in their ability to synthesize niacin from tryptophan. Cats, adapted to a diet high in amino acids, have approximately 50 times greater ACMSD activity than humans [52] and they demonstrate extremely poor utilization of tryptophan as a precursor of NAD [60]. Rats, on the other hand, are more efficient than humans in their use of tryptophan for NAD synthesis (in a ratio of about 33 mg tryptophan:1 mg niacin) [61]. Mice are resistant to niacin deficiency, even on diets containing as little as 6% casein, with 7% gelatin, a protein source lacking tryptophan (unpublished data). In the previous edition of this text, it was reported that guinea pigs are very susceptible to niacin deficiency, and eventually die on a niacin-free diet containing 20% casein [62]. This could be interpreted as a very poor conversion of tryptophan to niacin, and we decided to use guinea pigs for a series of experiments on niacin deficiency and neural function. We found that guinea pigs on a niacin-free 20% casein diet developed only a modest niacin deficiency, as assessed by tissue NAD levels [198]. However, these animals are very sensitive to environmental stressors and basically appeared to stop eating and die for no apparent metabolic reason. I apologize to anyone who attempted to use guinea pigs as a model of niacin deficiency after reading the previous edition of this chapter.

Absorption

Both nicotinamide and nicotinic acid can be absorbed through the stomach lining, but absorption in the small intestine is more rapid. For intact nucleotides, pyrophosphatase activity in the upper small intestine metabolizes NAD(P) to yield NMN, which is then quickly hydrolyzed to form nicotinamide riboside and eventually free nicotinamide.

Absorption of both nicotinic acid and nicotinamide at low concentrations appears to be via sodium-dependent facilitated diffusion [63], or by carrier-mediated transport making use of proton cotransporters [64] and anion antiporters [65]. Higher concentrations of both forms appear to be absorbed by passive diffusion. Once absorbed from the lumen into the enterocyte, nicotinamide may be converted to NAD or released into the portal circulation. Although some nicotinic acid moves into the blood in its native form, the bulk of nicotinic acid taken up by the enterocyte is converted via the Preiss–Handler pathway to NAD [63]. As required, NAD glycohydrolases in the enterocytes release nicotinamide from NAD into the plasma as the principal circulating form of niacin.

Distribution and Metabolism

Niacin compounds entering the portal circulation are either internalized by erythrocytes or transported to the liver. Erythrocytes take up nicotinic acid and nicotinamide effectively by facilitated diffusion, converting them to nucleotides to maintain a concentration gradient [66,67].

The liver is a central processing organ for niacin. Aside from its role in the conversion of tryptophan to NAD, it receives nicotinamide and some nicotinic acid via the portal circulation, as well as nicotinamide released from other extrahepatic tissues. In the liver, nicotinic acid and nicotinamide are metabolized to NAD or to yield compounds for urinary excretion, depending on the niacin status of the organism. The liver has some capacity for NAD storage. Because hepatic regulation of nicotinamide phosphoribosyltransferase by ATP and NAD (positive and negative, respectively) is less effective than in many other tissues, liver NAD concentrations increase significantly following dietary nicotinamide administration [63]. In rats, nicotinic acid and nicotinamide, at 1000 mg/kg diet, increase blood and liver NAD^+ to a similar and modest extent (about 50%) [68]. NAD glycohydrolases are thought to use hepatic NAD to produce nicotinamide [69], which is released for replenishment of extrahepatic tissues. The function of NAD glycohydrolases is controversial, however, and may be difficult to distinguish from mono-, poly-, and cyclic ADP-ribose formation and catabolism (see later sections).

The liver plays an important role in the preparation of niacin for urinary excretion, producing a variety of methylation and hydroxylation products of both nicotinic acid and nicotinamide. In humans, nicotinamide is primarily methylated to produce N^1-methylnicotinamide, whereas nicotinic acid is conjugated with glycine to form nicotinuric acid. Increasing levels of the untransformed vitamers can be found in the urine as the level of dietary niacin increases [63]. High levels of niacin intake can stress methyl donor status [45] and increase blood homocysteine levels [46].

BIOCHEMICAL FUNCTIONS

NAD Cofactors in Redox Reactions

Oxidation and reduction of the C-4 position on the pyridine ring of NAD coenzymes is the basis for hydrogen-transfer reactions important in oxidative phosphorylation and biosynthetic reactions. NAD^+ is reduced to NADH in glycolytic reactions, oxidative decarboxylation of pyruvate, oxidation of acetate in the TCA cycle, oxidation of alcohol, β-oxidation of fatty acids, and a large number of other cellular oxidation reactions. The electrons derived from these oxidation reactions are transferred to the electron transport chain through the oxidation of NADH. The energy resulting from these transfers is used to generate ATP. In contrast to the central role that NAD(H) plays in energy expenditure, NADP(H) is essential for the biosynthetic reactions involved in energy storage. NADPH is produced from reduction of $NADP^+$ in reactions of the pentose phosphate pathway and during the malate–pyruvate shuttle across the mitochondrial membrane. NADPH then acts as a reducing agent for fatty acid production, cholesterol synthesis, and manufacture of deoxyribonucleotides, as well as many other cellular macromolecules. NADPH is also notable for its involvement in glutathione regeneration, and therefore critical in oxidant defense and xenobiotic metabolism.

The extra phosphate group carried on NADP allows the cell to separate the oxidation and reduction activities of the nicotinamide cofactors by allowing most cellular enzymes to be specific for one of these coenzyme species. Because of this specificity, the majority of cellular NADP is maintained in the reduced state by the pentose phosphate pathway and reduction reactions are favored by mass action. Conversely, NAD is predominantly oxidized, improving the oxidant capabilities of this cofactor under cellular conditions. The role that NAD coenzymes play in redox reactions has been the function classically associated with niacin, since Warburg and Christian showed that nicotinamide was a component of NADP in 1935 and, in the following year, demonstrated the presence of nicotinamide in NAD [70]. It is probable that early researchers attributed the pathology associated with niacin deficiency to disruptions in redox cycling, since this was the only capacity for niacin known at that time. However, the distinctive clinical signs of pellagra (dementia, sun-sensitive dermatitis) may be better explained in relation to the functions of NAD described in the following sections.

NAD^+ as a Substrate

While the hydride-transfer chemistry of the pyridine nucleotides was initially described in the 1930s [70], the high-energy glycosidic linkage between nicotinamide and ADP-ribose received little attention before the discovery of mono- and poly(ADP-ribosyl)ation reactions in the 1960s. The energy provided by breaking this bond allows the addition of ADP-ribose to a variety of nucleophilic acceptors. These include glutamate side chains and hydroxyl groups of ribose for poly(ADP-ribose) synthesis; a variety of amino acid side chains in mono(ADP-ribosyl)ation reactions; and an internal ribose linkage for cyclic ADP-ribose synthesis (Figure 6.4). The catabolic activity of NAD glycohydrolase (if this reaction does exist in isolation) also represents an ADP-ribose transfer, in which water acts as the nucleophilic acceptor. NAD-dependent deacetylation reactions are also ADP-ribosylation reactions, forming *O*-acetyl-ADP-ribose as an end product.

ADP-Ribose Cyclization and NAADP Synthesis

In 1987, a metabolite of NAD^+ was found to cause intracellular calcium mobilization in sea urchin eggs [71] and was later identified as cyclic ADP-ribose [72]. Cells have several types of calcium channels, including the inositol-1,4,5-trisphosphate (IP_3) receptors and the ryanodine receptors, which regulate the release of calcium from internal stores. Evidence has accumulated that cyclic ADP-ribose is an endogenous messenger that controls type 2 and type 3 ryanodine receptors [73]. More recently, a contaminant of commercial NADP was found to mobilize calcium, and was identified as NAADP [74]. It is now accepted that control of intracellular calcium release is a result of overlapping signals from IP_3, cyclic ADP-ribose, and NAADP [75].

Calcium concentrations are about 10,000-fold higher outside cells than the levels in the cytoplasm or nucleoplasm. Transient increases in intracellular calcium are a major component of signaling in all the cells of the body. Calcium may move into a cell through the plasma membrane or it may be released from intracellular stores, including the endoplasmic or sarcoplasmic reticulum, mitochondria, lysosomes, and the nuclear envelope. When one stimulus causes calcium release, there is often a positive feedback leading to a much larger flow of calcium into the cytoplasm. The control of ryanodine receptors by cyclic ADP-ribose plays an important role in this calcium-induced calcium release (CICR), in conjunction with IP_3 and IP_3 receptors. As an example of this, an impulse traveling along a nerve axon arrives at a synapse, where voltage-gated channels allow a certain amount of calcium to cross the plasma membrane. This calcium initiates a variety of intracellular signals in the cytosol, including the formation of IP_3 and cyclic ADP-ribose, which bind to ryanodine and IP_3 receptors, causing more calcium release from intracellular stores. If the total calcium release reaches a certain threshold, the release of neurotransmitters will be sufficient to cause the impulse to be propagated across the synapse. Similar calcium release events occur in both

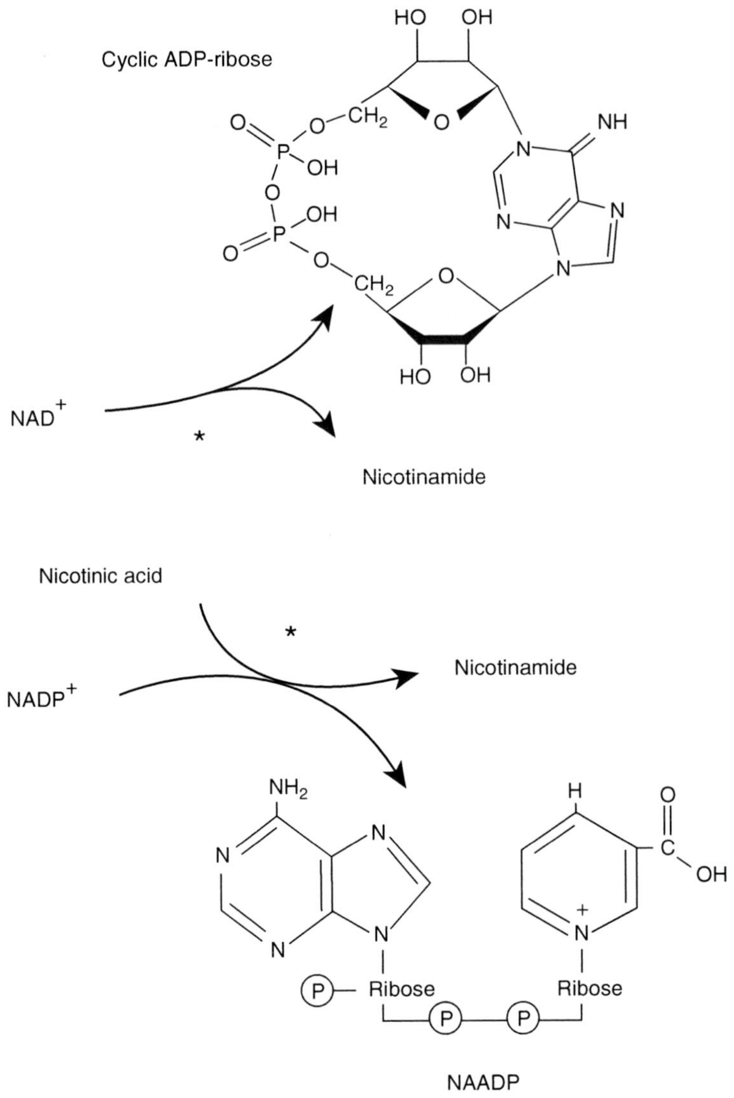

FIGURE 6.4 Structures and origin of cyclic ADP-ribose and NAADP.

the pre- and postsynaptic boutons, which enhance or dampen the strength of synapses and are involved in essentially all aspects of nervous system function. Analogous calcium-signaling events take place in all the cells of the body, including insulin release by beta cells, muscle cell contraction, T-lymphocyte activation, and so on.

ADP-ribosyl cyclases are enzymes that release nicotinamide from NAD^+ and form cyclic ADP-ribose (Figure 6.4). Cyclic ADP-ribose hydrolase is the activity responsible for degradation of cyclic ADP-ribose to linear ADP-ribose. NAD glycohydrolase, isolated from canine spleen, actually has both cyclase and hydrolase activities, leading to an overall reaction that appears to be NAD^+ glycohydrolysis [76]. The leukocyte cell-surface antigen CD38 also has both these activities [73]. It is likely that other enzymes previously identified as NAD glycohydrolases are actually cyclases and also likely that most cyclases have NAD glycohydrolase-like activity. The presence of both activities is probably useful given the rapid and transient nature of calcium signaling.

NAADP is the most potent of the calcium release agents, but does not appear to be involved in CICR. NAADP regulates intracellular calcium pools that are distinct from those controlled by IP_3 or cyclic ADP-ribose and it may play a role in the initial release that causes CICR. Surprisingly, NAADP appears to be formed by the same enzymes that make cyclic ADP-ribose, although the reaction mechanism seems quite different. This occurs in vitro by exchanging the nicotinamide on NADP with nicotinic acid (Figure 6.4). This reaction requires acidic pH and high levels of nicotinic acid and may function in vivo within a specialized vesicle or microenvironment, or may be an in vitro artifact. NAADP could be formed in vivo through phosphorylation of NAAD or deamination of NADP, although no enzymes with these activities have been identified [75]. In some cell types, NAADP causes release of calcium through type I ryanodine receptors whereas in other cells there appears to be a specialized receptor associated with an acidic vesicle [75]. NAADP is released at extremely low concentrations, but has been shown to accumulate during the response of pancreatic beta cells to glucose, smooth muscle cells to endothelin, and pancreatic acinar cells to cholecystokinin. Many other cell types have been shown to respond in vitro to exogenous NAADP [75], and the accumulated evidence strongly supports a physiological role for this molecule in cell signaling.

There are many questions to be answered concerning the roles of cyclic ADP-ribose and NAADP in cell signaling. ADP-ribosyl cyclase activities are widespread and many of these same enzymes have the potential to make NAADP. CD38 has been identified as an ectoenzyme in a wide variety of mammalian tissues, but is also internalized in lipid rafts and has also been found in the cytosol, endoplasmic reticulum, and nucleus [77], so there is much to learn about the regulation and function of CD38 [73]. As for non-CD38 enzymes, cyclases have been isolated from the cytosol of *Aplysia* and dog tissues [78], from the endoplasmic reticulum of canine spleen [76], and from skeletal muscle sarcoplasmic reticulum [79]. Of interest to the central nervous system (CNS) field, a cyclase has been found in synaptosomes from CD38-null mouse brains [80], which appears to be responsible for the majority of brain cyclic ADP-ribose formation. There may even be calcium-signaling roles for free linear ADP-ribose [81], which is created during the hydrolysis of cyclic, mono-, and poly(ADP-ribose).

To eventually understand the effect of niacin deficiency on these processes, we need to determine the subcellular localization of the active forms of these enzymes and their affinity for nucleotide substrates. Later in this chapter, we will try to integrate these functions with other NAD^+-utilizing reactions and consider how they might respond during niacin deficiency. We have recently found that niacin deficiency in rats, over a period of 4 weeks, causes 40% and 30% decreases in cortical–hippocampal NAD^+ and cyclic ADP-ribose, respectively [199], and we are proceeding to investigate neural function in this model. Researchers may find over the next few years that neural functions mediated by cyclic ADP-ribose and NAADP are impaired during niacin deficiency and are responsible for the unusual CNS disruptions and dementia of pellagra.

During niacin deficiency, altered levels of cyclic ADP-ribose and NAADP may affect processes other than neural function. Niacin deficiency causes genomic instability in bone marrow lineages [82], and it is logical to think of altered poly(ADP-ribose) metabolism [83]. However, many nuclear processes are controlled by calcium signals, and cyclic ADP-ribose and NAADP have been shown to liberate calcium from the inner surface of the nuclear envelope [84]. UV-induced skin cancer in mice is dramatically reduced by supraphysiological niacin intake, and this effect is related to immune surveillance [85]. This could be related to the role of CD38 in the function of lymphokine-activated killer cells [86].

NAD^+ Glycohydrolysis

NAD^+ glycohydrolase enzymes catalyze the donation of the ADP-ribose moiety of NAD^+ to water, resulting in free ADP-ribose and nicotinamide. There have been many reports of this activity in mammalian plasma membranes and in the cytosol [87]. However, difficulty in isolating the enzymes has prevented clear identification of their form and metabolic function. The function of these enzymes has never been clearly understood, but may become clearer with the discovery that cyclic ADP-ribose formation and hydrolysis are often catalyzed by the same enzyme, leading to the misleading appearance of simple NAD hydrolysis. It is possible that CD38 and other cyclase–hydrolase complexes are identical to the elusive membrane-bound NAD glycohydrolase [76]. To further complicate this issue, poly(ADP-ribose) polymerase (PARP) [88], bacterial ADP-ribosylating toxins [89], and endogenous mono(ADP-ribosyl) transferases [90] have the ability to use water as an acceptor of the ADP-ribose moiety, in lieu of a protein, thus leading to glycohydrolase-like activity. If true NAD glycohydrolase activities exist, their function may be related to the control of intracellular NAD levels and to the availability of nicotinamide for export from tissues such as the small intestine and liver [87].

Mono(ADP-Ribosyl)ation

Mono(ADP-ribosyl)ation is the transfer of a single ADP-ribose moiety, derived from NAD^+, to an amino acid residue on an acceptor protein [91,92]. Of these enzyme systems, the bacterial toxins are the best characterized. Cholera, pertussis, diphtheria, and *Pseudomonas* toxins use eukaryotic NAD^+ to ADP-ribosylate endogenous G-proteins, disrupting cellular function and allowing for virulent infection. Mono(ADP-ribosyl)ation of $G_{\alpha s}$ by cholera toxin results in the stimulation of adenylate cyclase activity, leading to disruption of ion transport in intestinal epithelial cells and the diarrhea which is characteristic of this disease. Pertussis toxin catalyzes the cysteine-specific ADP-ribosylation of several other forms of G-proteins, also leading to an uncoupling of their activities from the associated receptors. Diphtheria toxin and *Pseudomonas* exotoxin A ADP-ribosylate polypeptide elongation factor 2 (also a G-protein), halting protein synthesis. *Clostridium* toxins ADP-ribosylate various actin monomers to prevent actin polymerization.

The profound metabolic changes elicited by the bacterial toxins show that mono(ADP-ribosyl)ation is a powerful modulator of protein function. Mammalian cells are now known to contain a variety of endogenous mono-ADP-ribosyltransferases (ARTs) [92], although their functions are poorly understood. Like bacterial toxins, some of these enzymes regulate the function of G-proteins. There is also a broad spectrum of enzyme chemistry, with five or more amino acid side chains acting as ADP-ribose acceptors. There are two main groups of ARTs, as they are currently understood: those on the outer surface of cells or secreted from cells, known as ecto-ARTs and those expressed inside cells, known as endo-ARTs [92]. The four human ecto-ARTs are related gene products and were identified by sequence similarity to bacterial toxins. ART1 is expressed in muscle, heart, and lung, and has been shown to ADP-ribosylate integrins and control myogenesis. ART1 also ADP-ribosylates defensin, a small immune peptide, changing it from a bacterial toxin to a macrophage-signaling hormone. In vitro assays and ART-overexpressing cells have demonstrated other protein substrates, but these should be considered as potential substrates until they are identified in a naturally functioning system. ART2 has recently been shown to induce apoptosis through ADP-ribosylation of P_2X_7, an ATP-gated ion channel. T cells normally respond to ecto-NAD^+ by ADP-ribosylating cell-surface proteins, becoming resistant to activation and undergoing apoptosis. In ART2-null mice, all of these T-cell responses to NAD treatment are lost [93].

Other ecto-ARTs are highly expressed in testes and lymphatic tissues, but their roles are poorly understood. It is interesting to note that CD38 and ecto-ART enzymes are expressed on the outside of cells, where NAD^+ concentration is generally very low, and that they control overlapping areas of lymphoid differentiation, immune function, and apoptosis.

Several ideas have been proposed to rationalize the separation of ecto-enzyme and substrate, including NAD channels in the plasma membrane and NAD released from injured cells. These ideas suggest that NAD itself may be used as a signal of the metabolic state of a cell, or as a signal for the death of nearby cells, leading to signaling events which may be paracrine or autocrine in nature.

Endo-ARTs, acting in the cytosol or on inner membrane surfaces, are very poorly defined, and do not appear to have homology with ecto-ART genes. Some of the better characterized endo-ARTs are discussed later.

Heterotrimeric G-proteins are important components of cell signaling, and have been shown to be substrates for arginine-specific ADP-ribosylation. Following the stimulation of cell-surface receptors, linked G-protein β-subunits may be released and made available for further complex formation. It appears that an endo-ART on the inner surface of the plasma membrane may ADP-ribosylate and inactivate the excess β-subunits [92]. There is a hydrolase enzyme to remove the ADP-ribose and return the G-protein to an active pool. This mechanism could control any number of different pathways, depending on which cell-surface receptor the G-protein was linked to. Another G-protein that appears to be controlled by ADP-ribosylation is elongation factor 2, which is the site of attack for diphtheria and *Pseudomonas* toxins, although the endogenous enzyme appears to modify an arginine residue rather than diphthamide [94].

One of the most interesting proposed mechanisms of cellular regulation using mono-ADP-ribosylation involves the 78 kDa glucose-regulated-protein (GRP78). GRP78 is a molecular chaperone that aids in the correct folding of secreted proteins in the lumen of the endoplasmic reticulum. GRP78 may also bind incorrectly glycosylated proteins and prevent their secretion. When cells are under metabolic or environmental stress, GRP78 is mono(ADP-ribosyl)ated by a poorly characterized endo-ART. This modification is freely reversible, suggesting the presence of a hydrolase enzyme. The ADP-ribosylated form of GRP78 appears to be inactive in its chaperone functions, and the authors suggest that this is a mechanism to decrease the rate of protein secretion during times of nutritional stress [95], while preventing a total shutdown, which would eventually kill the cell [92].

There are potential artifacts in the study of mono(ADP-ribosyl)ation reactions. Free ADP-ribose reacts nonenzymatically with a variety of amino acid side chains, creating the illusion of mono(ADP-ribosyl)ation [94,96]. Careful determination of the enzymatic nature of proposed mono(ADP-ribosyl)ation reactions is necessary to avoid artifacts in the future. At the same time, it may turn out that nonenzymatic reactions of NAD or ADP-ribose with proteins are physiologically relevant and that these types of reactions could be affected by dietary niacin status. There are at least four human enzymes in the Nudix class of hydrolases that rapidly degrade free ADP-ribose [97], so there is some inclination that this intermediate presents a risk of toxicity to the cell, and it may be through spontaneous ADP-ribosylation reactions. At the same time, there is evidence that free ADP-ribose is released from the mitochondria during oxidant stress, leading to binding and opening of cell-surface TRPM2 channels, which initiate calcium signals [81]. Thus, free ADP-ribose may be considered the third calcium release agent derived from NAD metabolism. There is no real knowledge of the impact of dietary niacin status on mono-ADP-ribosyltransferase reactions. The potential for this is considered in a later section of this chapter.

Sirtuins, Genomic Stability, Caloric Restriction, and Aging

An additional role for NAD in genomic stability is through the action of SIR2 (rat) or SIRT1 (human), an NAD-dependent protein deacetylase [98]. This reaction is also in the ADP-ribosylation family, as the acetyl group is transferred from the protein to ADP-ribose, with the release of nicotinamide. Deacetylation of histones leads to a more compact chromatin structure and gene silencing. It also appears to protect sensitive areas of chromatin, like telomeres, against translocation events. In theory, niacin deficiency could lead to a more open DNA structure, with more active gene expression and greater sensitivity to damage and translocation events. It is clear from various models that SIR2–SIRT1 play central roles in the extended life span associated with caloric restriction [98]. SIR2 activity is sensitive to NAD^+ supply, but is also strongly inhibited by nicotinamide [99]. Some researchers have suggested that SIR2 is exquisitely designed to link control of chromatin structure to cellular energy status. Others feel that control of SIR2 occurs within a very small environment around sites of DNA damage, linked to PARP activation [99]. Activation of PARP-1/2 at strand breaks creates a localized depression in NAD^+ and an increase in nicotinamide. This inhibits SIR2 activity, allowing acetylation of histones, leading to chromatin relaxation [99]. This is quite similar to the effects of poly(ADP-ribosyl)ation around strand breaks (see chapter 16).

Another substrate for SIRT is p53, which is a central protein in genomic stability [100]. p53 controls cell cycle checkpoints, DNA repair, and apoptosis. The effects of p53 acetylation are not well understood, but acetylation appears to enhance p53 stability and accumulation by inhibiting ubiquitination [101]. Acetylation may also enhance transcriptional activation by p53, although this is controversial. The effect of niacin deficiency on p53 acetylation is not known. In our model of niacin deficiency in rats, we have observed an accumulation of slow mobility p53, and a disruption of p53-dependent processes, like cell cycle arrest, apoptosis, and DNA repair [200].

Poly(ADP-Ribosyl)ation

Poly(ADP-Ribose) Synthesis

The research field of ADP-ribosylation was born in 1966 with the discovery of poly(ADP-ribose) in liver nuclei by Mandel's group [102]. PARP (EC 2.4.2.30) was the first enzyme identified that had the ability to synthesize poly(ADP-ribose) (Figure 6.5). When the gene for this protein was disrupted in mice, and they were still found to synthesize a small amount of poly(ADP-ribose), a search for related enzymes led to a list of 18 PARP-like gene sequences [103]. The original enzyme is now referred to as PARP-1 and is responsible for the majority of poly(ADP-ribose) formation in mammalian cells. PARP-1 contains three functional domains [104]. The amino terminus contains two zinc fingers which allow the enzyme to bind specifically to strand breaks in DNA and signal the catalytic portion of the protein to initiate poly(ADP-ribose) synthesis [105]. The 55 kDa carboxy terminus region contains the NAD^+-binding and catalytic sites. Although more than 30 nuclear proteins may act as acceptors, most of the poly(ADP-ribose) is synthesized on PARP-1 itself (referred to as automodification). The middle section of the amino acid sequence of PARP-1 has been identified as the automodification domain. The synthesis of poly(ADP-ribose) on PARP-1 itself is critical in the regulation of its interactions with DNA.

Activated PARP-1 attaches the initial ADP-ribose unit to a glutamate or aspartate residue on an acceptor protein. A linear sequence of ADP-ribose units is synthesized on the initial protein-bound monomer. At intervals of 40 to 50 residues, branch points are created on the parent polymer chain and subsequently serve as sites for elongation [106]. These initiation, elongation, and branching reactions are all carried out by the catalytic domain at the carboxy terminus of PARP-1. Automodification of PARP-1 occurs by two PARP molecules working together as a dimer [107]. As PARP becomes more poly(ADP-ribosyl)ated, it takes on an increasingly negative charge because of the accumulation of phosphate groups. This creates electrostatic repulsion between automodified PARP and DNA, causing PARP to dissociate from the DNA nick and lose catalytic activity [108].

It is important to note that inhibition of PARP-1 activity by treatment with competitive inhibitors or removal of NAD from in vitro systems is very different from removing PARP

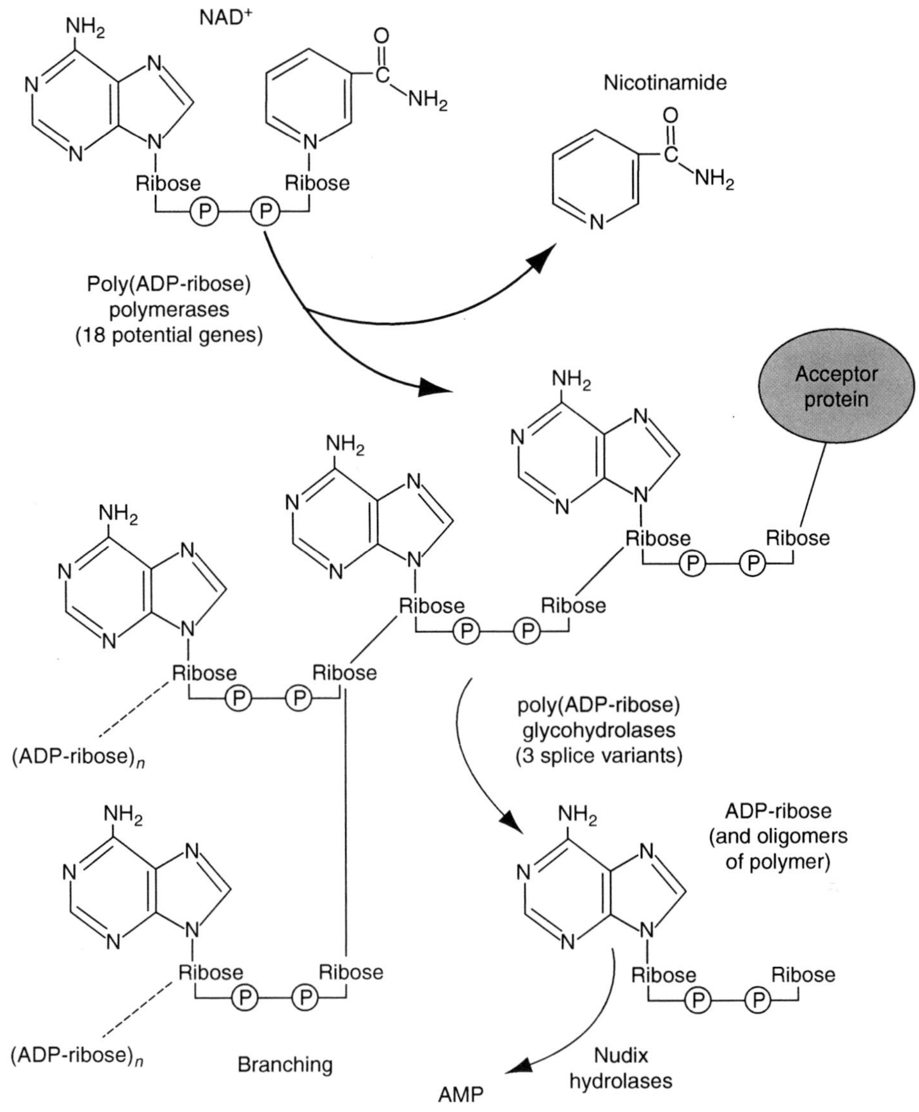

FIGURE 6.5 Synthesis and degradation of poly(ADP-ribose).

from the system. Inactive PARP binds to strand breaks, preventing access by repair enzymes, inhibiting DNA repair, and impeding the signals initiated by poly(ADP-ribose) formation. It is not known whether niacin deficiency in vivo will cause a similar situation. This will depend on the degree of depletion of NAD and the response of other aspects of poly(ADP-ribose) metabolism, including the rate of degradation of poly(ADP-ribose).

Alternate Poly(ADP-Ribose) Polymerase Genes

Eighteen putative PARP-encoding genes have been identified using homology with the catalytic region of PARP-1 [103]. Of the new PARP genes, PARP-2, PARP-3, vault-PARP (VPARP), tankyrase (TNKS), and tankyrase 2 (TNKS2) have been found as proteins and shown to have PARP activity [109]. They have highly varied distribution and function.

PARP-2 is the most similar to PARP-1, with an abbreviated DNA-binding domain. These are the only two PARPs known to bind to, and be activated by, DNA strand breaks. Both can hetero- and homodimerize, and both interact with XRCC1 in the regulation of base excision repair (BER) [110]. Both PARP-1 and PARP-2-null mice display genomic instability, and double knockouts die in utero, demonstrating a redundancy of activity between these two enzymes [111].

PARP-3 has a catalytic region similar to PARP-2, with a more abbreviated DNA-binding domain that appears to lack nick-sensing ability. PARP-3 tends to localize to the centrosome, and will heterodimerize with PARP-1, explaining the finding that PARP-1 will localize to the centrosome [109].

PARP-4, or VPARP, is found in association with vault particles, which are massive ribonucleoprotein particles found in the cytosol of mammalian cells. PARP-4 modifies a major vault protein and itself, when active, creating cytosolic poly(ADP-ribose) [109]. The role of PARP-4, and vault particles in general, is not understood.

TNKS and TNKS2 are related proteins found in association with telomeres, the repetitive sequences at the end of mammalian chromosomes [109]. TNKS and TNKS2 bind to a protein called telomeric-repeat binding factor 1 (TRF1), which in turn is bound to the repeated sequence of bases found in the telomere. If TNKS is activated (by phosphorylation events), it will poly(ADP-ribosyl)ate TRF1. The negative charge of the poly(ADP-ribose) forces the TRF1 away from the telomeric DNA, allowing telomerase access to the DNA terminus, which it elongates. Telomerase is required by dividing cells to prevent erosion and instability at the ends of the chromosome. Telomerase activity is critical to stem cell pools and also plays a key role in neoplastic development.

PARP-7, or dioxin-inducible PARP, is induced by activation of the aryl hydrocarbon receptor (AhR). It has the ability to poly(ADP-ribosyl)ate histones, and may play a role in the changes in gene expression caused by dioxins, PCBs, and other AhR agonists. PARP-10 can be found in the nucleus or cytoplasm, also has modifying activity toward histones, and interacts with the oncogenic signaling protein, Myc [109]. The remaining 10 PARP-related gene sequences have not been characterized as enzymes at this point.

Poly(ADP-Ribose) Degradation

There are several enzymes required to fully degrade poly(ADP-ribose). In spite of the fact that there are 18 possible PARP genes, there is only one poly(ADP-ribose) glycohydrolase, which cleaves the poly(ADP-ribose) in a combined endo- and exoglycosidic fashion to release free ADP-ribose units and some free oligomers, which are then substrates for further exoglycosidic action [112]. The one gene does produce three splice variants, which target the different forms of the enzyme to nuclear or cytosolic compartments [113].

ADP-ribosyl protein lyase appears to release the final ADP-ribose residue from the acceptor proteins, but this activity is poorly characterized [114]. Free ADP-ribose is rapidly degraded to AMP and ribose phosphate by the Nudix family of pyrophosphatase enzymes, which could be considered a third type of enzyme involved in poly(ADP-ribose) catabolism [97]. It is not certain why free ADP-ribose is catabolized so rapidly, although it may be to encourage the forward activity of glycohydrolase or to limit the nonenzymatic glycation of proteins, as discussed earlier [96]. As mentioned earlier, free ADP-ribose may also have calcium release properties [81], and rapid catabolism may be a reflection of its signaling activities.

Mechanisms of Action for Poly(ADP-Ribose)

The single-strand breaks required to activate PARP-1 and PARP-2 are produced in vivo through the processes of DNA replication, transcription, and repair [115]. The role played by poly(ADP-ribose) metabolism in these processes has been best characterized in DNA repair. In 1980, Durkacz et al. [116] demonstrated that poly(ADP-ribosyl)ation was required in order for cells in culture to repair DNA alkylation damage. This landmark study stimulated a wide variety of research to determine the roles which poly(ADP-ribose) metabolism plays in the DNA repair process, and provided new perspectives on the possible effects of niacin deficiency in the whole animal.

There are three general mechanisms proposed for the functions of poly(ADP-ribose). With the discovery of 18 possible PARP enzymes, this discussion has become more complex, but there are commonalities in the function of poly(ADP-ribose) in these different reactions. These mechanisms include polyanionic interactions, high-affinity poly(ADP-ribose)-binding sites, and control of enzyme activity.

Polyanionic interactions: The most obvious characteristic of the polymer is its strong negative charge, and its similarity in structure to DNA. It would appear that many functions of poly(ADP-ribose) are dependent on this anionic nature, which causes electrostatic repulsion from other polyanions such as DNA and attraction to cations such as basic DNA-binding proteins. Most of the poly(ADP-ribose) in whole cells and tissues is associated with PARP and histones. The extranucleosomal histone, H1, and histone H2B are modified, leading to localized disruption of the DNA–protein interactions within and among nucleosomes [115]. In a process referred to as "histone shuttling," the automodification of PARP may also contribute to chromatin relaxation by drawing nearby histones away from the DNA [108]. As a result of these modifications, poly(ADP-ribosylation) leads to a localized relaxation of nucleosomal structure. The exposed DNA is presumably available for interactions with other DNA-binding proteins such as helicases, topoisomerases, polymerases, and ligases involved in replication or repair [115]. The topic of niacin and chromatin structure is covered in more detail in chapter 16 of this volume. The repulsion between poly(ADP-ribose) and DNA may also serve the important purpose of keeping nonhomologous areas of DNA away from DNA strand breaks and telomeres, to decrease the occurrence of chromosomal translocations at these sensitive sites.

High-affinity poly(ADP-ribose)-binding sites: Thus, a poly(ADP-ribosyl)ated protein may be pushed away from DNA, and it may attract proteins with cationic DNA-binding sites. In an extension of this idea, there are sites on proteins specifically designed to interact noncovalently with poly(ADP-ribose). The first high-affinity poly(ADP-ribose)-binding sites were found on the tails of histones, and a consensus sequence was used to find other binding proteins. This search has generated a long list of nuclear proteins that are involved in DNA damage responses, including XRCC1, DNA ligase III, DNA polymerase ε, topoisomerases, p53, p21, NF-κB, and DNA-PK [117]. In each of these cases, noncovalent binding of the protein to poly(ADP-ribose) causes functional changes or changes in localization of the protein.

Control of enzyme activity by covalent poly(ADP-ribosyl)ation: A number of studies have also demonstrated poly(ADP-ribose) synthesis on enzymes involved in DNA repair [115]. Poly(ADP-ribosyl)ation of most enzymes, including DNA topoisomerases I and II and DNA polymerases α and β results in inhibition of their activities [115]. In addition, the poly(ADP-ribosyl)ation of Ca^{2+}- and Mg^{2+}-dependent endonuclease has been shown to suppress the rapid, nonspecific DNA-degrading activity of this enzyme [118] and this may be important in the regulation of apoptosis. In contrast, DNA ligase, the enzyme required to anneal the strand ends once excision repair is complete, appears to be stimulated by poly(ADP-ribosyl)ation [119]. Noncovalent association of PARP with DNA polymerase α has been found to stimulate the activity of DNA polymerase α [120].

Metabolic Roles of Poly(ADP-Ribosyl)ation

Many approaches have been used to determine the role of poly(ADP-ribose) metabolism in DNA repair, replication, and transcription. In some cases, investigators have created defined in vitro models, in which PARP activities can be added or removed, or controlled by the removal of NAD or the addition of inhibitors. However, these systems lack the complexity of chromatin structure and interactions with the nuclear matrix which exist in the whole cell. Lindahl and coworkers have used a simplified in vitro repair system to show that the combined addition of PARP-1 and NAD does not increase the rate of excision repair. However, in the absence of NAD, PARP effectively blocks repair because of its persistence at the site of damage [121]. These authors have suggested that PARP is not involved in excision repair directly, but may play a role in preventing nonhomologous recombination events between two sites of damage. In support of this, chemical inhibition of PARP in cells has been shown by others to increase homologous recombination and sister chromatid exchanges [122]. At the same time, it is apparent that the in vitro models do not contain the complexity of chromatin structure, including nucleosomal organization, DNA supercoiling, and nuclear matrix interactions seen in intact cells.

An excellent way to determine the role of a protein in the whole animal is to delete the gene using recombinant techniques and, if possible, create a fully homozygous animal lacking any functional expression of the gene. This is usually done in mice, and the modified strains are referred to as "knockouts." There have been a series of publications characterizing three new PARP-1 knockout mouse models [109]. PARP-1-null mice appear to be healthy and fertile, but they show sensitivity to radiation and alkylation injury, and demonstrate various forms of genomic instability. PARP-2 knockout mice also display genomic instability, and mice lacking PARP-1 and PARP-2 die in utero [111]. There is a clear overlap in function between PARP-1 and PARP-2 in the area of DNA repair. Of interest, PARP-1-null mice are dramatically protected from conditions like stroke, ischemic injury, septic shock, and other insults that cause widespread cell death through PARP-1 activation and NAD depletion. There may be great potential for pharmacological inhibition of PARP activity in many of these human conditions.

PARP-3 is not activated by DNA strand breaks, but it forms complexes with PARP-1, and contains a centrosome-targeting motif [109]. Centrosome function is critical to the genomic stability during cell division. The centrosomes need to duplicate once per cell cycle to accurately divide the chromosomes between the two daughter cells. The centrosomes must then accurately draw a single complement of chromosomes to each pole before cell division. These processes are highly controlled, with many checkpoints to slow the division process or induce apoptosis if problems occur. PARP-1, PARP-3, and TNKS all localize to the centrosome [109]; therefore, it is thought that poly(ADP-ribose) formation plays an important role in centrosome function.

PARP-4, or vault PARP, is a mystery, as are vault particles themselves. They appear to have a storage function, as they look like barrels, with a hollow center. The impact of PARP-4 modification of vault proteins is unknown. This observation has substantiated older reports on the existence of cytosolic poly(ADP-ribose), which were controversial. Cytosolic forms of the poly(ADP-ribose) glycohydrolase also support a story for cytosolic poly(ADP-ribose) function, and the details will probably become more clear in the coming years. Of interest, PARP-4 is also found in the nucleus, localized to the mitotic spindle, so it may also aid in the organized distribution of chromosomes during cell division [123].

TNKS and TNKS2 have related functions at the telomere. Poly(ADP-ribose) synthesis allows for telomerase activity by clearing TRF1 from the terminal area allowing the chromosome to be elongated [109]. This is dependent on expression of active telomerase components. Lengthening of telomeres is required for continued cell division, and overexpression of telomerase in cultured cells makes them immortal. Longer telomeres also prevent genomic instability events, like end-to-end fusions and telomeric translocations, which occur around eroded telomeres. As is the case with excision repair, there is more than one possible role for poly(ADP-ribose) synthesis at the telomere. At the site of a single- or double-strand break, or at the end of a chromosome, there is the potential for recombination events that lead to chromosomal translocations, which play a key role in carcinogenesis. The presence of poly(ADP-ribose) at these sites may be to repel other strands of DNA to prevent these dangerous recombination events.

Although the PARP enzymes described earlier appear to have very distinct functions, that may not be accurate. There are many surprising interactions between these PARP enzymes suggesting that they do work as a family. PARP-1 and PARP-2 have overlapping functions in excision repair [111]. TNKS, TNKS2, PARP-1, PARP-2, and PARP-4 all have roles in the maintenance and protection of telomeres [124]. PARP-1, PARP-3, PARP-4, and TNKS all appear to play a role in centrosome function [109]. During niacin deficiency, all these forms of PARP may be impaired, leading to a complex pattern of genomic instability [124].

Role of Poly(ADP-Ribose) Metabolism in Response to DNA Damage in Vivo

Given that poly(ADP-ribose) metabolism plays an important role in DNA repair, one would expect PARP activity to be important in the in vivo response to DNA damage. However, there are dramatically different models in use, with conflicting mechanisms, and potentially opposite conclusions. The first type of model uses very high levels of genotoxic stress, leading to widespread cell death and acute tissue injury. These models include chemically induced diabetes, septic shock, myocardial or cerebral ischemia, and other forms of inflammatory injury [125]. The second type of model focuses on spontaneous genomic instability, or lower levels of genotoxic stress, resulting in the long-term development of cancer. The high-stress, acute-damage models generally show PARP-1 to be a destructive influence, and PARP-1-null mice and animals treated with PARP-1 inhibitors show remarkable resistance to these pathologies. Conversely, basal levels of genomic instability, and the response to low levels of genotoxicity, tend to be enhanced when PARP-1 is ablated or inactive.

In the first type of model, PARP-1 acts as a destructive force by several mechanisms. The first of these to be appreciated was the suicidal NAD depletion effect. Excessive activation of PARP-1 causes a catastrophic drop in NAD and ATP, leading to widespread cell death [126]. In less drastic models, PARP-1 may mediate cell death in a slower progression of events involving inflammatory signaling. PARP-1 protein and catalytic activity play important roles in the activation of NFκB as a proinflammatory transcription factor [125]. In addition, PARP-1 activity enhances apoptosis through the action of apoptosis-inducing factor (AIF) [127]. The release of AIF from the mitochondria causes a caspase-independent cell death; this is controlled by PARP-1 activation and poly(ADP-ribose) synthesis and is greatly diminished in PARP-null mice [127]. The combination of NAD depletion, enhanced apoptosis, and inflammatory signaling can be quite devastating under certain circumstances.

An in vivo example of this type of model is the chemical induction of insulin-dependent diabetes mellitus (IDDM) in animals. Alloxan and streptozotocin are DNA-damaging agents, working via hydroxyl radical formation and base alkylation, respectively and are fairly selective pancreatic β-cell toxins. They are commonly used to induce IDDM in animal models. In these models, alloxan and streptozotocin induce poly(ADP-ribose) synthesis to the point of NAD depletion and cell death. Treatment with PARP inhibitors, including nicotinamide and 3-AB, results in conservation of pancreatic β-cells and maintenance of insulin secretion in rats treated with alloxan and streptozotocin [128]. However, the incidence of pancreatic β-cell tumors in these animals is essentially 100% later in life [129].

While this model illustrates the trade-off between short-term survival and long-term neoplastic development, it is probably overly pessimistic. Animal models of ischemic stroke and cardiac injury, septic shock, and other severe inflammatory conditions show dramatic benefit to inhibiting the catalytic activity and inflammatory signals generated by PARP-1 [125]. It is likely that PARP-inhibiting drugs will be an important tool in critical care medicine in the near future.

In contrast to these models, most human cancers result from a gradual accumulation of DNA damage under conditions in which poly(ADP-ribose) synthesis rates are low and NAD depletion is modest. Even very aggressive models of chemically induced carcinogenesis cause a high incidence of cancer initiation without severe depletion of NAD [130]. Cell culture models have a great contribution to make in understanding the relationship between niacin status and cellular defense as many parameters can be controlled and measured accurately, including NAD levels, degree of DNA damage, progression of apoptosis, and transformation to a neoplastic phenotype. However, researchers need to relate their in vitro models to the degree of NAD depletion and levels of DNA damage that are representative of the in vivo condition that they are modeling.

Dietary Niacin Deficiency, Poly(ADP-Ribose) Metabolism, and Carcinogenesis

The native population of the Transkei region in South Africa has a high risk for esophageal cancer [131]. A maize-based, low-protein diet is staple for these people and pellagra is common. Esophageal ulcerations and esophagitis, frequent in pellagrins, have been associated with development of carcinoma of the esophagus. Van Rensburg et al. [132] found a greater than fivefold increase in the risk of esophageal cancer in Zulu men who ate maize daily. Frequent consumption of maize by natives of the Henan province of China is also associated with increased esophageal cancer risk [133]. Consumption of maize in northeastern Italy was associated with increased risk of oral, pharyngeal, and esophageal cancers, especially with heavy consumption of alcohol [134]. The frequency of esophageal cancer appears to increase when maize replaces sorghum as a basic dietary component [131,135]. Low niacin intake in an American population, in western New York, was also associated with increased oral cancer risk, when controlled for smoking and alcohol consumption [136], which appeared to be the initiating factors in the disease. This is interesting in that the patients were not deficient in niacin to the degree of showing clinical symptoms of pellagra, and suggest that subclinical niacin deficiency may increase cancer risk. Most recently, Fenech et al. [137] have surveyed a population in Australia and found that lymphocyte micronucleus frequencies are 50% lower within the upper quartile of preformed niacin intake.

The Linxian province of northern China also has a very high rate of esophageal and gastric cancers. Recently a series of nutritional intervention trials were conducted in this area [138,139]. During 5 years of intervention, a combined supplement of β-carotene, vitamin E, and selenium decreased total mortality, total cancer mortality, and stomach cancer mortality. A parallel group receiving riboflavin and niacin did not show any benefits. The duration of the study was probably too short to examine the role of niacin during cancer initiation. In addition, the high esophageal cancer incidence in this population is associated with heavy contamination by fumonisin mycotoxins [140], which appear to promote carcinogenesis by a rather unique mechanism that may not be responsive to niacin status [141]. It is also uncertain whether niacin deficiency was prevalent in this population.

A limited number of animal experiments have been conducted to test whether niacin deficiency plays a causal role in the process of carcinogenesis. Miller and Burns [142] studied the interaction of niacin deficiency, protein energy malnutrition, and renal carcinogenesis in rats. The diets were low in tryptophan and total protein (25% of recommended intake), with nicotinamide at zero requirement or 10 times requirement levels. The diets did not affect tumor size or number, although death due to renal tumor burden may have been accelerated in the deficient animals. Unfortunately, pyridine nucleotides in the liver and kidney were not decreased by the deficient diet and it is difficult to determine if niacin deficiency had any impact in this experiment. This experiment highlights the difficulties in working with a nutrient that can be synthesized from an amino acid, requiring, in most species, an imbalanced amino acid diet to create the vitamin deficiency. Parameters must be controlled carefully to get the desired nutritional status.

Van Rensburg et al. [143] developed an animal model of malnutrition and esophageal cancer, induced by *N*-nitrosomethylbenzylamine (a DNA-alkylating agent) in corn-fed rats. Addition of 20 mg of nicotinic acid per kilogram of basal diet resulted in reduction of tumor incidence, size, and progression compared with that seen in rats fed the basal diet alone. NAD and poly(ADP-ribose) levels were not measured in this study. Another study has shown that lymphocytes from niacin-deficient rats were more susceptible to oxygen radical–induced DNA damage [144].

We have developed a model of niacin deficiency in rats, which maintains a positive growth rate. The diet is based on components with minimal niacin content and a mixture of casein (7%) and gelatin (6%) as sources of protein, designed to limit tryptophan content. Rats fed this diet develop clinical signs of deficiency, including dermatitis, diarrhea, and ataxia, and also have decreased hepatic NAD^+ and poly(ADP-ribose) levels [43]. However, following DNA damage, hepatic poly(ADP-ribose) accumulation was not affected by niacin deficiency, and there was no long-term effect of diet on the development of preneoplastic altered hepatic foci [145]. It is apparent that hepatic NAD^+ levels, which decreased from about 900 μM to about 600 μM in deficient rats, were still adequate to support the activity of PARP, which has a K_m in the range of 20–80 μM [146].

We have found that NAD depletion is not uniform in different organs and tissues during niacin deficiency [43,83]. The symptoms of pellagra also demonstrate tissue specificity, like most nutrient deficiencies. One factor that can cause more rapid nutrient depletion is cell turnover. The bone marrow has the most rapid rate of cell turnover in the body, with a doubling time of about 12 h, and these cells leave to other sites in the body, exporting nutrient resources with them. With this in mind, we have recently examined the effect of niacin status on NAD and poly(ADP-ribose) metabolism in the bone marrow of rats. We have found that NAD is decreased by 80% in the bone marrow and that basal poly(ADP-ribose) content is decreased to almost undetectable levels [83]. DNA damage–induced synthesis of poly(ADP-ribose) is almost completely blocked in the niacin-deficient marrow cells [83]. The most common problem with DNA damage to the bone marrow occurs during chemotherapy, so we started to treat niacin-deficient and control rats with nitrosourea drugs that are known to cause bone marrow suppression and induce leukemias in the long term. In this model of the side effects of chemotherapy drugs, niacin deficiency increased the severity of acute bone marrow suppression (anemia, leukopenia) [147] and increased the rate development of nitrosourea-induced leukemias [83]. There is a dramatic occurrence of genomic instability in niacin-deficient bone marrow; micronuclei and sister chromatid exchanges are increased with niacin deficiency alone and enhanced by deficiency combined with DNA damage [82]. In more recent studies, we have found that niacin deficiency delays strand break repair kinetics and increases chromosomal aberrations (unpublished data). These results may be very important to cancer patients, as many are niacin deficient [10,11], and bone marrow suppression and secondary leukemias are two serious problems in cancer therapy.

Many more experiments have been conducted on the effect of pharmacological supplementation of nicotinic acid or nicotinamide on various types of carcinogenesis [148]. Nicotinamide, alone, does not appear to present risk as a carcinogen. When used in conjunction with carcinogenic foods or compounds in animal experiments, nicotinamide has a confusing array of effects, suggesting varied mechanisms of action. When given with diethylnitrosamine, nicotinamide did not affect liver carcinogenesis, but it increased kidney neoplasms. Following streptozotocin treatment, nicotinamide decreased adenoma formation, but increased pancreatic islet cell tumors [129,148]. Conversely, nicotinamide has shown significant protective effects against bladder and intestinal cancers when provided in a diet containing bracken fern.

There is much less data on the effects of large doses of nicotinic acid on carcinogenesis. Surprisingly, the best information is probably from human studies, derived from the long-term use of this compound in the treatment of hypercholesterolemia. Nine years after a 6-year period of nicotinic acid use to treat hypercholesterolemic patients, there was a significant decrease in mortality in this group, but this did not appear to be due to a decrease in cancer incidence [149].

We have recently studied animals supplemented with nicotinamide or nicotinic acid and treated with diethylnitrosamine [68]. While both supplements increased liver NAD^+ to a modest extent in the absence of carcinogen treatment, only nicotinamide significantly increased basal poly(ADP-ribose) levels (before diethylnitrosamine), whereas only nicotinic acid increased poly(ADP-ribose) levels following diethylnitrosamine. Neither supplement affected the development of diethylnitrosamine-induced preneoplastic-altered hepatic foci. In contrast, we have found that pharmacological supplementation of both nicotinic acid and nicotinamide causes large increases in bone marrow NAD^+ and poly(ADP-ribose) in rats, and decreases the long-term development of leukemia [150]. We have recently repeated these experiments with a lower dose of nitrosourea and found a much larger protective effect of niacin supplementation (unpublished data). Pharmacological supplementation of nicotinamide in mouse diets caused a dramatic increase in skin NAD^+ and provided significant protection against skin cancer induced by ultraviolet radiation [138]. As with deficiency, it is not surprising that niacin supplementation affects cancer susceptibility in some tissues, like the marrow and skin, and not others, like the liver. We need to continue to build our knowledge of whole animal models to appreciate the complexities of niacin metabolism and allow accurate recommendations for human populations.

While some of the foregoing responses may have been due to changes in the functions associated with NAD^+ utilization, there are also a variety of pharmacological actions that are not related to NAD^+ synthesis. These may be responsible for the inconsistency of the responses, and some of the potential mechanisms will be discussed in a later section.

Niacin Status and Oxidant Lung Injury

Niacin supplementation can decrease the degree of lung injury and fibrosis from a variety of causes, including exposure to lipopolysaccharide, cyclophosphamide, and bleomycin. The best-defined model uses bleomycin, an antibiotic chemotherapy drug that intercalates with DNA and induces damage through the local production of oxygen radicals [151]. This is a very severe stress, which causes NAD and ATP depletion, perhaps leading to suicidal NAD depletion, as hypothesized by Berger [126]. Protection by niacin may be functioning through the maintenance of NAD levels, but nicotinamide is more effective in increasing NAD, while nicotinic acid is more potent in the reduction of lung pathology [152]. The protection of lung tissue with these supplements may allow much safer use of bleomycin as a chemotherapy agent, although it is not known whether they also protect tumor tissue.

Hyperoxia is another popular model of oxidant stress in the lung, and has clinical relevance to the care of premature infants and adult respiratory distress syndrome. Hyperoxia has been shown to induce poly(ADP-ribose) synthesis in the lung and, although poly(ADP-ribose) synthesis is decreased by niacin deficiency, the deficient state does not increase the severity of lung damage [153]. Consistent with this finding, pharmacological niacin supplementation is also ineffective in decreasing the severity of hyperoxic lung damage [154]. Why is this response different from that observed following bleomycin treatment? Bleomycin induces a more sudden and severe stress to pulmonary cells, and it targets DNA specifically as an intracellular target, leading to depletion of NAD and ATP. Hyperoxic damage occurs gradually over a period of 5 days or more [155] and does not cause NAD depletion [153]. The majority of oxygen radicals emanate from the mitochondria and endoplasmic reticulum and oxidative damage is distributed among the intracellular compartments. Perhaps of greatest interest in this model, hyperoxia actually increases lung NAD content in the niacin-deficient animal to almost that of niacin replete controls. This result strongly suggests that enzymes or transport systems involved in NAD turnover are regulated in response to certain aspects of cellular damage, perhaps via the oxidant stress response described for the induction of *fos* and *jun* [156]. The degree of oxidant stress and the time course of the stress, which differ between hyperoxia and bleomycin toxicity, are likely to be important in determining the ability of cells or tissues to adapt. In addition to this, poly(ADP-ribose) formation is known to enhance inflammatory responses and promote apoptotic cell death, so one might not be surprised to see hyperoxia respond well to PARP inhibitors [125].

Niacin Status and Skin Injury

Because of the sun sensitivity displayed by pellagrins, there has been a long-standing interest in the effect of niacin deficiency on skin health [157], although not very many studies have been conducted. Rainbow trout are more prone to ultraviolet light–induced skin damage when niacin deficient [158]. A relatively mild deficiency of niacin in mice increases their susceptibility to ultraviolet light-induced skin cancers [159].

On the other hand, many studies have been conducted using pharmacological doses of various forms of the vitamin. Nicotinic acid acts as a vasodilator in the skin, leading to an increase in blood flow through the microvasculature, which is caused by changes in prostaglandin production [160,161]. Over the years, a wide variety of treatment regimens and different forms of nicotinic acid have been used to treat various skin disorders [157]. The effects on blood flow occur only at supraphysiological levels of the vitamin and are not caused by modulation of NAD pools. However, nicotinic acid supplementation at 1 to 10 g/kg of diet was shown to dramatically decrease UV-induced skin cancers in mice [85]. The decrease was linear through the supplementation range, as was the increase in skin NAD content. This work shows that very large dietary doses of niacin may continue to influence cancer susceptibility through modulation of NAD pools. The underlying mechanisms may prove to be quite interesting, as the authors also showed that niacin supplementation was improving immune surveillance of tumors. This may be due to changes in mono- or cyclic ADP-ribose signaling events in immune cells [86,93].

Nicotinamide supplementation has also been shown to protect the skin from DNA-damaging agents in some animal models. Large doses of nicotinamide, given i.p., decreased the skin damage caused by the chemical warfare agent, sulfur mustard [162].

With the potential for niacin to improve skin health, especially in the face of ultraviolet exposure, niacin has been added to various skin creams. Topical application of natural forms of niacin provides little benefit as the water-soluble intermediates cannot cross the skin. Niadyne Incorporated has developed a derivative of nicotinic acid that crosses the skin and is released to support NAD synthesis (www.niadyne.com). Skin structure is changed by regular use of this product and it is under consideration by the National Cancer Institute as an agent for protection against skin cancer.

COMPETITION FOR NAD$^+$ DURING NIACIN DEFICIENCY

It seems obvious that the most critical cellular functions of the niacin-containing nucleotides are those of electron transport and energy metabolism. A loss in the capacity to deliver reducing equivalents to the electron transport chain would be similar to poisoning the cell with cyanide or suffocating from a lack of oxygen. It makes sense, then, that these functions are strongly protected when NAD levels start to deplete during niacin deprivation. Cultured cells, in the absence of DNA damage, can grow and divide with less than 5% of control NAD levels [116,163,164], leaving us with a variety of questions to be answered. How do the other pathways of NAD utilization, including poly, mono and cyclic ADP-ribose formation, compete for these limiting substrate pools? What is the nature of this competition at the cellular level with respect to compartmentalization between the nucleus, cytoplasm, and mitochondria? What is the role of extracellular NAD^+ in the function of mono(ADP-ribosyl)transferase and ADP-ribosyl cyclase enzymes on the outer surface of the cell? How are nicotinic acid and nicotinamide distributed among tissues during deficiency, and does this contribute to the distinctive signs and symptoms of pellagra? How do these interactions lead to the specific metabolic lesions that cause the sun-sensitive dermatitis, diarrhea, and dementia?

Possible mechanisms for unequal utilization of NAD at the subcellular level include (a) variation in the affinity of enzymes for NAD^+ (K_m) and (b) compartmentalization. K_m values are used to describe the affinity of an enzyme for its substrate and are defined as the concentration of substrate required to support 50% of the maximal activity. A lower K_m indicates a higher affinity and suggests that an enzyme will compete effectively with enzymes having a higher K_m as NAD^+ concentrations fall during deficiency. Some caution in interpretation is required; enzyme kinetics may change during purification, especially for membrane-bound proteins.

The K_m of PARP for NAD^+ is thought to be between 20 and 80 μM [146]. In certain cultured cells, the ability to synthesize poly(ADP-ribose) decreases when cellular NAD content drops to less than half of control levels [164], showing that the synthesis of poly (ADP-ribose) is one the most sensitive pathways of NAD utilization. This is similar to the proportionate decrease in NAD^+ during niacin deficiency in many tissues in vivo, but tissues vary in their absolute concentrations of NAD^+ and direct extrapolation to intact tissues could be problematic. For example, in rats, liver NAD^+ decreases by close to 50% during deficiency, but is still present at about 500 μM [43]. At this level of NAD^+, there was actually an increased poly(ADP-ribose) response to DNA damage [145], reminding us that PARP-1 is functioning in the nucleus, and there may be mechanisms to maintain nuclear NAD^+ during altered dietary status and in response to chronic DNA damage [165]. In our bone marrow model, control NAD^+ is estimated as 350 μM (much lower than liver) and likely around 100 μM during niacin deficiency [83]. This is in the range of the K_m of PARP-1 for NAD^+, and the synthesis of poly(ADP-ribose) in bone marrow cells is decimated during niacin deficiency [83].

It has been stated that poly(ADP-ribosyl)ation is the aspect of NAD^+ utilization, which is most sensitive to niacin deficiency because of a much higher K_m of PARP for NAD^+. Do the K_m values of other NAD^+-utilizing enzymes suggest that the sensitivity of poly(ADP-ribose) metabolism may be unique? There are scores of dehydrogenase enzymes that use NAD^+ as an electron acceptor, producing NADH for utilization in the electron transport chain. Glyceraldehyde phosphate dehydrogenase is a cytosolic enzyme, which is critical to the flow of substrates through glycolysis. It uses NAD^+ as an oxidant and has a K_m for this cofactor of 13 μM [166], smaller than that of PARP, indicating a higher affinity. Other cytosolic enzymes may have slightly higher affinities for NAD^+ than PARP, including alcohol and aldehyde dehydrogenases (17–110 μM and 16 μM, respectively) [166]. In the mitochondria, isocitrate is oxidatively decarboxylated in the TCA cycle by a dehydrogenase with a K_m for NAD^+ of 78 μM [166], which is similar to PARP. However, the mitochondrial form of malate dehydrogenase is also critical to the flow of substrate through the TCA cycle, and its K_m for NAD^+ has been reported as 540 μM [166]. If these data are correct, the TCA cycle appears to require compartmentalization of NAD^+ during niacin deficiency, and the role of the mitochondria in this regard will be discussed later. In the end, ATP production by the electron-transfer chain is only dependent on NADH levels. The fact that NADH is maintained during niacin deficiency, as NAD^+ declines, shows that the oxidative machinery of the cell can function at lower levels of NAD^+ and still maintain the flow of reducing equivalents to the electron transport chain.

With respect to cyclic ADP-ribose synthesis, the purified microsomal cyclase from canine spleen has a K_m of 10 μM for NAD^+ [76]. With access to cytosolic NAD pools, this enzyme should maintain its catalytic activity during niacin deficiency. The CD38 cyclase is reported to have a K_m of 15 μM for NAD^+ [167]. While this is a relatively high affinity for substrate, the curious aspect of this enzyme is that it faces the exterior of the cell. Does it have a requirement for extracellular NAD or access to intracellular pools? Cultured kidney epithelial cells synthesize cyclic ADP-ribose, but they require permeabilization to use NAD^+ in the medium and require over 500 μM for a half-maximal response [168]. There are several new concepts developing in this area, including the possibility that connexin channels deliver NAD^+ to ectoenzymes [169]. This could be a mechanism to regulate extracellular signals based on the energy status inside the cell. Another possibility is that areas of cell death lead to the local release of NAD^+, generating cyclic ADP-ribose signals that may play a role in inflammatory responses [170]. A cytosolic ADP-ribosyl cyclase has recently been described in mouse synaptosomes, and it represents the sort of enzyme that could explain the striking dementia of pellagra. It has a K_m of 21 μM [80] for NAD^+, and therefore should be relatively resistant to niacin deficiency. We have recently started measuring cyclic ADP-ribose levels in rat tissues, and have found them to be responsive to niacin status [199].

Mono(ADP-ribosyl)transferases are a very diverse group. The only published data on affinity for NAD^+ refers to the arginine-specific transferases. In a family of transferases from turkey erythrocytes, two cytosolic enzymes have K_m values of 7 and 36 μM, while a transferase from the membrane fraction has a K_m of 15 μM [171]. These enzymes would appear to compete with PARP under conditions of limiting NAD^+ pools, but a transferase from chicken liver nuclei has a K_m of between 200 and 500 μM, and a transferase from mammalian skeletal and heart muscle displays a K_m of 560 μM [171]. It appears that some mono(ADP-ribosyl)transferases may be quite sensitive to niacin deficiency. The resulting changes in cell signaling might not appear as problems in cell culture models, while presenting significant problems in the whole organism. As discussed earlier, there is a mono(ADP-ribosyl)transferase anchored to the outer surface of the plasma membrane, which, like CD38, appears to require extracellular NAD^+. This enzyme appears to cause the ADP-ribosylation of an intracellular protein, leading to a depression in T-cell proliferation. Although no attempt has been made to determine the K_m of this enzyme for NAD^+, levels of NAD^+ as low 1 μM in the culture medium are effective in decreasing cell proliferation [172].

It becomes apparent that the physical partitioning of NAD within the cell is a key factor in the availability of the molecule for various metabolic functions. The cytoplasmic pool provides substrate for soluble enzymes, as well as for those on the endoplasmic reticulum and on the inside of the plasma membrane. These would support a host of redox reactions and the activity of a variety of poorly defined mono(ADP-ribosyl)transferases and ADP-ribosylcyclases. The mitochondria isolate a pool of NAD^+ which is predominantly involved in electron transport, although mono(ADP-ribosyl)ation reactions have been reported in this organelle. Nuclear NAD^+ is probably used mainly for poly(ADP-ribosyl)ation reactions, but mono (ADP-ribosyl)transferases are also located here, and cyclic ADP-ribose is active in the release of calcium from the nuclear envelope. The least studied pool is extracellular NAD^+, which appears to play a role in some ADP-ribosylcyclase and mono(ADP-ribosyl)transferase activities. How distinct are these pools, and how do they respond to the progression of niacin deficiency?

Because of the presence of nuclear pores, it is not surprising that PARP-1 activation can deplete cytosolic NAD pools [173]. However, the final step in the synthesis of NAD^+ from nicotinamide is catalyzed predominantly by a nuclear enzyme, NMN adenylyltransferase-1 (Figure 6.3) [50]. In contrast, the last step in the conversion of nicotinic acid to NAD^+ occurs in the cytosol. This means that NAD^+ synthesized in the cell from newly arrived nicotinamide, or from nicotinamide released by any of the ADP-ribosylation reactions in the cell, may be directed toward nuclear reactions [174]. Nicotinic acid will lead to the production of cytosolic NAD^+, which may favor different patterns of utilization. Interestingly, certain mice express a mutant form of NMN adenylyltransferase that is overexpressed in the nucleus. They are protected from axonal cell death by a mechanism that is dependent on NAD synthesis and SIR2 function, illustrating the importance of nuclear NAD synthesis [175], even under conditions in which total cellular NAD is not enhanced.

The mitochondria are well equipped to regulate NAD levels. The inner mitochondrial membrane is essentially impermeable to all forms of NAD(P). Reducing equivalents in the form of NADH must be transformed via shuttle mechanisms to enter the mitochondria for ATP production. How does the mitochondrion produce or obtain NAD, and what levels does it maintain? Some researchers believe that mitochondria synthesize NAD [176], while others suggest that slow, high-affinity carriers bring the necessary NAD from the cytosol [177,178]. The net requirement is probably modest, as most of the reactions presently identified in this organelle do not degrade the cofactor. The important question concerns the ability of mitochondria to concentrate NAD^+, and it appears that they have potent mechanisms to accomplish this. NAD^+ levels in hepatocyte mitochondria appear to be about 10-fold higher than in the cytoplasm, with absolute concentrations in the neighborhood of 5 mM [179]. These NAD^+ concentrations would support enzymes with relatively low affinities for NAD^+, such as malate dehydrogenase [166]. With this ability to concentrate NAD^+, the mitochondrial pool could be well protected during niacin deficiency. As support for this thought, mitochondrial NAD is resistant to depletion by activated PARP-1 [173], until the failure of mitochondrial integrity associated with apoptosis. Prevention of mitochondrial permeability under these conditions can prevent or delay cell death [180].

The plasma pool of NAD^+ is poorly characterized. Levels of noncellular NAD^+ in blood samples are extremely low [31] and there is no information on the response of this pool to dietary niacin intake. Roles for extracellular NAD^+ likely involve localized situations, like regions of cell lysis [170].

In addition to the competition for NAD^+ at the cellular level, organs and tissues vary in their ability to conserve NAD pools or compete for precursors during the progression of niacin deficiency [43]. Some tissues, like the liver, also start with much higher levels of NAD^+, and these may act as reserves during deficiency. Blood $NADP^+$ is more stable than NAD^+ during niacin deficiency [36], but it may change in other tissues, and the impact of niacin deficiency on NAADP metabolism is not known. If NAADP is really synthesized in vivo from NADP and nicotinic acid, then it could be dramatically influenced by falling nicotinic acid levels during niacin deficiency. These are some of the concepts that must be appreciated as we progress toward a better understanding of the biochemical basis of the pathologies of pellagra, a disease whose clinical symptoms remain unexplained at the molecular level.

PHARMACOLOGY AND TOXICOLOGY

Levels of niacin in excess of the RDA have been used in attempts to treat Hartnup's disease, carcinoid syndrome, poor glucose tolerance, atherosclerosis, schizophrenia, hyperlipidemia, IDDM, and a variety of skin disorders. In some countries, during the shortages of proper medical supplies caused by World War II, nicotinic acid became a popular drug because the dramatic flushing reaction that it caused in the skin was interpreted as a sign of the potency of the treatment [181]. In recent years, nicotinic acid and nicotinamide have been used mainly in the prevention of cardiovascular disease and IDDM, respectively. Very few nutrients are prescribed medicinally for pharmacological purposes that are mechanistically distinct from their known nutrient functions. Both nicotinic acid and nicotinamide fall into this category, and the pharmacological effects of these two vitamers are surprisingly unrelated.

Nicotinic Acid

Nicotinic Acid and Hyperlipidemia

Historically, nicotinic acid has been administered to patients with a variety of disorders, often more for the dramatic skin reaction than proven curative powers. Its most successful use is for the treatment of hyperlipidemia. The mechanisms of action of high-dose nicotinic acid are unrelated to the formation of NAD(P) and unrelated to the actions of nicotinamide. The main effect is a decrease in lipolysis in adipose tissue due to an inhibition of adenylate cyclase activity. The resulting drop in cAMP levels leads to the decreased mobilization of fatty acids [182], which is at least partially responsible for a drop in VLDL formation by the liver and a subsequent drop in LDL levels, although there may also be direct effects on liver lipid metabolism. Unlike many treatments for hyperlipidemias, nicotinic acid also increases circulating levels of HDL [183], the beneficial lipoprotein that removes cholesterol from vascular tissue. In addition to the blood lipid effects, high-dose nicotinic acid causes a dramatic skin flush of the face and upper trunk.

All of these blood lipid effects appear to be due to the binding of nicotinic acid to a high-affinity receptor, which is in turn linked to an inhibitory G-protein, leading to decreased cAMP levels and inhibition of hormone-sensitive lipase [182]. This receptor is known as the niacin receptor or HM74A [184]. It is termed as an orphan receptor, as nicotinic acid is not thought to be its natural ligand, given the unphysiologically high doses required to activate it. The skin flush, which is mediated by prostaglandin formation, also appears to be caused by the binding of nicotininic acid to HM74A, in this case, on the surface of macrophages [185].

Nicotinic Acid Toxicity

There are a few drawbacks for using high levels of oral nicotinic acid. As mentioned earlier, the short-term side effects may include vasodilation, burning or stinging sensations in the face and hands, nausea, vomiting, and diarrhea. In the longer term, there may be varying degrees of hyperpigmentation of the skin, abnormal glucose tolerance, hyperuricemia, peptic ulcers, hepatomegaly, and jaundice [186]. Newer versions of time-release nicotinic acid have been reported to be safe and effective [182]. It should be noted that all drugs used in the treatment of hyperlipidemia have some side effects and many of these problems can be managed through changes in dose. Interestingly, nicotinic acid use for six years by patients with cardiovascular disease led to a decrease in all-cause mortality measured 8 years after the drug use was discontinued [149]. A lipid-soluble derivative of nicotinic acid, which is active in lowering blood cholesterol, and paradoxically, does not cause a skin flush reaction, is under development by Niadyne Incorporated (www.niadyne.com).

Nicotinamide

In the past, nicotinamide has been used in the treatment of schizophrenia [187], but more effective drugs have replaced it in this field. It has also been tested as a chemotherapy agent; in this application, nicotinamide potentiates the cytotoxic effects of chemotherapy and radiation treatment against tumor cells [188], an action that appears to be caused by increased blood flow and oxygenation of tumor tissue [189]. However, most of the recent interest in nicotinamide involves its potential use in the prevention or delay of onset of IDDM.

Nicotinamide and Insulin-Dependent Diabetes Mellitus

Interest in this area started with the finding that nicotinamide could prevent diabetes induced by the β-cell toxins alloxan and streptozotocin [128]. It was soon shown that the β-cells were killed by excessive activation of PARP, which depleted cellular NAD levels. Since nicotinamide is not a very high-affinity inhibitor of PARP [190], and cellular levels tend to stay low due to active conversion to NAD, it seems likely that protection in this model was due to the use of nicotinamide as a precursor of NAD synthesis, although PARP-1 may have been partially inhibited. We have shown that large oral doses of nicotinamide increase NAD^+ and poly(ADP-ribose) levels in the liver [68] and more recently, in the bone marrow [150]. Interestingly, animals protected from chemically induced diabetes by nicotinamide all developed insulin producing β-cell tumors [129], a form of cancer that is particularly lethal in humans [191]. It is not surprising that cells rescued from NAD depletion due to extreme DNA damage, either through inhibition of PARP or pharmacological support of NAD pools, would be at risk for neoplastic growth because of the survival of cells with significant levels of DNA damage.

In humans, the onset of IDDM occurs spontaneously by immune recognition of β-cell antigens. This is associated with leukocyte infiltration and the presence of anti-islet cell antibodies in the serum. The spontaneous occurrence of IDDM is similar in the nonobese diabetic (NOD) mouse. When nicotinamide is given to weaning NOD mice, the onset of diabetic symptoms is prevented or delayed [192]. As discussed in an earlier section, catalytically active PARP-1 is now recognized as an inflammatory mediator and as an inducer of apoptosis [125]. Inhibition or genetic ablation of PARP-1 has been shown to prevent diabetes in multiple low-dose streptozotocin and NOD animal models [193]. Recent studies more clearly implicate PARP-1 with the use of potent and specific inhibitors.

Clinical Trials

Encouraged by the type of data summarized above, a number of experiments have been conducted with human subjects. In the majority of these studies, patients were recruited in the early stages of clinically apparent diabetes. Since these subjects retain a varying degree of β-cell function, it is not surprising that the results have been inconsistent. However, a number of treatment protocols have been successful in inducing remission in some patients [194] and increasing the residual level of plasma insulin for up to 2 years after diagnosis [195].

The animal models show that nicotinamide treatment should start before the disease process is in an advanced stage. To do this in human populations, researchers must identify the susceptible population. Blood levels of islet cell antibodies, human leukocyte antigen, and family history are used as predictors of IDDM in recruiting subjects. These strategies were used in the organization of several large studies, including the European-Canadian Nicotinamide Diabetes Intervention Trial (ENDIT). Unfortunately, this large and well-designed study showed no benefit of nicotinamide supplementation [196]. It is quite possible that nicotinamide was not effective in PARP inhibition in the doses used in the human studies. If nicotinamide increased tissue NAD concentrations, it would have the potential to enhance the poly(ADP-ribose)-induced signals leading to inflammation and apoptosis. These effects would conflict with the possible benefits exerted by PARP inhibition. It is important to note that the use of potent PARP inhibitors in relatively healthy human populations may carry an unacceptable risk.

Nicotinamide Toxicity

The levels of nicotinamide that are used in the ENDIT trial (about 1–3 g/day) have not been reported to cause any adverse side effects on an acute basis. Larger doses (about 10 g/day) have been known to cause liver injury (parenchymal cell injury, portal fibrosis, and cholestasis) [197]. Chronic intake of nicotinamide can also induce a methyl-group deficiency state because of the methylation reactions involved in excretion [45].

SUMMARY

Niacin deficiency has the potential to alter redox reactions, poly and mono(ADP-ribose) synthesis, SIRT1 activity, and the formation of cyclic ADP-ribose and NAADP. During niacin deficiency, the metabolic changes that lead to the dramatic signs and symptoms of pellagra will likely be tissue-specific and reflect subcellular competition for NAD pools. The effect of chronic niacin undernutrition on human health, especially the process of carcinogenesis, appears to be an exciting area that deserves more attention. With a rapidly broadening perspective on the biochemical roles for niacin in metabolism, identification of optimal niacin nutriture should be possible in the coming decade.

Supplementation of nicotinic acid and nicotinamide above the dietary requirement may affect some of the same processes, but these compounds have distinctive pharmacological properties, some of which may be unrelated to their currently defined nutrient functions. Future research in models of niacin deficiency and supplementation may lead us to reevaluate the accepted metabolic roles of niacin and create new guidelines for niacin intake.

ACKNOWLEDGMENTS

The Cancer Research Society (Montreal, Canada) and the National Cancer Institute of Canada have supported our research on niacin status and ADP-ribose metabolism, which in turn has made the writing of this chapter possible. I would like to thank Drs. Janos Zempleni, Ralph Meyer, and Genevieve Young for critical reading of the manuscript and Lorman Ip for sharing his thoughts on high-leucine and high-fat diets, ketosis, and tryptophan metabolism.

REFERENCES

1. S. Harris, *Clinical Pellagra* (C.V. Mosby, St. Louis, 1941).
2. K.J. Carpenter, *Pellagra* (Hutchinson Ross, Stroudsburg, 1981).
3. S.R. Roberts, *Pellagra, History, Distribution, Diagnosis, Prognosis, Treatment, Etiology* (C.V. Mosby, St. Louis, 1914).
4. A.J. Bollet, Politics and pellagra: the epidemic of pellagra in the U.S. in the early twentieth century, *Yale J. Biol. Med. 65*, 211–221 (1992).
5. P. Malfait, A. Moren, J.C. Dillon, A. Brodel, G. Begkoyian, M.G. Etchegorry, G. Malenga, and P. Hakewill, An outbreak of pellagra related to changes in dietary niacin among Mozambican refugees in Malawi, *Int. J. Epidemiol. 22*, 504–511 (1993).
6. S.G. Kertesz, Pellagra in 2 homeless men, *Mayo Clin. Proc. 76*, 315–318 (2001).
7. M. Serdaru, C. Hausser-Hauw, D. Laplane, A. Buge, P. Castaigne, M. Goulon, F. Lhermitte, and J.J. Hauw, The clinical spectrum of alcoholic pellagra encephalopathy. A retrospective analysis of 22 cases studied pathologically, *Brain 111* (*Pt 4*), 829–842 (1988).
8. J.P. Monteiro, D.F. da Cunha, D.C. Filho, M.L. Silva-Vergara, S. dos, V.C.J. da, Jr., R.M. Etchebehere, J. Goncalves, S.F. de Carvalho da Cunha, A.A. Jordao, P.G. Chiarello, and

H. Vannucchi, Niacin metabolite excretion in alcoholic pellagra and AIDS patients with and without diarrhea, *Nutrition 20*, 778–782 (2004).
9. J.E. Prousky, Pellagra may be a rare secondary complication of anorexia nervosa: a systematic review of the literature, *Altern. Med. Rev. 8*, 180–185 (2003).
10. R.I. Inculet, J.A. Norton, G.E. Nichoalds, M.M. Maher, D.E. White, and M.F. Brennan, Water-soluble vitamins in cancer patients on parenteral nutrition: a prospective study, *J. Parenter. Enteral Nutr. 11*, 243–249 (1987).
11. S. Dreizen, K.B. McCredie, M.J. Keating, and B.S. Andersson, Nutritional deficiencies in patients receiving cancer chemotherapy, *Postgrad. Med. 87*, 163–167, 170 (1990).
12. H.P. Stevens, L.S. Ostlere, R.H. Begent, J.S. Dooley, and M.H. Rustin, Pellagra secondary to 5-fluorouracil, *Br. J.Dermatol. 128*, 578–580 (1993).
13. G.M. Shah, R.G. Shah, H. Veillette, J.B. Kirkland, J.L. Pasieka, and R.R. Warner, Biochemical assessment of niacin deficiency among carcinoid cancer patients, *Am. J. Gastroenterol. 100*, 2307–2314 (2005).
14. J.L. Spivak and D.L. Jackson, Pellagra: an analysis of 18 patients and a review of the literature, *Johns. Hopkins. Med. J. 140*, 295–309 (1977).
15. S. Pitsavas, C. Andreou, F. Bascialla, V.P. Bozikas, and A. Karavatos, Pellagra encephalopathy following B-complex vitamin treatment without niacin, *Int. J. Psychiatry Med. 34*, 91–95 (2004).
16. E.L. Jacobson, Niacin deficiency and cancer in women, *J. Am. Coll. Nutr. 12*, 412–416 (1993).
17. J. Goldberger, The relation of diet to pellagra, *JAMA 78*, 1676–1680 (1922).
18. C.A. Elvehjem, R.J. Madden, F.M. Strong, and D.M. Woolley, Relation of nicotinic acid and nicotinic acid amide to canine black tongue, *J. Am. Chem. Soc. 59*, 1767–1768 (1937).
19. W.A. Krehl, L.J. Teply, and C.A. Elvehjem, Corn as an etiological factor in the production of a nicotinic acid deficiency in the rat, *Science 101*, 283 (1945).
20. W.H. Sebrell, History of pellagra, *Fed. Proc. 40*, 1520–1522 (1981).
21. C. Heidelberger, E.P. Abraham, and S. Lepkovsky, Concerning the mechanism of the mammalian conversion of tryptophan into nicotinic acid, *J. Biol. Chem. 176*, 1461–1462 (1948).
22. J. Laguna and K.J. Carpenter, Raw versus processed corn in niacin-deficient diets, *J. Nutr. 45*, 21–28 (1951).
23. K.J. Carpenter, M. Schelstraete, V.C. Vilicich, and J.S. Wall, Immature corn as a source of niacin for rats, *J. Nutr. 118*, 165–169 (1988).
24. Buniva, Observations in pellagra: it would not appear to be contagious, *Pellagra*, K.J. Carpenter, ed. (Hutchinson Ross, Stroudsburg, 1981), 11–12.
25. T.D. Spies, W.B. Bean, and W.F. Ashe, Recent advances in the treatment of pellagra and associated deficiencies, *Pellagra*, K.J. Carpenter, ed. (Hutchinson Ross, Stroudsburg, 1981), 213–225.
26. A. Hoffer, Pellagra and schizophrenia, *Psychosomatics 11*, 522–525 (1970).
27. M. Freed, *Methods of Vitamin Assay* (The Association of Vitamin Chemists Inc., New York, 1966).
28. W. Friedrich, *Vitamins* (Walter de Gruyter, New York, 1988).
29. T.R. Guilarte and K. Pravlik, Radiometric–microbiologic assay of niacin using Kloeckera brevis: analysis of human blood and food, *J. Nutr. 113*, 2587–2594 (1983).
30. H.W. Huff and W.A. Perlzweig, The fluorescent condensation product of N^1-methylnicotinamide and acetone: II. A sensitive method for the determination of N^1-methylnicotinamide, *J. Biol. Chem. 167*, 157–167 (1947).
31. E.L. Jacobson, A.J. Dame, J.S. Pyrek, and M.K. Jacobson, Evaluating the role of niacin in human carcinogenesis, *Biochimie 77*, 394–398 (1995).
32. G.A. Smythe, O. Braga, B.J. Brew, R.S. Grant, G.J. Guillemin, S.J. Kerr, and D.W. Walker, Concurrent quantification of quinolinic, picolinic, and nicotinic acids using electron-capture negative-ion gas chromatography–mass spectrometry, *Anal. Biochem. 301*, 21–26 (2002).
33. J. Stein, A. Hahn, and G. Rehner, High-performance liquid chromatographic determination of nicotinic acid and nicotinamide in biological samples applying post-column derivatization resulting in bathmochrome absorption shifts, *J. Chromatogr. B Biomed. Appl. 665*, 71–78 (1995).
34. R. Roskoski, Determination of pyridine nucleotides by fluorescence and other optical techniques, *Pyridine Nucleotide Coenzymes: Chemical, Biochemical and Medical Aspects*, D. Dolphin, R. Poulson, and O. Avramovic, eds. (John Wiley & Sons, New York, 1987), 173–188.

35. D.P. Jones, Determination of pyridine dinucleotides in cell extracts by high-performance liquid chromatography, *J. Chromatogr. 225*, 446–449 (1981).
36. C.S. Fu, M.E. Swendseid, R.A. Jacob, and R.W. McKee, Biochemical markers for assessment of niacin status in young men: levels of erythrocyte niacin coenzymes and plasma tryptophan, *J. Nutr. 119*, 1949–1955 (1989).
37. K. Shibata, H. Shimada, and T. Kondo, Effects of feeding tryptophan-limiting diets on the conversion ratio of tryptophan to niacin in rats, *Biosci. Biotechnol. Biochem. 60*, 1660–1666 (1996).
38. J.B. Mason, N. Gibson, and E. Kodicek, The chemical nature of the bound nicotinic acid of wheat bran: studies of nicotinic acid-containing macromolecules, *Br. J. Nutr. 30*, 297–311 (1973).
39. E.G. Carter and K.J. Carpenter, The available niacin values of foods for rats and their relation to analytical values, *J. Nutr. 112*, 2091–2103 (1982).
40. The National Academy of Sciences, *Dietary Reference Intakes for Thiamin, Riboflavin, Niacin, Vitamin B_6, Folate, Vitamin B_{12}, Pantothenic Acid, Biotin and Choline* (National Academy Press, Washington, DC. 1999).
41. S.E. Sauberlich, Nutritional aspects of pyridine nucleotides, *Pyridine Nucleotide Coenzymes: Chemical, Biochemical and Medical Aspects*, D. Dolphin, R. Poulson, and O. Avramovic, eds. (John Wiley & Sons, New York, 1987), 599–626.
42. E.L. Jacobson and M.K. Jacobson, Tissue NAD as a biochemical measure of niacin status in humans, *Methods Enzymol. 280*, 221–230 (1997).
43. J.M. Rawling, T.M. Jackson, E.R. Driscoll, and J.B. Kirkland, Dietary niacin deficiency lowers tissue poly(ADP-ribose) and NAD^+ concentrations in Fischer-344 rats, *J. Nutr. 124*, 1597–1603 (1994).
44. L. Troppmann, K. Gray-Donald, and T. Johns, Supplement use: is there any nutritional benefit? *J. Am. Diet. Assoc. 102*, 818–825 (2002).
45. M.M. ApSimon, J.M. Rawling, and J.B. Kirkland, Nicotinamide megadosing increases hepatic poly(ADP-ribose) levels in choline-deficient rats, *J. Nutr. 125*, 1826–1832 (1995).
46. L.M. Stead, R.L. Jacobs, M.E. Brosnan, and J.T. Brosnan, Methylation demand and homocysteine metabolism, *Adv. Enzyme Regul. 44*, 321–333 (2004).
47. J.W. Foster and A.G. Moat, Nicotinamide adenine dinucleotide biosynthesis and pyridine nucleotide cycle metabolism in microbial systems, *Microbiol. Rev. 44*, 83–105 (1980).
48. J. Preiss and P. Handler, Biosynthesis of diphosphopyridine nucleotide I. Identification of intermediates, *J. Biol. Chem. 233*, 488–500 (1958).
49. L.S. Dietrich, L. Fuller, I.L. Yero, and L. Martinez, Nicotinamide mononucleotide pyrophosphorylase activity in animal tissues, *J. Biol. Chem. 241*, 188–191 (1966).
50. F. Berger, C. Lau, M. Dahlmann, and M. Ziegler, Subcellular compartmentation and differential catalytic properties of the three human nicotinamide mononucleotide adenylyltransferase isoforms, *J. Biol. Chem. 280*, 36334–36341 (2005).
51. A.G. Moat and J.W. Foster, Biosynthesis and salvage pathways of pyridine nucleotides, *Pyridine Nucleotide Coenzymes: Chemical, Biochemical and Medical Aspects, Part B*, D. Dolphin, M. Powanda, and R. Poulson, eds. (John Wiley & Sons, New York, 1982), 1–24.
52. M. Ikeda, H. Tsuji, S. Nakamura, A. Ichiyama, Y. Nishizuka, and O. Hayaishi, Studies on the biosynthesis of nicotinamide adenine dinucleotide. II. A role of picolinic carboxylase in the biosynthesis of nicotinamide adenine dinucleotide from tryptophan in mammals, *J. Biol. Chem. 240*, 1395–1401 (1965).
53. M.P. Heyes, C.Y. Chen, E.O. Major, and K. Saito, Different kynurenine pathway enzymes limit quinolinic acid formation by various human cell types, *Biochem. J. 326* (*Pt 2*), 351–356 (1997).
54. D.A. Bender, Effects of a dietary excess of leucine on the metabolism of tryptophan in the rat: a mechanism for the pellagragenic action of leucine, *Br. J. Nutr. 50*, 25–32 (1983).
55. N.V. Shastri, S.G. Nayudu, and M.C. Nath, Effect of high fat and high fat–high protein diets on biosynthesis of niacin from tryptophan in rats, *J. Vitaminol.* (*Kyoto*) *14*, 198–202 (1968).
56. N. Kimura, T. Fukuwatari, R. Sasaki, and K. Shibata, The necessity of niacin in rats fed on a high protein diet, *Biosci. Biotechnol. Biochem. 69*, 273–279 (2005).
57. S. Fukuoka, K. Ishiguro, K. Yanagihara, A. Tanabe, Y. Egashira, H. Sanada, and K. Shibata, Identification and expression of a cDNA encoding human alpha-amino-beta-carboxymuconate-epsilon-semialdehyde decarboxylase (ACMSD). A key enzyme for the tryptophan–niacine pathway and 'quinolinate hypothesis', *J. Biol. Chem. 277*, 35162–35167 (2002).

58. M.K. Horwitt, A.E. Harper, and L.M. Henderson, Niacin–tryptophan relationships for evaluating niacin equivalents, *Am. J. Clin. Nutr. 34*, 423–427 (1981).
59. A. Tanabe, Y. Egashira, S. Fukuoka, K. Shibata, and H. Sanada, Expression of rat hepatic 2-amino-3-carboxymuconate-6-semialdehyde decarboxylase is affected by a high protein diet and by streptozotocin-induced diabetes, *J. Nutr. 132*, 1153–1159 (2002).
60. A.C. Da Silva, R. Fried, and R.C. De Angelis, Domestic cat as laboratory animal for experimental nutrition studies; niacin requirements and tryptophan metabolism, *J. Nutr. 46*, 399–409 (1952).
61. L.V. Hankes, L.M. Henderson, W.L. Brickson, and C.A. Elvehjem, Effect of amino acids on the growth of rats on niacin–tryptophan deficient rations, *J. Biol. Chem. 174*, 873–881 (1948).
62. M.E. Reid, Nutritional studies with the guinea pig. VII. Niacin, *J. Nutr. 75*, 279–286 (1961).
63. L.M. Henderson, Niacin, *Annu. Rev. Nutr. 3*, 289–307 (1983).
64. S.M. Nabokina, M.L. Kashyap, and H.M. Said, Mechanism and regulation of human intestinal niacin uptake, *Am. J. Physiol. Cell Physiol. 289*, C97–C103 (2005).
65. H. Takanaga, H. Maeda, H. Yabuuchi, I. Tamai, H. Higashida, and A. Tsuji, Nicotinic acid transport mediated by pH-dependent anion antiporter and proton cotransporter in rabbit intestinal brush-border membrane, *J. Pharm. Pharmacol. 48*, 1073–1077 (1996).
66. S.J. Lan and L.M. Henderson, Uptake of nicotinic acid and nicotinamide by rat erythrocytes, *J. Biol. Chem. 243*, 3388–3394 (1968).
67. V. Micheli, H.A. Simmonds, S. Sestini, and C. Ricci, Importance of nicotinamide as an NAD precursor in the human erythrocyte, *Arch. Biochem. Biophys. 283*, 40–45 (1990).
68. T.M. Jackson, J.M. Rawling, B.D. Roebuck, and J.B. Kirkland, Large supplements of nicotinic acid and nicotinamide increase tissue NAD^+ and poly(ADP-ribose) levels but do not affect diethylnitrosamine-induced altered hepatic foci in Fischer-344 rats, *J. Nutr. 125*, 1455–1461 (1995).
69. C. Bernofsky, Physiology aspects of pyridine nucleotide regulation in mammals, *Mol. Cell Biochem. 33*, 135–143 (1980).
70. N.O. Kaplan, History of the pyridine nucleotides, *Pyridine Nucleotide Coenzymes: Chemical, Biochemical and Medical Aspects*, *Part A*, D. Dolphin, R. Poulson, and O. Avramovic, eds. (John Wiley & Sons, New York, 1987), 1–20.
71. D.L. Clapper, T.F. Walseth, P.J. Dargie, and H.C. Lee, Pyridine nucleotide metabolites stimulate calcium release from sea urchin egg microsomes desensitized to inositol trisphosphate, *J. Biol. Chem. 262*, 9561–9568 (1987).
72. H. Kim, E.L. Jacobson, and M.K. Jacobson, Position of cyclization in cyclic ADP-ribose, *Biochem. Biophys. Res. Commun. 194*, 1143–1147 (1993).
73. A.H. Guse, Second messenger function and the structure–activity relationship of cyclic adenosine diphosphoribose (cADPR), *FEBS J. 272*, 4590–4597 (2005).
74. H.C. Lee and R. Aarhus, A derivative of NADP mobilizes calcium stores insensitive to inositol trisphosphate and cyclic ADP-ribose, *J. Biol. Chem. 270*, 2152–2157 (1995).
75. M. Yamasaki, G.C. Churchill, and A. Galione, Calcium signalling by nicotinic acid adenine dinucleotide phosphate (NAADP), *FEBS J. 272*, 4598–4606 (2005).
76. H. Kim, E.L. Jacobson, and M.K. Jacobson, Synthesis and degradation of cyclic ADP-ribose by NAD glycohydrolases, *Science 261*, 1330–1333 (1993).
77. L. Sun, O.A. Adebanjo, A. Koval, H.K. Anandatheerthavarada, J. Iqbal, X.Y. Wu, B.S. Moonga, X.B. Wu, G. Biswas, P.J. Bevis, M. Kumegawa, S. Epstein, C.L. Huang, N.G. Avadhani, E. Abe, and M. Zaidi, A novel mechanism for coupling cellular intermediary metabolism to cytosolic Ca^{2+} signaling via CD38/ADP-ribosyl cyclase, a putative intracellular NAD^+ sensor, *FASEB J. 16*, 302–314 (2002).
78. H.C. Lee, R. Graeff, and T.F. Walseth, Cyclic ADP-ribose and its metabolic enzymes, *Biochimie 77*, 345–355 (1995).
79. I. Bacher, A. Zidar, M. Kratzel, and M. Hohenegger, Channelling of substrate promiscuity of the skeletal-muscle ADP-ribosyl cyclase isoform, *Biochem. J. 381*, 147–154 (2004).
80. C. Ceni, N. Pochon, M. Villaz, H. Muller-Steffner, F. Schuber, J. Baratier, M. De Waard, M. Ronjat, and M.J. Moutin, The CD38-independent ADP-ribosyl cyclase from mouse brain synaptosomes: a comparative study of neonate and adult brain, *Biochem. J. 395 (2)*, 417–426 (2006).
81. A.L. Perraud, C.L. Takanishi, B. Shen, S. Kang, M.K. Smith, C. Schmitz, H.M. Knowles, D. Ferraris, W. Li, J. Zhang, B.L. Stoddard, and A.M. Scharenberg, Accumulation of free

ADP-ribose from mitochondria mediates oxidative stress-induced gating of TRPM2 cation channels, *J. Biol. Chem. 280*, 6138–6148 (2005).
82. J.C. Spronck and J.B. Kirkland, Niacin deficiency increases spontaneous and etoposide-induced chromosomal instability in rat bone marrow cells in vivo, *Mutat. Res. 508*, 83–97 (2002).
83. A.C. Boyonoski, J. C. Spronck, L.M. Gallacher, R.M. Jacobs, G.M. Shah, G.G. Poirier, and J.B. Kirkland, Niacin deficiency decreases bone marrow poly(ADP-ribose) and the latency of ethylnitrosourea-induced carcinogenesis in rats, *J. Nutr. 132*, 108–114 (2002).
84. O. Gerasimenko and J. Gerasimenko, New aspects of nuclear calcium signalling, *J. Cell Sci. 117*, 3087–3094 (2004).
85. H.L. Gensler, T. Williams, A.C. Huang, and E.L. Jacobson, Oral niacin prevents photocarcinogenesis and photoimmunosuppression in mice, *Nutr. Cancer 34*, 36–41 (1999).
86. S.Y. Rah, K.H. Park, M.K. Han, M.J. Im, and U.H. Kim, Activation of CD38 by interleukin-8 signaling regulates intracellular Ca^{2+} level and motility of lymphokine-activated killer cells, *J. Biol. Chem. 280*, 2888–2895 (2005).
87. J. Yamauchi and S. Tanuma, Occurrence of an NAD^+ glycohydrolase in bovine brain cytosol, *Arch. Biochem. Biophys. 308*, 327–329 (1994).
88. Y. Desmarais, L. Menard, J. Lagueux, and G.G. Poirier, Enzymological properties of poly(ADP-ribose) polymerase: characterization of automodification sites and NADase activity, *Biochim. Biophys. Acta 1078*, 179–186 (1991).
89. R. Antoine and C. Locht, The NAD-glycohydrolase activity of the pertussis toxin S1 subunit. Involvement of the catalytic HIS-35 residue, *J. Biol. Chem. 269*, 6450–6457 (1994).
90. C. Bourgeois, I. Okazaki, E. Cavanaugh, M. Nightingale, and J. Moss, Identification of regulatory domains in ADP-ribosyltransferase-1 that determine transferase and NAD glycohydrolase activities, *J. Biol. Chem. 278*, 26351–26355 (2003).
91. S.P. Yates, R. Jorgensen, G.R. Andersen, and A.R. Merrill, Stealth and mimicry by deadly bacterial toxins, *Trends Biochem. Sci.* (2006).
92. M. Di Girolamo, N. Dani, A. Stilla, and D. Corda, Physiological relevance of the endogenous mono(ADP-ribosyl)ation of cellular proteins, *FEBS J. 272*, 4565–4575 (2005).
93. W. Ohlrogge, F. Haag, J. Lohler, M. Seman, D.R. Littman, N. Killeen, and F. Koch-Nolte, Generation and characterization of ecto-ADP-ribosyltransferase ART2.1/ART2.2-deficient mice, *Mol. Cell Biol. 22*, 7535–7542 (2002).
94. M. Bektas, R. Nurten, K. Ergen, and E. Bermek, Endogenous ADP-ribosylation for eukaryotic elongation factor 2: evidence of two different sites and reactions, *Cell Biochem. Funct. 24 (4)*, 369–380 (2005).
95. B.E. Ledford and G.H. Leno, ADP-ribosylation of the molecular chaperone GRP78/BiP, *Mol. Cell Biochem. 138*, 141–148 (1994).
96. E.L. Jacobson, D. Cervantes-Laurean, and M.K. Jacobson, Glycation of proteins by ADP-ribose, *Mol. Cell Biochem. 138*, 207–212 (1994).
97. A.L. Perraud, B. Shen, C.A. Dunn, K. Rippe, M.K. Smith, M.J. Bessman, B.L. Stoddard, and A.M. Scharenberg, NUDT9, a member of the Nudix hydrolase family, is an evolutionarily conserved mitochondrial ADP-ribose pyrophosphatase, *J. Biol. Chem. 278*, 1794–1801 (2003).
98. G. Blander and L. Guarente, The Sir2 family of protein deacetylases, *Annu. Rev. Biochem. 73*, 417–435 (2004).
99. M. Kruszewski and I. Szumiel, Sirtuins (histone deacetylases III) in the cellular response to DNA damage—facts and hypotheses, *DNA Repair (Amst) 4*, 1306–1313 (2005).
100. H. Vaziri, S.K. Dessain, E.N. Eaton, S.I. Imai, R.A. Frye, T.K. Pandita, L. Guarente, and R.A. Weinberg, hSir2(SIRT1) functions as an NAD-dependent p53 deacetylase, *Cell 107*, 149–159 (2001).
101. C.L. Brooks and W. Gu, Ubiquitination, phosphorylation and acetylation: the molecular basis for p53 regulation, *Curr. Opin. Cell Biol. 15*, 164–171 (2003).
102. P. Chambon, J.D. Weill, J. Doly, M.T. Strosser, and P. Mandel, On the formation of a novel adenylic compound by enzymatic extracts of liver nuclei, *Biochem. Biophys. Res. Commun. 25*, 638–643 (1966).
103. J.C. Ame, C. Spenlehauer, and G. de Murcia, The PARP superfamily, *Bioessays 26*, 882–893 (2004).

104. I. Kameshita, Z. Matsuda, T. Taniguchi, and Y. Shizuta, Poly(ADP-ribose) synthetase. Separation and identification of three proteolytic fragments as the substrate-binding domain, the DNA-binding domain, and the automodification domain, *J. Biol. Chem. 259*, 4770–4776 (1984).
105. M. Ikejima, S. Noguchi, R. Yamashita, T. Ogura, T. Sugimura, D.M. Gill, and M. Miwa, The zinc fingers of human poly(ADP-ribose) polymerase are differentially required for the recognition of DNA breaks and nicks and the consequent enzyme activation. Other structures recognize intact DNA, *J. Biol. Chem. 265*, 21907–21913 (1990).
106. C.C. Kiehlbauch, N. Aboul-Ela, E.L. Jacobson, D.P. Ringer, and M.K. Jacobson, High resolution fractionation and characterization of ADP-ribose polymers, *Anal. Biochem. 208*, 26–34 (1993).
107. H. Mendoza-Alvarez and R. Alvarez-Gonzalez, Poly(ADP-ribose) polymerase is a catalytic dimer and the automodification reaction is intermolecular, *J. Biol. Chem. 268*, 22575–22580 (1993).
108. F.R. Althaus, L. Hofferer, H.E. Kleczkowska, M. Malanga, H. Naegeli, P. Panzeter, and C. Realini, Histone shuttle driven by the automodification cycle of poly(ADP-ribose) polymerase, *Environ. Mol. Mutagen. 22*, 278–282 (1993).
109. A. Burkle, Poly(ADP-ribose). The most elaborate metabolite of NAD^+, *FEBS J. 272*, 4576–4589 (2005).
110. V. Schreiber, J.C. Ame, P. Dolle, I. Schultz, B. Rinaldi, V. Fraulob, J. Menissier-de Murcia, and G. de Murcia, Poly(ADP-ribose) polymerase-2 (PARP-2) is required for efficient base excision DNA repair in association with PARP-1 and XRCC1, *J. Biol. Chem. 277*, 23028–23036 (2002).
111. A. Huber, P. Bai, J.M. de Murcia, and G. de Murcia, PARP-1, PARP-2 and ATM in the DNA damage response: functional synergy in mouse development, *DNA Repair* (*Amst*) *3*, 1103–1108 (2004).
112. S. Desnoyers, G.M. Shah, G. Brochu, J.C. Hoflack, A. Verreault, and G.G. Poirier, Biochemical properties and function of poly(ADP-ribose) glycohydrolase, *Biochimie 77*, 433–438 (1995).
113. M.L. Meyer-Ficca, R.G. Meyer, D.L. Coyle, E.L. Jacobson, and M.K. Jacobson, Human poly(-ADP-ribose) glycohydrolase is expressed in alternative splice variants yielding isoforms that localize to different cell compartments, *Exp. Cell Res. 297*, 521–532 (2004).
114. J. Oka, K. Ueda, O. Hayaishi, H. Komura, and K. Nakanishi, ADP-ribosyl protein lyase. Purification, properties and identification of the product, *J. Biol. Chem. 259*, 986–995 (1984).
115. D. D'Amours, S. Desnoyers, I. D'Silva, and G.G. Poirier, Poly(ADP-ribosyl)ation reactions in the regulation of nuclear functions, *Biochem. J. 342* (*Pt 2*), 249–268 (1999).
116. B.W. Durkacz, O. Omidiji, D.A. Gray, and S. Shall, $(ADP\text{-ribose})_n$ participates in DNA excision repair, *Nature 283*, 593–596 (1980).
117. M. Malanga and F.R. Althaus, The role of poly(ADP-ribose) in the DNA damage signaling network, *Biochem. Cell Biol. 83*, 354–364 (2005).
118. M.F. Denisenko, V.A. Soldatenkov, L.N. Belovskaya, and I.V. Filippovich, Is the NAD-poly (ADP-ribose) polymerase system the trigger in radiation-induced death of mouse thymocytes? *Int. J. Radiat. Biol. 56*, 277–285 (1989).
119. Y. Ohashi, K. Ueda, M. Kawaichi, and O. Hayaishi, Activation of DNA ligase by poly(ADP-ribose) in chromatin, *Proc. Natl. Acad. Sci. USA 80*, 3604–3607 (1983).
120. C.M. Simbulan, M. Suzuki, S. Izuta, T. Sakurai, E. Savoysky, K. Kojima, K. Miyahara, Y. Shizuta, and S. Yoshida, Poly(ADP-ribose) polymerase stimulates DNA polymerase alpha by physical association, *J. Biol. Chem. 268*, 93–99 (1993).
121. M.S. Satoh and T. Lindahl, Role of poly(ADP-ribose) formation in DNA repair, *Nature 356*, 356–358 (1992).
122. T.J. Jorgensen, J.C. Leonard, P.J. Thraves, and A. Dritschilo, Baseline sister chromatid exchange in human cell lines with different levels of poly(ADP-ribose) polymerase, *Radiat. Res. 127*, 107–110 (1991).
123. V.A. Kickhoefer, A.C. Siva, N.L. Kedersha, E.M. Inman, C. Ruland, M. Streuli, and L.H. Rome, The 193-kD vault protein, VPARP, is a novel poly(ADP-ribose) polymerase, *J. Cell Biol. 146*, 917–928 (1999).
124. S.L. Oei, C. Keil, and M. Ziegler, Poly(ADP-ribosylation) and genomic stability, *Biochem. Cell Biol. 83*, 263–269 (2005).

125. K. Erdelyi, E. Bakondi, P. Gergely, C. Szabo, and L. Virag, Pathophysiologic role of oxidative stress-induced poly(ADP-ribose) polymerase-1 activation: focus on cell death and transcriptional regulation, *Cell Mol. Life Sci. 62*, 751–759 (2005).
126. N.A. Berger, Poly(ADP-ribose) in the cellular response to DNA damage, *Radiat. Res. 101*, 4–15 (1985).
127. S.J. Hong, T.M. Dawson, and V.L. Dawson, Nuclear and mitochondrial conversations in cell death: PARP-1 and AIF signaling, *Trends Pharmacol. Sci. 25*, 259–264 (2004).
128. H. Okamoto, The role of poly(ADP-ribose) synthetase in the development of insulin-dependent diabetes and islet β-cell regeneration, *Biomed. Biochim. Acta 44*, 15–20 (1985).
129. T. Yamagami, A. Miwa, S. Takasawa, H. Yamamoto, and H. Okamoto, Induction of rat pancreatic B-cell tumors by the combined administration of streptozotocin or alloxan and poly (adenosine diphosphate ribose) synthetase inhibitors, *Cancer Res. 45*, 1845–1849 (1985).
130. J.M. Rawling, E.R. Driscoll, G.G. Poirier, and J.B. Kirkland, Diethylnitrosamine administration in vivo increases hepatic poly(ADP-ribose) levels in rats: results of a modified technique for poly(ADP-ribose) measurement, *Carcinogenesis 14*, 2513–2516 (1993).
131. G.P. Warwick and J.S. Harington, Some aspects of the epidemiology and etiology of esophageal cancer with particular emphasis on the Transkei, South Africa, *Adv. Cancer Res. 17*, 121–131 (1973).
132. S.J. Van Rensburg, E.S. Bradshaw, D. Bradshaw, and E.F. Rose, Oesophageal cancer in Zulu men, South Africa: a case-control study, *Br. J. Cancer 51*, 399–405 (1985).
133. J. Wahrendorf, J. Chang-Claude, Q.S. Liang, Y.G. Rei, N. Munoz, M. Crespi, R. Raedsch, D. Thurnham, and P. Correa, Precursor lesions of oesophageal cancer in young people in a high-risk population in China [see comments], *Lancet 2*, 1239–1241 (1989).
134. S. Franceschi, E. Bidoli, A.E. Baron, and C. La Vecchia, Maize and risk of cancers of the oral cavity, pharynx, and esophagus in northeastern Italy, *J. Natl. Cancer Inst. 82*, 1407–1411 (1990).
135. S.J. Van Rensburg, Epidemiologic and dietary evidence for a specific nutritional predisposition to esophageal cancer, *J. Natl. Cancer Inst. 67*, 243–251 (1981).
136. J.R. Marshall, S. Graham, B.P. Haughey, D. Shedd, R. O'Shea, J. Brasure, G.S. Wilkinson, and D. West, Smoking, alcohol, dentition and diet in the epidemiology of oral cancer, *Eur. J. Cancer B Oral Oncol. 28B*, 9–15 (1992).
137. M. Fenech, P. Baghurst, W. Luderer, J. Turner, S. Record, M. Ceppi, and S. Bonassi, Low intake of calcium, folate, nicotinic acid, vitamin E, retinol, beta-carotene and high intake of pantothenic acid, biotin and riboflavin are significantly associated with increased genome instability—results from a dietary intake and micronucleus index survey in South Australia, *Carcinogenesis 26*, 991–999 (2005).
138. G.Q. Wang, S.M. Dawsey, J.Y. Li, P.R. Taylor, B. Li, W.J. Blot, W.M. Weinstein, F.S. Liu, K.J. Lewin, and H. Wang, Effects of vitamin/mineral supplementation on the prevalence of histological dysplasia and early cancer of the esophagus and stomach: results from the General Population Trial in Linxian, China, *Cancer Epidemiol. Biomarkers Prev. 3*, 161–166 (1994).
139. W.J. Blot, J.Y. Li, P.R. Taylor, W. Guo, S. Dawsey, G.Q. Wang, C.S. Yang, S.F. Zheng, M. Gail, and G.Y. Li, Nutrition intervention trials in Linxian, China: supplementation with specific vitamin/mineral combinations, cancer incidence, and disease-specific mortality in the general population [see comments], *J. Natl. Cancer Inst. 85*, 1483–1492 (1993).
140. H. Wang, H. Wei, J. Ma, and X. Luo, The fumonisin B1 content in corn from North China, a high-risk area of esophageal cancer, *J. Environ. Pathol. Toxicol. Oncol. 19*, 139–141 (2000).
141. R.T. Riley, E. Enongene, K.A. Voss, W.P. Norred, F.I. Meredith, R.P. Sharma, J. Spitsbergen, D.E. Williams, D.B. Carlson, and A.H. Merrill, Jr., Sphingolipid perturbations as mechanisms for fumonisin carcinogenesis, *Environ. Health Perspect. 109* (*Suppl 2*), 301–308 (2001).
142. E.G. Miller and H. Burns, Jr., *N*-Nitrosodimethylamine carcinogenesis in nicotinamide-deficient rats, *Cancer Res. 44*, 1478–1482 (1984).
143. S.J. Van Rensburg, J.M. Hall, and P.S. Gathercole, Inhibition of esophageal carcinogenesis in corn-fed rats by riboflavin, nicotinic acid, selenium, molybdenum, zinc, and magnesium, *Nutr. Cancer 8*, 163–170 (1986).
144. J.Z. Zhang, S.M. Henning, and M.E. Swendseid, Poly(ADP-ribose) polymerase activity and DNA strand breaks are affected in tissues of niacin-deficient rats, *J. Nutr. 123*, 1349–1355 (1993).

145. J.M. Rawling, T.M. Jackson, B.D. Roebuck, G.G. Poirier, and J.B. Kirkland, The effect of niacin deficiency on diethylnitrosamine-induced hepatic poly(ADP-ribose) levels and altered hepatic foci in the Fischer-344 rat, *Nutr. Cancer 24*, 111–119 (1995).
146. K. Ueda, M. Kawaichi, and O. Hayshi, Poly(ADP-ribose) synthetase, *ADP-ribosylation Reactions, Biology and Medicine*, O. Hayashi and K. Ueda, eds. (Academic Press, New York, 1982), 118–155.
147. A.C. Boyonoski, L.M. Gallacher, M.M. ApSimon, R.M. Jacobs, G.M. Shah, G.G. Poirier, and J.B. Kirkland, Niacin deficiency in rats increases the severity of ethylnitrosourea-induced anemia and leukopenia, *J. Nutr. 130*, 1102–1107 (2000).
148. G.T. Bryan, The influence of niacin and nicotinamide on in vivo carcinogenesis, *Advances in Experimental Medicine and Biology. Vol 206—Essential Nutrients in Carcinogenesis*, L.A. Poirier, P.M. Newberne, and M.W. Pariza, eds. (Plenum Press, New York, 1986), 331–338.
149. P.L. Canner, K.G. Berge, N.K. Wenger, J. Stamler, L. Friedman, R.J. Prineas, and W. Friedewald, Fifteen year mortality in Coronary Drug Project patients: long-term benefit with niacin, *J. Am. Coll. Cardiol. 8*, 1245–1255 (1986).
150. A.C. Boyonoski, J.C. Spronck, R.M. Jacobs, G.M. Shah, G.G. Poirier, and J.B. Kirkland, Pharmacological intakes of niacin increase bone marrow poly(ADP-ribose) and the latency of ethylnitrosourea-induced carcinogenesis in rats, *J. Nutr. 132*, 115–120 (2002).
151. S.N. Giri, R. Blaisdell, R.B. Rucker, Q. Wang, and D.M. Hyde, Amelioration of bleomycin-induced lung fibrosis in hamsters by dietary supplementation with taurine and niacin: biochemical mechanisms, *Environ. Health Perspect. 102* (*Suppl 10*), 137–147 (1994).
152. A. Nagai, H. Matsumiya, M. Hayashi, S. Yasui, H. Okamoto, and K. Konno, Effects of nicotinamide and niacin on bleomycin-induced acute injury and subsequent fibrosis in hamster lungs, *Exp. Lung Res. 20*, 263–281 (1994).
153. J.M. Rawling, M.M. ApSimon, and J.B. Kirkland, Lung poly(ADP-ribose) and NAD^+ concentrations during hyperoxia and niacin deficiency in the Fischer-344 rat, *Free Radic. Biol. Med. 20*, 865–871 (1996).
154. S.G. Jenkinson, R.A. Lawrence, and D.L. Butler, Inability of niacin to protect from in vivo hyperoxia or in vitro microsomal lipid peroxidation, *J. Toxicol. Clin. Toxicol. 19*, 975–985 (1982).
155. J.D. Crapo, Morphologic changes in pulmonary oxygen toxicity, *Annu. Rev. Physiol. 48*, 721–731 (1986).
156. S. Bergelson, R. Pinkus, and V. Daniel, Intracellular glutathione levels regulate *fos/jun* induction and activation of glutathione *S*-transferase gene expression, *Cancer Res. 54*, 36–40 (1994).
157. J.K. Wilkin, T.B. Bentley, D.L. Latour, and E.W. Rosenberg, Nicotinic acid treatment of skin disorders, *Br. J. Dermatol. 100*, 471–472 (1979).
158. H.A. Poston and M.J. Wolfe, Niacin requirement for optimum growth, feed conversion and protection of rainbow trout, *Salmo gairdneri*, from ultraviolet-B radiation, *J. Fish Dis. 8*, 451–460 (1985).
159. G.M. Shah, Y. Le Rhun, I. Sutarjono, and J.B. Kirkland, Niacin deficient SKH-1 mice are more susceptible to ultraviolet B radiation-induced skin carcinogenesis, *Cancer Res. 131*(*11S*), 3150S (2002).
160. J.D. Morrow, J.A. Awad, J.A. Oates, and L.J. Roberts, Identification of skin as a major site of prostaglandin D2 release following oral administration of niacin in humans, *J. Invest. Dermatol. 98*, 812–815 (1992).
161. J.K. Wilkin, G. Fortner, L.A. Reinhardt, O.V. Flowers, S.J. Kilpatrick, and W.C. Streeter, Prostaglandins and nicotinate-provoked increase in cutaneous blood flow, *Clin. Pharmacol. Ther. 38*, 273–277 (1985).
162. J.J. Yourick, J.S. Dawson, C.D. Benton, M.E. Craig, and L.W. Mitcheltree, Pathogenesis of 2,2′-dichlorodiethyl sulfide in hairless guinea pigs, *Toxicology 84*, 185–197 (1993).
163. C.M. Whitacre, H. Hashimoto, M.L. Tsai, S. Chatterjee, S.J. Berger, and N.A. Berger, Involvement of NAD-poly(ADP-ribose) metabolism in p53 regulation and its consequences, *Cancer Res. 55*, 3697–3701 (1995).
164. E.L. Jacobson, V. Nunbhakdi-Craig, D.G. Smith, H.Y. Chen, B.L. Wasson, and M.K. Jacobson, ADP-ribose polymer metabolism: implications for human nutrition, *ADP-Ribosylation Reactions*, G.G. Poirier and P. Moreau, eds. (Springer-Verlag, New York, 1992), 153–162.

165. J.C. Spronck, A.P. Bartleman, A.C. Boyonoski, and J.B. Kirkland, Chronic DNA damage and niacin deficiency enhance cell injury and cause unusual interactions in NAD and poly(ADP-ribose) metabolism in rat bone marrow, *Nutr. Cancer 45*, 124–131 (2003).
166. T.E. Barnum, ed., *Enzyme Handbook* (Springer-Verlag, New York, NY, 1969).
167. R.M. Graeff, T.F. Walseth, K. Fryxell, W.D. Branton, and H.C. Lee, Enzymatic synthesis and characterizations of cyclic GDP-ribose. A procedure for distinguishing enzymes with ADP-ribosyl cyclase activity, *J. Biol. Chem. 269*, 30260–30267 (1994).
168. K.W. Beers, E.N. Chini, H.C. Lee, and T.P. Dousa, Metabolism of cyclic ADP-ribose in opossum kidney renal epithelial cells, *Am. J. Physiol. 268*, C741–C746 (1995).
169. A. De Flora, E. Zocchi, L. Guida, L. Franco, and S. Bruzzone, Autocrine and paracrine calcium signaling by the CD38/NAD^+/cyclic ADP-ribose system, *Ann. NY Acad. Sci. 1028*, 176–191 (2004).
170. A. Zolkiewska, Ecto-ADP-ribose transferases: cell-surface response to local tissue injury, *Physiology (Bethesda) 20*, 374–381 (2005).
171. A. Zolkiewska, I.J. Okazaki, and J. Moss, Vertebrate mono-ADP-ribosyltransferases, *Mol. Cell Biochem. 138*, 107–112 (1994).
172. J. Wang, E. Nemoto, A.Y. Kots, H.R. Kaslow, and G. Dennert, Regulation of cytotoxic T cells by ecto-nicotinamide adenine dinucleotide (NAD) correlates with cell surface GPI-anchored/arginine ADP-ribosyltransferase, *J. Immunol. 153*, 4048–4058 (1994).
173. W. Ying, C.C. Alano, P. Garnier, and R.A. Swanson, NAD^+ as a metabolic link between DNA damage and cell death, *J. Neurosci. Res. 79*, 216–223 (2005).
174. M.Y. Kim, T. Zhang, and W.L. Kraus, Poly(ADP-ribosyl)ation by PARP-1: 'PAR-laying' NAD^+ into a nuclear signal, *Genes Dev. 19*, 1951–1967 (2005).
175. T. Araki, Y. Sasaki, and J. Milbrandt, Increased nuclear NAD biosynthesis and SIRT1 activation prevent axonal degeneration, *Science 305*, 1010–1013 (2004).
176. H. Grunicke, H.J. Keller, B. Puschendorf, and A. Benaguid, Biosynthesis of nicotinamide adenine dinucleotide in mitochondria, *Eur. J. Biochem. 53*, 41–45 (1975).
177. J.L. Purvis and J.M. Lowenstein, The relationship between intra- and extramitochondrial pyridine nucleotides, *J. Biol. Chem. 236*, 2794–2803 (1961).
178. A. Behr, H. Taguchi, and R.K. Gholson, Apparent pyridine nucleotide synthesis in mitochondria: an artifact of NMN and NAD glycohydrolase activity? *Biochem. Biophys. Res. Commun. 101*, 767–774 (1981).
179. M.E. Tischler, D. Friedrichs, K. Coll, and J.R. Williamson, Pyridine nucleotide distributions and enzyme mass action ratios in hepatocytes from fed and starved rats, *Arch. Biochem. Biophys. 184*, 222–236 (1977).
180. C.C. Alano, W. Ying, and R.A. Swanson, Poly(ADP-ribose) polymerase-1-mediated cell death in astrocytes requires NAD^+ depletion and mitochondrial permeability transition, *J. Biol. Chem. 279*, 18895–18902 (2004).
181. M. Weiner and J. van Eys, *Nicotinic Acid: Nutrient-Cofactor-Drug* (Marcel Dekker, New York, 1983).
182. L.A. Carlson, Nicotinic acid: the broad-spectrum lipid drug. A 50th anniversary review, *J. Intern. Med. 258*, 94–114 (2005).
183. J.D. Alderman, R.C. Pasternak, F.M. Sacks, H.S. Smith, E.S. Monrad, and W. Grossman, Effect of a modified, well-tolerated niacin regimen on serum total cholesterol, high density lipoprotein cholesterol and the cholesterol to high density lipoprotein ratio, *Am. J. Cardiol. 64*, 725–729 (1989).
184. A. Wise, S.M. Foord, N.J. Fraser, A.A. Barnes, N. Elshourbagy, M. Eilert, D.M. Ignar, P.R. Murdock, K. Steplewski, A. Green, A.J. Brown, S.J. Dowell, P.G. Szekeres, D.G. Hassall, F.H. Marshall, S. Wilson, and N.B. Pike, Molecular identification of high and low affinity receptors for nicotinic acid, *J. Biol. Chem. 278*, 9869–9874 (2003).
185. H.J. Knowles, R.T. Poole, P. Workman, and A.L. Harris, Niacin induces PPAR-gamma expression and transcriptional activation in macrophages via HM74 and HM74a-mediated induction of prostaglandin synthesis pathways, *Biochem. Pharmacol. 71*, 646–656 (2006).
186. J.R. DiPalma and W.S. Thayer, Use of niacin as a drug, *Annu. Rev. Nutr. 11*, 169–187 (1991).
187. A. Hoffer, Megavitamin B_3 therapy for schizophrenia, *Can. Psychiatr. Assoc. J. 16*, 499–504 (1971).

188. M.R. Horsman, Nicotinamide and other benzamide analogs as agents for overcoming hypoxic cell radiation resistance in tumours. A review, *Acta Oncol. 34*, 571–587 (1995).
189. D.J. Chaplin, M.R. Horsman, and M.J. Trotter, Effect of nicotinamide on the microregional heterogeneity of oxygen delivery within a murine tumor, *J. Natl. Cancer Inst. 82*, 672–676 (1990).
190. P.W. Rankin, E.L. Jacobson, R.C. Benjamin, J. Moss, and M.K. Jacobson, Quantitative studies of inhibitors of ADP-ribosylation in vitro and in vivo, *J. Biol. Chem. 264*, 4312–4317 (1989).
191. J.A. Norton, J.L. Doppman, and R.T. Jensen, Cancer of the endocrine system, *Cancer: Principles and Practice of Oncology*, V.T. DeVita, S. Hellman, Jr., and S.A. Rosenberg, eds. (J.B. Lippincott Co., Philadelphia, 1989), 1324–1331.
192. S. Reddy, N.J. Bibby, and R.B. Elliott, Early nicotinamide treatment in the NOD mouse: effects on diabetes and insulitis suppression and autoantibody levels, *Diabetes Res. 15*, 95–102 (1990).
193. C. Szabo, Roles of poly(ADP-ribose) polymerase activation in the pathogenesis of diabetes mellitus and its complications, *Pharmacol. Res. 52*, 60–71 (2005).
194. P. Vague, R. Picq, M. Bernal, V. Lassmann-Vague, and B. Vialettes, Effect of nicotinamide treatment on the residual insulin secretion in type 1 (insulin-dependent) diabetic patients, *Diabetologia 32*, 316–321 (1989).
195. P. Pozzilli, N. Visalli, R. Buzzetti, M.G. Baroni, M.L. Boccuni, E. Fioriti, A. Signore, C. Mesturino, L. Valente, and M.G. Cavallo, Adjuvant therapy in recent onset type 1 diabetes at diagnosis and insulin requirement after 2 years, *Diabetes Metab. 21*, 47–49 (1995).
196. E.A. Gale, P.J. Bingley, C.L. Emmett, and T. Collier, European Nicotinamide Diabetes Intervention Trial (ENDIT): a randomised controlled trial of intervention before the onset of type 1 diabetes, *Lancet 363*, 925–931 (2004).
197. S.L. Winter and J.L. Boyer, Hepatic toxicity from large doses of vitamin B_3 (nicotinamide), *N. Engl. J. Med. 289*, 1180–1182 (1973).
198. S.L. Thorn, G.S. Young, and J.B. Kirkland, The guinea pig is a poor animal model for studies of niacin deficiency and presents challenges in any study using purified diets, *Br. J. Nutr.* (in press).
199. G.S. Young, E.L. Jacobson, and J.B. Kirkland, Water maze performance in young male Long-Evans rats is inversely affected by dietary intakes of niacin and may be linked to levels of the NAD+ metabolite cADPR, *J. Nutr.* (in press).
200. J.C. Spronck, J.L. Nickerson, and J.B. Kirkland, Niacin deficiency alters p53 expression and impairs etoposide-induced cell cycle arrest and apoptosis in rat bone marrow cells, *Nutr. Cancer*, (in press).

7 Riboflavin (Vitamin B_2)

Richard S. Rivlin

CONTENTS

INTRODUCTION

Within the last few years, much has been learned about the role of riboflavin in intermediary metabolism and in several categories of disease. The relationship of riboflavin to other B vitamins has undergone further clarification. Like many of the B vitamins, its metabolically active forms are as coenzyme derivatives, the formation of which is regulated by the nutritional state, hormones, drugs, and other stimuli. There are now new approaches to riboflavin supplementation for specific purposes.

Several recent reviews have emphasized the role of riboflavin in health (1), the regulation of riboflavin metabolism (2), and the inborn errors of riboflavin metabolism with neurological sequelae (3).

HISTORY

Perhaps the earliest scientific studies showing prevention of a deficiency state by riboflavin and other factors were those of McCollum and Kennedy (4), who observed its efficacy against a pellagra-like condition. In later studies, a heat-labile and heat-stable fraction were identified. The heat-stable fraction contained a yellow growth factor that was able to fluoresce. After purification, the factor was named riboflavin (5). This heat-stable fraction contained a number of other essential nutrients, including niacin (variably called vitamin B_3) and vitamin B_6.

The physiological role of the yellow growth factor was shown later by Warburg and Christian (6) who described the factor as "old yellow enzyme," composed of an apoenzyme and a yellow cofactor as coenzyme. The coenzyme was found to have an isoalloxazine ring (7) and a phosphate-containing side chain (8).

Riboflavin was synthesized by Kuhn et al. (9) and Karrer et al. (10). The structure of the first coenzyme formed sequentially from riboflavin, riboflavin-5′-phosphate, also called flavin mononucleotide (FMN), was established by Theorell (11). The structure of the second coenzyme formed, flavin adenine dinucleotide (FAD), was established by Warburg and Christian (12). This coenzyme was synthesized from its coenzyme precursor, FMN.

CHEMISTRY

FMN and FAD serve as coenzymes for enzymes in a wide variety of reactions in intermediary metabolism. There are also tissue forms of FAD, which are covalently linked from the 8-alpha position of the isoalloxazine portion of the flavin via N(1) or N(3) of histidyl or the S of cysteinyl residues within specific enzymes that have a number of significant roles in metabolism (13). Those mammalian enzymes with covalently bound flavins include sarcosine dehydrogenase, succinic dehydrogenase, monoamine oxidase, and L-gulonolactone oxidase (14). L-gulonolactone oxidase synthesizes ascorbic acid from its precursors and is not present as a functional holoenzyme in human tissues.

The planar isoalloxazine ring forms the basic structure for riboflavin, FMN, and FAD, as shown in Figure 7.1. The sequence of events in the synthesis of the flavin coenzymes from riboflavin and its control by thyroid hormones are shown in Figure 7.2. Thyroid hormones regulate the activities of the flavin biosynthetic enzymes (15), the synthesis of the flavoproteins apoenzymes, and the formation of covalently bound flavins (16). The first biosynthetic enzyme, flavokinase, catalyzes the initial phosphorylation of riboflavin from ATP to form FMN. A fraction of FMN is directly used in this form as a coenzyme. The largest fraction of FMN, however, combines with a second molecule of ATP to form FAD, the predominant tissue flavin, in a reaction catalyzed by FAD synthetase, also called FAD pyrophosphorylase. The covalent attachment of flavins to specific tissue proteins occurs after FAD has been synthesized. A sequence of phosphatases returns FAD to FMN, and FMN, in turn, to riboflavin (15). Most flavoproteins use FAD rather than FMN as coenzyme for a wide variety of metabolic reactions.

Microsomal NADPH-cytochrome P450 reductase is the first mammalian enzyme shown to contain both FMN and FAD as coenzymes and in equimolar ratios. Human novel reductase 1, like other diflavin reductases, also contains both FMN and FAD as prosthetic groups (17,18). In addition, nitric oxide synthase (19) and methionine synthase (20) also contain both FMN and FAD as coenzymes.

Riboflavin is yellow in color and has a high degree of natural fluorescence when excited by UV light, a property that can be used conveniently in its assay. There are a number of variations in structure in the naturally occurring flavins. Riboflavin and its coenzymes are sensitive to alkali and to acid, particularly in the presence of UV light. Under alkaline conditions, riboflavin is photodegraded to yield lumiflavin (7,8,10-trimethylisoalloxazine), which is inactive biologically. Riboflavin is photodegraded under acidic conditions to lumichrome (7,8-dimethylalloxazine), a product that is also biologically inactive. Thus, an important physical property of riboflavin and its derivatives is their sensitivity to UV light, resulting in rapid inactivation. Therefore, phototherapy of neonatal jaundice and of certain skin disorders has the potential to promote systemic riboflavin deficiency. The structure–function relationships of the various biologically active flavins have been comprehensively reviewed (21).

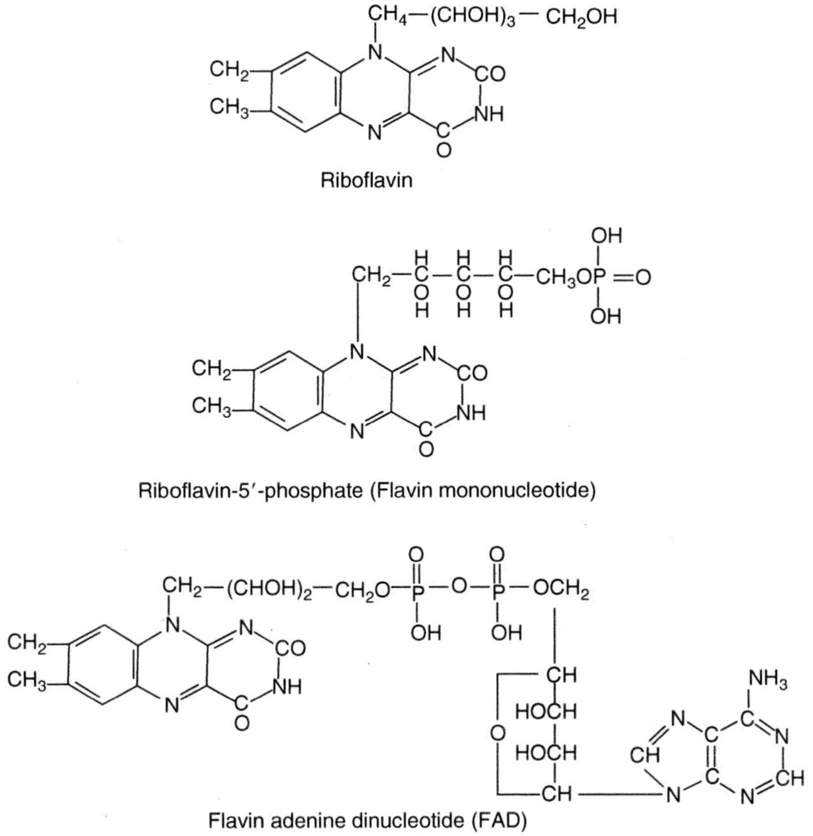

CH_4—$(CHOH)_3$— CH_2OH
N N CO
CH_2 CH_3
N C NH
O

Riboflavin

OH
CH_2—C—C—C—CH_3OP =O
H H H
O O O
H H H
OH
N N CO
CH_2 CH_3
N C NH
O

Riboflavin-5′-phosphate (Flavin mononucleotide)

O O
CH_2—$(CHOH)_2$—CH_2O—P—O—P—OCH_2
OH OH
N N CO
CH_2 CH_3
N C NH
O
CH
HOCH
O
HOCH
CH
NH_3
N C C N
CH C N CH
N

Flavin adenine dinucleotide (FAD)

FIGURE 7.1 Structural formulas of riboflavin and the two coenzymes derived from riboflavin, FMN and FAD. FMN is formed from riboflavin by the addition in the 5′ position of a phosphate group derived from adenosine triphosphate. FAD is formed from FMN after combination with a second molecule of adenosine triphosphate.

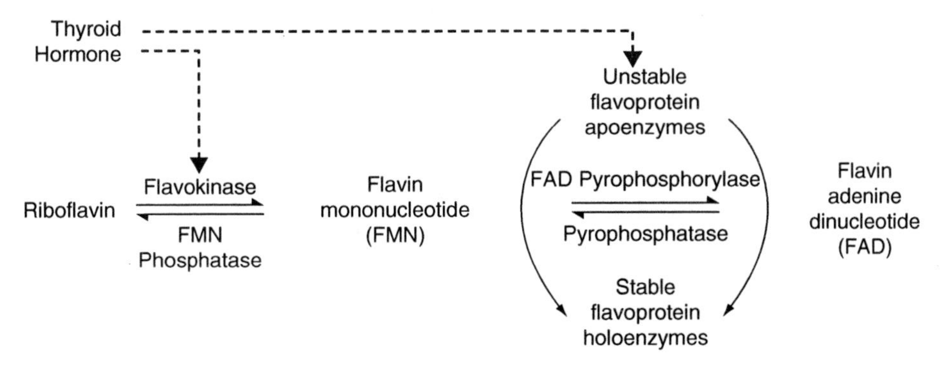

FIGURE 7.2 Metabolic pathway of conversion of riboflavin into FMN, FAD, and covalently bound flavin, together with its control by thyroid hormones. (From Rivlin, R.S., *N. Engl. J. Med.*, 283, 463, 1970.)

RIBOFLAVIN DEFICIENCY AND FOOD-RELATED ISSUES

RIBOFLAVIN DEFICIENCY

Isolated clinical deficiency of riboflavin is not recognizable at the bedside by any unique or characteristic physical feature. The classical glossitis, angular stomatitis, and dermatitis observed in advanced cases are not specific to riboflavin deficiency and may be due to other vitamin deficiencies as well. In fact, when deficiency of riboflavin does occur, it is almost invariably in association with multiple nutrient deficits (22).

With the onset of riboflavin deficiency, one of the adaptations that occurs is a fall in the hepatic free riboflavin pool to nearly undetectable levels, with relative sparing of the pools of FMN and FAD that are needed to fulfill critical metabolic functions (23). Another adaptation to riboflavin deficiency in its early stages is an increase in the de novo synthesis of reduced glutathione (GSH) from its amino acid precursors, in response to the diminished conversion of oxidized glutathione back to GSH (24). This may represent a compensatory reaction resulting from depressed activity of glutathione reductase, a key FAD-requiring enzyme, as shown in Figure 7.3.

Dietary inadequacy is not the only cause of riboflavin deficiency. Certain endocrine abnormalities, such as adrenal and thyroid hormone insufficiency, specific drugs, and diseases may interfere significantly with vitamin utilization (24,25). Psychotropic agents, such as chlorpromazine; antidepressants, including imipramine and amitriptyline (26); cancer

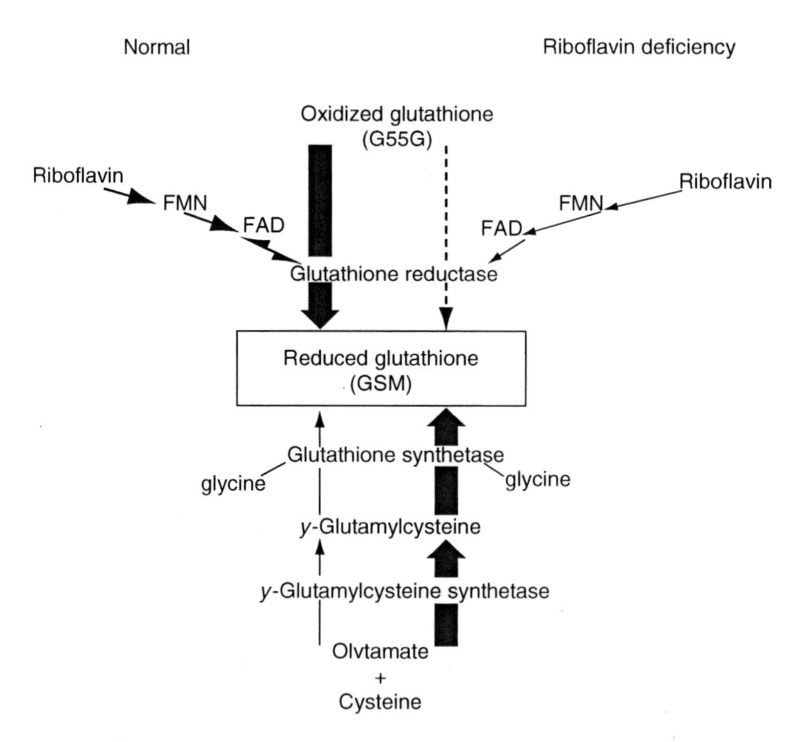

FIGURE 7.3 Regeneration of reduced glutathione (GSH) under normal and riboflavin-deficient conditions. The diagram represents two major pathways for the formation of GSH in erythrocytes, that is, reduction of oxidized glutathione (GSSG) via the glutathione reductase pathway and de novo biosynthesis via glutamylcysteine synthetase and glutathione synthetase. Bold arrows are used to emphasize the predominant pathways, thin arrows represent pathways that are operating below maximal levels, and the dotted arrow indicates diminished enzymatic activity.

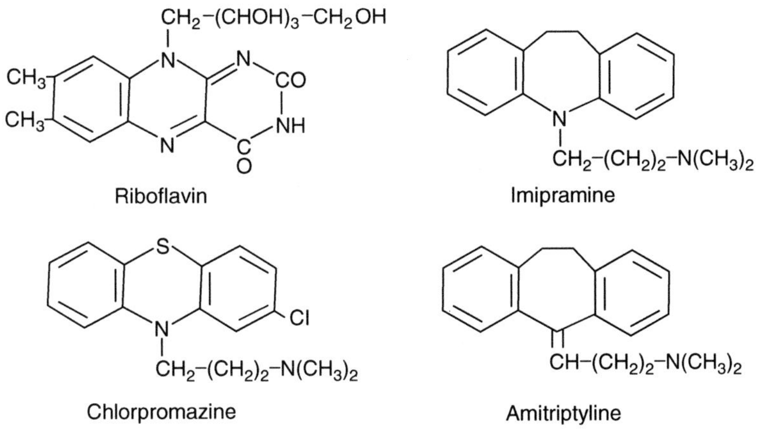

Riboflavin

Imipramine

Chlorpromazine

Amitriptyline

FIGURE 7.4 Structural formulas of riboflavin, chlorpromazine, imipramine, and amitriptyline showing their similarities.

chemotherapeutic drugs, for example, adriamycin; and some antimalarial agents, for example, quinacrine (27), impair riboflavin utilization by inhibiting the conversion of this vitamin into its active coenzyme derivatives. Figure 7.4 shows the structural similarities among riboflavin, imipramine, chlorpromazine, and amitriptyline. There is evidence that alcohol causes riboflavin deficiency by inhibiting both its digestion from dietary sources and its intestinal absorption (28).

In approaching riboflavin deficiency, as well as other nutrient deficiencies, it may be useful to think in terms of risk factors. That is to say, the consequences of a poor diet may be intensified if the patient is also abusing alcohol, using certain drugs for prolonged periods, is elderly, or has malabsorption or other underlying illnesses affecting vitamin metabolism (24).

In experimental animals, hepatic architecture is markedly disrupted in riboflavin deficiency. Mitochondria in riboflavin-deficient mice increase greatly in size, and cristae increase in both number and size (29). These structural abnormalities may disturb energy metabolism by interfering with the electron transport chain and metabolism of fatty acids. Villi decrease in number in the rat small intestine; villus length increases, as does the rate of transit of developing enterocytes along the villus (30). These structural abnormalities, together with the accelerated rate of intestinal cell turnover (31), may help to explain why dietary riboflavin deficiency leads to both decreased iron absorption and increased iron loss from the intestine.

There are many other effects of riboflavin deficiency on intermediary metabolism, particularly in lipid, protein, and vitamin metabolism. Of particular relevance is the impaired conversion of vitamin B_6 to its coenzyme derivative, pyridoxal-5′-phosphate (32). Riboflavin deficiency has been studied in many animal species and has several vital effects, foremost of which is failure to grow. Other effects include loss of hair, skin disturbances, degenerative changes in the nervous system, and impaired reproduction. Congenital malformations occur in the offspring of female rats that are riboflavin-deficient. The conjunctivae become inflamed, and the cornea is vascularized and eventually opaque with cataract formation (33).

Changes in the skin consist of scaliness and incrustation of red–brown material consistent with changes in lipid metabolism. Alopecia may develop, lips become red and swollen, and filiform papillae on the tongue deteriorate. During late deficiency, anemia develops. Fatty degeneration of the liver occurs. Important metabolic changes occur, so that deficient rats require 15% to 20% more energy than control animals to maintain the same body weight

(34,35). Thus, in all species studied, riboflavin deficiency causes profound structural and functional changes in an ordered sequence. Early changes are very readily reversible. Later anatomical changes, such as formation of cataract, are largely irreversible despite treatment with riboflavin.

In humans, as noted earlier, the clinical features of human riboflavin deficiency do not have absolute specificity. Early symptoms may include weakness, fatigue, mouth pain and tenderness, burning and itching of the eyes, and possible personality changes. More advanced deficiency may give rise to cheilosis, angular stomatitis, dermatitis, corneal vascularization, anemia, and brain dysfunction. Thus, the syndrome of dietary riboflavin deficiency in humans has many similarities to that in animals, with one notable exception. The spectrum of congenital malformations observed in rodents (33) with maternal riboflavin deficiency has not been clearly identified in humans.

The role of riboflavin in cataract has been the subject of recent renewed interest. For some time, higher intake of riboflavin has been associated with reduced cataract formation (36). The use of riboflavin for a 5 year period in the Nurses Health Study was associated with a decreasing rate of development of lens opacification (37). In another study of patients who already had keratoconus, riboflavin administered in eye drops delayed its progression (38). Treatment of keratoconus with riboflavin and UV light increases the stiffness of the cornea, increases the cross-linking of collagen, and in this manner may inhibit progression of the disorder. UVA light reduces the activity of glutathione reductase in the lens because of the light sensitivity of its FAD coenzyme (39).

Food-Related Issues

The most significant dietary sources of riboflavin in the United States today are meat and meat products, including poultry and fish, as well as milk and dairy products, such as eggs and cheese. In developing countries, plant sources contribute most of the dietary riboflavin intake. Green vegetables, such as broccoli, collard greens, and turnip greens, are reasonably good sources of riboflavin. Natural grain products tend to be relatively low in riboflavin, but fortification and enrichment of grains and cereals has led to a considerable increase in riboflavin intake from these food items.

The food sources of riboflavin are similar to those of other B vitamins. Therefore, it is not surprising that if a given individual's diet has inadequate amounts of riboflavin, it is very likely to be inadequate in other vitamins as well. A primary deficiency of dietary riboflavin has wide implications for other vitamins, as flavin coenzymes are involved in the metabolism of folic acid, pyridoxine, vitamin K, niacin, and vitamin D (22).

Several factors in food preparation and processing may influence the amount of riboflavin that is actually bioavailable from dietary sources. In view of the light sensitivity of riboflavin noted earlier, it is not surprising that appreciable amounts of riboflavin may be lost with exposure to UV light, particularly during cooking and processing. Prolonged storage of milk in clear bottles or containers may result in flavin degradation (40). Fortunately, most milk is no longer sold in clear bottles. There has been some controversy as to whether opaque plastic containers provide greater protection than do cartons, particularly when milk is stored on a grocery shelf exposed to continuous fluorescent lighting. Milk must be perfectly protected against light; otherwise significant amounts of riboflavin and vitamin A will be lost and the flavor will deteriorate (41).

It is highly likely that large amounts of riboflavin are lost during the sun-drying of fruits and vegetables. The precise magnitude of the loss is not known but varies with the duration of exposure. The practice of adding sodium bicarbonate as baking soda to green vegetables to make them appear fresh can result in accelerated photodegradation of riboflavin. The riboflavin content of common food items with the highest amounts is shown in Table 7.1.

TABLE 7.1
Top Sources of Riboflavin and Their Caloric Content

Top Food Sources	Riboflavin (mg/100 g)	Energy (kcal/100 g)	Top Food Sources	Riboflavin (mg/100 g)	Energy (kcal/100 g)
Yeast baker's dry (active)	5.41	282	Cheese, pasteurized, process American	3.53	375
Liver, lamb, broiled	5.11	261	Liver, chicken, simmered	1.75	165
Yeast, torula	5.06	277	Corn flakes, with added nutrients	1.40	380
Kidneys, beef, braised	4.58	252	Almonds, shelled	0.93	598
Liver, hog, fried in margarine	4.36	241	Cheese, natural, Roquefort	0.59	369
Yeast, brewer's, debittered	4.28	283	Eggs, chicken, fried	0.54	210
Liver, beef or calf, fried	4.18	242	Beef, tenderloin steak, broiled	0.46	224
Brewer's yeast, tablet form	4.04	—	Mushrooms, raw	0.46	28
Cheese, pasteurized, process American	3.53	375	Cheese, natural Swiss (American)	0.40	372
Turkey, giblets, cooked (some gizzard fat), simmered	2.72	233	Wheat flour, all-purpose, enriched	0.40	365
Kidneys, lamb, raw	2.42	105	Turnip greens, raw	0.39	28
Kidneys, calf, raw	2.40	113	Cheese, natural Cheddar	0.38	402
Eggs, chicken, dried, white powder	2.32	372	Wheat bran	0.35	353
Whey, sweet, dry	2.21	354	Soybean flour	0.35	333
Eggs, chicken, dried, white flakes	2.16	351	Bacon, cured, cooked, drained, sliced medium	0.34	575
Liver, turkey, simmered	2.09	174	Pork, loin, lean, broiled	0.33	391
Whey, acid dry	2.06	339	Lamb, leg, good or choice, separable lean roasted	0.30	186
Heart, hog, braised	1.89	195	Corn meal, degermed, enriched	0.26	362
Milk, cow's dry, skim, solids, instant	1.78	353	Chicken, dark meat without skin, fried	0.25	220
Liver, chicken, simmered	1.75	165	Bread, white, enriched	0.24	270
Liver, beef or calf, fried	4.18	242	Milk, cow's, whole, 3.7%	0.17	66

Source: From Ensminger, A.M., Ensminger, M.E., Konlande, J.E., and Robson, J.R.K. in *Food and Nutrition Encyclopedia*, CRC Press, Boca Raton, FL, p. 1927, 1994.

Figures are given in terms of the riboflavin and calorie amounts in 100 g (approximately 3.5 oz) of the items as usually consumed. Portion size and moisture content differ among food items.

PHYSIOLOGY

Absorption, Transport, Storage, Turnover, and Excretion

Since dietary sources of riboflavin are largely in the form of their coenzyme derivatives, these molecules must be hydrolyzed before absorption. Very little dietary riboflavin is found as free riboflavin from sources in nature. Under ordinary circumstances, the main sources of free riboflavin are commercial multivitamin preparations, which are consumed increasingly by the general public.

The absorptive process for flavins occurs in the upper gastrointestinal tract by specialized transport involving a dephosphorylation–rephosphorylation mechanism, rather than by passive diffusion. This process is sodium-dependent and involves an ATPase-active transport system that can be saturated (35). It has been estimated that under normal conditions the upper limit of intestinal absorption of riboflavin at any one time is approximately 25 mg (34). This amount represents approximately 15 times the recommended dietary allowance (RDA). Therefore, the common practice of some megavitamin enthusiasts to consume massive doses of multivitamins has little benefit with respect to riboflavin, as the additional amounts would be passed in the stool. Dietary covalent-bound flavins are largely inaccessible as nutritional sources. In experimental animals, the uptake of riboflavin from the intestine is increased in dietary riboflavin deficiency (35), which likely represents an adaptive mechanism to vitamin deficiency.

A number of physiological factors influence the rate of intestinal absorption of riboflavin (24). Diets high in psyllium gum decrease the rate of riboflavin absorption, whereas wheat bran has no detectable effect. The time from oral administration to peak urinary excretion of riboflavin is prolonged by the antacids, aluminum hydroxide, and magnesium hydroxide. Total urinary excretion is unchanged by these drugs, however, and their major effects appear to be delaying the rate of intestinal absorption rather than inhibiting net absorption. As noted earlier, alcohol interferes with both the digestion of food flavins into riboflavin and the direct intestinal absorption of the vitamin (28). This observation suggests that the initial rehabilitation of malnourished alcoholic patients may be accomplished more rapidly and efficiently with vitamin supplements containing riboflavin rather than with food sources comprising predominantly phosphorylated flavin derivates. This hypothesis needs to be tested directly.

There is evidence that the magnitude of intestinal absorption of riboflavin is increased by the presence of food. This effect of food may be due to decreasing the rates of gastric emptying and intestinal transit, thereby permitting more prolonged contact of dietary riboflavin with the absorptive surface of the intestinal mucosal cells. In general, delaying the rate of gastric emptying tends to increase the intestinal absorption of riboflavin. Bile salts also increase the rate of intestinal absorption of riboflavin (24).

A number of metals and drugs form chelates or complexes with riboflavin and riboflavin-5′-phosphate that may affect their bioavailability (42). Among the agents in this category are the metals, copper, zinc, and iron; the drugs, caffeine, theophylline, and saccharin; and the vitamins, nicotinamide and ascorbic acid; as well as tryptophan and urea. The clinical significance of this complex formation is not known with certainty in most instances and deserves further study.

In human blood, the transport of flavins involves loose binding to albumin and tight binding to a number of globulins. The major binding of riboflavin and its phosphorylated derivatives in serum is to several classes of immunoglobulins, that is, IgA, IgG, and IgM (42). In human erythrocytes, there is very little free riboflavin, compared with the much larger amounts of FMN and FAD (43). Following supplementation of human subjects with 1.6 mg/day of riboflavin, the concentrations of riboflavin in serum and FMN in erythrocytes are increased more than 80% compared with levels in placebo-fed controls (43).

Pregnancy induces the formation of flavin-specific binding proteins initially found in birds (44). Riboflavin-binding proteins have also been found in sera from pregnant cows, monkeys, and humans. A comprehensive review of riboflavin-binding proteins covers the nature of the binding proteins in various species and provides evidence that, as in birds, these proteins are crucial for successful mammalian reproduction (13). Pregnancy-specific binding proteins may help transport riboflavin to the fetus.

Serum riboflavin-binding proteins appear to influence placental transfer and fetal or maternal distribution of riboflavin. There are differential rates of uptake of riboflavin at the maternal and fetal surfaces of the human placenta (45). Riboflavin-binding proteins regulate the activity of flavokinase, the first biosynthetic enzyme in the riboflavin-to-FAD pathway (21).

Urinary excretion of flavins occurs predominantly in the form of riboflavin; FMN and FAD are not found in urine. McCormick (13) has identified and described a large number of flavins and their derivatives in human urine. Besides the 60% to 70% of urinary flavins contributed by riboflavin itself, other major derivatives include 7-hydroxymethylriboflavin (10% to 15%), 8α-sulfonylriboflavin (5% to 10%), 8-hydroxymethylriboflavin (4% to 7%), riboflavinyl peptide ester (5%), and 10-hydroxyethylflavin (1% to 3%), representing largely metabolites from covalently bound flavoproteins and intestinal riboflavin degradation by microorganisms. Traces of lumiflavin and other derivatives have also been found.

Accidental ingestion of boric acid greatly increases urinary excretion of riboflavin (24). This agent when consumed forms a complex with the side chain of riboflavin and other molecules that have polyhydroxyl groups, such as glucose and ascorbic acid. In rodents, riboflavin treatment greatly ameliorates the toxicity of administered boric acid. This treatment should also be effective in humans with accidental exposure of boric acid, although in practice it may be difficult to provide adequate amounts of riboflavin because of its low solubility and limited absorptive capacity from the intestinal tract.

Urinary excretion of riboflavin in rats is also greatly increased by chlorpromazine (46). Levels are twice those of age- and sex-matched pair-fed control rats. In addition, chlorpromazine accelerates urinary excretion of riboflavin during dietary deficiency. Urinary concentrations of riboflavin are increased within 6 h of treatment with this drug.

SPECIFIC FUNCTIONS

The major function of riboflavin, as noted earlier, is to serve as the precursor of the flavin coenzymes, FMN and FAD, and of covalently bound flavins. These coenzymes are widely distributed in intermediary metabolism and catalyze numerous oxidation–reduction reactions. As FAD is part of the respiratory chain, riboflavin is central to energy production. Other major functions of riboflavin include drug and steroid metabolism, in conjunction with cytochrome P450 enzymes, and lipid metabolism. The redox functions of flavin coenzymes include both one-electron transfers and two-electron transfers from the substrate to the flavin coenzymes (13).

Flavoproteins catalyze dehydrogenation reactions as well as hydroxylations, oxidative decarboxylations, dioxygenations, and reductions of oxygen to hydrogen peroxide. Thus, many different kinds of oxidative and reductive reactions are catalyzed by flavoproteins.

Antioxidant Activity

In the wake of contemporary interest in dietary antioxidants, one vitamin that is often not appreciated sufficiently as a member of this category is riboflavin. Riboflavin has little, if any, significant antioxidant action per se, but powerful antioxidant activity is derived from its role as a precursor to FMN and FAD. A major protective role against lipid peroxides is provided by the glutathione redox cycle (47). Glutathione peroxidase breaks down reactive lipid peroxides. This enzyme requires GSH, which in turn is regenerated from its oxidized form (GSSG) by the FAD-containing enzyme glutathione reductase. Thus, riboflavin nutrition may be critical in regulating the rate of inactivation of lipid peroxides. Diminished glutathione reductase activity would be expected to lead to diminished concentrations of GSH that serve as substrate for glutathione peroxidase and glutathione S-transferase, and therefore would limit the rate of degradation of lipid peroxides and xenobiotic substances (48).

Furthermore, the reducing equivalents provided by NADPH, the other substrate required by glutathione reductase, are primarily generated by an enzyme of the pentose monophosphate shunt, glucose-6-phosphate dehydrogenase. Taniguchi and Hara (49), as well as Dutta et al. (50), have found that the activity of glucose-6-phosphate dehydrogenase is significantly diminished during riboflavin deficiency. This observation provides an additional mechanism to explain the diminished glutathione reductase activity in vivo during riboflavin deficiency and the eventual decrease in antioxidant activity.

There have been reports (51,52) indicating that riboflavin deficiency is associated with compromised oxidant defense and furthermore that supplementation of riboflavin and its active analogs improves oxidant status. Riboflavin deficiency is associated with increased hepatic lipid peroxidation and riboflavin supplementation limits this process (49–52). In our laboratory, we have shown that feeding a riboflavin-deficient diet to rats increases basal as well as stimulated lipid peroxidation (48).

Riboflavin and Malaria

There is increasing evidence that riboflavin deficiency may be protective against malaria both in experimental animals and in humans (53,54). With dietary riboflavin deficiency, parasitemia is decreased dramatically, and symptomatology of infection may be diminished. In a study with human infants suffering from malaria, normal riboflavin nutritional status was associated with high levels of parasitemia. In similar fashion, supplementation with iron and vitamins that included riboflavin resulted in increased malaria parasitemia (55,56).

Further evidence for a beneficial role of riboflavin deficiency in malaria is provided by studies using specific antagonists of riboflavin, for example, galactoflavin and 10-(4′-chlorophenyl)-3-methylflavin (57,58). These flavin analogs as well as newer isoalloxazines derivatives are glutathione reductase inhibitors and possess clear antimalarial efficacy. The exact mechanism by which riboflavin deficiency appears to inhibit malarial parasitemia is not yet established. One possibility relates to effects on the redox status of erythrocytes, which is an important determinant of growth of malaria parasites. Protection from malaria is afforded by several oxidant drugs, vitamin E deficiency, and specific genetic abnormalities in which oxidative defense is compromised (47).

It is well known that malaria parasites (*Plasmodium berghei*) are highly susceptible to activated oxygen species. Parasites are relatively more susceptible than erythrocytes to the damaging effects of lipid peroxidation (47). We have hypothesized that the requirement of parasites for riboflavin should be higher than that of the host cells and therefore that marginal riboflavin deficiency should be selectively detrimental to parasites. Support for this hypothesis comes from the finding that the uptake of riboflavin and its conversion to FMN and FAD are significantly higher in parasitized than in unparasitized erythrocytes and furthermore that the rate of uptake of riboflavin is proportional to the degree of parasitemia (59). These results strongly suggest that parasites have a higher requirement for riboflavin than do host erythrocytes.

In a recent report of malaria patients in Gabon (60), plasma levels of FAD, FMN, and riboflavin were normal, but the authors point out that because of the high degree of hemolysis, dehydration, and liver and kidney problems in these patients, plasma flavin levels may not be comparable with values found in other population groups.

Riboflavin and Homocysteine

An emerging role for riboflavin lies in its regulation of homocysteine metabolism. Homocysteine is involved in the pathogenesis of vascular disease, including cardiovascular, cerebrovascular, and peripheral vascular disorders (61). Blood levels of folic acid sensitively determine serum homocysteine concentrations (62). *N*-5-methyltetrahydrofolate is a cosubstrate with homocysteine in its inactivation by conversion to methionine. Methylcobalamin is also a coenzyme in this enzymatic reaction. Vitamin B_6 is widely recognized for its importance in the inactivation of homocysteine by serving as coenzyme for two degradative enzymes, cystathionine β-synthase and cystathioninase.

As we pointed out in the previous edition of this volume (2), it is not widely appreciated that riboflavin also has a vital function in homocysteine metabolism. The flavin coenzyme, FAD, is required by methyltetrahydrofolate reductase, the enzyme responsible for converting *N*-5,10-methylenetetrahydrofolate into *N*-5-methyltetrahydrofolate. Thus, the efficient utilization of dietary folic acid requires adequate riboflavin nutrition.

A mutation leading to a heat-sensitive form of methylenetetrahydrofolate reductase has been identified (63). This genetic variation is found in approximately 10% to 15% of the population of Europe and North America (64). Homozygous individuals are especially sensitive to folate, and those with folate levels in the lower part of the so-called normal range tend to have elevated serum levels of homocysteine.

It is now evident that riboflavin also shares the property of stabilizing this enzyme variation (64,65). Furthermore, there are now a number of reports (66,67) that the state of riboflavin nutrition governs homocysteine metabolism in patients who are homozygous for this genetic variation. It seems likely that patients with this genotype would respond more rapidly and effectively to riboflavin supplementation than those individuals without this genetic variation (63).

Furthermore, dietary intake of riboflavin in food is inversely related to serum homocysteine concentrations in the United States (69). Consistent with this finding is the observation that riboflavin improves the genomic instability of the genetic variant of methylenetetrahydrofolate reductase (68,70–72). Other investigators have suggested that folate and riboflavin together lower plasma homocysteine concentrations regardless of genotype (69).

The results of previous studies demonstrating thyroid hormone control of riboflavin metabolism (15,16,22,24) predict that, as a consequence, thyroid hormone status would regulate serum homocysteine levels. This prediction has been borne out and thyroid hormone status has been shown to affect phenotypic expression of the genetic variant of methylenetetrahydrofolate reductase. With treatment of hyperthyroidism, serum concentrations of flavin cofactors fall as expected and homocysteine levels rise (73).

Inborn Errors of Metabolism

The important role of riboflavin in fat metabolism has been highlighted by demonstrations that in certain rare inborn errors administration of riboflavin may be therapeutic. In acyl-CoA dehydrogenase deficiency, infants present with recurrent hypoglycemia, lipid storage myopathy, and increased urinary excretion of organic acids. Clinical improvement has occurred rapidly after riboflavin supplementation (74,75). Three varieties of the disorder occur, all of which involve flavoproteins of various types. Five patients with a mitochondrial disorder associated with NADH dehydrogenase deficiency were improved by riboflavin treatment (75). A form of riboflavin-responsive glutaric aciduria (type II) can present as a leukodystrophy (76).

The genetic disorder known as riboflavin-responsive, multiple acylcoenzyme A dehydrogenase deficiency is characterized by a lipid storage myopathy and decreased β-oxidation. There are also defects in the respiratory chain. An uncoupling protein (UCP3) is increased in concentration in both this disorder and in normal rodents fasted and may mediate the underlying metabolic abnormalities (77). At present, Type B lactic acidosis occurs in association with HIV treatment and also responds to riboflavin (78,79). This observation, if confirmed and extended, may be of widespread clinical significance.

PHARMACOLOGY, TOXICOLOGY, AND CARCINOGENESIS

There is general agreement that dietary riboflavin intake at many times the RDA is without demonstrable toxicity (13,80–82). Because riboflavin absorption is limited to a maximum of about 25 mg at any one time (13), the consumption of megadoses of this vitamin would not be expected to increase the total amount absorbed significantly. Furthermore, classical animal investigations showed an apparent upper limit to tissue storage of flavins that cannot be exceeded under ordinary circumstances (83). The tissue storage capacity for flavins is probably limited by the availability of proteins capable of providing binding sites. Thus, protective mechanisms prevent tissue accumulation of excessive amounts of the vitamin. Because riboflavin has very low solubility, even intravenous administration of the vitamin would not introduce large amounts into the body. FMN is more water-soluble than riboflavin but is not ordinarily available for clinical use.

Nevertheless, the photosensitizing properties of riboflavin raise the possibility of some potential risks. Phototherapy in vitro leads to degradation of DNA and increase in lipid peroxidation, which may have implications for carcinogenesis, mutagenesis, and other disorders. Irradiation of rat erythrocytes in the presence of FMN increases potassium loss (84). Topical administration of riboflavin to the skin may increase melanin synthesis by stimulation of free-radical formation. Riboflavin forms an adduct with tryptophan and accelerates the photooxidation of this essential amino acid (85). Further research is needed to explore the full implications of the photosensitizing capabilities of riboflavin and its phosphorylated derivatives.

The photosensitization of vinca alkaloids by riboflavin may distort results of efficacy testing of cytotoxic drugs if the studies are carried out in the presence of visible light, as is usually done (86). This property of riboflavin needs to be considered in drug evaluations, inasmuch as cell death will occur even without the addition of the drug.

Riboflavin is capable of reacting with chromate, forming a complex, and then increasing DNA breaks because of a chromium-induced free-radical mechanism (87). Treatment of mouse FM3A cells with riboflavin greatly increases the frequency of mutation and the extent of cellular DNA damage in the presence of light (88). There is increasing evidence that in the presence of visible light, riboflavin and its degradative products may enhance mutagenicity (89).

On the other hand, other studies (90) confirm earlier reports (91) that riboflavin deficiency may enhance carcinogenesis by increasing activation of carcinogens, particularly nitrosamines. Riboflavin may provide protection against damage to DNA caused by certain carcinogens through its action as a coenzyme with a variety of cytochrome P450 enzymes.

It is important to establish the role of riboflavin as a dietary factor capable of preventing carcinogenesis while determining the full implications of the photosensitizing actions of riboflavin on mutagenesis and carcinogenesis. There are reports raising the possibility that deficient riboflavin nutritional status, together with shortages of other vitamins, may possibly enhance development of precancerous lesions of the esophagus in China (92,93) and in Russia (94). These population groups require further long-term follow-up.

REQUIREMENTS AND ASSESSMENT

There are a variety of methods available for analysis of riboflavin and its derivatives in biological samples. Bioassays (95) measure the growth effect of vitamins but lack the precision of more sensitive analytical procedures. Fluorometric procedures take advantage of the inherent fluorescent properties of flavins (96). Some degree of purification of the urine or tissues may be required before analysis is performed as there is often significant interference by other natural substances that lead to quenching of fluorescence and methodological artifacts.

A procedure has been developed for measuring riboflavin by competitive protein binding, which is applicable to studies in human urine (97). Riboflavin binds specifically to the avian egg white riboflavin-binding protein and thereby provides the basis for quantitative analysis (98). Other procedures based on binding to specific apoenzymes, such as D-amino acid oxidase, are also in use. Currently, procedures using high-pressure liquid chromatography (HPLC) are widely applied as they have great precision and can be used for analysis of riboflavin in pure form as well as in biological fluids and tissues (99). HPLC is the method most widely employed at this time for determination of flavins in blood and other tissues.

In clinical studies that involve individual patients as well as population groups, the status of riboflavin nutrition is generally evaluated by determining urinary excretion of riboflavin (100) and the erythrocyte glutathione reductase activity coefficient (EGRAC). Urinary riboflavin determinations are made in the basal state, in random samples, in 24 h collections, or after a riboflavin load test. Normal urinary excretion of riboflavin is approximately 120 μg/g creatinine/24 h or higher. It is useful to express urinary excretion in terms of creatinine to verify the completeness of the collection and to relate excretion to this biological parameter. Expressed in terms of the total amount of urinary flavins in the normal adult (not taking supplements), excretion is about 1.5–2.5 mg/day, which is very close to the RDA of the National Academy of Sciences. Riboflavin excretion per se is only about 1.0–1.5 mg/day. Flavin metabolites account for an appreciable portion of total urinary flavins, as noted earlier.

In deficient adult individuals, urinary riboflavin excretion is reduced to about 40 μg/g creatinine/24 h. Thus, deficient individuals have reduced urinary excretion, reflecting diminished dietary intake and depleted body stores. Normal urinary excretion is reduced with age, may be reduced by physical activity (as discussed later), and is stimulated by elevated body temperature, treatment with certain drugs, and various stressful conditions associated with negative nitrogen balance (99). Interpretation of urinary riboflavin excretion must be made with these factors in mind.

Another potential drawback to using urinary riboflavin excretion as an assessment of nutritional status of this vitamin is that the amount excreted reflects recent intake very sensitively. Thus, if an individual has been depleted of riboflavin for a long time but consumes a food item high in riboflavin, urinary excretion determined a few hours later may not be in the deficient range, but is likely to be normal or even elevated.

It is for this reason that attention has been directed to the development of assessment techniques that more accurately reflect long-term riboflavin status. The method most widely employed that largely meets these needs is the EGRAC assay, as noted earlier. The principle of the method is that the degree of saturation of the apoenzyme with its coenzyme, FAD, should reflect the body stores of FAD. In deficient individuals, relative unsaturation of the apoenzyme with FAD leads to decreased basal activity of the enzyme. Therefore, the addition of FAD to the enzyme contained in a fresh erythrocyte hemolysate from deficient individuals will increase activity in vitro to a greater extent than that observed in a preparation from well-nourished individuals in whom the apoenzyme is more saturated with FAD.

The EGRAC is the ratio of in vitro enzyme activity with the addition of FAD to that without it. In general, most studies propose that an activity coefficient of 1.2 or less indicates adequate riboflavin status, 1.2–1.4 borderline-to-low status, and greater than 1.4 a clear riboflavin deficiency (100,101).

It must be kept in mind that a number of physiological variables influence the results of this determination. In the inherited disorder of glucose-6-phosphate dehydrogenase deficiency, associated with hemolytic anemia, the apoenzyme has a higher affinity for FAD than that of the normal erythrocyte and will affect the measured EGRAC. Thyroid function affects glutathione reductase activity, with the coefficient elevated in hypothyroidism and decreased in hyperthyroidism (102), reflecting that hypothyroidism has many biochemical features in common with those of riboflavin deficiency (24).

The latest RDAs issued by the Food and Nutrition Board (80) call for adult males aged 19–50 years to consume 1.3 mg/day. Adult females from 19 to 50 years of age should consume 1.1 mg/day. It is recommended that intake be increased to 1.4 mg/day during pregnancy and to 1.6 mg/day in lactation.

There has been some concern as to whether these figures are applicable to other population groups around the world. Chinese tend to excrete very little riboflavin, and their requirement may be lower than that of Americans (103). Adults in Guatemala have similar requirements in individuals older than 60 compared with those 51 years or younger (104). This finding may not necessarily be relevant to populations of other countries. The requirements of various national groups require further study. Environmental factors, protein-calorie intake, physical activity, and other factors may have an impact on riboflavin requirements. More research is needed on the requirements of the extremely old, who form an increasingly large proportion of the population. They are also the population group that consumes the largest number of prescribed and over-the-counter medications.

In women aged 50–67 who exercise vigorously for 20–25 min/day, 6 days a week, both a decrease in riboflavin excretion and a rise in the EGRAC were noted, findings consistent with a marginal riboflavin-deficient state (105). Supplementation with riboflavin did not, however, improve exercise performance. These investigators observed compromised riboflavin status as well in young women exercising vigorously (106). Similar observations of reduced urinary riboflavin excretion and elevated EGRAC were made in young Indian males who exercised actively (107).

To determine whether the status of riboflavin nutrition influences metabolic responses to exercise, blood lactate levels were determined in a group of physically active college students from Finland before and after an exercise period. A number of the students were initially in a state of marginal riboflavin deficiency. Following supplementation with vitamins, including riboflavin, which produced improvement in the elevated EGRAC, the blood lactate levels were unaffected and were related only to the degree of exercise (108).

Thus, to date, while exercise clearly produces biochemical abnormalities in riboflavin metabolism, it has not been shown that these abnormalities lead to impaired performance, nor has it been shown that riboflavin supplementation under these conditions leads to improved exercise performance.

ACKNOWLEDGMENTS

This research was supported in part by the Clinical Nutrition Research Unit grant (P30-CA29502) from the National Institutes of Health and by grants from the Sunny and Abe Rosenberg Foundation, American Institute for Cancer Research (AICR), the Ronald and Susan Lynch Foundation, the editor C. Blum Foundation, and the Heisman Trophy Trust.

REFERENCES

1. Powers, H.J. Riboflavin (vitamin B_2) and health. *Am. J. Clin. Nutr.*, 77, 1352, 2003.
2. Rivlin, R.S. and Pinto, J.T. Riboflavin, in *Present Knowledge in Nutrition*, 8th ed. Bowman, B and Russell, R., eds., ILSI Press, Washington, DC, pp. 1313–1332, 2001.
3. Baxter, P. Vitamin responsive conditions in paediatric neurology, in *International Review of Child Neurology Series*. Baxter, P., ed., MacKeith Press, London, 60, p. 181, 2003.
4. McCollum, E.V. and Kennedy, C. The dietary factors operating in the production of polyneuritis. *J. Biol. Chem.*, 24, 491, 1916.
5. Emmett, A.D. and Luros, G.O. Water soluble vitamins. I. Are the antineuritic and the growth-promoting water-soluble B vitamins the same? *J. Biol. Chem.*, 43, 265, 1920.
6. Warburg, O. and Christian W. Uber ein neues Oxydationsferment und sein Absorptionsspetrum. *Biochem., Z.* 254, 438, 1932.
7. Stern, K.G. and Holiday, E.R. Zur Konstitution des Photo-flavins; Versuche in der Alloxazine-Reihe. Ber. *Dtsch. Chem. Gesellsch.*, 67, 1104, 1934.
8. Theorell, H. Reindarstellung (Kristallisation) des gelben Atmungsfermentes und die reversible Spaltung desselben. *Biochem., Z.* 272, 155, 1934.
9. Kuhn, R. et al. Synthetisches 6,7-Dimethyl-9-d-riboflavin. *Naturwissenschaften* 23, 260, 1935.
10. Karrer, P., Scopp, K., and Benz, F. Synthesis of flavins IV. *Helv. Chim. Acta*, 18, 426, 1935.
11. Theorell, H. Die freie Eiweisskomponente des gelben Ferments und ihre Kupplung mit Lactoflavinphosphorsaure. *Biochem., Z.* 290, 293, 1937.
12. Warburg, O. and Christian, W. Co-Ferment der d-Aminosaure-Deaminase. *Biochem., Z.* 295, 261, 1938.
13. McCormick, D.B. Riboflavin, in *Modern Nutrition in Health and Disease*, 8th ed. Shils, M.E., Olson, J.A., and Shike, M., eds., Lea and Febiger, Philadelphia, p. 366, 1994.
14. Yagi, K. et al. Incorporation of riboflavin into covalently-bound flavins in rat liver. *J. Biochem.*, 79, 841, 1976.
15. Rivlin, R.S. Medical progress: riboflavin metabolism. *N. Engl. J. Med.*, 283, 463, 1970.
16. Pinto, J.T. and Rivlin, R.S. Regulation of formation of covalently bound flavins in liver and cerebrum by thyroid hormones. *Arch. Biochem. Biophys.*, 194, 313, 1979.
17. Paine, M.J. et al. Cloning and characterization of a novel human dual flavin reductase. *J. Biol. Chem.*, 275, 1471, 2000.
18. Finn, R.D. et al. Determination of the redox potentials and electron transfer properties of the FAD- and FMN-binding domains of the human oxidoreductase NRI. *Eur. J. Biochem.*, 270, 1164, 2003.
19. Bredt, D.S. et al. Cloned and expressed nitric oxide synthase structurally resembles cytochrome P-450 reductase. *Nature* 351, 714, 1991.
20. Dignam, J. and Strobel, H. Preparation of homogeneous NADPH-cytochrome P-450 reductase from rat liver. *Biochim. Biophys. Res. Commun.*, 63, 845, 1975.
21. Merrill, A.H. Jr. et al. Formation and mode of action of flavoproteins. *Annu. Rev. Nutr.*, 1, 281, 1981.
22. Rivlin, R.S. Vitamin deficiency, in *Conns' Current Therapy*. Rakel, R.E., ed., W.B. Saunders, Philadelphia, p. 551, 1994.
23. Fass, S. and Rivlin, R.S. Regulation of riboflavin-metabolizing enzymes in riboflavin deficiency. *Am. J. Physiol.*, 217, 988, 1969.
24. Rivlin, R.S. Disorders of vitamin metabolism: deficiencies, metabolic abnormalities and excesses, in *Cecil Textbook of Medicine*, 19th ed., Wyngaarden, J.H., Smith, L.H. Jr., Bennett, J.C., and Plum, F., eds., W.B. Saunders, Philadelphia, 1170, 1991.
25. Cimino, J.A. et al. Riboflavin metabolism in the hypothyroid human adult. *Proc. Soc. Exp. Biol. Med.*, 184, 121, 1987.
26. Pinto, J.T., Huang, Y.P., and Rivlin, R.S. Inhibition of riboflavin metabolism in rat tissues by chlorpromazine, imipramine and amitriptyline. *J. Clin. Invest.*, 67, 1500, 1981.
27. Dutta, P., Pinto, J.T., and Rivlin, R.S. Antimalarial effects of riboflavin deficiency. *Lancet* 2, 1040, 1985.
28. Pinto, J.T., Huang, J.P., and Rivlin, R.S. Mechanisms underlying the differential effects of ethanol upon the bioavailability of riboflavin and flavin adenine dinucleotide. *J. Clin. Invest.*, 79, 1343, 1987.

29. Tandler, B., Erlandson, R.A., and Wynder, E.L. Riboflavin and mouse hepatic cell structure and function. I. Ultrastructural alterations in simple deficiency. *Am. J. Pathol.*, 52, 69, 1968.
30. Williams, E.A., Rumsey, R.D.E., and Powers, H.J. Cytokinetic and structural responses of the rat small intestine to riboflavin depletion. *Br. J. Nutr.*, 75, 315, 1996.
31. Powers, H.J. et al. A proposed intestinal mechanism for the effect of riboflavin deficiency on iron loss in the rat. *Br. J. Nutr.*, 69, 551, 1993.
32. McCormick, D.B. Two interconnected B vitamins: riboflavin and pyridoxine. *Physiol. Rev.*, 69, 1170, 1989.
33. Goldsmith, G.A. Riboflavin deficiency, in *Riboflavin*. Rivlin, R.S., ed., Plenum Press, NY, p. 221, 1975.
34. Zempleni, J., Galloway, J.R., and McCormick, D.B. Pharmacokinetics of orally and intravenously administered riboflavin in healthy humans. *Am. J. Clin. Nutr.*, 63, 54, 1996.
35. Said, H.M. and Mohammadkhani, R. Uptake of riboflavin across the brush border membrane of rat intestine: regulation by dietary vitamin levels. *Gastroenterology* 105, 1294, 1993.
36. Jacques, P.F. Nutritional antioxidants and prevention of age-related eye disease, in *Antioxidants and Disease Prevention*. Garewal, H.S., ed., CRC Press, Boca Raton, FL, p. 149, 1997.
37. Jacques, P.F. et al. Long-term nutrient intake and 5-year change in nuclear lens opacities. *Arch. Ophthalmol.*, 123, 517, 2005.
38. Sandner, D. et al. Collagen crosslinking by combined riboflavin/ultraviolet-A (UVA) treatment can stop progression of keratoconus. *Invest. Ophthalmol. Vis. Sci.*, 45, E-abstract, 2887, 2004.
39. Linetsky, M. et al. Studies on the mechanism of the UVA light-dependent loss of glutathione reductase activity in human lenses. *Invest. Ophthalmol. Vis. Sci.*, 44, 3920, 2003.
40. Wanner, R.L. Effects of commercial processing of milk and milk products on their nutrient content, in *The Nutritional Evaluation of Food Processing*. Harris, R.S. and Loesecke, H.V., eds., John Wiley, NY, p. 173, 1960.
41. Mestdagh, F. et al. Protective influence of several packaging materials on light oxidation of milk. *J. Dairy Sci.*, 88, 499, 2005.
42. McCormick, D.B. Riboflavin, in *Present Knowledge in Nutrition*, 6th ed. Brown, M.L., ed., International Life Sciences Institute, Washington, DC, p. 146, 1990.
43. Hustad, S. et al. Riboflavin, flavin mononucleotide and flavin adenine dinucleotide in human plasma and erythrocytes at baseline and after low-dose riboflavin supplementation. *Clin. Chem.*, 48, 157, 2002.
44. Clagett, C.O. Genetic control of the riboflavin carrier protein. *Fed. Proc.*, 30, 127, 1971.
45. Dancis, J., Lehanka, J., and Levitz, M. Placental transport of riboflavin: differential rates of uptake at the maternal and fetal surfaces of the perfused human placenta. *J. Obstet. Gynecol.*, 158, 204, 1988.
46. Pelliccione, N.J. et al. Accelerated development of riboflavin deficiency by treatment with chlorpromazine. *Biochem. Pharmacol.*, 32, 2949, 1983.
47. Dutta, P. Disturbances in glutathione metabolism and resistance to malaria: current understanding and new concepts. *J. Soc. Pharm. Chem.*, 23, 11, 1993.
48. Rivlin, R.S. and Dutta, P. Vitamin B_2 (riboflavin). Relevance to malaria and antioxidant activity. *Nutr. Today* 30, 62, 1995.
49. Taniguchi, M. and Hara, T. Effects of riboflavin and selenium deficiencies on glutathione and related enzyme activities with respect to lipid peroxide content of rat livers. *J. Nutr. Vitaminol.* 29, 283, 1983.
50. Dutta, P. et al. Acute ethanol exposure alters hepatic glutathione metabolism in riboflavin deficiency. *Alcohol* 12, 43, 1995.
51. Miyazawa, T., Tsuchiya, K., and Kaneda, T. Riboflavin tetrabutyrate: an antioxidative synergist of alpha-tocopherol as estimated by hepatic chemiluminescense. *Nutr. Rep. Int.*, 29, 157, 1984.
52. Miyazawa, T., Sato, C., and Kaneda, T. Antioxidative effects of α-tocopherol and riboflavin-butyrate in rats dosed with methyl linoleate hydroperoxide. *Agric. Biol. Chem.*, 47, 1577, 1983.
53. Kaikai, P. and Thurnham, D.I. The influence of riboflavin deficiency on *Plasmodium berghei* infections in rats. *Trans. R. Soc. Trop. Med. Hyg.*, 77, 680, 1983.
54. Das, B.S. et al. Riboflavin deficiency and severity of malaria. *Eur. J. Clin. Nutr.*, 42, 227, 1988.
55. Thurnham, D.I., Oppenheimer, S.J., and Bull, R. Riboflavin status and malaria in infants in Papua New Guinea. *Trans. R. Soc. Trop. Med. Hyg.*, 77, 423, 1983.

56. Oppenheimer, S.J., Bull, R., and Thurnham, D.I. Riboflavin deficiency in Madang infants. *Papua N. Guinea Med. J.*, 26, 17, 1983.
57. Becker, K. et al. Flavin analogs with antimalarial activity as glutathione reductase inhibitors. *Biochem. Pharmacol.*, 39, 59, 1990.
58. Schonleben-Jana, A. et al. Inhibition of human glutathione reductase by 10-arylisoalloxazines: crystallographic, kinetic and electrochemical studies. *J. Med. Chem.*, 39, 1549, 1996.
59. Dutta, P. Enhanced uptake and metabolism of riboflavin in erythrocytes infected with *Plasmodium falciparium. J. Protozool.*, 38, 479, 1991.
60. Traunmuller, F. et al. Normal riboflavin status in malaria patients in Gabon. *Am. J. Trop. Med. Hyg.*, 68, 182, 2003.
61. Graham, I.A. et al. Plasma homocysteine as a risk factor for vascular disease. The European concerted project. *JAMA* 277, 1775, 1997.
62. Boushey, C.J. et al. A quantitative assessment of plasma homocysteine as a risk factor for vascular disease. *JAMA* 274, 1049, 1995.
63. Frosst, P. et al. A candidate genetic risk factor for vascular disease: a common mutation in methylenetetrahydrofolate reductase. *Nat. Genet.*, 10, 111, 1995.
64. Jacques, P.F. et al. Relation between folate status, a common mutation in methylenetetrahydrofolate reductase and plasma homocysteine concentration. *Circulation* 93, 7, 1996.
65. McNulty, H. et al. Impaired functioning of thermolabile methylenetetrahydrofolate reductase is dependent on riboflavin status: implications for riboflavin requirements. *Am. J. Clin. Nutr.*, 76, 436, 2002.
66. Rozen, R. Methylenetetrahydrofolate reductase: a link between folate and riboflavin. *Am. J. Clin. Nutr.*, 76, 301, 2002.
67. Yamada, K. et al. Effects of common polymorphisms on the properties of recombinant human methyltetrahydrofolate reductase. *Proc. Natl. Acad. Sci., USA* 98, 14853, 2001.
68. Hustad, S. et al. Riboflavin as a determinant of plasma total homocysteine: effect modification by the methylenetetrahydrofolate reductase C677T polymorphism. *Clin. Chem.*, 46, 1065, 2000.
69. Ganji, G. and Kafai, M.R. Frequent consumption of milk, yogurt, cold breakfast cereals, peppers and cruciferous vegetables and intakes of dietary folate and riboflavin but not vitamins B_{12} and B_6 are inversely associated with serum total homocysteine concentrations in the US population. *Am. J. Clin. Nutr.*, 80, 1500, 2004.
70. Kimura, M. et al. Methylenetetrahydrofolate reductase C677T polymorphism, folic acid and riboflavin are important determinants of genome stability in cultured human lymphocytes. *J. Nutr.*, 134, 48, 2004.
71. Stern, L.L. et al. Combined marginal folate and riboflavin status affect homocysteine methylation in cultured immortalized lymphocytes from persons homozygous for the MTHFR C677T mutation. *J. Nutr.*, 133, 2716, 2003.
72. Moat, S.J. et al. Effect of riboflavin status on the homocysteine-lowering effect of folate in relation to the MTHFR (C677T) genotype. *Clin. Chem.*, 49, 295, 2003.
73. Hustad, S. et al. Phenotypic expression of the methylenetetrahydrofolate reductase C677T polymorphism and flavin cofactor availability in thyroid dysfunction. *Am. J. Clin. Nutr.*, 80, 1050, 2004.
74. Bernsen, P.L.J.A. et al. Treatment of complex I deficiency with riboflavin. *J. Neurol. Sci.*, 118, 181, 1993.
75. Walker, U.A. and Byrne, E. The therapy of respiratory chain encephalomyopathy: a critical review of the past and present perspective. *Acta Neurol. Scand.*, 92, 273, 1995.
76. Uziel, G. et al. Riboflavin-responsive glutaric aciduria type II presenting as a leukodystrophy. *Pediatr. Neurol.*, 13, 333, 1995.
77. Russell, A.P. et al. Decreased fatty acid β-oxidation in riboflavin-responsive, multiple acylcoenzyme A dehydrogenase–deficient patients is associated with an increase in uncoupling protein-3. *J. Clin. Endocrinol. Metab.*, 8, 5921, 2003.
78. Vasseur, B.G. et al. Type B lactic acidosis: a rare complication of antiretroviral therapy after cardiac surgery. *Ann. Thorac. Surg.*, 74, 1151, 2002.
79. Bowens, J.H. and Bert-Moreno, A. Treatment of HAART-induced lactic acidosis with B vitamin supplements. *Nutr. Clin. Prac.*, 19, 375, 2004.

80. Food and Nutrition Board. Institute of Medicine. Riboflavin, Chapter 5, in *Dietary Reference Intakes for Thiamin, Riboflavin, Niacin, Vitamin B_6, Folate, Vitamin B_{12}, Pantothenic Acid, Biotin and Choline*, National Academy Press, Washington, DC, p. 87, 2000.
81. Rivlin, R.S. Effect of nutrient toxicities (excess) in animals and man: riboflavin, in *Handbook of Nutrition and Foods*. Recheigl, M., ed., CRC Press, Boca Raton, FL, p. 25, 1979.
82. Cooperman, J.M. and Lopez, R. Riboflavin, in *Handbook of Vitamins: Nutritional, Biochemical and Clinical Aspects*. Machlin, L.J., ed., Marcel Dekker, NY, p. 299, 1984.
83. Burch, H.B. et al. Effects of riboflavin deficiency and realimentation on flavin enzymes of tissues. *J. Biol. Chem.*, 223, 29, 1956.
84. Ghazy, F.S. et al. The photodynamic action of riboflavin on erythrocytes. *Life Sci.*, 21, 1703, 1977.
85. Salim-Hanna, M., Edwards, A.M., and Silva, E. Obtention of a photo-induced adduct between a vitamin and an essential amino acid. Binding of riboflavin to tryptophan. *Int. J. Vitam. Nutr. Res.*, 57, 155, 1987.
86. Granzow, C, Kopun, M., and Krober, T. Riboflavin-mediated photosensitization of vinca alkaloids distorts drug sensitivity assays. *Cancer Res.*, 55, 4837, 1995.
87. Sugiyama, M. et al. Potentiation of sodium chromate (VI)-induced chromosomal aberrations and mutation by vitamin B_2 in Chinese hamster V79 cells. *Mutat. Res.*, 283, 211, 1992.
88. Bessho, T. et al. Induction of mutations in mouse FM3A cells by treatment with riboflavin plus visible light and its possible relation with formation of 8-hydroxyguanine (7,8-dihydro-8-oxoguanine) in DNA. *Carcinogenesis* 14, 1069, 1993.
89. Kale, H. et al. Assessment of the genotoxic potential of riboflavin and lumiflavin. B. Effect of light. *Mutat. Res.*, 298, 17, 1992.
90. Webster, R.P., Gawde, M.D., and Bhattacharya, R.K. Modulation of carcinogen-induced DNA damage and repair enzyme activity by dietary riboflavin. *Cancer Lett.*, 98, 129, 1996.
91. Rivlin, R.S. Riboflavin and cancer: a review. *Cancer Res.*, 33, 1997, 1973.
92. Munoz, N. et al. Vitamin intervention on precancerous lesions of the esophagus in a high-risk population in China. *Ann. N.Y. Acad. Sci.*, 534, 618, 1988.
93. Wahrendorf, J. et al. Blood retinol and zinc riboflavin status in relation to precancerous lesions of the esophagus: findings from a vitamin intervention trial in the People's Republic of China. *Cancer Res.*, 48, 2280, 1988.
94. Zaridze, D.G. et al. Relationship between esophageal mucosa pathology and vitamin deficit in population with high frequency of esophageal cancer. *Vop. Onkol.* 35, 939, 1989.
95. Baker, H. and Frank, O. Analysis of riboflavin and its derivatives in biologic fluids and tissues, in *Riboflavin*. Rivlin, R.S., ed., Plenum Press, NY, p. 49, 1975.
96. Bessey, O.A, Lowry, O.H., and Love, R.H. Fluorometric measure of the nucleotides of riboflavin and their concentration in tissues. *J. Biol. Chem.*, 180, 755, 1949.
97. Fazekas, A.G. et al. A competitive protein-binding assay for urinary riboflavin. *Biochem. Med.*, 9, 167, 1974.
98. Kim, M.J. et al. Homogeneous assays for riboflavin mediated by the interaction between enzyme–biotin and avidin–riboflavin conjugates. *Anal. Biochem.*, 231, 400, 1995.
99. Chastain, J.L. and McCormick, D.B. Flavin catabolites: identification and quantitation in human urine. *Am. J. Clin. Nutr.*, 46, 830, 1987.
100. Sauberlich, H.E. et al. Application of the erythrocyte glutathione reductase assay in evaluating riboflavin nutritional status in a high school student population. *Am. J. Clin. Nutr.*, 25, 756, 1972.
101. Rivlin, R.S. *Riboflavin: in Present Knowledge in Nutrition*. Ziegler, E.E. and Filer, L.J. Jr., eds., ILSI press, Washington, DC, p. 167, 1966.
102. Menendez, C.E. et al. Thyroid hormone regulation of glutathione reductase activity in rat erythrocytes and liver. *Am. J. Physiol.*, 226, 1480, 1974.
103. Brun, T.A. et al. Urinary riboflavin excretion after a load test in rural China as a measure of possible riboflavin deficiency. *Eur. J. Clin. Nutr.*, 44, 195, 1990.
104. Boisvert, W.A. et al. Riboflavin requirement of healthy elderly humans and its relationship to macronutrient composition of the diet. *J. Nutr.*, 123, 915, 1993.
105. Trebler-Winters, L.R. et al. Riboflavin requirements and exercise adaptation in older women. *Am. J. Clin. Nutr.*, 56, 526, 1992.

106. Belko, A.Z. et al. Effects of aerobic exercise and weight loss on riboflavin requirements of moderately obese, marginally deficient young women. *Am. J. Clin. Nutr.*, 40, 553, 1984.
107. Soares, M.J. et al. The effects of exercise on the riboflavin status of adult men. *Br. J. Nutr.*, 69, 541, 1993.
108. Fogelholm, M. et al. Lack of association between indices of vitamin B_1, B_2 and B_6 status and exercise-induced blood lactate in young adults. *Int. J. Sport. Nutr.*, 3, 165, 1993.
109. Ensminger, A.M., Ensminger, M.E., Konlande, J.E., and Robson, J.R.K. *Food and Nutrition Encyclopedia*, CRC Press, Boca Raton, FL, p. 1927, 1994.

8 Thiamine

Chris J. Bates

CONTENTS

HISTORY

The story of the discovery of thiamine, as the preventative and curative agent of the human disease, beriberi, or kakke, is a fascinating one [1]. The disease had become increasingly common in many far-eastern, rice-dependent countries, especially during the nineteenth century. At this time, it was widely believed to be caused by a toxin or an infection.

However, in 1885 Dr. K. Takaki, surgeon-general of the Japanese navy, introduced extra rations of protein-rich foods such as meat and the replacement of rice by wheat flour or barley in the diet of the beriberi-prone lower naval ranks, since higher-ranking officers, whose diets contained more protein, seldom suffered from beriberi. This intervention was successful.

Dr. Christiaan Eijkman, a Dutch medical researcher working in Batavia (now Jakarta) in the Dutch East Indies (now Indonesia) during the late nineteenth century, made the next advance. He found that chickens fed exclusively on white rice from human diets in the local military hospital developed a polyneuritic condition that resembled dry beriberi in humans. Other chickens, fed less-purified red or brown rice from which the silverskin (containing the aleurone layer) had not been removed by machine milling, did not develop polyneuritis. These observations enabled his successor, Gerrit Grijns, and then Fraser and Stanton in Malaya, to reach, eventually, the correct conclusion that highly polished white rice lacked an essential organic trace nutrient, which could be extracted from rice polishings, parboiled rice, or the silverskin layer of rice by water or alcohol. Such an extract could convert the disease-causing polished white rice into a more adequate food that did not result in polyneuritis in chickens. Observations on the prevalence of human beriberi in Javanese prisons during the mid-1890s, by Adolphe Vorderman, a friend of Eijkman, indicated that diets based on heavily milled white rice were associated with a high prevalence of the disease in humans also, whereas brown rice, with a higher proportion of the silverskin and embryo, was protective [1]. Although the chicken polyneuritis model was not identical to human beriberi, there were many common features.

Thus, steam-powered rice mills removed not only the husk, but also the vitamin-rich aleurone layer of cells (silverskin) between the starchy endosperm and the husk, and the vitamin-rich embryo and its associated scutellum layer. Less aggressive polishing, or parboiling (which redistributes some of the vitamin content to the endosperm), and avoidance of leaching during cooking, could reduce the risk of beriberi.

In the following decades, Grijns, Casimir Funk (who coined the name vitamine, now shortened to vitamin, to describe a whole new class of essential organic micronutrients), and Roger Williams, a chemist working in Manila in the Philippines, all attempted further purification of the beriberi-preventative factor in rice polishings. In 1926, Jansen and Donath, two chemists working in Java, succeeded in purifying and crystallizing the active substance (see section Isolation, Chemical Synthesis, and Biosynthesis). They used ricebirds (*Munia maja*), which developed the pathological symptoms of deficiency more rapidly and reliably than chickens did. Roger Williams thus obtained ca. 100 mg of pure, crystalline antineuritic material from 600 kg rice polishings from which he determined the structure of the active component, thiamine, and then achieved its synthesis from defined chemical precursors by defined chemical reactions.

CHEMISTRY

Structure and Nomenclature

The empirical formula of the hydrochloride salt of thiamine is $C_{12}H_{17}N_4OSCl.HCl$ and its chemical name is 3-(4′-amino-2′-methyl-pyrimidin-5′-ylmethyl)-5-(2-hydroxyethyl)-4-methylthiazolium chloride hydrochloride. Figure 8.1 shows the molecular structure. The essential key features of the molecule are the linked pyrimidine and thiazole rings, the hydroxyethyl side chain at position 5 of the thiazole ring, which becomes phosphorylated in the cell (Figure 8.1), the unsubstituted carbon at position 2 of the thiazole ring, which

Free thiamine base

Thiamine chloride hydrochloride crystalline salt

Thiamine monophosphate

Thiamine diphosphate

Thiamine triphosphate

Ring numbering convention

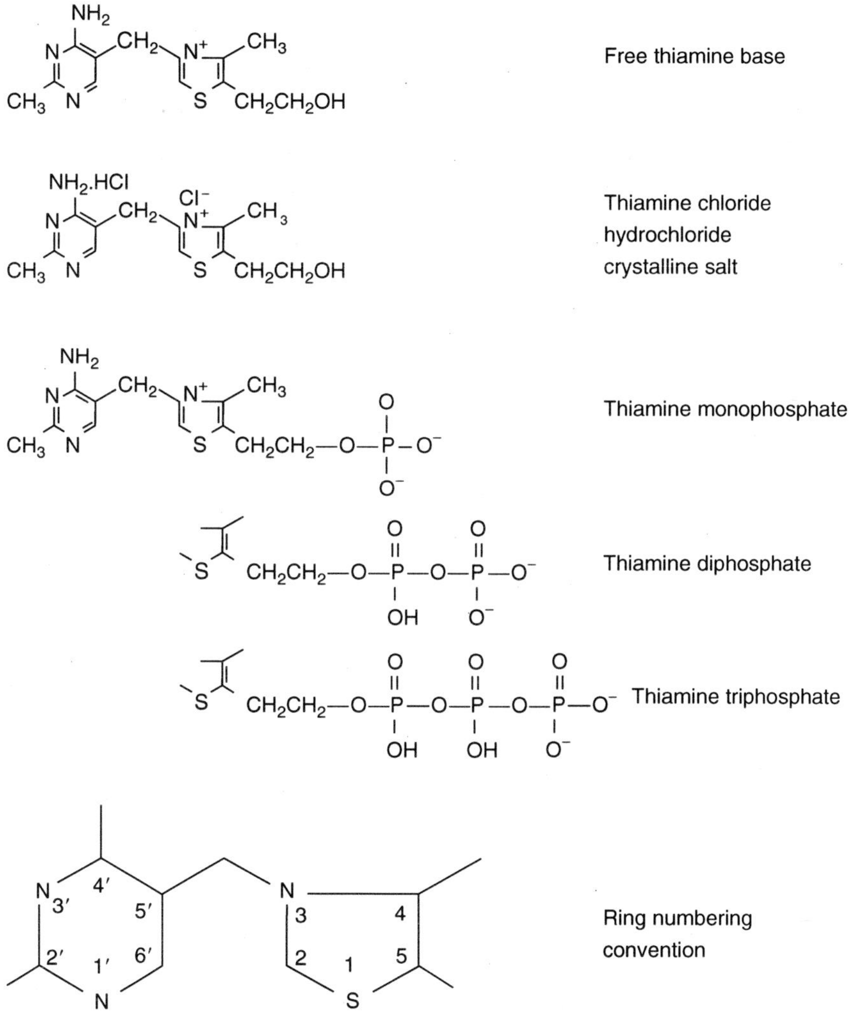

FIGURE 8.1 Structures of thiamine and thiamine phosphates. The names thiamine diphosphate and thiamine pyrophosphate are used interchangeably. Cocarboxylase is an older name for the same substance.

is capable of forming a carbanion, and the amino group at position 4′ of the pyrimidine ring. The crystalline vitamin salts that are most widely produced commercially are the hydrochloride and the mononitrate.

The name thiamine (with or without the final "e") is used interchangeably with the older alternative name, vitamin B_1. During the early years of investigation, the name aneurin(e) was also used, especially in the United Kingdom, to emphasize the antineuritic properties of the vitamin.

Isolation, Chemical Synthesis, and Biosynthesis

As noted in section History, Jansen and Donath [2] achieved the first recorded isolation of a crystalline thiamine salt in 1926. Their purification steps included precipitation with silver nitrate, phosphotungstic acid, platinic chloride, acetone, and picrolinic acid, redissolving at each stage in barium hydroxide. Isolation was greatly assisted when they found that a hydrated aluminium silicate, known as Fuller's earth, would adsorb the vitamin from dilute aqueous solutions, from which it could be eluted in a partially purified state with hot acidic potassium chloride solution. This Fuller's earth purification step continued to be used for many years as the second step, after extraction, in thiamine assay procedures. It was usually followed by open-column chromatography, using a cation-exchange resin, or by paper or thin-layer chromatography, to achieve further purification [3].

The chemical characterization and synthesis of thiamine was carried out during the 1930s, with Roger Williams playing a major role [4]. Once the empirical formula had been correctly established by elemental analysis, he made an important advance by splitting the two halves of the molecule apart by treatment with sulfite. This permitted physical separation of two simpler components, and comparison of each against known compounds with known structures. The correct chemical structure for the intact molecule was proposed in 1936, and the stage was then set for a complete chemical synthesis, which was achieved almost simultaneously by Williams and two other groups in 1936–1937 [3,4]. In the preferred synthesis pathway [3] the pyrimidine ring is built first, largely from organic nitrile compounds, then the thiazole ring is added by reaction with a chloro-ketone, carbon disulfide and ammonia, and finally an oxidation step with hydrogen peroxide removes a sulfur atom and introduces a ring double bond so as to complete the thiazole ring.

Thiamine cannot be synthesized within the tissues of any animal species, as far as we know, and is thus a universally essential dietary component throughout the animal kingdom. All higher plants can make the vitamin, thereby providing a dietary source for animals, and it is produced also by yeasts. In plant tissues, the pyrimidine and thiazole moieties are synthesized separately; the pyrimidine is converted to its mono- or diphosphate and the thiazole to its monophosphate; then the two rings are condensed together by thiamine phosphate synthetase to yield thiamine monophosphate. This is then phosphorylated by ATP to the diphosphate or dephosphorylated to free thiamine [3,5]. Some, but not all, microorganisms can make thiamine de novo, and small amounts of thiamine are produced in the mammalian large intestine by the gut flora there; however, it is very poorly absorbed in this region of the intestine, and becomes available to the host only if the feces are recycled by coprophagy.

Physical and Chemical Properties

Thiamine chloride hydrochloride (the name is often shortened to thiamine hydrochloride) is a colorless, crystalline, hygroscopic, and highly water-soluble substance. Thiamine mononitrate is an alternative commercially available salt that is less hygroscopic than the chloride and is often preferred for use in food fortification. These two thiamine salts are moderately soluble in alcohol and acetone, from which they can be crystallized, but they are essentially insoluble in nonpolar solvents. They have a characteristic pungent odor. In aqueous solution at pH 5, thiamine exhibits two UV-light absorption maxima, at 235 and 267 nm, and at lower pH, around 3, it has a single absorption maximum at 246 nm and a molar extinction coefficient of 11,305. This property of UV-light absorption can be used (albeit with limited sensitivity and specificity) for detection and quantitation, for example, in liquid chromatographic analysis of pharmaceutical preparations, or of fortified or rich food sources, or for calibration of the concentration of pure solutions.

Free thiamine base unstable and very easily oxidized. When dry, thiamine salts are much more stable and survive at temperatures exceeding 100°C. In aqueous solution the hydrochloride is acidic (pH ca. 3.5 at 5% w/v concentration), and at acidic pH values, below about pH 5, it is stable even at autoclave temperatures of 120°C–130°C, and is not readily oxidized. However, at neutral pH it is less stable, and is destroyed (largely by oxidation), especially at high temperatures. At pH 8 and above, thiamine solutions rapidly turn yellow and form complex degradation products. In the presence of an oxidant such as potassium ferricyanide in strongly alkaline solutions, thiamine is converted almost quantitatively to the oxidized, tricyclic, highly fluorescent product, thiochrome (Figure 8.2). Its excitation maximum is at 375 nm and its emission maximum is at 432–435 nm. This reaction is widely used in the detection and quantitative analysis of thiamine and its phosphate esters in food and tissue extracts, which is made possible because virtually no other naturally occurring compound can undergo conversion to such a strongly fluorescent product with similar optical characteristics, under the same chemical conditions. Thiamine can also be converted to various colored products that can be used for its quantitation by spectrophotometry; for example,

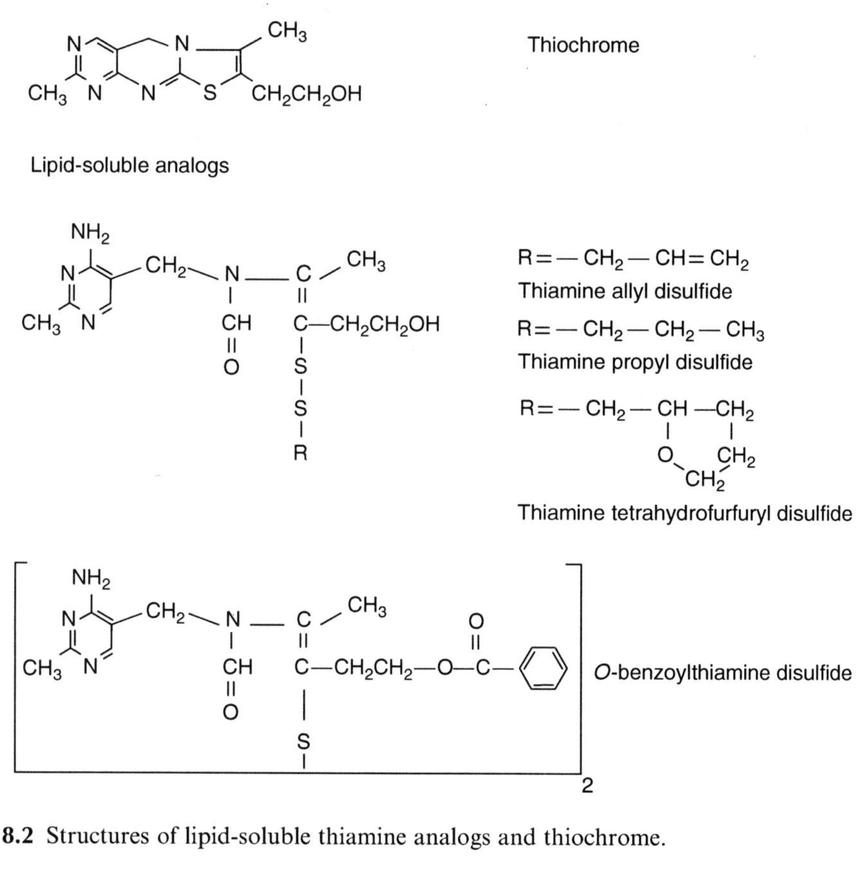

Thiochrome

Lipid-soluble analogs

$R = -CH_2-CH=CH_2$ Thiamine allyl disulfide

$R = -CH_2-CH_2-CH_3$ Thiamine propyl disulfide

Thiamine tetrahydrofurfuryl disulfide

O-benzoylthiamine disulfide

FIGURE 8.2 Structures of lipid-soluble thiamine analogs and thiochrome.

it yields pink- or red-colored derivatives with diazotized sulfanilic acid and formaldehyde, or with *p*-aminoacetophenone. However, none of these alternative assays can compete with the thiochrome reaction, especially in terms of sensitivity of detection.

Solutions containing sulfite at pH 6 or above rapidly and irreversibly cleave thiamine at its methylene bridge, thus splitting apart the pyrimidine and thiazole moieties. This chemical inactivation has major significance for the food industry, because sulfite is widely used as an antioxidant in food preservation. Exposure to chlorine (e.g., from chlorinated tap water) also increases the rate of cleavage and hence irreversible inactivation of thiamine.

Thiamine Phosphates and Lipid-Soluble Thiamine Derivatives

Figure 8.1 includes the structures of the biologically significant phosphate esters of thiamine: firstly thiamine monophosphate (TMP), secondly thiamine diphosphate (TDP), also known as thiamine pyrophosphate (TPP) (and originally named cocarboxylase, because of its function as the coenzyme for carboxylase, the enzyme that is now known as pyruvate dehydrogenase), and thirdly, thiamine triphosphate (TTP). Of these three esters, only thiamine diphosphate has well-defined biological functions, acting as an essential coenzyme in five key enzyme systems in mammals (see sections Pyruvate Dehydrogenase Complex, Alpha-Ketoglutarate Dehydrogenase and Branched-Chain Alpha-Keto Acid Dehydrogenase Complexes, Transketolase, and Peroxisomal Alpha-Oxidation of 3-Methyl Branched-Chain Fatty Acids and Cleavage of 2-Hydroxylated Fatty Acids). The biological significance of thiamine triphosphate is poorly understood; one theory is that it may have a functional role in the brain (section Thiamine-Dependent Reactions in the Nervous System). The monophosphate is a transport form and breakdown intermediate, but has no known cofactor roles.

Depicted in Figure 8.2 are four relatively lipid-soluble substances known as allithiamines (thiamine allyl disulfide, thiamine propyl disulfide, thiamine tetrahydrofurfural disulfide and *O*-benzoylthiamine disulfide) that can act as precursors of thiamine, and hence as alternative delivery routes for absorbed thiamine in man and animals, because reduction of their disulfide bridge structure is followed by spontaneous thiazole ring formation to generate thiamine within the body. Some allithiamines occur naturally in plants, especially in the genus *Allium* (garlic) where they contribute to the characteristic odor; others are synthetic compounds, developed especially by the Japanese pharmaceutical industry, mainly for the purpose of bypassing the readily saturable intestinal absorption step that limits the entry of thiamine (see section Metabolism: Bioavailability, Absorption, Tissue Distribution, Turnover). As they are more completely absorbed than thiamine at high doses, and also more efficiently retained in the body, where they are then converted slowly to thiamine, these precursors can be useful, especially in the treatment of alcoholics, whose body stores are diminished, whose absorption efficiency is compromised, and in whom there is a need for rapid restoration of thiamine-dependent functions, despite frequent poor compliance with conventional therapy. About half of an oral dose of the tetrahydrofurfural disulfide derivative is hydrolyzed in the gastrointestinal tract [6], and it may therefore be more efficient to deliver the allithiamines intravenously than orally. Once absorbed, they enter the red cells and are there slowly reduced by glutathione, which results in spontaneous ring closure to produce free thiamine; this then exits to the plasma and is distributed to the rest of the body [7].

Thiamine Analogs That Act as Antagonists

Figure 8.3 shows the structures of three compounds that all have somewhat similar structures to thiamine, but lack thiamine-replacement activity, and instead act as antagonists, thereby selectively inducing functional thiamine deficiency states in animals or bacteria, even when dietary supplies of thiamine would otherwise be adequate.

Oxythiamine is an example of a group of compounds with intact pyrimidine and thiazole rings, but with alterations to the substituent groups attached to the two rings. A key difference from thiamine is that it lacks the pyrimidine 4′-NH_2 group, which is essential for the release of aldehyde adducts from carbon-2 of the thiazole ring, after splitting a carbon–carbon bond in the course of the reactions that are catalyzed by thiamine diphosphate enzymes [3]. Because it has a hydroxyethyl group substituent on the thiazole ring, as does thiamine itself, it can form a diphosphate by the shared enzymic pyrophosphorylation reaction, and then binds to thiamine diphosphate-requiring enzymes, resulting in an inactive complex. Since the displacement of thiamine diphosphate at key enzyme sites is rapid, the time lag to onset of pathology is shorter than that required for a deficiency state to be achieved by simply removing thiamine from the diet. Another important difference from the result of simple thiamine deficiency is that oxythiamine does not penetrate the blood–brain barrier, and it therefore does not affect pyruvate dehydrogenase or other thiamine-dependent enzymes in the brain; nor does it produce neurological dysfunction symptoms of thiamine deficiency, such as ataxia or convulsions [3].

The second thiamine antagonist shown in Figure 8.3, pyrithiamine, is an example of a different group of antagonists, all of which have ring modifications in either the pyrimidine or the thiazole rings, instead of, or in addition to, any changes in the attached (i.e., substituent) groups. In contrast to oxythiamine, pyrithiamine does penetrate the blood–brain barrier. It severely reduces both pyruvate dehydrogenase and alpha-ketoglutarate dehydrogenase activities in brain tissue and it induces ataxia and convulsions (much more rapidly and efficiently than by simple dietary thiamine deficiency) [3]. Unlike oxythiamine, pyrithiamine increases urinary thiamine excretion and general tissue thiamine depletion. However, it is not readily converted to a pyrophosphate derivative; instead it inhibits the conversion of thiamine to thiamine diphosphate and thereby deprives the tissues, especially brain, of thiamine diphosphate. It does not readily cause anorexia or weight loss, and its efficacy in producing the nonneurological symptoms of thiamine deficiency is low by comparison with oxythiamine or dietary thiamine deprivation. Pyrithiamine is widely used for research into experimental

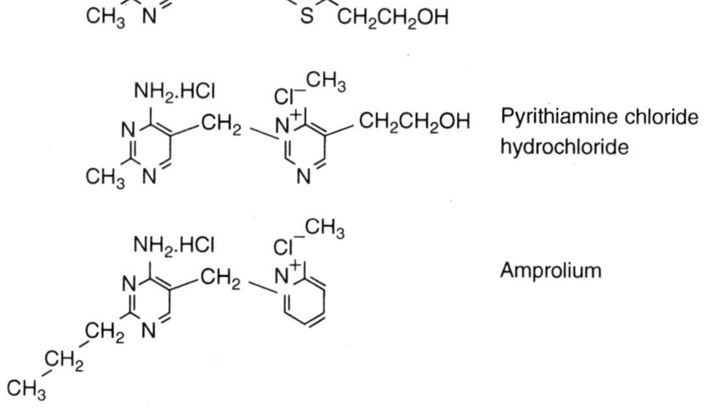

FIGURE 8.3 Structures of thiamine and selected antagonists.

animal and cell culture models of thiamine deficiency, especially when the neurological effects of deficiencies of the thiamine-cofactor-dependent pathways are studied.

The third thiamine antagonist shown in Figure 8.3, amprolium (usually supplied in the bromide form), is the most widely used member of a group of compounds that are employed in veterinary practice to treat coccidial infections, especially in farmed birds such as chickens. Amprolium, like pyrithiamine, has a pyridine ring structure in place of the thiazole of thiamine, and therefore lacks the sulfur atom. However, the amprolium series do not have a hydroxyethyl side chain on the pyridine ring, and they are therefore unable to form diphosphate derivatives, which makes them relatively weak antithiamine antagonists in the birds, except at high doses, where they can reduce thiamine absorption. However, in most bacteria, they reduce thiamine absorption very efficiently, thereby achieving a useful therapeutic ratio by starving bacterial pathogens of an essential nutrient.

ANALYTICAL PROCEDURES

UNITS AND RANGE OF PROCEDURES

Before the isolation of pure thiamine, assay methods used international units, where one unit is now equivalent to 3 μg thiamine chloride hydrochloride, to calibrate animal assays for thiamine. The thiamine content of foods and pharmaceuticals is now expressed in μg/g (= mg/kg) or as mg/100 g, and body fluid or tissue concentrations are in SI units, for example, as μmol/L or nmol/L. The molecular weight of free thiamine base is 266.4, but that of the chloride hydrochloride salt is 26% higher at 337.3. Fortified foods mainly contain thiamine; nonfortified foods often mainly contain thiamine diphosphate, which needs to be converted to thiamine for analysis. Quantitation is then achieved by microbiological or chromatographic assays. High-performance liquid chromatography has replaced open-column ion-exchange resin-based and paper chromatographic or thin-layer separation methods. The historically important animal assays were usually based on the cure of pathological deficiency signs such as bradycardia, or reversal of impaired growth.

EXTRACTION

To liberate thiamine, food samples of animal origin can be autoclaved in 0.1 N hydrochloric acid for 30 min at ca. 121°C. Free thiamine is best extracted at 108°C–109°C [8]. Rice flour can be extracted with 0.1N hydrochloric acid in 40% aqueous methanol for 30 min at 60°C [9]. To ensure that thiamine phosphates are completely hydrolyzed and that interference by protein is minimized, enzyme digestion with fungal diastase preparations containing phosphatase may be used.

MICROBIOLOGICAL ASSAY

Thiamine assays have traditionally used *Lactobacilli* species: *L. viridescens* (ATCC 12706), which is preferred, or *L. fermenti* (ATCC 9338) [8]. Detection of nanogram amounts is feasible, and the assay is specific and robust. Thiamine diphosphate is 130% as active as free thiamine in the *L. fermenti* assay [7]. An alternative, highly sensitive and specific protozoon-based assay, using *Ochromonas danica*, has been developed by Baker et al. [10] for blood-based thiamine status assays.

FLUORIMETRIC ASSAYS AND HIGH-PERFORMANCE LIQUID CHROMATOGRAPHY

Fluorimetric thiamine assays require extraction, oxidation of thiamine to thiochrome, which is then extracted into isobutanol, and measurement of its fluorescence with a blank correction that is achieved by omitting the oxidant. An officially adopted procedure [11] for foods containing thiamine diphosphate required acid digestion, enzymatic hydrolysis, partial purification by cation-exchange open-column chromatography, conversion of thiamine to fluorescent thiochrome by reaction with alkaline potassium hexacyanoferrate, extraction of the thiochrome into isobutanol, and measurement of fluorescence.

HPLC-based assays for thiamine in foods have been available since the 1980s [8,12]. Fluorescence detection is usually preferred. Conversion of thiamine to thiochrome can be performed either before the chromatographic separation, or else between the column and the detector by using an effluent–reagent mixing coil. Precolumn conversion can achieve better resolution, but may expose the column to a caustic mobile phase that shortens its working life.

Most HPLC methods use C_{18} (octadecyl silica) reverse-phase column-packing materials; many also use ion-pairing agents to interact with the positively charged nitrogen atom of thiamine [12]. External quality assurance schemes and calibrated materials for interlaboratory exchange and assay verification are essential to achieve harmonization of results between different laboratories.

FOOD CONTENT OF THIAMINE AND THIAMINASE ENZYMES

Thiamine in Food

In most animal products, 95%–98% of the thiamine present is in the phosphorylated form, with around 80%–85% as the diphosphate, whereas in plant foods, and especially in commercially fortified foods, a higher proportion of nonphosphorylated thiamine may be found [3]. Some of the best dietary sources of thiamine include yeast extract, offal, pork and ham, wheat germ and wheat bran, most nuts and some legumes, and fortified foods such as breakfast cereals and bread (Table 8.1). Pork meat contains considerably more thiamine than the muscle of other farm animals. Egg yolk is a rich source of the vitamin, whereas egg white is a poor source—although the difference is much smaller with food energy as the denominator. Raw peanuts are a good source, but roasted peanuts contain much less due to heat destruction during roasting.

About 17%–18% of the thiamine in the diet of U.S. adults came from bread and bread products in 1995 [13]. Although the thiamine content of green vegetables on a weight basis is comparatively low (Table 8.1), on an energy basis they make an important contribution (see also Gubler [3]). Legumes are better sources than leafy vegetables. Wholemeal foods tend to contain more thiamine than the corresponding white versions, unless the latter are fortified. The amount present in unfortified rice as eaten depends enormously on the method of removal of the husk; heavily (mechanically) milled rice has the lowest content (e.g., only ca. 0.02 mg/100 g cooked rice [5]). Thiamine can be partly redistributed within the rice grain by parboiling before dehusking, a process that originated in Bengal. This requires preliminary soaking and steaming of the grain within the husk and then drying before milling, which facilitates the separation of the husk, and gelatinizes the vitamin-rich layers, allowing the vitamin to diffuse from the silverskin into the endosperm, thus reducing subsequent losses during milling.

Highly refined white flour has a low thiamine content, and many western countries, including the United Kingdom and the United States, have introduced mandatory fortification of some types of bread. In the United Kingdom, thiamine must be added at not less than 0.24 mg/100 g flour that is used commercially for making white or brown bread.

Alkaline pH, for example, use of bicarbonate during cooking to preserve the green color of vegetables, increases the rate of thiamine destruction, and large volumes of cooking water that are then discarded cause substantial losses of all the water-soluble vitamins, including

TABLE 8.1
Thiamine and Energy Contents of Selected Foods from UK Food Composition Tables

Food Description	Thiamine (mg/100 g)	Energy (kcal/100 g)
Meat and offal		
Pork muscle (loin chops, lean, grilled)	0.78	184
Beef muscle (rump steak, grilled)	0.13	177
Pig's liver, stewed	0.21	189
Ox liver, stewed	0.18	198
Pig's kidneys, stewed	0.21	153
Ox kidney, stewed	0.18	138
Chicken, roast, average	0.07	177
Fish		
Cod, baked	0.03	96
Haddock, steamed	0.04	89
Sardines in oil (drained)	0.01	220
Dairy products		
Cow's milk, whole	0.03	66
Human milk	0.02	69
Yoghurt, whole milk	0.06	79
Egg white (chicken, raw)	0.01	36
Egg yolk (chicken, raw)	0.30	339
Cereals, cereal products		
Cornflakes (fortified, breakfast cereal, dry)	1.20	376
Porridge as eaten, with milk (not fortified)	0.09	113
White rice, raw (fortified, easy cook)	0.41	383
Brown rice, raw	0.59	357
Brown rice, boiled	0.14	141
White bread (sliced)	0.24	219
Wholemeal bread	0.25	217
Vegetables		
Potatoes, new, boiled	0.09	75
Broccoli, boiled	0.05	24
Cauliflower, boiled	0.07	28
Courgette, boiled	0.08	19
Onions, fried	0.08	164
Tomatoes, raw	0.09	17
Tomato puree	0.40	76
Fruits		
Apples, eating	0.03	47
Pears	0.02	41
Oranges	0.11	37
Blackcurrants	0.03	28
Cherries	0.03	48
Strawberries	0.03	27
Other foods		
Baker's yeast, dry	2.33	169
Peanuts, uncooked	1.14	563
Peanuts, roasted	0.18	589

Source: From Food Standards Agency in *McCance and Widdowson's The Composition of Foods*, 6th Summary Edition, Royal Society of Chemistry, Cambridge, 2002. With permission.

thiamine, by leaching. Stir-frying in fat or the use of cooking water in soups or stews minimizes losses. Rice should be cooked in an amount of water that it absorbs. Heat sterilization of milk causes greater losses (30%–50%) than pasteurization (10%–20%), and use of sulfite to preserve fruit, fruit juices, and minced meat can cause major losses. UV light and oxygen are also destructive. However, binding to protein or starch provides some protection.

Antithiamine Compounds in Food

Some foods contain thiamine-splitting enzymes (thiaminases) [5]. The threat to health and life that can be posed by such enzymes is graphically illustrated by an ill-fated expedition led by Burke and Wills, which set out to explore the center of Australia from 1860 to 1861 [14]. During their return journey, the explorers were compelled to eat inadequately cooked freshwater mussels and flour from Nardoo ferns. Both foods contain high amounts of thiaminase, and four of five members of the expedition perished from beriberi.

Thiaminase type I occurs in the visceral organs of freshwater fish, shellfish, ferns, certain seawater fish, and in some species of microorganisms. Other species of microorganisms produce thiaminase type II, which is less common. Both enzymes split thiamine into its two component rings, each by a different mechanism. Thiaminase I acts by base-exchange between the thiazole ring of thiamine and various nitrogenous bases; thiaminase II acts by simple hydrolysis. When present in intact cells the thiaminases are inactive, but they become activated when intracellular contents are liberated by cell membrane disruption. They can destroy thiamine either during food storage, or during its preparation, or even within the gastrointestinal tract. However, they can usually be inactivated by thorough cooking, and are not a major problem in most human diets.

Polyphenolic compounds such as tannic acid, chlorogenic acid, and caffeic acid, which occur in tea, coffee, betel nuts, and ferns, have also been reported to impair thiamine status in human subjects. However, some of the research on these effects has later proved misleading, either because there was interference by polyphenols with the thiochrome assay, or because the products of polyphenol treatment of thiamine could be reconverted to thiamine within the body [1], and the practical importance of heat-stable antithiamine substances is controversial.

In ruminant animals the rumen microflora may exert complex effects on the thiamine supply to the host animal. Some species of rumen bacteria synthesize and release thiamine, which can then be absorbed by the host animal; others have surface enzymes that destroy it, especially at low pH [15]. Severe destruction of thiamine arises especially with high-concentration diets. Cerebrocortical necrosis in ruminants is almost certainly caused by thiamine deficiency whose origin is a thiaminase from the rumen bacteria [7]. Bracken or endophyte-infected fescue grass can antagonize thiamine, and high sulfate intakes can give rise to sulfite by reduction processes in the rumen; this can then destroy the vitamin.

METABOLISM: BIOAVAILABILITY, ABSORPTION, TISSUE DISTRIBUTION, TURNOVER

Body stores of thiamine are not generally maintained above functional requirements. Rates of catabolism and loss imply that if the dietary intake falls to near zero, functional and clinical abnormalities begin to become apparent in humans within a few weeks, that is, more rapidly than for most other micronutrients.

About half the total amount of thiamine in the body is present in muscle, and the total amount of thiamine in a well-nourished adult human is about 30 mg, of which about four-fifths occurs as the enzyme cofactor, thiamine diphosphate.

Adenosine triphosphate (ATP) provides the diphosphate moiety for the synthesis of thiamine diphosphate from free thiamine by the action of thiamine pyrophosphokinase. Thiamine diphosphate can be metabolized either by dephosphorylation to form thiamine monophosphate, catalyzed by thiamine pyrophosphatase, or by further phosphorylation to give thiamine triphosphate, catalyzed by thiamine diphosphate–ATP phosphoryltransferase [3,5]. To a limited extent, free thiamine can be converted to thiamine monophosphate by an intestinal membrane alkaline phosphatase, in the presence of phosphate donors [16].

Bioavailability and Intestinal Absorption

Thiamine phosphate esters in food are mostly converted to free thiamine by digestive enzymes (phosphatases) before the vitamin is absorbed. Any excess vitamin that escapes absorption in the ileum is metabolized or degraded by the gut flora of the large bowel.

Both free thiamine and thiamine monophosphate can be actively absorbed by the intestinal mucosa; thiamine is transported more efficiently of the two forms [16]. In all animal species that have been studied, which include rat, mouse, frog, chicken, and human, thiamine absorption in the intestine takes place by two parallel mechanisms, saturable active transport, which comes into play at low luminal thiamine concentrations (e.g., $<1.25\ \mu mol/L$) and simple diffusion at higher luminal thiamine concentrations. Because the low-concentration pathway is saturable, it ensures that when intakes are modest, almost all the available thiamine is efficiently absorbed; however, its saturation at higher intakes ensures that energy is not wasted by transferring excessive amounts when gut luminal concentrations are high.

The low-concentration, saturable pathway in the apical brush border of the epithelium of the intestine is an energy-dependent process, which is most active in the duodenal region [3,17,18]. It is now known to be linked to the counter-transport of hydrogen ions, and is not sodium dependent, as was once believed [16]. In a study of human intestinal biopsies [19], it was found to exhibit Michaelis–Menten-type kinetics, with an apparent K_m for thiamine of 4.4 $\mu mol/L$; other studies have yielded slightly different K_m values. The active transport process is competitively inhibited by all three types of thiamine analogs that are represented, respectively, by oxythiamine, pyrithiamine, and amprolium (see section Thiamine Analogs that Act as Antagonists and Figure 8.3).

The efficiency of transport appears to change with increasing age in a rat model [20], thus raising the question whether there may also be an age-dependency in humans? For the active transport process in rats the affinity for substrate declines with age, but the number of transporter sites increases, and passive transport declines. Transport is also modulated via various different mechanisms, by factors such as the diabetic state, by hormones such as thyroxin and calmodulin, by ethanol exposure, and by calcium [16]. Exploration of these important control mechanisms, especially those mediated by hormones, is, however, incomplete.

Once inside the intestinal cells, phosphorylation of thiamine to its phosphate esters (mainly the diphosphate) occurs to a considerable extent. Transfer from the intestinal cell cytoplasm to the portal circulation requires the release of thiamine from these intracellular phosphate esters, followed by transport by an outward facilitative thiamine transporter across the basolateral cell membrane. This basolateral transporter, like the brush border transporter, is pH-dependent and electroneutral, but may differ from the brush border inward transporter because unlike the latter, it was reported to be sodium–potassium–ATPase-dependent in rats [21], although no such dependence was found in a study of humans [22]. Like the brush border transporter, the basolateral transporter is relatively specific for thiamine and some of its structural analogs.

Important advances have been made during the past few years in characterizing the active thiamine transporter proteins that are present in the intestine and in a number of other mammalian tissues. These proteins, and the genes that encode them, have been sequenced, their genes have been transfected into cells that do not normally contain them, and their properties, including control by promoter regions of the genome, have been studied [23]. Specific gene knockout models in mice have helped to define the functions of the transporters, and to determine whether and how they may be essential for avoidance of pathology [23–25]. There are two well-characterized microtubule-associated transporter proteins that are specific for free thiamine and some of its analogs; these are designated ThTr1 and ThTr2, respectively (see Table 8.2 for a comparison of some of their reported characteristics). The corresponding genes are designated *SLC19A2* and *SLC19A3*, respectively, and their chromosome loci are 1q23.3 and 2q37 [25]. The promoter region of the *SLC19A2* gene has been partially explored [26]. The SLC19A2 messenger (for ThTr1) is expressed in all gastrointestinal tissues. The ThTr1 messenger RNA concentration, when compared between different tissues, showed the following relative concentrations in humans: liver > stomach > duodenum > jejunum > colon > cecum > rectum > ileum [26]. Expression of SLC19A3 messenger (for ThTr2) occurs throughout the human gastrointestinal tract, but maximally in the proximal small intestine [27]. The specific functions of different parts of these transporter proteins are explored, thus amino acid no. 138 in the protein sequence of ThTr1 is essential for transporter activity [28]; other identifiable regions of the molecule determine whether or not it is expressed at the cell surface, a property that is essential for functional activity, and yet others determine the characteristics of intracellular trafficking mechanisms [29].

In the *ThTr1* gene, 14 distinct mutations have been identified in a series of patients with the rare genetic disease, thiamine-responsive megaloblastic anemia (TRMA, or Roger's disease) [30]. The pathology associated with this condition, however, differs radically

TABLE 8.2
Summary of Reported Characteristics of ThTr1 and ThTr2 Thiamine Transporters in Human and Mouse Tissues [16,23,27,31,145]

Species	Location and Characteristics	ThTr1	ThTr2
Human and mouse	Transporter expressed at apical intestinal brush border surface?	Yes	Yes
Human	Transporter expressed in basolateral membrane of intestinal cells?	Yes	No
Human	Apparent K_m	Micromolar range	Nanomolar range
Mouse	Transporter protein, mRNA, and functional activity upregulated by thiamine deficiency in intestine?	No	Yes
Human and mouse	Transporter expressed in renal tubular brush border epithelium?	Yes	Yes
Mouse	Transporter protein, mRNA, and functional activity upregulated by thiamine deficiency in kidney?	Yes	Yes
Human transfected in mouse	Transfected promoter region of genome (human → mouse), evidence for regulation by thiamine status at transcriptional level in humans?	No (intestine), Yes (renal)	Yes (intestine + renal)
Human and mouse	Transporters expressed at other sites: liver, brain, muscle (including heart), placenta, red blood cells, fibroblasts, etc?	Yes	Not yet sufficient info[a]
Human	Defects reported in Roger's disease (TRMA)?	Yes	No

[a] Reported to be present in brain and heart [31]; little information is available about ThTr2 at other sites, but it may be absent from red blood cells and fibroblasts [16].

from that of dietary thiamine deficiency seen in genetically normal people. It is characterized by megaloblastic anemia, sensorineural deafness, and diabetes. A mouse *ThTr1* gene knock-out mutant exhibits pathologies that are similar to the human TRMA condition [24]. However, these mice have normal plasma thiamine levels, suggesting that an additional pathway, possibly using ThTr2, can compensate for the absence of the ThTr1 transporter at the sites of intestinal absorption. Said et al. [27] have recently shown, in a human (Caco) intestinal cell line, that both human ThTr1 and ThTr2 transporters contribute to thiamine transport. They found that if either gene product were knocked out (i.e., silenced) by treatment with a small interfering RNA, only about half the transport activity was lost, but if both were silenced, essentially all the activity was lost. The location pattern of ThTr1 differed from that of ThTr2 in this study; the former was found at both the brush border and basolateral membranes, whereas the latter was detected only at the brush border. Moreover, the apparent K_m of human ThTr2 was in the nanomolar range (27.1 ± 7.6 nmol/l) whereas existing estimates for the K_m of human ThTr1 were in the micromolar range (see earlier).

From a recent study in mice, it has been reported that thiamine deficiency results in the upregulation of the intestinal mRNA and transporter protein for mouse ThTr2, but does not affect those for ThTr1 [31]. Transgenic mice containing promoters of the transporter genes of human origin likewise exhibited an increase in the promoter activity of the gene for ThTr2 but not that for ThTr1, in the thiamine-deficient state. Previous to this report, evidence had already been obtained to suggest that thiamine transport activity may be upregulated when body thiamine stores are low, derived from observations on a rat jejunal sac model [32] and on a duodenal biopsy from a thiamine-deficient human subject [19].

A third gene, which exhibits considerable structural homology to the two thiamine transporter genes, is designated *SLC19A1*, which encodes a reduced folate transporter (RFT) protein. This protein transports not only 5-methyltetrahydrofolate and other reduced folate species, but also, to a limited extent, the mono- and diphosphates of thiamine (but not free thiamine). The in vivo significance of this transporter protein, with respect to functional transport of thiamine phosphates, is not yet known. However, it is known that thiamine monophosphate can be actively transported across the intestinal mucosa, and that it can also be transported across the blood–brain barrier [16]. Rapid progress has been made in the characterization of thiamine transporter proteins and their encoding genes, and ongoing studies are exploring their links with the physiological aspects of thiamine economy.

Thiamine Transport in Other Tissues

Saturable active transport of thiamine also occurs in the brush border of the renal tubular epithelium [33], which helps to ensure, as with other essential nutrients, that when the plasma concentrations of the vitamin are below the upper limit of tubular reabsorption, essentially all of it will be returned to the plasma following filtration in the glomerulus. The saturable nature of the renal tubular transporter ensures that if plasma concentrations are increased considerably above the requirements of the tissues, the excess is rapidly excreted in the urine. This property determines the shape of the thiamine intake:urinary excretion relationship, whereby a gradual rise in excretion rate with increasing intake below the renal threshold is followed by a steep rise at higher intakes [34]. However, if high doses of thiamine are given intravenously, then although most of the excess is excreted rapidly in the urine, some additional phosphorylated thiamine derivatives also accumulate within the cells, at concentrations above their usual levels [35]. In the renal brush border, the expression of both ThTr1 and ThTr2 transporters and of both their transgenically inserted human promoter activities were upregulated by thiamine deficiency [31].

Active transport of thiamine also takes place in the placenta [36], thus apparently ensuring that the developing fetus is preferentially supplied, even when maternal intakes and plasma levels are low. Exchange of thiamine for H^+ has been studied in human placental epithelium [16].

Breast milk thiamine concentrations vary with the stage of lactation [37]. However, they are clearly dependent also on the thiamine status of the mother, because there are many reports of over thiamine deficiency in apparently fully breast-fed infants in populations where beriberi is endemic. Moreover, a recent study has reported nearly a twofold difference in mature breast milk thiamine concentrations between two groups of Spanish lactating women with low versus high thiamine intakes and biochemical status indices [38]. In well-nourished lactating women, between 0.1 and 0.2 mg thiamine is secreted into breast milk each day at peak lactation, which implies an additional thiamine requirement for at least this amount in the maternal diet during lactation.

Active transport of thiamine has also been studied in erythrocytes, and these cells, too, exhibit both saturable and nonsaturable thiamine transport pathways [16]. People with TRMA lack the erythrocyte-active thiamine transporter. Cultured fibroblasts from people with TRMA cannot survive without increased thiamine supplementation, which indicates the probable importance of the ThTr1 pathway in these cells also. Rat liver sinusoidal membranes likewise contain a pH-dependent saturable thiamine transporter [16]. Clearly, similar mechanisms for active thiamine transport are shared between a wide range of tissues and cell types.

Thiamine is nonspecifically bound to several proteins, especially albumin, in the plasma. There has also been a report that treatment of pregnant rats with an antibody to a plasma estrogen-inducible thiamine carrier protein that had been isolated from chickens resulted in fetal resorption in the rat, suggesting a possible role for this carrier, in thiamine transport to the fetus [39].

The levels to which thiamine and its esters are concentrated at particular tissue sites vary considerably between species [3]. For instance, pig muscle contains 0.7–1.2 mg/100 g, compared with 0.05–0.4 mg/100 g in muscle from most other species. Mouse liver contains 1.3 mg/100 g whereas cod liver contains only 0.03 mg/100 g. Analysis of distribution between subcellular fractions has shown that in most tissues, about 50% of the thiamine (plus its esters) occurs in the soluble fraction, 35% in mitochondria, 10% in the nuclei, and 5% in the microsomal fraction.

Degradation and Turnover of Thiamine

A study of thiamine turnover in man, using a radioactively labeled thiamine probe [40], estimated the half-life to be 9.5–18.5 days. The rate of thiamine degradation, mainly to water-soluble products that are excreted in the urine, has been reported to be approximately constant within an individual, not varying greatly with variations in thiamine intakes and body stores. Therefore, the ratio of intact thiamine to its breakdown products in the urine increases steeply with increasing thiamine intake and hence increasing plasma thiamine levels. Of around 20–30 different metabolites of thiamine that have been identified in rat and human urine following ingestion of radioactively labeled thiamine only a minority have been studied [3,41]. For instance, 2-methyl-4-amino-5-pyrimidinecarboxylic acid was identified in rat and human urine [42]. 4-methylthiazole-5-acetic acid, together with a thiamine-containing peptide, molecular weight ca. 25,000 was also characterized in human urine [40]. 5-(2-hydroxyethyl)-4-methylthiazole was reported to occur in rat urine [43], and some thiamine disulfide and thiochrome may be present. It has been suggested [44] that the measurement of urinary thiamine metabolites might offer a better insight into tissue thiamine reserves than urinary intact thiamine, because the metabolites continue to be excreted even when tissue thiamine stores become depleted. Many of the urinary thiamine metabolites were found to contain part, at least, of both rings of the vitamin [45]. Small amounts of intact thiamine are also lost in sweat. However, little is known about the factors that determine the rate of thiamine turnover in mammals.

BIOCHEMICAL FUNCTIONS

The four enzyme complexes in animal tissues that have, for many years, been known to require thiamine diphosphate as an essential cofactor comprise three closely related dehydrogenase systems, which catalyze oxidative decarboxylation reactions: pyruvate dehydrogenase complex, alpha-ketoglutarate dehydrogenase complex, and branched-chain ketoacid dehydrogenase complex, together with one enzyme that catalyzes a somewhat different type of reaction, namely transketolase, which catalyzes a glycolaldehyde moiety transfer reaction between sugars. Studies that paved the way for our understanding of these key biochemical pathways began in the 1920s and 1930s [46]. Much more recently, a fifth thiamine diphosphate-requiring enzyme has been added: this is a peroxisomal enzyme that catalyzes thiamine diphosphate-dependent cleavage following the alpha-oxidation of 3-methyl branched-chain fatty acids such as phytanic acid [47], and also the cleavage of 2-hydroxy straight-chain fatty acids to yield formate [48].

Thiamine diphosphate has a special relationship with magnesium ions at the active site of all thiamine diphosphate-requiring enzymes: this divalent cation is universally required to achieve binding of the anionic thiamine diphosphate cofactor to its apoenzymes.

Pyruvate Dehydrogenase Complex

The reactions catalyzed by the pyruvate dehydrogenase complex are shown in Figure 8.4. Pyruvate, produced from glucose by the Embden–Meyerhof (glycolytic) pathway, can either be reduced to lactate, or else committed to complete oxidation in the citric acid (Krebs) cycle via pyruvate dehydrogenase, which is thus a key enzyme in the overall oxidative metabolism of carbohydrates. The reaction product, acetyl coenzyme A, is also a key intermediate in fatty

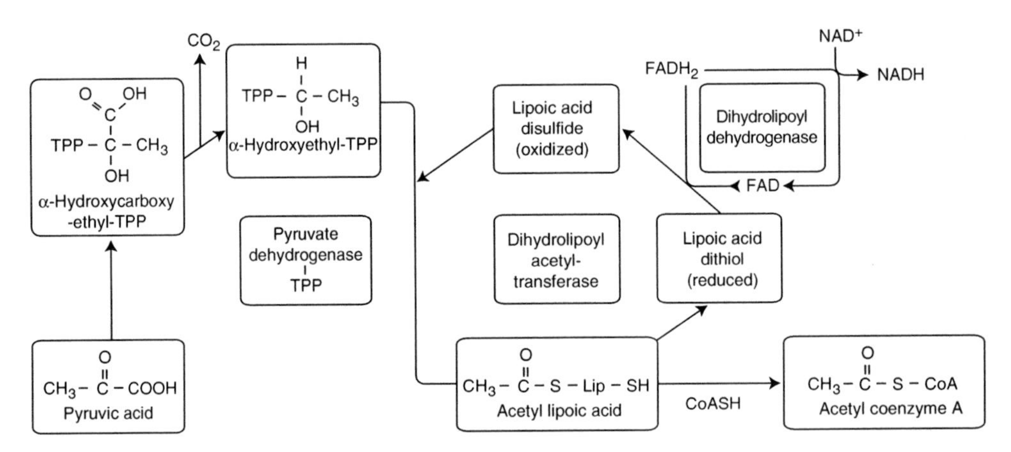

FIGURE 8.4 Reactions of the pyruvate dehydrogenase enzyme complex. The names of the three principal component enzymes of the complex are highlighted in bold type. Pyruvate dehydrogenase catalyzes the first (decarboxylation) step. Lipoic acid, in its oxidized disulfide form, bound as lipoamide to dihydrolipoyl acetyltransferase, then reacts with the product of pyruvic acid decarboxylation, by which it is converted to its reduced, dithiol form. Its reoxidation to the disulfide form releases two reducing equivalents via FAD to NAD^+, catalyzed by dihydrolipoyl dehydrogenase.

acid and steroid synthesis and, of course, in a myriad of acetylation reactions. The first enzyme in the sequence, pyruvate dehydrogenase (E1), is sometimes called pyruvate decarboxylase. It catalyzes the initial conversion of pyruvate to a hydroxyethyl carboxy derivative bound at position 2 of the thiazole ring of the thiamine diphosphate coenzyme and decarboxylation. The hydroxyethyl product then passes on to a lipoamide–protein complex in the second enzyme, dihydrolipoyl acetyltransferase (E2), which produces acetyl coenzyme A. Reoxidation of the reduced lipoamide requires the third enzyme, dihydrolipoyl dehydrogenase (E3). Two reducing equivalents are captured, via FAD to NAD^+. The same sequence of E1 (thiamine pyrophosphate-dependent decarboxylase), E2 (lipoamide-containing acyltransferase), and E3 (FAD-dependent dihydrolipoyl dehydrogenase generating NADH from NAD^+) occurs in alpha-ketoglutarate dehydrogenase and branched-chain alpha-keto acid dehydrogenase. E3 is identical in all three complexes.

A central feature, especially of the pyruvate dehydrogenase complex, is a metabolite-driven regulation mechanism involving reactants and products of the pathway, ensuring that its activity is rapidly and flexibly responsive to changing levels of these metabolites in vivo [49]. Pyruvate dehydrogenase activity is partly controlled by end-product inhibition [5], thus it is inhibited by the end-products, acetyl CoA and NADH. Further fine-tuning regulation is achieved by a phosphorylation–dephosphorylation cycle, involving serine residues in the alpha subunit of pyruvate dehydrogenase. The fully dephosphorylated form is by far more active, with an affinity for the thiamine diphosphate coenzyme that is enhanced at least 12-fold. There are three different serine phosphorylation sites within the dehydrogenase, each with a different degree of interaction with thiamine diphosphate and with the lipoyl groups of the acetyltransferase enzyme, and there are four different isoenzymes of the kinase (phosphorylating) enzyme, each with different specificities for the three serine phosphorylation sites, thus providing flexibility of regulation [50]. The pyruvate dehydrogenase complex in eukaryotes has a multiunit structure containing 20–30 heterotetramers of E1, each tetramer with two alpha and two beta subunits. Each 20–30 tetramers of E1 are associated with 60 units of acetyltransferase (E2), with 12 units of a dihydrolipoyl dehydrogenase-binding protein, with 6–12 homodimers of the dihydrolipoyl dehydrogenase enzyme (E3), and with the regulatory (kinase–phosphatase) enzyme system, which consists of 1–2 homo or heterodimers of pyruvate dehydrogenase kinase and 2–3 heterodimers of phosphopyruvate dehydrogenase phosphatase [51]. The subunit composition differs between different tissues and between species. The pyruvate dehydrogenase kinase activity is stimulated by the end-products of the pathway, NADH and acetyl CoA, and it is inhibited by ADP, pyruvate, CoA, NAD^+, thiamine diphosphate, and by intracellular free calcium. The phosphatase activity is stimulated by calcium and inhibited by NADH; the NADH inhibition can be reversed by NAD^+.

Genetic defects in the pyruvate decarboxylase complex, for example, Leigh's disease (section Thiamine-Dependent Reactions in the Nervous System) can lead to lethal lactic acidosis, psychomotor retardation, central nervous system damage, ataxia, muscle fiber atrophy, and developmental delay [52].

Alpha-Ketoglutarate Dehydrogenase and Branched-Chain Alpha-Keto Acid Dehydrogenase Complexes

These two dehydrogenase enzyme complexes resemble pyruvate dehydrogenase, both in the sequence of reactions that achieve oxidative decarboxylation and in possessing a multienzyme unit structure. The thiamine diphosphate cofactor is, however, more tightly bound here than in pyruvate dehydrogenase.

In the alpha-ketoglutarate dehydrogenase reaction, the equilibrium in the conversion of alpha-ketoglutarate to succinyl CoA lies far in the direction of succinyl CoA. Although alpha-ketoglutarate dehydrogenase apparently does not possess the same kinase–phosphatase control mechanism that acts on pyruvate dehydrogenase and branched-chain alpha-keto acid dehydrogenase, it is, nevertheless, subject to control through inhibition by ATP, GTP, NADH, and succinyl CoA and through stimulation by calcium ions [5,53]. The enzyme is considered to be vulnerable to oxidative stress, and is also claimed to be a contributor to such stress by generating hydrogen peroxide as a side reaction when the NADH:NAD^+ ratio is high [54].

There is an alternative pathway of alpha-ketoglutarate turnover that increases its throughput if the thiamine-dependent conversion to succinate is inhibited, for instance by a deficiency of thiamine. This pathway is known as the GABA shunt, and it gives rise to gamma-aminobutyric acid (via glutamate), which can be transaminated to give succinic semialdehyde and then oxidized to succinate. When this pathway increases in the hypothalamus, the feeding stimulus is reduced and anorexia results. This is one of the first functional lesions that is observed in thiamine-deficient animals such as rodents. Increased throughput for the GABA shunt in thiamine-deficient rats has been demonstrated by studies using labeled glutamate [55].

The third thiamine diphosphate-dependent dehydrogenase complex, which is based on the branched-chain alpha-keto acid dehydrogenase, forms part of the sequence of enzyme-catalyzed reactions that oxidize three branched-chain amino acids, valine, leucine, and isoleucine, so as to liberate energy from them when they are present in excess of requirements for protein synthesis [5]. Following transamination of these amino acids to give the corresponding alpha-keto acids, the dehydrogenase complex effects oxidative decarboxylation to liberate carbon dioxide and to reduce NAD^+ to NADH. The reaction products of this pathway are isobutyryl CoA, isovaleryl CoA, and alpha-methyl-butyryl CoA, respectively. Subsequently, pathways of fatty acid oxidation yield acetyl CoA or propionyl CoA from these intermediates; propionyl CoA is converted to succinyl CoA, and complete oxidation is then achieved by the tricarboxylic acid cycle. The branched-chain dehydrogenase enzyme, like pyruvate dehydrogenase, is regulated by protein phosphorylation–dephosphorylation, but here it appears to involve just a single serine residue (amino acid 292 of the E1b subunit) [56]. Phosphorylation generates a disordered loop that prevents E1b binding to the lipoyl-bearing domain of the E2b subunit, thereby inhibiting the entire reaction sequence. Thiamine deficiency (in rats) increases the proportion of the hepatic branched-chain dehydrogenase that is in the active, dephosphorylated state, thus helping to maintain its activity [57]. Therefore, paradoxically, the activities of the branched-chain dehydrogenase and of alpha-ketoglutarate dehydrogenase may respond in opposite directions in rat liver during thiamine depletion and repletion [57].

Maple syrup urine disease (branched-chain keto-aciduria) is a rare human genetic abnormality that results from various mutations of the genes for the first two of the three enzymes of the branched-chain dehydrogenase complex. In addition to ketoacidosis, there may also be mental retardation, ataxia, and sometimes blindness. Amelioration of some of these symptoms has been achieved by high thiamine intakes, in those individuals where increased tissue thiamine levels can counteract a reduced apoenzyme affinity for the thiamine cofactor [58–60].

Transketolase

Transketolase catalyzes two key reactions of the pentose phosphate pathway, one of whose functions is to generate pentose sugars, especially for synthesis of nucleic acids, their precursors, and related metabolites. It interconverts sugars with chain lengths between C_3 and C_7, of which C_3 and C_6 can enter the glycolytic sequence. The pentose phosphate pathway also generates the reduced form of NADP, which in turn is required for a wide range of biosynthetic reactions, including the synthesis of fatty acids. The fundamental reaction that transketolase catalyzes is a two-carbon (glycolaldehyde group) transfer from one sugar phosphate to another, resulting in the lengthening of the carbon chain of one of the sugar phosphates at the expense of the other:

$$\text{Xylulose-5-phosphate } (C_5) + \text{ribose-5-phosphate } (C_5) \leftrightarrow \text{glyceraldehyde-3-phosphate } (C_3) + \text{sedoheptulose-7-phosphate } (C_7)$$

and

$$\text{Xylulose-5-phosphate } (C_5) + \text{erythrose-4-phosphate } (C_4) \leftrightarrow \text{glyceraldehyde-3-phosphate } (C_3) + \text{fructose-6-phosphate } (C_6)$$

Transketolase acts in conjunction with the enzyme transaldolase, a non-thiamine diphosphate-requiring enzyme that catalyze

$$\text{Sedoheptulose-7-phosphate } (C_7) + \text{glyceraldehyde-3-phosphate } (C_3) \leftrightarrow \text{erythrose-4-phosphate}(C_4) + \text{fructose-6-phosphate } (C_6)$$

The pentose phosphate pathway is especially active in adipose tissue, mammary glands, and adrenal cortex, but less so in skeletal muscle and liver. Transketolase is found in most tissues and cell types. It is found in surprisingly high concentrations (10% of total soluble protein) in the cornea [61]. The highly active pentose phosphate pathway that is present in erythrocytes is thought to be necessary to generate NADPH rapidly, so as to maintain reduced glutathione levels in an oxidizing environment. Erythrocyte transketolase becomes partially depleted of its cofactor, thiamine diphosphate, during a period of dietary thiamine deficiency. The resulting apoenzyme can then be reactivated by an excess of the cofactor added in vitro, and the resulting increase in activity forms the basis for a commonly used test of thiamine status, the erythrocyte transketolase test (see section Erythrocyte Transketolase Assay).

Under thiamine-deficient conditions, several different types of cultured human cells were found to respond by reducing the synthesis of the messenger RNAs (i.e., there was transcriptional control) for transketolase and also for the beta subunit of pyruvate dehydrogenase, but not for alpha-ketoglutarate dehydrogenase. Thus, thiamine status may regulate gene expression for some thiamine diphosphate enzymes but not others [62].

Peroxisomal Alpha-Oxidation of 3-Methyl Branched-Chain Fatty Acids and Cleavage of 2-Hydroxylated Fatty Acids

A relative newcomer to the list of mammalian enzyme systems which requires thiamine diphosphate is a peroxisomal enzyme complex that catalyzes the alpha-oxidation and cleavage of 3-methyl fatty acids such as phytanic acid, and the cleavage of 2-hydroxy straight-chain fatty acids such as 2-hydroxyoctadecanoic acid that occurs in brain cerebrosides and sulfatides. Alpha-oxidation shortens them by a single carbon atom and thus enables them to enter the beta-oxidation pathway [47,48,63].

There are four sequential reactions in the alpha-oxidation pathway of 3-methyl fatty acids: firstly, activation of the 3-methyl fatty acid to its CoA derivative; secondly, hydroxylation at the 2-carbon; thirdly, thiamine diphosphate-dependent cleavage of the 1-carbon (to liberate formyl CoA and hence generate formate); and fourthly, dehydrogenation of the resulting long-chain aldehyde to an acyl group. The dependence of the third step on thiamine diphosphate was the first thiamine-cofactor-requiring reaction to be recognized in the peroxisomes. Clinically, this sequence of reactions is significant mainly for the occurrence of pathology linked to mutations in the gene for the second (hydroxylase) enzyme.

For the 2-hydroxy straight-chain fatty acids, formation of the CoA derivative is followed by thiamine diphosphate-dependent cleavage to formate and to an aldehyde with one less carbon than the original 2-hydroxy fatty acid [48]. Oxythiamine inhibits the latter reaction in cultured fibroblasts. Dependence on ATP, Mg^{2+}, and NAD^{+}, as well as thiamine diphosphate, has been demonstrated [48].

Thiamine-Dependent Reactions in the Nervous System

The polyneuritis of thiamine deficiency, characteristic of dry beriberi (section Dry Beriberi), and the neurological pathology of the Wernicke–Korsakoff syndrome (section Wernicke–Korsakoff Syndrome) have indicated that there is likely to be some special vulnerability of the nervous system (both central and peripheral regions) to the effects of thiamine depletion. Brain tissue, unlike other tissues, cannot use fatty acids for energy release and is wholly dependent on glucose as an energy source. However, despite a large body of research, the precise nature of the links between the biochemical and the functional vulnerability has remained elusive. There are indications that, whereas acute severe thiamine deficiency affects mainly the central nervous system, a chronic milder deficiency is more likely to result in pathology (such as polyneuritis) in the slower-responding peripheral nerves [64]. The hypothesis that thiamine may play a role in nervous tissue that is independent of its well-established coenzyme functions in other tissues was proposed, with some supporting evidence, by von Muralt [65].

One approach to this problem has focused on thiamine triphosphate that occurs in nerve cells. Bettendorff et al. [66–68] showed that chloride uptake was correlated with formation of thiamine triphosphate in membrane vesicles from brain and that neuroblastoma cells in culture respond (irreversibly) to the triphosphate by activating a large conductance chloride ion channel. It was proposed that a key protein within the channel becomes phosphorylated, and is thus activated, by thiamine triphosphate. The genetic disease, subacute necrotizing encephalomyopathy (Leigh's disease, see section Pyruvate Dehydrogenase Complex), which presents with dendrite and myelin lesions of the brain stem and third ventricle, and a range of neurological signs and symptoms, was reported to be accompanied by a reduction in levels of thiamine triphosphate but not of the diphosphate, and the presence of a compound in body fluids, which specifically inhibits the synthesis of thiamine triphosphate in the central nervous system [69–71]. This inhibition could be overcome by high oral doses of thiamine. There was also some evidence that thiamine triphosphate can act as the phosphate donor for phosphorylation of synaptic proteins [72], and that it could modify ion transport, especially sodium transport [73]. However, in the brains of thiamine-deficient rats, in which thiamine diphosphate levels had fallen as low as 26% of control levels in the pons region, thiamine triphosphate levels were unaffected, suggesting that the triphosphate may be relatively resistant to depletion, at least at this site [74]. Clearly the putative roles and significance of the triphosphate, in the brain and elsewhere, remain controversial and unresolved.

Studies on severely thiamine-deficient rats [75] have shown that the turnover of acetylcholine, the synthesis of catecholamines, the normal metabolism of serotonin, and the concentration of some functionally important amino acids (glutamate, aspartate, glutamine, gamma-aminobutyric acid) are all disturbed, thus identifying neurotransmitter metabolism as an area of potential vulnerability to deficiency. Malfunction of the blood–brain barrier has been reported in thiamine-deficient mice [76]; however, it is unclear whether this is a primary, or a later, secondary, defect.

Studies by Gibson and others of the neurological sequelae of thiamine deficiency in human subjects, in animal models, and in cultured cells have focused particularly on the oxidative stress and oxidant damage that accompanies thiamine depletion [77,78].

In Wernicke–Korsakoff syndrome in humans, neurodegeneration becomes apparent, initially as a reversible lesion and later irreversibly in very specific areas of the brain, notably the submedial thalamic nucleus and parts of the cerebellum, especially the superior cerebellar vermis [79]. Lactic acid accumulates in the medial thalamus, but not in the frontal cortex, in thiamine deficiency [80]. Many of the biochemical changes resulting from thiamine deficiency can affect both neurons and nonneuronal brain cells (e.g., astrocytes, microglial cells, endothelial cells, and neutrophils), and some of the changes were described as characteristic of oxidative stress. For instance, the disappearance of neurons and the elevation of markers of neurodegeneration during thiamine deficiency coincide with changes in microglial (resident immune) brain cells that include increases in redox active iron, nitric oxide synthase, and heme-oxygenase 1, all of which are markers of inflammation and oxidative stress [78]. Oxidation damage markers such as 4-hydroxynonenal, advanced glycation endproducts, and fragmentation damage to DNA have been observed in cultured neurons that are deprived of thiamine. Some of these changes are preventable by traditional antioxidants such as vitamin E or butylated hydroxyanisole [81].

It has been proposed that in the early stages of thiamine deficiency, biochemical changes in the (relatively robust) nonneuronal cells of the brain can be neuroprotective, but at the later stages of deficiency they are likely to exacerbate neuronal degeneration [78]. Another possible clue relating to neuronal cell vulnerability is that apoptosis of thiamine-deprived neuronal cells in culture has been linked to the decline of a specific regulatory protein kinase, Jnk1 [82].

Although neuronal cells have been most extensively studied with respect to oxidative stress-linked degeneration during thiamine deficiency, there is also some evidence of a similar type of damage in lens fiber cells in thiamine-deficient mice [83]. Increased expression of Alzheimer precursor protein, amyloid beta protein peptides, and presenilin 1 damage markers was detected.

The oxidant damage hypothesis, the concept that some cell types, especially neuronal cells, are especially vulnerable to irreversible damage and apoptosis during thiamine deficiency, and the complex interaction between different cell types during the course of deficiency represent approaches that may help to provide fresh perspectives on this difficult area of research; however, many key questions still remain unanswered.

PATHOGENESIS OF DEFICIENCY AND HIGH-RISK CONDITIONS

Beriberi in Infants

In thiamine-deficient infants, edema and right-sided heart failure are frequently accompanied by increased pulse rate and blood pressure. There may be gastrointestinal malfunction, with loss of appetite, vomiting, diarrhea, and oliguria, and convulsions may occur. The child may either cry loudly, or suffer hoarseness or even aphonia due to paralysis of the recurrent laryngeal nerve. Four subtypes have been described [5]. Causes include low thiamine levels in breast milk and weaning foods.

Wet Beriberi in Older Children and Adults

Edema and heart failure are common. In a rat model, ATP concentrations were reduced in the heart, but not in other tissues [84]. Cardiac blood output in deficient humans may be normal, high, or low. Where it is low, myocardial damage is suspected, and where high, vasomotor depression has been proposed [5]. A severe form is known as acute pernicious (fulminating) beriberi or shoshin beriberi, and accounted for ca. 26,000 deaths/year in Japan in the 1920s. There was heart failure, and circulating lactic acid levels were high. Its occurrence declined, but it then reappeared years later, in adolescents [85].

Dry Beriberi

A diet that is moderately deficient in thiamine may result in a symmetrical ascending peripheral polyneuritis, without cardiac symptoms. A chronic marginal deficiency can thus produce a different pathological syndrome from an acute, severe deficiency [64].

Weakness and numbness in the legs are followed by loss of the ankle jerk reflex and of control of the muscles of the foot, then the calf, and then the thigh. Foot and hand droop occur. Hyperaesthesia (abnormally increased sensation) in a glove and stocking pattern is followed by surface anesthesia, together with deep muscular pain. Axonal degeneration with flattened sacs or tubules of the axoplasm of large myelinated fibers is seen, which returns toward normal after treatment with thiamine [86]. In a rat model there is axonal degeneration with increased mitochondrial and endoplasmic reticulum vesicle counts, followed by disruption of the neurotubules, neurofilaments, and myelin sheaths [87]. Prolonged nerve degeneration may become resistant to repair.

Wernicke–Korsakoff Syndrome

Chronic alcohol abuse is frequently associated with Wernicke's encephalopathy, Korsakoff psychosis, or a combination, known as Wernicke–Korsakoff syndrome. Alcoholics often have poor diets, and hence a low intake of thiamine, impaired absorption (because ethanol reduces thiamine transport at both the brush border and the basolateral membrane of the intestinal mucosa), and impaired utilization of the vitamin, especially if there is fibrotic liver damage. Thiamine supplements frequently produce dramatic clinical improvement, but some types of damage may be irreversible.

Diagnosis of Wernicke's encephalopathy classically depends on the presence of ataxia, paralysis of eye movements, and abnormal motor function [88]. If amnesia or apathy and confabulation are present, Wernicke–Korsakoff syndrome is diagnosed. Magnetic resonance imaging [89,90] for diagnosis is being developed.

Alcoholic neuropathy and thiamine-deficiency neuropathy can be distinguished [91]. Sural nerve specimens from alcoholic neuropathy had small fiber-predominant axonal loss, whereas thiamine-deficiency neuropathy exhibited large fiber axonal loss. In Australia, mandatory addition of thiamine to bread flour in 1991 was followed by some improvement [92–94].

Possible variations in genetic susceptibility have been considered [95]. One study [96] reported that transketolase from skin fibroblasts from people with Korsakoff's psychosis had an affinity for thiamine diphosphate that was 10-fold lower than that of controls. Another reported that in alcoholics (men and their sons) transketolase exhibited reduced affinity for its cofactor [97]. However, the original finding could not be confirmed in several other studies [98,99]. Thiamine-dependent hysteresis of transketolase has been described [100], which might cause interindividual variation. In one Wernicke–Korsakoff patient, a transketolase assembly defect was present [101]. Thus, research on predisposing factors is continuing.

Alzheimer's Disease and Other Neurodegenerative Conditions

A potential association between thiamine-dependent enzyme defects and neurodegenerative diseases such as Alzheimer's and Parkinson's diseases has been proposed. A modest (18%–21%) reduction in thiamine diphosphate levels was seen in two studies of Alzheimer brain [102,103]. Gibson and Zhang [77] have summarized the evidence that all thiamine-dependent enzyme activities, especially that of the alpha-ketoglutarate dehydrogenase complex, are severely impaired in the brains of Alzheimer's, Parkinson's, and other degenerative brain disease sufferers, and have proposed that this impairment may be directly linked to the pathophysiology of the disease. Although thiamine supplementation studies have so far failed to provide convincing evidence of benefit in Alzheimer's sufferers [104,105] further investigation seems warranted [77].

Other High-Risk Groups

In western society, certain older adults are at risk of suboptimum thiamine status. In the United Kingdom, older people in nursing homes were found to have especially poor biochemical status [106,107]. Low erythrocyte thiamine diphosphate concentrations, below 140 nmol/L, were found in 16% of 225 subjects aged 65 years and over [108], and poor status was also seen in older people in the United States [109]. Thiamine-cofactor concentrations in the human brain may decline with increasing age [110]. Use of diuretic drugs by older people may increase urinary losses of thiamine, although the evidence is not conclusive [111].

Others at risk include people receiving parenteral nutrition, especially if their main energy source is glucose without added thiamine. Patients with intestinal resection, in whom the major sites of thiamine absorption have been damaged or removed, postgastrectomy patients, people who are treated with the cancer chemotherapy drug 5-flurouracil, and pregnant women with prolonged hyperemesis gravidarum, especially if treated with intravenous glucose without added thiamine. People with HIV are likely to have poor status [112].

Sporadic outbreaks of beriberi occur in developing countries. In The Gambia, in West Africa, hard physical work and a monotonous rice-based diet, especially during the rainy season, have led to beriberi in adult men, with a number of deaths [113]. Postpartum women in a Thai Karen refugee camp [114] and their infants [115] have developed beriberi, and other outbreaks have been reported from Indonesia, the Seychelles, and the Amazonian Indians of South America [116–118]. Thiamine deficiency may increase the risk of cerebral complications of malaria [119]. Tropical neuropathies are suspect. An outbreak of optical and peripheral neuropathy affected ca. 50,000 people in Cuba in 1993, after food availability and quality had deteriorated, following severance of trading partnerships with the Soviet Union [120]. A high intake of sugar (a local cash crop) and alcohol was accompanied by poor biochemical thiamine status [121]. The increased neuropathy prevalence subsided with a countrywide multivitamin supplementation program. Sporadic outbreaks of deficiency can arise, especially in the tropics, in conditions of stress coupled with poor diet.

ASSESSMENT OF THIAMINE STATUS

Nutrient status assessment of individuals and population groups is based on a combination of clinical investigations and biochemical index measurements. Clinical observations are especially important in situations where deficiency is believed to be severe. Where an intervention, such as vitamin supplementation, is planned, they form an essential part of the process of monitoring its efficacy. However, clinical signs may be difficult to interpret, especially where there are multiple insults. The strength of biochemical status tests is that they can be made very specific for a particular insult, such as thiamine deficiency in the presence of other nutrient deficiencies and disease processes, and they can detect mild, subclinical deficiencies, which can then act as an early warning of suboptimum nutrition, of the risk of future clinical deterioration, and they can help to clarify the etiology of pathologies with multiple causation.

Measurement of biochemical status in a sample of body fluid is less demanding of subject cooperation than an accurate long-term dietary history, and it is able to detect tissue depletion that is caused by factors other than low dietary intake, such as impaired absorption (see section Metabolism: Bioavailability, Absorption, Tissue Distribution, Turnover).

For thiamine, the principal options available for biochemical status measurement are urinary thiamine excretion rates, whole blood or erythrocyte total thiamine concentrations,

TABLE 8.3
Biochemical Tests of Thiamine Status: Interpretative Guidelines

Status Assay (Units)	Sample Required	Age-Group	Interpretation		
			Deficient	Marginal	Normal
Urinary thiamine excretion: μg/g creatinine (μmol/mol creatinine)	24 h or single urine samples[a]	1–3 years	<120 (<51)	120–175 (51–75)	>175 (>75)
		4–6 years	<85 (<36)	85–120 (36–51)	>121 (>51)
		7–9 years	<70 (<30)	70–180 (30–77)	>181 (>77)
		10–12 years	<60 (<25)	60–180 (25–77)	>181 (>77)
		13–15 years	<50 (<21)	50–150 (21–64)	>151 (>64)
		Adult	<27 (<12)	27–65 (12–28)	>66 (>28)
Erythrocyte thiamine diphosphate[b]: nmol/L	Washed erythrocytes	All ages	<120	120–150	>150
Erythrocyte transketolase activation coefficient: ETKAC:enzyme activity ratio; without units	Washed erythrocytes	All ages	>1.25	1.16–1.24	1.00–1.15

Source: From Sauberlich, H.E. in *Laboratory Tests for the Assessment of Nutritional Status*, CRC Press, Boca Raton, 1999, 37–53. With permission.

[a] Here, 24 h urine samples are preferred, but their collection is more demanding than for single-void samples.
[b] Tentative interpretation, because relevant studies are scarce.

and the erythrocyte transketolase activation test (Table 8.3). Other, less frequently-used options include serum or plasma thiamine concentrations and thiamine in cerebrospinal fluid. Serum (or plasma) and cerebrospinal fluid both contain free thiamine and its monophosphate, but not the higher phosphates [122], whereas red cells (like most intact cells) contain mainly thiamine diphosphate. Horwitt and Kreisler historic carbohydrate metabolism index [123], which is an interesting example of a functional test at whole body rather than specific enzyme level, is included for completeness.

Urinary Thiamine Excretion

The rate of excretion of thiamine in the urine has for many years been recognized as reflecting the thiamine supply to the individual, and hence as providing an indirect index of tissue status, and it underpinned some of the earliest studies of human thiamine requirements in the 1940s and 1950s. A dataset that illustrates covariance of thiamine excretion rates with group thiamine intakes in healthy adults in the United States [34,124] reveals that above a certain threshold of thiamine intake, which is around 0.3–0.4 mg/1000 kcal in adults, urinary concentrations increase steeply. This necessarily occurs when plasma thiamine concentrations reach a level at which renal tubular reabsorption approaches saturation. Urinary excretion rates reflect variations in thiamine intake in the adequate range, but they are less sensitive to variations in intake at very low intakes where tissue deficiency occurs. At an adequate intake of 0.5 mg/1000 kcal, the daily excretion rate was at least 100 μg [125,126]; at a marginal intake of 0.2 mg/1000 kcal the daily excretion rate was only 5–25 μg [4,125,126], and in cases of beriberi it was 0–15 μg [4]. Large within- and between-subject variabilities of urinary thiamine for a given thiamine intake are encountered, so that this test is more useful to characterize groups of people than it is for individuals.

Early studies quantitated thiamine in urine either by microbiological assay procedures or by chemical conversion to thiochrome followed by extraction into a less-polar solvent (typically isobutanol) and direct measurement of the thiochrome fluorescence (see section Analytical Procedures). More recently, the use of HPLC with precolumn or postcolumn conversion to thiochrome has made the assay much more specific and accurate, thereby permitting more reliable assays, especially of samples from deficient subjects. Although 24 h urine collections are preferable, because they overcome the problem of diurnal fluctuations in intake and excretion, the cost of a 24 h collection and limitations of subject compliance have meant that they are relatively difficult to obtain, and it is cumbersome to verify the completeness of collection in population surveys. Therefore, a more extensive body of data is available for single or spot urine samples. Variable urine dilution can be corrected for by using urinary creatinine as the denominator, but it is important to be aware that creatinine excretion rates differ markedly between age-groups. Pearson [127] found that in children, urinary thiamine:creatinine ratios are much higher than those in adults, so that age-specific interpretative guidelines are needed [34], see Table 8.3.

A thiamine load test (e.g., 5 mg given parenterally, followed by the measurement of urinary excretion over a 4 h postdose period, which yields <20 μg excreted by deficient subjects) is occasionally used as a confirmatory diagnostic test in individuals with suspected deficiency, but this test is too cumbersome for survey use.

Thiamine Concentrations in Serum or Plasma, Whole Blood, or Erythrocytes

The measurement of thiamine in serum or plasma has been used as a status assay, but this has not become popular, partly because extracellular levels of nutrients such as thiamine generally reflect recent intakes rather than long-term status, and because the concentrations encountered are much lower than those in erythrocytes, making them more difficult to measure accurately and more susceptible to contamination by leakage of thiamine from cells during sample preparation. About 80% of total blood thiamine is found in the erythrocytes; only about 10% is in the plasma [128].

The direct assay of thiamine in whole blood or washed red cells is generally recognized as useful as an index of status, and indeed is preferred over other approaches by several laboratories, but the details of the procedures vary widely, including the choice of denominator, often making it difficult to compare results between laboratories. Moreover, there are no universally accepted interpretative guidelines available to define the normal and the deficient ranges of whole blood or red cell thiamine. Table 8.3 shows some tentative guidelines for the interpretation of erythrocyte thiamine diphosphate concentrations. There is on average about twice as much total thiamine in the red cells (or whole blood) of well-nourished subjects as in those with signs of deficiency.

The measurement of total thiamine in whole blood has been the preferred choice of procedure in a number of laboratories, but variations in hematocrit need to be corrected for. It is, of course, possible to measure the thiamine concentration in both whole blood and separated plasma and then to calculate the concentration in the red cells, based on the hematocrit, as is common practice for red cell folate assays. However, this rather cumbersome approach has not gained favor for thiamine. Alternatively, washed erythrocyte preparations may be assayed, and the thiamine content then expressed as a ratio to hemoglobin [129] or as a concentration in the intracellular fluid. This approach has the advantage that the white cells (which contain a higher concentration of thiamine than erythrocytes) can be removed. Since erythrocytes contain mainly phosphorylated thiamine, whereas free thiochrome formation requires the free vitamin, phosphatase treatment may need to be included when total thiamine in whole blood or erythrocyte preparations is measured. However, of the 19 published HPLC assay methods listed by Lynch and Young [12] for thiamine assay in biological fluids, more than half estimate the individual phosphate esters and the free thiamine separately. Baines and Davies [130], Kuriyama et al. [131], and Talwar et al. [129] have reported that the concentration of total thiamine or thiamine diphosphate in erythrocytes correlates well with erythrocyte transketolase-based status measurements, but there is disagreement about which of the two status assays is preferable. Studies providing data to define a lower limit of the normal range for thiamine diphosphate concentrations in erythrocytes have generally suggested around 140–150 nmol/L [132–134], but more data are needed to confirm this estimate. Talwar et al. [129] have quoted a normal range (mean $\pm$ 2SD) of 280–590 ng TDP/g hemoglobin in washed erythrocytes from 147 Scottish subjects.

Erythrocyte Transketolase Assay

Since the original development of the erythrocyte transketolase assay as an index of thiamine status by Brin in the early 1960s [135], this enzyme activation-based assay has proved robust insofar that it is highly specific for thiamine and sensitive to progressive tissue thiamine depletion in the marginal-to-deficient range. As it is a ratio of two enzyme activities, there is no possibility of variable interlaboratory choices in the choice of denominator. The test is analogous to the erythrocyte glutathione reductase assay for riboflavin status and erythrocyte aminotransferase assay for vitamin B_6 status, which are further examples of in vitro erythrocyte enzyme activation assays.

Transketolase activity (see section Transketolase) is measured simultaneously in two identical subsamples of the washed erythrocyte hemolysate from each subject, one of which contains no added cofactor and the other contains sufficient thiamine diphosphate cofactor to saturate and reactivate any transketolase apoenzyme that may be present. It can be measured by a colorimetric end-point assay, which in the original assay by Brin was based on disappearance of pentose (orcinol reaction) and the formation of hexose (anthrone reaction) after a standard incubation. A later version of the colorimetric end-point assay measured the formation of sedoheptulose phosphate by its reaction with sulfuric acid and cysteine. These older colorimetric assays have now been superseded by a pyridine nucleotide-based assay of the formation, from ribose-5-phosphate, of glyceraldehyde-3-phosphate, which is further converted to dihydroxyacetone phosphate and then to glycerol-1-phosphate by two added enzymes (triose phosphate isomerase and glycerol-1-phosphate dehydrogenase), where the final enzymic step is linked to the oxidation of NADH [136]. This is usually measured by spectrophotometric monitoring of the intact enzyme reaction mixture at 340 nm wavelength. It is often monitored as a rate reaction, and is compatible with several automated clinical chemistry analyzers (provided that they are flexibly programmable and operationally compatible with the long incubation time that is required) [137,138]. Microtitre plate assay technology is also potentially feasible. The extent of in vitro activation of the enzyme by its cofactor, thiamine diphosphate, is expressed either as a percentage of the basal enzyme activity (= thiamine pyrophosphate effect) or else as an activation coefficient (ETKAC), which is the fractional ratio of stimulated to unstimulated activity. Thus, a thiamine pyrophosphate effect of 10% translates to an ETKAC of 1.10. Interpretative guidelines, based on Brin's studies, are shown in Table 8.3.

In some situations, prolonged chronic deficiency of thiamine can reduce the transketolase apoenzyme concentration in the red cells in vivo, and thereby result in low basal activity but minimal activation by thiamine diphosphate in vitro [5]. It is therefore often recommended that the basal activity of erythrocyte transketolase should also be measured (e.g., substrate conversion per unit time per unit of hemoglobin in a sample without added thiamine diphosphate), since this index, in addition to ETKAC, may reveal abnormal status and the need for intervention. Low apoenzyme levels have been reported in certain disease states, including diabetes and uremia. In contrast, in some situations where red cell turnover rates are increased (e.g., iron deficiency or pernicious anemia), basal ETK activity may be increased because of an increase in the proportion of younger cells, but ETKAC remains normal, provided that tissue thiamine status is normal.

TABLE 8.4
Erythrocyte Transketolase Activation Coefficient Values in Four Age-Groups: Percentages of Values in the Abnormal Range in the UK National Diet and Nutrition Survey Series

	ETKAC: Male Subjects			ETKAC: Female Subjects		
Survey	**Base No.**	**% >1.15**	**% >1.25**	**Base No.**	**% >1.15**	**% >1.25**
Young people aged 4–18 years (a)	561	22	0	534	23	2
Adults aged 19–64 years (b)	628	46	3	672	34	1
People aged 65+ years: free-living (c)	454	57	8	439	51	9
People aged 65+ years: in institutions (c)	134	57	11	117	54	15

Source: (a) From Gregory, J., Lowe, S., Bates, C.J., Prentice, A., Jackson, L.V., Smithers, G., Wenlock, R., and Farron, M., in *Volume 1: Report of the Diet and Nutrition Survey*, The Stationery Office, London, 2000; (b) From Ruston, D., Hoare, J., Henderson, L., Gregory, J., Bates, C.J., Prentice, A., Birch, M., Swan, G., and Farron, M., in *Volume 4: Nutritional Status (Anthropometry and Blood Analytes), Blood Pressure and Physical Activity*, The Stationery Office, London, 2004; (c) From Finch, S., Doyle, W., Lowe, C., Bates, C.J., Prentice, A.M., Smithers, G., and Clarke, P.C., in *Volume 1: Report of the Diet and Nutrition Survey*, The Stationery Office, London, 1998.

The preparation of washed red cells for the ETKAC assay is time consuming and requires specialized equipment, so it may not be feasible under fieldwork conditions at remote sites, in which case, the use of whole blood can be an acceptable alternative.

As an example of the use of ETKAC in population surveillance, Table 8.4 shows the percentages of values for ETKAC above 1.15 and 1.25 in four nationally representative samples of subjects, living in mainland UK in the final decade of the twentieth century, derived from reports of the National Diet and Nutrition Surveys. Except in the subgroup of older people living in institutions such as nursing homes, only a small percentage of subjects had ETKAC values above 1.25, which are indicative of severe biochemical deficiency. However, the proportion of subjects with values above 1.15, indicative of mild biochemical deficiency, was much greater, and it increased progressively with age. In the 19–64 year age-group, fewer women than men had ETKAC values above 1.15, which is consistent with a more frequent use of dietary supplements by women [139].

Carbohydrate Metabolism Index

Thiamine deficiency increases blood pyruvate and lactate concentrations, especially after a glucose load and exercise. Horwitt and Kreisler [123] made use of this effect to devise a functional test known as the carbohydrate metabolism index, in which pyruvate and lactate levels are assayed after an oral dose of glucose plus mild exercise. Although a true functional test, which measures biochemical function by an end-product of a key pathway, it is now considered impractical because it is not sufficiently specific for thiamine deficiency, and it is too cumbersome to be used for population studies.

HUMAN REQUIREMENTS AND RECOMMENDED INTAKES

Many of the biochemical functions of thiamine are linked to the release of energy from energy-providing substrates. Depending on the preference of individual expert committees, human thiamine requirements and recommendations have been expressed both on an absolute daily basis and as a ratio to dietary energy. In the Dietary Reference Values for the United Kingdom published in 1991 [140] the Reference Nutrient Intakes for thiamine have been given in both ways. A more recent appraisal in the United States for the Dietary Reference Intakes in 1998 [13] concluded that it is better to express thiamine requirements in absolute daily amounts. This was because under normal conditions, variations in physical activity did not appear to influence thiamine requirements, although there was some published evidence that they may be increased by very heavy physical work.

A comparison of the current UK Reference Dietary Intakes and U.S. Recommended Dietary Allowances (Table 8.5) indicates reasonably close conformity between the two sets of recommendations.

TABLE 8.5
U.S. Dietary Reference Intakes [13] and UK Dietary Reference Values [140] for Thiamine

	U.S. DRIs (mg/day)			UK DRVs (mg/1000 kcal)			UK DRVs (mg/day)
Age-Groups	AI[a]	EAR[b]	RDA[c]	LRNI[d]	EAR[b]	RNI[e]	RNI[e]
Children							
0–6 months	0.2			0.2	0.23	0.3	0.2
7–9 months	0.3			0.2	0.23	0.3	0.2
10–12 months	0.3			0.2	0.23	0.3	0.2
1–3 years		0.4	0.5	0.23	0.3	0.4	0.5
4–6 years				0.23	0.3	0.4	0.7
4–8 years		0.5	0.6				
7–10 years				0.23	0.3	0.4	0.7
Males							
9–13 years		0.7	0.9				
11–14 years				0.23	0.3	0.4	0.9
14–18 years		1.0	1.2				
15–18 years				0.23	0.3	0.4	0.1
19+ years		1.0	1.2				
19–50 years				0.23	0.3	0.4	1.0
50+ years				0.23	0.3	0.4	0.9
Females							
9–13 years		0.7	0.9				
11–14 years				0.23	0.3	0.4	0.7
14–18 years		0.9	1.0				
15–18 years				0.23	0.3	0.4	0.8
19+ years		0.9	1.1				
19–50 years				0.23	0.3	0.4	0.8
50+ years				0.23	0.3	0.4	0.8
Pregnancy		1.2	1.4	0.23	0.3	0.4	0.9 (third trimester)
Lactation		1.2	1.4	0.23	0.3	0.4	1.0

Source: Extracted from Food and Nutrition Board, *Institute of Medicine, Dietary Reference Intakes: Thiamine, Riboflavin, Niacin, Vitablin B_6, Folate, Vitamin B_{12}, Pantothemic Acid, Biotin and choline, Eds.*, National Academy Press, Washington DC, 1998, 58–86. With permission; Extracted from Department of Health, *Report on Health and Social Subjects No. 41. Dietary Reference Values for Food Energy and Nutrients for the United Kingdom. Report of the Panel on Dietary Reference Values of the Committee on Medical Aspects of Food Policy*, HMSO, London, 1991, 90–93. With permission.

[a] Adequate intake.

[b] Estimated average requirement.

[c] Recommended dietary allowance.

[d] Lower reference nutrient intake.

[e] Reference nutrient intake. In the U.S. and the UK tables, the RDA and the RNI are each intended to meet the needs of the majority of healthy people in the population group described.

For suckled infants, the UK estimated average requirement is based on an estimate of the mean thiamine content of human milk from UK mothers, 0.16 mg/L, which equates to 0.23 mg/1000 kcal [141]. Artificial feeds for young infants in the United Kingdom have been recommended to contain not less than 0.2 mg thiamine/1000 kcal [141].

PHARMACOLOGY, HIGH DOSES, TOXICITY

Thiamine is generally well tolerated, even at high oral intakes, partly because of the brush border limit on excessive absorption. Commercial multivitamin supplements for prevention of deficiency typically contain 1–5 mg thiamine/daily dose; those used for treatment of deficiency often provide 10–35 mg/day and thiamine as a single nutrient is available at up to 300 mg/day dosage. Frank beriberi is frequently treated by 50–100 mg thiamine daily, given intramuscularly or intravenously for 7–14 days, followed by an oral maintenance dose. As noted in the section Chemistry, synthetic allithiamine compounds are readily absorbed and then converted to thiamine, thereby achieving high concentrations for rapid therapy. For instance, 50 mg thiamine propyl disulfide, given orally to Wernicke patients, efficiently restored their low biochemical status and reversed their clinical deficiency signs [142]. Very large doses of thiamine given intravenously to animals can cause vasodilatation, a fall in blood pressure, bradycardia, and respiratory depression or arrhythmia, and can suppress transmission of nerve impulses at the neuromuscular junction [3]. In humans, very high parenteral doses of thiamine are sometimes toxic, possibly due to anaphylaxis [143]. Death in one instance and clinical signs including respiratory distress, nausea, abdominal pain, shock, and pruritus have been recorded following parenteral or intramuscular administration of large doses, but no upper limit on oral intake has been set [13]

An apparently unexplained observation was the occurrence of extremely high serum thiamine concentrations in infants who succumbed to sudden infant death syndrome (SIDS) [7]. There was no indication that the biochemical anomaly was responsible for the deaths.

CONCLUSION

Just over a century ago, the discovery of the dietary cause of beriberi, followed in the next quarter century by the isolation of thiamine, the determination of its structure and its chemical synthesis, were major advances in nutritional science. Elucidation of the role of thiamine diphosphate as an essential cofactor in several key enzyme reactions of carbohydrate and fatty acid metabolism was a second important milestone. However, the links between the catalysis of specific biochemical reactions and the signs and symptoms of thiamine deficiency diseases, especially in nerve tissues, remain only partly understood, even today. The relationships between thiamine deficiency, prooxidant damage, and apoptosis, especially in neurons in the brain, and the complex interactions that occur between different cell types represent a new area of research, which is vigorously explored. Possible roles of thiamine in certain common degenerative diseases affecting the brain, especially in older people, deserve exploration. In recent years, the specific thiamine transporter proteins in the gastrointestinal tract and elsewhere, and their genes and promoters, have been intensively studied, and important advances have been made in this area. Thiamine degradation within the body and factors affecting its turnover, however, are topics that have received less attention.

The burden of disease that is attributable to thiamine deficiency or thiamine-responsive conditions, worldwide, is poorly documented. In parts of the world where diet quality is especially poor and lacking in thiamine, sporadic outbreaks of beriberi continue to affect especially young infants, women in late pregnancy and during lactation, and adults, especially men, with high levels of energy expenditure. Chronic alcoholics are especially at risk in some affluent countries. New imaging techniques are developed for human studies, particularly for Wernicke's encephalopathy, to help diagnose and characterize subtle clinical abnormalities. Public health intervention, which may include fortification of a staple food, or careful identification of high-risk individuals for individual treatment, needs to be tailored to the specific problem areas.

ACKNOWLEDGMENT

Updated by: C.J. Bates, MRC Human Nutrition Research, Elsie Widdowson Laboratory, Fulbourn Road, Cambridge, CB1 9NL, UK, from the chapters on thiamine in the two previous editions, by C.J. Gubler and V. Tanphaichitr.

REFERENCES

1. Carpenter, K.J., *Beriberi, White Rice and Vitamin B: A Disease, a Cause and a Cure*, University of California Press, Berkeley, CA, 2000.
2. Jansen, B.C.P. and Donath, W.F., On the isolation of anti-beriberi vitamin, *Proc. K. Ned. Akad. Wet.*, 29, 1390, 1926.
3. Gubler, C.J., Thiamin, in *Handbook of Vitamins*, 2nd edn., Machlin, L.J., ed., Marcel Dekker, Inc., NY, 1991, 233.
4. Williams, R.R., *Toward the Conquest of Beriberi*, Harvard University Press, Cambridge, MA, 1961.
5. Tanphaichitr, V., Thiamine, in *Handbook of Vitamins*, 3rd edn., Rucker, R.B., Suttie, J.W., McCormick, D.B., and Machlin, L.J., eds., Marcel Dekker, Inc., NY, 2001, 275.
6. Lonsdale, D., Thiamine tetrahydrofurfuryl disulfide: a little known therapeutic agent, *Med. Sci. Monit.*, 10, RA199, 2004.
7. Davis, R.E. and Icke, G., Clinical chemistry of thiamin, *Adv. Clin. Chem.*, 23, 93, 1983.
8. Ball, G.F.M., Thiamin (Vitamin B_1), in *Bioavailability and Analysis of Vitamins in Foods*, Chapman and Hall, London, 1998, 267.
9. Ohta, H., Maeda, M., and Nogata, Y., A simple determination of thiamine in rice (*Oryza sativa* L.) by high performance liquid chromatography with post-column derivatisation, *J. Liq. Chromatogr.*, 16, 2617, 1993.
10. Baker, H. et al., A method for assessing thiamine status in man and animals, *Am. J. Clin. Nutr.*, 14, 197, 1964.
11. AOAC, Thiamin (vitamin B_1) in foods. Fluorimetric method. Final action. 942.23, in *AOAC Official Methods of Analysis*, 15th edn., Helrich, K., ed., Association of Official Analytical Chemists, Inc., Arlington, VA, 1990.
12. Lynch, P.L.M. and Young, I.S., Determination of thiamine by high-performance liquid chromatography, *J. Chromatogr. A*, 881, 267, 2000.
13. Food and Nutrition Board, Institute of Medicine, ed., *Dietary Reference Intakes: Thiamin, Riboflavin, Niacin, Vitamin B_6, Folate, Vitamin B_{12}, Pantothenic Acid, Biotin and Choline*, National Academy Press, Washington DC, 1998, 58–86.
14. Earl, J.W. and McCleary, B.V., Mystery of the poisoned expedition, *Nature*, 368, 683, 1994.
15. Harmeyer, J. and Kollenkirchen, U., Thiamin and niacin in ruminant nutrition, *Nutr. Res. Rev.*, 2, 201, 1989.
16. Rindi, G. and Laforenza, U., Thiamine intestinal transport and related issues: recent aspects, *Proc. Soc. Exp. Biol. Med.*, 224, 246, 2000.
17. Rindi, G. and Ventura, U., Thiamine intestinal transport, *Physiol. Rev.*, 52, 821, 1972.
18. Gregory, J.F., Bioavailability of thiamin, *Eur. J. Clin. Nutr.*, 51 (Suppl 1), S34, 1997.
19. Laforenza, U. et al., Thiamine uptake in human biopsy specimens, including observations from a patient with acute thiamine deficiency, *Am. J. Clin. Nutr.*, 66, 320, 1997.
20. Gastaldi, G. et al., Age-related thiamine transport by small intestinal microvillous vesicles of rat, *Biochim. Biophys. Acta*, 1103, 271, 1992.

21. Laforenza, U., Gastaldi, G., and Rindi, G., Thiamin outflow from the enterocyte: a study using basolateral membrane vesicles from rat small intestine, *J. Physiol. Lond.*, 468, 401, 1993.
22. Dudeja, P.K. et al., Evidence for a carrier-mediated mechanism for thiamine transport to human jejunal basolateral membrane vesicles, *Dig. Dis. Sci.*, 48, 109, 2003.
23. Said, H.M., Recent advances in carrier-mediated intestinal absorption of water-soluble vitamins, *Annu. Rev. Physiol.*, 66, 419, 2004.
24. Oishi, K. et al., Targeted disruption of Slc19a2, the gene encoding the high-affinity thiamin transporter Thtr-1, causes diabetes mellitus, sensorineural deafness and megaloblastosis in mice, *Hum. Mol. Genet.*, 11, 2951, 2002.
25. Ganapathy, V., Smith, S.B., and Prasad, P.D., SLC19: the folate/thiamine transporter family, *Eur. J. Physiol.*, 447, 641, 2004.
26. Reidling, J.C. et al., Expression and promoter analysis of *SLC19A2* in the human intestine, *Biochim. Biophys. Acta*, 1561, 180, 2002.
27. Said, H.M. et al., Expression and functional contribution of *hTHTR-2* in thiamin absorption in human intestine, *Am. J. Physiol.*, 286, G491, 2004.
28. Balamuragan, K. and Said, H.M., Functional role of specific amino acid residues in human thiamine transporter SLC19A2: mutational analysis, *Am. J. Physiol.*, 283, G37, 2002.
29. Subramanian, V.S. et al., Cell biology of the human thiamine transporter-1 (hTHTR1). Intracellular trafficking and membrane targeting mechanisms, *J. Biol. Chem.*, 278, 3976, 2003.
30. Neufeld, E.J. et al., Thiamine-responsive megaloblastic anemia syndrome: a disorder of high-affinity thiamine transport, *Blood Cells Mol. Dis.*, 27, 135, 2001.
31. Reidling, J.C. and Said, H.M., Adaptive regulation of intestinal thiamin uptake: molecular mechanism using wild-type and transgenic mice carrying *hTHTR-1* and *-2* promoters, *Am. J. Physiol.*, 288, G1127, 2005.
32. Patrini, C. et al., Thiamine transport by rat small intestine in vitro: influence of endogenous thiamine content of jejunal tissue, *Acta Vitaminol. Enzymol.*, 3, 17, 1981.
33. Verri, A. et al., Molecular characteristics of small intestinal and renal brush border thiamin transporters in rats, *Biochim. Biophys. Acta*, 1558, 187, 2002.
34. Sauberlich, H.E., Vitamin B_1 (Thiamin), in *Laboratory Tests for the Assessment of Nutritional Status*, CRC Press, Boca Raton, 1999, 37–53.
35. Zempleni, J. et al., Utilization of intravenously infused thiamin hydrochloride in healthy adult males, *Nutr. Res.*, 16, 1479, 1996.
36. Grassl, S.M., Thiamine transport in human placental brush border membrane vesicles, *Biochim. Biophys. Acta*, 1371, 213, 1998.
37. Bates, C. and Prentice, A., Vitamins, minerals and essential trace elements, in *Drugs and Human Lactation*, 2nd edn., Bennett, P.N., ed., Elsevier Science Publishers, Amsterdam, 1996, 533.
38. Ortega, R.M. et al., Thiamin status during the third trimester of pregnancy and its influence on thiamin concentrations in transition and mature breast milk, *Br. J. Nutr.*, 92, 129, 2004.
39. Adiga, P.R. and Munyappa, K., Estrogen induction and functional importance of carrier proteins for riboflavin and thiamin in the rat during gestation, *J. Steroid Biochem.*, 9, 829, 1978.
40. Ariaey-Nejad, M.R. et al., Thiamin metabolism in man, *Am. J. Clin. Nutr.*, 23, 764, 1970.
41. Neal, R.A. and Sauberlich, H.E., Thiamine, in *Modern Nutrition in Health and Disease*, 5th edn., Goodhart, S. and Shils, M.E., eds., Lea & Febiger, Philadelphia, PA, 1973, 186.
42. Neal, R. and Pearson, W., Studies of thiamine metabolism in the rat. II. Isolation and identification of 2-methyl-4-amino-5-pyrimidinecarboxylic acid as a metabolite of thiamine in rat urine, *J. Nutr.*, 83, 351, 1964.
43. Iacono, J. and Johnson, B., Thiamine metabolism. I. The metabolism of thiazole-2-C14-thiamine in the rat, *J. Am. Chem. Soc.*, 79, 6321, 1957.
44. Pearson, W. et al., Excretion of metabolites of ^{14}C-pyrimidine-labeled thiamine by the rat at different levels of thiamine intake, *J. Nutr.*, 89, 133, 1966.
45. Balaghi, M. and Pearson, W., Comparative studies of the metabolism of ^{14}C-pyrimidine-labelled thiamine, ^{14}C-thiazole-labeled thiamine and ^{35}S-labeled thiamine in the rat, *J. Nutr.*, 91, 9, 1967.
46. Peters, R.A., *Biochemical Lesions and Lethal Synthesis*, Pergamon Press, Oxford, 1963.
47. Casteels, M. et al., Alpha-oxidation of 3-methyl-substituted fatty acids and its thiamine dependence, *Eur. J. Biochem.*, 270, 1619, 2003.

48. Foulon, V. et al., Breakdown of 2-hydroxylated straight chain fatty acids via peroxisomal 2-hydroxyphytanoyl-CoA lyase: a revised pathway for the alpha-oxidation of straight chain fatty acids, *J. Biol. Chem.*, 280, 9802, 2005.
49. Behal, H. et al., Regulation of the pyruvate dehydrogenase multienzyme complex, *Annu. Rev. Nutr.*, 13, 497, 1993.
50. Patel, M.S. and Korotchkina, L.G., Regulation of mammalian pyruvate dehydrogenase complex by phosphorylation: complexity of multiple phosphorylation sites and kinases, *Exp. Mol. Med.*, 33, 191, 2001.
51. Patel, M.S. and Roche, T.E., Molecular biology and biochemistry of pyruvate dehydrogenase complexes, *FASEB J.*, 4, 3224, 1990.
52. Robinson, B.H., Lactic acidemia (disorders of pyruvate carboxylase, pyruvate dehydrogenase). Chapter 44, in *The Metabolic and Molecular Bases of Inherited Disease*, 7th edn., Scriver, C.R., ed., McGraw-Hill, Inc., NY, 1995, 1479.
53. Olson, M.S., Bioenergetics and oxidative metabolism, in *Textbook of Biochemistry with Clinical Correlations*, 3rd edn., Devlin, T.M., ed., Wiley-Liss, NY, 1992, 237.
54. Tretter, L. and Adam-Vizi, V., Generation of reactive oxygen species in the reaction catalyzed by alpha-ketoglutarate dehydrogenase, *J. Neurosci. Res.*, 24, 7771, 2004.
55. Page, M.G. et al., Brain glutamate and γ-aminobutyrate (GABA) metabolism in thiamin deficient rats, *Brit. J. Nutr.*, 62, 245, 1989.
56. Wynn, R.M. et al., Molecular mechanism for regulation of the human mitochondrial branched-chain alpha-ketoacid dehydrogenase complex by phosphorylation, *Structure (Camb)*, 12, 2185, 2004.
57. Blair, P.V. et al., Dietary thiamin level influences levels of its diphosphate form and thiamin-dependent enzymic activities of rat liver, *J. Nutr.*, 129, 641, 1999.
58. Scriver, C.R. et al., Thiamine-responsive maple-syrup-urine disease, *Lancet*, 1, 310, 1971.
59. Duran, M. and Wadman, S.K., Thiamine-responsive inborn errors of metabolism, *J. Inherit. Metab. Dis.*, 8, 70, 1985.
60. Ames, B.N., Elson-Schwab, I., and Silver, E.A., High-dose vitamin therapy stimulates variant enzymes with coenzyme binding affinity (increased K_m): relevance to genetic disease and polymorphisms, *Am. J. Clin. Nutr.*, 75, 616, 2002.
61. Sax, C.M. et al., Transketolase is a major protein in the mouse cornea, *J. Biol. Chem.*, 271, 3568, 1996.
62. Pekovich, S.R., Martin, P.R., and Singleton, C.K., Thiamin deficiency decreases steady-state transketolase and pyruvate dehydrogenase but not α-ketoglutarate dehydrogenase mRNA levels in three human cell types, *J. Nutr.*, 128, 683, 1998.
63. Foulon, V. et al., Purification, molecular cloning, and expression of 2-hydroxyphytanoyl-CoA lyase, a peroxisomal thiamine pyrophosphate-dependent enzyme that catalyses the carbon–carbon bond cleavage during alpha-oxidation of 3-methyl-branched fatty acids, *Proc. Natl. Acad. Sci., USA*, 96, 10039, 1999.
64. Carpenter, K.J., Acute versus marginal deficiencies of nutrients, *Nutr. Rev.*, 60, 277, 2002.
65. von Muralt, A., The role of thiamine in neurophysiology, *Ann. N.Y. Acad. Sci.*, 98, 499, 1962.
66. Bettendorff, L. et al., Metabolism of thiamine triphosphate in rat brain: correlation with chloride permeability, *J. Neurochem.*, 60, 423, 1993.
67. Bettendorff, L. et al., Chloride permeability of rat brain membrane vesicles correlates with thiamine triphosphate content, *Brain Res.*, 652, 157, 1994.
68. Bettendorff, L., Kolb, H.A., and Schoffeniels, E., Thiamine triphosphate activates an anion channel of large unit conductance in neuroblastoma cells, *J. Membr. Biol.*, 136, 281, 1993.
69. Murphy, J.V., Craig, L.J., and Glew, R.H., Leigh's disease: biochemical characteristics of the inhibitor, *Arch. Neurol.*, 31, 220, 1974.
70. Montpetit, V.J.A. et al., Sub-acute necrotizing encephalomyelopathy, a review and a study of two families, *Brain*, 94, 1, 1971.
71. Cooper, J.R., Itokawa, Y., and Pincus, J.H., Thiamin triphosphate deficiency in sub-acute necrotizing encephalomyelopathy, *Science*, 164, 74, 1969.
72. Nghiem, H.O., Bettendorff, L., and Changeux, J.P., Specific phosphorylation of Torpedo 43K rapsyn by endogenous kinase(s) with thiamine triphosphate as the phosphate donor, *FASEB. J.*, 14, 543, 2000.

73. Barchi, R.L., The nonmetabolic role of thiamine in excitable membrane function, in *Thiamine*, Gubler, C.J., ed., Wiley, NY, 1976, 283.
74. Pincus, J.H. and Grove, I., Distribution of thiamine phosphate esters in thiamine deficient brains, *Exp. Neurol.*, 28, 477, 1970.
75. Haas, R.H., Thiamin and the brain, *Annu. Rev. Nutr.*, 8, 483, 1988.
76. Harata, N. and Iwasaki, Y., The blood–brain barrier and selective vulnerability in experimental thiamine-deficiency encephalopathy in the mouse, *Metab. Brain Dis.*, 11, 55, 1996.
77. Gibson, G.E. and Zhang, H., Interactions of oxidative stress with thiamine homeostasis promote neurodegeneration, *Neurochem. Int.*, 40, 493, 2002.
78. Ke, Z.-J. and Gibson, G.E., Selective response of various brain cell types during neurodegeneration induced by mild impairment of oxidative metabolism, *Neurochem. Int.*, 45, 361, 2004.
79. Martin, P.R., Singleton, C.K., and Hiller-Sturmhofel, S., The role of thiamine deficiency in alcoholic brain disease, *Alcohol Res. Health*, 27, 134, 2003.
80. Kruse, M. et al., Increased brain endothelial nitric oxide synthase expression in thiamine deficiency: relationship to selective vulnerability, *Neurochem. Int.*, 45, 49, 2004.
81. Pannunzio, P. et al., Thiamine deficiency results in metabolic acidosis and energy failure in cerebellar granule cells: an in vitro model for the study of cell death mechanisms in Wernicke's encephalopathy, *J. Neurosci. Res.*, 62, 286, 2000.
82. Wang, J.J.-L. et al., JNK1 is inactivated during thiamine deficiency-induced apoptosis in human neuroblastoma cells, *J. Nutr. Biochem.*, 11, 208, 2000.
83. Frederikse, P.H., Farnsworth, P., and Zigler, J.S.J., Thiamine deficiency in vivo produces fiber cell degeneration in mouse lenses, *Biochem. Biophys. Res. Commun.*, 258, 703, 1999.
84. McCandless, D.W. et al., Cardiac metabolism in thiamine deficiency in rats, *J. Nutr.*, 106, 1144, 1970.
85. Kawai, C. et al., Reappearance of beriberi heart disease in Japan, *Am. J. Med.*, 69, 383, 1980.
86. Takahashi, K., Kittagawa, T., and Shimao, M., Acute polyneuritis associated with edema: a recent revival of beriberi neuropathy in Japan, *Jpn. J. Med.*, 15, 214, 1976.
87. Pawlik, F., Bischoff, A., and Bitsch, I., Peripheral nerve changes in thiamine deficiency and starvation, an electron microscopic study, *Acta Neuropathol. (Berl.)*, 39, 211, 1977.
88. Victor, M. and Martin, J.B., Nutritional and metabolic diseases of the nervous system, in *Harrison's Principles of Internal Medicine*, 13th edn., Isselbacher, K.J., Braunwald, E., Wilson, J.D., Martin, J.B., Fauci, A.S., and Kasper, D.L., eds., McGraw-Hill, NY, 1994, 2238.
89. Pagnan, L., Berlot, G., and Pozzi-Mucelli, R.S., Magnetic resonance imaging in a case of Wernicke's encephalopathy, *Eur. Radiol.*, 8, 977, 1998.
90. Weidauer, S. et al., Wernicke encephalopathy: MR findings and clinical presentation, *Eur. Radiol.*, 13, 1001, 2003.
91. Koike, H. et al., Alcoholic neuropathy is clinicopathologically distinct from thiamine-deficiency neuropathy, *Ann. Neurol.*, 54, 19, 2003.
92. Harper, C. et al., An international perspective on the prevalence of the Wernicke–Korsakoff syndrome, *Metabol. Brain Dis.*, 10, 17, 1995.
93. Rolland, S. and Truswell, A.S., Wernicke–Korsakoff syndrome in Sydney hospitals after 6 years of thiamin enrichment of bread, *Public Health Nutr.*, 1, 117, 1998.
94. Harper, C.G. et al., Prevalence of Wernicke–Korsakoff syndrome in Australia: has thiamine fortification made a difference? *Med. J. Aust.*, 168, 542, 1998.
95. Zubaran, C., Fernandes, J.G., and Rodnight, R., Wernicke–Korsakoff syndrome, *Postgrad. Med. J.*, 73, 27, 1997.
96. Blass, J.P. and Gibson, G.E., Abnormality of a thiamine-requiring enzyme in patients with Wernicke–Korsakoff syndrome, *New Engl. J. Med.*, 297, 1367, 1977.
97. Mukherjee, A.B., Svoronos, S., and Ghazanfari, A., Transketolase abnormality in cultured fibroblasts from familial chronic alcoholic men and their male offspring, *J. Clin. Invest.*, 79, 1039, 1987.
98. Nixon, P.F. et al., An erythrocyte tranketolase isoenzyme pattern associated with the Wernicke–Korsakoff syndrome, *Eur. J. Clin. Invest.*, 14, 278, 1984.
99. McCool, S.G. et al., Cloning of human transketolase cDNAs and comparison of the coding region in Wernicke–Korsakoff and non-Wernicke–Korsakoff individuals, *J. Biol. Chem.*, 268, 1397, 1993.
100. Singleton, C.K. et al., The thiamin-dependent hysteretic behavior of human transketolase: implications for thiamin deficiency, *J. Nutr.*, 125, 189, 1995.

101. Wang, J.J.-L., Martin, P.R., and Singleton, C.K., A transketolase assembly defect in a Wernicke–Korsakoff syndrome patient, *Alcohol. Clin. Exp. Res.*, 21, 576, 1997.
102. Mastrogiacomo, F. et al., Brain thiamine, its phosphate esters, and its metabolising enzymes in Alzheimer's disease, *Ann. Neurol.*, 39, 585, 1996.
103. Heroux, M. et al., Alterations of thiamine phosphorylation and of thiamine-dependent enzymes in Alzheimer's disease, *Metabol. Brain Dis.*, 11, 81, 1996.
104. Kanofsky, J.D., Thiamin status and cognitive impairment in the elderly, *J. Am. Coll. Nutr.*, 15, 197, 1996.
105. Mimori, Y., Katsuoka, H., and Nakamura, S., Thiamine therapy in Alzheimer's disease, *Metab. Brain Dis.*, 11, 89, 1996.
106. O'Rourke, N. et al., Thiamin status of healthy and institutionalised elderly subjects: analysis of dietary intake and biochemical indices, *Age Ageing*, 19, 325, 1990.
107. Finch, S., Doyle, W., Lowe, C., Bates, C.J., Prentice, A.M., Smithers, G., and Clarke, P.C., National Diet and Nutrition Survey: People aged 65 years and over. *Volume 1: Report of the Diet and Nutrition Survey*, The Stationery Office, London, 1998.
108. Wilkinson, T.J. et al., The response to treatment of subclinical thiamin deficiency in the elderly, *Am. J. Clin. Nutr.*, 66, 925, 1997.
109. Iber, F.L. et al., Thiamin in the elderly—relation to alcoholism and to neurological degenerative disease, *Am. J. Clin. Nutr.*, 6, 1067, 1982.
110. Bettendorff, L. et al., Thiamine, thiamine phosphates and their metabolizing enzymes in human brain, *J. Neurochem.*, 66, 250, 1996.
111. Suter, P.M. and Vetter, W., Diuretics and vitamin B_1: are diuretics a risk factor for thiamin malnutrition? *Nutr. Rev.*, 58, 319, 2000.
112. Muri, R.M. et al., Thiamin deficiency in HIV-positive patients: evaluation by erythrocyte transketolase activity and thiamin pyrophosphate effect, *Clin. Nutr.*, 18, 375, 2000.
113. Tang, C.M. et al., Outbreak of beri-beri in The Gambia, *Lancet*, 2, 206, 1989.
114. McGready, R. et al., Postpartum thiamine deficiency in a Karen displaced population, *Am. J. Clin. Nutr.*, 74, 808, 2001.
115. Luxemburger, C. et al., Beri-beri: the major cause of infant mortality in Karen refugees, *Trans. R. Soc. Trop. Med. Hyg.*, 97, 251, 2003.
116. Djoenaidi, W., Notermans, S.L.H., and Verbeek, A.L.M., Subclinical beriberi polyneuropathy in the low income group: an investigation with special tools on possible patients with suspected complaints, *Eur. J. Clin. Nutr.*, 50, 549, 1996.
117. Bovet, P. et al., Blood thiamin status and determinants in the population of Seychelles (Indian Ocean), *J. Epidemiol. Community Health*, 52, 237, 1998.
118. San Sebastian, M. and Jativa, R., Beriberi in a well-nourished Amazonian population, *Acta Trop.*, 70, 193, 1998.
119. Krishna, S. et al., Thiamine deficiency and malaria in adults from southeast Asia, *Lancet*, 353, 546, 1999.
120. Roman, G.C., An epidemic in Cuba of optic neuropathy, sensorineural deafness, peripheral sensory neuropathy and dorsolateral myeloneuropathy, *J. Neurol. Sci.*, 11, 11, 1994.
121. Macias-Matos, C. et al., Biochemical evidence of thiamine depletion during the Cuban neuropathy epidemic, 1992–1993, *Am. J. Clin. Nutr.*, 64, 347, 1996.
122. Tallaksen, C.M.E., Bohmer, T., and Bell, H., Concentrations of the water-soluble vitamins thiamin, ascorbic acid, and folic acid in serum and cerebrospinal fluid of man, *Am. J. Clin. Nutr.*, 56, 559, 1992.
123. Horwitt, M.K. and Kreisler, O., The determination of early thiamine-deficient state by estimation of blood lactic and pyruvic acids after glucose administration and exercise, *J. Nutr.*, 37, 411, 1949.
124. Interdepartmental Committee on Nutrition for National Defense, *Manual for Nutrition Surveys*, 2nd edn., U.S. Government Printing Offices, Washington DC, 1963.
125. Pearson, W.H., Blood and urine vitamin levels as potential indices of body stores, *Am. J. Clin. Nutr.*, 20, 514, 1967.
126. Sauberlich, H.E. et al., Thiamin requirement of the adult human, *Am. J. Clin. Nutr.*, 32, 2237, 1979.
127. Pearson, W.H., Biochemical appraisal of the vitamin nutritional status in man, *JAMA*, 180, 49, 1962.

128. Schrijver, J. et al., A reliable semiautomated method for the determination of total thiamine in whole blood by the thiochrome method with high-performance liquid chromatography, *Ann. Clin. Biochem.*, 19, 52, 1982.
129. Talwar, D. et al., Vitamin B_1 status assessed by direct measurement of thiamin pyrophosphate in erythrocytes or whole blood by HPLC: comparison with erythrocyte transketolase assay, *Clin. Chem.*, 46, 704, 2000.
130. Baines, M. and Davies, G., The evaluation of erythrocyte thiamin diphosphate as an indicator of thiamin status in man, and its comparison with erythrocyte transketolase activity measurements, *Ann. Clin. Biochem.*, 25, 698, 1988.
131. Kuriyama, M. et al., Blood vitamin B_1, transketolase and thiamine pyrophosphate (TPP) effect in beriberi patients, with studies employing discriminant analysis, *Clin. Chim. Acta*, 108, 159, 1980.
132. Wagner, P.I., Beriberi heart disease. Physiologic data and difficulties in diagnosis, *Am. Heart J.*, 69, 200, 1965.
133. Warnock, L.G., Prudhomme, C.R., and Wagner, C., The determination of thiamin pyrophosphate in blood and other tissues and its correlation with erythrocyte transketolase activity, *J. Nutr.*, 108, 421, 1978.
134. Bailey, A.L. and Finglas, P.M., A normal phase high-performance liquid chromatographic method for the determination of thiamin in blood and tissue samples, *J. Micronutr. Anal.*, 7, 147, 1990.
135. Brin, M., Thiamine deficiency and erythrocyte metabolism, *Am. J. Clin. Nutr.*, 12, 107, 1963.
136. Smeets, E.H.J., Muller, H., and de Wael, J., A NADH dependent transketolase assay in erythrocyte hemolysates, *Clin. Chim. Acta*, 33, 379, 1971.
137. Mak, Y.T. and Swaminathan, R., Assessment of vitamin B_1, B_2 and B_6 status by coenzyme activation of red cell enzymes using a centrifugal analyzer, *J. Clin. Chem. Clin. Biochem.*, 24, 213, 1988.
138. Vuilleumier, J.P., Keller, H.E., and Keck, E., Clinical chemical methods for the routine assessment of the vitamin status in human populations. Part III. The apoenzyme stimulation tests for vitamin B_1, B_2 and B_6 adapted to the Cobas-Bio analyzer, *Int. J. Vitam. Nutr. Res.*, 60, 126, 1990.
139. Hoare, J. et al., National Diet and Nutrition Survey: Adults aged 19 to 64 years. *Volume 5: Summary Report*, The Stationery Office, London, 2003.
140. Department of Health, *Report on Health and Social Subjects No. 41. Dietary Reference Values for Food Energy and Nutrients for the United Kingdom. Report of the Panel on Dietary Reference Values of the Committee on Medical Aspects of Food Policy*, HMSO, London, 1991, 90–93.
141. Department of Health and Social Security, *The Composition of Mature Human Milk. Report on Health and Social Subjects No. 12*, HMSO, London, 1977.
142. Baker, H. and Frank, O., Absorption, utilization, and clinical effectiveness of allithiamines compared to water-soluble thiamines, *J. Nutr. Sci. Vitaminol.*, 22 (Suppl), 63, 1976.
143. Stephen, J.M., Grant, R., and Yeh, C.S., Anaphylaxis from administration of intravenous thiamine, *Am. J. Emerg. Med.*, 10, 61, 1992.
144. Food Standards Agency, *McCance and Widdowson's The Composition of Foods, 6th Summary Edition*, Royal Society of Chemistry, Cambridge, 2002.
145. Boulware, M.J. et al., Polarized expression of members of the solute carrier SLC19A gene family of water-soluble multivitamin transporters: implications for physiological function, *Biochem. J.*, 376 (Pt 1), 43, 2003.
146. Gregory, J., Lowe, S., Bates, C.J., Prentice, A., Jackson, L.V., Smithers, G., Wenlock, R., and Farron, M., National Diet and Nutrition Survey: Young people aged 4 to 18 years. *Volume 1: Report of the Diet and Nutrition Survey*, The Stationery Office, London, 2000.
147. Ruston, D., Hoare, J., Henderson, L., Gregory, J., Bates, C.J., Prentice, A., Birch, M., Swan, G., and Farron, M., National Diet and Nutrition Survey: Adults aged 19 to 64 years. *Volume 4: Nutritional Status (Anthropometry and Blood Analytes), Blood Pressure and Physical Activity*, The Stationery Office, London, 2004.

9 Pantothenic Acid

Robert B. Rucker and Kathryn Bauerly

CONTENTS

INTRODUCTION AND HISTORY

The discovery of pantothenic acid followed the same path that led to the discovery of other water-soluble vitamins evolving from studies using bacteria and single-cell eukaryotic organisms (e.g., yeast) and eventually animal models [1–23]. Although the widespread occurrence of pantothenic acid in food makes a dietary deficiency unlikely, the use of experimental animal models [5–14], antagonistic analogs, such as ω-methyl-pantothenate [24–29], and in the past several decades, the feeding of semisynthetic diets free of pantothenic acid [25,30–34] have helped to define pantothenate's functions. Largely the efforts of research groups associated with R.J. Williams, C.A. Elvehjem, and T.H. Jukes led to the identification of pantothenic acid as an essential dietary factor. R.J. Williams and coworkers established that pantothenic acid was required for the growth of certain bacteria and yeast [1,17,20,22,23]. Next, Elvehjem and associates [21] and Jukes and associates demonstrated that pantothenic acid was a growth factor for rats and chicks [2,16,35,36]. Early nutritional studies in animals also demonstrated that there was loss of fur color in black and brown rats and an usual dermatitis that occurred in chickens fed pantothenate-deficient diets; thus, at one point pantothenate was known as the antigray or antidermatitis factor [37].

Williams coined the name pantothenic acid from the Greek meaning "from everywhere" to indicate its widespread occurrence in foodstuffs. The eventual characterization and synthesis of pantothenic acid by Williams in 1940 took advantage of observations that the antidermatitis factor present in acid extracts of various food sources, i.e., pantothenic acid, did not bind to fuller's earth (a highly adsorbent claylike substance consisting of hydrated aluminum silicates) under acidic conditions [22,23]. Using chromatographic and fractionation procedures, which were typical of the 1930s and 1940s (solvent-dependent chemical partitioning), Williams isolated several grams of pantothenic acid for structural determination from 250 kg of liver as starting material [22,23]. With this information, a number of research groups contributed to the chemical synthesis and commercial preparation of pantothenic acid. Pantothenate and its derivatives are now produced mainly through chemical synthesis and the global market in the past decade was $>7 \times 10^6$ kg/year [38].

As emphasized throughout this chapter, pantothenic acid, which is sometimes designated as vitamin B_5, is the core of the structure of coenzyme A (CoA), an essential cofactor in pathways important to oxidative respiration, lipid metabolism, and the synthesis of many secondary metabolites such as steroids, acetylated compounds (e.g., acetylated amino acids, carbohydrates), and prostaglandins and prostaglandin-like compounds. In addition, the phosphopantetheine moiety (a pantothenic acid derivative derived from CoA metabolism) is incorporated into the prosthetic group of the acyl carrier proteins (ACP) used in fatty acid synthases, polyketide synthases, lysine synthesis in yeast and bacteria, and nonribosomal peptide synthetases. Coenzyme A was discovered as the cofactor essential for the acetylation of sulfonamides and choline in the early 1950s [39–42]. In the mid-1970s, pantothenic acid was identified as a component of ACP in the fatty acid synthesis (FAS) complex [43–46]. These developments, in addition to a steady series of observations throughout this period on the effects of pantothenic acid deficiency in humans and other animals, provide the foundation for our current understanding of this vitamin.

CHEMICAL PERSPECTIVES AND NOMENCLATURE

Pantothenic acid [β-alanine-*N*-4-dihydroxy-3,3-dimethyl-1-oxobutyl)-(R); vitamin B_5; CAS Registry Number 79-83-4] is synthesized by microorganisms via an amide linkage of pantoic acid and β-alanine subunits (Figure 9.1). Pantothenic acid is an essential metabolite for all biological systems; however, the biosynthesis of pantothenic acid is limited to plants, bacteria, eubacteria, and archaea (Figure 9.2). It is worth noting that the biosynthesis pathway for pantothenic acid in microorganisms and plants is also viewed as a strong candidate for the discovery of novel antibiotic and herbicidal compounds [38].

Pure pantothenic acid is water soluble, viscous, and yellow. It is stable at neutral pH, but is readily destroyed by acid, alkali, and heat. Calcium pantothenate, a white, odorless, crystalline substance, is the form of pantothenic acid usually found in commercial vitamin supplements due to greater stability than the pure acid. The structure elucidation of pantothenate was based on the identification of a lactone formed by degradation of pantothenate. Initial analytical work revealed an α-hydroxy acid that was readily lactonized. Stiller et al. [17] identified the lactone as α-hydroxy-β,β-dimethyl-χ-butyrolactone (pantoyl lactone or pantolactone), which aided in the structural elucidation of pantothenate.

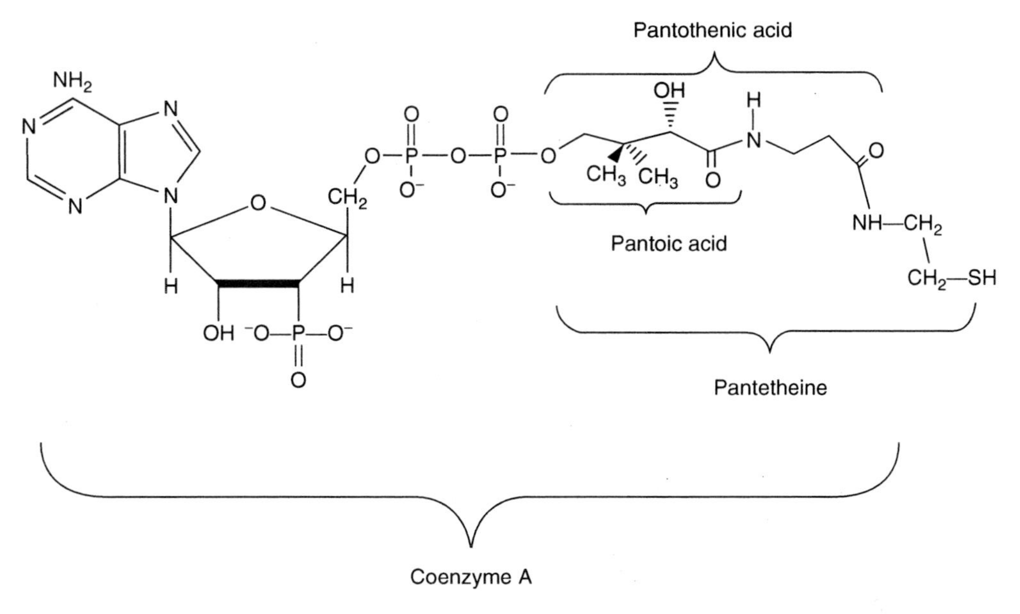

FIGURE 9.1 Structural components of coenzyme A.

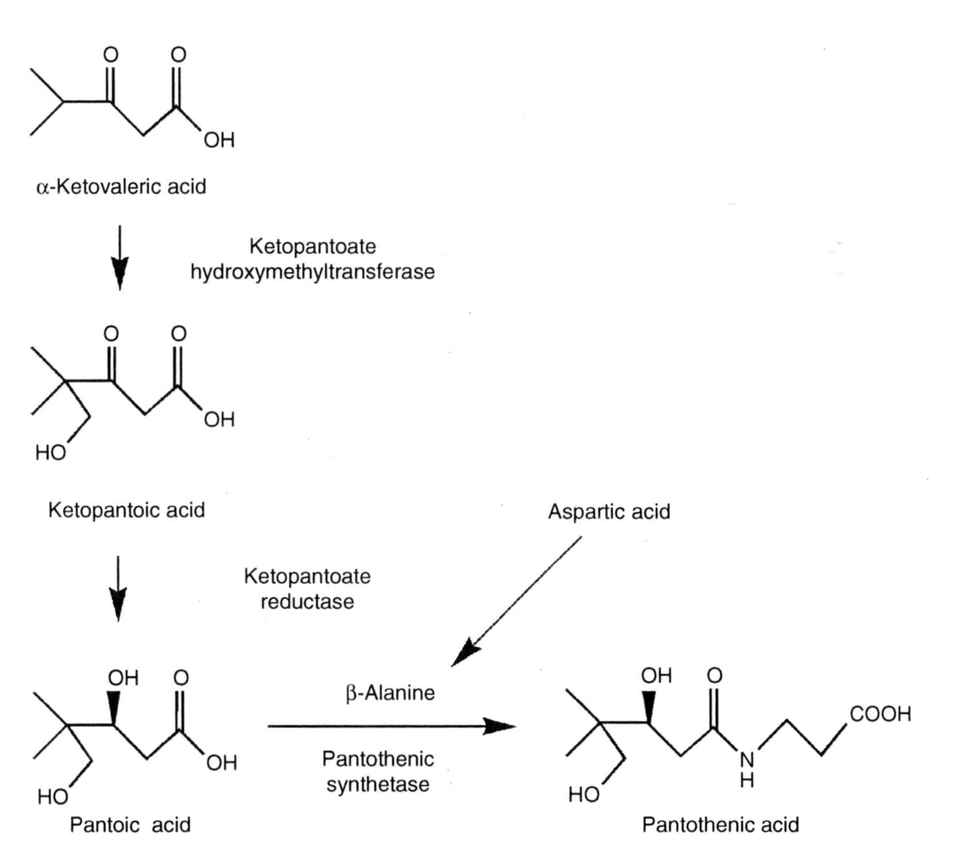

FIGURE 9.2 Pathway for the biosynthesis of pantothenic acid found in plants, bacteria (including archaea), and eubacteria.

FOOD SOURCES AND REQUIREMENTS

Pantothenic Acid Requirements

Although limited, available data suggest that at intakes of 4–6 mg of pantothenic acid per day, serum levels of pantothenic acid are maintained in young adults and no known signs of deficiency are observed. The U.S. recommended dietary allowance (RDA) for pantothenic acid, which is used for determining daily percent values on nutritional supplement and food labels, is 10 mg/day [47].

Pantothenic acid is found in edible animal and plant tissues ranging from 10 to 50 μg/g of tissue. Thus, it is possible to meet the current daily recommended intake for adults with a mixed diet containing as little as 100 to 200 g of solid food; i.e., the equivalent of a mixed diet corresponding to 600 to 1200 kcal or 2.4 to 4.8 MJ. In this regard, the typical Western diet usually contains 6 mg or more of available pantothenic acid [37,48]. Table 9.1 gives the current recommended amounts of pantothenic acid for humans, expressed as dietary reference intakes (DRI) [47]. Moreover, when expressed on a per energy intake equivalent basis, the need for pantothenic acid is remarkably constant across species [49]. Although in mice small amounts of pantothenic acid are synthesized by intestinal bacteria, the contribution of bacterial synthesis to human pantothenic acid status is not known and probably small [28,50]. Regrettably, relatively little quantitative information on the enteric synthesis of pantothenic acid exists.

Food Sources

Chicken, beef, potatoes, oat cereals, tomatoes, eggs, broccoli, and whole grains are major sources of pantothenic acid. Refined grains have a lower content. Table 9.2 contains some typical values for pantothenic acid in selected food. The processing and refining of grains

TABLE 9.1
Pantothenic Acid Dietary Reference Intakes (RDI)[a]

Category	Recommendation
0 through 6 months	1.7 mg/day ~0.2 mg/kg
7 through 12 months	1.8 mg/day ~0.2 mg/kg
Children	
1 through 3 years	2 mg/day
4 through 8 years	3 mg/day
Girls and boys	
9 through 13 years	4 mg/day
14 through 18 years	5 mg/day
Women and men	
19 years and older	5 mg/day
Pregnancy	
14 through 50 years	6 mg/day
Lactation	
14 through 50 years	7 mg/day

Note: There is no evidence of toxicity associated; thus, the lowest observed adverse-effect level (LOAEL) and an associated no observed adverse-effect level (NOAEL) have not been determined.

[a] Recommendation of the Food and Nutrition Board of the Institute of Medicine of the U.S. National Academy of Sciences.

TABLE 9.2
Pantothenic Content in Selected Foods

Ingredient	~Amount (mg/100 g or mL of Edible Portion)
Beer	<0.1
Soft drinks	<0.03
Wine	0.02–0.04
Wheat bran	2–3
Boiled rice	0.2–0.3
Soy flour	1.5–2.5
Raw eggs	1.5–2.0
Cooked fish	0.2–0.5
Lobster	1.5
Oysters	0.5
Salmon	0.5
Tuna	0.4
Apples	0.05
Apricots, bananas	0.1–0.2
Dates	0.8
Grapes	0.04
Lemon and orange juice	0.1
Plums	0.2
Prunes	0.5
Strawberries	0.3
Beef	0.5–1.2
Chicken boiled	0.3–1.0
Liver	5–7
Kidney	4–6
Pork	0.5–1.0
Cheese	1.5
Milk (bovine)	1
Milk (human)	0.3–0.4
Almonds	2–3
Peanuts	2–3
Walnuts	1
Peanut butter	5–8

can produce as much as a 50% loss of pantothenic acid [51–53]. In keeping with the proposed requirements for humans, human milk contains ~5–6 mg of pantothenic acid per 1000 kcal [54–56]. It has been estimated that for every milligram of pantothenic acid consumed in the diet, ~0.4 mg can be transported into milk when lactation is active. Because the pantothenic content of milk correlates well with maternal intakes of pantothenic acid, the possibility does exist that pantothenic acid deficiency may occur in infants consuming milk produced by mothers deficient in the vitamin (e.g., those who consume predominantly refined cereals). Because of the widespread distribution of pantothenic acid in foods and apparently the diets of adults have to be markedly devoid of pantothenic acid to induce deficiency, the need for aggressive fortification of pantothenic acid may never become a high priority.

INTESTINAL ABSORPTION AND MAINTENANCE

The vast majority of pantothenic acid in food is present as CoA or 4′-phosphopantetheine. In order to be absorbed, these substances must first be hydrolyzed [50]. This occurs in the intestinal lumen by the sequential activity of two hydrolases, pyrophosphatase and phosphatase, with pantotheine as the product. Intestinal phosphatases and nucleosidases are capable of very efficient hydrolysis of CoA so that near-quantitative release of pantothenic acid occurs as a normal part of digestion. Pantotheine is either absorbed as is, or further metabolized to pantothenic acid by a third intestinal hydrolase, pantothenase [57–60]. In rats, pantothenic acid absorption was initially found to be absorbed in all sections of the small intestine by simple diffusion [28,50,61]. However, subsequent work in rats and chicks indicated that at low concentrations, the vitamin is absorbed by a saturable, sodium-dependent transport mechanism [62]. Further, the overall K_m for pantothenic acid intestinal uptake is 10–20 μM. At an intake of ~10–15 mg of coenzyme A, the amount of coenzyme A in a typical meal, the pantothenic acid concentration in luminal fluid would be ~1–2 μM. At this concentration, pantothenic acid would not saturate the transport system and should be efficiently and actively absorbed [61].

Researchers have demonstrated that pantothenic acid shares a common membrane transport system in the small intestine with another vitamin, biotin [61,63–67]. Experiments using Caco-2 cell monolayers as a model of intestinal absorption have established that pantothenic acid uptake is inhibited competitively by biotin and vice versa [61,63–67]. Similar relationships were observed in transport experiments involving the blood–brain barrier [61,68,69], heart [70–73], and placenta [74–77]. For example, membrane transport pathways for transplacental transfer of pantothenate were investigated by Grassl [77] assessing the possible presence of a Na^+–pantothenate cotransport mechanism in the maternal facing membrane of human placental epithelial cells. The presence of Na^+–pantothenate cotransport was determined from radiolabeled tracer flux measurements of pantothenate uptake using preparations of purified brush-border membrane vesicles. Compared with other cations, the imposition of an inward Na^+ gradient stimulated vesicle uptake of pantothenate to levels ~40-fold greater than those observed at equilibrium. The effect of biotin on the kinetics of Na^+-dependent pantothenate uptake and the effect of pantothenate on the kinetics of Na^+-dependent biotin uptake suggest that placental absorption of biotin and pantothenate from the maternal circulation also occurs by a common Na^+ cotransport mechanism.

After absorption, pantothenic acid enters the circulation from which it is taken up by cells in a manner similar to that of intestinal absorption (see the following section). The vitamin is excreted in the urine primarily as pantothenic acid [27,78–85]. This occurs after its release from CoA by a series of hydrolysis reactions that cleave off the phosphate and β-mercaptoethylamine moieties.

CELLULAR REGULATION OF PANTOTHENIC ACID, CoA, AND THE IMPORTANCE OF PANTOTHENIC KINASE

Cellular Transport and Maintenance

Said and others [61,63–67] have observed that similar to enterocytes, other epithelial cells take up pantothenic acid in a manner that is inhibited by Na-K-ATPase inhibitors, such as ouabain, and is in competition with biotin. In most instances, activity of this transporter is sensitive to phosphokinase C (PKC)- and A (PKA)-mediated activation and inhibition. For example, pretreatment of epithelial cells with phorbol 12-myristate 13-acetate (PMA), but not with its negative control (4α-PMA) or with 1,2-dioctanoyl-*sn*-glycerol, both activators of PKC, causes significant inhibition in uptake, whereas pretreatment of cells with staurosporine and chelerythrine, inhibitors of PKC, promotes stimulation in uptake [67]. These findings point toward the involvement of a PKC-mediated pathway in the regulation of biotin and pantothenic acid uptake by epithelial cells.

Pantothenic Acid Kinase

Following uptake, the maintenance of pantothenic acid cellular concentration depends on its incorporation into CoASH and pantotheine. The most important control step in this process is the phosphorylation of pantothenic acid to 4′-phosphopantothenic acid by pantothenic acid kinase [86–101] (Figure 9.3). There are four members in the human PanK family: PanK1, PanK2, PanK3, and PanK4, which are located on chromosomes 10q23.31, 20p13, 5q35, and 1p36.32, respectively [98]. Pantothenic acid kinases possess a broad pH optimum (between pH 6 and 9). The K_m for pantothenic acid in the liver enzyme of most animals is ~20 μM. Mg-ATP is the nucleotide substrate for this phosphorylation reaction with a K_m of ~0.6 mM [88,102–112].

The relationships involving the various isoforms are complex. Two murine PanK1s exist, mPanK1α and mPanK1β [86,88,95,97,100]. These two transcripts are the result of an alternate splicing of the same gene. PanK1 localizes predominantly in heart, liver, and kidney [86,88,95,97,100]. PanK2 is ubiquitously expressed with the highest levels in retinal and infant basal ganglia [95,113–115]. PanK3 is limited to the liver, but expressed at a high level [88,95]. The expression of PanK4 occurs in most tissues with a high concentration in muscle [88,95]. Metabolic labeling experiments in rat heart support the role of PanK in controlling the flux of the CoA biosynthesis. For example, enhanced mPanK1β expression reduced the intracellular pantothenate pool and triggered a 13-fold increase in intracellular CoA content. PanK1β activity in vitro was stimulated by CoA and strongly inhibited by acetyl CoA, illustrating the differential modulation of mPanK1β activity by pathway end products and supporting the concept that the expression or activity of PanK is a determining factor in the physiological regulation of the intracellular CoA concentration [100].

Pantothenic acid kinase is activated and inhibited nonspecifically by various anions. More significantly, feedback inhibition of the kinase by CoA or CoA derivatives governs flux through the subsequent steps in the CoA synthesis pathway and defines the upper threshold for intracellular CoA cofactor levels. Inhibition by acetyl CoA is slightly greater than that of free CoA. The inhibition by free CoA is uncompetitive with respect to pantothenate concentration; K_i for inhibition of 0.2 μM. Interestingly, L-carnitine, important for the transport of fatty acids into mitochondria, is a nonessential activator of pantothenic acid kinase. Carnitine

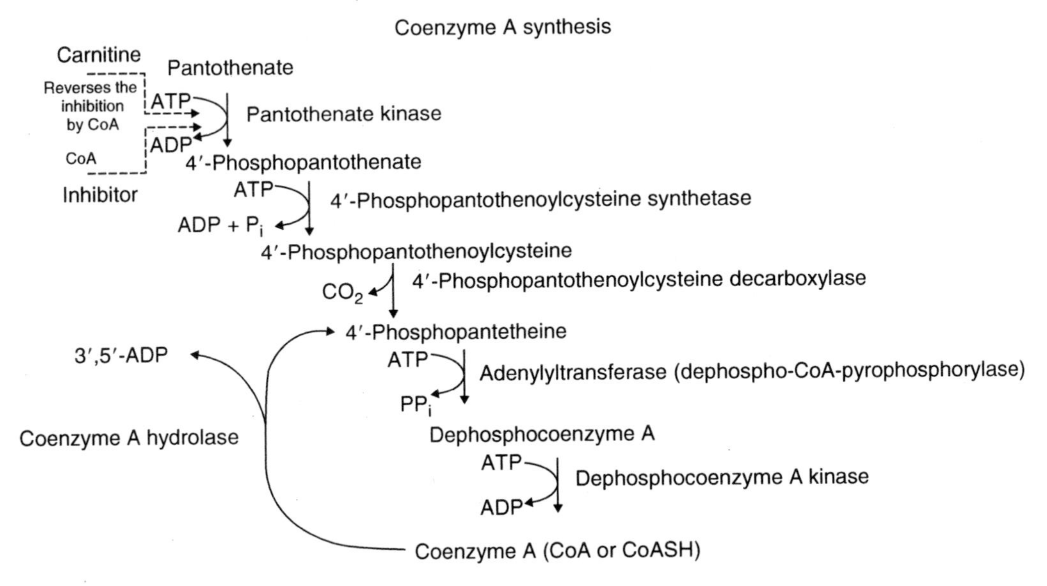

FIGURE 9.3 Coenzyme A metabolism and importance of pantothenic acid kinase.

has no effect by itself, but specifically reverses the inhibition by CoA. In heart, the free carnitine content varies directly with the phosphorylation of pantothenic acid. Thus, these properties of the kinase provide a potential mechanism for the control of CoA synthesis and regulation of cellular pantothenic acid content, i.e., feedback inhibition by CoA and its acyl esters that is reversed by changes in the concentration of free carnitine [71,107,108,111,116].

In this regard, it is important to underscore that the free concentration of acyl CoA in cells is low and variable because the bulk of acyl derivatives are protein bound. Moreover, similar to CoA, carnitine exists in both free and acylated forms and reversal of kinase inhibition by CoA does not occur when carnitine is acylated [107]. The ratio of free to acylated carnitine varies considerably depending on feeding and hormonal influences, with insulin of particular importance. Fasting and diabetes (states of low insulin) increase pantothenic acid kinase activity and the total content of CoA [102,105,110]. Perfusion of heart preparations or incubation of liver cells with glucose, pyruvate, or palmitate markedly inhibits pantothenic acid phosphorylation because of reduction in free carnitine and increases in the free and acylated forms of CoA [116].

CoA Formation

For CoA synthesis, the additional steps include the addition of adenine and ribose 3′-phosphate to produce CoA composed of 4′-phosphopantetheine linked by an anhydride bond to adenosine 5′-monophosphate, modified by a 3′-hydroxyl phosphate (Figure 9.3). In yeast and perhaps higher organisms (for which details of the pathway require further resolution), these steps are carried out on a protein complex with multifunctional catalytic sites [117–120]. Important enzymatic features of this complex in yeast include dephospho-CoA-pyrophosphorylase activity, which catalyzes the reaction between 4′-phosphopantetheine and ATP to form 4′-dephospho-CoA; dephospho-CoA-kinase activity, which catalyzes the ATP-dependent final step in CoA synthesis; and CoA hydrolase activity, which catalyzes the hydrolysis of CoA to 3′,5′-ADP and 4′-phosphopantetheine. This sequence of reactions is referred to as the CoA/4′-phosphopantetheine cycle and provides a mechanism by which the 4′-phosphopantetheine can be recycled to form CoA [107–110]. Each turn of the cycle utilizes two molecules of ATP and produces one molecule of ADP, one molecule of pyrophosphate, and one molecule of 3′,5′-ADP. Although some enzymes of the pathway were identified relatively rapidly, it was not possible to identify all enzymes using traditional methods. Hence, the use of bacterial mutants and the application of molecular biology have been essential in resolving key features of the pathway shown in Figure 9.3.

As CoA holds a central position in cellular metabolism, it may therefore be assumed to be an ancient molecule [119]. Starting from the known *Escherichia coli* pathway and known human enzymes required for the biosynthesis of CoA, phylogenetic profiles and chromosomal proximity methods have led to the conclusion that the topology of CoA synthesis from common precursors is essentially conserved across the three domains of life [119].

CoA Regulation

In animal tissue, the levels of CoA cover a wide range and change in response to signals arising from hormones, nutrients, and cellular metabolites. Hepatic CoA levels are among the most responsive to such changes, ranging from 100 to 500 nmol/g liver. In decreasing order: heart > kidney > diaphragm > skeletal muscle contain CoA in concentrations ranging from 100 to 50 nmol/g [43,103,106,108,121,122]. Fasting results in high levels of long-chain fatty acyl CoA thioesters, whereas glucose feeding results in nonacylated CoA derivatives. The total CoA levels decrease in response to insulin, but increase in response to glucagon. The transfer of activated acyl moieties across organelle membranes, to and from the CoA pools in mitochondria, cytosol, and peroxisomes occurs through the carnitine transferase system and ABC-like transporters [123–125].

The concentration of nonacylated CoA determines the rate of oxidation-dependent energy production in both mitochondria and peroxisomes, and the interorganelle transport of CoA-linked metabolites helps to maintain CoA availability. Although much remains to be investigated regarding the relative roles, various compartments play a role in CoA regulation; available evidence suggests that mitochondria are the principle sites of CoA synthesis. For example, PanK2s localization in mitochondria is proposed to initiate intramitochondrial CoA biosynthesis.

CoA synthase is also of importance in this process. 4′-phosphopantetheine adenylyltransferase and dephospho CoA kinase activities are both catalyzed by CoA synthase [126]. The full-length CoA synthase is associated with the mitochondrial outer membrane, whereas the removal of the N-terminal region relocates the enzyme to the cytosol. Phosphatidylcholine and phosphatidylethanolamine, which are principle components of the mitochondrial outer membrane, are potent activators of both enzymatic activities of CoA synthase. Taken together, it may be inferred that CoA synthesis is regulated by phospholipids and intimately linked to mitochondrial function [118]. At steady state, cytosolic CoA concentrations range from 0.02 to 0.15 mM, mitochondrial concentrations range from 2 to 5 mM, and peroxisomal concentration are ~0.5 mM CoA [106,108].

Acyl Carrier Protein

ACP is also referred to as a "macro-cofactor" because in bacteria, yeast, and plants, it is composed of a dissociable polypeptide chain (MW ~8500–8700 Da) to which 4′-phosphopantetheine is attached [43,44,127]. However, in higher animals, ACP is most often associated with a fatty acid synthase complex that is composed of two very large protein subunits (MW ~250,000 Da each). The carrier segment or domain of the fatty acid synthetic complex is also called ACP, i.e., one of seven functional or catalytic domains on each of the two subunits that comprise fatty acid synthase (Table 9.3).

In addition to fatty acid production and catabolism, in yeast, bacteria, and plants, capable of essential amino acid synthesis, proteins with 4′-phosphopantetheine attachment sites are utilized. An example is aminoadipic acid reductase (e.g., LYS2 in yeast). The pantetheine transferase (LYS5), which aids in the activation of aminoadipic acid reductase, has also been isolated and cloned from a human source, i.e., a putative human homolog to the LYS5 gene [128].

Regarding ACP assembly to form holo-ACP, apo-ACP is posttranslationally modified via transfer of 4′-phosphopantetheine from CoA to a serine residue on apo-ACP [126,127,129]. The resulting holo-ACP is then active as the central coenzyme of fatty acid biosynthesis, either as individual subunit in bacterial systems or as a specific domain in the fatty acid synthetase complex in higher animals (Figure 9.4). Moreover, the transfer of the 4′-phosphopantetheine moiety of CoA to acyl carrier proteins may also serve as an alternate to CoA degradation or catabolism, i.e., ACP formation has the potential of providing an additional strategy for coordination of CoA levels [117,118,129].

In summary, the regulation of pantothenic acid kinase is complex and occurs via allosteric and transcriptional mechanisms. Multiple approaches to regulating this important enzyme are of obvious importance given the central roles and importance of both ACP and CoA to intermediary metabolism, protein processing, and gene regulation. In addition to the allosteric controls, transcriptional regulation by peroxisome proliferator activated receptor transcription factors, sterol regulatory element binding proteins (SREBP), and interaction with the glucose response element [95] are also essential.

TABLE 9.3
Catalytic Sites Associated with the Fatty Acid Synthase Complex

Catalytic Site	Function
Acetyl transferase	Catalyzes the transfer of an activated acetyl group on CoA to the sulfidryl group of 4′-phosphopantetheine (ACP domain). In the next step, the acetyl group is transferred to a second cysteine-derived sulfidryl group near active site of 3-oxoacyl synthase (see step 3) leaving the 4′-phosphopantetheine sulfhydryl group free for step 2
Malonyl transferase	Catalyzes the transfer of successive incoming malonyl groups to 4′-phosphopantetheine
3-Oxoacyl synthetase	Catalyzes the first condensation reaction in the process. The acetyl moiety (transferred in step 1) occurs with decarboxylation and condensation to yield a 3-oxobutryl (acetoacetyl) derivative. In the subsequent series of cycles, the newly formed acyl moieties react with the malonyl group added at each cycle (see step 6)
Oxoacyl reductase	Catalyzes reductions of acetoacetyl or 3-oxoacyl intermediates. The first cycle of this reaction generates D-hydroxybutyrate, and in subsequent cycles, hydroxyfatty acids
3-Hydroxyacyl dehydratase	Catalyzes the removal of a molecule of water from the 3-hydroxyacyl derivatives produced in step 4 to form enoyl derivatives
Enoyl reductase	Catalyzes the reduction of the enoyl derivatives (step 5). This acyl group is transferred to the sulfidryl group adjacent to 3-oxoacyl synthase, as described in step 1, until a 16-carbon palmitoyl group is formed. This group, still attached to the 4′-phosphopantetheine arm, is high-affinity substrate for the remaining enzyme of the complex, thioester hydrolase
Thioester hydrolase	This enzyme liberates palmitic acid (step 6) from the 4′-phosphopantetheine arm

SELECTED PHYSIOLOGIC FUNCTIONS OF ACP AND CoA

To reiterate, the functions of pantothenic acid as a vitamin are inexorably linked to processes that utilize CoA as a substrate and cosubstrate, particularly given that the bulk of 4′-phosphopantotheine incorporated into ACP also derives from transfer reactions that require CoA as substrate. Descriptions of the hundreds of reactions involving CoA in acetyl and acyl transfers are beyond the scope of a chapter specifically focused on pantothenic acid. However, the following descriptions (Table 9.4) were chosen to underscore how pantothenic acid as a component of CoA and ACP is central to virtually all aspects of metabolism.

CoA AND ACP AS HIGH-ENERGY INTERMEDIATES

Intermediates arising from the transfer reactions catalyzed by CoA and 4′-phosphopantetheine in ACP are "high-energy" compounds [130]. Thioesters (–S–CO–R) are thermodynamically

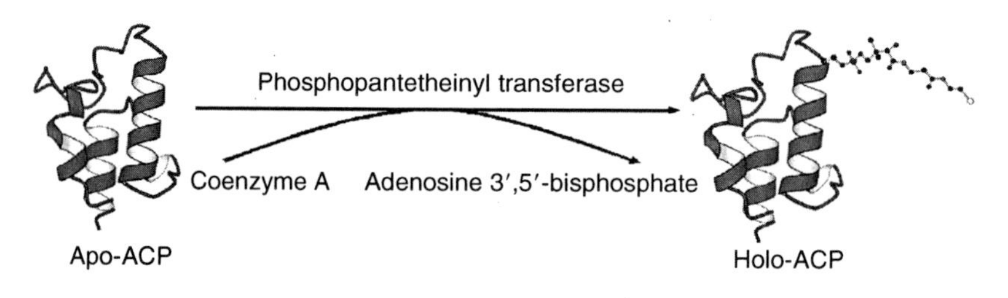

FIGURE 9.4 Pantethenylation of acyl carrier protein.

TABLE 9.4
Functions of CoA and ACP

Function	Importance
Carbohydrate-related citric acid cycle transfer reactions	Oxidative metabolism
Acetylation of sugars (e.g., *N*-acetylglucosamine)	Production of carbohydrates important to cell structure
Lipid-related	
Phospholipid biosynthesis	Cell membrane formation and structure
Isoprenoid biosynthesis	Cholesterol and bile salt production
Steroid biosynthesis	Steroid hormone production
Fatty acid elongation	Ability to modify cell membrane fluidity
Acyl (fatty acid) and triacyl glyceride synthesis	Energy storage
Protein-related	
Protein acetylation	Altered protein conformation; activation of certain hormones and enzymes, e.g., adrenocorticotropin transcriptional regulation, e.g., acetylation of histone
Protein acylation (e.g., myristic and palmitic acid, and prenyl moiety additions)	Compartmentalization and activation of hormones and transcription factors

less stable than typical esters (–O–CO–R) or amides (–N–CO–R). The double-bond character of the C=O bond in –S–C=O–R does not extend significantly into the C–S bond, i.e., in thiol esters the d-orbitals of sulfur do not overlap with the p-orbitals of carbon. This causes thioesters to have relatively high-energy potential, and for most reactions involving CoA or ACP, no additional energy, for example, from ATP hydrolysis, is required for transfer of the acetyl or acyl group. At pH 7.0, the $-\Delta G$ of hydrolysis is ~7.5 kcal for acetyl coenzyme A and 10.5 kcal for acetoacetyl CoA, compared with 7–8 kcal for the hydrolysis of adenosine triphosphate to AMP plus PP_i or ADP plus P_i. CoA or ACP also reacts with acetyl or acyl groups to form thioesters. The pK_a of the thiol in CoA–SH is ~10 (ROH ~ 16); at physiological pH, reasonable amounts of CoA–S– can be formed. CoA–SH is a potent nucleophile and more nucleophilic than RO–; moreover, RS– is a much better leaving group than RO–. Therefore, there is no mesomeric effect that makes the carbonyl group more polar than in regular ester [R–O–CO–R′] or amide bonds [R–N–CO–R′].

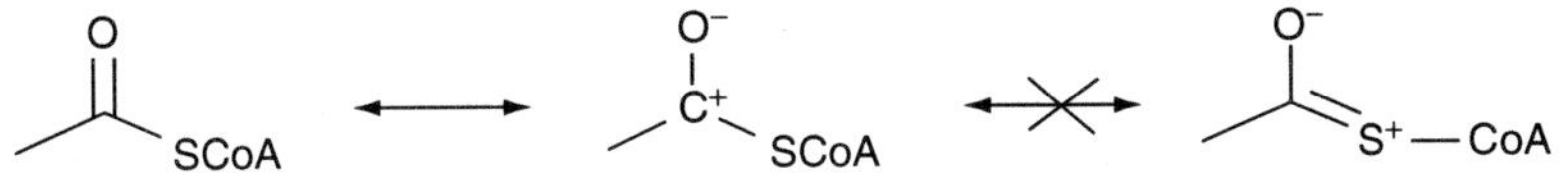

O SCoA ⟷ O⁻ C+ SCoA ⟷(crossed) O⁻ S+—CoA

Their reactivity toward nucleophiles lies between esters and anhydrides. Thiol esters are easier to enolize than esters, i.e., the α-hydrogens are more acidic.

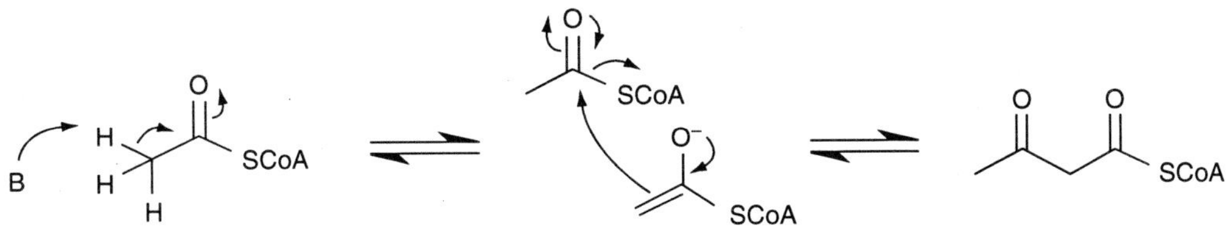

B H H H O SCoA ⇌ O SCoA O⁻ SCoA ⇌ O O SCoA

As such, acetyl CoA is involved in Claisen condensations, which is the basis of fatty acid, polyketide, phenol, terpene, and steroid biosynthesis. Coenzyme A is also central to the balance between carbohydrate metabolism and fat metabolism. Carbohydrate metabolism needs some CoA for the citric acid cycle to continue, and fat metabolism needs a larger amount of CoA for breaking down fatty acid chains during β-oxidation [120].

Synthetic Versus Catabolic Processes Involving Pantetheine

As a fundamental distinction, CoA is involved in a broad array of acetyl and acyl transfer reactions and processes related to primarily oxidative metabolism and catabolism, whereas ACP is involved in synthetic reactions (Table 9.4). The adenosyl moiety of CoA provides a site for tight binding to CoA-requiring enzymes, while allowing the 4′-phosphopantetheine portion to serve as a flexible arm to move substrates from one catalytic center to another [43,120]. Similarly, when pantothenic acid (as 4′-phosphopantetheine) in ACP is used in transfer reactions, it also functions as a flexible arm that allows for an orderly and systematic presentation of thiol ester derivatives to each of the active centers of the FAS complex described in the previous section. A FAS system also exists in mitochondria [131]. The mitochondrial FAS pathway is novel in that it is similar to the FAS pathway in bacteria (designated the "type ii" pathway), for example, discrete soluble protein catalyzes each step of the reaction cycle rather than a multidomain complex.

Acetylations as Regulatory Signals

The addition of an acetyl group into an amino acid –[NH_2] or –[C=O–OH] function can markedly alter chemical properties. The same is true for biogenic amines, carbohydrates, complex lipids and hormones, xenobiotics, and drugs [132–137]. Specific compounds range from acetylcholine to melatonin to structural carbohydrates which are subject to O-linked acetylations. Examples include acetylated sialic acids (under the control of two groups of enzymes, *O*-acetyltransferases and 9-*O*-acetylesterases), cell surface antigens, and a wide variety of lipopolysaccharides, and *N*-acetylgangliosides. Acetylation is critical to cell–cell surface and cell surface protein–protein interactions (e.g., antigenic sites and determinants).

Of the hundreds of examples of covalently modified proteins, acetylation may be the most common [138,139]. Acetylations are catalyzed by a wide range of acetyltransferases that transfer acetyl groups from acetyl CoA to amino groups. Acetylation can alter enzymatic activity, stability, DNA binding, protein–protein/peptide interactions [140–145].

Amino-terminal acetylations occur cotranslationally and posttranslationally on processed eukaryotic regulatory peptides [140–150]. Proteins with serine and alanine termini are the most frequently acetylated, although methionine, glycine, and threonine may also be targets. This type of acetylation is usually irreversible and occurs shortly after the initiation of translation. The biological significance of amino-terminal modification varies in that some proteins require acetylation for function whereas others do not have an absolute requirement. In some cases, the process may be promiscuous, given the large number of proteins that may be acetylated. For example, it is estimated that over 50% of all proteins are acetylated [149].

Lysine residues are also target for acetylations [143]. Lysine acetylations also occur posttranslationally. Histones, transcription factors, cotranscriptional activators, nuclear receptors, and α-tubulin are proteins in which acetylation of specific lysyl residues modulates or alters function [147,148,150]. Acetylation occurs on internal lysine residues within these proteins, and is balanced by the action of a large number of deacetylases [141]. The deacetylases are NAD-dependent. Instead of water, the NAD-dependent deacetylases use a highly reactive ADP-ribose intermediate as a recipient for the acetyl group. The products of the reaction are nicotinamide, acetyl ADP-ribose, and a deacetylated substrate [145]. As an example of an important function, regions of chromatin that are inactive exist as hypo-acetylated heterochromatin-like (tightly packaged) domains. Therefore, acetylation–deacetylation results in different states of chromatin configuration and is an important regulator of gene expression [145].

Other nonhistone proteins and transcription fractions that are reversibly acetylated have been implicated in protein–protein interactions and have been shown to facilitate specific binding of regulatory proteins, such as steroid hormone receptors or that modulate transcription by altering protein–protein interactions (e.g., high-mobility group proteins: HMG1 and HMG2). From a regulatory perspective, although there is no clear evidence that acetyltransferases act in classical cascade sequences (e.g., similar to phosphorylation or dephosphorylation signals), acetylations do alter the charge of the targeted lysyl group in a given protein. Such modifications can markedly influence or cause changes in protein structure.

Acylation Reactions

Another type of CoA facilitated posttranslational modification is acylation. Acylations occur by covalent attachment of lipid groups to change the polarity and strengthen the association of an acylated protein with membranes, both intra- and extracellularly. To date, the best characterized acylation pathways are those involving S-acyl linkages to proteins. Work with Ras proteins has shown that the S-acylation–deacylation cycle along with prenylation and carboxylmethylation may regulate the cycling of Ras between intracellular membrane compartments [151,152]. Indeed, many signaling proteins (e.g., receptors, G-proteins, protein tyrosine kinases, and other cell membrane "scaffolding" molecules) are acylated. Examples of acylations include S-acylation [153] (predominately the addition of a palmitoyl group), N-terminal myristoylations [109], and C-terminal prenylations and internal prenylations [154].

PANTOTHENIC ACID DEFICIENCY, CLINICAL RELATIONSHIPS, AND POTENTIAL INTERACTIONS INVOLVING POLYMORPHISMS

Pantothenic acid deficiency would be expected to result in generalized malaise, perturbations in CoA and lipid metabolism, and mitochondrial dysfunction. In turn, altered homeostasis of CoA would be expected to be associated with a number of disease states; indeed CoA has been described as a component of diabetes, alcoholism, and Reye syndrome [37,43]. Changes in or responses to hormones important to lipid metabolism (e.g., glucocorticoids, insulin, glucagon, and PPAR agonists, such as clofibrate) also occur with either pantothenic acid deficiency or in response to pantothenic acid kinase inhibitors. To reiterate, severe deficiencies of pantothenate are difficult to achieve (e.g., even commercial "vitamin-free" casein can contain up to 3 mg pantothenate/kg [155]). Nevertheless, under conditions of mild pantothenate deficiency in which weight differences between groups are not observed, serum triglyceride and free fatty acid levels are elevated, a reflection of reduced CoA levels.

In deficient states, pantothenate is reasonably conserved, particularly when there is prior exposure to the vitamin. For example, in studies using rodent embryos explanted at 9.0, 9.5, and 10.5 days and cultured for periods of 2 days or more in vitamin-free serum, some type of vitamin augmentation was necessary for normal growth [156]. However, lack of vitamins has a more marked effect on the younger embryos than on those explanted at 10.5 days. Experiments with media deficient in individual vitamins show that for normal development, 9.0 day embryos required a number of vitamins and biofactors (e.g., pantothenic acid, riboflavin, inositol, folic acid, and niacinamide); however, 10.5 day embryos need only riboflavin added to serum using growth and closure of the hindbrain as indices. In animals, the classical signs of deficiency include growth retardation and dermatitis as a secondary consequence of altered lipid metabolism [6,7,9,12,13,29,157–167]. Neurological, immunological [6,167], hematological, reproductive [29,162,168], and gastrointestinal pathologies

TABLE 9.5
Effects of Pantothenic Acid Deficiency in Selected Species

Species	Symptoms
Chicken	Dermatitis around beak, feet, and eyes; poor feathering; spinal cord myelin degeneration; involution of the thymus; fatty degeneration of the liver
Fish	Anorectic behavior; listlessness; fused gill lamellae; reproductive failure
Rat	Dermatitis; loss of hair color with alopecia; hemorrhagic necrosis of the adrenals; duodenal ulcer; spastic gait; anemia; leukopenia; impaired antibody production; gonadal atrophy with infertility
Dog	Anorexia; diarrhea; acute encephalopathy; coma; hypoglycemia; leukocytosis; hyperammonemia; hyperlactemia; hepatic steatosis; mitochondrial enlargement
Pig	Dermatitis; hair loss; diarrhea with impaired sodium, potassium, and glucose absorption; lachrymation; ulcerative colitis; spinal cord and peripheral nerve lesions with spastic gait

[169] have been reported. The effects of pantothenic acid deficiency in different species are summarized in Table 9.5.

What is known about pantothenic acid deficiency in humans comes primarily from two sources. First, during World War II, malnourished prisoners of war in Japan, Burma, and the Philippines experienced numbness and burning sensations in their feet. While these individuals suffered multiple deficiencies, numbness and burning sensations were only reversed on pantothenic acid supplementation [170]. Second, experimental pantothenic acid deficiency has been induced in both animals and humans by administration of the pantothenic acid kinase inhibitor, ω-methylpantothenate, in combination with a diet low in pantothenic acid [24,159,171–175]. Observed symptoms in humans also included numbness and burning of the hands and feet, as well as some of the other symptoms listed in Table 9.5. Another pantothenic acid antagonist, calcium hopantenate, has been shown to induce encephalopathy with hepatic steatosis and a Reye-like syndrome in both dogs and humans [176].

With respect to temporal expression of pantothenic acid deficiency, if 5 mg or more is needed per day by humans, it may be predicted that with a severe deficiency of pantothenic acid, ~6 weeks would be required in an adult before clear signs of deficiency are observed. A daily loss of 4–6 mg of pantothenic acid represents a 1%–2% loss of the body pool of pantothenic acid in humans. For example, for many water-soluble vitamins (at a loss of 1%–2% of the body pool) 1–2 months of depletion results in deficiency signs [37,49]. In this regard, from the limited studies on pantothenic acid depletion ~6 weeks of severe depletion are required before urinary pantothenic acid decreases to a basal level of excretion [79,177,178].

With regard to clinical applications, claims for pantothenic acid range from prevention and treatment of graying hair (based on the observation that pantothenic acid deficiency in rodents causes fur to gray) to improved athletic performance. Several studies have indicated that pantetheine, in doses ranging from 500 to 1200 mg/day, may lower total serum cholesterol, low-density lipoprotein cholesterol, and triacylglycerols [25,179–189]. Oral administration of pantothenic acid and application of pantothenol ointment to the skin seems to accelerate the closure of skin wounds and increase the strength of scar tissue in animal models [190–192].

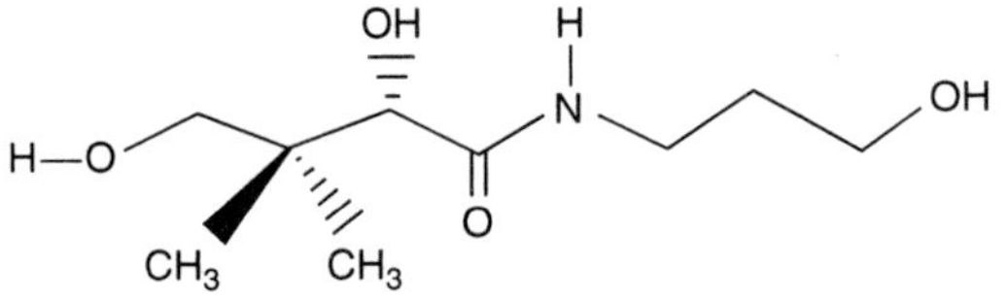

OH H
H—O N OH
O
CH_3 CH_3

Structure of pantothenol

However, the results are equivocal in humans. In a randomized, double-blind study examining the effect of supplementing patients undergoing surgery for tattoo removal with pantothenic acid did not demonstrate any significant improvement in the wound-healing process [191]. Papers may also be found on lupus erythematosus and pantothenic acid deficiency. Procainamide, hydralazine, and isoniazid are known to cause drug-induced lupus erythematosus. Because these drugs are metabolized via CoA-dependent acetylation, it is argued that there is an increased demand for CoA, which causes a pantothenic acid deficit. However, clinical trials involving pantothenic acid supplementation and given diseases, lupus in particular, have yet to show promise [193–199].

Polymorphisms or gene defects in enzymes involved in CoA synthesis pathway exist, and result in disease states, such as Hallervorden–Spatz syndrome or pantothenate kinase–associated neurodegeneration [89,91,96,113–115]. This disease results from mutations in PanK2, which is the most abundantly expressed form in the brain and localized in mitochondria. This autosomal recessive neurodegenerative disorder is characterized clinically by dystonia and optic atrophy or pigmentary retinopathy with iron deposits in the basal ganglia and globus pallidus [114,115].

PHARMACOLOGY

Several pantothenate-related compounds have been recommended as inhibitors of *Staphylococcus aureus* infections or proliferation of malarial parasites. Most of these analogs retain the 2,4-dihydroxy-3,3-dimethylbutyramide core of pantothenic acid. Many analogs are relatively specific, inhibiting the proliferation of human cells only at concentrations several fold higher than those required for inhibition of parasite or bacterial growth. The structures and chemical characteristics of selected analogs are provided in Figure 9.5.

Some classic observations utilizing pantothenic acid antagonists such as ω-methyl-pantothenic acid and calcium hopantenate were mentioned in the previous section. Tragic lessons were learned utilizing these compounds. In moderate doses, ω-methyl-pantothenic acid can be potentially lethal [24]. Similarly, calcium hopantenate administration may cause fatal and acute encephalopathy ([176]).

As was noted in the previous section, pantothenic acid supplementation has also been associated with lipid-lowering effects, but pantothenic acid administration does not compete with the excellent drugs that are currently available, although it is conceivable that the

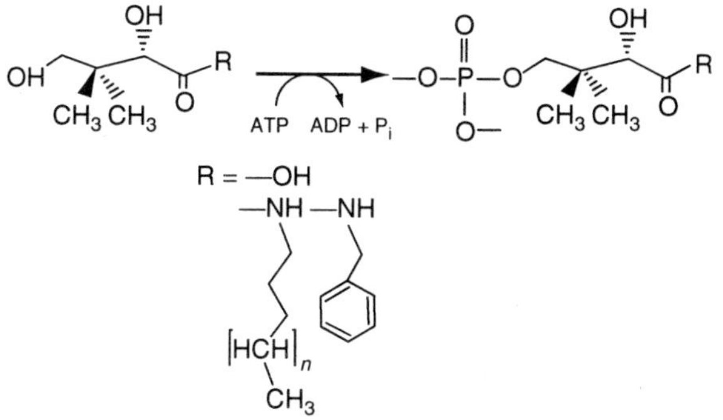

OH
OH
CH3 CH3
O
R
ATP
ADP + Pi
—O—P—O
O
O—
OH
CH3 CH3
O
R
R = —OH
—NH —NH
HCH n
CH3

FIGURE 9.5 Pantothenic acid analogs that have potential as CoA synthesis inhibitors. Modifying the carboxyl moiety of pantothenic acid by the addition of an aromatic or acyl group in amide linkage results in a derivative that is effective as an inhibitor of 4′-phosphopantothenoylcysteine synthetase and subsequent transferases (see Figure 9.2).

combination of pantetheine and an appropriate peroxisomal activated regulator receptor agonists or coactivator may be of utility in normalizing lipid metabolism [95,179].

Regarding other applications, amelioration of the adverse effects of valproic acid on ketogenesis and liver CoA metabolism by cotreatment with pantothenate and carnitine has proven successful in developing mice. Valproic acid ($CH_3–CH_2–CH_2]_2=CH–COOH$) is a Food and Drug Administration (FDA)-approved drug used in the treatment of epilepsy and has been used in the treatment of manic episodes associated with bipolar disorder. Considering the side effects of valproic acid (nausea, tremors, and liver failure), pantothenic acid supplementation has been suggested to have some promise in modulating such symptoms when valproic acid is the drug chosen [200–205].

TOXICITY

Pantothenic acid is generally safe, even at extremely high doses. Excesses are mostly excreted in the urine. Very high oral doses (>1 g/day) of pantothenic acid may be associated with diarrhea and gastrointestinal disturbances. However, there are no reports of acute toxic effects in humans, or commonly available pharmaceutical forms of pantothenic acid, other than gastrointestinal disturbance. Indeed, no data are available that suggest neurotoxicity, carcinogenicity, genotoxicity, or reproductive toxicity. Calcium pantothenate, sodium pantothenate, and panthenol are not mutagenic in bacterial tests.

In animals, young rats fed 50 mg/day (~0.5 g/kg bw/day) as calcium pantothenate for 190 days had no adverse effects. When bred, their offspring were maintained using the same diets with no signs of abnormal growth or gross pathology. Similar studies in mice (both oral and i.p.) have led to the same conclusions. In the early 1940s, Unna and Greslin [15,18] reported acute and chronic toxicity tests with D-calcium pantothenate in mice, rats, dogs, and monkeys. Acute oral LD_{50} values were 10,000 mg/kg bw, mice, and rats, with lethal doses producing death by respiratory failure. An oral dose of 1000 mg/kg bw produced no toxic signs in dogs or in one monkey. Oral dosing (500 or 2000 mg/kg bw/day to rats, 50 mg/kg bw/day to dogs, 200–250 mg/kg bw/day to monkeys) for 6 months produced no toxic signs, weight loss, or evidence of histopathological changes at autopsy [206].

In humans, Welsh [193,195] reported that giving patients high doses of pantothenic acid derivatives ($\leq$10–15 g) with the goal of treating symptoms of lupus erythematosus (see previous section) had no side effects other than transient nausea and gastric distress. Likewise, Goldman [207] described the use of panthenol for the treatment of lupus erythematosus at various dosage levels up to 8–10 g/day, for periods ranging from 5 days to 6 months with few side effects. Webster [70] carried out a randomized, double-blind, placebo-controlled, crossover study to assess the effects of pantothenic acid on exercise performance in six highly trained cyclists. For each subject, two testing (cycling performance) sessions were carried out, separated by a 21 day washout period. One testing session was carried out immediately after 7 days supplementation with pantotheine derivatives at ~2 g/day or placebo. No significant differences were identified between assessed parameters of cycling performance and no side effects of the therapy were reported. In summary, high doses of pantothenic acid, 100–500 times the normal requirements, appear well tolerated.

STATUS DETERMINATION

Whole blood concentration and urinary excretion reflects pantothenic acid status. In humans, whole blood concentrations typically range from 1.6 to 2.7 μmol/L [37,47,85,208] and a value <1 μmol/L is considered low. Urinary excretion is considered a more reliable indicator of status because it is more closely related to dietary intake [79]. Excretion of <1 mg pantothenic acid per day in urine is considered low. Plasma level of the vitamin is a poor indicator of status because it is not highly correlated with changes in intake or status.

Pantothenic acid concentrations in whole blood, plasma, and urine are measured by microbiological assay employing *Lactobacillus plantarum*. For whole blood, enzyme pretreatment is required to convert CoA to free pantothenic acid since *L. plantarum* does not respond to CoA. Other methods that have been employed to assess pantothenic acid status include radioimmunoassay, ELISA, and gas chromatography [52,53,84,85,209,210].

ACKNOWLEDGMENT

Preparation was supported in part by NIH training grant DK07355-24.

REFERENCES

1. Williams, R.J., Lyman, C.M., Goodyear, G.H., Truesdail, J.H., Holaday, D.: Pantothenic acid, a growth determinant of universal biological occurrence. *J. Am. Chem. Soc.*, 1933, 55:2912–2927.
2. Jukes, T.H.: The pantothenic acid requirements of the chick. *J. Biol. Chem.*, 1939, 129:225–231.
3. Jukes, T.H.: The pantothenic acid requirement of the chick. *J. Biol. Chem.*, 1939, 120:225–231.
4. SubbaRow, Y., Hitchings, G.H.: Pantothenic acid as a factor in rat nutrition. *J. Am. Chem. Soc.*, 1939, 61:1615–1618.
5. Milligan, J.L., Briggs, G.M.: Replacement of pantothenic acid by panthenol in chick diets. *Poult. Sci.*, 1949, 28:202–205.
6. Ludovici, P.P., Axelrod, A.E., Carter, B.B.: Circulating antibodies in vitamin efficiency states; pantothenic acid deficiency. *Proc. Soc. Exp. Biol. Med.*, 1949, 72:81–83.
7. Becker, E.R., Brodine, C.E., Marousek, A.A.: Eyelid lesion of chicks in acute dietary deficiency resulting from blood-induced *Plasmodium lophurae* infection; role of pantothenic acid and biotin. *J. Infect. Dis.*, 1949, 85:230–238.
8. Kratzer, F.H., Williams, D.E.: The pantothenic acid requirement for poultry and early growth. *Poult. Sci.*, 1948, 27:518–523.
9. Wintrobe, M.M., Follis, R.H., Alcayaga, R., Paulson, M., Humphreys, S.: Pantothenic acid deficiency in swine with particular reference to the effects on growth and on the alimentary tract. *Bull. Johns Hopkins Hospital*, 1943, 73:313–319.
10. Schock, N.W., Sebrall, W.H.: The effects of changes in concentration of pantothenate on the work output of perfused frog muscles. *Am. J. Physiol.*, 1944, 142:274–278.
11. Glusman, M.: The syndrome "burning feet" (nutritional melagia) as a manifestation of nutritional deficiency. *Am. J. Med.*, 1947, 3:211–223.
12. Sullivan, M., Nicholls, J.: Nutritional dermatoses in the rat. VI. The effects of pantothenic acid deficiency. *Arch. Dermatol. Syphilol.*, 1942, 45:917–932.
13. Schaefer, A.E., McKibbin, J.M., Elvehjem, C.A.: Pantothenic acid deficiency in dogs. *J. Biol. Chem.*, 1942, 143:321–330.
14. Francis, J.P., Axelrod, A.E., Elvehjem, C.E.: The metabolism of pyruvate by liver from pantothenic acid and biotin deficient rats. *J. Biol. Chem.*, 1942, 145:237–340.
15. Unna, K., Greslin, J.G.: Studies on the toxicity and pharmacology of pantothenic acid. *J. Pharmacol. Exp. Ther.*, 1941, 73:85–90.
16. Spies, T.D., Stanberry, S.R., Williams, R.J., Jukes, T.H., Babcock, S.H.: Pantothenic acid in human nutrition. *J. Am. Med. Assoc.*, 1940, 115:523–524.
17. Stiller, E.T., Harris, S.A., Finkelstein, J., Keresztesy, J.C.: Pantothenic acid. VIII. The total synthesis of pure pantothenic acid. *J. Am. Chem. Soc.*, 1940, 62:1785–1790.
18. Unna, K., Greslin, J.G.: Toxicity of pantothenic acid. *Proc. Soc. Exp. Biol. Med.*, 1940, 45:311–312.
19. Williams, R.J., Major, R.T.: The structure of pantothenic acid. *J. Am. Chem. Soc.*, 1940, 61:1615.
20. Williams, R.J., Major, R.T.: The structure of pantothenic acid. *Science*, 1940, 91:246–248.
21. Wooley, D.W., Waisman, H.A., Elvehjem, C.A.: Nature and partial synthesis of the chick antidermatitic factor. *J. Am. Chem. Soc.*, 1939, 61:977–978.

22. Williams, R.J., Truesdail, J.H., Weinstock, H.H., Jr., Rohrmann, E., Lyman, C.M., McBurney, C.H.: Pantothenic acid. II. Its concentration and purification from liver. *J. Am. Chem. Soc.*, 1939, 60:2719–2723.
23. Williams, R.J.: Pantothenic acid—vitamin. *Science*, 1939, 89:486.
24. Hodges, R.E., Bean, W.B., Ohlson, M.A., Bleiler, R.: Human pantothenic acid deficiency produced by omega-methyl pantothenic acid. *J. Clin. Invest.*, 1959, 38:1421–1425.
25. Kimura, S., Furukawa, Y., Wakasugi, J., Ishihara, Y., Nakayama, A.: Antagonism of L(−)pantothenic acid on lipid metabolism in animals. *J. Nutr. Sci. Vitaminol.*, (*Tokyo*) 1980, 26:113–117.
26. Pietrzik, K., Hesse, C., Hotzel, D.: [Influencing of acetylation and corticosterone biosynthesis through long-term pantothenic acid deficiency in rats]. *Int. J. Vitam. Nutr. Res.*, 1975, 45:251–261.
27. Pietrzik, K., Hesse, C.H., Zur Wiesch, E.S., Hotzel, D.: [Urinary excretion of pantothenic acid as a measurement of nutritional requirements]. *Int. J. Vitam. Nutr. Res.*, 1975, 45:153–162.
28. Stein, E.D., Diamond, J.M.: Do dietary levels of pantothenic acid regulate its intestinal uptake in mice? *J. Nutr.*, 1989, 119:1973–1983.
29. Drell, W., Dunn, M.S.: Production of pantothenic acid deficiency syndrome in mice with methylpantothenic acid. *Arch. Biochem.*, 1951, 33:110–119.
30. McDowell, M.E., Leveille, GA: Feeding experiments with algae. *Fed. Proc.*, 1963, 22:1431–1438.
31. Sarett, H.P., Barboriak, J.J.: Inhibition of D-pantothenate by L-pantothenate in the rat. *Am. J. Clin. Nutr.*, 1963, 13:378–384.
32. Wells, I.C., Hogan, J.M.: Effects of dietary deficiencies of lipotropic factors on plasma cholesterol esterification and tissue cholesterol in rats. *J. Nutr.*, 1968, 95:55–62.
33. Williams, M.A., Chu, L.C., McIntosh, D.J., Hincenbergs, I.: Effects of dietary fat level on pantothenate depletion and liver fatty acid composition in the rat. *J. Nutr.*, 1968, 94:377–382.
34. Pietrzik, K., Hesse, C., Schulze zur Wiesch, E., Hotzel, D.: [Experimental pantothenic acid deficiency in the rat]. *Nahrung*, 1974, 18(5):491–502.
35. Emerson, G.A.: Agnes Fay Morgan and early nutrition discoveries in California. *Fed. Proc.*, 1977, 36:1911–1914.
36. Jukes, T.H.: Dilworth Wayne Woolley (1914–1966)—a biographical sketch. *J. Nutr.*, 1974, 104:507–511.
37. Bender, D.A.: Optimum nutrition: thiamin, biotin and pantothenate. *Proc. Nutr. Soc.*, 1999, 58:427–433.
38. Webb, M., Abeil C: Biosynthesis of pantothenate. *Nat. Prod. Rep.*, 2004, 21:695–721.
39. Chantrenne, H., Lipmann, F.: Coenzyme A dependence and acetyl donor function of the pyruvate–formate exchange system. *J. Biol. Chem.*, 1950, 187:757–767.
40. Lipmann, F., Kaplan, N.O., Novelli, G.D., Tuttle, L.C., Guirard, B.M.: Isolation of coenzyme A. *J. Biol. Chem.*, 1950, 186:235–243.
41. Lipmann, F.: On chemistry and function of coenzyme A. *Bacteriol. Rev.*, 1953, 17:1–16.
42. Lipmann, F., Jones, M.E., Black, S., Flynn, R.M.: The mechanism of the ATP-CoA-acetate reaction. *J. Cell. Physiol.*, 1953, 41(Suppl 1):109–112.
43. Tahiliani, A.G., Beinlich, C.J.: Pantothenic acid in health and disease. *Vitam. Horm.*, 1991, 46:165–228.
44. Roncari, D.A.: Mammalian fatty acid synthetase. II. Modification of purified human liver complex activity. *Can. J. Biochem.*, 1975, 53:135–142.
45. Prescott, D.J., Vagelos, P.R.: Acyl carrier protein. *Adv. Enzymol. Relat. Areas Mol. Biol.*, 1972, 36:269–311.
46. Knudsen, J.: Acyl-CoA-binding protein (ACBP) and its relation to fatty acid-binding protein (FABP): an overview. *Mol. Cell. Biochem.*, 1990, 98:217–223.
47. Panel on Folate OBV, and Choline, Subcommittee on Upper Reference Levels of Nutrients FNB, IOM: Dietary Reference Intakes for Thiamin, Riboflavin, Niacin, Vitamin B_6, Folate, Vitamin B_{12}, Pantothenic Acid, Biotin, and Choline. Washington, DC: National Academy Press, 2000, 1998:1–592.
48. Tarr, J.B., Tamura, T., Stokstad, E.L.: Availability of vitamin B_6 and pantothenate in an average American diet in man. *Am. J. Clin. Nutr.*, 1981, 34:1328–1337.
49. Rucker, R.B., Steinberg, F.M.: Vitamin requirements: relationship to basal metabolic need and functions. *Biochem. Mol. Biol. Educ.*, 2002, 30:86–89.

50. Shibata, K., Gross, C.J., Henderson, L.M.: Hydrolysis and absorption of pantothenate and its coenzymes in the rat small intestine. *J. Nutr.*, 1983, 113:2107–2115.
51. Schroeder, H.A.: Losses of vitamins and trace minerals resulting from processing and preservation of foods. *Am. J. Clin. Nutr.*, 1971, 24:562–573.
52. Walsh, J.H., Wyse, B.W., Hansen, R.G.: Pantothenic acid content of 75 processed and cooked foods. *J. Am. Diet. Assoc.*, 1981, 78:140–144.
53. Walsh, J.H., Wyse, B.W., Hansen, R.G.: Pantothenic acid content of a nursing home diet. *Ann. Nutr. Metab.*, 1981, 25:178–181.
54. Nichols, E.L., Nichols, V.N.: Human milk: nutritional resource. *Prog. Clin. Biol. Res.*, 1981, 61:109–146.
55. Johnston, L., Vaughan, L., Fox, H.M.: Pantothenic acid content of human milk. *Am. J. Clin. Nutr.*, 1981, 34(10):2205–2209.
56. Deodhar, A.D., Ramakrishnan, C.V.: Studies on human lactation (Relation between the dietary intake of lactating women and the chemical composition of milk with regard to vitamin content). *J. Trop. Pediatr.*, 1960, 6:44–47.
57. Airas, R.K.: Kinetic study on the reaction mechanism of pantothenase: existence of an acyl-enzyme intermediate and role of general acid catalysis. *Biochemistry*, 1978, 17:4932–4938.
58. Airas, R.K.: Pantothenase. *Methods Enzymol.*, 1979, 62:267–275.
59. Airas, R.K.: Pantothenase-based assay of pantothenic acid. *Anal. Biochem.*, 1983, 134(1):122–125.
60. Airas, R.K.: Pantothenase-based assay of pantothenic acid. *Methods Enzymol.*, 1986, 122:33–35.
61. Said, H.M.: Cellular uptake of biotin: mechanisms and regulation. *J. Nutr.*, 1999, 129(Suppl):490S–493S.
62. Fenstermacher, D.K., Rose, R.C.: Absorption of pantothenic acid in rat and chick intestine. *Am. J. Physiol.*, 1986, 250:G155–G160.
63. Balamurugan, K., Ortiz, A., Said, H.M.: Biotin uptake by human intestinal and liver epithelial cells: role of the SMVT system. *Am. J. Physiol. Gastrointest. Liver Physiol.*, 2003, 285:G73–G77.
64. Balamurugan, K., Vaziri, N.D., Said, H.M.: Biotin uptake by human proximal tubular epithelial cells: cellular and molecular aspects. *Am. J. Physiol. Renal Physiol.*, 2005, 288:F823–F831.
65. Chatterjee, N.S., Kumar, C.K., Ortiz, A., Rubin, S.A., Said, H.M.: Molecular mechanism of the intestinal biotin transport process. *Am. J. Physiol.*, 1999, 277:C605–C613.
66. Dey, S., Subramanian, V.S., Chatterjee, N.S., Rubin, S.A., Said, H.M.: Characterization of the 5′ regulatory region of the human sodium-dependent multivitamin transporter, hSMVT. *Biochim. Biophys. Acta*, 2002, 1574:187–192.
67. Said, H.M., Ortiz, A., McCloud, E., Dyer, D., Moyer, M.P., Rubin, S.: Biotin uptake by human colonic epithelial NCM460 cells: a carrier-mediated process shared with pantothenic acid. *Am. J. Physiol.*, 1998, 275:C1365–C1371.
68. Park, S., Sinko, P.J.: The blood–brain barrier sodium-dependent multivitamin transporter: a molecular functional in vitro–in situ correlation. *Drug Metab. Dispos.*, 2005, 33:1547–1554.
69. Spector, R., Sivesind, C., Kinzenbaw, D.: Pantothenic acid transport through the blood–brain barrier. *J. Neurochem.*, 1986, 47:966–971.
70. Webster, M.J.: Physiological and performance responses to supplementation with thiamin and pantothenic acid derivatives. *Eur. J. Appl. Physiol. Occup. Physiol.*, 1998, 77(6):486–491.
71. Beinlich, C.J., Naumovitz, R.D., Song, W.O., Neely, J.R.: Myocardial metabolism of pantothenic acid in chronically diabetic rats. *J. Mol. Cell. Cardiol.*, 1990, 22(3):323–332.
72. Beinlich, C.J., Robishaw, J.D., Neely, J.R.: Metabolism of pantothenic acid in hearts of diabetic rats. *J. Mol. Cell Cardiol.*, 1989, 21(7):641–649.
73. Lopaschuk, G.D., Michalak, M., Tsang, H.: Regulation of pantothenic acid transport in the heart. Involvement of a Na^+-cotransport system. *J. Biol. Chem.*, 1987, 262(8):3615–3619.
74. Wang, H., Huang, W., Fei, Y.J., Xia, H., Yang-Feng, T.L., Leibach, F.H., Devoe, L.D., Ganapathy, V., Prasad, P.D.: Human placental Na^+-dependent multivitamin transporter. Cloning, functional expression, gene structure, and chromosomal localization. *J. Biol. Chem.*, 1999, 274:14875–14883.
75. Prasad, P.D., Wang, H., Kekuda, R., Fujita, T., Fei, Y.J., Devoe, L.D., Leibach, F.H., Ganapathy, V.: Cloning and functional expression of a cDNA encoding a mammalian sodium-dependent vitamin transporter mediating the uptake of pantothenate, biotin, and lipoate. *J. Biol. Chem.*, 1998, 273:7501–7506.

76. Prasad, P.D., Ramamoorthy, S., Leibach, F.H., Ganapathy, V.: Characterization of a sodium-dependent vitamin transporter mediating the uptake of pantothenate, biotin and lipoate in human placental choriocarcinoma cells. *Placenta*, 1997, 18:527–533.
77. Grassl, S.M.: Human placental brush-border membrane Na(+)–pantothenate cotransport. *J. Biol. Chem.*, 1992, 267:22902–22906.
78. Cohenour, S.H., Calloway, D.H.: Blood, urine, and dietary pantothenic acid levels of pregnant teenagers. *Am. J. Clin. Nutr.*, 1972, 25:512–517.
79. Fry, P.C., Fox, H.M., Tao, H.G.: Metabolic response to a pantothenic acid deficient diet in humans. *J. Nutr. Sci. Vitaminol.*, (*Tokyo*) 1976, 22:339–346.
80. Srinivasan, V., Belavady, B.: Nutritional status of pantothenic acid in Indian pregnant and nursing women. *Int. J. Vitam. Nutr. Res.*, 1976, 46:433–438.
81. Tao, H.G., Fox, H.M.: Measurements of urinary pantothenic acid excretions of alcoholic patients. *J. Nutr. Sci. Vitaminol.*, (*Tokyo*) 1976, 22:333–337.
82. Duke, M.L., Kies, C, Fox, H.M.: Niacin and pantothenic acid excretions of humans fed a low-methionine, plant-based diet. *J. Nutr. Sci. Vitaminol.*, (*Tokyo*) 1977, 23:481–489.
83. Pietrzik, K., Hotzel, D.: Studies for the evaluation of pantothenic acid requirement. *Nutr. Metab.*, 1977, 21(Suppl 1):23–24.
84. Eissenstat, B.R., Wyse, B.W., Hansen R.G.: Pantothenic acid status of adolescents. *Am. J. Clin. Nutr.*, 1986, 44:931–937.
85. Song, W.O., Wyse, B.W., Hansen, R.G.: Pantothenic acid status of pregnant and lactating women. *J. Am. Diet Assoc.*, 1985, 85:192–198.
86. Virga, K.G., Zhang, Y.M., Leonardi, R., Ivey, R.A., Hevener, K., Park, H.W., Jackowski, S., Rock, C.O., Lee, R.E.: Structure–activity relationships and enzyme inhibition of pantothenamide-type pantothenate kinase inhibitors. *Bioorg. Med. Chem.*, 2006, 14:1007–1020.
87. Li, Y., Chang, Y., Zhang, L., Feng, Q., Liu, Z., Zhang, Y., Zuo, J., Meng, Y., Fang, F.: High glucose upregulates pantothenate kinase 4 (PanK4) and thus affects M2-type pyruvate kinase (Pkm2). *Mol. Cell. Biochem.*, 2005, 277:117–125.
88. Zhang, Y.M., Rock, C.O., Jackowski, S.: Feedback regulation of murine pantothenate kinase 3 by coenzyme A and coenzyme A thioesters. *J. Biol. Chem.*, 2005, 280:32594–32601.
89. Kapoor, S., Hortnagel, K., Gogia, S., Paul, R., Malhotra, V., Prakash, A.: Pantothenate kinase associated neurodegeneration (Hallervorden–Spatz syndrome). *Indian J. Pediatr.*, 2005, 72:261–263.
90. Brand, L.A., Strauss, E.: Characterization of a new pantothenate kinase isoform from *Helicobacter pylori*. *J. Biol. Chem.*, 2005, 280:20185–20188.
91. Le Gall, J.Y., Jouanolle, A.M., Fergelot, P., Mosser, J., David, V.: Genetics of hereditary iron overload. *Bull. Acad. Natl. Med.*, 2004, 188:247–262; discussion 262–243.
92. Vadali, R.V., Bennett, G.N., San, K.Y.: Applicability of CoA/acetyl-CoA manipulation system to enhance isoamyl acetate production in *Escherichia coli*. *Metab. Eng.*, 2004, 6:294–299.
93. Healy, D.G., Abou-Sleiman, P.M., Wood, N.W.: PINK, PANK, or PARK? A clinician's guide to familial parkinsonism. *Lancet Neurol.*, 2004, 3:652–662.
94. Lin, H., Vadali, R.V., Bennett, G.N., San, K.Y.: Increasing the acetyl-CoA pool in the presence of overexpressed phosphoenolpyruvate carboxylase or pyruvate carboxylase enhances succinate production in *Escherichia coli*. *Biotechnol. Prog.*, 2004, 20:1599–1604.
95. Ramaswamy, G., Karim, M.A., Murti, K.G., Jackowski, S.: PPARalpha controls the intracellular coenzyme A concentration via regulation of PANK1 alpha gene expression. *J. Lipid Res.*, 2004, 45:17–31.
96. Cossu, G., Melis, M., Floris, G., Hayflick, S.J., Spissu, A.: Hallervorden Spatz syndrome (pantothenate kinase associated neurodegeneration) in two Sardinian brother with homozygous mutation in PANK2 gene. *J. Neurol.*, 2002, 249:1599–1600.
97. Rock, C.O., Karim, M.A., Zhang, Y.M., Jackowski, S.: The murine pantothenate kinase (Pank1) gene encodes two differentially regulated pantothenate kinase isozymes. *Gene*, 2002, 291:35–43.
98. Ni, X., Ma, Y., Cheng, H., Jiang, M., Ying, K., Xie, Y., Mao, Y.: Cloning and characterization of a novel human pantothenate kinase gene. *Int. J. Biochem. Cell. Biol.*, 2002, 34:109–115.
99. Yun, M., Park, C.G., Kim, J.Y., Rock, C.O., Jackowski, S., Park, H.W.: Structural basis for the feedback regulation of *Escherichia coli* pantothenate kinase by coenzyme A. *J. Biol. Chem.*, 2000, 275(36):28093–28099.

100. Rock, C.O., Calder, R.B., Karim, M.A., Jackowski, S.: Pantothenate kinase regulation of the intracellular concentration of coenzyme A. *J. Biol. Chem.*, 2000, 275:1377–1383.
101. Calder, R.B., Williams, R.S., Ramaswamy, G., Rock, C.O., Campbell, E., Unkles, S.E., Kinghorn, J.R., Jackowski, S: Cloning and characterization of a eukaryotic pantothenate kinase gene (panK) from *Aspergillus nidulans*. *J. Biol. Chem.*, 1999, 274:2014–2020.
102. Reibel, D.K., Wyse, B.W., Berkich, D.A., Neely, J.R.: Regulation of coenzyme A synthesis in heart muscle: effects of diabetes and fasting. *Am. J. Physiol.*, 1981, 240:H606–H611.
103. Reibel, D.K., Wyse, B.W., Berkich, D.A., Palko, W.M., Neely, J.R.: Effects of diabetes and fasting on pantothenic acid metabolism in rats. *Am. J. Physiol.*, 1981, 240:E597–E601.
104. Halvorsen, O., Skrede, S.: Regulation of the biosynthesis of CoA at the level of pantothenate kinase. *Eur. J. Biochem.*, 1982, 124:211–215.
105. Robishaw, J.D., Berkich, D., Neely, J.R.: Rate-limiting step and control of coenzyme A synthesis in cardiac muscle. *J. Biol. Chem.*, 1982, 257:10967–10972.
106. Robishaw, J.D., Neely, J.R.: Pantothenate kinase and control of CoA synthesis in heart. *Am. J. Physiol.*, 1984, 246:H532–H541.
107. Fisher, M.N., Robishaw, J.D., Neely, J.R.: The properties and regulation of pantothenate kinase from rat heart. *J. Biol. Chem.*, 1985, 260:15745–15751.
108. Robishaw, J.D., Neely, J.R.: Coenzyme A metabolism. *Am. J. Physiol.*, 1985, 248:E1–E9.
109. Shoji, S., Kubota, Y.: [Function of protein myristoylation in cellular regulation and viral proliferation]. *Yakugaku Zasshi*, 1989, 109:71–85.
110. Kirschbaum, N., Clemons, R., Marino, K.A., Sheedy, G., Nguyen, M.L., Smith, C.M.: Pantothenate kinase activity in livers of genetically diabetic mice (db/db) and hormonally treated cultured rat hepatocytes. *J. Nutr.*, 1990, 120:1376–1386.
111. Renstrom, B., Liedtke, A.J., Nellis, S.H.: The effects of pantothenic acid, cysteine and dithiothreitol in intact, reperfused pig hearts. *Mol. Cell. Biochem.*, 1991, 105:27–35.
112. Saleheen, D., Nazir, A., Khanum, S., Haider, S.R., Frossard, P.: A novel mutation in a patient with pantothenate kinase–associated neurodegeneration. *Can. Med. Assoc. J.*, 2006, 13:173–174.
113. Kuo, Y.M., Duncan, J.L., Westaway, S.K., Yang, H., Nune, G., Xu, E.Y., Hayflick, S.J., Gitschier, J.: Deficiency of pantothenate kinase 2 (Pank2) in mice leads to retinal degeneration and azoospermia. *Hum. Mol. Genet.*, 2005, 14:49–57.
114. Gordon, N.: Pantothenate kinase-associated neurodegeneration (Hallervorden–Spatz syndrome). *Eur. J. Paediatr. Neurol.*, 2002, 6:243–247.
115. Hayflick, S.J.: Unraveling the Hallervorden–Spatz syndrome: pantothenate kinase-associated neurodegeneration is the name. *Curr. Opin. Pediatr.*, 2003, 15:572–577.
116. Lopaschuk, G.D., Hansen, C.A., Neely, J.R.: Fatty acid metabolism in hearts containing elevated levels of CoA. *Am. J. Physiol.*, 1986, 250:H351–H359.
117. Stuible, H.P., Meier, S., Wagner, C., Hannappel, E., Schweizer, E.: A novel phosphopantetheine:protein transferase activating yeast mitochondrial acyl carrier protein. *J. Biol. Chem.*, 1998, 273:22334–22339.
118. Zhyvoloup, A., Nemazanyy, I., Panasyuk, G., Valovka, T., Fenton, T., Rebholz, H., Wang, M.L., Foxon, R., Lyzogubov, V., Usenko, V., et al.: Subcellular localization and regulation of coenzyme A synthase. *J. Biol. Chem.*, 2003, 278:50316–50321.
119. Genschel, U.: Coenzyme A biosynthesis: reconstruction of the pathway in archaea and an evolutionary scenario based on comparative genomics. *Mol. Biol. Evol.*, 2004, 21:1242–1251.
120. Leonardi, R., Zhang, Y.M., Rock, C.O., Jackowski, S.: Coenzyme A: back in action. *Prog. Lipid Res.*, 2005, 44:125–153.
121. Shiau, S.Y., Hsu, C.W.: Dietary pantothenic acid requirement of juvenile grass shrimp, *Penaeus monodon*. *J. Nutr.*, 1999, 129:718–721.
122. Wittwer, C.T., Schweitzer, C., Pearson, J., Song, W.O., Windham, C.T., Wyse, B.W., Hansen, R.G.: Enzymes for liberation of pantothenic acid in blood: use of plasma pantetheinase. *Am. J. Clin. Nutr.*, 1989, 50:1072–1078.
123. Hettema, E.H., van Roermund, C.W., Distel, B., van den Berg, M., Vilela, C., Rodrigues-Pousada, C., Wanders, R.J., Tabak, H.F.: The ABC transporter proteins Pat1 and Pat2 are required for import of long-chain fatty acids into peroxisomes of *Saccharomyces cerevisiae*. *EMBO J.*, 1996, 15:3813–3822.

124. Webb, E., Claas, K., Downs, D.: thiBPQ encodes an ABC transporter required for transport of thiamine and thiamine pyrophosphate in *Salmonella typhimurium*. *J. Biol. Chem.*, 1998, 273:8946–8950.
125. Neubauer, H., Pantel, I., Lindgren, P.E., Gotz, F.: Characterization of the molybdate transport system ModABC of *Staphylococcus carnosus*. *Arch. Microbiol.*, 1999, 172:109–115.
126. Aghajanian, S., Worrall, D.M.: Identification and characterization of the gene encoding the human phosphopantetheine adenylyltransferase and dephospho-CoA kinase bifunctional enzyme (CoA synthase). *Biochem. J.*, 2002, 365:13–18.
127. Lornitzo, F.A., Qureshi, A.A., Porter, J.W.: Subunits of fatty acid synthetase complexes. Enzymatic activities and properties of the half-molecular weight nonidentical subunits of pigeon liver fatty acid synthetase. *J. Biol. Chem.*, 1975, 250:4520–4529.
128. Praphanphoj, V., Sacksteder, K.A., Gould, S.J., Thomas, G.H., Geraghty, M.T.: Identification of the alpha-aminoadipic semialdehyde dehydrogenase-phosphopantetheinyl transferase gene, the human ortholog of the yeast LYS5 gene. *Mol. Genet. Metab.*, 2001, 72:336–342.
129. Bucovaz, E.T., Macleod, R.M., Morrison, J.C., Whybrew, W.D.: The coenzyme A-synthesizing protein complex and its proposed role in CoA biosynthesis in bakers' yeast. *Biochimie*, 1997, 79:787–798.
130. Srivastava, D.K., Bernhard, S.A.: Biophysical chemistry of metabolic reaction sequences in concentrated enzyme solution and in the cell. *Annu. Rev. Biophys. Biophys. Chem.*, 1987, 16:175–204.
131. Schneider, R., Brors, B., Massow, M., Weiss, H.: Mitochondrial fatty acid synthesis: a relic of endosymbiotic origin and a specialized means for respiration. *FEBS. Lett.*, 1997, 407:249–252.
132. Randy, L., Rose, E.H.: Metabolism of toxicants. In: *A Textbook of Modern Toxicology*, Ernest Hodgson, ed., New York: John Wiley & Sons, 2004, 111–148.
133. Gilroy, D.W., Perretti, M.: Aspirin and steroids: new mechanistic findings and avenues for drug discovery. *Curr. Opin. Pharmacol.*, 2005, 5:405–411.
134. Seiler, N.: Catabolism of polyamines. *Amino Acids*, 2004, 26:217–233.
135. Caldovic, L., Tuchman, M.: *N*-Acetylglutamate and its changing role through evolution. *Biochem. J.*, 2003, 372(Pt 2):279–290.
136. Baker, R.R.: Lipid acetylation reactions and the metabolism of platelet-activating factor. *Neurochem. Res.*, 2000, 25:677–683.
137. King, C.M., Land S.J., Jones, R.F., Debiec-Rychter, M., Lee, M.S., Wang, C.Y.: Role of acetyltransferases in the metabolism and carcinogenicity of aromatic amines. *Mutat. Res.*, 1997, 376:123–128.
138. Yan, S.C., Grinnell, B.W., Wold, F.: Post-translational modifications of proteins: some problems left to solve. *Trends Biochem. Sci.*, 1989, 14:264–268.
139. Rucker, R.B., Wold, F.: Cofactors in and as posttranslational protein modifications. *FASEB J.*, 1988, 2:2252–2261.
140. Grant, P.A., Berger, S.L.: Histone acetyltransferase complexes. *Semin. Cell Dev. Biol.*, 1999, 10:169–177.
141. Fu, M., Wang, C., Wang, J., Zafonte, B.T., Lisanti, M.P., Pestell, R.G.: Acetylation in hormone signaling and the cell cycle. *Cytokine Growth Factor Rev.*, 2002, 13:259–276.
142. Lo, W.S., Henry, K.W., Schwartz, M.F., Berger, S.L.: Histone modification patterns during gene activation. *Methods Enzymol.*, 2004, 377:130–153.
143. Yang, X.J.: The diverse superfamily of lysine acetyltransferases and their roles in leukemia and other diseases. *Nucleic Acids Res.*, 2004, 32:959–976.
144. Nemajerova, A., Erster, S., Moll, U.M.: The post-translational phosphorylation and acetylation modification profile is not the determining factor in targeting endogenous stress-induced p53 to mitochondria. *Cell Death Differ.*, 2005, 12:197–200.
145. Yasui, K., Matsuyama, T., Ito, T.: [Transcriptional regulation by post-translational modification of histone]. *Seikagaku*, 2005, 77:498–504.
146. Wallis, N.G., Perham, R.N.: Structural dependence of post-translational modification and reductive acetylation of the lipoyl domain of the pyruvate dehydrogenase multienzyme complex. *J. Mol. Biol.*, 1994, 236:209–216.
147. Kozminski, K.G., Diener, D.R., Rosenbaum, J.L.: High level expression of nonacetylatable alpha-tubulin in *Chlamydomonas reinhardtii*. *Cell Motil. Cytoskeleton*, 1993, 25:158–170.

148. Edde, B., Rossier, J., Le Caer, J.P., Berwald-Netter, Y., Koulakoff, A., Gros, F., Denoulet, P.: A combination of posttranslational modifications is responsible for the production of neuronal alpha-tubulin heterogeneity. *J. Cell. Biochem.*, 1991, 46:134–142.
149. Stadtman, E.R.: Covalent modification reactions are marking steps in protein turnover. *Biochemistry*, 1990, 29:6323–6331.
150. Troitskii, G.V.: [Post-synthetic modification of proteins]. *Ukr. Biokhim. Zh.*, 1985, 57:81–98.
151. Desrosiers, R.R., Gauthier, F., Lanthier, J., Beliveau, R.: Modulation of Rho and cytoskeletal protein attachment to membranes by a prenylcysteine analog. *J. Biol. Chem.*, 2000, 275:14949–14957.
152. Rowinsky, E.K., Windle, J.J., Von Hoff, D.D.: Ras protein farnesyltransferase: a strategic target for anticancer therapeutic development. *J. Clin. Oncol.*, 1999, 17:3631–3652.
153. Smotrys, J.E., Linder, M.E.: Palmitoylation of intracellular signaling proteins: regulation and function. *Annu. Rev. Biochem.*, 2004, 73:559–587.
154. Maurer-Stroh, S., Washietl, S., Eisenhaber, F.: Protein prenyltransferases: anchor size, pseudogenes and parasites. *Biol. Chem.*, 2003, 384:977–989.
155. Wittwer, C.T., Beck, S., Peterson, M., Davidson, R., Wilson, D.E., Hansen, R.G.: Mild pantothenate deficiency in rats elevates serum triglyceride and free fatty acid levels. *J. Nutr.*, 1990, 120:719–725.
156. Cockroft, D.L.: Changes with gestational age in the nutritional requirements of postimplantation rat embryos in culture. *Teratology*, 1988, 38:281–290.
157. Nelson, M.M., Sulon, E., Becks, H., Wainwright, W.W., Evans, H.M.: Changes in endochondral ossification of the tibia accompanying acute pantothenic acid deficiency in young rats. *Proc. Soc. Exp. Biol. Med.*, 1950, 73:31–36.
158. Krehl, W.A.: Pantothenic acid in nutrition. *Nutr. Rev.*, 1953, 11(8):225–228.
159. Bean, W.B., Hodges, R.E.: Pantothenic acid deficiency induced in human subjects. *Proc. Soc. Exp. Biol. Med.*, 1954, 86:693–698.
160. Macdonald, R.A., Jones, R.S., Pechet, G.S.: Folic acid deficiency and hemochromatosis. *Arch. Pathol.*, 1965, 80:153–160.
161. Brown, R.V.: Vitamin deficiency and voluntary alcohol consumption in mice. *Q. J. Stud. Alcohol.*, 1969, 30:592–597.
162. Gries, C.L., Scott, M.L.: The pathology of thiamin, riboflavin, pantothenic acid and niacin deficiencies in the chick. *J. Nutr.*, 1972, 102:1269–1285.
163. Moran, J.R., Greene, H.L.: The B vitamins and vitamin C in human nutrition. II. 'Conditional' B vitamins and vitamin C. *Am. J. Dis. Child.*, 1979, 133:308–314.
164. Wilson, R.P., Bowser, P.R., Poe, W.E.: Dietary pantothenic acid requirement of fingerling channel catfish. *J. Nutr.*, 1983, 113:2124–2128.
165. Blair, R., Newsome, F.: Involvement of water-soluble vitamins in diseases of swine. *J. Anim. Sci.*, 1985, 60:1508–1517.
166. Masumoto, T., Hardy, R.W., Stickney, R.R.: Pantothenic acid deficiency detection in rainbow trout (*Oncorhynchus mykiss*). *J. Nutr.*, 1994, 124:430–435.
167. Axelrod, A.E.: Immune processes in vitamin deficiency states. *Am. J. Clin. Nutr.*, 1971, 24:265–271.
168. Gontzea, I.: [Congenital malformations due to defective diet. II. Etiopathogenetic considerations]. *Nutr. Dieta Eur. Rev. Nutr. Diet.*, 1969, 11:145–156.
169. Nelson, R.A.: Intestinal transport, coenzyme A, and colitis in pantothenic acid deficiency. *Am. J. Clin. Nutr.*, 1968, 21:495–501.
170. Davenport, R.E., Spaide, J., Hodges, R.E.: An evaluation of various survival rations. *Am. J. Clin. Nutr.*, 1971, 24:513–523.
171. Bean, W.B., Hodges, R.E., Daum, K.: Pantothenic acid deficiency induced in human subjects. *J. Clin. Invest.*, 1955, 34:1073–1084.
172. Thornton, G.H., Bean, W.B., Hodges, R.E.: The effect of pantothenic acid deficiency of gastric secretion and motility. *J. Clin. Invest.*, 1955, 34:1085–1091.
173. Hodges, R.E., Ohlson, M.A., Bean, W.B.: Pantothenic acid deficiency in man. *J. Clin. Invest.*, 1958, 37:1642–1657.
174. Hodges, R.E., Bean, W.B., Ohlson, M.A., Bleiler, RE.: Factors affecting human antibody response. III. Immunologic responses of men deficient in pantothenic acid. *Am. J. Clin. Nutr.*, 1962, 11:85–93.

175. Hodges, R.E., Bean, W.B., Ohlson, M.A., Bleiler, R.E: Factors affecting human antibody response. V. Combined deficiencies of pantothenic acid and pyridoxine. *Am. J. Clin. Nutr.*, 1962, 11:187–199.
176. Shimizu, S., Miura, M., Kawaguchi, T., Nakamura, Y., Takei, M., Miyahara, H., Furuta, K., Sodeyama, T., Kiyosawa, K., Furuta, S.: [A case of Reye's syndrome occurred during administration of calcium hopantenate]. *Nippon Shokakibyo Gakkai Zasshi*, 1990, 87:2540–2544.
177. Annous, K.F., Song, W.O.: Pantothenic acid uptake and metabolism by red blood cells of rats. *J. Nutr.*, 1995, 125:2586–2593.
178. Fox, H.M., Linkswiler, H.: Pantothenic acid excretion on three levels of intake. *J. Nutr.*, 1961, 75:451–454.
179. Binaghi, P., Cellina, G., Lo Cicero, G., Bruschi, F., Porcaro, E., Penotti, M.: [Evaluation of the cholesterol-lowering effectiveness of pantethine in women in perimenopausal age]. *Minerva Med.*, 1990, 81:475–479.
180. Nieman, D.C., Underwood, B.C., Sherman, K.M., Arabatzis, K., Barbosa, JC., Johnson, M., Shultz, T.D.: Dietary status of Seventh-Day Adventist vegetarian and non-vegetarian elderly women. *J. Am. Diet. Assoc.*, 1989, 89:1763–1769.
181. Cighetti, G., Del Puppo, M., Paroni, R., Galli Kienle, M.: Modulation of HMG-CoA reductase activity by pantetheine/pantethine. *Biochim. Biophys. Acta*, 1988, 963:389–393.
182. Eto, M., Watanabe, K., Chonan, N., Ishii, K.: Lowering effect of pantethine on plasma beta-thromboglobulin and lipids in diabetes mellitus. *Artery*, 1987, 15:1–12.
183. Cighetti, G., Del Puppo, M., Paroni, R., Fiorica, E., Galli Kienle, M.: Pantethine inhibits cholesterol and fatty acid syntheses and stimulates carbon dioxide formation in isolated rat hepatocytes. *J. Lipid Res.*, 1987, 28:152–161.
184. Arsenio, L., Bodria, P., Bossi, S., Lateana, M., Strata, A.: [Clinical use of pantethine by parenteral route in the treatment of hyperlipidemia]. *Acta Biomed. Ateneo Parmense*, 1987, 58:143–152.
185. Cighetti, G., Del Puppo, M., Paroni, R., Galli, G., Kienle, M.G.: Effects of pantethine on cholesterol synthesis from mevalonate in isolated rat hepatocytes. *Atherosclerosis*, 1986, 60:67–77.
186. Bertolini, S., Donati, C., Elicio, N., Daga, A., Cuzzolaro, S., Marcenaro, A., Saturnino, M., Balestreri, R.: Lipoprotein changes induced by pantethine in hyperlipoproteinemic patients: adults and children. *Int. J. Clin. Pharmacol. Ther. Toxicol.*, 1986, 24:630–637.
187. Arsenio, L., Bodria, P., Magnati, G., Strata, A., Trovato, R: Effectiveness of long-term treatment with pantethine in patients with dyslipidemia. *Clin. Ther.*, 1986, 8:537–545.
188. Miccoli, R., Marchetti, P., Sampietro, T., Benzi, T., Tognarelli, M., Navalesi, R.: Effects of pantethine on lipids and apolipoproteins in hypercholesterolemic diabetic and nondiabetic patients. *Curr. Ther. Res.*, 1984, 36:545–549.
189. Gaddi, A., Descovich, G.C., Noseda, G., Fragiacomo, C., Colombo, L., Craveri, A., Montanari, G., Sirtori, C.R.: Controlled evaluation of pantethine, a natural hypolipidemic compound, in patients with different forms of hyperlipoproteinemia. *Atherosclerosis*, 1984, 50:73–83.
190. Vaxman, F., Olender, S., Lambert, A., Nisand, G., Aprahamian, M., Bruch, J.F., Didier, E., Volkmar, P., Grenier, J.F.: Effect of pantothenic acid and ascorbic acid supplementation on human skin wound healing process. A double-blind, prospective and randomized trial. *Eur. Surg. Res.*, 1995, 27:158–166.
191. Vaxman, F., Olender, S., Lambert, A., Nisand, G., Grenier, J.F.: Can the wound healing process be improved by vitamin supplementation? Experimental study on humans. *Eur. Surg. Res.*, 1996, 28:306–314.
192. Weimann, B.I., Hermann, D.: Studies on wound healing: effects of calcium D-pantothenate on the migration, proliferation and protein synthesis of human dermal fibroblasts in culture. *Int. J. Vitam. Nutr. Res.*, 1999, 69:113–119.
193. Welsh, A.L.: Lupus erythematosus treatment by combined use of massive amounts of calcium pantothenate or panthenol with synthetic vitamin E. *AMA Arch. Derm. Syphilol.*, 1952, 65:137–148.
194. Cochrane, T., Leslie, G.: The treatment of lupus erythematosus with calcium pantothenate and panthenol. *J. Invest. Dermatol.*, 1952, 18:365–367.
195. Welsh, A.L.: Lupus erythematosus: treatment by combined use of massive amounts of pantothenic acid and vitamin E. *AMA Arch. Derm. Syphilol.*, 1954, 70:181–198.

196. Slepyan, A.H., Frost, D.V., Overby, L.R., Fredrickson, R.L., Osterberg, A.E.: The diagnosis of lupus erythematosus; probable significance of pantothenate blood levels. *AMA Arch. Derm.*, 1957, 75:845–850.
197. Tishchenko, L.D.: Combined treatment of lupus erythematosus patients with resochin and calcium pantothenate. *Vestn. Dermatol. Venerol.*, 1963, 37:16–20.
198. Rodesch, P.: The smooth tongue of the aged. *Acta Stomatol. Belg.*, 1968, 65:155–187.
199. Leung, L.H.: Systemic lupus erythematosus: a combined deficiency disease. *Med. Hypotheses*, 2004, 62:922–924.
200. Dawson, J.E., Raymond, A.M., Winn, L.M.: Folic acid and pantothenic acid protection against valproic acid-induced neural tube defects in CD-1 mice. *Toxicol. Appl. Pharmacol.*, 2006, 211:124–132.
201. Baggot, P.J., Kalamarides, J.A., Shoemaker, J.D.: Valproate-induced biochemical abnormalities in pregnancy corrected by vitamins: a case report. *Epilepsia*, 1999, 40:512–515.
202. Sato, M., Shirota, M., Nagao, T.: Pantothenic acid decreases valproic acid-induced neural tube defects in mice (I). *Teratology*, 1995, 52:143–148.
203. Thurston, J.H., Hauhart, R.E.: Vitamins to prevent neural-tube defects. *N. Engl. J. Med.*, 1993, 328:1641–1642.
204. Thurston, J.H., Hauhart, R.E.: Reversal of the adverse chronic effects of the unsaturated derivative of valproic acid—2-*n*-propyl-4-pentenoic acid—on ketogenesis and liver coenzyme A metabolism by a single injection of pantothenate, carnitine, and acetylcysteine in developing mice. *Pediatr. Res.*, 1993, 33:72–76.
205. Thurston, J.H., Hauhart, R.E.: Amelioration of adverse effects of valproic acid on ketogenesis and liver coenzyme A metabolism by co-treatment with pantothenate and carnitine in developing mice: possible clinical significance. *Pediatr. Res.*, 1992, 31:419–423.
206. Scientific Committee on Food: Opinion of the Scientific Committee on Food on the tolerable upper intake level of pantothenic acid. Report of the European Commission: Health and consumer protection directorate-general, SCF/CS/NUT/UPPLEV/61 Final: 1–6.
207. Goldman, L.: Intensive panthenol therapy of lupus erythematosus. *J. Invest. Dermatol.*, 1950, 15:291–293.
208. Sauberlich, H.: Pantothenic acid. In: *Laboratory Tests for the Assessment of Nutritional Status*, 2nd edn. Boca Raton: CRC Press, 1999, 175–183.
209. Gonthier, A., Boullanger, P., Fayol, V., Hartmann D.J.: Development of an ELISA for pantothenic acid (vitamin B_5) for application in the nutrition and biological fields. *J. Immunoassay*, 1998, 19:167–194.
210. Rychlik, M.: Pantothenic acid quantification by a stable isotope dilution assay based on liquid chromatography–tandem mass spectrometry. *Analyst*, 2003, 128:832–837.

10 Vitamin B_6

Shyamala Dakshinamurti and Krishnamurti Dakshinamurti

CONTENTS

INTRODUCTION

The B vitamins provide cofactors or prosthetic groups to various enzymatic reactions. Among the B vitamins, vitamin B_6 is unique in that it is involved in the metabolism of all three macronutrients, proteins, lipids, and carbohydrates. The enzymes involved in the metabolism of amino acids use pyridoxal phosphate as the cofactor. Because of the extensive nature of these reactions, the requirement of this vitamin is related to the protein content of the diet. Through the amino acid decarboxylase reactions that generate monoamine neurotransmitters, vitamin B_6 is intimately associated with the function of the nervous system. It also has an obligatory role in immune and endocrine systems. This chapter attempts to review the biological role of vitamin B_6 in health and in disease.

Paul Gyorgy (1) identified vitamin B_6 as a factor distinct from riboflavin and the pellagra-preventive factor (niacin) of Goldberger. The isolation of crystalline vitamin B_6 was reported by Gyorgy (2) and Lepkovsky (3). The chemical structure was identified as 3-hydroxy-4,5-hydroxymethyl-2-methyl pyridine and its synthesis was reported by Harris and Folkers (4) and Kuhn et al. (5). Gyorgy first referred to this compound as pyridoxine. In the years that followed, natural materials were found to have more "vitamin B_6 activity" than could be accounted for by its pyridoxine content. This led to the identification of the derivatives of vitamin B_6, which we now refer to as "vitamin B_6 vitamers." The term generally used, "vitamin B_6" now refers to the group of naturally occurring pyridine derivatives represented by pyridoxine (pyridoxol), pyridoxal, and pyridoxamine and their phosphorylated derivatives with similar physiological actions. They are referred to as vitamin B_6 vitamers. The term vitamin B_6 is generically used to refer to all these related chemicals.

The term "pyridoxine" specifically refers to the alcohol form, "pyridoxal" to the aldehyde form, and "pyridoxamine" to the amine form. The natural free forms of the vitamers could be converted to the key coenzymatic form, pyridoxal-5′-phosphate (PLP) by the action of two enzymes, a kinase and an oxidase. The kinase phophorylates the hydroxymethyl group of all three vitamers and the oxidase catalyzes the oxidation of pyridoxine-5′-phosphate (PNP) and pyridoxamine-5′-phosphate (PMP) to PLP. Phosphatases catalyze the dephosphorylation of the vitamer phosphate derivatives (Figure 10.1).

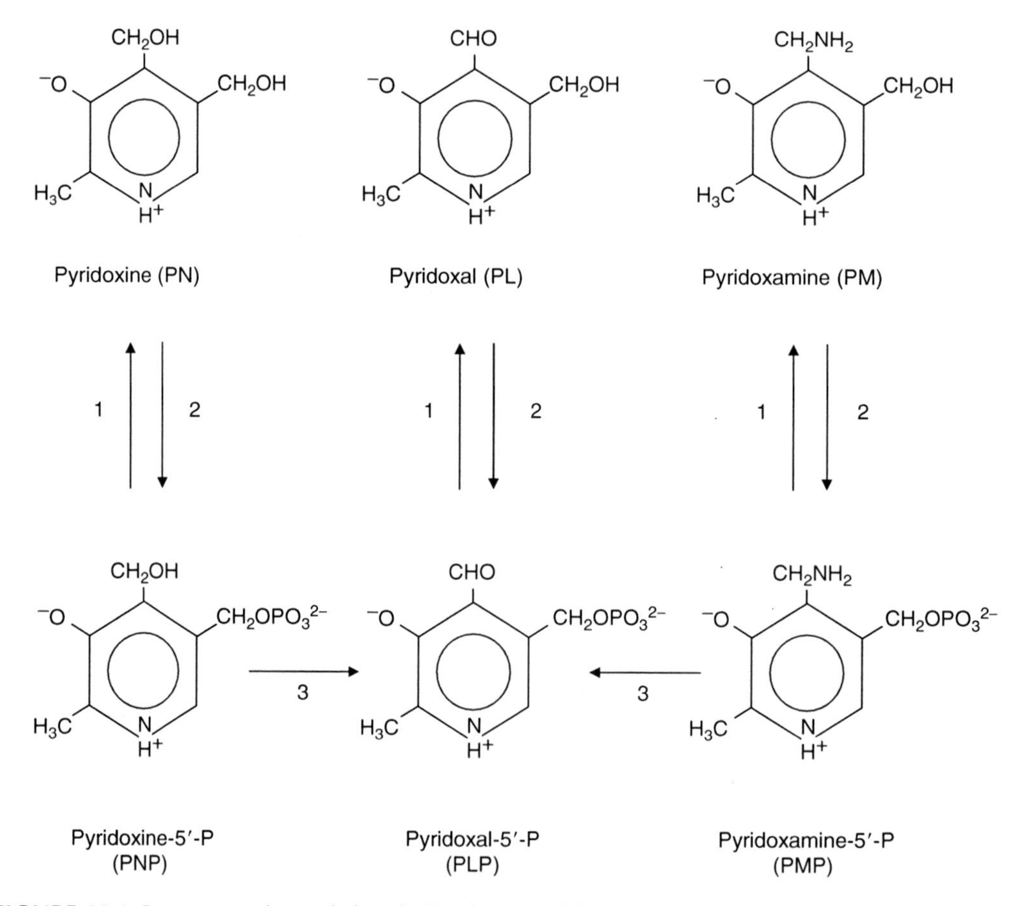

FIGURE 10.1 Interconversions of vitamin B_6 vitamers. (1) Phosphatase, (2) kinase, and (3) pyridoxine phosphate oxidase.

The kinases of most higher organisms use Zn^{2+} rather than Mg^{2+} as the ATP-chelated cofactor and there is an additional activation by K^+ (6–9). Pyridoxal kinase is inhibited by carbonyl reagents (10). The mammalian kinase is a benzodiazepine-binding protein (11). The PNP oxidase has been purified from various tissue sources as well as from *Escherichia coli* (12–16). By comparing primary sequence of PNP (PMP) oxidase from various organisms, McCormick and Chen (8) have pointed out that all known sequences of PNP (PMP) oxidases contain protein kinase c phosphorylation sites, casein kinase phosphorylation sites, and tyrosine kinase phosphorylation sites. PLP and PMP account for most of the vitamin content of various tissues (17,18). The oxidase is developmentally regulated in liver and brain (19). In the rat brain, the level of PLP rises from roughly 36% of adult level at birth to 65% by 6 days of age and to 82% by 30 days of age. In contrast, PMP remains at approximately 25% of adult level for the first 10 days of age and rises to 80% by 23 days of age. Pyridoxal kinase increases during brain maturation from 30% of adult levels at 5 days of age to 95% at 30 days of age (17). The activity of this enzyme in red blood cells of American blacks is approximately 50% lower than that of American whites. There is no difference between the enzymes from these two sources with respect to properties such as heat stability, chromatographic mobility, K_m for pyridoxine, and inhibition by analogs such as 4-deoxypyridoxine. The activity of the enzyme in lymphocytes, granulocytes, and fibroblasts is the same in both racial groups. It is suggested (20) that a structural gene mutation coding for an enzyme of approximately one-third the usual activity has reached a population frequency of 1.0 in the African population. Unanswered yet is the question whether this large decrease in enzyme activity leads to any decrease in the levels of phosphorylated pyridoxine vitamers in various tissues of the African and Afro-American population. In terms of metabolic regulation, inverse relationships between the activity of the kinase and the concentration of brain PLP as well as the concentrations of brain monoamines have been reported (21,22).

PNP oxidase is inhibited by PLP. Unbound PLP is hydrolyzed by an alkaline phosphatase (23). A large part of the PLP in muscle and liver is protein bound. Thus, the feedback regulation of the enzymes of PLP synthesis as well as the sequestration of PLP by protein binding serves to regulate the concentration of active-unbound PLP in tissues.

PYRIDOXAL-5′-PHOSPHATE-DEPENDENT ENZYMES

Since its identification as the active cofactor form of vitamin B_6, there has been extensive research aimed at understanding the versatility of the reactions catalyzed by PLP-dependent enzymes. There are over 140 enzymatic reactions, which are PLP dependent. PLP-dependent enzymes are found in all organisms. They are involved in reactions that synthesize, degrade, and interconvert amino acids. In view of the versatility of its catalysis, PLP-dependent enzymes are involved in linking carbon and nitrogen metabolism, replenishing the pool of one-carbon units and forming biogenic amines. It has been pointed out that PLP enzymes belong to five of the six enzyme classes as defined by the Enzyme Nomenclature Committee of the International Union of Biochemistry and Molecular Biology (24).

Pyridoxal is a carbonyl compound and reacts with primary amines to form a Schiff base referred to as the external aldimine. The fully formed carbanion is referred to as the quinonoid intermediate. The structural features that facilitate this first step leading to a variety of molecular transformations in PLP-mediated enzyme catalysis have been listed (25). The 2-methyl group brings the pK_a of the proton of the pyridine ring into the physiological range. The phenoxide oxygen in position 3 helps in the expulsion of the nucleophile at position 4. The phosphate in position 5 prevents hemiacetal formation and drain of electrons from the ring. The protonated nitrogen helps in regulating the pK_a of the 3-hydroxyl group. Delocalization of the negative charge through the P_i system of PLP facilitates the stabilization of the C_α anion. PLP alone can catalyze many of the enzymatic reactions in the absence of the enzyme, although the rates of these reactions would be extremely slow. The protein apoenzyme enhances the catalytic potential of PLP, the selectivity of the substrate binding, and the reaction type (26).

With delineation of the structures of most PLP enzymes, they have been found to belong to one of five fold types. Fold Type I is the largest group, the aspartate amino transferase family. They function as homodimers or higher order oligomers with two active sites per dimer. Fold Type II is the tryptophan synthase family. The enzymes are similar to Fold Type I but the proteins are distinct. The active sites are in one monomer. Fold Type IV is the D-amino acid aminotransferase family. They are functional homodimers. Fold Type III is the alanine racemase family and Fold Type V is the glycogen phosphorylase family. The fold type of the enzyme protein does not determine the reaction type catalyzed by the enzyme. The reaction types are classified into three groups depending on the site of elimination and replacement of the substituents. Reactions occurring at the α-carbon atom include enzymes such as transaminase, racemases of α-amino acid, amino acid α-decarboxylases, and enzymes catalyzing condensation of glycine and the α–β cleavage of β-hydroxy amino acids such as δ-aminolevulinic acid synthetase, serine hydroxy methylase, and sphingosine synthetase. Reactions occurring at the β-carbon atom of the substrate include enzymes such as serine and threonine dehydrases, cystathionine synthetase, tryptophanase, and kynureninase. Reactions occurring at the γ-carbon atom of the substrate include enzymes such as homoserine dehydrase and γ-cystathionase.

Glycogen phosphorylase catalyzes the first step in the degradation of glycogen. Although the reaction catalyzed is reversible, the enzyme acts in vivo in the direction of phosphorolysis. The physiological role of phosphorylase in skeletal muscle is as an energy source as this enzyme in the inactive phosphorylase b form comprises about 2% of the total soluble protein of muscle tissue. Phosphorylase b is under regulatory control with AMP and IMP as activators and ATP, ADP, purines, flavins, D-glucose, and UDP-glucose as inhibitors. The catalytic site in the phosphorylase b monomer is located in a deep crevice between the N-terminal and C-terminal domains with binding sites for glucose-1-phosphate, P_i, and glycogen. PLP, the cofactor necessary for activity is part of the active site. Phosphorylase can be reversibly resolved into an enzymatically inactive apophosphorylase and free PLP (27).

In other PLP enzymes, the cofactor is bound as a Schiff base with the ε-amino group of corresponding lysine residue of the protein moiety. Hence reduction of the aldimine bond with sodium borohydride causes loss of enzyme activity. Although PLP in phosphorylase is connected to lysine 680 through an aldimine bond reduction of this bond with sodium borohydride results in an enzyme form with over 60% of the activity of the native enzyme (28). Thus, the free aldehyde group is not involved in catalysis. Helmreich (28a) has proposed that the phosphate group of PLP functions in the phosphorylase in the form of dianion as a proton donor–acceptor. In the forward reaction, phosphorolysis of α-1,4-glycoside bond in oligo- or polysaccharides occurs followed by stabilization of the incipient oxocarbonium ion and subsequent covalent binding to form α-glucose-1-phosphate. In the reverse direction, protonation of the phosphate of glucose-1-phosphate destabilizes the glycosidic bond and promotes the formation of a glucosyl carbonium ionphosphate anion pair. The involvement of the phosphate group rather than the carbonyl group is a novel feature of the role of PLP in the phosphorylase reaction and thus, the mechanism of action is completely different from other PLP-dependent enzymes. A structural role for PLP in glycogen phosphorylase has been documented (29). The dissociation of PLP from phosphorylase b causes structural rearrangement in the phosphorylase molecule in the contact area of monomers in the dimer, in the region of the glycogen storage site, and in the region of the allosteric inhibitor site. Reconstruction of the holoenzyme from the apoenzyme and PLP causes restoration of the affinity for glycogen and for flavin mononucleotide (FMN). Thus, PLP plays an important role in maintaining the quaternary structure and conformation of the enzyme (29a). A reservoir function for PLP in muscle phosphorylase has also been suggested (6).

In determining the activity of PLP-dependent enzymes, two parameters can be established. The enzyme activity without the in vitro addition of PLP gives an estimate of the holoenzyme. Enzyme activity in presence of an excess of in vitro PLP in the incubation system gives an estimate of the availability of the apoenzyme. The percentage saturation of the enzyme with the coenzyme might, in some instances, reflect the vitamin B_6 status of the organism. This should take into account the tightness of binding of PLP to various apoproteins. PLP cannot practically be dissociated from glutamic oxaloacetic transaminase whereas it is easily dissociated from kynurenine transaminase.

From the point of molecular evolution, most enzymes depend on the nonprotein component, either inorganic ions or small molecular weight organic compounds. PLP interacts with amino acid substrates in the absence of enzyme and catalyzes the transformations although at a very slow rate. These transformations have been made more efficient through association with protein during the transition from prebiotic to biotic evolution. It has been suggested that "specialization of the catalytic apparatus for reaction specificity may be assumed to require more extensive structural adaptations than specialization for specific substrate. For the organization of metabolism in the uncompartmented progenote cell, the development of catalysts that accelerate one particular reaction of diverse substrates seems more important than the development of catalysts that act only on one substrate" (24). PLP is a prime example of this concept.

VITAMIN B_6 VITAMERS—DETERMINATION, SOURCES, AND BIOAVAILABILITY

Traditionally, microbiological methods were used for the determination of vitamin B_6 in foods and biological samples (30,31). Much of the data currently available on the total vitamin B_6 content of foods are based on microbiological methods, using the growth of *Saccharomyces uvarium* (ATCC 9080). Enzymatic and radioenzymatic techniques have been used for the assay of PLP (32). Currently, the most commonly used methods are based on ion-exchange or paired-ion reverse-phase HPLC techniques with postcolumn derivatization (33–35).

The three vitamers and their phosphorylated forms are present in most foods. Pyridoxine, pyridoxamine, and their phosphorylated forms are the major forms of vitamin B_6 present in plant foods whereas pyridoxal and PLP are the major forms found in animal foods. Glycosylated forms of pyridoxine, such as 5′-0-(β-D-glucopyranosyl)pyridoxine and 5′-0-(6-0-malonyl-β-D-glucopyranosyl)pyridoxine are present in plant foods (36,37). The vitamin B_6 content of selected foods and the percentage distribution of the three vitamers have been listed (38).

The B_6 vitamers and their phosphorylated derivatives are photosensitive. Food processing, including heat sterilization, results in loss of vitamin activity. Heat-sterilized infant formula was responsible for the epidemic of seizures caused by vitamin B_6 deficiency in infants fed such formula diet (39). The phosphorylated vitamers are hydrolyzed by an alkaline phosphatase in the intestines. There is a gradient of decreasing rates of uptake, with a saturable component, from the proximal to the distal part of the intestine (40). The bioavailability of vitamin B_6 present in various foods depends on the chemical nature of the vitamin B_6 derivative present. The low bioavailability of vitamin B_6 in plant foods is related to the content of glycosylated vitamin B_6 in these foods (41).

The absorption of vitamin B_6 occurs following the hydrolysis of the phosphorylated forms in the lumen of intestine. Earlier it was believed to occur via simple diffusion. Recent studies have provided evidence for the existence of a specialized, Na^+-dependent carrier-mediated system for the uptake of pyridoxine (42).

Once absorbed, there is interconversion of the various forms of the vitamin B_6 vitamers. Pyridoxine hydrochloride is the most commonly available form of vitamin B_6. It is sold as a vitamin supplement or as a component of multivitamin preparations. Orally administered pyridoxine hydrochloride is less efficiently utilized than intravenous infusion. Intravenously infused PN is rapidly spread in its volume of distribution. PN does not bind to proteins of blood plasma and so has a large rate constant of elimination. In spite of this there is a significant build up of PL, PLP, and 4-pyridoxic acid (4-PA) in blood plasma. Thus, there is an efficient utilization of PN (43). Pyridoxal (PL) is converted to 4-pyridoxic acid (PA) by either of two pathways—using an NAD-dependent dehydrogenase or a FAD-dependent aldehyde oxidase. In livers of humans, only the aldehyde oxidase has been detected. The conversion of PL to PA is an irreversible reaction. The concentrations of PL and PLP in the erythrocyte are 2.6- and 1.8-fold higher than in blood plasma. This is explained by the easy penetration of erythrocyte membrane by PL and the higher affinity of PL to hemoglobin than to albumin. PLP, synthesized in the erythrocytes themselves, is also bound to hemoglobin with an affinity greater than that of PL. In view of this, the concentration of PMP is very low in spite of the ease of conversion of PLP and PMP by transamination (44). The kinase, oxidase, and transaminase are all present in the erythrocytes. In view of these interconversions, PL and PLP in blood plasma and PL in erythrocytes are the forms in which they are transported to all tissues following hepatic metabolism. In the muscle, vitamin B_6 is present mostly as PLP bound to glycogen phosphorylase (45). About two-thirds of the total vitamin B_6 is associated with glycogen phosphorylase. About half the total vitamin B_6 of the body seems to be associated with a single enzyme, muscle phosphorylase. Muscle was initially considered to be a storage organ for vitamin B_6 (45). A specific protease, which might be involved in this function, is known (46). Although both PLP and glycogen phosphorylase levels in muscle responded positively to a diet high in vitamin B_6 (47), it was found that these levels decreased only in response to a caloric deficit in the diet and not to a depletion of vitamin B_6 in the diet (48).

Assessment of Vitamin B_6 Status and Requirement

A variety of methods have been used to assess the vitamin B_6 (pyridoxine) status in humans. This is based on the availability of body fluids or effluents as against tissue samples for the determination of vitamin B_6 content. Direct assessment would comprise the measurement of total vitamin B_6, including the distribution of the vitamers in blood plasma and erythrocytes. 4-PA is the final oxidized metabolite of vitamin B_6 and is excreted in the urine. As such it is a measure of the total vitamin B_6 metabolized in the body, although a relationship between graded dietary intake of vitamin B_6 and the excretion of 4-PA in urine has still not been established.

Although erythrocyte transaminase activities (alanine amino transferase and aspartate amino transferase) have been used in the assessment of vitamin B_6 status of individuals (49), there are questions as to the reliability. Measurement of activation coefficients (ratio of activity in presence of excess in vitro added PLP to activity with no in vitro added PLP) is complicated by the high affinity of the transaminases for PLP. The levels of blood plasma and erythrocyte contents of PL and PLP are indicatives of the acute vitamin B_6 status of the individual rather than the status of overall tissue stores.

As vitamin B_6 participates as a coenzyme in various metabolic pathways, determination of the effectiveness of a metabolic pathway under specified conditions, including after a metabolic challenge, can be used to indicate the status of the individual with respect to vitamin B_6. Tryptophan and methionine load tests fall in this category. Determination of urinary excretion of xanthurenic acid following an oral dose of 5 g L-tryptophan has been used to assess vitamin B_6 status. In normal individuals with adequate tissue stores of vitamin B_6, there is no increase in the excretion of urinary xanthurenic acid under these conditions. Here again, the effects of protein intake, stress, and hormonal imbalances on the metabolism of tryptophan must be taken into consideration (50,51). The excretion of cystathionine following an oral load of methionine offers much promise, as cystathionase seems to be quite sensitive to tissue levels of PLP (52).

In view of the fact that vitamin B_6 coenzyme is involved extensively in amino acid metabolism, the establishment of a requirement for vitamin B_6 is based on protein intake. The initial studies aimed at determining the requirement were of the depletion–repletion design (53). There was much variation in the duration of depletion and the amount of vitamin B_6 in the diet during this depletion period. Again, in terms assessment of vitamin B_6 status, various indices such as plasma total vitamin B_6, plasma PLP, urinary 4-PA excretion, xanthurenic acid excretion following a load of tryptophan and erythrocyte transaminase activation were used. In addition only two levels of protein intake, a high and a low level, were considered. These studies were all done on male volunteers. In more recent studies, efforts have been made to include other indices of vitamin B_6 function such as EEG studies and immune function. In addition a broader cross section of age groups, including both the sexes as well as more levels of protein intake, was included (54–56). Recommendation about the requirement would depend on which biochemical or functional impairment is to be reversed. Also to be taken into consideration in these determinations is the availability of vitamin from the food source, particularly plant foods. Physiological requirements depend on the age, sex, body size, extent of physical activity, and protein intake in the diet.

Oral contraceptive drug use has been associated with many clinical side effects that are normally associated with pregnancy. The altered tryptophan metabolism produced by estrogens, glucocorticoids, and pregnancy is related to the induction of tryptophan-2, 3-dioxygenase, the rate-limiting enzyme of tryptophan metabolism in the liver. The effect of these metabolic alterations on brain monoamine status as well as the impact of this on the physiology and behavior of the individual needs further investigation. It is recognized that the requirement in women during lactation and of adolescents during the rapid phase of muscle mass increase would be high. The current recommended dietary allowance (RDA) recommendations are set at 2.0 mg for adult males and females, 0.9 mg for children in the age group of 4–6 years, and 1.2 mg for children in the age group of 7–10 years.

CLINICAL MANIFESTATIONS OF VITAMIN B_6 DEFICIENCY AND SECONDARY VITAMIN B_6 DEFICIENCY

Impairment of somatic growth, a pellagra-like dermatitis, and ataxia have been reported in all species of vitamin B_6-deficient animals. Anemia occurs in all species except the rat (57,58). Among the most outstanding symptoms are those related to the nervous system. Ataxia, hyperacousis, hyperirritability, impaired alertness, abnormal head movements, and convulsions are observed in a variety of species studied such as the chicken, duck, turkey, rat, guinea pig, pig, cow, and human (32,59). Snyderman et al. (60) reported on the development of vitamin B_6 deficiency in a 2-month-old hydrocephalic child fed a deficient diet for 76 days. The biochemical correlates of vitamin B_6 deficiency were present and the child had convulsive seizures, which were relieved by intravenous administration of pyridoxine. The widespread occurrence of vitamin B_6 deficiency induced convulsive seizures in infants receiving a heat-sterilized proprietary milk formula has been reported (39). Electroencephalogram (EEG) techniques were used to monitor the effectiveness of treatment. Marked improvement in the waveform and normalization of the amplitude and frequency were seen on the EEG following treatment with pyridoxine.

Clinically recognized signs of vitamin B_6 deficiency due to a primary dietary deficiency are rarely seen. However, a variety of conditions are recognized in which a relative deficiency of vitamin B_6 is caused by factors such as increased requirement, poor availability of the vitamin, or formation of inactive complexes between the vitamin and various drugs.

Such a condition of relative vitamin B_6 deficiency has been recognized in pregnant woman, based on the tryptophan load test (61). In view of the complexities introduced by hormonal influence on the metabolism of tryptophan, it was doubted whether there was a real vitamin B_6 deficiency. This was proved to be so, in a later study based on measurement of vitamin B_6 vitamer levels. The blood levels of PLP were significantly lower during pregnancy whereas the fetal cord blood levels were high (62). In another study (63), erythrocyte glutamic oxaloacetic transaminase activation was used in assessing the vitamin B_6 status of 493 pregnant women. About 50% of them had suboptimal coenzyme saturation as compared with nonpregnant women. Even on a daily intake of 2.0–2.5 mg pyridoxine per day pregnant women had a relative deficiency of vitamin B_6, based on determinations of plasma PLP and erythrocyte aspartate aminotransferase activation (64). When maternal vitamin B_6 levels were low, the PLP levels of cord blood were significantly decreased (65). The differences in PL and PLP levels between the umbilical vein and artery indicate extensive utilization of the vitamers transported across the placenta. Premature infants have very low levels of plasma PLP at birth (66). Plasma PLP of pregnant women with hyperemesis gravidarum was as low as that of healthy pregnant women during the last trimester of pregnancy (67).

Oral contraceptive drugs have been associated with clinical side effects that are the same as those associated with pregnancy. These are related to hormonal induction of tryptophan-2,3-dioxygenase and hence an altered tryptophan metabolism. The biochemical abnormalities are corrected by administration of 25 mg pyridoxine. Perioral dermatosis and neuropsychiatric disorders including depression and sleep disorder associated with oral contraceptive use in some women are corrected by supplements of pyridoxine.

A functional deficiency of vitamin B_6 might exist in uremic patients. Symptoms such as neuromuscular irritability, central nervous system depression, convulsions, and peripheral neuritis seen in these patients are indicative of vitamin B_6 deficiency as both plasma PLP and erythrocyte glutamic oxaloacetate transaminase levels are low in both undialyzed and dialyzed uremic patients (68). Various causes such as impaired intestinal absorption, tissue phosphorylation, increased phosphatase activity, or inactivation of PLP by complexing with amines in blood could contribute to the deficiency of vitamin B_6.

PLP is chemically a very active compound and forms a Schiff base with compounds that have an $-NH_2$ group. Such a complex could reduce the concentration of biologically active form of vitamin B_6 or could even bind irreversibly to the apoenzyme. Some therapeutic drugs such as isonicotinic acid hydrazide (isoniazid), cycloserine, and penicillamine have an anti-vitamin B_6 action (Figure 10.2).

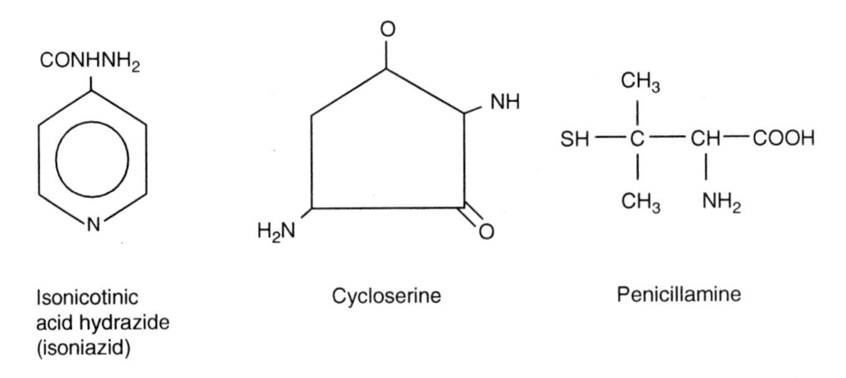

FIGURE 10.2 Antipyridoxine compounds.

Isonicotinic acid hydrazide has been used for long in the treatment of pulmonary tuberculosis. Peripheral neuropathy has been one of the commonly reported side effects of this treatment. Increased excretions of xanthurenic acid following a tryptophan load and of cystathionine following a load of methionine have been reported. The low saturation of erythrocyte transaminase is indicative of deficiency. Supplementation with 50 mg pyridoxine resulted in an optimum state of vitamin B_6. The need for routine pyridoxine supplementation in patients with newly discovered tuberculosis was emphasized (68,69). White leghorn fertile eggs injected with isoniazid had a high level of embryonic mortality and developmental alterations at the level of the neural epithelium (70). These effects of isoniazid were countered by concurrent administration of pyridoxine. Cycloserine is used effectively in the treatment of human tuberculosis, in cases resistant to the streptomycin-*p*-aminosalicylate-isoniazid regimen. The toxicity symptoms include neuropsychiatric manifestations. There was considerable loss of pyridoxine-like material in the urine. The neurological side effects were greatly reduced by the concurrent administration of 50 mg pyridoxine to these patients (71).

Penicillamine has been used in the treatment of Wilson's disease in view of its copper-chelating action and also for cystinuric patients to prevent formation of urinary cystine stones. Epileptic seizures were reported in several of the treated patients. A moderate supplement of pyridoxine corrected the neurological abnormality and normalized their EEG pattern (72).

NEUROBIOLOGY OF VITAMIN B_6

The biochemical reactions involving PLP as the coenzyme are of diverse types as over 140 enzymes are PLP dependent. Most are involved in catabolic reactions of amino acids. The crucial role played by vitamin B_6 in the nervous system is evident from the fact that the putative neurotransmitters, dopamine (DA), norepinephrine (NE), serotonin (5-HT), and γ-aminobutyric acid (GABA) as well as taurine, sphingolipids, and polyamines are synthesized by PLP-dependent enzymes. There is considerable variation in the affinities of the various apoenzymes for PLP. This explains the observed differential susceptibility of various PLP enzymes to decrease during vitamin B_6 depletion in animals and humans. Of the PLP enzymes those involved in the decarboxylations, respectively, of glutamic acid, 5-hydroxytrytophan, and ornithine are of considerable significance and can explain most of the neurological defects of vitamin B_6 deficiency in all species studied.

L-Aromatic Amino Acid Decarboxylase

The enzyme L-aromatic amino acid decarboxylase (AADC, EC 4.1.1.28) lacks substrate specificity and has been considered to be involved in the formation of the catecholamines and serotonin. This has been considered to be a single protein entity, based on immunological evidence (73). The established immunological cross-reactivity of dihydroxyphenylalanine (DOPA) decarboxylase and histidine decarboxylase using antibodies against these enzymes suggests the presence of similar antigenic recognition sites inside the native molecules of the decarboxylases that are exposed when the enzymes are denatured (74).

The best evidence for a "single protein" hypothesis has been reported by Albert et al. (75). They purified AADC to homogeneity, using DOPA as the substrate, produced antibodies against it and isolated the cDNA clone complementary to bovine adrenal AADC mRNA. A single form of AADC was detected in rat and bovine tissues and the proteins were indistinguishable from one another biochemically and immunochemically in brain, liver, kidney, and adrenal medulla. By in situ hybridization, a single 2.3 kb mRNA was detected in bovine adrenal, kidney, and liver. Southern blot analyses were consistent with the presence of a single gene coding for AADC.

However, there are many differences in the optimal conditions for enzyme activity, including kinetics, affinity for PLP, activation and inhibition by specific chemicals, and regional differences in the distribution of DOPA and 5-hydroxytryptophan (5-HTP) decarboxylation activities (76–78). Nonparallel changes in brain monoamines in the vitamin B_6-deficient rat have been reported (79). Brain content of dopamine and norepinephrine were not decreased during deficiency whereas serotonin was significantly decreased. Decreased availability of the precursor 5-HTP or increased catabolism of 5-HT was excluded as contributing to this. The decarboxylation step was shown to be the site of difference between vitamin B_6-replete and vitamin B_6-deficient rats in regard to the decrease of serotonin (80). It has been reported that brain serotonergic neurons can take up DOPA, decarboxylate it to dopamine and, at least in vitro, release dopamine in a stimulus-dependent fashion (81). On the other hand, intracisternal injection of 6-hydroxydopamine into rats pretreated with pargyline caused a marked decrease in DOPA decarboxylation in upper and lower brain stem regions while not affecting 5-HTP decarboxylation (82). The decarboxylation of 5-HTP actually increased in the hypothalamus, cerebellum, and lateral pons medulla.

Research has shown that the neurotoxin, 1-methyl-4-phenyl-1,2,3,6-tetrahydropyridine (MPTP) and its oxidation product, MPP^+, enhance 5-HTP decarboxylase activity but not DOPA decarboxylase (DDC) activity in the brain and liver of the cat (83). Rat liver DDC activity is preferentially inactivated by sodium dodecyl sulfate treatment and 5-HTP decarboxylase activity by urea (84). The selective inhibition of brain AADC by subacute α-monofluoromethyl-*p*-tyrosine administration led to a decrease in brain catecholamines but not of brain serotonin (85). Carbidopa has been reported to differentially affect DOPA and 5-HTP decarboxylations (86). High concentrations of aminooxyacetic acid inhibited more than 95% of the DDC activity of rat brain whereas the 5-HTP decarboxylase activity was inhibited only to about 40%. AADC is considered to be localized in the cellular soluble fraction. However, a population of the decarboxylase has been found to be associated with the cellular membrane fraction (87).

AADC is expressed in nonneuronal tissues such as liver and kidney although its function in these tissues is not known. The rat genomic DNA encoding AADC was isolated. Two separate promoters specific for the transcription of neuronal and nonneuronal forms of AADC were identified. Transcription initiating at distinct promoters followed by alternate splicing might be responsible for the expression of the neuronal and nonneuronal forms of the enzyme (88,89).

The single copy of the gene encoding for the enzyme is located on chromosome 7, in close proximity to the epidermal growth factor gene, and is composed of 15 exons spanning more than 85 kb (90). An alternative transcript of the enzyme lacking exon 3 was identified (91). This splicing event leads to the production of two distinct DDC protein isoforms, with the shorter transcript predominating in the neuronal tissues (92). Both alternative mRNA splice variants were identified in human placenta. There is still considerable discussion about the substrate specificity and structure of AADC (93).

The decrease in serotonin in various brain areas of the vitamin B_6-deficient rat has physiological consequences (Figure 10.3). The decrease in the synaptic release of serotonin in the deficient rat brain regions was indicated by the increase in the postsynaptic receptor density (93). The B_{max} and binding affinities of the ligands to respective D-1 and D-2 receptors were not affected in synaptosomal membrane preparations from vitamin B_6-deficient rat striatum, in keeping with the data on dopamine levels.

γ-Aminobutyric Acid

GABA is present almost exclusively in the nervous system of invertebrates and vertebrates. It is formed from glutamic acid through the action of glutamic acid decarboxylase (GAD)

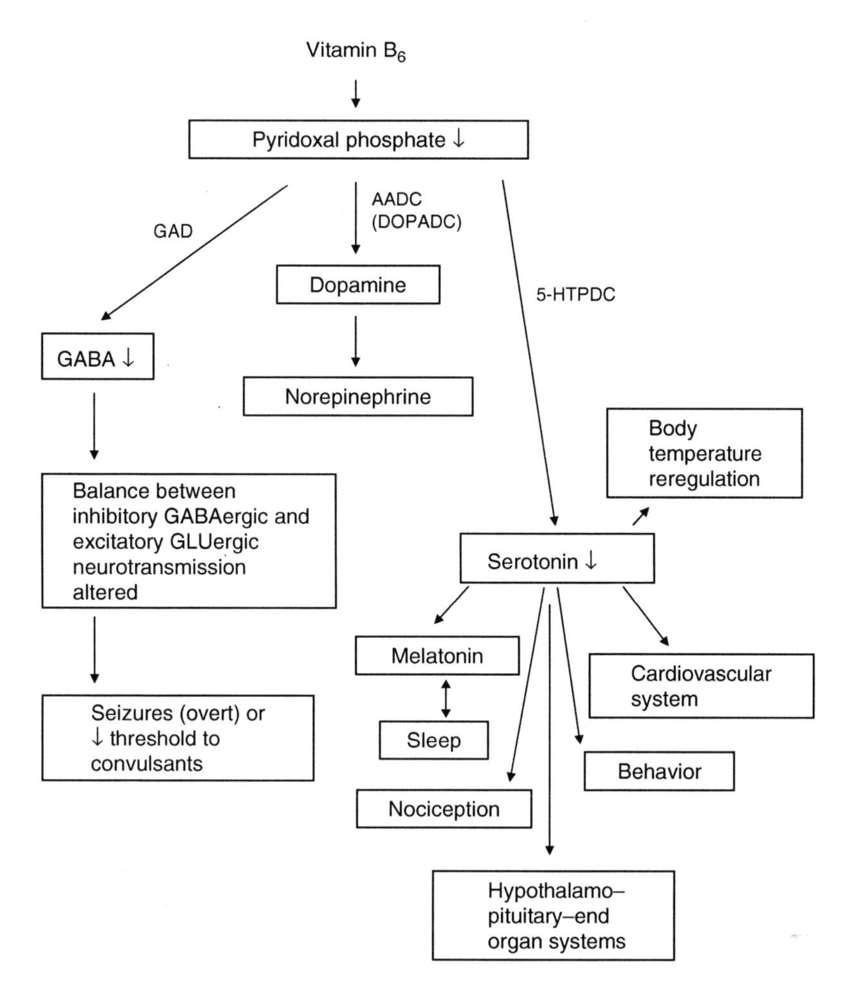

FIGURE 10.3 Physiological consequences of vitamin B_6 deficiency.

and is catabolized by transamination catalyzed by GABA transaminase (GABA-T) to yield succinic semialdehyde (SSA). Both GAD and GABA-T are PLP enzymes. SSA is oxidized by SSA dehydrogenase to succinic acid. GABA is an inhibitory neurotransmitter whereas glutamic acid is an excitatory neurotransmitter.

GABA, GAD, and GABA-T are localized predominantly in the regions of the brain that are inhibitory in function. The concentration of GABA in the cerebellum is particularly high in the Purkinje cells. The destruction of Purkinje cells resulted in a 70% decrease in both GABA and GAD activity of the dorsal part of the Dieter's nucleus of the brain, where Purkinje cell axon terminals synapse (94).

The neurophysiological action of GABA studied by iontophoretic application resembles that observed in postsynaptic inhibition produced by electrical stimulation (95). When GABA is injected in young chicks, it produces abolition of photically evoked responses (96). During sleep, GABA was detected in cerebral cortex perfusates with a decrease in glutamic acid release (97). GABA is involved in the etiology of convulsive seizures (98). Apart from the involvement of GABA in the etiology of certain convulsive seizures, abnormalities in GABAergic neuronal pathways contributing to other CNS disorders such as depression, anxiety, and panic disorders have been recognized. In Huntington's chorea, a disease marked by the onset of dementia and choreiform movements, there is a marked decrease in the concentration of GABA as well as in the activity of GAD in the basal ganglia. In Parkinson's disease, the main neurochemical lesion is associated with degeneration of the dopaminergic neurons in the substantia nigra. In addition to this, decreases are observed in both GABA and GAD in the basal ganglia, indicating an interrelationship between these two neuronal systems.

Molecular cloning studies indicate that in the adult brain GAD exists as two major isoforms referred to as GAD65 and GAD67 based on their molecular masses. They are the products of two independently regulated genes located on the chromosomes 2 and 10, respectively in humans (99). The two GAD genes are coexpressed in most GABA-containing neurons. GAD65 is more responsive than GAD67 to the cofactor PLP and it accounts for the majority of apoGAD. GAD65 is the major isoform present in most brain regions in the rat. Available evidence indicates that GAD67 might be involved in GABA synthesis for general metabolic activity and GAD65 might be involved in synaptic transmission (100). The expression of these two isoforms of GAD is regulated by distinct intracellular mechanisms.

Although all neurotransmitter monoamine-synthesizing decarboxylases are PLP-dependent enzymes, the affinities of the apodecarboxylases for PLP vary considerably. In view of this, during a moderate deficiency of vitamin B_6 and consequent decrease in PLP, the activities of the decarboxylases with low affinities for PLP would decrease whereas the decarboxylases with high affinities for PLP would not be affected. Thus, in the moderately vitamin B_6-deficient rat there is biologically significant decrease in the activities of GAD65 and AADC (5-HTP-DC) acting on 5-HTP leading to decreases in neurotransmitters GABA and serotonin (5-HT). DDC activity is not affected during PLP depletion, resulting in no change or even in an increase in catecholamine levels in the nervous system. The biological correlates of the nonparallel changes in brain monoamines are indicated in Figure 10.3. Decreased brain serotonin in the vitamin B_6-deficient rat is implicated in physiological changes such as decreased deep body temperature and altered sleep pattern with shortening of deep slow-wave sleep and rapid eye movement (REM) sleep. The effects of vitamin B_6 depletion on sleep parallel the effects of experimental serotonergic deficit (101).

NEUROENDOCRINOLOGY OF VITAMIN B_6 DEFICIENCY

HYPOTHALAMUS–PITUITARY–END ORGAN RELATIONSHIP

The hypothalamus is one of the areas of the brain of vitamin B_6-deficient rats with significant decreases in PLP and serotonin compared with vitamin B_6-replete controls. There is no decrease in the contents of dopamine and norepinephrine. The secretion by the anterior pituitary of ACTH, growth hormone, prolactin (PRL), thyroid-stimulating hormone (TSH), and the gonadotropins is regulated by releasing factors and in some instances by the release of inhibitory factors from the hypothalamus. The concept of the regulatory role of the hypothalamus through the neurotransmitters is generally accepted. Regulation of the release of stimulatory or inhibitory factors by the hypothalamus involves complex neural circuitry in which the serotonergic and dopaminergic neurons represent links in the control mechanisms (102). The hypothalamus of the normal animal has high concentrations of both dopamine and serotonin, which are essentially antagonistic in their effects on pituitary hormone regulation.

We have examined the hypothalamus–pituitary–thyroid relationship in vitamin B_6 deficiency. The secretion of TSH is directly controlled by two factors: a negative feedback signal indicating serum thyroid status and a stimulatory factor, thyrotropin-releasing hormone (TRH), released from the hypothalamus (Figure 10.4).

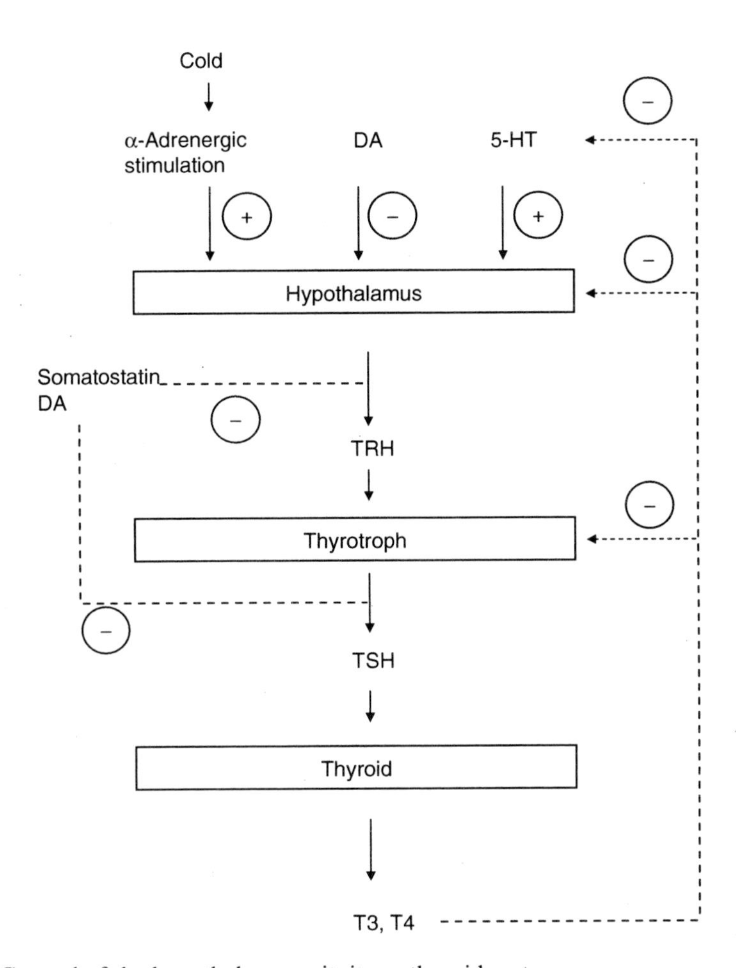

FIGURE 10.4 Control of the hypothalamus–pituitary–thyroid system.

Injection of serotonin into the third ventricle caused a rapid increase in serum TSH, an effect completely reversed by pretreatment of rats with the serotonin receptor antagonist, cyproheptadine (103). Serotonin stimulates TRH release from superfused hypothalamus (104). A direct relationship between hypothalamic serotonin turn over and TSH release has been reported (105). Dopaminergic neurons exert an inhibitory effect on the secretion of TSH. This effect is at the level of the pituitary as bromocriptine blunts the stimulatory effect of TRH in euthyroid subjects. The inhibitory effect of dopamine is abolished by dopamine receptor antagonists such as domperidone. The cold-induced secretion of TSH is mediated by norepinephrine. Studies using inhibitors of norepinephrine synthesis or α-adrenergic blockers have established a stimulatory role for norepinephrine in the control of TRH-mediated TSH secretion (106). Thus, it appears that serotonergic neurons have a stimulatory effect on hypothalamic control of pituitary secretion of TSH in situations where central control is natural, such as in timing of the circadian rhythm and, possibly, in the pulsatile secretion of TSH.

We compared the thyroid status of vitamin B_6-deficient and pair-fed vitamin B_6-replete young and adult rats. Serum concentration of thyroxin (T_4) and triiodothyronine (T_3) of the deficient rats were significantly lower in comparison with normal control rats (106). There was no significant change in the concentration of serum TSH in the deficient rats.

However, the pituitary content of TSH in the deficient rats was significantly decreased. Pyridoxine treatment restored the hypothalamic levels of PLP and serotonin to normal.

In determining the locus of the biochemical lesion leading to the hypothyroid state in vitamin B_6 deficiency, various possibilities such as primary with a defective thyroid gland, secondary with defective pituitary thyrotroph, or tertiary with defective hypothalamus were considered. If the defect were only at the level of the thyroid gland, low serum T_4 and T_3 levels would be coupled with a compensatory increase in serum TSH, which was not seen. With a defective pituitary, the low levels of serum T_3 and T_4 would be coupled with a sharp decrease in serum TSH as well as unresponsiveness to TRH, which again was not seen (107). Hypothalamic hypothyroidism is due to deficient TRH secretion. The administration of TRH to deficient rats significantly increased serum TSH as well as serum T_4 and T_3 in both vitamin B_6-deficient and vitamin B_6-replete rats. The chronic deficiency of TRH in the deficient rat is indicated by an increase in the number of TRH receptors with no change in receptor affinity (108). These results are consistent with a hypothalamic type of hypothyroidism in the vitamin B_6-deficient rat caused by the specific decrease in hypothalamic serotonin level.

Pineal Melatonin Secretion

The pineal gland tranduces photoperiodic information and hence has a crucial role in the temporal organization of various metabolic, physiological, and behavioral processes. Melatonin is the major secretory product of the pineal gland. Tryptophan is hydroxylated in the pinealocyte to 5-HTP and decarboxylated to yield serotonin. Serotonin is converted to *N*-acetylserotonin (NAS) by the enzyme *N*-acetyltransferase (NAT). NAS is converted to melatonin by hydroxyindole-*O*-methyltransferase. Melatonin synthesis is stimulated by β-adrenergic postganglionic sympathetic fibers from the superior cervical ganglion, which are stimulated in the dark. Melatonin levels in tissues and body fluids show both circadian and seasonal rhythms.

We have examined the effect of a moderate deficiency of vitamin B_6 on indolamine metabolism in the pineal gland of adult rats (109). Melatonin and NAS showed significant circadian variation in both vitamin B_6-deficient and vitamin B_6-replete control animals. However, the peak nighttime levels of pineal melatonin and NAS were also significantly lower in the deficient animals. Pineal levels of 5-HT and 5-hydroxy indole acetic acid (5-HIAA) were significantly lower in the deficient rats. Treatment of deficient rats with pyridoxine restored the levels of 5-HT, NAS, and melatonin to levels seen in vitamin B_6-replete controls. Such reversal was evident both during day and night periods. There was no difference in pineal NAT between deficient and control animals. However, pineal 5-HTP decarboxylase activity was significantly decreased in vitamin B_6-deficient rats. Tryptophan hydroxylation is considered to be the rate-limiting step in the syntheses of serotonin. Several studies indicate that a decrease in pineal 5-HT can reduce melatonin synthesis. In vivo administration of AADC inhibitors such as benserazide or monofluoromethyl dopa results in a reduction in the synthesis of pineal 5-HT and melatonin levels without altering pineal NAT activity. Thus, 5-HT availability, in addition to other known factors, could be important in the regulation of the synthesis of melatonin. The best understood endocrinological function of the pineal is the antigonadotropic action of melatonin (110). Melatonin acts at the level of the hypothalamus regulating the formation of releasing factors for anterior pituitary hormones. Melatonin might act through the serotonergic pathway (111), although direct effects of melatonin on pituitary, adrenals, and thyroid are also indicated.

Prolactin Secretion

The secretion of PRL is controlled by both stimulatory and inhibitory factors of hypothalamic origin. The inhibitory control is exerted primarily by dopamine, which is released from the tuberoinfundibular dopaminergic (TIDA) neurons into the pituitary portal circulation (112). Evidence based on peripheral administration of serotonin precursors, agonists or antagonists, intraventricular injection of serotonin, and electrical stimulation of the raphe nucleus indicates that central serotonergic projections to the hypothalamus are involved in the stimulation of PRL (113). The stimulatory effect of serotonin could be achieved either by increasing a PRL-releasing factor or by reducing the activity of the TIDA neurons. In view of the nonparallel changes in brain dopamine and serotonin during vitamin B_6 depletion, we investigated the effect of deficiency on PRL secretion (112). Plasma concentration of PRL was significantly reduced in vitamin B_6-deficient as compared with vitamin B_6-replete control adult male rats. The reduction in plasma PRL in deficient rats corresponded with the significantly reduced hypothalamic contents of PLP and serotonin in these rats. Administration of pyridoxine to deficient rats resulted in a significant increase in plasma PRL. Administration of the 5-HT_{1A} agonist, 8-hydroxy-2-*n*-dipropylaminotetralin, also resulted in a significant increase in plasma PRL whereas administration of 5-HT_{1A} antagonist spiroxatrine had the opposite effect. These results support our suggestion (102) about the neuroendocrine consequences of moderate vitamin B_6 deficiency and extend it to decreases in function of both pituitary thyrotrophs and lactotrophs.

VITAMIN B_6—SEIZURES AND NEUROPROTECTION

Although a statistical relationship between poor central nervous system function and physical signs of undernutrition in children had been recognized for long, these studies implicated low protein intake or imbalance between protein and carbohydrate as the causative (114). It was the general belief that if the nutrition of the mother was adequate for conception and maintenance of pregnancy, the intrauterine mechanisms for active transport and concentration would supply the necessary nutrients for the normal development of her unborn child (115). In view of the clinical and biochemical manifestations of vitamin B_6 deficiency in young and adult animals, it was of interest for us to produce and characterize vitamin B_6 deficiency in the very young rat. The report of the existence of a critical period in the development of the central nervous system indicated the importance of inducing deficiency during or prior to this period (116).

Female Holtzman rats were mated and the sperm-positive rats continued to be maintained on a vitamin B_6-replete diet during the first week of gestation. Following this, they were divided into two groups. One group was continued on the vitamin B_6-supplemented diet and the other was fed the vitamin B_6-deficient diet until the delivery of the pups and also during the nursing period. There was a small, but significant decrease in the body weight of the deficient litters even at birth. However, there was no significant difference in the brain weights between the two groups. Deficient pups had a significantly lower content of PLP in their brains. There was no difference between the vitamin B_6-replete and vitamin B_6-deficient groups in the concentration of GAD apoenzyme (enzyme activity in the presence of excess added PLP). However, the enzyme activity measured as such in the absence of externally added PLP was significantly reduced in the vitamin B_6-deficient group. Related to this observation was the occasional finding, among the vitamin B_6-deficient group, of pups with spontaneous convulsions that became noticeable at about 3–4 days of postnatal age. These fits were characterized by a high-pitch scream followed by generalized convulsions of a few seconds duration and repeated many times within a 1–3 min time period. It was noticed that when one neonate of a dam was affected with convulsions, all or a majority of other pups were also afflicted. The motility, perception, and alertness of the deficient neonates were inferior to that of the controls. This was the first report of the production of congenital pyridoxine deficiency (32). In view of the high mortality of the deficient pups, we could not use them in studies on the development of the central nervous systems, which in the rat extends from tenth to the twenty-first day after birth. In a further study, female rats were fed a vitamin B_6-deficient diet from the first postpartum day and the pups were fed the deficient diet from the time they were weaned till they were 5–6 weeks of age. The induction of pyridoxine deficiency during the most intense period of development of the CNS resulted in a decrease in both body and brain weights of the pups. The lower content of PLP found in the brains of deficient pups confirmed their vitamin B_6-deficient status. The lower GABA levels in the brains of deficient pups are directly related to the decrease in the activity of the GAD holoenzyme. The GAD apoenzyme levels were quite significantly increased, possibly due to stimulation of the apoprotein synthesis by the low concentration of GABA (117). We examined the effect of deficiency on various electrophysiological parameters. The bursts of high-voltage spikes during spontaneous EEG activity, as well as the spontaneous convulsions observed, reflect the decrease in cerebral GABA concentration in deficient rats. The more complicated changes in cortical auditory evoked potentials in the vitamin B_6-deficient rats are the results of the retardation of the normal ontogenetic development of the CNS of these rats (117). The inability of the cerebral cortex of the deficient pups to follow the increasing frequency of any kind of repetitive stimulus as well as a marked decrease in the amplitude of evoked potentials were quite apparent and correlated with decreases in both PLP and GABA levels in various brain areas. There was a significant increase in the maximal binding (B_{max}) of both $GABA_A$ and $GABA_B$ receptors, with no difference in the binding affinities (K_d), suggesting a supersensitivity of both these receptors, which correlated negatively with the concentration of GABA in these brain areas (118).

In further work (119–121), we investigated the effects of vitamin B_6 deficiency in adult rats. It is recognized that the thalamus acts as a relay station for various peripheral and central inputs to the cerebral cortex. We studied the electroresponsiveness of thalamic ventroposterior lateral (VPL) neurons in normal control and vitamin B_6-deficient adult rats in response to local administration of convulsants such as picrotoxin or pentylene tetrazole. The extent of neuronal recovery following intrathalamic administration of either GABA or pyridoxine or systemic administration of pyridoxine was assessed using computerized EEG analysis. The results demonstrated an antiepileptic effect of exogenously applied GABA and pyridoxine on thalamic VPL neurons, with pyridoxine having a much slower effect than GABA. Brain levels of PLP, GAD, and GABA responded to the systemic administration of pyridoxine. Even in normal rats, GAD is unsaturated with respect to the cofactor PLP (117,119). Brain levels of glutamate were significantly increased following administration of picrotoxin or pentylene tetrazole. Excitatory neurotransmitters such as glutamate are linked to the initiation and spread of seizure discharge and GABA is responsible for the termination of seizure activity (122–124). Neuronal recovery following pyridoxine is related to the synthesis of GABA through activation of GAD.

Domoic acid, a rigid structural analog of glutamate, is an excitatory neurotransmitter. It was identified as the toxic contaminant of cultivated mussels responsible for the outbreaks of acute food poisoning characterized by gastrointestinal and neurologic symptoms (125). The hippocampal CA-3 region was chosen for the study of seizure activity as this region has minimum seizure threshold as compared with other cerebral areas. We reported that acute intrahippocampal administration of picomole amounts of domoic acid led to EEG epileptiform seizure discharge activity. Domoic acid was 125 times more potent than kainic acid, a well-known neuroexcitant (126). Local administration of GABA or pyridoxine attenuated the seizure activity (119,127). Following domoic acid injection, GABA levels decreased significantly in various brain regions. Domoic acid inhibited GAD activity. As tissue levels of glutamate do not represent the neuronal pool of glutamate, we studied the effect of domoic acid on the in vitro release of glutamate in tissue superfusion experiments. The KCl-induced depolarization leads to the release of neurotransmitter glutamate. This was augmented by domoic acid. The direct application of GABA to the hippocampus of rats exhibiting domoic acid-induced seizure activity resulted in suppression of spike discharges. The slower effect of pyridoxine is related to the augmented PLP-dependent formation of GABA from glutamate. Similar observations have been reported by others (128).

Seizure discharge activity, following microinjection of domoic acid in the ipsilateral rat hippocampal CA-3 region, was attenuated by the microinjection of the serotonin 5-HT_{1A} agonist, 8-hydroxy-2-(di-*N*-propylamino) tertralin [8-(OH)-DPAT] and augmented by the specific 5-HT_{1A} antagonist, spiroxatrine, in the contralateral hippocampal CA-3 region (129). Serotonin-dependent signal transduction by 8-(OH)-DPAT is routed through 5-HT_{1A} receptor activation postsynaptically via second messenger cyclic GMP and calcium across the neuronal membrane. It has been reported that serotonin functions in the stabilization of brain regional GABAergic neurons and in seizure control. Serotonin has been shown to have a stimulatory effect on brain GABAergic neurotransmission. The neuroprotective action of pyridoxine flows from its effect on the synthesis of both GABA and serotonin. Hippocampal changes in developing mice at postnatal age of 10–30 days following intrauterine exposure to a single dose of domoic acid at day 13 of gestation were studied (130). The mice exhibited age-related developmental neurotoxicity. Brain regional GABA levels were significantly reduced and glutamate levels increased in these mice. Neuronal death was apparent in the offspring at 30 days of chronological age. This delayed neurotoxicity cannot be attributed to the acute effect of domoic acid and might be related to the increased sensitivity of hippocampal cells to the high concentration of endogenous glutamate.

In other experiments, electroencephalographic recordings in cerebral cortex of adult mice given a single subconvulsive dose of domoic acid exhibited typical spike and wave discharges. Administration of drugs such as sodium valproate or nimodipine or pyridoxine simultaneously with or after domoic aid treatment resulted in significantly less spike and wave activity. Administration of these same drugs 45 min prior to the administration of domoic acid also significantly decreased domoic acid-induced EEG background (131). Mechanistically, sodium valproate and pyridoxine significantly attenuated the domoic acid-induced increase in the levels of glutamate, increase in calcium c-*fos*, *jun*-B, and *jun*-D. Pyridoxine, acting through PLP, appears to decrease intracellular levels of glutamate by increasing influx, decrease in levels of GABA and increase in levels of the proto-oncogenes GAD activity, and decrease calcium influx through its action on cell surface calcium channels. Such actions of PLP were established in smooth muscle and in cardiac sarcolemma (see section on Vitamin B_6 and cardiovascular function). In the former, voltage-gated L-type calcium channels were the major calcium transporters whereas in cardiac sarcolemma purinergic P2X receptors activated by ATP seem to be the major pathway of calcium transfer. PLP inhibits both calcium transport mechanisms and is central to the neuroprotective action of pyridoxine.

These studies in whole animals were followed by experiments where primary cultures of hippocampal neurons were exposed to domoic acid. This resulted in apoptotic changes. ^{1}H-NMR proton spectra of domoic acid-treated neuronal cultures exhibited significantly increased glutamate and reduced GABA levels. Pretreatment of cells with PLP prior to domoic acid exposure reduced glutamate and increased GABA levels. Exposure of cells to domoic acid or Bay-K 8644 increased the calcium influx into neurons. This was again significantly decreased by preincubating hippocampal cells with either nimodipine or PLP. The domoic acid-induced proto-oncogene expression was also significantly suppressed by preincubation of the cell culture with either nimodipine or PLP (131). These results would suggest that domoic acid-induced apoptosis might occur through increased calcium influx, proto-oncogene induction, and intranucleosomal DNA fragmentation. Similar results were obtained by exposure of cultures of neuroblastoma/glioma 108/15 cells to domoic acid and to pyridoxine, respectively.

PYRIDOXINE-DEPENDENCY SEIZURES

For about half a century, pyridoxine dependency has been recognized as an inborn abnormality (132). Infants present, generally soon after birth, with seizures that are resistant to the commonly used antiepileptic drugs and respond only to pharmacologic doses of pyridoxine. It is a rare autosomal recessive genetic disorder. In view of the prevalence of atypical variants of this disorder, it is thought to be underrecognized. A pyridoxine-dependent condition has to be considered in all children with intractable epilepsy up to 3 years of age (133). A variety of seizure types such as myoclonic seizures, atonic seizures, partial and generalized seizures, as well as infantile spasms are all associated with this condition. The unusual rhythmic in utero movements reported retrospectively by some mothers might represent fetal seizures (134). At present, there is no biochemical test to confirm pyridoxine-dependency seizures and clinical diagnosis is the only mode of recognition. Response to pyridoxine monotherapy and recurrence of seizures following withdrawal of treatment is the only confirmatory test. Such testing is fraught with difficulty due to ethical considerations. Pyridoxine dependency is to be distinguished from vitamin B_6 deficiency, first reported in infants fed on commercial milk formula where autoclaving destroyed the vitamin B_6 content (39).

The intravenous administration of 50–100 mg of pyridoxine results, generally, in a dramatic cessation of seizures. In some cases, doses up to 500 mg as well as repeated dosings might be needed. This additional requirement of pyridoxine is for life. Once the initial seizures are controlled, the minimum dose necessary for maintenance of a seizure-free state can be titrated. This is about 15 mg/kg body weight per day. Delay in achieving milestones, developmental defects, as well as permanent brain damage are the concomitants of untreated pyridoxine-dependency condition. Most patients have some degree of cognitive impairment, particularly, in language expression. Brain imaging studies indicate gray and white matter atrophy in these patients. The progressive magnetic resonance imaging (MRI) changes are suggestive of selective neuronal loss (135,136). Magnetic resonance spectroscopy is complementary to MRI and shows the presence of various metabolites in the samples. Such study revealed a decrease in *N*-acetylaspartate to creatine ratio in the frontal and parieto-occipital cortices indicative of neuronal loss (137), as reported in pathologic studies (138). Recent studies (133,139) indicate that increasing the dose of pyridoxine in pyridoxine-dependent children without seizures could improve their IQ, indicating a role for pyridoxine in normal brain development and in functions other than controlling the excitable state.

There is no conclusive resolution of the etiology of pyridoxine-dependent seizures. Autopsy studies showed elevated glutamate and decreased GABA levels in the frontal and occipital cortices (137). Similar observations in the cerebrospinal fluid (CSF) of affected patients point to a defect in the conversion of glutamate to GABA (140,141). GABA is an inhibitory neurotransmitter. Its precursor, glutamic acid, which itself is an excitatory neurotransmitter, undergoes decarboxylation by the enzyme GAD. PLP is the coenzyme of GAD. An abnormality of this enzyme has been presumed to be responsible for the impairment in the synthesis of GABA from glutamate. Of the two isoforms of GAD, GAD-65 is PLP dependent and the defective binding of PLP to this enzyme was suggested to be the cause of the decreased synthesis of GABA in vitamin B_6-dependent seizures. Studies using cultured fibroblasts obtained from affected patients showed a reduction in the PLP-dependent GABA synthesis (142). A biochemical defect related to the interaction between PLP and GAD is indicated. More recent studies, however, have excluded a mutation in either of the two isoforms of GAD as the molecular defect responsible for pyridoxine-dependent seizures (143,144). Other proteins involved in GABA metabolism such as GABA-T, plasma membrane GABA transporter GAT-1, and pyridoxal kinase have also been ruled out in the search for the etiology of this genetic defect. However, a linkage to markers on chromosome 5q31 has been reported (145). The report of elevated blood and CSF levels of pipecolic acid, a precursor to a PLP-dependent reaction in the pathway of the metabolic conversion of lysine to glutaryl CoA, is significant as it has been shown that a high concentration of pipecolic acid inhibits GABA uptake (146). We can only speculate that a defective glutamate–GABA conversion in association with other, not well defined, abnormalities contributes to the pathology of vitamin B_6-dependent seizures.

There are other seizure conditions in which pyridoxine therapy finds a place. Infantile spasms (spastic convulsions), in combination with diffuse electroencephalographic abnormalities (hypsarrhythmia), is referred to as "West Syndrome." Mental retardation is associated with this condition (147,148). Adrenocorticotropic hormone (ACTH) is effective for the short-term treatment of infantile spasms. In view of the elevated therapy associated morbidity (149), valproic acid and vigabatrin have been used (150). Following reports of beneficial effects of high doses of pyridoxine, initial treatment for 1–2 weeks with high doses of pyridoxine is the established therapy in some European countries and in Japan (151,152). Combined therapy with high-dose pyridoxine in association with low-dose corticotrophin has also been reported as a promising therapy for seizure control, normalized EEG, and intellectual outcome (153).

VITAMIN B_6 AND CARDIOVASCULAR FUNCTION

Hypertension is one of the major causes of chronic illness in Western Societies, where about 20%–30% of the adult population has some degree of elevation of blood pressure. As in most of these patients, a causative has not been recognized and they are referred to as those that have "essential hypertension." Various rat and dog models such as uninephrectomized deoxycorticosterone acetate (DOCA)–saline-treated rats, adrenal regeneration in rats, Goldblatt renal hypertension in dogs, obese rat strains, and spontaneously hypertensive rats (SHRs) have been used in the study of hypertension. We have introduced the moderately vitamin B_6-deficient male rat as an additional animal model (154–157).

Male Sprague–Dawley rats were fed a vitamin B_6-deficient diet for up to 12 weeks (32) and compared with a group pair-fed a pyridoxine-supplemented diet. Systolic blood pressure (SBP) was measured indirectly in conscious restrained animals trained to this procedure, by tail-cuff plethysmography. These values were comparable with those obtained directly from a cannula placed in the right carotid artery in anesthetized animals (155). The blood pressure changes in the vitamin B_6-deficient rat can be classified into three phases: prehypertensive (1–4 weeks), hypertensive (5–11 weeks), and posthypertensive (from the 12th week). During the hypertensive phase, the rats were only moderately vitamin B_6 deficient and have been biochemically characterized in terms of tissue vitamin B_6 levels. They were functionally deficient in neurotransmitters serotonin and GABA. Treatment of the hypertensive vitamin B_6-deficient rats with dietary pyridoxine corrected both the deficiency state and the hypertensive condition. After 11 weeks of vitamin B_6 depletion, the rats were at an advanced state of vitamin B_6 depletion but were not hypertensive. They were generally hypotensive and could be titrated with very small dietary vitamin B_6 supplements to a hypertensive state. The "moderately vitamin B_6-deficient" rat is an animal model of moderate hypertension. Using drugs such as phenytoin, valproic acid, and diltiazem, it was shown that the hypertension was not the result of a hyperexcitable state in these animals.

We examined the possibility that the reversible hypertension was related to sympathetic stimulation. The concentration of norepinephrine (NE) in plasma is a valid reflection of sympathetic activity. To draw blood samples from the conscious animal without trauma, we developed a technique of implanting a vascular-access port (VAP) with catheterization to the jugular vein (158). We showed (159) that both epinephrine and norepinephrine levels in the plasma of hypertensive vitamin B_6-deficient rats were threefold higher than controls.

Significantly, NE turn over in the hearts of deficient hypertensive rats was threefold higher than that in controls. Treatment of the rats with pyridoxine returned both the blood pressure and catecholamine levels to normal within 24 h. Pyridoxine administration to control rats had no significant effect on any of these parameters. The complete reversibility of hypertension in such a short time would preclude permanent structural damage to the vessel wall of the vitamin B_6-deficient rat. The lesion could be at the level of neurotransmitter regulation.

Cardiovascular Effects of Serotonin

Serotonergic neurotransmission in the central nervous system controls a wide variety of functions such as blood pressure, emotional behavior, endocrine secretion, perception of pain, and sleep (Figure 10.3). In addition, there are effects on peripheral neurons and nonneural tissues. Serotonin, when administered into the brain elicits complex cardiovascular responses. Depressor, pressor, or biphasic responses are reported, which reflects the non-homogenous nature of brain 5-HT neurons subserving different functions. The receptors that mediate the diverse effects of serotonin have been categorized into major families and subtypes. The development of specific agonists for serotonin such as the centrally acting 8-hydroxy-2-(di-*n*-propylamino)tetralin (8-OH-DPAT), ipsapirone, and flesinoxan with specificity to 5-HT_A subtype receptors has led to the recognition that 5-HT_{1A} receptors are involved in the central control of autonomic flow (160).

The decrease in neuronal 5-HT and the consequent changes in its receptors, particularly 5-HT_{1A}, may cause hypertension in vitamin B_6 deficiency. This was investigated in vitamin B_6-deficient rats after they had developed peak hypertension by examining the effects of various 5-HT_{1A} agonists. They all had an acute hypotensive effect in these rats. When doses that caused a fall in SBP of 20 mmHg were compared, the following rank order was established: 8-OH-DPAT > flesinoxan > 5-methylurapidil > urapidil (161). The affinity of the agonists for the 5-HT_{1A} receptor site correlated with the order of their antihypertensive activity indicating that this effect is mediated through the 5-HT_{1A} receptor site (162). The selective 5-HT_{1A} receptor antagonist spiroxatrine (161) dose-dependently antagonized the hypotensive activity of 5-HT_{1A} receptor agonists.

The moderately vitamin B_6-deficient hypertensive rats have a low concentration of serotonin in various brain areas and correspondingly an increased 5-HT_{1A} receptor number in membrane preparations from the tissues. What is the mechanism of the hypotensive action of the 5-HT_{1A} agonists? The hypertension of the moderately vitamin B_6-deficient rat is characterized by central sympathetic stimulation as seen in other animal models of hypertension. When the α_2-adrenoreceptors in the nucleus tractus solitarii (NTS) are stimulated, inhibitory neurons of the vasomotor center are activated. Sympathetic outflow, which originates from the vasomotor center and innervates the peripheral vasculature, heart, and kidney, is reduced. As a result, peripheral vascular tone, heart rate, and renin release are decreased, resulting in a decrease in total peripheral resistance and cardiovascular output. Drugs such as clonidine, an α_2-agonist, exert their cardiovascular effect through stimulation of the α_2-adrenoreceptors in the brain stem. Activation of central α_2-adrenoreceptors in the NTS requires a serotonergic input through the 5-HT_{1A} receptor (163). Hence it results in the hypotensive action of 5-HT_{1A} receptor agonists as well as the hypertensive response in the serotonin-deficient, moderately vitamin B_6-deficient rat.

Pyridoxal-5′-Phosphate and Calcium Channels

The end result of centrally mediated sympathetic stimulation is an increase in peripheral resistance. This is reflected in elevations of both resting and stimulated vascular tone in the resistance arteries of the moderately vitamin B_6-deficient hypertensive rats (164).

Elevated peripheral resistance is the hall mark of hypertension as seen in other models of hypertension. The increase in tone of caudal artery segments from the hypertensive vitamin B_6-deficient rat is calcium dependent. The decrease in tone following the addition to the medium of the calcium-channel antagonist, nifedipine, indicates that the increased peripheral resistance resulting from increased permeability of smooth muscle plasma membrane to Ca^{2+} might be central to the development of hypertension in the vitamin B_6-deficient rat (164).

The initiation of smooth muscle contraction is principally dependent on the short-term increase in cytosolic Ca^{2+}. Calcium moves in and out of the cell and intracellular storage sites in response to chemical, electrical, pressure, and other physical stimuli (165). Calcium influx occurs through plasma membrane Ca^{2+} channels, which are voltage-operated or receptor-mediated. Voltage-sensitive calcium channels open on depolarization of the cell membrane resulting in an inward movement of calcium ions. ATP is an important extracellular nucleotide that mediates its effect via plasma membrane-bound P2 receptors. The P2 purinoceptors belong to two different families P2X and P2Y, respectively, which differ in their molecular structure and transduction mechanisms. P2X receptors are agonist-gated nonselective cation channels that mediate a rapid depolarization through influx of both Ca^{2+} and Na^{+}. P2Y receptors act via G-protein-coupled receptors.

The slow channel (L-type) is the major pathway by which Ca^{2+} enters the cell during excitation for initiation and regulation of the force of contraction of cardiac and skeletal muscle. Vascular smooth muscle also contains the L-type channel. We evaluated the possibility that in the vitamin B_6-deficient hypertensive rat a higher concentration of cytosolic free Ca^{2+} might be responsible for the higher tension in the vascular smooth muscle. The high cytosolic free Ca^{2+} could result from an increase in the permeability of dihydropyridine-sensitive L-type calcium channel of the vascular smooth muscle plasma membrane. We determined the intracellular calcium uptake by caudal artery segments of vitamin B_6-deficient hypertensive and control rats using the lanthanum-resistant calcium [$^{45}Ca^{2+}$] uptake as an index. In the hypertensive, deficient rats, the [$^{45}Ca^{2+}$] influx into the vascular smooth muscle was significantly increased to twice that of the control (164).

We investigated the alterations in $[Ca^{+2}]_i$ induced by KCl in vitamin B_6-deficient hypertensive and control rats. $[Ca^{2+}]_i$ was measured in isolated cardiomyocytes using the Fura-2 fluorescent technique. The KCl-induced $[Ca^{2+}]_i$ increase was significantly higher in cardiomyocyte isolated from vitamin B_6-deficient hypertensive rats. A single injection of vitamin B_6 (10 mg/kg body weight) to the deficient animal completely reversed the KCl-induced changes in $[Ca^{2+}]_i$ due to vitamin B_6 deficiency (166).

The defects in the calcium channel of vitamin B_6-deficient hypertensive rats were examined further by studying the effect of calcium-channel antagonists on the SBP of conscious hypertensive rats (167). All the calcium-channel antagonists were effective in lowering the SBP of the vitamin B_6-deficient hypertensive rats with a rank order of potency: nifedipine $>$ (−)202–791 $>$ (±)verapamil $>$ diltiazem. The specificity of the effect was demonstrated as the dihydropyridine agonist, BAY K 8644 antagonized the hypotensive effect of nifedipine.

In further experiments, we examined the relationship between vitamin B_6 levels in the diet and some dietarily induced hypertensive conditions. Low levels of calcium in the diet potentiated the hypertension induced by the vitamin B_6-deficient diet (168). In addition high dietary calcium reduced the SBP of vitamin B_6-deficient hypertensive rats, similar to the observations in other hypertensive animal models (169,170).

Chronic ingestion of simple carbohydrates such as sucrose or fructose has been shown to increase the SBP in several rat strains (171). This was attenuated by the inclusion of a vitamin B_6 supplement (five times the normal intake) in the diet (172). In further work, we investigated whether a dietary supplement of vitamin B_6 could attenuate the elevation of SBP in genetically hypertensive animal models such as the Zucker obese or the SHR. Male Zucker obese rats (*fa/fa*) fed a commercial rat chow developed hypertension in 3–4 weeks.

The inclusion of a dietary vitamin B_6 supplement (five times the normal intake) resulted in a complete attenuation of the hypertension in the obese strain, which was reversible (172). In contrast to the effect seen in the Zucker obese rats, there was no response to the inclusion of a dietary vitamin B_6 supplement in SHRs. The changes in SBP in the Zucker as well as in the sucrose- or fructose-fed rats correlated with the changes in the uptake of calcium by the caudal artery segments in these groups.

In view of the earlier results, we investigated the possibility that pyridoxine or more particularly PLP could directly modulate the cellular calcium uptake process. BAY K 8644, a DHP-sensitive calcium-channel agonist (173) stimulated calcium [$^{45}Ca^{2+}$] entry into artery segments from control rats. PLP dose-dependently reduced the BAY K 8644-stimulated calcium uptake by control artery segments (174,175). The basal uptake of [$^{45}Ca^{2+}$] by caudal artery segments from vitamin B_6-deficient hypertensive rats was at least twice the uptake by artery segments from control normal rats. PLP or nifedipine added to the incubation medium significantly decreased the [$^{45}Ca^{2+}$] uptake by artery segments from the vitamin B_6-deficient hypertensive rats. However, in the presence of BAY K 8644 in the incubation medium, both PLP and nifedipine were much less effective in attenuating the [$^{45}Ca^{2+}$] uptake by artery segments from the deficient hypertensive rats. These in vitro direct antagonisms indicate the possibility that the calcium-channel agonist BAY K 8644, the calcium-channel antagonist nifedipine and PLP might all act at the same site on the calcium channel. We examined the effect of PLP on the binding of tritiated nitrendipine, a dihydropyridine calcium-channel antagonist, to membrane preparation from caudal artery of normal rats. PLP treatment of crude membranes of caudal artery resulted in a significant decrease in the number of [3H]nitrendipine-binding sites (166).

In a further study, we examined the influence of PLP on the ATP-induced contractile activity of the isolated rat heart and the ATP-mediated increase in $[Ca^{2+}]_i$ in freshly isolated adult rat cardiomyocytes as well as on the specific binding of ATP to cardiac sarcolemmal membrane to determine if PLP is an effective antagonist of ATP receptors in the myocardium. The contractile activity of the isolated perfused rat heart was monitored on infusion with 50 μm ATP in the presence or absence of 50 μm PLP. The infusion of ATP caused an immediate increase (within seconds) in left ventricular diastolic pressure (LVDP), $+dP/dt$, and $-dP/dt$. This effect was completely blocked in the hearts pretreated with PLP for 10 min. The antagonistic effect of PLP was concentration dependent. The specificity of the effect of PLP was established as propranolol, which prevented the positive inotropic action of isoproterenol showed no effect on the positive inotropic action of ATP. Conversely, the contractile activity of isoproterenol was unaffected by PLP (166,176).

The ATP-induced increase in $[Ca^{2+}]_i$ was significantly decreased in cardiomyocytes following pretreatment with PLP. We also examined the effect of PLP on both the high- and low-affinity binding sites for ATP on cardiac sarcolemma. PLP almost completely blocked the low-affinity binding whereas the high-affinity binding was decreased by about 60%. Other purinergic P2X antagonists such as suramin, cibacron blue, and 4,4′-diisothiocyanatostilbene-2,2′-disulfonic acid (DIDS) inhibited ATP binding at both high- and low-affinity sites.

Agents such as propranolol (β-adrenoreceptor blocker), prazosin (α-adrenoreceptor blocker), verapamil (L-type Ca^{2+}-channel blocker), and ryanodine (sarcoplasmic reticulum Ca^{2+}-release channel blocker) did not show any significant effect on the high- or low-affinity ATP-binding sites. PLP is a weak antagonist of P_2 receptors (177). Synthetic polyanionic diazo derivative of PLP such as pyridoxal-α^5-phosphate-6-azophenyl-2′,4′-disulfonic acid (PPADS) and 2,5-disulfonate isomer of PPADS (iso-PPADS) are P2 receptor antagonists, with a preference for P2X receptor (178–181).

PLP in vitro attenuates the influx of extracellular calcium. This effect is achieved through modulation of ligand binding. This is analogous to the effect of PLP on steroid hormone activity (182). The action of drugs at the calcium channels would indicate that endogenous factors or ligands might serve as physiological regulators, a function that is mimicked by synthetic calcium-channel agonists or antagonists. The KCl-induced increase in $[Ca^{2+}]_i$ was increased in cardiomyocytes from vitamin B_6-deficient rats. Administration of vitamin B_6 to the deficient rats abolished this condition. It is possible that the augmentation of KCl-induced increase in $[Ca^{2+}]_i$ in the deficient rat is related to an increase in Ca^{2+} influx through the sarcolemmal calcium channels. An increase in Ca^{2+} influx in smooth muscle cells causes an increase in tone of the smooth muscle and hence, hypertension in the deficient animal (155,174).

Studies in humans have identified an independent association between low plasma vitamin B_6 concentration and a higher risk of coronary artery disease (CAD) (183). In addition to a role for vitamin B_6 in atherosclerosis, other potential explanations have been considered. These include the role of PLP in platelet aggregation through inhibition of adenosine-5′-diphosphate receptors (184), downregulation of glycoprotein IIb gene expression (185), and the association between low PLP and inflammatory markers (186,187). Low plasma concentration of PLP has been inversely related to C-reactive protein (CRP) in the Framingham Heart Study Cohort (188). The relation between plasma PLP and major markers of acute-phase reactions in affecting CAD was evaluated in a cohort of subjects who were characterized by angiography for severe coronary atherosclerosis and a control group of CAD-free individuals (189). They determined plasma PLP, fibrinogen, high-sensitivity CRP (hs-CRP), serum lipid concentrations, and all major biochemical CAD risk factors including total homocysteine. A significant, inverse-graded relation was observed between PLP and both hs-CRP and fibrinogen. The CAD risk as a result of low PLP was additive when considered in combination with elevated hs-CRP concentration or with an increased ratio of low-density lipoprotein (LDL) to high-density lipoprotein (HDL). Low plasma PLP concentrations were inversely associated with major markers of inflammation and independently associated with increased CAD risk (188). The association of low PLP concentration with higher risk of CAD remained even after the inclusion, in a multivariate logistic regression model, of hs-CRP, fibrinogen, and variables related to homocysteine metabolism. It has been suggested that the association of low PLP with CAD risk is mainly due to the effect of inflammation on plasma PLP concentration (190). Friso et al. (191) contend that the additive effect of low PLP to that conferred by hs-CPR was seen in the progressive increase in the estimate of CAD risk across increasing hs-CRP quintiles. This is supported by the observation of Kelly et al. (192) that a low PLP status was associated with stroke and only partially mediated via inflammation, as expressed by the major inflammation marker hs-CRP.

Our observations on the role of PLP in both the major calcium channels for the influx of extracellular calcium might proffer a viable biochemical explanation for the association between low PLP concentration and the risk for CAD. The increase in $[Ca^{2+}]_i$ in cardiomyocytes in the vitamin B_6-deficient rat might contribute to heart dysfunction and increased susceptibility to myocardial infarction (166) and explain the beneficial effect of vitamin B_6 in patients with hypertension (193) and myocardial infarction (166). PLP also antagonizes the cardiac action of ATP by blocking purinoceptors on the myocardium. This is consistent with pharmacological studies showing the antagonistic effect of PLP on ATP-induced changes in rat vagus and vas deferens (177). It is significant that PLP has an inhibitory effect on both the major channels, the L-type as well as the ATP-mediated, for the influx of extracellular calcium into the cell.

HYPERHOMOCYSTEINEMIA—CARDIOVASCULAR IMPLICATIONS

Homocysteine is a sulfur-containing amino acid formed during the metabolism of methionine, an essential amino acid. These two amino acids undergo interconversion through the demethylation and remethylation pathways. This "methionine cycle" is important in the conservation

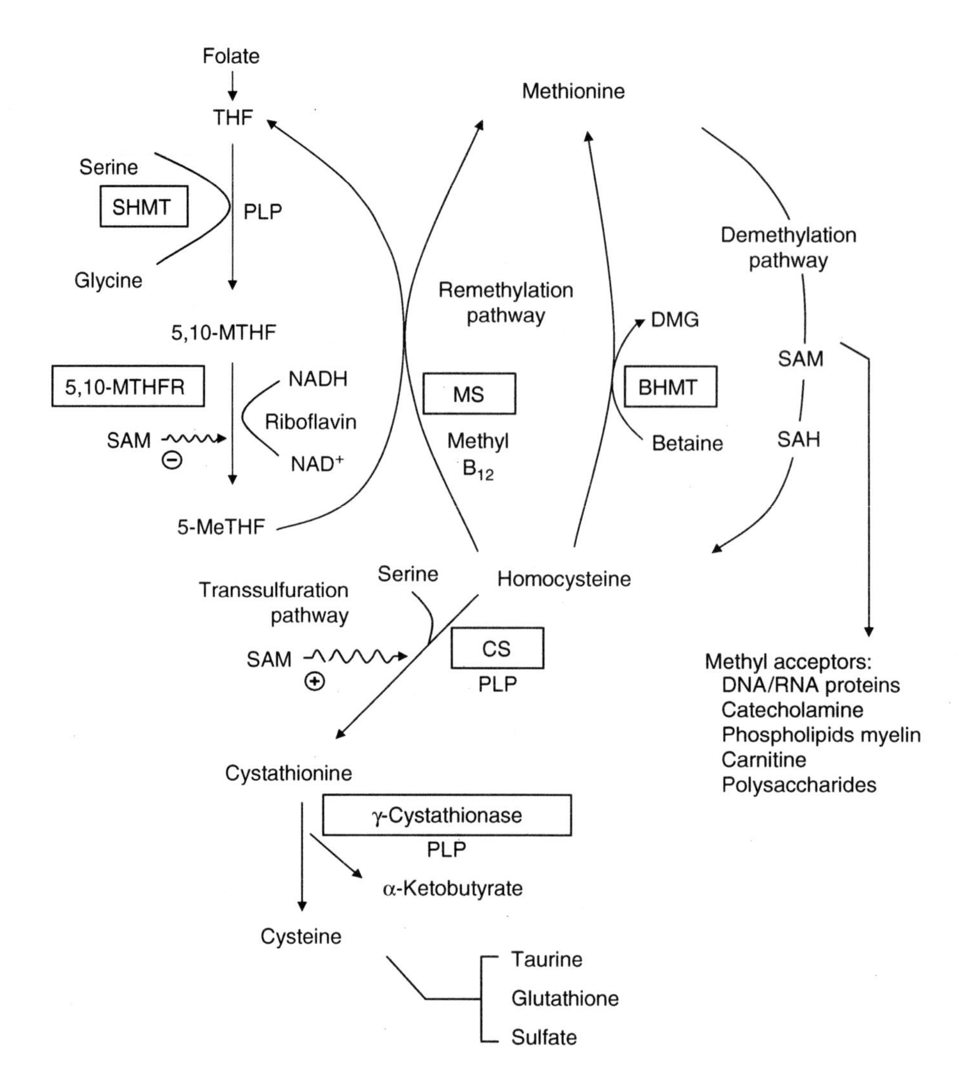

FIGURE 10.5 Metabolism of methionine–homocysteine. SHMT, Serine hydroxyl methyl transferase; 5,10-MTHFR, 5,10-methylene tetrahydrofolate reductase; MS, methionine synthetase; BHMT, betaine homocysteine methyltransferase; CS, cystathionine synthetase; THF, tetrahydrofolate; 5,10-MTHF, 5,10-methylene tetrahydrofolate; 5-MeTHF, 5-methyltetrahydrofolate; SAM, *S*-adenosylmethionine; SAH, *S*-adenosylhomocysteine; methyl B_{12}, methylcobalamin; DMG, dimethyl glycine.

of methionine and occurs in all tissues. In the demethylation pathway, methionine is stepwise converted through *S*-adenosylmethionine (SAM) and *S*-adenosylhomocysteine (SAH) to homocysteine. SAM is an universal methyl donor, and the methyl acceptors are DNA, RNA, proteins, catecholamines, phospholipids, myelin, carnitine, and polysaccharides (Figure 10.5).

The product, homocysteine, is converted back to methionine, for conservation of this essential amino acid, by the remethylation pathways. In the significant remethylation pathway, methionine synthetase adds the methyl group to homocysteine with 5-methyltetrahydrofolate (5-MeTHF) as the methyl donor. This reaction requires methylcobalamin. The other product of this reaction, tetrahydrofolate is converted back to 5-MeTHF through successive steps. The first step is catalyzed by serine hydroxymethyl transferase, a PLP-dependent enzyme. The product 5,10-methylenetetrahydrofolate (5,10-MTHF) is reduced to 5-MeTHF by 5,10-MTHF reductase, a flavin enzyme that uses NADH as the reducing potential. 5-MeTHF is restored as the methyl source in the "methionine cycle." A minor pathway of remethylation uses betaine as the methyl source.

Homocysteine is catabolized by the transsulfuration pathway in which homocysteine is converted to cystathionine by cystathionine synthetase (CS), a PLP enzyme. Cystathionine is further degraded to cysteine by γ-cystathionase, another PLP enzyme. Cysteine contributes to the syntheses of taurine and more significantly of glutathione. The sulfur is terminally degraded to inorganic sulfate. The smooth operation of these metabolic pathways ensures normal tissue and plasma concentrations of methionine and homocysteine.

Two features of the methionine–homocysteine metabolic pathways are to be noted. The first relates to the control of methionine–homocysteine metabolism. SAM, the product of the demethylation pathway inhibits 5,10-MTHFR and activates CS, under conditions of cellular methionine excess. The second feature of the metabolic pathways is the number of vitamins involved. In the remethylation pathway, dietary folate is the source of 5-MeTHF of the methyl transferase reaction, which also requires methylcobalamin (methyl-B_{12}). The formation of 5,10-MTHF from THF requires PLP (vitamin B_6). The reduction of 5,10-MTHF to 5-MeTHF requires riboflavin and niacinamide. The key steps of the "transsulfuration" pathway are catalyzed by CS and γ-cystathionase, respectively. Both require PLP (vitamin B_6). Hence the interrelationships occur among water-soluble vitamins particularly folate, vitamin B_{12}, and vitamin B_6 and homocysteine metabolism (194,195). High homocysteine concentrations (hyperhomocysteinemia, homocysteinuria) are the result of genetic defects, deficiencies of folate, vitamins B_{12}, and B_6 (196), or renal failure (197). In the Framingham study, inadequate vitamin status was associated with more than two-thirds of the cases of hyperhomocysteinemia (198).

The vascular pathology of hyperhomocysteinemia implicating it in the pathogenesis of arteriosclerosis was first proposed by McCully (199) based on autopsy evidence of precocious arterial thrombosis and atherosclerosis in a homocysteinuric patient. Although dormant for decades, this hypothesis has received much clinical and experimental evidence. Even mild hyperhomocysteinemia has been shown to be an independent risk factor for arthrosclerosis and thromboembolic diseases (200–203). In hyperlipidemic patients with atherosclerotic disease, hyperhomocysteinemia is an independent predictor of atherosclerotic events (204).

The pathological mechanisms of hyperhomocysteinemia include its effect on blood pressure (205,206). The effects involve the stimulation of smooth muscle cell proliferation as well as the alteration of the elastic properties of the vascular wall. There is evidence to suggest that hyperhomocysteinemia mediates atherosclerosis through endothelial dysfunction (207), generation of reactive oxygen species, and increased susceptibility of LDL to oxidation (208). The oxidation products of reduced homocysteine include H_2O_2 and superoxide anions (209). The impairment of vasodilation in homocysteinemia is due to the decreased availability of nitric oxide (NO), through formation of peroxynitrite in the reaction between superoxide anion and NO (210). Homocysteine increases the thickness of vascular intima, endothelial cell desquamation, and monocyte adhesion to vessel wall (206). The regulation of collagen expression is mediated by a redox-sensitive homocysteine receptor. Homocysteine activates nuclear factor kappa-B (NF-κB), which contributes to the mitogenic effect by activating cyclin D_1 expression. This leads to increase in vascular smooth muscle proliferation contributing to constrictive collagen remodeling. Homocysteine enhances collagen synthesis (211). The resultant reduction in the elastin–collagen ratio would contribute to the changes in the vessel wall characteristics leading to increased systemic vascular resistance.

In view of the established connection between hyperhomocysteinemia and vascular dysfunction, there have been efforts to study clinically and experimentally the effect of decreasing homocysteine concentration on vascular function. A strong inverse association between homocysteinemia and plasma folate was established in the adult survivors of the Framingham Heart Study. In this study, a weaker inverse association with plasma vitamin B_{12} and PLP was also seen. Inadequate plasma concentrations of one or more, among folate, vitamin B_{12}, and vitamin B_6 contributed to 67% of the cases of hyperhomocysteinemia (198). In various studies, therapy of homocysteinemia with a combination of folate and vitamin B_6 resulted in normalization of plasma homocysteine concentration. Glueck et al. (204) treated patients for 15 weeks with folic acid (5 mg/day) and pyridoxine (100 mg/day), resulting in a normalization of plasma homocysteine. Similar results have been reported by others (201,202). In one study, Till et al. (212) used carotid intima–media thickness (IMT) as a marker of atherosclerotic changes and studied the effect of multiple vitamin treatment. In a double-blind randomized trial, patients received 2.5 mg folic acid, 25 mg pyridoxine, and 0.5 mg vitamin B_{12} or placebo daily for 1 year. There was a significant decrease in plasma homocysteine as well as in IMT in the treated group. In another study (213), vitamin B_{12} and vitamin B_6 were effective in lowering plasma homocysteine even after an initial lowering of homocysteine by folic acid treatment. Marcucci et al. (214) studied 310 nonvalvular atrial fibrillation (NVAF) patients on oral anticoagulant treatment and 310 controls. Hyperhomocysteinemia (highest quartile) and vitamin B_6 deficiency (lowest quartile) were independently associated with NVAF after multivariate analysis. Various reports indicate that homocysteine and vitamin B_6 are independent and additive cardiovascular risk factors (215). Within the framework of a large Austrian study on recurrent venous thromboembolism (VTE), the impact of hyperhomocysteinemia on VTE was assessed. Homocysteinemia due to genetic factors or vitamin deficiency was an independent risk factor of recurring VTE and low vitamin B_6 levels were associated with an increased risk of first venous thrombosis.

Patients with inflammatory bowel disease (IBD) are at increased risk for thrombosis and vitamin deficiencies. Low plasma levels of vitamin B_6 are an independent risk factor for thrombosis and low levels of vitamin B_6 were significantly more frequent in patients with active IBD than in patients with the quiescent disease. Low vitamin B_6 levels were significantly correlated with serum concentrations of C-reactive protein (inflammation marker) and also homocysteine (216). In experiments using the rat, a vitamin B_6-deficient diet induced hyperhomocysteinemic condition compared with a normal vitamin B_6 diet. This hyperhomocysteinemia induced by vitamin B_6 deficiency was increased 10-fold in rats fed a high polyunsaturated fatty acid diet. It is significant that PLP is a cofactor of δ-6-desaturase, which is involved in polyunsaturated fatty acid metabolism (217).

There is evidence to suggest that a deficiency of vitamin B_6 leads to hyperhomocysteinemia. The relationship of hyperhomocysteinemia to various cardiovascular and thromboembolic diseases is well established. Hyperhomocysteinemia is attenuated by treatment with folate, vitamin B_{12}, and vitamin B_6. The reduction in homocysteine concentration following folate treatment of hyperhomocysteinemia is further augmented by treatment with vitamin B_6. In addition to its relationship to cardiovascular diseases through the homocysteine connection, it has been shown that vitamin B_6 deficiency is an independent risk factor for various cardiovascular diseases. This relationship could be through the development of hypertension in vitamin B_6 deficiency. The specific decrease in the neurotransmitter serotonin in the central nervous system and its connection to sympathetic stimulation is well established. Hence, the connection between PLP and calcium entry into the vascular cell and cardiomyocytes occurs, controlling vascular tone.

ADVANCED GLYCATION END PRODUCT INHIBITORS—PYRIDOXAMINE

The implication of advanced glycation end products (AGEs) on the pathogenesis of diabetic and uremic complications as well as on aging and atherosclerosis has been recognized recently leading to investigations on the inhibition of the formation of AGEs.

Nonenzymatic glycation involves the Schiff-base condensation of the carbonyl group of sugar aldehydes with the N terminus or free amino groups of proteins. This is reversible process and is referred to as the Maillard reaction. It is dependent on the concentration of glucose. The Schiff bases are later rearranged to intermediate ketamine Amadori products. This is a partially reversible reaction. In the later phase, over a period of weeks and months, glucose-independent reactions including rearrangements, condensation, dehydration, polymerization, and fragmentation lead to a host of metabolites that are referred to as "advanced glycation end products" (AGEs). Lipid peroxidation of polyunsaturated fatty acids gives rise to corresponding "advanced lipoxidation end products" (ALEs). AGEs comprise a vast range of molecular species including aminoacids (carboxymethyllysine, CML), glyoxal-derived lysine dimers (GOLD), methylglyoxal-derived lysine dimers (MOLD), carbohydrates (pentosidine), and lipids (malondialdehyde-lysine, 4-hydroxynonenal protein adducts).

High tissue levels of glucose as in diabetes accelerate the formation of AGEs. These compounds, because of their low molecular weight, are cleared by the kidney. Hence, under conditions of renal impairment the serum concentration of AGEs builds up. Oxidative stress and carbonyl stress contribute to the formation of AGEs and ALEs. An imbalance between reactive oxygen and nitrogen species or free radicals and antioxidants in favor of free radicals is referred to as oxidative stress. The overproduction of carbonyl compounds caused by increased formation or decreased clearance of reactive carbonyls is referred to as carbonyl stress (218). Carbonyl compounds are formed from carbohydrates, lipids, and amino acids by oxidative and nonoxidative pathways, which are detoxified by several enzymes and are excreted by the kidneys. Carbonyl compounds react nonenzymatically with amino groups of proteins to give rise to Schiff base, which rearrange to Amadori products and eventually to AGEs.

Tissue accumulation of AGEs results in toxic effects. AGEs can directly damage the structure of extracellular matrix and change its physical, chemical, and metabolic properties. This happens through cross-linking, quench reactions of nitric oxide, lipoperoxidations or through AGE-specific receptors. AGE receptors (RAGE) are expressed on the surface of various cells such as monocytes, macrophage, mesangial cells, neurons, endothelial cells, smooth muscle cells, and fibroblasts. Following the interaction of AGEs with RAGE, signaling involving $P21^{ras}$, MAP kinase, and NF-κB are activated (219). This results in stimulation of transcription of genes for cytokines, growth factors (TNF, IL-1, PDGF, IGF-1, interferon), and adhesion molecules (ICAM-1, VCAM-1). Stimulation of cell proliferation, increase in vascular permeability, induction of migration of macrophages, stimulation of endothelin-1 formation, downregulation of thrombomodulin, increased synthesis of collagen, fibronectin, and proteoglycans, as well as procoagulant tissue factors ensue (219,220).

Thus, AGEs and ALEs are involved in the pathogenetic mechanisms leading to the complications of diabetes such as nephropathy, angiopathy, neuropathy, retinopathy, and renal failure. Even in nondiabetic conditions such as aging, atherosclerosis, dialysis-related amyloidosis, neurodegenerative diseases, osteoporosis, and rheumatoid arthritis, the increased formation of AGEs leads to complications (219). Hence, the design of drugs to inhibit the formation of AGEs and ALEs is a major challenge in the treatment of microvascular complications of chronic disease states such as diabetes and uremia. These inhibitors trap low molecular weight reactive intermediates of AGE and ALE formation.

Amino guanidine (AG) is the prototype AGE inhibitor (221). It has been shown to be effective in the abatement of a wide range of diabetic complications such as nephropathy, neuropathy, retinopathy, and vasculopathy in various animal models of diabetes. These positive effects are achieved without any effect on blood glucose concentration, indicating that AG acts as an inhibitor of advanced glycation reactions. In addition to the inhibition of AGE formation, AG has other effects such as both anti- and prooxidant effects on lipid peroxidation, chelation of redox-active mental ions, and inhibition of inducible nitric oxide synthase. These effects are independent of the formation of AGE. Clinical trials of AG indicate that the usefulness of AG is compromised by its hepatotoxicity. AG reacts with PLP and so, adversely affects vitamin B_6 metabolism (222).

In view of the toxicity of AG, the AGE inhibitory activity of analogs of vitamins such as thiamine and vitamin B_6, involved in the metabolism of carbonyl compounds, was examined. Thiamine pyrophosphate potently inhibited AGE formation and was more potent than AG. Pyridoxal and PLP competitively inhibit Schiff-base condensation of aldehydes with protein amino groups at glycation sites. PLP produced a stronger inhibition than AG (223).

Pyridoxamine (PM), a vitamer of vitamin B_6, is a potent scavenger of reactive carbonyls and inhibits the later stages of glycation reactions leading to AGE formation (224). In contrast to AG, PM is a more potent inhibitor of AGE formation from glycated proteins. Because it inhibits formation of AGE from Amadori-modified proteins, PM is referred to as a post-Amadori inhibitor of AGE formation (amadorin). PM also prevents protein modification by products of lipid peroxidation and thus, prevents formation of ALEs.

Various mechanisms of action of PM have been indicated (222). PM reacts with keto-aldehydes formed from glucose during Maillard reactions. PM also reacts with protein-bound dicarbonyl compounds that are formed from Amadori adducts and are the precursors of AGEs. PM cleaves α-dicarbonyl compounds and so, could be an AGE-breaker. It is an inhibitor of the chemical modification of proteins by polyunsaturated fatty acids.

In cell culture studies, both pyridoxamine and pyridoxine (which is not an inhibitor of AGE formation) decrease superoxide generation and protect red cells against oxidative stress. PM also protects against oxidative damage to DNA during the growth of umbilical vein endothelial cells in a high glucose medium (225).

PM has been shown to be a potent inhibitor of the development of renal disease in diabetic rats. It has positive effects on major microvascular lesions in diabetes such as retinopathy. PM provides protection against a wide range of pathologies associated with chronic diabetes, functioning, at least in part, as an inhibitor of AGE and ALE formation in vivo. The function of PM is not related to its role as a vitamin B_6 vitamer. PM, in combination therapy, might find a use in the treatment of a wide range of chronic diseases in which oxidative stress, inflammation, and tissue damage lead to an increase in chemical modification of proteins (222).

VITAMIN B_6—GENE EXPRESSION AND ANTICANCER EFFECT

In rats fed a diet adequate in vitamin B_6, the fraction of total PLP found in the nuclei of liver cells was 21% and this increased to 39% in rats fed a vitamin B_6-deficient diet indicating a conservation of the vitamin in the nuclear compartment during deficiency (226). This is analogous to the distribution of biotin in biotin-replete and biotin-deficient animals (227). PLP in the cell nucleus is protein bound and this protein has an apparent molecular mass of 50 to 55 kDa. Cells grown in the presence of 5 mM pyridoxine have a decreased glucocorticoid-dependent induction of enzymes such as tyrosine aminotransferase. Vitamin B_6 regulates transcriptional activation of human glucocorticoid receptors in the HeLa cells. The modulatory role in transcription is not restricted to the glucocorticoid receptor but extends to other members of the steroid hormone superfamily (228). The intracellular concentration of PLP could have a profound influence on steroid hormone-induced gene expression, with increased PLP levels resulting in a decreased transcriptional response to various steroid hormones and vice versa (229). The possibility of an interaction between vitamin B_6 and steroid hormone has been known for sometime. Kondo and Okada (230) found that the induction of aspartate aminotransferase in rat liver cytosol (cAspAT) of adrenalectomized vitamin B_6-deficient rats by hydrocortisone was suppressed by the administration of pyridoxine. Oka et al. (231) have reported that the level of cAspAT mRNA in the liver of vitamin B_6-deficient rats was several fold higher than that of controls. The administration of hydrocortisone induced the expression of hepatic cAspAT mRNA. This induction was suppressed by the simultaneous administration of pyridoxine. Using an oligonucleotide probe of glucocorticoid-response elements (GREs), the binding of nuclear extract to oligonucleotide was assessed. The binding of nuclear extracts prepared from liver of vitamin B_6-deficient rats was greater than that of control rats. The preincubation of nuclear extracts with PLP resulted in a significant decrease in the binding of the extract to GREs.

The level of steroid-induced gene expression from simple promoters containing only hormone response elements and a TATA sequence was not affected by changes in the vitamin B_6 status. However, the modulatory influence of vitamin B_6 status was restored when a binding site for a transcription factor, nuclear factor I (NFI) was included within the hormone-responsive promoter indicating that PLP modulates gene expression through its influence on a functional interaction between the steroid hormone receptors and transcription factor NFI (232).

A general increase in gene expression that includes housekeeping genes such as β-action is seen in livers of vitamin B_6-deficient rats. This has been ascribed to the activation of RNA polymerase II and I in the deficient liver. Among the vitamin B_6-independent proteins, the expression of the albumin gene is increased in vitamin B_6 deficiency. Serum albumin is the most abundant protein synthesized and secreted by the liver. The level of albumin mRNA in vitamin B_6-deficient rat livers was increased sevenfold over control levels (233). A 170 nucleotide region immediately upstream of the transcription initiation site of the albumin gene is sufficient for tissue-specific expression of this gene. This region contains various transcription factors such as HNF-1 and C/EBP. Oligonucleotides that interacted with HNF-1 and C/EBP were synthesized and the binding activity of liver nuclear extracts to each of these olignonucleotides was assessed. Binding activity of extracts prepared from vitamin B_6-deficient rat livers was greater than that prepared from vitamin B_6-replete rat livers. The lower binding activity of extracts from vitamin B_6-replete rat liver was suggested to be due to inactivation of tissue-specific factors by PLP. In further work (232), recombinant HNF-1 was produced in *E. coli* and the site of PLP binding in vitro was examined. PLP was bound to lysine 197 of HNF-1. Lysine 197 lies in the homeodomain of HNF-1. Hence PLP binding to this lysine residue renders the HNF-1 less accessible to the HNF-1 binding site of the albumin gene.

diSorbo et al. (234) reported that the growth of B_{16} melanoma in vitro was inhibited by 5 mM of pyridoxine or pyridoxal. Treatment of mice with 0.5 g pyridoxal per kilogram body weight reduced the growth of both new and established B_{16} melanoma. Topical administration of pyridoxal exhibited selective toxicity for melanoma and also resulted in the necrosis and regression of murine B_{16}-C_3 melanomas in mice (235,236). Pyridoxal supplementation was shown to reduce cell proliferation and DNA synthesis in estrogen-dependent and independent mammary carcinoma cell lines (237). Natori et al. (232) have shown that the growth of hepatoma HepG2 cells was inhibited by the addition of pyridoxine or pyridoxal to the culture medium. There was concurrent inhibition of protein synthesis and secretion of albumin. They also reported that the growth of MH-134 hepatoma cells, transplanted into C3H/He mice, was significantly reduced by the administration of large amounts of pyridoxine to mice. Other reports (235) indicate that vitamin B_6 suppressed azoxymethane-induced colon cancer. High dietary intake of vitamin B_6 has also been shown to suppress herpes simplex virus type 2 transformed (H-238) cell-induced tumor growth in BALB/c mice (238).

Epidemiological studies including the "Seven country study" indicate a reduced risk of lung and colorectal cancer in older men ingesting high doses of vitamin B_6 (239,240). An inverse relationship between vitamin B_6 status and incidence of prostate cancer has been reported. This relationship is supported by experimental work in mice (241). It has been suggested that inhibition of angiogenesis might be responsible for the anticancer effect of high doses of vitamin B_6. Vitamin B_6 was shown to suppress angiogenesis in a rat aortic ring angiogenesis model (242). Pyridoxal and PLP were shown to suppress human umbilical vein endothelial cell (HUVEC) proliferation without affecting HUVEC tube formation (243). Of the vitamin B_6 vitamers, PLP was reported to be a strong inhibitor of DNA polymerase α and ε from phylogenetically wide range of organisms from protists, plants, insects, and fish to mammals (244). These polymerase classes are related to DNA replication (245). Treatment with pharmacological doses of vitamin B_6 suppressed the expression of cell proliferation-related genes, c-*myc* and c-*fos*, in colon epithelium of mice treated with azoxymethane (241). PLP has also been shown to inhibit DNA topoisomerase I and II (246). DNA topoisomerase is ubiquitous and needed for strand separation, replication, and recombination. Inhibition of DNA topoisomerase arrests cell cycle and induces apoptosis (243). PLP has been shown to be an effective inhibitor of many enzymes that have binding sites for phosphate-containing substrates or effectors including RNA polymerase, reverse transcriptase, and DNA polymerase (247).

The preventive effects of vitamin B_6 on tumorigenesis might also derive from the strong antioxidant effect of vitamin B_6 (248). The expressions of c-*myc* and c-*fos* are induced by oxidative stress and suppressed by vitamin B_6 (249). Vitamin B_6 deficiency in animals on a high fat diet lends to increased lipid peroxidation (248). Nitric oxide (NO) plays an important role in colon carcinogenesis by elevating cyclooxygenase-2 and angiogenesis. The production of NO and the expression on iNOS mRNA are increased by oxidative stress and suppressed by pharmacological doses of vitamin B_6 (235). These observations highlight the potential use of pharmacological doses of vitamin B_6 in cancer therapy.

VITAMIN B_6 AND IMMUNITY

The early work of Stoerk and Eisen (250) and Axelrod et al. (251) was focused on the requirement of vitamin B_6 in antibody production. Over the years, the evidence for this connection has accumulated. The thymus of rats made vitamin B_6 deficient was depleted of lymphocytes and there was atrophy of lymph nodes. Thymic epithelial cells of moderately vitamin B_6-deficient rats were unable to induce maturation of lymphoid precursors from neonatally thymectomized donors. The T lymphocytes were reduced. Vitamin B_6 deficiency induced dietarily with or without a supplement of the antipyridoxine drug, deoxypyridoxine, resulted in impaired antibody formation following exposure to various antigens and this was associated with a reduction in the number of antibody-forming cells in the spleens of the deficient rats (252–254).

Cell-mediated immunity is also impaired in vitamin B_6-deficient rats. Thoracic duct lymphocytes from vitamin B_6-deficient rats had a decreased ability to respond in mixed lymphocyte culture and to incorporate uridine into DNA. The delayed type hypersensitivity (DTH) skin response is reduced in vitamin B_6-deficient animals. The rejection of a homologous transplant is due to cellular immune response of the recipient to antigens of the donor tissues. Immunosuppression is associated with depletion of vitamin B_6 and this facilitates induction of immune tolerance (255,256). Thus successful skin homografts could be achieved in vitamin B_6-deficient rats. Trakatellis et al. (256) have highlighted the role of serine hydroxymethyl transferase in this transplantation. Serine hydroxymethyl transferase has a significant role in the production of one-carbon units used in the syntheses of nucleotides and purines. Thus, in vitamin B_6 deficiency or when the enzyme is inhibited by antipyridoxine compounds such as deoxypyridoxine, the decreased production of one-carbon units impairs the synthesis of DNA, which is evident particularly in rapidly proliferating cells. They postulate that this metabolic impairment underlies the decreased humoral and cellular responses in the vitamin B_6-deficient state.

The effect of a supplement of vitamin B_6 on the development of tumors and on the in vitro response associated with cell-mediated immunity was assessed. It was found that peripheral blood and splenic lymphocyte proliferative responses to T-cell mitogens such as phytohemagglutinin and concanavalin A were higher in mice fed the highest levels of pyridoxine. High intake of vitamin B_6 also suppressed tumor development (235).

A decline in immune response is almost a concomitant of the aging process in animals and in humans, with the most significant effect on cell-mediated immunity, through a decrease in the number of T lymphocytes and also changes in T-cell surface receptors. The effect of pyridoxine supplements on lymphocyte responses in elderly persons was studied. Lymphocyte proliferative response to both T- and B-cell antigens was reduced. Lymphocyte subpopulations were augmented in the supplemented group and correlated with plasma PLP levels. Similar findings have been reported (257,258).

Macrophage activation by gram-negative bacterial endotoxin (lipopolysaccharide, LPS) is central to the mammalian inflammatory response to this agent. The expression of P2 purinergic receptors that bind extracellular adenine nucleotides has been shown to serve as markers of macrophage differentiation in response to LPS and various cytokines. P2X purinergic receptors participate in the nucleotide-induced modulation of LPS-stimulated inflammatory mediator production. Pretreatment of RAW 264.7 macrophages with a P2X receptor antagonist such as PPADS substantially inhibits LPS-stimulated functions such as NO production and iNOS expression (259). PPAPDS and PLP have similar biological activity.

Disease states such as uremia and arthritis are associated with immunological abnormalities. Treatment of uremic patients with pharmacologic doses of pyridoxine (260) resulted in a significant increase in lymphocyte reactivity in mixed lymphocyte cultures. Plasma PLP was found to be 50% lower in patients with rheumatoid arthritis than in controls matched for age, gender, race, and weight (261). All groups had similar intakes of the B vitamins. The plasma levels of PLP inversely correlated with production of tumor necrosis factor by unstimulated peripheral blood mononuclear cells.

Vitamin B_6 deficiency is widely prevalent among HIV-infected persons (262) despite an adequate dietary intake and quite often, supplementation with multivitamins. It is suggested that this might be related to the HIV-related enteropathy. The relationship of PLP to activation of CD4 T cells by antigen-presenting cells has been investigated. CD4 T cells are mediators in the initiation and continuation of the immune response causing autoimmune diseases and allogenic transplant rejection.

The CD4 glycoprotein is the characteristic surface receptor of all helper T cells. The extracellular part of CD4 molecules comprises four domains D1–D4. CD4 binds to MHC class II through the D1 and D2 domains. It has been shown that PLP binds very tightly to the D1 domain on CD4 (263) and thus interferes with the CD4–MHC II interaction. Nonincorporation of CD4 into the activation complex could lead to T-cell apoptosis. Further, the tight association of D1 and PLP would prevent protein–protein interaction of CD4 itself, its dimerization, or the interaction of the dimer with other molecules on the T-cell surface leading to apoptosis. PLP has been shown to be an anion-channel blocker in a variety of cells (264). It has been suggested (265) that PLP might have a role in the treatment of autoimmunity and in transplant rejection. In addition, as the interaction of HIV gp120 and CD4 occurs through the D1 domain, PLP may have an anti-HIV effect as well. High concentrations of PLP inhibit viral coat protein (envelope glycoprotein) binding and infection of $CD4^+$ T cells by isolates of HIV-1 in vitro (266). Thus PLP might function not only as an immune stimulator by increasing CD4 T-cell count but also protect uninfected CD4 T cells from infection by HIV-1 (267). These effects of PLP are seen at a concentration of 50–70 μM (266). At issue is the mechanism of increasing the tissue concentration of PLP to therapeutic levels. The rapid hydrolysis of PLP by tissue nonspecific alkaline phosphatase is a major problem. Levamisole (2,3,5,6-tetrahydro-b-phenylimidazo [2,1-b]thiazole), an antihelminthic drug, is an inhibitor of this enzyme (268). A combination of phosphatase inhibitor with high-ingested doses of pyridoxine might maintain the required high tissue concentrations of PLP to afford protection of uninfected CD4 T cells against HIV-1 (267). Further work along these lines is warranted.

TOXICITY OF PYRIDOXINE

Concern about the toxicity of pyridoxine was the result of the controversy associated with the use of Bendectin (doxylamine plus pyridoxine) by pregnant women and the subsequent occurrence of birth defects in some offsprings. Later studies have consistently ruled out any teratogenic effect of pyridoxine (269). Concerns about its toxicity resurfaced following reports of reversible sensory neuropathy in persons ingesting gram quantities of pyridoxine for long periods of time extending to years (270). The significant feature to note in these reports is that the reported sensory neuropathy is reversible, indicating no permanent structural damage to the nervous system. High doses of pyridoxine ingested for several years has been in vogue for a long time in the treatment of various clinical conditions, significant among them are homocysteinemia, pyridoxine-dependent convulsions, autism, and Down's syndrome (271,272). It is to be noted that pyridoxine administration up to 750 mg/day in patients homozygous for homocysteinemia treated up to 24 years has been safe without any report of sensory neuropathy (273). There has been no report of adverse effects associated with these treatments. An assessment of available clinical data attests to the general low toxicity of pyridoxine. Bendich and Cohen (274) conclude that doses of 500 mg/day of pyridoxine for up to 2 years are not associated with neuropathy whereas doses about 1000 mg/day for variable periods of time might be been associated with neuropathy. There is no report of permanent damage to the nervous system following ingestion of large doses of pyridoxine over long time periods, as the reported neuropathy is reversible following withdrawal of the pyridoxine supplement.

CONCLUDING REMARKS

The diversity of the chemical reactions involving vitamin B_6 is because of the participation of PLP in determining the three-dimensional structure of PLP-dependent enzymes as well as in determining the sites of elimination and replacement of substituents. Apart from its role in phospholipid metabolism through the synthesis of sphingosine and in glycogen metabolism through its structural role in glycogen phosphorylase, PLP participates in the metabolism of amino acids. The formation of monoamine neurotransmitters through PLP-dependent decarboxylation of the precursors highlights the role of vitamin B_6 in the function of the nervous system. There is a range in the affinity of PLP to the apodecarboxylases with the result that during mild or moderate vitamin B_6 deficiency, the formation of some monoamine neurotransmitters is impaired whereas those of others are not. Thus, the nonparallel effect on monoamine neurotransmitter syntheses leads to significant alterations in the function of neuro and neuroendocrine systems. A moderate depletion of vitamin B_6 is characterized by significant decreases in the synthesis and secretion of GABA and serotonin with no change in the catecholamines. In addition, even under conditions not associated with a depletion of vitamin B_6, administration of pyridoxine to animals results in the augmented synthesis of some neurotransmitters, with significant biological effects. PLP also has significant effects on calcium transport, both through the voltage-dependent and the ATP-dependent pathways. As calcium is at the center of much metabolic regulation, this results in wide-ranging effects in the functioning of the organism. Here again, the administration of pyridoxine to animals, not associated with a vitamin-depleted state, have significant calcium-mediated biological effects indicating a continuum of effects of pyridoxine administration. It is to be noted that ingestion of very high doses of pyridoxine does not have irreversible toxic effects. The associated neuropathy is reversed on withdrawal of the huge supplement. The beneficial effects of a supplement of pyridoxine (vitamin B_6) on the nervous and cardiovascular systems and related disease processes and the protection afforded by pyridoxine under these conditions need further study.

Apart from its cofactor role, the affinity of PLP to diverse proteins is at the center of its noncofactor biological role. PLP modulates gene expression through its influence on the interaction between steroid hormone receptors and the corresponding transcription factors. PLP binding to tissue-specific transcription factors makes them less accessible to their binding site on the target gene. The binding of PLP to the D1 domain of CD4 glycoprotein surface receptors of helper T cells seems to regulate cell-mediated immunity. The binding of PLP to cell surface calcium transport systems such as the L-type and the ATP-mediated calcium channels is the basis of cellular calcium changes mediated by PLP. The study of the mechanism of these protein–PLP interactions should provide valuable information and newer approaches to the therapeutic potential of PLP-related compounds.

REFERENCES

1. P. Gyorgy, Vitamin B_2 and the pellagra-like dermatitis of rats. *Nature*, 133: 448–449 (1934).
2. P. Gyorgy, Crystalline vitamin B_6. *J. Am. Chem. Soc.*, 60: 983–984 (1938).
3. S. Lepkovsky, Crystalline factor 1. *Science* 87: 169–170 (1938).
4. S.A. Harris and K. Folkers, Synthesis of vitamin B_6. *J. Am Chem. Soc.*, 61: 1245–1247 (1939).
5. R. Kuhn, K. Westphal, G. Wendt, and O. Westphal, Synthesis of adermin. *Naturewissenschaften* 27: 469–470 (1939).
6. D.B. McCormick and E.E. Snell, Pyridoxal kinase of human brain and its inhibition by hydrazine derivatives. *Proc. Natl. Acad. Sci., USA* 45: 1371–1379 (1959).
7. D.B. McCormick and E.E. Snell, Pyridoxal phosphokinase II. Effects of inhibitors. *J. Biol. Chem.*, 236: 2085–2088 (1961).
8. D.B. McCormick and H. Chen, Update on interconversions of vitamin B_6 with its coenzyme. *J. Nutr.*, 129: 325–327 (1999).
9. D.B. McCormick, Biochemistry of coenzymes. In: *Encyclopedia of Molecular Biology and Molecular Medicine* (R.A. Meyers, ed.), Vol. 1, pp. 396–406, VCH, Weinheim, Germany (1996).
10. D.B. McCormick, B.M. Guirard, and E.E. Snell, Comparative inhibition of pyridoxal kinase and glutamic acid decarboxylase by carbonyl reagents. *Proc. Soc. Exp. Biol. Med.*, 104: 554–557 (1960).
11. M.C. Hanna, A. Turner, and E.F. Kirkness, Human pyridoxal kinase. cDNA cloning, expression and modulation by ligands of the benzodiazepine receptor. *J. Biol. Chem.*, 272: 10756–10760 (1997).
12. H. Wada and E.E. Snell, The enzymatic oxidation of pyridoxine and pyridoxamine phosphates. *J. Biol. Chem.*, 236: 2089–2095 (1961).
13. M.N. Kazarinoff and D.B. McCormick, Rabbit liver pyridoxamine (pyridoxine) 5′-phosphate oxidase. Purification and properties. *J. Biol. Chem.*, 250: 3436–3442 (1975).
14. D.B. McCormick and A.H. Merrill, Jr., Pyridoxamine (pyridoxine) phosphate oxidase. In: *Vitamin B_6 Metabolism and Role in Growth* (H.P. Tryfiates, ed.), pp. 1–26, Food and Nutrition Press, Westpoint, CT (1980).
15. B.B. Bowman and D.B. McCormick, Pyridoxine uptake by rat renal proximal tubular cells. *J. Nutr.*, 119: 745–749 (1989).
16. G. Zhao and M.E. Winkler, 4-Phospho-hydroxy-L-threonine is an obligatory intermediate in pyridoxal 5′-phosphate coenzyme biosynthesis in *Escherichia coli* K-12. *FEMS Microbiol. Lett.*, 135: 275–280 (1996).
17. Y.H. Loo, Levels of B_6 vitamins and of pyridoxal phosphokinase in rat brain during maturation. *J. Neurochem.*, 19: 1835–1837 (1972).
18. H.G. Tiselius, Metabolism of tritium-labelled pyridoxine and pyridoxine 5′-phostphate in central nervous system. *J. Neurochem.*, 20: 937–946 (1973).

19. K. Dakshinamurti, B Vitamins and nervous system function. In: *Nutrition and the Brain* (R.J. Wurtman and J.J. Wurtman, eds.), pp. 249–318, Raven Press, New York (1977).
20. C.J. Chern and E. Beutler, Pyridoxal kinase: decreased activity in red blood cells of Afro-Americans. *Science*, 187: 1084–1086 (1975).
21. M.S. Ebadi, E.E. McCoy, and R.B. Kugel, Interrelationships between the activity of pyridoxal kinase and the level of biogenic amines in rabbit brain. *J. Neurochem.*, 15: 659–665 (1968).
22. J.T. Neary, R.L. Meneely, M.R. Grever, and W.F. Diven, The interaction between biogenic amines and pyridoxal, pyridoxal phosphate and pyridoxal kinase. *Arch. Biochem. Biophys.*, 151: 42–47 (1972).
23. T.K. Li and L. Lumeng, Regulation of hepatic pyridoxal phosphate content: a role of alkaline phosphatase. *Fed. Proc.*, 33: 1546 (1974).
24. P. Christen and P.K. Mehta, From cofactor to enzymes. The molecular evolution of pyridoxal-5′-phosphate-dependent enzymes. *Chem. Rec.*, 1: 436–447 (2001).
25. D.I. Leussing, Model reactions. In: *Coenzymes and Cofactors*, Vol. 1. Vitamin B_6 Pyridoxal Phosphate (D. Dolphin, R. Poulson, and O. Avramovic, eds.), pp. 69–115, John Wiley & Sons, New York (1986).
26. A.C. Eliot and J.F. Kirsch, Pyridoxal phosphate enzymes: Mechanistic, structural and evolutionary considerations. *Annu. Rev. Biochem.*, 73: 383–415 (2004).
27. C.F. Cori and B. Illingworth, The prosthetic group of phosphorylase. *Proc. Natl. Acad. Sci., USA* 43: 547–552 (1957).
28. E.H. Fischer, A.B. Kent, E.R. Snyder, and E.G. Krebs, The reaction of sodium borohydride with muscle phosphorylase. *J. Am. Chem. Soc.*, 80: 2906–2907 (1958).
28a. E.J.M. Helmreich., How pyridoxal 5′-phosphate could function in glycogen phosphorylase catalysis. *BioFactors*, 3: 159–172 (1992).
29. J.L. Hedrick, The role of pyridoxal 5′-phosphate in the structure and function of glycogen phosphorylase. *Adv. Biochem. Psychopharmacol.*, 4: 23–27 (1972).
29a. N.B. Livanova, N.A. Chebotareva, T.B. Eronina, and B.I. Kurganov, Pyridoxal 5′-phosphate as a catalytic and conformational cofactor of muscle glycogen phosphorylase b. *Biochemistry (Moscow)*, 67: 1089–1098 (2002).
30. C.A. Storvick, E.M. Benson, M.A. Edwards, and M.J. Woodring, Chemical and microbiological determination of vitamin B_6. *Methods Biochem. Anal.*, 12: 183.
31. M. Polansky, Microbiological assay of vitamin B_6 in foods. In: *Methods in Vitamin B_6 Nutrition* (J.E. Leklem and R.D. Reynolds, eds.), pp. 21–44, Plenum Press, New York (1981).
32. K. Dakshinamurti and M.C. Stephens, Pyridoxine deficiency in the neonate rat. *J. Neurochem.*, 16: 1515–1522 (1969).
33. J.F. Gregory, Methods for determination of vitamin B_6 in foods and other biological materials: a critical review. *J. Food Comp. Anal.*, 1: 105–123 (1988).
34. K. Tadera and Y. Naka, Isocratic paired-ion high-performance liquid chromatographic method to determine B_6 vitamers and pyridoxine glucoside in food. *Agric. Biol. Chem.*, 55: 562–564 (1991).
35. S.K. Sharma and K. Dakshinamurti, Determination of vitamin B_6 vitamers and pyridoxic acid in biological samples. *J. Chromatography*, 578: 45–51 (1992).
36. K. Yasumoto, H. Tsuji, K. Iwanii, and H. Metsuda, Isolation from rice bran of a bound form of vitamin B_6 and its identification as 5′-*O*-(β-D-glucopyranosyl) pyridoxine. *Agric. Biol. Chem.*, 41: 1061–1067 (1977).
37. K. Tadera, E. Mori, F. Yagi, A. Kobayashi, K. Imada, and M. Imabeppu, Isolation and structure of a minor metabolite of pyridoxine in seedling of *Pisum sativwri* L. *J. Nutri. Sci. Vitaminol.*, 31: 403–408 (1985).
38. J.E. Leklem, Vitamin B_6. In: *Handbook of Vitamins*, 3rd Edition (R.B. Rucker, J.W. Suttie, D.B. McCormick, and L.J. Machlin, eds.), pp. 339–396, Marcel Dekker, New York (2001).
39. D.B. Coursin, Convulsive seizures in infants with pyridoxine-deficient diet. *JAMA*, 154: 406–408 (1954).
40. H.M. Middleton, Uptake of pyridoxine by in vivo perfused segments of rat small intestine: a possible role for intracellular vitamin metabolism. *J. Nutr.*, 115: 1079–1088 (1985).
41. J.F. Gregory, P.R. Trumbo, and L.B. Bailey, Bioavailability of pyridoxine 5′-β-D-glucoside determined in humans by stable-isotope methods. *J. Nutr.*, 121: 177–186 (1991).

42. H.M. Said, Recent advances in carrier-mediated intestinal absorption of water-soluble vitamins. *Annu. Rev. Physiol.*, 66: 419–446 (2004).
43. J. Zempleni and W. Kubler, The utilization of intravenously infused pyridoxine in humans. *Clin. Chim. Acta*, 229: 27–36 (1994).
44. L.R. Solomon, Vitamin B_6 metabolism in human red cells: limitation in cofactor activities of pyridoxal and pyridoxal 5′-phosphate. *Enzyme* 28: 242–250 (1982).
45. E.G. Krebs and E.H. Fischer, Phosphorylase and related enzymes of glycogen metabolism. *Vitam. Horm.*, 22: 399–410 (1964).
46. N. Katunama, Enzyme degradation products and its regulation by group-specific proteases in various organs of rats. *Curr. Top. Cell Regul.*, 8: 175–203 (1973).
47. A.L. Black, B.M. Guirard, and E.E. Snell, Increased muscle phosphorylase in rats fed high levels of vitamin B_6. *J. Nutr.*, 107: 1962–1968 (1977).
48. A.L. Black, B.M. Guirard, and E.E. Snell, The behavior of muscle phosphorylase as a reservoir for vitamin B_6 in the rat. *J. Nutr.*, 108: 670–677 (1978).
49. H. Kishi, T. Kishi, R.H. Williams, and K. Folkers, Human deficiencies of vitamin B_6. I. Studies on parameters of the assay of glutamic oxaloacetic transaminase by the CAS principle. *Res. Commun. Chem. Pathol. Pharmacol.*, 12: 557–569 (1975).
50. J.G. Canham, E.M. Baker, R.S. Harding, H.E. Sauberlich, and I.C. Plaugh, Dietary protein: its relationship to vitamin B_6 requirement and function. *Ann. N.Y. Acad. Sci.*, 166: 16–29 (1968).
51. W.W. Coon and E. Nagler, The tryptophan load as a test for pyridoxine deficiency in hospitalized patients. *Ann. N.Y. Acad. Sci.*, 166: 29–43 (1968).
52. H.M. Linkswiler, Methionine metabolite excretion as affected by a vitamin B_6 deficiency. In: *Methods in Vitamin B_6 Nutrition* (J.E. Leklem and R.D. Reynolds, eds.), pp. 373–381, Plenum Press, New York (1981).
53. L.T. Miller, J.E. Leklem, and T.D. Shultz, The effect of dietary protein on the metabolism of vitamin B_6 in humans. *J. Nutr.*, 115: 1663–1672 (1985).
54. J.D. Ribaya-Mercado, R.M. Russel, N. Sahyoun, F.D. Morrow, and S.N. Gershoff, Vitamin B_6 requirements of elderly men and women. *J. Nutr.*, 121: 1062–1074 (1991).
55. M.J. Kretsch, H.E. Sauberlich, J.H. Skala, and H.L. Johnson, Vitamin B_6 requirement and status assessment: young women fed a depletion diet followed by plant-or-animal-protein diet with graded amounts of vitamin B_6. *Am. J. Clin. Nutr.*, 61: 1091–1101 (1995).
56. Y.C. Huang, W. Chan, M.A. Evans, M.E. Mitchell, and T.D. Shultz, Vitamin B_6 requirement and status assessment of young women fed a high-protein diet with various levels of vitamin B_6. *Am. J. Clin. Nutr.*, 67: 208–220 (1998).
57. J.W. Harris and D.L. Horrigan, Pyridoxine-responsive anemia-prototype and variations on the theme. *Vitam. Horm.*, 22: 721–753 (1964).
58. C.L. Gries and M.L. Scott, The pathology of pyridoxine deficiency in chicks. *J. Nutr.*, 102: 1259–1267 (1972).
59. D.B. Tower, Neurochemical aspects of pyridoxine metabolism and function. *Am. J. Clin. Nutr.*, 4: 329–345 (1956).
60. S.E. Snyderman, L.E. Holt, Jr., R. Carretero, and K. Jacobs, Pyridoxine deficiency in the human infant. *Am. J. Clin. Nutr.*, 1: 200–207 (1953).
61. M. Wachstein and A. Gudaitis, Disturbance of vitamin B_6 metabolism in pregnancy. III Abnormal vitamin B_6 load test. *Am. J. Obstet. Gynecol.*, 62: 1207–1213 (1953).
62. S.F. Contractor and B. Shane, Blood and urine levels of vitamin B_6 in the mother and fetus before and after loading of the mother with vitamin B_6. *Am. J. Obstet. Gynecol.*, 107: 635–640 (1970).
63. S. Heller, R.M. Salkeld, and W.F. Korner, Vitamin B_6 status in pregnancy. *Am. J. Clin. Nutr.*, 26: 1339–1348 (1973).
64. A. Hamfelt and T. Tuvemo, Pyridoxal phosphate and folic acid concentration in blood and erythrocyte aspartate aminotransferase activity during pregnancy. *Clin. Chem. Acta*, 41: 287–298 (1972).
65. R.E. Cleary, L. Lumeng, and T.K. Li, Maternal and fetal plasma levels of pyridoxal phosphate at term: adequacy of vitamin B_6 supplementation during pregnancy. *Am. J. Obstet. Gynecol.*, 121: 25–28 (1975).

66. L. Reinken and B. Mangold, Pyridoxal phosphate values in premature infants. *Int. J. Vitam. Nutr. Res.*, 43: 472–478 (1973).
67. L. Reinken and H. Gart, Vitamin B_6 nutrition in women with hyperemesis gravidarum during the first trimester of pregnancy. *Clin. Chem. Acta*, 55: 101–102 (1974).
68. H.W.F. Dobbelstein, W. Korner, H. Mempel, W. Grosse, and H.H. Edel, Vitamin B_6 deficiency in uremia and its implications for the depression of immune response. *Kidney Int.*, 5: 233–239 (1974).
69. M.E. Visser, C. Texeira-Swiegelaar, and G. Maartens, The short-term effects of anti-tuberculosis therapy on plasma pyridoxine levels in patients with pulmonary tuberculosis. *Int. J. Tuberc. Lung Dis.*, 8: 260–262 (2004).
70. M.A. Castellano, J.L. Tortora, N.I. Geronimo, F. Rama, and C. Ohanian, The effects of isonicotinic acid hydrazide on the early chick embryo. *J. Embryol. Exp. Morphol.*, 29: 209–219 (1973).
71. A.A. Cohen, Pyridoxine in the prevention and treatment of convulsions and neurotoxicity due to cycloserine. *Ann. N.Y. Acad. Sci.*, 166: 346–349 (1968).
72. D.B. Smith and B.B. Gallagher, The effect of penicillamine on seizure threshold: the role of pyridoxine. *Arch. Neurol.*, 23: 59–62 (1970).
73. J.G. Christenson, W. Dairman, and S. Undenfriend, On the identity of DOPA decarboxylase and 5-hydroxytryptophan decarboxylase. *Proc. Natl. Acad. Sci., USA* 69: 343–347 (1972).
74. M.H. Ando-Yamamoto, Y. Hayashi, H. Taguchi, T. Fukui, T. Watanabe, and H. Wada, Demonstration of immunohistochemical cross-reactivity of L-histidine and L-DOPA decarboxylase using antibodies against the two enzymes. *Biochem. Biophys. Res. Commun.*, 141: 306–312 (1986).
75. V.A. Albert, J.M. Allen, and T.H. Joh, A single gene codes for aromatic L-amino-acid decarboxylase in both neural and non-neural tissues. *J. Biol. Chem.*, 262: 9404–9411 (1987).
76. K.L. Sims, G.A. Davis, and F.F. Bloom, Activities of 3,4-dihydroxy-L-phenylalanine and 5-hydroxy-L-tryptophan decarboxylases in rat brain: assay characteristics and distribution. *J. Neurochem.*, 20: 449–464 (1973).
77. Y.L. Siow and K. Dakshinamurti, Effect of pyridoxine deficiency on aromatic L-amino acid decarboxylase in adult rat brain. *Exp. Brain Res.*, 59: 575–581 (1985).
78. Y.L. Siow and K. Dakshinamurti, Effect of 1-methyl-4-phenyl-1,2,3,6-tetrahydrophyridine and 1-methyl-4-phenyl-pyridinium on aromatic L-amino acid decarboxylase in rat brain. *Biochem. Pharmacol.*, 35: 2640–2641 (1986).
79. K. Dakshinamurti, W.D. Leblancq, R. Herchl, and V. Havlicek, Nonparallel changes in brain monoamines of pyridoxine-deficient growing rats. *Exp. Brain Res.*, 26: 355–366 (1976).
80. Y.L. Siow and K. Dakshinamurti, Neuronal DOPA decarboxylase. *Ann. N.Y. Acad. Sci.*, 585: 173–188 (1990).
81. L.K.Y. Ng, T.N. Chase, R.W. Colburn, and I.J. Kopin, A possible mechanism of action. *Neurology (Minneap)*, 22: 688–696 (1972).
82. K.L. Sims and F.E. Bloom, Rat brain L-3,4-dihydroxy-phenylalanine and L-5-hydroxy tryptophan decarboxylase activities: differential effects of 6-hydroxydopamine. *Brain Res.*, 49: 165–175 (1973).
83. S. Bouchard, C. Bousquet, and A.G. Roberge. Characteristics of dihydroxy phenylalanine/5-hydroxy tryptophan decarboxylase activity in brain and liver of the cat. *J. Neurochem.*, 37: 781–787 (1981).
84. D.A. Bender and W.F. Coulson, Variation in aromatic amino acid decarboxylase activity toward DOPA and 5-hydroxy tryptophan caused by pH changes and denaturation. *J. Neurochem.*, 19: 2801–2810 (1972).
85. M.J. Jung, J.M. Horsperger, F. Gerhart, and J. Wagner, Inhibition of aromatic amino acid decarboxylase and depletion of biogenic amines in brain of rats treated with α-monofluoromethyl *p*-tyrosine: similitudes and differences with the effect of α-monofluoromethyl dopa. *Biochem. Pharmacol.*, 33: 327–330 (1984).
86. C. Borri-Voltattorni, A. Minelli, P. Vecchini, A. Fiori, and C. Turano, Purification and characterization of L-3,4-dihydroxy-phenylalanine decarboxylase from pig kidney. *Eur. J. Biochem.*, 93: 181–188 (1979).
87. P. Poulikako, D. Vassilacopoulou, and E.G. Fragoulis, L-Dopa decarboxylase: association with membranes in mouse brain. *Neurochem. Res.*, 26: 479–485 (2001).

88. J.W. Jahng, T.C. Wessel, T.A. Houpt, J.H. Sin, and T.H. Joh, Alternate promoters in the rat aromatic L-amino acid decarboxylase gene for neuronal and nonneuronal expression: an in situ hybridization study. *J. Neurochem.*, 66: 14–19 (1996).
89. C. Sumi-Ichinose, S. Hasegawa, H. Ichinose, H. Sawada, K. Kobayashi, M. Saki, T. Fujii, H. Nomura, T. Nomura, I. Nagatsu, Y. Hagino, K. Fujita, and T. Nagatsu, Analysis of the alternate promoters that regulate tissue-specific expression of human aromatic L-amino acid decarboxylase. *J. Neurochem.*, 64: 514–524 (1995).
90. S.P. Craig, A.L. Thai, N. Weber, and J.W. Craig, Localization of the gene for human aromatic L-amino acid decarboxylase (DDC) to chromosome 7p13–p11 by in situ hybridization. Cytogenet. *Cell Genet.*, 61: 114–116 (1992).
91. K.L. O'Malley, S. Harmon, M. Moffat, A. Vhland-Smith, and S. Wong, The human aromatic L-amino acid decarboxylase gene can be alternatively spliced to generate unique protein isoforms. *J. Neurochem.*, 65: 2409–2416 (1995).
92. Y.T. Chang, G. Mues, and K. Hyland, Alternative splicing in the coding region of human aromatic L-aminoacid decarboxylase mRNA. *Neurosci. Lett.*, 202: 157–160 (1996).
93. M.-Z. Siaterli, D. Vassilacopoulou, and E.G. Fragoulis, Cloning, and expression of human placental L-Dopa decarboxylase. *Neurochem. Res.*, 28: 797–803 (2003).
94. C.S. Paulose, and K. Dakshinamurti, Effect of pyridoxine deficiency in young rats on high-affinity serotonin and dopamine receptors. *J. Neurosci. Res.*, 12: 263–270 (1985).
95. K. Krnjevic, and S. Schwartz, The action of γ-aminobutyric acid on cortical neurons. *Exp. Brain Res.*, 3: 320–336 (1967).
96. E. Roberts, and K. Kuriyama, Biochemical–physiological correlations in studies of the γ-aminobutyric acid system. *Brain Res.*, 8: 1–35 (1968).
97. H.H. Jasper, R.T. Khan, and K.A.C. Elliott, Amino acids released from the cerebral cortex in relation to its state of activation. *Science*, 147: 1448–1449 (1965).
98. R. Tapia and H. Pasantees, Relationships between pyridoxal phosphate availability, activity of vitamin B_6-dependent enzymes and convulsions. *Brain Res.*, 29: 111–112 (1971).
99. J.-J. Soghomonian and D.L. Martin, Two isoforms of glutamate decarboxylase: why? *Trends Pharmacol. Sci.*, 19: 500–505 (1998).
100. D.L. Martin and K. Rimvall, Regulation of γ-aminobutyric acid synthesis in the brain. *J. Neurochem.*, 60: 395–407 (1993).
101. K. Dakshinamurti, Neurobiology of pyridoxine. In: *Advances in Nutrition Research* (H.H. Draper, ed.), Vol. 4, pp. 143–179, Plenum Press, New York (1982).
102. K. Dakshinamurti, C.S. Paulose, M. Viswanathan, and Y.L. Siow, Neuroendocrinology of pyridoxine deficiency. *Neurosci. Biobehav. Rev.*, 12: 189–193 (1988).
103. D. Jordan, C. Poncet, R. Monex, and G. Ponsin, Participation of serotonin in thyrotropin release. I. Evidence for the action of serotonin on thyrotropin releasing hormone release. *Endocrinology*, 103: 414–419 (1978).
104. Y.F. Chen and V.D. Ramire. Serotonin stimulates thyrotropin-releasing hormone release from superfused rat hypothalami. *Endocrinology*, 108: 2359–2366 (1981).
105. G.A. Smythe, J.E. Bradshaw, C.Y. Cai, and R.J. Simons, Hypothalamic serotonergic stimulation of thyrotropin secretion and related brain-hormone and drug interactions in the rat. *Endocrinology*, 111: 1181–1191 (1982).
106. P. Mannisto, T. Ranta, and J. Tuomisto, Dual action of adrenergic system on the regulation of thyrotropin secretion in the male rat. *Acta Endocrinol.* (Copenhagen) 90: 249–258 (1979).
107. K. Dakshinamurti, C.S. Paulose, and J. Vriend, Thyroid function in pyridoxine-deficient young rats. *J. Endocrinol.*, 104: 339–349 (1985).
108. K. Dakshinamurti, C.S. Paulose, and J. Vriend, Hypothyroidism of hypothalamic origin in pyridoxine-deficient rats. *J. Endocrinol.*, 109: 345–349 (1986).
109. M. Viswanathan, Y.L. Siow, C S. Paulose, and K. Dakshinamurti, Pineal indoleamine metabolism in pyridoxine-deficient rats. *Brain Res.*, 473: 37–42 (1988).
110. J.P. Prolock, The pineal gland: basic implications and clinical correlations. *Endocrinol. Rev.*, 5: 282–308 (1984).
111. A.R. Smith and J.A. Kapper, Effect of pinealectomy, gonadectomy, pCPA and pineal extracts on rat-parvocellular neurosecretory hypothalamic system, a fluorescence histochemical investigation. *Brain Res.*, 86: 353–371 (1975).

112. S.K. Sharma and K. Dakshinamurti, Effects of serotonergic agents on plasma prolactin levels in pyridoxine-deficient adult male rats. *Neurochem. Res.*, 19: 687–692 (1994).
113. L.D. Van de Kar, Neuroendocrine pharmacolocy of serotonergic neurons. *Ann. Rev. Pharmacol. Toxicol.*, 31: 289–320 (1991).
114. J. Cravito and E. Delicardie, Micro environmental factors in severe protein-caloric malnutrition. *Basic Life Sci.*, 7: 25–35 (1976).
115. E. Eberle and S. Eiduson, Effect of pyridoxine deficiency on aromatic L-amino acid decarboxylase in the developing rat liver and brain. *J. Neurochem.*, 15: 1071–1083 (1968).
116. A.N. Davidson and J. Dobbin, Myelination as a vulnerable period in brain development. *Brit. Med. Bull.*, 22: 40–44 (1966).
117. M.C. Stephens, V. Havlicek, and K. Dakshinamurti, Pyridoxine deficiency and development of the central nervous system in the rat. *J. Neurochem.*, 18: 2407–2416 (1971).
118. C.S. Paulose and K. Dakshinamurti, Enhancement of high affinity γ-amino butyric acid receptor binding in cerebellum of pyridoxine-deficient rat. *Neurosci. Lett.*, 48: 311–316 (1984).
119. S.K. Sharma and K. Dakshinamurti, Seizure activity in pyridoxine-deficient adult rats. *Epilepsia*, 33: 235–247 (1992).
120. K. Dakshinamurti, S.K. Sharma, and K.J. Lal, Pyridoxine deficiency: animal model for CNS serotonin and GABA depletion. In: *Neuromethods, V22: Animal Models of Neurological Disease* (A. Boulton, G. Baker, and R. Butterworth, eds.), pp. 299–327, The Humani Press, New York (1992).
121. S.K. Sharma, B. Bolster, and K. Dakshinamurti, Picrotoxin and pentylene tetrazole induces seizure activity in pyridoxine-deficient rats. *J. Neurolog. Sci.*, 121: 1–9 (1994).
122. M. Hiramatsu, R. Edamatsu, H. Kabuto, Y. Higashihare, and A. Mori, Increased seizure susceptibility induced by guanidino-ethane sulfonate in E I mice and its relation to glutamatergic neurons. *Neurochem. Res.*, 14: 85–89 (1989).
123. R.J. Lee, A. Depaulis, P. Loamx, and R.W. Olsen, Anticonvulsive effects of muscimol injected into the thalamus of spontaneously epileptic Mongolian gerbils. *Brain Res.*, 487: 363–367 (1989).
124. B.S. Meldrum, GABA-ergic mechanisms in the pathogenesis and treatment of epilepsy. *Br. J. Clin. Pharmacol.*, 27: 3S–11S (1989).
125. J.S. Teitelbaum, R.J. Zatorre, S. Carpenter, D. Gendron, A.C. Evans, A. Gjedde, and N.R. Cashman, Neurologic sequelae of domoic acid intoxication due to ingestion of contaminated mussels. *N. Engl. J. Med.*, 322: 1781–1787 (1990).
126. G. Sperk, H. Lassman, and H. Barn, Kainic acid induced seizures: neurochemical and histopathological changes. *Neuroscience* 10: 1301–1315 (1983).
127. K. Dakshinamurti, S.K. Sharma, and M. Sundaram, Domoic acid induced seizures activity in rats. *Neurosci. Lett.*, 127: 193–197 (1991).
128. S.M. Strain and R.A.R. Tasker, Hippocampal damage produced by systemic injections of domoic acid in mice. *Neuroscience* 44: 343–352 (1991).
129. S.K. Sharma and K. Dakshinamurti, Suppression of domoic acid-induced seizures by 8-(OH)-DPAT. *J. Neural Transm.*, 93: 87–98 (1993).
130. K. Dakshinamurti, S.K. Sharma, M. Sundaram, and T. Watanabe, Hippocampal changes in developing postnatal mice following intrauterine exposure to domoic acid. *J. Neurosci.* 13: 4486–4495 (1993).
131. K. Dakshinamurti, S.K. Sharma, and J.D. Geiger, Neuroprotective actions of pyridoxine. *Biochim. Biophys. Acta*, 1647: 225–229 (2003).
132. A.D. Hunt, J. Stokes, M.D. Wallace, W. McCrory, and H.H. Stroud, Pyridoxine dependency: report of a case of intractable convulsions in an infant controlled by pyridoxine. *Pediatrics* 13: 140–145 (1954).
133. S.M. Gospe, Jr., Pyridoxine-dependent seizures: findings from recent studies pose new question. *Pediatr. Neurol.*, 26: 181–185 (2002).
134. M. Bejsovec, Z. Kulenda, and E. Ponca, Familial intrauterine convulsions in pyridoxine dependency. *Arch. Dis. Child.*, 42: 201–207 (1967).
135. S.M. Gospe, Jr. and S.T. Hecht, Longitudinal MRI findings in pyridoxine-dependent seizures. *Neurology*, 51: 74–78 (1998).
136. A. Sigirci, I. Orkan, and C. Yakinci, Pyridoxine-dependent seizures: magnetic resonance spectroscopy findings. *J. Child. Neurol.*, 19: 75–78 (2004).

137. A. Alkan, K. Sarac, and R. Kutlu, Early and late state subacute sclerosing panencephalitis: chemical shift imagining and single voxel MR spectroscopy. *Am. J. Neuroradiol.*, 24: 501–506 (2003).
138. I.T. Lott, T. Coulombe, and R.V. DiPaolo, Vitamin B_6-dependent seizures: pathology and chemical findings in brain. *Neurology*, 28: 47–54 (1978).
139. P. Baxter, Pyridoxine-dependent seizures: a clinical and biochemical conundrum. *Biochim. Biophys. Acta*, 1647: 36–41 (2003).
140. G. Kurlemann, R. Ziegler, and M. Grunelberg, Disturbance of GABA metabolism in pyridoxine-dependent seizures. *Neuropediatrics*, 23: 257–259 (1992).
141. A. Kelly and C.A. Stanley, Disorders of glutamate metabolism, *MRDD Res. Rev.*, 7: 287–295 (2001).
142. S.M. Gospe, Jr., Current perspectives on pyridoxine-dependent seizures. *J. Pediatr.*, 132: 919–923 (1998).
143. S. Kure, J. Sakata, and S. Miyabashi, Mutation and polymorphic marker anaylsis of 65K- and 67K-glutamate decarboxylase genes in two families with pyridoxine-dependent epilepsy. *J. Hum. Genet.*, 43: 128–131 (1998).
144. G. Battaglioli, D.R. Rosen, S.M. Gospe, Jr., and D.L. Martin, Glutamate decarboxylase is not genetically linked to pyridoxine-dependent seizures. *Neurology*, 55: 309–311 (2000).
145. V. Cormier-Daire, N. Dagoneua, and R. Nabbout, A gene for pyridoxine-dependent epilepsy maps to chromosome 5q31. *Am. J. Hum. Genet.*, 67: 991–993 (2000).
146. B. Plecko, S. Stockler-Ipsiroglu, E. Paske, W. Erwa, E.A. Struys, and C. Jacobs, Pipecolic acid elevation in plasma and cerebrospinal fluid of two patients with pyridoxine-dependent epilepsy. *Ann. Neurol.*, 48: 121–125 (2000).
147. J.M. Pellock, The classification of childhood seizures and epilepsy syndromes. *Neurol. Clin.*, 8: 619–631 (1990).
148. M.A. Mikati, G.A. Lepejian, and G.L. Holmes, Medical treatment of patients with infantile spasms. *Clin. Neuropharmacol.*, 25: 61–70 (2002).
149. O.M. Debus, J. Kohring, B. Fiedler, M. Franssen, and G. Kurlemann, Add-on treatment with pyridoxine and sulthiame in 12 infants with West syndrome: an open clinical study. *Seizure*, 11: 381–383 (2002).
150. N. Fejerman, R. Cers-Simo, and R. Caraballo, Vigabatrin as a first-choice drug in the treatment of West syndrome. *J. Child Neurol.*, 15: 161–165 (2000).
151. Y. Ohtsuka, M. Matsuda, T. Ogino, K. Kobayashi, and S. Ohtahara, Treatment of the West syndrome with high-dose pyridoxal phosphate. *Brain Dev.*, 9: 418–421 (1987).
152. J. Pietz, C. Benninger, H. Schafer, D. Sontheimer, G. Mittermaier, and D. Rating, Treatment of infantile spasms with high-dosage vitamin B_6. *Epilepsia*, 34: 757–763 (1993).
153. Y. Takuma and T. Seki, Combination therapy of infantile spasms with high-dose pyridoxal phosphate and low-dose corticotrophin. *J. Child Neurol.*, 11: 35–40 (1996).
154. C.S. Paulose, K. Dakshinamurti, S. Packer, and N.L. Stephens, Hypertension in pyridoxine deficiency. *J. Hypertens.*, 4, Suppl., 5: S174–S175 (1986).
155. C.S. Paulose, K. Dakshinamurti, S. Packer, and N.L. Stephens, Sympathetic stimulation and hypertension in pyridoxine-deficient adult rat. *Hypertension*, 11: 387–391 (1988).
156. K. Dakshinamurti and K.J. Lal, Vitamins and hypertension. *World Rev. Nutr. Diet.*, 69: 40–73 (1992).
157. K. Dakshinamurti and S. Dakshinamurti, Blood pressure regulation and micronutrients. *Nutr. Res. Rev.*, 14: 3–43 (2001).
158. C.S. Paulose and K. Dakshinamurti, Chronic catheterization using vascular access port in rats: blood sampling with minimal stress fro plasma catecholamine determination. *J. Neurosci. Methods*, 22: 141–146 (1987).
159. M. Viswanathan, C.S. Paulose, K.J. Lal, and K. Dakshinamurti, Alterations in brain stem α adrenoreceptor activity in pyridoxine-deficient rat model of hypertension. *Neurosci. Lett.*, 111: 201–205 (1990).
160. P. Schoeffler and D. Hoyer, Centrally acting hypotensive agents with affinity for $5HT_{1A}$ binding sites inhibit forskolin-stimulated adenyl cyclase activity in calf hippocampus. *Brit. J. Pharmacal.*, 95: 975–985 (1988).
161. K.J. Lal and K. Dakshinamurti, Hypotensive action of 5-HT receptor agonists in the vitamin B_6-deficient hypertensive rat. *Eur. J. Pharmacol.*, 234: 183–189 (1993).

162. G. Gorz, G. Hantt, and N. Kolassa, Urapidil and some analogs with hypotensive properties show high affinities for 5-HT binding sites of the 5 HT_{1A} subtype for α_1-adrenoceptor binding sites. *Naunyn-Schmiedberg's Arch. Pharmacol.*, 336: 597–601 (1987).
163. A. Rappaport, F. Strutz, and P. Guicheney, Regulation of central α-adrenoreceptor by serotonergic denervation. *Brain Res.*, 344: 158–161 (1985).
164. M. Viswanathan, R. Bose, and K. Dakshinamurti, Increased calcium influx in caudal artery of rats made hypertensive with pyridoxine deficiency. *Am. J. Hypertens.*, 4: 252–255 (1991).
165. S. Dakshinamurti, J. Geiger, and K. Dakshinamurti, Control of intracellular calcium levels. In: *Nutrients and Cell Signaling* (J. Zempleni and K. Dakshinamurti, eds.), pp. 589–620, CRC Press, Boca Raton, FL (2005).
166. K. Dakshinamurti, K.J. Lal, N.S. Dhalla, S. Musat, and X. Wang, Pyridoxal 5′-phosphate and calcium channels. In: *Biochemistry and Molecular Biology of Vitamin B_6 and PQQ-dependent proteins* (A. Iriarte, H.M. Kagan, and M. Martinez-Carrion, eds.), pp. 307–315, Birkhauser Verlag, Basel (2000).
167. K.J. Lal and K. Dakshinamurti, Calcium channels in vitamin B_6 deficiency-induced hypertension. *J. Hypertens.*, 11: 1357–1362 (1993).
168. K.J. Lal and K. Dakshinamurti, The relationship between low-calcium-induced increase in systolic blood pressure and vitamin B_6. *J. Hypertens.*, 13: 327–332 (1995).
169. D.E. Grobbee and H.J. Waal-Manning, The role of calcium supplementation in the treatment of hypertension. Current evidence. *Drugs*, 39: 7–18 (1990).
170. I. Porsti, Arterial smooth muscle contraction in spontaneously hypertensive rats on a high calcium diet. *J. Hypertens.*, 10: 255–263 (1992).
171. M. Zein, J.L. Areas, and H.G. Preus, Long-term effects of excess sucrose ingestion on three strains of rats. *Am. J. Hypertens.*, 3: 560–562 (1990).
172. K.J. Lal, K. Dakshinamurti, and J. Thliveris, The effects of vitamin B_6 on the systolic blood pressure of rats in various animal models of hypertension. *J. Hypertens.*, 14: 355–363 (1996).
173. H. Yamamoto, O.K. Hwang, and C. Van Breeman, BAY K 8644 differentiates between potential and receptor operated Ca^{2+} channels. *Eur. J. Pharmacol.*, 102: 555–557 (1984).
174. K.J. Lal, S.K. Sharma, and K. Dakshinamurti, Regulation of calcium influx into vascular smooth muscle by vitamin B_6. *Clin. Exp. Hypertens.*, 15: 489–500 (1993).
175. K. Dakshinamurti, K.J. Lal, and P.K. Ganguly, Hypertension, calcium channels and pyridoxine (vitamin B_6). *Mol. Cell. Biochem.*, 188: 137–148 (1998).
176. X. Wang, K. Dakshinamurti, S. Musat, and N.S. Dhalla, Pyridoxal 5′-phosphate is an ATP-receptor antagonist in freshly isolated rat cardiomyocytes. *J. Mol. Cell Cardiol.*, 31: 1063–1072 (1999).
177. D.J. Trezise, N.J. Bell, B.S. Khakh, A.D. Michel, and R.A. Humphrey, P2 purinoceptor antagonist properties of pyridoxal 5-phosphate. *Eur. J. Pharmacol.*, 259: 295–300 (1994).
178. G. Lambrecht, T. Friebe, U. Grimm, U. Windscheif, E. Bungardt, C. Hildebrandt, H.G. Baumert, G. Spatz-Kumbel, and E. Mutschler, PPADS, a novel functionally selective antagonist of P2 purinoceptor-mediated responses. *Eur. J. Pharmacol.*, 217: 217–219 (1992).
179. G. Lambrecht, Design and pharmacology of selective P2-purinoceptor antagonists. *J. Auton. Pharmacol.*, 16: 341–344 (1996).
180. K.A. Jacobson, Y.C. Kim, S.S. Wildmann, A. Mohanram, T.K. Harden, J.L. Boyer, B.F. King, and G. Burnstock, A pyridoxine cyclic phosphate and its 6-axoaryl derivative selectively potentiate and antagonize activities of P2X receptors. *J. Med. Chem.*, 41: 2201–2206 (1996).
181. G. Lambrecht, Agonists and antagonists acting at P2X receptors: selectivity profiles and functional implications. *Nauyn-Schmiedeberg's Arch. Pharmacol.*, 362: 340–350 (2000).
182. G. Litwack, The glucocorticoid receptor at the protein level. *Cancer Res.*, 48: 2636–2640 (1988).
183. K. Robinson, K. Arheart, and H. Refsum, Low circulating folate and vitamin B_6 concentrations: risk factors for stroke, peripheral vascular disease, and coronary artery disease. *Circulation*, 97: 437–443 (1998).
184. N.W. Schoene, P. Chanmugam, and R.D. Reynolds, Effect of oral vitamin B_6 supplementation on in vitro platelet aggregation. *Am. J. Clin. Nutr.*, 43: 825–830 (1986).
185. S.J. Chang, H.J. Chuang, and H.H. Chen, Vitamin B_6 down-regulates the expression of human GPIIb gene. *J. Nutr. Sci. Vitaminol.*, (Tokyo) 45: 471–479 (1999).

186. R. Roubenoff, R.A. Roubenoff, and J. Selhub, Abnormal vitamin B_6 status in rheumatoid cachexia. Association with spontaneous tumor necrosis factor alpha production and markers of inflammation. *Arthritis Rheum.*, 38: 105–109 (1995).
187. S. James, H.H. Vorster, and C.S. Venter, Nutritional status influences fibrinogen concentration: evidence from the THUSA survey. *Thromb. Res.*, 98: 388–394 (2000).
188. S. Friso, P.F. Jacques, P.W. Wilson, I.H. Rosenberg, and J. Selhub, Low circulation vitamin B_6 is associated with elevation of the inflammation marker C-reactive protein independently of plasma homocysteine levels. *Circulation* 103: 2788–2791 (2001).
189. S. Friso, D. Girelli, N. Martinelli, O. Oliveri, V. Lotto, C. Bozzini, F. Pizzolo, G. Faccini, F. Beltrame, and R. Corrocher, Low plasma vitamin B_6 concentrations and modulation of coronary artery disease risk. *Am. J. Clin. Nutr.*, 79: 992–998 (2004).
190. J. Dierkes, K. Hoffmann, K. Klipstein-Grobusch, C. Weikert, H. Boeing, B.-C. Zyriax, E. Windler, and J. Kratzsch, Low plasma pyridoxal-5′-phosphate and cardiovascular disease risk in women: results from the coronary Risk Factors for Atherosclerosis in Women Study. *Am. J. Clin. Nutr.*, 81: 725–727 (2005).
191. S. Friso, D. Girelli, N. Martinelli, O. Olivieri, and R. Corrocher, Reply to J. Dierkes et al. *Am J. Clin. Nutr.*, 81: 727–728 (2005).
192. P.J. Kelly, J.P. Kistler, and V.E. Shih, Inflammation, homocysteine, and vitamin B_6 status after ischemic stroke. *Stroke*, 35: 12–15 (2004).
193. M. Aybak, A. Sermet, M.O. Ayyildiz, and A.Z. Karakilcik, Effect of oral pyridoxine hydrochloride supplementation on arterial blood pressure in patients with essential hypertension. *Arzneim-Forsch/Drug Res.*, 45: 1271–1273 (1995).
194. W. Li, T. Zheng, J. Wang, B.T. Altura, and B.M. Altura, Extracellular magnesium regulates effects of vitamin B_6, B_{12} and folate on homocysteinemia-induced depletion of intracellular free magnesium ions in canine cerebral vascular smooth muscle cells: possible relationship to $[Ca^{2+}]_i$, atherogenesis and stroke. *Neurosci. Lett.*, 274: 83–86 (1999).
195. P.C. Choy, D. Mymin, Q. Zhu, K. Dakshinamurti, and O. Karmin, Atherosclerosis risk factors: the possible role of homocysteine. *Mol. Cell. Biochem.*, 207: 143–150 (2000).
196. A. Von Eckardstein, M.R. Malinow, B. Upson, J. Heinrich, H. Schulte, R. Schonfeld, E. Kohler, and G. Assman, Effects of age, lipoproteins, and hemostatic parameters on the role of homocysteinemia as a cardiovascular risk factor in men. *Arterioscler. Thromb.*, 14: 460–464 (1994).
197. M. Amadottir, C. Brattstrom, O. Simonsen, H. Thysell, B. Hultberg, A. Anderson, and P. Nilsson-Ehle, The effect of high dose pyridoxine and folic acid supplementation on serum lipid and plasma homocysteine concentration in dialysis patients. *Clin. Nephrol.*, 40: 236–240 (1993).
198. J. Selhub, P.F. Jacque, P.W. Wilson, D. Rush, and I.H. Rosenberg, Vitamin status and intake as primary determinants of homocysteinemia in an elderly population. *JAMA*, 270: 2693–2698 (1993).
199. K.S. McCully, Vascular pathology of homocysteinemia: implications for the pathogenesis of arteriosclerosis. *Am. J. Pathol.*, 56: 111–128 (1969).
200. B.M. Coull, M.R. Malinow, N. Beamer, G. Sexton, F. Nordt, and P. deGarmo, Elevated plasma homocysteine concentration as a possible independent risk factor for stroke. *Stroke*, 21: 572–576 (1990).
201. J.B. Ubbink, W.J.K. Vermaak, J.M. Bennett, P.J. Becker, D.A. Staden, and S. Bissbort, The prevalence of homocysteinemia and hypercholesterolemia in angiographically defined coronary heart disease. *Wien Klin. Wochenschr.*, 69: 527–534 (1991).
202. L. Braltstrom, B. Israelsson, and B. Norrving, Impaired homocysteine metabolism in early onset cerebral and peripheral occlusive arterial disease: effects of pyridoxine and folic acid treatment. *Atherosclerosis*, 81: 51–60 (1990).
203. G.H.J. Boers, Mild hyperhomocysteinemia is an independent risk factor of arterial vascular disease. *Semin. Thromb. Hemost.*, 26: 291–295 (2000).
204. C.J. Glueck, P. Shaw, J.E. Long, T. Tracy, L. Sieve-Smith, and Y. Wang, Evidence that homocysteine is an independent risk factor for atherosclerosis in hyperlipidemic patients. *Am. J. Cardiol.*, 75: 132–136 (1995).

205. K. Sutton-Tyrell, A. Bostom, H. Selhub, and C. Zeigler-Johnson, High homocysteine levels are independently related to isolated systolic hypertension in older adults. *Circulation*, 96: 1745–1749 (1997).
206. R. Rodrigo, W. Passalacquo, A. Araya, M. Orellana, and G. Rivera, Homocysteine and essential hypertension. *J. Clin. Pharmacol.*, 43: 1299–1306 (2003).
207. G. Blundell, B.G. Jones, F.A. Rose, and N. Tudball, Homocysteine-mediated endothelial cell toxicity and its amelioration. *Atherosclerosis*, 122: 163–172 (1996).
208. B. Halvorsen, I. Brude, C.A. Drevon, J. Nysom, L. Ose, and E.N. Christiansen, Effect of homocysteine on copper ion-catalyzed azo compound-initiation and mononuclear cell-mediated oxidative modification of low density lipoprotein. *J. Lipid Res.*, 37: 1591–1600 (1996).
209. D.W. Jacobson, Homocysteine and vitamins in cardiovascular disease. *Clin. Chem.*, 44: 1833–1843 (1998).
210. C.G. Schanackenberg, Oxygen radicals in cardiovascular-renal disease. *Curr. Opin. Pharmacol.*, 2: 121–125 (2002).
211. A. Majors, L.A. Ehrhard, and E.H. Pezacka, Homocysteine as a risk factor for vascular disease: enhanced collagen production and accumulation by smooth muscle cells. *Arterioscler. Thromb. Vasc. Biol.*, 17: 2074–2081 (1997).
212. U. Till, P. Rohl, A. Jentsch, H. Till, A. Muller, K. Bellstedt, D. Plonne, H.S. Fink, R. Vollandt, U. Siwka, F.H. Herrmann, H. Petermann, and R. Riezler, Decrease of carotid intima-media thickness in patients at risk to cerebral ischemia after supplementation with folic acid, vitamin B_6 and B_{12}. *Atherosclerosis*, 181: 131–135 (2005).
213. J.J. Strain, L. Dowey, M. Ward, K. Pentieva, and H. McNulty, B-Vitamins, homocysteine metabolism and CVD. *Proc. Nutr. Soc.*, 63: 597–603 (2004).
214. R. Marcucci, I. Betli, E. Cecchi, D. Poli, B. Giusti, S. Fedi, I. Lapini, R. Abbate, G.F. Gensini, and D. Prisco, Hyperhomocysteinemia and vitamin B_6 deficiency: new risk markers for nonvalvular atrial fibrillation? *Am. Heart J.*, 148: 456–461 (2004).
215. R. DeCaterina, A. Zampolli, R. Madonna, P. Fioretti, and D. Vanuzzo, New cardiovascular risk factors: homocysteine and vitamins involved in homocysteine metabolism. *Ital. Heart J.*, 5, Suppl. 6: 19S–24S (2004).
216. S. Saibeni, M. Cattaneo, M. Vecchi, M.L. Zighetti, A. Lecchi, R. Lombardi, G. Meucci, L. Spina, and R. de Franchis, Low vitamin B_6 plasma levels, a risk factor for thrombosis, in inflammatory bowel disease: role of inflammation and correlation with acute phase reactants. *Am. J. Gastroenterol.*, 98: 112–117 (2003).
217. L. Cabrini, D. Bochicchio, A. Bordoni, S. Sassi, M. Marchetti, and M. Maranesi, Correlation between dietary polyunsaturated fatty acids and plasma homocysteine concentration in vitamin B_6-deficient rats. *Nutr. Metab. Cardiovasc. Dis.*, 15: 94–99 (2005).
218. J.W. Baynes and S.R. Thorpe, Role of oxidative stress in diabetic complications. *Diabetics*, 48: 1–9 (1999).
219. M. Kalousova, T. Zima, V. Tesar, S. Stipek, and S. Sulkova, Advanced glycation end products in clinical nephrology. *Kidney Blood Press. Res.*, 27: 18–28 (2004).
220. T. Kislinger, C. Fu, B. Huber, W. Qu, A. Taguchi, S.D. Yan, M. Hofmann, S.F. Yan, M. Pischensrieder, D. Stern, and A.M. Schmidt, Ne-(carboxymethyl) lysine adducts of proteins are ligands for receptor for advanced glycation end products that activate cell signaling pathways and modulate gene expression. *J. Biol. Chem.*, 274: 31740–31749 (1999).
221. B.O. Nilsson., Biological effects of aminoguanidine: an update. *Inflamm. Res.*, 48: 509–515 (1999).
222. T.O. Metz, N.L. Alderson, S.R. Thorpe, and J.W. Baynes. Pyridoxamine, an inhibitor of advanced glycation and lipoxidation reactions: a novel therapy for treatment of diabetic complications. *Arch. Biochem. Biophys.*, 419: 41–49 (2003).
223. A.A. Booth, R.G. Khalifah, and B.G. Hudson, Thiamine pyrophosphate and pyridoxamine inhibit the formation of antigenic advanced glycation end-products: comparison with aminoguanidine. *Biochem. Biophys. Res. Commun.*, 220: 113–119 (1996).
224. A. Stitt, T.A. Gardiner, N.L. Anderson, P. Canning, N. Frizzell, N. Duffy, C. Boyle, A.J. Januszewski, M. Chachich, J.W. Baynes, and S.R. Thorpe. The AGE inhibitor pyridoxamine inhibits development of retinopathy in experimental diabetes. *Diabetes* 51: 2828–2832 (2002).

225. K. Shimoi, A. Okitsu, M.H. Green, J.E. Lowe, T. Ota, K. kaji, H. Terato, H. Ide, and N. Kinae, Oxidative DNA damage induced by high glucose and its suppression in human umbilical vein endothelial cells. *Mutat. Res.*, 480–481: 371–378 (2001).
226. N.T. Meisler and J.W. Thanassi, Pyridoxine-derived B_6 vitamers and pyridoxal 5′-phosphate-binding protein in cytosolic and nuclear fractions of HTC cells. *J. Biol. Chem.*, 265: 1193–1198 (1990).
227. K. Dakshinamurti, Vitamin receptors. In: *Encyclopedia of Molecular Biology and Molecular Medicine*, 2nd Edition (R.A. Meyers, ed.), Vol. 15, pp. 505–535, Wiley-VCH Verlag GmbH & Co, KGaA, Weinheim (2005).
228. V.E. Allgood and J.A. Cidlowski, Vitamin B_6 modulates transcriptional activation by multiple members of the steroid hormone receptor superfamily. *J. Biol. Chem.*, 267: 3819–3824 (1992).
229. D.B. Tully, V.E. Allgood, and J.A. Cidlowski, Modulation of steroid receptor-mediated gene expression by vitamin B_6. *FASEB J.*, 8: 343–349 (1994).
230. T. Kondo and M. Okada, Effect of pyridoxine administration on the induction of cytosolic aspartate amino-transferase in the liver of rats treated with hydrocortisone. *J. Nutr. Sci. Vitaminol.*, 31: 509–517 (1985).
231. T. Oka, N. Komori, M. Kuwahata, Y. Hiroi, T. Shimoda, M. Okada, and Y. Natori, Pyridoxal 5′-phosphate modulates expression of cytosolic aspartate amino-transferase gene by inactivation of glucocorticoid receptor. *J. Nutr. Sci. Vitaminol.*, 41: 363–375 (1995).
232. Y. Natori, T. Oka, and M. Kuwahata, Modulation of gene expression by vitamin B_6. In: *Biochemistry and Molecular Biology of Vitamin B_6 and PQQ-dependent proteins* (A. Iriarte, H.M. Kagan, and M. Martinez-Carrion, eds.), pp. 301–306, Birkhauser Verlag, Basel (2000).
233. Y. Natori and T. Oka, Vitamin B_6 modulation of gene expression. *Nutr. Res.*, 17: 1199–1207 (1997).
234. D.M. diSorbo, R. Wagner, and L. Nathanson, In vivo and in vitro inhibition of B_{16} melanoma growth by vitamin B_6. *Nutr. Cancer*, 38: 281–286 (2000).
235. S. Komatsu, N. Yanaka, K. Matsubara, and N. Kato, Antitumor effect of vitamin B_6 and its mechanisms. *Biochim. Biophys. Acta*, 1647: 127–130 (2003).
236. A.B. Maksymowych, N.M. Robertson, and G. Litwack, Effect of pyridoxal treatment in controlling the growth of melanoma in cell culture and an animal pilot study. *Anticancer Res.*, 13: 1925–1938 (1993).
237. B.A. Davis and B.E. Cowing, Pyridoxal supplementation reduces cell proliferation and DNA synthesis in estrogen-dependent and independent mammary carcinoma cell lines. *Nutr. Cancer*, 38: 281–286 (2000).
238. D.S. Gridley, D.R. Stickney, R.L. Nutter, J.M. Slater, and T.D. Shultz, Suppression of tumor growth and enhancement of immune status with high levels of dietary vitamin B_6 in BALB/c mice. *J. Natl. Cancer Inst.*, 78: 951–959 (1987).
239. M.C. Jansen, H.B. Beuno-de-Mesquita, R. Buzina, F. Fidanza, A. Minotti, H. Blackburn, A.M. Nissenen, F.J. Kok, and D. Kromhout, Dietary fiber and plant foods in relation to colorectal cancer mortality: the seven countries study. *Int. J. Cancer*, 81: 174–179 (1999).
240. T.J. Hartman, K. Woodson, R. Stolzenberg-Solomon, J. Virtamo, J. Selhub, M.J. Barrett, and D. Albanes, Association of the B vitamins, pyridoxal 5′-phosphate, B_{12}, and folate with lung cancer risk in older men. *Am. J. Epidemiol.*, 153: 688–693 (2001).
241. S. Komatsu, H. Watanabe, T. Oka, H. Tsuge, and N. Kato, Dietary vitamin B_6 suppresses colon tumorigenesis, 8-hydroxyguanosine, 4-hydroxynonenal-inducible nitric oxide synthase protein in azoxymethane-treated mice. *J. Nutr. Sci. Vitaminol.*, 48: 65–68 (2002).
242. K. Matsubara, M. Mori, Y. Matsuura, and N. Kato, Pyridoxal 5′-phosphate and pyridoxal inhibit angiogenesis in the serum-free rat aortic ring assay. *Int. J. Mol. Med.*, 8: 505–508 (2001).
243. K. Matsubara, H. Matsumoto, Y. Mizushina, J.S. Lee, and N. Kato, Inhibitory effect of pyridoxal 5′-phosphate on endothelial cell proliferation, replicative DNA polymerase and DNA topoisomerase. *Int. J. Mol. Med.*, 12: 51–55 (2003).
244. Y. Mizushina, X. Yu, K. Matsubara, C. Murakami, I. Kuriyama, M. Oshiga, M. Takemura, N. Kato, H. Yoshida, and K. Sakaguchi, Pyridoxal 5′-phosphate is a selective inhibitor in vivo of DNA polymerase α and ε. *Biochim. Biophys. Res. Commun.*, 312: 1025–1032 (2003).

245. H. Hubscher, G. Maga, and S. Spadari. Eukaryotic DNA polymerase. *Annu. Rev. Biochem.*, 71: 133–163 (2002).
246. J.J. Vermeersch, S. Christmann-Frank, L.V. Karabashyan, S. Fermandjian, G. Mirambeau, and P. Arsene Der Garabedian, Pyridoxal 5′-phosphate inactivates DNA topoisomerase IB by modifying the lysine general acid. *Nucleic Acid Res.*, 32: 5649–5657 (2004).
247. K. Matsubara, S.-I. Komatsu, T. Oka, and N. Kato, Vitamin B_6-mediated suppression of colon tumorigenesis, cell proliferation and angiogenesis. *J. Nutr. Biochem.*, 14: 246–250 (2003).
248. S.K. Jain and G. Lim, Pyridoxine and pyridoxamine inhibits superoxide radicals and prevents lipid peroxidation, protein glycosylation and (Na^+, K^+)–ATPase activity reduction in high glucose-treated human erythrocytes. *Free Radic. Biol. Med.*, 30: 232–237 (2001).
249. V. Ravichandran and R. Selvam, Increased lipid peroxidation by vitamin B_6-deficient rats. *Biochem. Int.*, 21: 599–605 (1990).
250. H.C. Stoerk and H.N. Eisen, Suppression of circulating antibodies in pyridoxine deficiency. *Proc. Soc. Exp. Biol. Med.*, 62: 88–89 (1946).
251. A.E. Axelrod, B.B Carter, B.H. McCoy, and R. Geisinger, Circulating antibodies in vitamin deficiency states: pyridoxine, riboflavin and pantothenic acid deficiencies. *Proc. Soc. Exp. Biol. Med.*, 66: 137–140 (1947).
252. M. Kumar and A.E. Axelrod, Cellular antibody synthesis in Vitamin B_6 deficient rats. *J. Nutr.*, 96: 39–45 (1968).
253. A.E. Axelrod and A.C. Trakatellis, Relationship of pyridoxine to immunological phenomenon. *Vitam. Horm.*, 22: 591–607 (1964).
254. S. Doke, N. Inagaki, T. Hayakawa, and H. Tsuge, Effect of Vitamin B_6 deficiency on antibody production in mice, *Biosci. Biotech. Biochem.*, 61: 1331–1336 (1997).
255. A. Trakatellis, M. Exindari, C.S. Haitoglou, and A. Dimitriadou, Serine hydroxyl methyltransferase (SHMT) as a precise indication of antiproliferative or immunosuppressive potency of various compounds. *Int. J. Immunopathol. Pharmacol.*, 8: 31–37 (1995).
256. A. Trakatellis, A. Dimitriadou, and M. Trakatellis, Pyridoxine deficiency: new approaches in immunosuppression and chemotherapy. *Postgrad. Med. J.*, 73: 617–622 (1997).
257. S.N. Meydani, J.D. Ribaya-Mercado, R.M. Russel, N. Sahyoun, F.D. Morrow, and S.N. Gershoff, Vitamin B_6 deficiency impairs interleukin 2 production and lymphocyte proliferation in elderly adults. *Am. J. Clin. Nutr.*, 53: 1275–1280 (1991).
258. H.-K. Kwak, C.M. Hansen, J.E. Leklem, K. Hardin, and T.D. Shultz, Improved vitamin B_6 status is positively related to lymphocyte proliferation in young women consuming a controlled diet. *J. Nutr.*, 132: 3308–3313 (2002).
259. Y. Hu, P.L Fisette, L.C. Denlinger, A.G. Guadarrama, J.A. Sommer, R.A. Procter, and P.J. Bertics, Purinergic receptor modulation of lipopolysaccharide signaling and inducible nitric-oxide synthase expression in RAW 264.7 macrophages. *J. Biol. Chem.*, 273: 27170–27175 (1998).
260. W.J. Stone, L.G. Warnock, and C. Wagner, Vitamin B_6 deficiency in uremia. *Am. J. Clin. Nutr.*, 28: 950–957 (1975).
261. R. Roubenoff, R.A. Roubenoff, and J. Selhub, Abnormal vitamin B_6 status in rheumatoid cachexia: association with spontaneous tumor necrosis factor alpha production and markers of inflammation. *Arthritis Rheum.*, 38: 105–109 (1995).
262. M.K. Baum, E. Mantero-Atienze, G. Shor-Posner, M.A. Fletcher, R. Morgan, C. Eisdorfer, H.E. Sauberlich, P.E. Cornwall, and R.S. Beach, Association of Vitamin B_6 status with parameters of immune function in early HIV-1 infection. *J. Acquir. Immune Defic. Syndr.*, 4: 1122–1132 (1991).
263. J.M. Salhany and L.M. Schopper. Pyridoxal 5-phosphate binds specifically to soluble CD4 protein, the HIV-1 receptor. Implications for AIDS therapy. *J. Biol. Chem.*, 268: 7643–7645 (1993).
264. H.M. Korchak, B.A. Eisenstar, S.T. Hoffstein, P.B. Dunham, and G. Weissman, Anion channel blockers inhibit lysosomal enzyme secretion from human neutrophils without affecting generation of superoxide anion. *Proc. Natl. Acad. Sci., USA* 77: 2721–2725 (1990).
265. M.R. Niazi, Pyridoxal 5′-phosphate as a novel weapon against auto immunity and transplant rejection. *FASEB J.*, 17: 2184–2186 (2003).
266. L. Guo, N.K. Heinzinger, M. Stevenson, L.M. Schoffer, and J.M. Salfany, Inhibition of gp 120-CD4 interaction and human immunodeficiency virus type 1 infection in vitro by pyridoxal 5-phosphate. *Antimicrob. Agents Chemother.*, 38: 2483–2487 (1994).

267. J.M. Salhany and M. Stevenson, Hypothesis: potential utility of pyridoxal 5-phosphate (vitamin B_6) and levamisole in immune modulation and HIV-1 infections. AID patient care STDs 10: 353–356 (1996).
268. G. Renoux, Modulation of immunity by levamisole. *J. Pharmacol. Ther.*, A2: 397–423 (1978).
269. W.A. Check, CDC study: no evidence for teratogenicity of Bendectin. *JAMA*, 242: 2518 (1979).
270. H. Schaumburg, J. Kaplan, A. Windebank, N. Vick, S. Rasmus, D. Pleasure, and M.J. Brown. Sensory neuropathy from pyridoxine abuse. A new megavitamin syndrome. *N. Engl. J. Med.*, 309: 445–448 (1983).
271. G.W. Barber and G.L. Spaeth, The successful treatment of homocystinuria with pyridoxine. *J. Pediatr.*, 75: 463–478 (1969).
272. B. Rimland, E. Calloway, and P. Dreyfus, The effects of high doses of vitamin B_6 on autistic children: a double-blind crossover study. *Am. J. Psychiatry*, 135: 472–475 (1978).
273. C. Mpofus, S.M. Alani, C. Whitehouse, B. Fowler, and J.E. Wraith, No sensory neuropathy during pyridoxine treatment in homocystinuria. *Arch. Dis. Child*, 66: 1081–1082 (1991).
274. A. Bendich and M. Cohen, Vitamin B_6 safety issues. *Ann. N.Y. Acad. Sci.*, 585: 320–330 (1990).

11 Biotin

Donald M. Mock

CONTENTS

HISTORY OF DISCOVERY

Although a growth requirement for the "bios" fraction had been demonstrated in yeast, Boas was the first to demonstrate the requirement for biotin in a mammal. In rats fed protein derived from egg white, Boas observed a syndrome of severe dermatitis, hair loss, and neuromuscular dysfunction known as "egg-white injury." A factor present in liver cured the egg-white injury and was named "protective factor X." The critical event in this "egg-white injury" of both humans and rats is the highly specific and very tight binding ($K_d = 10^{-15}$ M) of biotin by avidin, a glycoprotein found in egg white [1]. This very high-affinity, high-specificity interaction is used in an extraordinary range of biochemical, biological, and pharmaceutical applications. From an evolutionary standpoint, avidin probably serves as a bacteriostat in egg white; consistent with this hypothesis is the observation that avidin is resistant to a broad range of bacterial proteases in both the free and biotin-bound form. Because avidin is also resistant to pancreatic proteases, avidin in dietary egg white binds to dietary biotin preventing absorption, thus carrying the biotin through the gastrointestinal tract. Biotin is also synthesized by many intestinal microbes; the contribution of microbial biotin to absorbed biotin in the absence of egg-white feeding is unknown, but any biotin released from intestinal microbes is also bound by avidin, preventing absorption. Cooked egg white does not cause biotin deficiency because cooking denatures avidin, rendering it susceptible to cleavage by pancreatic proteases and unable to interfere with absorption of biotin.

CHEMISTRY OF BIOTIN

STRUCTURE

As reviewed by Bhatia et al. [2] and Bonjour [3], the structure of biotin (Figure 11.1) was independently elucidated by Kogl and du Vigneaud in the early 1940s. Because biotin has three asymmetric carbons in its structure, eight stereoisomers exist. Of these, only one (designated D-(+)-biotin) is found in nature and is enzymatically active. This compound is generally referred to simply as biotin or D-biotin. Biocytin (ε-*N*-biotinyl-L-lysine) is about as active as biotin on a mole basis in mammalian growth studies.

Biotin is a bicyclic compound. One of the rings contains a ureido group (–N–CO–N–) and the other is a tetrahydrothiophene ring. The tetrahydrothiophene ring has a valeric acid side chain. On the basis of biotin analog binding to avidin and the X-ray crystallographic structure of the biotin:avidin complex [1], the ureido ring of biotin is the most important region for the extraordinarily tight binding of biotin to avidin. Biotin also binds tightly to streptavidin, a protein secreted by *Streptomyces avidinii*. Other studies [1] suggest that the length of the side chain or the apolar nature of the $-CH_2-$ moieties in the side chain also play a role in the binding of biotin to the hydrophobic site on (strept)avidin.

CHEMICAL SYNTHESIS OF BIOTIN

The structure of biotin was confirmed by de novo chemical synthesis by Harrison and coworkers in the 1940s [3]. The stereospecific synthesis was developed by Goldberg and Sternbach in 1949 in the laboratories of Hoffman-LaRoche [4]. Additional stereospecific methods of synthesis have been published [5,6].

PHYSIOLOGY OF BIOTIN

DIGESTION OF PROTEIN-BOUND BIOTIN

The content of biotin is highly variable among foods [7]. Likewise, the proportion of free and protein-bound biotin likely varies substantially even within food groups [8,9]. "Free biotin" is defined functionally in most studies as water extractable and dialyzable [10]. "Bound biotin" is usually defined as biotin that is sedimentable after a water extraction of the homogenized

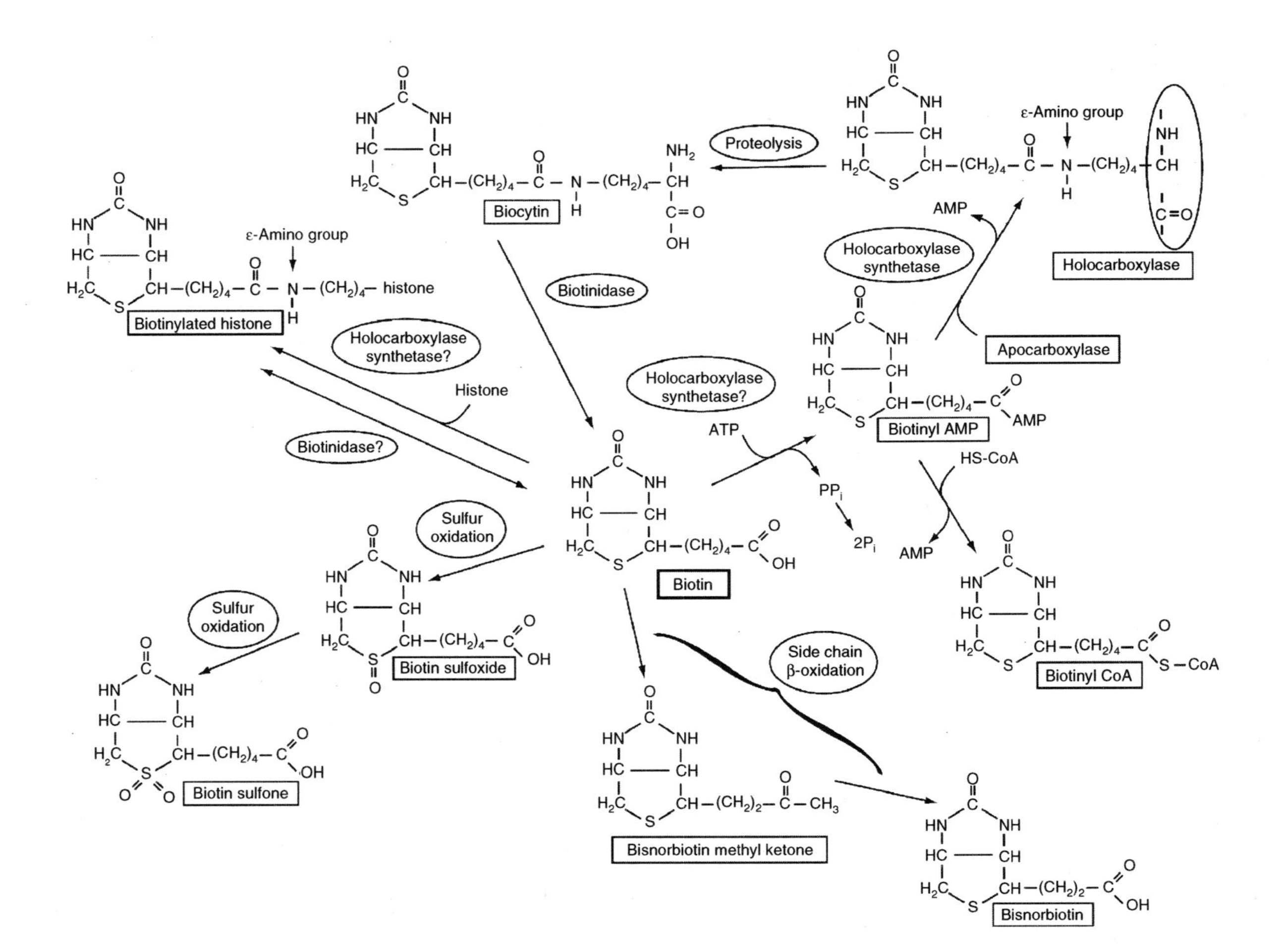

FIGURE 11.1 Metabolism, degradation, and recycling of biotin as well as biotinylated enzymes and histones. Ovals denote enzymes or enzyme systems; rectangles denote biotin, intermediates, metabolites, and substrates in pathways (which can also be enzymes); AMP, adenosine monophosphate; ATP, adenosine triphosphate; CoA, coenzyme A; PP_i, pyrophosphate.

food [11,12]. Bound biotin must be released to render the biotin fully detectable by either microbial or avidin-binding assays. Release has generally been accomplished by enzymatic or acid-catalyzed proteolysis; these methods have likely resulted in incomplete biotin release, destruction of biotin, or both as discussed in the sections Requirement and Assessment and Dietary Sources of Biotin.

Proteolytic degradation of dietary protein likely yields biocytin and biotinyl oligopeptides. Neither the exact mechanism of the intestinal hydrolysis of protein-bound biotin nor the relationship of digestion of protein-bound biotin to its bioavailability has been clearly elucidated, but Wolf and coworkers have postulated that biotinidase (EC 3.5.1.12, an amide hydrolase) in pancreatic secretions cleaves biocytin [13,14]. Given the observation that biocytin uptake is substantially less active than that of biotin [15], this cleavage of biocytin by biotinidase may substantially enhance the bioavailability of bound biotin.

Intestinal Absorption of Biotin

Intestinal absorption of biotin has been the subject of an excellent recent review by Said [16]. His studies are the source of a substantial amount of the information concerning intestinal biotin absorption.

The nutritional significance of biotin synthesized by the normal intestinal microflora remains uncertain. However, a considerable amount of the bacterially synthesized biotin appears to be in the free (absorbable) form, and studies in humans, rats, and mini-pigs have shown that the large intestine is capable of absorbing luminally introduced biotin. Moreover, studies utilizing human-derived colonic epithelial cells have shown that these cells posses an efficient, Na^+-dependent, carrier-mediated mechanism for biotin uptake [16].

Absorption of free biotin in the small intestine has been studied using several intestinal preparations including isolated loops, intestinal cells in culture, and brush-border membrane vesicles in vitro. Biotin is absorbed from the lumen at the brush border by an Na^+-dependent carrier. The carrier is structurally specific, requiring both a free carboxyl group on the valeric acid side chain and an intact ureido ring [17,18]. The transport of biotin is temperature dependent and occurs against a concentration gradient. At high concentrations, biotin transport also occurs by simple diffusion.

Based on a study in which biotin was administered orally in pharmacologic amounts, the bioavailability of biotin is ~100% [19]. This observation provides a rational basis for the pharmacologic doses used in the treatment of biotin-responsive inborn errors of metabolism and for predicting that the bioavailability of free biotin is likely to be high for physiologic doses as well.

Substantial evidence indicates that the intestinal biotin transporter is encoded by the *sodium-dependent multivitamin transporter* (*SMVT*) gene [16]. *SMVT* expression generally parallels biotin transport. Biotin uptake is competitively inhibited by pantothenic acid and lipoic acid; this observation is consistent with studies of the overexpressed *SMVT*, which indicate that *SMVT* transports pantothenic acid and lipoic acid in addition to biotin. Hence the origin of the name sodium-dependent multivitamin transporter. In addition, studies using gene-specific siRNA to silence the *SMVT* gene in human intestinal epithelial cells indicate that *SMVT* is the main (if not the only) biotin uptake system that operates in these cells.

Biotin transport is regulated by multiple factors including biotin nutritional status, enterocyte maturity, anatomic location, and ontogeny. Upregulation of biotin transport occurs in response to biotin deficiency. The mechanism for most of the change appears to be an increased V_{max} (presumably mediated by an increased number of carriers) rather than change in the carrier affinity. Biotin transport is more active in the villus cells than in the crypt cells. Transport is most active in the upper small intestine and progressively less active aborally into the colon.

The intestinal biotin uptake process appears to be under the regulation of intracellular protein kinase C and Ca^{2+}–calmodulin-mediated pathways. Transcription of the *SMVT* gene of rats appears to be driven by three distinct promoters whereas that of humans appears to involve two distinct promoters. Said has identified four distinct variants (I, II, III, IV) in the rat small and large intestine, which have significant heterogeneity in the 5′ untranslated region [16].

The exit of biotin from the polarized enterocyte occurs by transport across the basolateral membrane. Basolateral transport is also carrier-mediated but is independent of Na^+. Basolateral transport is electrogenic and does not accumulate biotin against a concentration gradient. The gene is yet to be identified.

Transport of Biotin from the Intestine to Peripheral Tissues

Biotin concentrations in plasma are small relative to those of other water-soluble vitamins. Most biotin in plasma is free and dissolved in the aqueous phase of plasma. However, small amounts are reversibly bound and covalently bound to plasma protein (~7% and 12%, respectively); binding to human serum albumin likely accounts for most of the reversible binding [10,11]. Biotinidase has been proposed as a specific biotin-binding protein or biotin-carrier protein for the transport into cells [20,21]. A biotin-binding immunoglobulin has recently been identified in human serum. An approximately fivefold higher concentration of this biotin-binding immunoglobulin was reported in patients with Graves, disease than in normal and healthy controls [22].

Transport of Biotin into the Liver

Studies of 3T3-L1 fibroblasts [23] rat hepatocytes isolated by collagenase profusion [18,24], basolateral membrane vesicles from human liver [25,26], and HepG2 human hepatoma cells [27,28], indicate that uptake of free biotin is mediated both by diffusion and by a specialized carrier system that is dependent on an Na^+ gradient, temperature, and energy. Transport is electroneutral (Na^+ to biotin 1:1) and specific for a free carboxyl group, but transport is not strongly specific for the structure in the region of the thiophene ring [27]. Recent work from Said and coworkers provides evidence that the primary, and perhaps only, transporter for biotin into hepatocytes is coded by the *SMVT* gene [28]. At physiologic nanomolar concentrations, biotin transport into HepG2 cells was inhibited by siRNA specific to the human *SMVT*; pantothenic acid uptake was also effectively inhibited by *hSMVT*-specific siRNA.

Studies in cultured rat hepatocytes have demonstrated trapping of biotin [29], presumably covalently bound in holocarboxylase enzymes and histones. These studies confirm earlier studies by McCormick and recapitulate the importance of metabolic trapping of water-soluble vitamins as a mechanism for an intracellular vitamin accumulation [18].

After entering the hepatocyte, biotin diffuses into the mitochondria via a pH-dependent process leading to the hypothesis that biotin enters the mitochondria in the neutral, protonated form and dissociates into the anionic form in the alkaline mitochondrial environment, thus becoming trapped by the charge [30]. Biliary excretion of biotin and metabolites is quantitatively negligible based on a rat study [31].

Transport of Biotin into the Central Nervous System

Using in situ rat brain perfusion, Spector and Mock [32] demonstrated that biotin is transported across the blood–brain barrier by a saturable system; the apparent K_m is $\approx$100 μmol/L (a value several orders of magnitude greater than the concentration of free biotin in plasma). Transport was structurally specific. Transfer of biotin directly into the cerebral spinal fluid

(CSF) via the choroid plexus did not appear to be important for biotin entry into the central nervous system (CNS). Additional studies using either intravenous or intraventricular injection of ^{3}H-biotin into rabbits [33] indicated that biotin was cleared from the CSF more rapidly than mannitol, suggesting specific transport systems for biotin uptake into the neurons after biotin crosses the blood–brain barrier; further, biotin entry did not depend on the subsequent metabolism of biotin or immediate trapping by incorporation into brain proteins.

Ozand et al. have described 10 patients in Saudi Arabia with a novel biotin-responsive basal ganglia disease. Patients presented with subacute encephalopathy, confusion, disartria, and dysphasia progressing to cogwheel rigidity, distonia, and quadriparesis. These findings improved dramatically within days in response to 5–10 mg biotin per kilogram body weight per day. The symptoms recurred if biotin was discontinued [34]. Zeng et al. working in collaboration with this group mapped the genetic defect to chromosome 2q36.3 [35]. Each affected member of the family kindreds displayed one of two missense mutations. Both mutations alter the coding sequence for the SLC19A3 transporter. SLC19A3 codes for a protein previously identified as a thiamine transporter and designated THTR-2. These investigators have speculated that SLC19A3 may be responsible for biotin transport or recycling in the CNS [35], although the possibility remains that biotin responsiveness is secondary to an effect on thiamine transport. Vlasova and Mock have identified SLC19A3 as a gene that is highly responsive to biotin status in peripheral blood leukocytes in culture [36]; SLC19A3 is also responsive to experimental biotin deficiency induced in vivo in human subjects [37].

Mardach et al. have reported an 18 month old boy with sudden onset biotin-responsive coma [38]. This child had a profound biotin-transporter defect in both normal and EBV-transformed lymphocytes; the parents of this child had intermediate biotin transporter activities consistent with heterozygous status. Despite possessing a biotin-responsive pattern of organic aciduria consistent with multiple carboxylase deficiency, this child had normal holocarboxylase synthetase and biotinidase activities; pantothenic acid transport and *SMVT* gene coding sequence were normal. The gene defect of this subject is under active investigation.

Mock has measured the concentrations of free "biotin" (i.e., total avidin-binding substances) in human CSF and ultrafiltrates of plasma; the ratio was 0.85 ± 0.5 for 11 subjects [39]. This result is similar to the CSF:plasma ratios determined for biotin by Spector and Mock in rabbits, a species that has a specific system for biotin transport across the blood–brain barrier [33]. Livaniou and coworkers have also measured CSF concentrations of biotin of normal adults and adults with a variety of neurologic disorders [40]. Both studies provide evidence that biotin is not highly concentrated in normal CSF. Livaniou and coworkers also reported a significant reduction in CSF biotin in epileptics and subjects with multiple sclerosis.

Renal Handling of Biotin

Specific systems for the reabsorption of water-soluble vitamins from the glomerular filtrate likely contribute importantly to conservation of the water-soluble vitamins [17]. A biotin transport system has been identified in brush-border membrane vesicles from human kidney cortex [41,42]. Uptake by brush-border membrane vesicles was electroneutral, structurally specific, saturable, occurred against a biotin concentration gradient, and was dependent on an inwardly directed Na^+ gradient.

Biotin uptake by human-derived proximal tubular epithelial HK-2 cells is dependent on temperature, energy, and an inwardly directed Na^+ gradient [43] and is inhibited by both pantothenic acid and lipoate, suggesting the involvement of *SMVT*. Said and coworkers demonstrated that *SMVT* is expressed as both mRNA and protein in HK-2 cells. In their study, silencing of the *SMVT* gene by specific siRNA led to specific and significant inhibition of biotin uptake. Studies with protein kinase C and Ca^{2+}–calmodulin modulators provided evidence that renal biotin uptake is under regulation via these pathways. Uptake was also adaptively regulated by biotin deficiency consistent with previous studies demonstrating reduced biotin excretion early in experimentally induced biotin deficiency in human subjects [44,45].

The renal clearance of biotin in normal adults and children who are not receiving biotin supplementation is ~0.4 when expressed as biotin to creatinine clearance ratio [41,46,47]. In patients with biotinidase deficiency, renal wasting of biotin and biocytin occurs; biotin to creatinine clearance ratios typically exceed 1, and half-lives for biotin clearance are about half of the normal value. The mechanism for the increased renal excretion of biotin in biotinidase deficiency has not been defined, but this observation suggests that there may also be a role for biotinidase in the renal handling of biotin.

Placental Transport of Biotin

Biotin concentrations are 3–17-fold greater in plasma from human fetuses than their mothers in the second trimester, consistent with active placental transport. Specific systems for transport of biotin from the mother to the fetus have been reported [48–50]. Studies using microvillus membrane vesicles and cultured trophoblasts [48,49] detected a saturable transport system for biotin, which was dependent on Na^+ and actively accumulated biotin within the placenta with slower release into the fetal compartment. However, in the isolated, perfused single cotyledon [48,49] transport of biotin across the placenta is slow relative to placental accumulation. Studies using fetal facing (basolateral) membrane vesicles detected a saturable, Na^+-dependent, electroneutral, carrier-mediated uptake process, which was not as active as the biotin uptake system in the maternal facing (apical) membrane vesicles [50]. *SMVT* was originally discovered in human chorionic carcinoma cells [51] and is expressed in normal human placenta [52]. Biotin supply affects the rates of cell proliferation, biotinylation of carboxylases and histones, expression of *SMVT*, and progesterone secretion in chorionic carcinoma cells [53].

Transport of Biotin into Human Milk

Greater than 95% of the biotin in human milk is free in the aqueous phase of the skim fraction [54]. A steady increase in the biotin concentration is observed during the first 18 days postpartum in about half of the women; after 18 days postpartum, biotin concentrations vary substantially [55]. Bisnorbiotin accounts for about half of the total biotin plus metabolites in early and transitional human milk; biotin sulfoxide accounts for about 10%. With postpartum maturation, the absolute concentration of biotin increases as well as the proportion of the total due to biotin; however, bisnorbiotin and biotin sulfoxide still account for about 25% and 8% of the total at 5 weeks postpartum [56].

The concentration of biotin in human milk exceeds the plasma concentration by 10–100-fold [56], implying that a transport system exists. The location and the nature of the biotin transport system for human milk have yet to be elucidated.

SPECIFIC FUNCTIONS

In mammals, biotin serves as an essential cofactor for five carboxylases; each enzyme catalyzes a critical step in intermediary metabolism [57,58]. All five of the mammalian carboxylases catalyze the incorporation of bicarbonate into a substrate as a carboxyl group. Four similar carboxylases, two other carboxylases, two decarboxylases, and a transcarboxylase are found in nonmammalian organisms. Each works by a similar mechanism.

Incorporation into Carboxylases and Histones

Attachment of the biotin to the apocarboxylase (Figure 11.1) is a condensation reaction catalyzed by holocarboxylase synthetase. The holocarboxylase synthetase reaction is driven thermodynamically by hydrolysis of ATP to pyrophosphate and onto inorganic phosphate. An amide bond is formed between the carboxyl group of the valeric acid side chain of biotin and the ε-amino group of a specific lysyl residue in the apocarboxylase. The lysine residue is consistently found within a biotin acceptor sequence (A/Bio) MKM that is at the center of a 60 to 80 amino acid domain. One interpretation concerning conservation of this amino acid sequence is that these residues allow the biotinylated peptide to swing the carboxyl (or acetyl) group from the site of activation to the receiving substrate [59].

Much of our knowledge of the reaction mechanisms for holocarboxylase synthetase comes from studies of BirA in the analogous *Escherichia coli* acetyl CoA carboxylase (ACC) [60]. BirA acts not only as a biotin transfer enzyme and a carboxylase, but this protein also acts as a repressor of the operand for the biosynthesis of biotin [60,61]. Biotin is transferred via a two-step reaction involving biotinyl 5′AMP. This intermediate remains bound to BirA producing a conformational shift that stabilizes the complex preventing unproductive release of biotinyl 5′AMP [62,63]. Biotin is then transferred to a biotin carboxyl-carrier protein (BCCP) of ACC with the release of AMP.

Human holocarboxylase synthetase (HCLS, EC 6.3.4.10) has been cloned [64–67]. HCLS is located on chromosome 21q22.1 and consists of 14 exons and 13 entrons in a span of 240 kb. Comparison with BirA indicates substantial homology in some regions. Studies of human mutant HCLS indicate that all forms of holocarboxylase synthetase are likely encoded by one gene.

Biotinylation of histones is emerging as an important histone modification; biotinylation likely interacts with other covalent modification of histones. Elsewhere in this text, see an excellent review of vitamin-dependent modifications of chromatin by Zempleni and coworkers. Briefly, the relative importance in biotinidase and HCLS in the biotinylation and debiotinylation of histones has yet to be elucidated and is under active investigation [68–70]. HCLS is present in the nucleus in greater quantities than in the cytosol or the mitochondria [68]. Gravel and Narang have produced exciting evidence that HCLS likely acts in the nucleus to catalyze the biotinylation of histones [68] and have hypothesized that biotinidase acts primarily to catalyze the debiotinylation of histones producing a biotin regeneration cycle similar to that observed for the biotinylation of apocarboxylases and the regeneration of biotin during turnover of mitochondrial proteins (Figure 11.1). As fibroblasts from patients with HCLS deficiency are severely deficient in histone biotinylation [71], a direct or indirect role for biotinidase in histone biotinylation is likely. Genetic deficiencies of holocarboxylase synthetase and biotinidase cause two types of multiple carboxylase deficiency. These inborn errors bear some phenotypic resemblance to biotin deficiency, especially biotinidase deficiency, but are not identical. See the excellent recent review by Wolf in *The Metabolic and Molecular Basis of Inherited Disease* for a more detailed discussion [14]. Some clinical findings and biochemical abnormalities of biotinidase deficiency resemble those of biotin deficiency (dermatitis, alopecia, conjunctivitis, ataxia, developmental delay) suggesting that they are caused by biotin deficiency [72,73]. However, the signs and symptoms of biotin deficiency and biotinidase deficiency are not identical. Seizures, irreversible neurosensory hearing loss, and optic atrophy have been observed in biotinidase deficiency, but not in biotin deficiency. The gene for human biotinidase has been cloned, sequenced, and characterized [14]. The biotinidase gene is a single copy gene of 1629 bases encoding a 543 amino acid protein; the mRNA is present in multiple tissues including heart, brain, placenta, liver, lung, skeletal muscle, kidney, and pancreas. Biotinidase activity is greatest in serum, the liver, the kidney, and the adrenal gland. The liver is thought to be the source of serum biotinidase.

Five Mammalian Carboxylases

The five biotin-dependent carboxylases are propionyl CoA carboxylase (PCC), methylcrotonyl CoA carboxylase (MCC), pyruvate carboxylase (PC), acetyl CoA carboxylase 1 (ACC1), and acetyl CoA carboxylase 2 (ACC2). All except ACC2 are mitochondrial enzymes. In the carboxylase reaction, the carboxyl moiety is first attached to biotin at the ureido nitrogen opposite the side chain. Next, the carboxyl group is transferred to the substrate. The reaction is driven by the hydrolysis of ATP to ADP and inorganic phosphate.

ACC1 and ACC2 both catalyze the incorporation of bicarbonate into acetyl CoA to form malonyl CoA (Figure 11.2). ACC1 is located in the cytosol and produces the malonyl CoA, which is the rate-limiting substrate in fatty acid synthesis (elongation). ACC2 is located on the outer mitochondrial membrane and controls fatty acid oxidation in mitochondria through the inhibitory effect of malonyl CoA on fatty acid transport into mitochondria.

Pyruvate carboxylase (PC, EC 6.4.1.1) catalyzes the incorporation of bicarbonate into pyruvate to form oxaloacetate, an intermediate in the tricarboxylic acid cycle (Figure 11.2). Thus, PC catalyzes an anapleurotic reaction. In gluconeogenic tissues (i.e., liver and kidney), the oxaloacetate can be converted to glucose. Deficiency of PC is probably the cause of the lactic acidemia (Figure 11.2), and CNS lactic acidosis observed in biotin deficiency and biotinidase deficiency and may contribute to abnormalities in glucose regulation.

Methylcrotonyl CoA carboxylase (MCC, EC 6.4.1.4) catalyzes an essential step in the degradation of the branch-chained amino acid leucine (Figure 11.2). Deficient activity of MCC (whether due to the isolated MCC deficiency, HCLS deficiency, or biotin deficiency per se) leads to metabolism of its substrate 3-methylcrotonyl CoA by an alternate pathway to

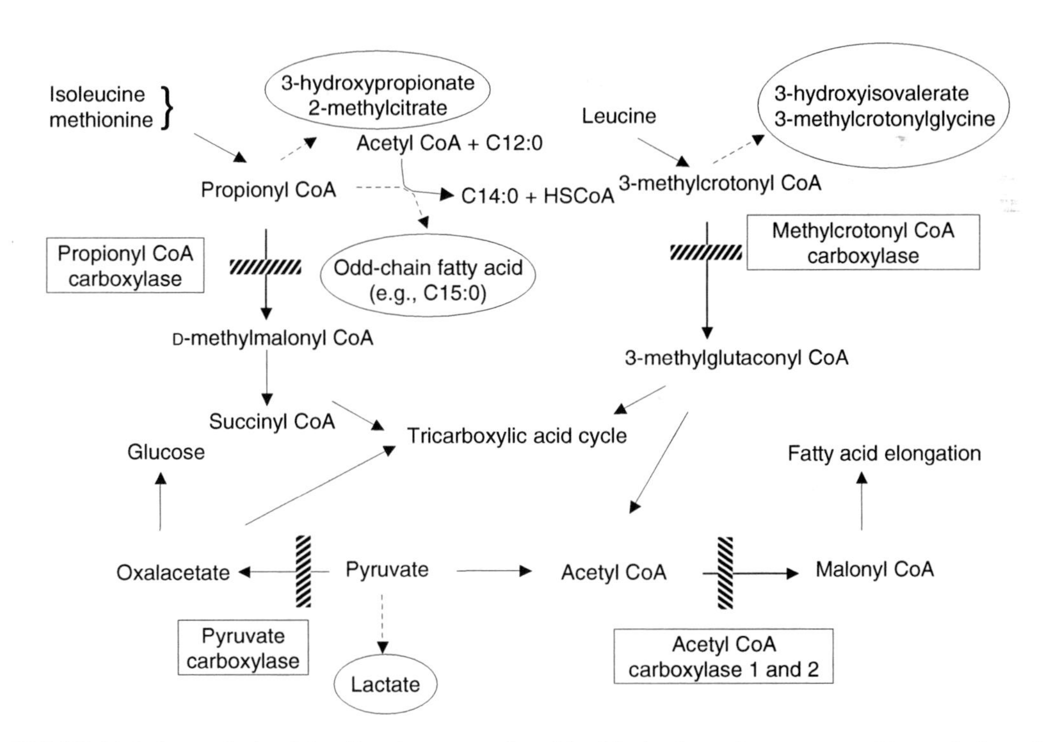

FIGURE 11.2 Interrelationship of pathways catalyzed by biotin-dependent enzymes (shown in boxes). Organic acids and odd-chain fatty acids accumulate because biotin deficiency causes reduced activity of biotin-dependent enzymes. Hatched bars denote metabolic blocks at deficient carboxylases. Ovals denote accumulation of products from alternative pathways, which are denoted by dashed arrows.

3-hydroxyisovaleric acid, 3-methylcrotonylglycine, and related organic acids (Figure 11.2). Thus, increased urinary excretion of these abnormal metabolites in the urine reflects deficient activity of MCC.

Propionyl CoA carboxylase (PCC, EC 6.4.1.3) catalyzes the incorporation of bicarbonate into propionyl CoA to form methylmalonyl CoA (Figure 11.2). Methylmalonyl CoA undergoes isomerization to succinyl CoA and enters the tricarboxylic acid cycle. Deficiency of PCC leads to increased urinary excretion of 3-hydroxypropionic acid and 2-methylcitric acid (Figure 11.2).

Biotin Catabolism

Instead of incorporation into carboxylases or histones, biotin may be catabolized. Biotin, possibly in the form of biotinyl CoA, can be oxidized to bisnorbiotin and tetranorbiotin (metabolites with two and four fewer carbons in the valeric acid side chain, respectively; Figure 11.1). The sulfur can be oxidized to sulfoxide and possibly sulfone. Biotin, bisnorbiotin, and biotin sulfoxide are present in mole ratios of ~3:2:1 in human urine and plasma. Biotin catabolism is induced during pregnancy, with cigarette smoking, and with anticonvulsant therapy, thereby increasing the ratio of biotin catabolites to biotin [74,75] and likely contributing to biotin depletion.

REQUIREMENT AND ASSESSMENT

Circumstances Leading to Deficiency

The requirement for biotin by the normal human has been clearly documented in three situations: prolonged consumption of raw egg white, parenteral nutrition without biotin supplementation in patients with short-gut syndrome [39], and infant feeding with an elemental formula devoid of biotin. As in Japan biotin could not legally be added as a supplement to infant formulas until 2003, all reports related to infant formula have come from Japan [76]. The most recent report by Fujimoto and colleagues describes the ninth such infant and provides an excellent summary of the results of the other eight infants [76]. The infants generally developed the classic cutaneous manifestations of biotin deficiency as well as the characteristic pattern of organic aciduria. Often feeding of an elemental formula was instituted because of chronic diarrhea in the infant. Biotinidase deficiency and zinc deficiency were ruled out in most of the infants. An undiagnosed deficiency of holocarboxylase synthetase deficiency was functionally ruled out in most infants by the gradual weaning of biotin supplementation at an age when the infant would be introduced to biotin-containing foods [76].

On the basis of lymphocyte carboxylase activity and plasma biotin levels, biotin deficiency likely also occurs in children with severe protein energy malnutrition; biotin deficiency may contribute to the clinical syndrome of protein energy malnutrition [77,78].

Long-term anticonvulsant therapy in adults can lead to biotin depletion [79,80]. The depletion can be severe enough to interfere with leucine metabolism and cause increased urinary excretion of 3-hydroxyisovaleric acid [75,81]. The mechanism of biotin depletion during anticonvulsant therapy is not known, but may involve accelerated biotin catabolism based on increased urinary excretion of biotin catabolites [75,82]. Impaired biotin absorption [83,84], impaired biotin transport in plasma, or impaired renal reclamation biotin [20] may also contribute to biotin depletion.

Studies of biotin status during pregnancy provide evidence that a marginal degree of biotin deficiency develops in at least one-third of women during normal pregnancy [85,86]. Although the degree of biotin deficiency was not severe enough to produce overt manifestations of biotin deficiency, the deficiency was sufficiently severe to produce metabolic derangements. A similar marginal degree of biotin deficiency causes high rates of fetal malformations in some mammals [87]. Moreover, data from a multivitamin supplementation study provide significant, although indirect, evidence that the marginal degree of biotin deficiency that occurs spontaneously in normal human gestation is teratogenic [88].

Biotin deficiency has also been reported or inferred in several other clinical circumstances. These include Leiner's disease, sudden infant death syndrome, renal dialysis, gastrointestinal diseases, and alcoholism [39].

Clinical Findings of Frank Deficiency

Whether caused by egg-white feeding or omission of biotin from total parenteral nutrition, the clinical findings of frank biotin deficiency in adults and older children have been quite similar to those reported by Sydenstricker in his pioneering study of egg-white feeding [39,89]. Typically, the findings began to appear gradually after several weeks to months for egg-white feeding. Six months to three years typically elapsed between the initiation of total intravenous feeding without biotin and the onset of the findings of biotin deficiency [39,90]. Thinning of hair, often with loss of hair color, was reported in most patients. A skin rash described as scaly (seborrheic) and red (eczematous) was present in the majority; in several, the rash was distributed around the eyes, nose, and mouth. Depression, lethargy, hallucinations, and paresthesias of the extremities were prominent neurologic symptoms in the majority of adults.

In infants who developed biotin deficiency, the signs and symptoms of biotin deficiency began to appear within 3 to 6 months after initiation of total parenteral nutrition or biotin-free formula. This earlier onset may reflect an increased biotin requirement because of growth. The rash typically appeared first around the eyes, nose, and mouth; ultimately, the ears and perineal orifices were involved (periorificial). The appearance of the rash was similar to that of cutaneous candidiasis (i.e., an erythematous base and crusting exudates); typically, *Candida* could be cultured from the lesions. The rash of biotin deficiency is similar, but not identical to the rash of zinc deficiency [76]. In infants, hair loss, including eyebrows and lashes, can occur after 6 to 9 months of parenteral nutrition. These cutaneous manifestations, in conjunction with an unusual distribution of facial fat, have been dubbed "biotin deficiency facies." The most striking neurologic findings in biotin-deficient infants were hypotonia, lethargy, and developmental delay. A peculiar withdrawn behavior was noted and may reflect the same CNS dysfunction diagnosed as depression in the adult patients.

Laboratory Findings of Biotin Deficiency

Methodology for Measuring Biotin

Methods for measuring biotin at pharmacologic and physiologic concentrations have been reviewed [39]. For measuring biotin at physiologic concentrations found in plasma and urine (i.e., 100 pmol/L to 100 nmol/L), a variety of assays have been proposed, and a limited number have been used to study biotin nutriture. All the published studies of biotin nutriture have used one of three basic types of biotin assays: (a) bioassays (most studies), (b) avidin-binding assays (several recent studies), or (c) fluorescent derivative and complex assays (a few published studies).

Bioassays generally have adequate sensitivity to measure biotin in blood and urine. Radiometric bioassays offer both sensitivity and precision. However, the bacterial bioassays (and perhaps the eukaryotic bioassays as well) suffer interference from unrelated substances and variable growth response to biotin analogs; these bioassays can give conflicting results if biotin is bound to protein [39].

Avidin-binding assays generally measure the ability of biotin to do one of the following: (a) to compete with radiolabeled biotin for binding to avidin (isotope dilution assays),

(b) to bind to ^{125}I-avidin and thus prevent ^{125}I-avidin (or enzyme-coupled avidin) from binding to a biotinylated protein adsorbed to plastic (sequential, solid phase assay), or (c) to prevent the binding of a biotinylated enzyme to avidin and thereby prevent the consequent inhibition of an enzyme activity. Other methods detect the postcolumn enhancement of fluorescence activity caused either by the mixing of the column eluate with fluorescent-labeled avidin or derivatization of biotin and metabolites by a fluorescent agent before separation by HPLC [91–93]. Avidin-binding assays using novel detection systems such as electrochemical detection [94], bioluminescence linked through glucose-6-phosphate dehydrogenase [95], or a double antibody technique [96] have been published and may offer some advantages in terms of sensitivity. Avidin-binding assays have been criticized for remaining cumbersome, requiring highly specialized equipment or reagents, or performing poorly when applied to biological fluids. Avidin-binding assays detect all avidin-binding substances, although the relative detectability of biotin and analogs varies between analogs and between assays, depending on how the assay is conducted (e.g., competitive vs. sequential). Assays that couple chromatographic separation of biotin analogs with subsequent avidin-binding assays of the chromatographic fractions are more sensitive and chemically specific [85,91,93]. These assays have been used in several studies that provide new insights into biotin nutrition [44,74,97–99].

A problem in the area of biotin analytical technology that remains unaddressed is the disagreement among the various bioassays and avidin-binding assays concerning the true concentration of biotin in human plasma. Reported mean values range from ~500 to >10,000 pmol/L.

Although commonly used to assess biotin status in a variety of clinical populations, the putative indexes of biotin status had not been previously studied during progressive biotin deficiency. To address this issue, Mock and coworkers [44] induced progressive biotin deficiency by feeding egg white. The urinary excretion of biotin declined dramatically with time on the egg-white diet, reaching frankly abnormal values in eight of nine subjects by day 20 of egg-white feeding. Bisnorbiotin excretion declined in parallel with urinary biotin, providing evidence for regulation of catabolism of the biotin metabolic pools. By day 14 of egg-white feeding, 3-hydroxyisovaleric acid excretion was abnormally increased in all nine subjects, providing evidence that biotin depletion decreases the activity of the biotin-dependent enzyme MCC and alters intermediary metabolism of leucine earlier in the course of experimental biotin deficiency than previously appreciated. Serum concentrations of free biotin as measured by HPLC separation and avidin-binding assay decreased to abnormal values in less than half of the subjects. Thus, these studies provide objective confirmation of the impression of many investigators in this field [100] that blood biotin concentration is not an early or sensitive indicator of impaired biotin status.

Plasma concentrations of biotin (i.e., total avidin-binding substances) are higher in term infants than older children and, for reasons that are not simply related to dietary intake, decline after 3 weeks of breast feeding or feeding a formula containing 11 μg/L of biotin. Infant formulas supplemented with 300 μg/L produce plasma concentrations ~20-fold greater than normal [101]; consequences of these higher levels, if any, are unknown.

Odd-chain fatty acid accumulation is a marker of biotin deficiency [102–105]. Several groups have independently demonstrated increases in the percentage composition of odd-chain fatty acids (e.g., 15:0, 17:0, etc.) in hepatic, cardiac, or serum phospholipids in the biotin-deficient rat and chick. Moreover, Mock and coworkers detected accumulation of odd-chain fatty acids in red cell membranes and plasma lipids of subjects in whom biotin deficiency was induced experimentally [99] and in the plasma of patients who developed biotin deficiency during parenteral nutrition [106]. The accumulation of odd-chain fatty acid is thought to result from PCC deficiency, based on the observation that the isolated genetic deficiency of PCC and related disorders cause an accumulation of odd-chain fatty acids in plasma, red blood cells, and liver [107,108]. Apparently, the accumulation of propionyl CoA leads to the substitution of propionyl CoA moiety for acetyl CoA in the ACC reaction, and hence, to the ultimate incorporation of a three carbon, rather than a two carbon, moiety during fatty acid elongation [109].

Biochemical Pathogenesis

The mechanisms by which biotin deficiency produces specific signs and symptoms remain to be completely delineated. However, several recent studies have given new insights into the biochemical pathogenesis of biotin deficiency. The assumption of most studies is that the clinical findings of biotin deficiency result directly or indirectly from deficient activities of the five biotin-dependent carboxylases. However, the recently elucidated role of biotin as a covalent modifier of histones and other evolving roles of the effects of biotin open the possibility that these mechanisms may also contribute to the phenotype of biotin deficiency.

Sander and coworkers initially suggested that the CNS effects of biotinidase deficiency (and, by implication, biotin deficiency) might be mediated through deficiency of PC and the attendant CNS lactic acidosis. As brain PC activity declined more slowly than hepatic PC activity during progressive biotin deficiency in the rat, these investigators discounted this mechanism. However, subsequent studies suggest their original hypothesis is correct. Diamantopoulos et al. [110] expanded the hypothesis by proposing that deficiency of brain biotinidase (which is already quite low in the normal brain) [111] combined with biotin deficiency leads to a deficiency of brain pyruvate carboxylase and, in turn, to CNS accumulation of lactic acid. This CNS lactic acidosis is postulated to be the primary mediator of the hypotonia, seizures, ataxia, and delayed development seen in biotinidase deficiency. Additional support for the CNS lactic acidosis hypothesis has come from direct measurements of CSF lactic acid in children with either biotinidase deficiency or isolated pyruvate carboxylase deficiency and from the rapid resolution of lactic acidemia and CNS abnormalities in patients who have developed biotin deficiency during parental nutrition [39]. The work of Suchy and coworkers has provided evidence against an etiologic role for disturbances in brain fatty acid composition in the CNS dysfunction [103,112].

Several studies have demonstrated abnormalities in metabolism of fatty acids in biotin deficiency and have suggested that these abnormalities are important in the pathogenesis of the skin rash and hair loss. The cutaneous manifestations of biotin deficiency and essential fatty acid deficiency are similar but not identical and the pathogenesis likely involves impaired lipid synthesis. For example, Munnich et al. [113] described a 12 year old boy with multiple carboxylase deficiency; in retrospect, the enzymatic defect was almost certainly biotinidase deficiency [114]. The child presented with alopecia and periorificial scaly dermatitis. Oral administration of "unsaturated fatty acids composed of 11% C18:1, 71% C18:2, 8% C18:3, and 0.3% C20:4" at a rate of "2–400 mg/day" plus twice daily topical administration of the same mixture of fatty acids "resulted in dramatic improvement of the dermatologic condition" and hair growth. Lactic acidosis and organic aciduria remained the same.

Three studies in the rat support the possibility of abnormal polyunsaturated fatty acid (PUFA) metabolism as a cause of the cutaneous manifestations of biotin deficiency. Kramer et al. [102] and Mock et al. [104] have reported significant abnormalities in the *n*-6 phospholipids of blood, liver, and heart. Watkins and Kratzer also found abnormalities of *n*-6 phospholipids in liver and heart of biotin-deficient chicks [115]. Several investigators have speculated [103–109,111,114,116,117] that these abnormalities in PUFA composition might result in abnormal composition or metabolism of the prostaglandins and related substances derived from these PUFAs. However, these studies did not directly address the question of an etiologic role. To address that question, Mock [118] examined the effect of supplementation of the n-6 PUFA (as intralipid) on the cutaneous manifestations of biotin deficiency in a nutrient interaction experiment. Supplementation of n-6 PUFA prevented the development of the cutaneous manifestations of biotin deficiency in a group of rats that were as biotin deficient (based on biochemical measurements) as the biotin-deficient control group. The rats not receiving the supplemental n-6 fatty acids did develop the classic rash and hair loss. This study provides evidence that an abnormality in n-6 PUFA metabolism plays a pathogenic role in the cutaneous manifestations of biotin deficiency and that the effect of the n-6 PUFA cannot be attributed to biotin sparing.

Other Effects of Deficiency

Subclinical biotin deficiency has been shown to be teratogenic in several species including chicken, turkey, mouse, rat, and hamster [39]. Fetuses of mouse dams with degrees of biotin deficiency too mild to produce the characteristic cutaneous or CNS findings developed micrognathia, cleft palate, and micromelia [119–123]. The incidence of malformation increased with the degree of biotin deficiency to a maximum incidence of ~90%. Differences in teratogenic susceptibility among rodent species have been reported; a corresponding difference in biotin transport from the mother to the fetus has been proposed as the cause [124]. Bain et al. have hypothesized that biotin deficiency affects bone growth by affecting synthesis of prostaglandins from n-6 fatty acid [125]. This effect on bone growth might be the mechanism for the skeletal malformations caused by biotin deficiency.

On the basis of studies of cultured lymphocytes in vitro and of rats and mice in vivo, biotin is required for normal function of a variety of immunological cells. These functions include production of antibodies, immunological reactivity, protection against sepsis, macrophage function, differentiation of T and B lymphocytes, afferent immune response, and cytotoxic T-cell response [126–131]. However, in rats in which only moderate biotin deficiency was induced, immune function was not strikingly impaired. Specifically, neither phenotype nor organ redistribution of lymphocytes occurred, and mitogen T-cell proliferation, mitogen-induced interferon-γ, and interleukin-4, and IgG antibody responses and natural killer cell activity were not affected by moderate biotin deficiency [123]. In humans, Okabe et al. [132] have reported that patients with Crohn's disease have depressed natural killer activity caused by biotin deficiency and are responsive to biotin supplementation. In patients with biotinidase deficiency, Cowan et al. [133] have demonstrated defects in both T-cell and B-cell immunity. However, supplementation of 750 μg of biotin per day for 14 days in normal subjects actually caused a significant decrease in peripheral blood monocyte proliferation as well as release of interleukin-1β and interleukin-2 [122].

Evidence is accumulating that biotin has stimulatory effects on genes whose actions favor lowering blood glucose concentrations; these include insulin, insulin receptor, and both pancreatic and hepatic glucokinase. Biotin also decreases expression of hepatic phosphoenolpyruvate carboxykinase, a key enzyme in gluconeogenesis by the liver. Thus, the net effect observed from biotin in whole animal and cell culture studies favors hypoglycemia. These observations are in accord with studies detecting impaired glucose tolerance and decreased glucose utilization in biotin-deficient rats. Recently, pharmacologic amounts of biotin have been reported to lower postprandial glucose concentrations and improve tolerance to glucose in genetically diabetic mice strains and in individuals with Type I and Type II diabetes. In a similar fashion, older studies indicating that biotin deficiency interferes with lipid metabolism and pharmacologic biotin therapy improves hyperglycemia have been confirmed in recent studies in individuals with hypertriglyceridemia. This topic is the subject of an excellent recent review by Fernandez-Mejia [134].

Diagnosis of Biotin Deficiency

The diagnosis of biotin deficiency has been established by demonstrating reduced PCC activity in peripheral blood lymphocytes [135,136], reduced urinary excretion of biotin [44,45], increased urinary excretion of the characteristic organic acids discussed earlier [45,99], and resolution of the signs and symptoms of deficiency in response to biotin supplementation. Plasma and serum levels of biotin, whether measured by bioassay or avidin-binding assay, have not uniformly reflected biotin deficiency [44,85,100]. The clinical response to administration of biotin has been dramatic in all well-documented cases of biotin deficiency. Within a few weeks, healing of the rash has been striking, and growth of healthy hair was generally present after 1–2 months of biotin supplementation. In infants, hypotonia, lethargy, and depression generally resolved within 1–2 weeks of biotin supplementation; accelerated mental and motor development followed.

Requirements and Allowances

Data providing an accurate estimate of the biotin requirement for infants, children, and adults are lacking [137]; as a result, recommendations often conflict among countries [39]. Data providing an accurate estimate of the requirement for biotin administered parenterally are also lacking. For parenteral administration, uncertainty about the true metabolic requirement for biotin is compounded by lack of information concerning the effects of infusing biotin systemically and continuously (rather than the usual postprandial absorption into intestinal portal blood). Despite these limitations, recommendations for biotin supplementation have been formulated for oral and parenteral intake from preterm infants through adults [137–139]. These recommendations are given in Table 11.1. One published study describes infants parenterally supplemented [140]; normal plasma levels of biotin were detected in term infants supplemented at 20 μg/day and increased plasma levels of biotin were detected in preterm infants supplemented at 13 μg/day (note that the units for plasma biotin should be picogram per milliliter in this publication [140]).

TABLE 11.1
Recommended Intake of Biotin

Age	Safe and Adequate Daily Oral Intakes (μg)	Daily Parenteral Intakes (μg)
Preterm infants	5	5–8 $\mu g\ kg^{-1}$
Infants up to 6 months	5	20
Infants 7–12 months	6	20
Children 1–3 years	8	20
Children 4–8 years	12	20
Children 9–13 years	20	20
Children 14–18 years	25	20
Adults	30	60
Pregnancy	30	—
Lactation	35	—

Sources: National Research Council in *Recommended Dietary Allowances*, 11th ed., Food and Nutrition Board Institute of Medicine National Academy Press, Washington, DC, 1998, 374–389; Greene, H.L., Hambridge, K.M., Schanler, R., and Tsang, R.C., *Am. J. Clin. Nutr.*, 48, 1324, 1988; Greene, H.L. and Smidt, L.J. in *Nutritional Needs of the Preterm Infant*, Tsang, R.C., Lucas, A., Uauy, R., and Zlotkin, S., eds., Williams & Wilkins, Baltimore, MD, 1993, 121–133.

An important factor in the current uncertainty concerning the biotin requirement is the possibility that biotin synthesized by intestinal bacteria may contribute significantly to absorbed biotin. If so, the required intake would be reduced and might be dependent on factors that influence the density and species distribution of intestinal flora. Unfortunately, few data are available for assessing the actual magnitude of the absorbed microbial biotin.

Dietary Sources of Biotin

There is no published evidence that biotin can be synthesized by mammals; thus, the higher animals must derive biotin from other sources. The ultimate source of biotin appears to be de novo synthesis by bacteria, primitive eukaryotic organisms such as yeast, molds, and algae, and some plant species.

Most measurements of the biotin content of various foods have used bioassays [141–145]. Recent publications [12,146] provide evidence that the values are likely to contain substantial errors. However, some worthwhile generalizations can still be made. Biotin is widely distributed in natural foodstuffs, but the absolute content of even the richest sources is low when compared with the content of most other water-soluble vitamins. Foods relatively rich in biotin include egg yolk, liver, nuts, legumes, and some vegetables [12,146]. The average daily dietary biotin intake has been estimated to be ~35–70 μg using a microbial assay [141,147–149].

PHARMACOLOGY AND TOXICITY

Treatment of Biotin Deficiency

Pharmacologic doses of biotin (e.g., 1–20 mg) have been used to treat most patients with biotin deficiency and biotin-related inborn errors. For two patients, parenteral administration of physiologic amounts of biotin (100 μg/day) was adequate to cause resolution of the signs and symptoms of biotin deficiency and to prevent their recurrence [39]. However, abnormal organic aciduria persisted for at least 10 weeks in one patient receiving 100 μg/day, suggesting that this dose may not have been adequate to restore tissue biotin levels to normal over that time. In pregnant women with increased 3-hydroxyisovaleric acid excretion treatment with 300 μg of biotin for 2 weeks resulted in decreased 3-hydroxyisovaleric acid excretion in every woman, but 3-hydroxyisovaleric acid excretion did not return to normal in 3 of 13 women. Likely, this organic aciduria indicates that biotin status at the tissue level was not restored entirely to normal. Whether this degree of deficiency is sufficient to cause significant, subtle morbidity is currently not known.

Toxicity

Daily doses up to 200 mg orally and up to 10–20 mg intravenously for over 6 months have been given to treat biotin-responsive inborn errors of metabolism and acquired biotin deficiency; toxicity has not been reported [14].

Pharmacology

Mounting reports of biotin deficiency in commercial animals and humans have led to several studies of plasma levels, pharmacokinetics, and bioavailability after acute or chronic oral, intramuscular, or intravenous administration of biotin in cattle [150], swine [151,152], and human subjects [19,153,154].

Doses greater than 300 μg result in high biotin concentrations in blood and the urinary excretion of a large proportion as the unchanged vitamin [153–155]. Increased blood concentrations of bisnorbiotin and biotin sulfoxide [155] and urine excretion rates [156] of bisnorbiotin and biotin sulfoxide are also observed. These observations are consistent with the metabolites originating from human tissues rather than enteric bacteria.

ACKNOWLEDGMENTS

With appreciation to Maribeth Mock, Nell Matthews Mock, and Cindy Henrich for graphic and processing support.

REFERENCES

1. Green, N.M., Avidin and streptavidin, in *Methods in Enzymology*, Wilchek, M. and Bayer, E., eds., Academic Press, New York, 1990, Vol. 186, pp. 51–67.
2. Bhatia, D., Borenstein, B., Gaby, S., Gordon, H., Iannarone, A., Johnson, L., Machlin, L.J., Mergens, W., Scheiner, J., Scott, J., and Waysek, E., Vitamins, Part XIII: Biotin, in *Encyclopedia of Food Science and Technology*, Hui, Y.U., ed., John Wiley & Sons, New York, 1992, pp. 2764–2770.
3. Bonjour, J.-P., Biotin, in *Handbook of Vitamins*, 2nd ed., Machlin, L.J., ed., Marcel Dekker, New York, 1991, pp. 393–427.
4. Sternbach, L.H., Biotin, in *Comprehensive Biochemistry*, Florkin, M. and Stotz, E.G., eds., Elsevier, New York, 1963, pp. 66–81.
5. Miljkovic, D., Velimirovic, S., Csanadi, J., and Popsavin, V., Studies directed towards stereospecific synthesis of oxybiotin, biotin, and their analogs. Preparation of some new 2,5,anhydro-xylitol derivatives, *J. Carbohydr. Chem.*, 8, 457–467, 1989.
6. Deroose, F.D. and DeClercq, P.J., Novel enantioselective syntheses of (+)-biotin, *J. Org. Chem.*, 60, 321–330, 1995.
7. Lampen, J.O., Bahler, G.P., and Peterson, W.H., The occurrence of free and bound biotin, *J. Nutr.*, 23, 11–21, 1942.
8. Combs, G.F., Biotin, in *The Vitamins: Fundamental Aspects in Nutrition and Health*, Academic Press, San Diego, 1992, pp. 329–343.
9. Frigg, M., Bio-availability of biotin in cereals, *Poult. Sci.*, 55, 2310–2318, 1976.
10. Mock, D.M. and Malik, M.I., Distribution of biotin in human plasma: Most of the biotin is not bound to protein, *Am. J. Clin. Nutr.*, 56, 427–432, 1992.
11. Mock, D.M. and Lankford, G., Studies of the reversible binding of biotin to human plasma, *J. Nutr.*, 120, 375–381, 1990.
12. Staggs, C.G., Sealey, W.M., McCabe, B.J., and Mock, D.M., Determination of the biotin content of select foods using accurate and sensitive HPLC/avidin binding, *J. Food Composit. Anal.*, 17, 767–776, 2004.
13. Wolf, B., Heard, G., McVoy, J.R.S., and Raetz, H.M., Biotinidase deficiency: The possible role of biotinidase in the processing of dietary protein-bound biotin, *J. Inherit. Metab. Dis.*, 7 (Suppl 2), 121–122, 1984.
14. Wolf, B., Disorders of biotin metabolism, in *The Metabolic and Molecular Basis of Inherited Disease*, 8th ed., Scriver, C.R., Beaudet, A.L., Sly, W.S., and Valle, D., eds., McGraw-Hill, New York, 2001, pp. 3151–3177.
15. Said, H.M., Thuy, L.P., Sweetman, L., and Schatzman, B., Transport of the biotin dietary derivative biocytin (*N*-biotinyl-L-lysine) in rat small intestine, *Gastroenterology*, 104, 75–80, 1993.
16. Said, H.M., Recent advances in carrier-mediated intestinal absorption of water-soluble vitamins, *Annu. Rev. Physiol.*, 66 (January), 419–446, 2004.
17. Bowman, B.B., McCormick, D.B., and Rosenberg, I.H., Epithelial transport of water-soluble vitamins, *Ann. Rev. Nutr.*, 9, 187–199, 1989.
18. McCormick, D.B. and Zhang, Z., Cellular assimilation of water-soluble vitamins in the mammal: Riboflavin, B_6, biotin, and C, *Proc. Soc. Exp. Biol. Med.*, 202, 265–270, 1993.

19. Zempleni, J. and Mock, D.M., Bioavailability of biotin given orally to humans in pharmacologic doses, *Am. J. Clin. Nutr.*, 69, 504–508, 1999.
20. Chauhan, J. and Dakshinamurti, K., Role of human serum biotinidase as biotin-binding protein, *Biochem. J.*, 256, 265–270, 1988.
21. Wolf, B., Biotinidase: Its role in biotinidase deficiency and biotin metabolism, *J. Nutr. Biochem.*, 16 (7), 441–445, 2005.
22. Nagamine, T., Takehara, K., Fukui, T., and Mori, M., Clinical evaluation of biotin-binding immunoglobulin in patients with Graves' disease, *Clin. Chim. Acta*, 226 (1), 47–54, 1994.
23. Cohen, N.D. and Thomas, M., Biotin transport into fully differentiated 3T3-L1 cells, *Biochem. Biophys. Res. Commun.*, 108 (4), 1508–1516, 1982.
24. Boumendil-Podevin, E.F. and Podevin, R.A., Nicotinic acid transport by brush border membrane vesicles from rabbit kidney, *Am. J. Physiol. Renal Fluid Electrolyte Physiol.*, 240, F185–F191, 1989.
25. Said, H.M., Korchid, S., and Horne, D.W., Transport of biotin in basolateral membrane vesicles of rat liver, *Am. J. Physiol.*, 259, G865–G872, 1990.
26. Said, H.M., Hoefs, J., Mohammadkhani, R., and Horne, D., Biotin transport in human liver basolateral membrane vesicles: A carrier-mediated, Na^+ gradient-dependent process, *Gastroenterology*, 10, 2120–2125, 1992.
27. Said, H.M., Ma, T.Y., and Kamanna, V.S., Uptake of biotin by human hepatoma cell line, Hep G(2): A carrier-mediated process similar to that of normal liver, *J. Cell Physiol.*, 161 (3), 483–489, 1994.
28. Balamurugan, K., Ortiz, A., and Said, H.M., Biotin uptake by human intestinal and liver epithelial cells: Role of the SMVT system, *Am. J. Physiol. Gastrointest. Liver Physiol.*, 285 (1), G73–G77, 2003.
29. Weiner, D. and Wolf, B., Biotin uptake, utilization, and efflux in normal and biotin-deficient rat hepatocytes, *Biochem. Med. Metab. Biol.*, 46, 344–363, 1991.
30. Said, H.M., McAlister-Henn, L., Mohammadkhani, R., and Horne, D.W., Uptake of biotin by isolated rat liver mitochondria, *Am. J. Physiol.*, 263, G81–G86, 1992.
31. Zempleni, J., Green, G.M., Spannagel, A.U., and Mock, D.M., Biliary excretion of biotin and biotin metabolites is quantitatively minor in rats and pigs, *J. Nutr.*, 127, 1496–1500, 1997.
32. Spector, R. and Mock, D.M., Biotin transport through the blood–brain barrier, *J. Neurochem.*, 48, 400–404, 1987.
33. Spector, R. and Mock, D.M., Biotin transport and metabolism in the central nervous system, *Neurochem. Res.*, 13 (3), 213–219, 1988.
34. Ozand, P.T., Gascon, G.G., Al Essa, M., Joshi, S., Al Jishi, E., Bakheet, S., Al Watban, J., Al-Kawi, M.Z., and Dabbagh, O., Biotin-responsive basal ganglia disease: A novel entity, *Brain*, 121, 1267–1279, 1999.
35. Zeng, W., Al-Yamani, E., Acierno, J., Slaugenhaupt, S., Gillis, T., Macdonald, M., Ozand, P., and Gusella, J., Biotin-responsive basal ganglia disease maps to 2q36.3 and is due to mutations in SLC19A3., *Am. J. Hum. Genet.*, 77 (1), 16–26, 2005.
36. Vlasova, T.I. and Mock, D.M., Biotin deficiency reduces expression of SLC19A3, a potential biotin transporter, and decreases expression of several biotin-related genes in the peripheral blood mononuclear cells (PBMC) of normal humans, in *Experimental Biology, 2004*, Washington, DC, FASEB, select.biosis.org/faseb/eb2004_data/FASEB009278.html, 2004.
37. Vlasova, T.I., Stratton, S.L., Wells, A.M., Mock, N.I., and Mock, D.M., Biotin deficiency reduces expression of SLC19A3, a potential biotin transporter, in leukocytes from human blood, *J. Nutr.*, 135 (1), 42–47, 2005.
38. Mardach, R., Zempleni, J., Wolf, B., Cress, S., Boylan, J., Roth, S., Cederbaum, S., and Mock, D., Biotin dependency due to a defect in biotin transport, *J. Clin. Invest.*, 109 (12), 1617–1623, 2002.
39. Mock, D.M., Biotin, in *Present Knowledge in Nutrition*, 6th ed., Brown, M., ed., International Life Sciences Institute—Nutrition Foundation, Blacksburg, VA, 1990, pp. 189–207.
40. Livaniou, E., Nyalala, J., Anagnostouli, M., Papageorgiou, C., Evangelatos, G., and Ithakissios, D., Determination of biotin levels in cerebrospinal fluid samples, *J. Pharm. Biomed. Anal.*, 21 (4), 875–879, 1999.
41. Baumgartner, E.R., Suormala, T., and Wick, H., Biotinidase deficiency associated with renal loss of biocytin and biotin, *J. Inherit. Metab. Dis.*, 7 (Suppl 2), 123–125, 1985.
42. Baur, B. and Baumgartner, E.R., Na(+)-dependent biotin transport into brush-border membrane vesicles from human kidney cortex, *Pflugers Archiv: Eur. J. Physiol.*, 422, 499–505, 1993.

43. Chatterjee, N.S., Kumar, C.K., Ortiz, A., Rubin, S., and Said, H.M., Molecular mechanism of the intestinal biotin transport process, *Am. J. Physiol.*, 277 (*Cell Physiol.*, 46), C605–C613, 1999.
44. Mock, N.I., Malik, M.I., Stumbo, P.J., Bishop, W.P., and Mock, D.M., Increased urinary excretion of 3-hydroxyisovaleric acid and decreased urinary excretion of biotin are sensitive early indicators of decreased status in experimental biotin deficiency, *Am. J. Clin. Nutr.*, 65, 951–958, 1997.
45. Mock, D.M., Henrich, C.L., Carnell, N., and Mock, N.I., Indicators of marginal biotin deficiency and repletion in humans: Validation of 3-hydroxyisovaleric acid excretion and a leucine challenge, *Am. J. Clin. Nutr.*, 76, 1061–1068, 2002.
46. Baumgartner, E.R., Suormala, T., and Wick, H., Biotinidase deficiency: Factors responsible for the increased biotin requirement, *J. Inherit. Metab. Dis.*, 8 (Suppl 1), 59–64, 1985.
47. Baumgartner, E.R., Suormala, T., and Wick, H., Biotin-responsive multiple carboxylase deficiency (MCD): Deficient biotinidase activity associated with renal loss of biotin, *J. Inherit. Metab. Dis.*, 8 (Suppl 1), 59–64, 1985.
48. Karl, P.I. and Fisher, S.E., Biotin transport in microvillous membrane vesicles, cultured trophoblasts and the isolated perfused cotyledon of the human placenta, *Am. J. Physiol.*, 262, C302–C308, 1992.
49. Schenker, S., Hu, Z., Johnson, R.F., Yang, Y., Frosto, T., Elliott, B.D., Henderson, G.I., and Mock, D.M., Human placental biotin transport: Normal characteristics and effect of ethanol, *Alcohol. Clin. Exp. Res.*, 17 (3), 566–575, 1993.
50. Hu, Z.-Q., Henderson, G.I., Mock, D.M., and Schenker, S., Biotin uptake by basolateral membrane of human placenta: Normal characteristics and role of ethanol, *Proc. Soc. Biol. Exp. Med.*, 206 (4), 404–408, 1994.
51. Prasad, P.D., Ramamoorthy, S., Leibach, F.H., and Ganapathy, V., Characterization of a sodium-dependent vitamin transporter mediating the uptake of pantothenate, biotin and lipoate in human placental choriocarcinoma cells, *Placenta*, 18, 527–533, 1997.
52. Wang, H., Huang, W., Fei, Y.J., Xia, H., Fang-Yeng, T.L., Leibach, F.H., Devoe, L.D., Ganapathy, V., and Prasad, P.D., Human placental Na^+-dependent multivitamin transporter, *J. Biol. Chem.*, 274, 14875–14883, 1999.
53. Crisp, S., Griffin, J., White, B., Toombs, C., Camporeale, G., Said, H.M., and Zempleni, J., Biotin supply affects rates of cell proliferation, biotinylation of carboxylases and histones, and expression of the gene encoding the sodium-dependent multivitamin transporter in JAr choriocarcinoma cells, *Eur. J. Nutr.*, 43 (1), 23–31, 2004.
54. Mock, D.M., Mock, N.I., and Langbehn, S.E., Biotin in human milk: Methods, location, and chemical form, *J. Nutr.*, 122, 535–545, 1992.
55. Mock, D.M., Mock, N.I., and Dankle, J.A., Secretory patterns of biotin in human milk, *J. Nutr.*, 122, 546–552, 1992.
56. Mock, D.M., Stratton, S.L., and Mock, N.I., Concentrations of biotin metabolites in human milk, *J. Pediatr.*, 131 (3), 456–458, 1997.
57. McMahon, R.J., Biotin in metabolism and molecular biology, *Annu. Rev. Nutr.*, 22, 221–239, 2002.
58. Mock, D., Biotin: Physiology, dietary sources and requirements, in *Encyclopedia of Human Nutrition*, 2nd ed., Caballero, B., Allen, L., and Prentice, A., eds., Academic Press, London, 2004.
59. Browner, M.F., Taroni, F., Sztul, E., and Rosenberg, L.B., Sequence analysis, biogenesis, and mitochondrial import of the alpha-subunit of rat liver propionyl-CoA carboxylase, *J. Biol. Chem.*, 264, 12680–12685, 1989.
60. Chapman-Smith, A. and Cronan, J., The enzymatic biotinylation of proteins: A post-translational modification of exceptional specificity, *Trends Biochem. Sci.*, 24 (9), 359–363, 1999.
61. Cronan, J.E., Jr., The *E. coli* bio operon: Transcriptional repression by an essential protein modification enzyme, *Cell*, 58, 427–429, 1989.
62. Xu, Y. and Beckett, D., Kinetics of biotinyl-5′-adenylate synthesis catalyzed by the *Escherichia coli* repressor of biotin biosynthesis and the stability of the enzyme-product complex, *Biochemistry*, 33, 7354–7360, 1994.
63. Beckett, D., The *Escherichia coli* biotin regulatory system: A transcriptional switch, *J. Nutr. Biochem.*, 16 (7), 411–415, 2005.

64. Suzuki, Y., Aoki, Y., Ishida, Y., Chiba, Y., Iwamatsu, A., Kishino, T., Niikawa, N., Matsubara, Y., and Narisawa, K., Isolation and characterization of mutations in the human holocarboxylase synthetase cDNA, *Nat. Genet.*, 8 (2), 122–128, 1994.
65. Leon-Del-Rio, A., Leclerc, D., Akerman, B., Wakamatsu, N., and Gravel, R., Isolation of a cDNA encoding human holocarboxylase synthetase by functional complementation of a biotin auxotroph of *Escherichia coli*, *Proc. Natl. Acad. Sci., USA*, 92 (10), 4626–4630, 1995.
66. Campeau, E. and Gravel, R.A., Expression in *Escherichia coli* of N- and C-terminally deleted human holocarboxylase synthetase. Influence of the N-terminus on biotinylation and identification of a minimum functional protein, *J. Biol. Chem.*, 276 (15), 12310–12316, 2001.
67. Yang, X., Aoki, Y., Li, X., Sakamoto, O., Hiratsuka, M., Kure, S., Taheri, S., Christensen, E., Inui, K., Kubota, M., Ohira, M., Ohki, M., Kudoh, J., Kawasaki, K., Shibuya, K., Shintani, A., Asakawa, S., Minoshima, S., Shimizu, N., Narisawa, K., Matsubara, Y., and Suzuki, Y., Structure of human holocarboxylase synthetase gene and mutation spectrum of holocarboxylase synthetase deficiency, *Hum. Genet.*, 109 (5), 526–534, 2001.
68. Gravel, R. and Narang, M., Molecular genetics of biotin metabolism: Old vitamin, new science, *J. Nutr. Biochem.*, 16 (7), 428–431, 2005.
69. Ballard, T., Wolff, J., Griffin, J., Stanley, J., van Calcar, S., and Zempleni, J., Biotinidase catalyzes debiotinylation of histones, *Eur. J. Nutr.*, 41 (2), 78–84, 2002.
70. Stanley, C., Hymes, J., and Wolf, B., Identification of alternatively spliced human biotinidase mRNAs and putative localization of endogenous biotinidase, *Mol. Genet. Metab.*, 81 (4), 300–312, 2004.
71. Narang, M.A., Dumas, R., Ayer, L.M., and Gravel, R.A., Reduced histone biotinylation in multiple carboxylase deficiency patients: A nuclear role for holocarboxylase synthetase, *Hum. Mol. Genet.*, 13 (1), 15–23, 2004.
72. Wolf, B., Heard, G.S., McVoy, J.R.S., and Grier, R.E., Biotinidase deficiency, *Ann. N.Y. Acad. Sci.*, 447, 252–262, 1985.
73. Mock, D.M., Delorimer, A.A., Liebman, W.M., Sweetman, L., and Baker, H., Biotin deficiency complicating parenteral alimentation, in *Biotin*, Dakshinamurti, K. and Bhagavan, H., eds., *New York Academy of Science*, New York, 1985, pp. 314–334.
74. Mock, D.M., Quirk, J.G., and Mock, N.I., Marginal biotin deficiency during normal pregnancy, *Am. J. Clin. Nutr.*, 75, 295–299, 2002.
75. Mock, D.M. and Dyken, M.E., Biotin catabolism is accelerated in adults receiving long-term therapy with anticonvulsants, *Neurology*, 49 (5), 1444–1447, 1997.
76. Fujimoto, W., Inaoki, M., Fukui, T., Inoue, Y., and Kuhara, T., Biotin deficiency in an infant fed with amino acid formula, *J. Dermatol.*, 32 (4), 256–261, 2005.
77. Velazquez, A., Martin-del-Campo, C., Baez, A., Zamudio, S., Quiterio, M., Aguilar, J.L., Perez-Ortiz, B., Sanchez-Ardines, M., Guzman-Hernandez, J., and Casanueva, E., Biotin deficiency in protein-energy malnutrition, *Eur. J. Clin. Nutr.*, 43, 169–173, 1988.
78. Velazquez, A., Teran, M., Baez, A., Gutierrez, J., and Rodriguez, R., Biotin supplementation affects lymphocyte carboxylases and plasma biotin in severe protein-energy malnutrition, *Am. J. Clin. Nutr.*, 61, 385–391, 1995.
79. Krause, K.-H., Berlit, P., and Bonjour, J.-P., Impaired biotin status in anticonvulsant therapy, *Ann. Neurol.*, 12, 485–486, 1982.
80. Krause, K.-H., Berlit, P., and Bonjour, J.-P., Vitamin status in patients on chronic anticonvulsant therapy, *Int. J. Vitam. Nutr. Res.*, 52 (4), 375–385, 1982.
81. Krause, K.-H., Kochen, W., Berlit, P., and Bonjour, J.-P., Excretion of organic acids associated with biotin deficiency in chronic anticonvulsant therapy, *Int. J. Vitam. Nutr. Res.*, 54, 217–222, 1984.
82. Mock, D.M., Mock, N.I., Lombard, K.A., and Nelson, R.P., Disturbances in biotin metabolism in children undergoing long-term anticonvulsant therapy, *J. Pediatr. Gastroenterol. Nutr.*, 26 (3), 245–250, 1998.
83. Said, H.M., Mock, D.M., and Collins, J.C., Regulation of biotin intestinal transport in the rat: Effect of biotin deficiency and supplementation, *Am. J. Physiol.*, 256 (2 Pt 1), G306–G311, 1989.
84. Said, H.M., Redha, R., and Nylander, W., Biotin transport and anticonvulsant drugs, *Am. J. Clin. Nutr.*, 49, 127–131, 1989.
85. Mock, D.M., Stadler, D.D., Stratton, S.L., and Mock, N.I., Biotin status assessed longitudinally in pregnant women, *J. Nutr.*, 127 (5), 710–716, 1997.

86. Mock, N.I., Evans, T.T., and Mock, D.M., Biotin supplementation during pregnancy reverses depleted biotin status as assessed by excretion of urinary 3-hydroxyisovaleric acid (3HIA), *FASEB J.*, 13 (5), A923, 1999.
87. Mock, D.M., Mock, N.I., Stewart, C.W., LaBorde, J.B., and Hansen, D.K., Marginal biotin deficiency is teratogenic in ICR mice, *J. Nutr.*, 133, 2519–2525, 2003.
88. Zempleni, J. and Mock, D.M., Marginal biotin deficiency is teratogenic, *Proc. Soc. Exp. Biol. Med.*, 223 (1), 14–21, 2000.
89. Sydenstricker, V.P., Singal, S.A., Briggs, A.P., DeVaughn, N.M., and Isbell, H., Observations on the 'egg white injury' in man, *JAMA*, 118, 1199–1200, 1942.
90. Mock, D.M., Water-soluble vitamin supplementation and the importance of biotin, in *Textbook on Total Parenteral Nutrition in Children: Indications, Complications, and Pathophysiological Considerations*, Lebenthal, E., ed., Raven Press, New York, 1986, pp. 89–108.
91. Przyjazny, A., Hentz, N.G., and Bachass, L.G., Sensitive and selective liquid chromatographic postcolumn reaction detection system for biotin and biocytin using a homogeneous fluorophore-linked assay, *J. Chromatogr.*, 654, 79–86, 1993.
92. Stein, J., Hahn, A., Lembcke, B., and Rehner, G., High-performance liquid chromatographic determination of biotin in biological materials after crown ether-catalyzed fluorescence derivatization with panacyl bromide, *Anal. Biochem.*, 200, 89–94, 1992.
93. Lahely, S., Ndaw, S., Arella, F., and Hasselmann, C., Determination of biotin in foods by high-performance liquid chromatography with post-column derivatization and fluorimetric detection, *Food Chem.*, 65, 253–258, 1999.
94. Sugawara, K., Tanaka, S., and Nakamura, H., Electrochemical determination of avidin–biotin binding using an electroactive biotin derivative as a marker, *Bioelectrochem. Bioenerg.*, 33, 205–207, 1994.
95. Terouanne, B., Bencheich, M., Balaguer, P., Boussioux, A.M., and Nicolas, J.C., Bioluminescent assays using glucose-6-phosphate dehydrogenase: Application to biotin and streptavidin detection, *Anal. Biochem.*, 180, 43–49, 1989.
96. Thuy, L.P., Sweetman, L., and Nyhan, W.L., A new immunochemical assay for biotin, *Clin. Chim. Acta*, 202 (3), 191–198, 1991.
97. Mock, N.I., Evans, T., and Mock, D.M., Urinary 3-hydroxypropionic acid is not an early indicator of biotin deficiency, *FASEB J.*, 12, A247, 1998.
98. Stratton, S.L., Bogusiewicz, A., Mock, M.M., Mock, N.I., Wells, A.M., and Mock, D.M., Lymphocyte propionyl-CoA Carboxylase and its activation by biotin are sensitive indicators of marginal biotin deficiency in humans, *Am. J. Clin. Nutr.*, 84, 384–388, 2006.
99. Mock, D.M., Henrich-Shell, C.L., Carnell, N., Stumbo, P., and Mock, N.I., 3-hydroxypropionic acid and methylcitric acid are not reliable indicators of marginal biotin deficiency, *J. Nutr.*, 134, 317–320, 2004.
100. Bonjour, J.-P., Biotin in human nutrition, in *Biotin*, Dakshinamurti, K. and Bhagavan, H., eds., *New York Academy of Sciences*, New York, 1985, pp. 97–104.
101. Livaniou, E., Mantagos, S., Kakabakos, S., Pavlou, V., Evangelatos, G., and Ithakissios, D.S., Plasma biotin levels in neonates, *Biol. Neonate*, 59, 209–212, 1991.
102. Kramer, T.R., Briske-Anderson, M., Johnson, S.B., and Holman, R.T., Effects of biotin deficiency on polyunsaturated fatty acid metabolism in rats, *J. Nutr.*, 114, 2047–2052, 1984.
103. Suchy, S.F., Rizzo, W.B., and Wolf, B., Effect of biotin deficiency and supplementation on lipid metabolism in rats: Saturated fatty acids, *Am. J. Clin. Nutr.*, 44, 475–480, 1986.
104. Mock, D.M., Mock, N.I., Johnson, S.B., and Holman, R.T., Effects of biotin deficiency on plasma and tissue fatty acid composition: Evidence for abnormalities in rats, *Pediatr. Res.*, 24 (3), 396–403, 1988.
105. Watkins, B.A. and Kratzer, F.H., Tissue lipid fatty acid composition of biotin-adequate and biotin-deficient chicks, *Poult. Sci.*, 66, 306–313, 1987.
106. Mock, D.M., Johnson, S.B., and Holman, R.T., Effects of biotin deficiency on serum fatty acid composition: Evidence for abnormalities in humans, *J. Nutr.*, 118, 342–348, 1988.
107. Wendel, U., Baumgartner, R., van der Meer, S.B., and Spaapen, L.J.M., Accumulation of odd-numbered long-chain fatty acids in fetuses and neonates with inherited disorders of propionate metabolism, *Pediatr. Res.*, 29 (4), 403–405, 1991.

108. Kishimoto, Y., Williams, M., Moser, H.W., Hignite, C., and Biemann, K., Branched-chain and odd-numbered fatty acids and aldehydes in the nervous system of a patient with deranged vitamin B_{12} metabolism, *J. Lipid Res.*, 14, 69–77, 1973.
109. Fenton, W. and Rosenberg, L.E., Disorders of propionate and methylmalonate metabolism, in *The Metabolic and Molecular Bases of Inherited Disease*, Scriver, C.R., Beaudet, A.L., Sly, W.S., and Valle, D., eds., McGraw-Hill, New York, 1995, pp. 1423–1449.
110. Diamantopoulos, N., Painter, M.J., Wolf, B., Heard, G.S., and Roe, C., Biotinidase deficiency: Accumulation of lactate in the brain and response to physiologic doses of biotin, *Neurology*, 36, 1107–1109, 1986.
111. Suchy, S.F., McVoy, J.R.S., and Wolf, B., Neurologic symptoms of biotinidase deficiency: Possible explanation, *Neurology*, 35, 1510–1511, 1985.
112. Suchy, S.F., Brown, S.B., Goodman, S.I., and Wolf, B., Diagnosis of biotin deficiency prior to the appearance of cutaneous symptoms, *Pediatr. Res.*, 16, 179A, 1982.
113. Munnich, A., Saudubray, J.M., Coude, F.K., Charpentier, C., Saurat, J.H., and Frezal, J., Fatty-acid-responsive alopecia in multiple carboxylase deficiency, *Lancet*, 1 (8177), 1080–1081, 1980.
114. Wolf, B., Grier, R.E., Allen, R.J., Goodman, S.I., and Kien, C.L., Biotinidase deficiency: An enzymatic defect in late-onset multiple carboxylase deficiency, *Clin. Chim. Acta*, 131, 273–281, 1983.
115. Watkins, B.A. and Kratzer, F.H., Effect of oral dosing of lactobacillus strains on gut colonization and liver biotin in broiler chicks, *Poult. Sci.*, 62, 2088–2094, 1983.
116. Marshall, M.W., The nutritional importance of biotin an update, *Nutr. Today*, 22 (6), 26–30, 1987.
117. Watkins, B.A. and Kratzer, F.H., Dietary biotin effects on polyunsaturated fatty acids in chick tissue lipids and prostaglandin E_2 levels in freeze-clamped hearts, *Poult. Sci.*, 66, 1818–1828, 1987.
118. Mock, D.M., Evidence for a pathogenic role of ω6 polyunsaturated fatty acid in the cutaneous manifestations of biotin deficiency, *J. Pediatr. Gastroenterol. Nutr.*, 10, 222–229, 1990.
119. Watanabe, T. and Endo, A., Teratogenic effects of maternal biotin deficiency in mouse embryos examined at midgestation, *Teratology*, 42, 295–300, 1990.
120. Watanabe, T., Dietary biotin deficiency affects reproductive function and prenatal development in hamsters, *J. Nutr.*, 123 (12), 2101–2108, 1993.
121. Watanabe, T., Dakshinamurti, K., and Persaud, T.V.N., Biotin influences palatal development of mouse embryos in organ culture, *J. Nutr.*, 125, 2114–2121, 1995.
122. Zempleni, J., Helm, R.M., and Mock, D.M., In vivo biotin supplementation at a pharmacologic dose decreases proliferation rates of human peripheral blood mononuclear cells and cytokine release, *J. Nutr.*, 131 (5), 1479–1484, 2001.
123. Helm, R.M., Mock, N.I., Simpson, P., and Mock, D.M., Certain immune markers are not good indicators of mild to moderate biotin deficiency in rats, *J. Nutr.*, 132, 3231–3236, 2001.
124. Watanabe, T. and Endo, A., Species and strain differences in teratogenic effects of biotin deficiency in rodents, *J. Nutr.*, 119, 255–261, 1989.
125. Bain, S.D., Newbrey, J.W., and Watkins, B.A., Biotin deficiency may alter tibiotarsal bone growth and modeling in broiler chicks, *Poult. Sci.*, 67, 590–595, 1988.
126. Rabin, B.S., Inhibition of experimentally induced autoimmunity in rats by biotin deficiency, *J. Nutr.*, 113, 2316–2322, 1983.
127. Pruzansky, J. and Axelrod, A.E., Antibody production to diphtheria toxoid in vitamin deficiency states, *Proc. Soc. Exp. Biol. Med.*, 89, 323–325, 1955.
128. Petrelli, F., Moretti, P., and Campanati, G., Studies on the relationships between biotin and the behaviour of B and T lymphocytes in the guinea pig, *Experientia*, 37, 1204–1206, 1981.
129. Kung, J.T., MacKenzie, C.G., and Talmage, D.W., The requirement for biotin and fatty acids in the cytotoxic T-cell response, *Cell Immunol.*, 48, 100–110, 1979.
130. Kumar, M. and Axelrod, A.E., Cellular antibody synthesis in thiamin, riboflavin, biotin and folic acid-deficient rats, *Proc. Soc. Exp. Biol. Med.*, 157, 421–423, 1978.
131. Báez-Saldaña, A., Díaz, G., Espinoza, B., and Ortega, E., Biotin deficiency induces changes in subpopulations of spleen lymphocytes in mice, *Am. J. Clin. Nutr.*, 67, 431–437, 1998.
132. Okabe, N., Urabe, K., Fujita, K., Yamamoto, T., and Yao, T., Biotin effects in Crohn's disease, *Dig. Dis. Sci.*, 33 (11), 1495–1496, 1988.
133. Cowan, M.J., Wara, D.W., Packman, S., Yoshino, M., Sweetman, L., and Nyhan, W., Multiple biotin-dependent carboxylase deficiencies associated with defects in T-cell and B-cell immunity, *Lancet*, 2 (8134), 115–118, 1979.

134. Fernandez-Mejia, C., Pharmacologic effects of biotin, *J. Nutr. Biochem.*, 16, 424–427, 2005.
135. Mock, D.M., Henrich, C.L., Carnell, N., Mock, N.I., and Swift, L., Lymphocyte propionyl-CoA carboxylase and accumulation of odd-chain fatty acid in plasma and erythrocytes are useful indicators of marginal biotin deficiency, *J. Nutr. Biochem.*, 13 (8), 462–470, 2002.
136. Mock, D.M., Mock, M.M., Bogy, C.D., Mock, N.I., and Stratton, S.L., Lymphocyte propionyl-CoA carboxylase (PCC) and activation of PCC by biotin are useful indicators of marginal biotin deficiency in humans, *FASEB J.*, 19 (4), A55, 2005.
137. National Research Council, Dietary reference intakes for thiamin, riboflavin, niacin, vitamin B_6, folate, vitamin B_{12}, pantothenic acid, biotin, and choline, in *Recommended Dietary Allowances*, 11th ed., Food and Nutrition Board Institute of Medicine National Academy Press, Washington, DC, 1998, pp. 374–389.
138. Greene, H.L., Hambridge, K.M., Schanler, R., and Tsang, R.C., Guidelines for the use of vitamins, trace elements, calcium, magnesium, and phosphorus in infants and children receiving total parenteral nutrition: Report of the Subcommittee on Pediatric Parenteral Nutrient Requirements for the Committee on Clinical Practice Issues of The American Society for Clinical Nutrition, *Am. J. Clin. Nutr.*, 48, 1324–1342, 1988.
139. Greene, H.L. and Smidt, L.J., Water soluble vitamins: C, B_1, B_2, B_6, niacin, pantothenic acid, and biotin, in *Nutritional Needs of the Preterm Infant*, Tsang, R.C., Lucas, A., Uauy, R., and Zlotkin, S., eds., Williams & Wilkins, Baltimore, MD, 1993, pp. 121–133.
140. Moore, M.C., Greene, H.L., and Phillips, B., Evaluation of a pediatric multiple vitamin preparation for total parenteral nutrition in infants and children: I. Blood levels of water-soluble vitamins, *Pediatrics*, 77, 530–538, 1986.
141. Hardinge, M.G. and Crooks, H., Lesser known vitamins in food, *J. Am. Diet. Assoc.*, 38, 240–245, 1961.
142. Wilson, J. and Lorenz, K., Biotin and choline in foods—Nutritional importance and methods of analysis: A review, *Food Chem.*, 4, 115–129, 1979.
143. Hoppner, K. and Lampi, B., The biotin content of breakfast cereals, *Nutr. Rep. Int.*, 28 (4), 793–798, 1983.
144. Pennington, J.A.T., Biotin, in *Bowes and Church's Food Values of Portions Commonly Used*, 15th ed., Lippincott, Philadelphia, 1989.
145. Guilarte, T.R., Analysis of biotin levels in selected foods using a radiometric-microbiological method, *Nutr. Rep. Int.*, 32 (4), 837–845, 1985.
146. Teague, A.M., Sealey, W.M., McCabe-Sellers, B., and Mock, D., Biotin is stable in frozen foods, *FASEB J.*, 18 (4), A143 (abst), 2004.
147. Hoppner, K., Lampi, B., and Smith, D.C., An appraisal of the daily intakes of vitamin B_{12}, pantothenic acid and biotin from a composite Canadian diet, *Can. Inst. Food Sci. Technol. J.*, 11 (2), 71–74, 1978.
148. Bull, N.L. and Buss, D.H., Biotin, pantothenic acid and vitamin E in the British household food supply, *Hum. Nutr.: Appl. Nutr.*, 36A, 125–129, 1982.
149. Lewis, J. and Buss, D.H., Trace nutrients: Minerals and vitamins in the British household food supply, *Br. J. Nutr.*, 60, 413–424, 1988.
150. Frigg, M., Straub, O.C., and Hartmann, D., The bioavailability of supplemental biotin in cattle, *Int. J. Vit. Nutr. Res.*, 63, 122–128, 1993.
151. Bryant, K.L., Kornegay, E.T., Knight, J.W., and Notter, D.R., Uptake and clearance rates of biotin in pig plasma following biotin injections, *Int. J. Vit. Nutr. Res.*, 60, 52–57, 1989.
152. Misir, R. and Blair, R., Biotin bioavailability from protein supplements and cereal grains for weanling pigs, *Can. J. Anim. Sci.*, 68, 523–532, 1988.
153. Bitsch, R., Salz, I., and Hötzel, D., Studies on bioavailability of oral biotin doses for humans, *Int. J. Vit. Nutr. Res.*, 59, 65–71, 1989.
154. Clevidence, B., Marshall, M., and Canary, J.J., Biotin levels in plasma and urine of healthy adults consuming physiological levels of biotin, *Nutr. Res.*, 8, 1109–1118, 1988.
155. Mock, D.M. and Mock, N.I., Serum concentrations of bisnorbiotin and biotin sulfoxide increase during both acute and chronic biotin supplementation, *J. Lab. Clin. Med.*, 129, 384–388, 1997.
156. Mock, D.M. and Heird, G.M., Urinary biotin analogs increase in humans during chronic supplementation: The analogs are biotin metabolites, *Am. J. Physiol. Endocrinol. Metab.*, 272, 83–87, 1997.

12 Folic Acid

Lynn B. Bailey

CONTENTS

INTRODUCTION

The isolation, structure identification, and synthesis of folic acid, which took place in the 1940s, led to the widespread therapeutic use of this water-soluble vitamin for the treatment of megaloblastic anemia. During the next 50 years, the basic aspects of folate metabolism and the biochemical functions were investigated and the key role of folate coenzymes in one carbon metabolism established. Since the early 1990s, the links between folate intake and birth outcome or chronic disease risk were explored. One of the most important public health discoveries of this century is that daily supplemental folic acid taken periconceptionally significantly reduces the risk of neural tube defects (NTDs). The conclusive evidence related to folic acid and NTD risk reduction led to the implementation of global public health policies including mandatory folic acid fortification in North America. The identification of genetic polymorphisms that affect the structure–function of folate-related enzymes and proteins has served as the catalyst for the ongoing search for links between these polymorphisms and increased risk for birth defects or chronic disease.

This chapter highlights the current knowledge of folate nutrition including key aspects of the chemistry, food sources, intake recommendations, methods of analysis and status assessment, metabolism, biochemical functions, and genetic polymorphisms. An overview of the association between folate status and health-related risks provides the foundation for new research efforts to address challenging new questions that have evolved from research efforts to date.

CHEMISTRY

STRUCTURE AND NOMENCLATURE

Folate consists of a family of compounds that differ in a variety of ways including the oxidation state of the molecule, the length of the glutamate side chain, and the specific one carbon units attached to the molecule. The folate molecule, tetrahydrofolate (THF), is derived from 5,6,7,8-tetrahydropteroylglutamate, which consists of a 2-amino-4-hydroxy-pteridine (pterin) moiety linked via a methylene group at the C-6 position to a *p*-aminobenzoylglutamic acid (*p*ABG) (Figure 12.1). The pyrazine ring in THF is fully reduced at the 5,6,7, and 8 positions and reduction at positions 7 and 8 only yields dihydrofolate. The monoglutamate form of the vitamin contains one glutamic acid molecule, which can be converted to a glutamate chain by the addition of glutamate residues by γ-peptide linkage. In the majority of naturally occurring folates, the number of glutamate units in the side chain varies from 5 to 8. The fully oxidized monoglutamate form of the vitamin is referred to as folic acid and is the form used commercially in supplements and fortified foods. In contrast to polyglutamyl folate, folic acid rarely occurs naturally in food. Specific one

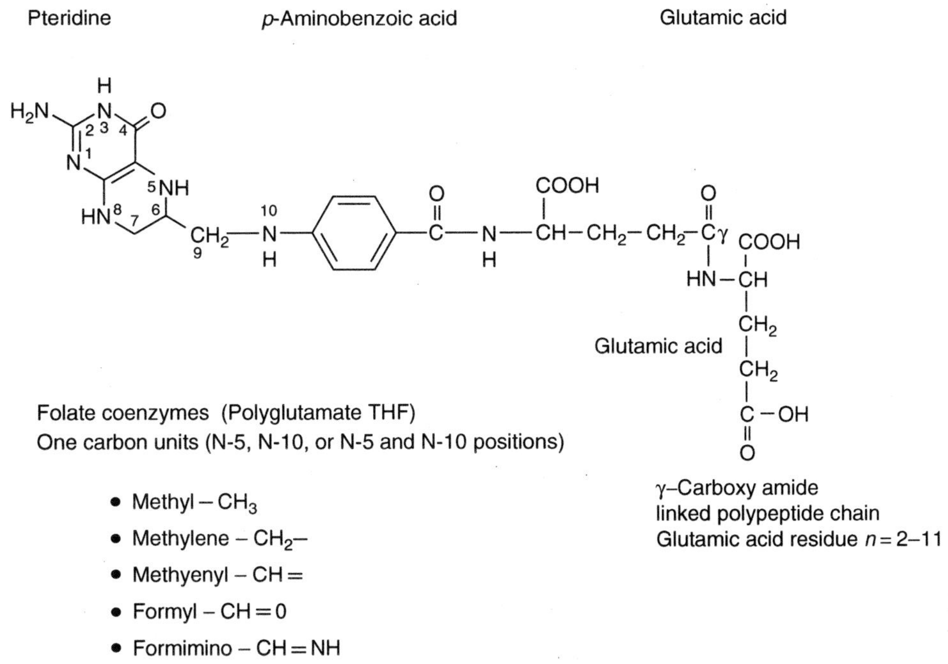

Pteridine *p*-Aminobenzoic acid Glutamic acid

H_2N H N O 2 3 4 N 1 5 NH HN 8 7 6 CH_2—N— 10 H 9 O C—N—H COOH CH–CH_2–CH_2–Cγ O COOH HN–CH CH_2 CH_2 C–OH O

Glutamic acid

Folate coenzymes (Polyglutamate THF)
One carbon units (N-5, N-10, or N-5 and N-10 positions)

- Methyl – CH_3
- Methylene – CH_2–
- Methyenyl – CH=
- Formyl – CH=0
- Formimino – CH=NH

γ–Carboxy amide
linked polypeptide chain
Glutamic acid residue $n = 2–11$

FIGURE 12.1 Folic acid structure. Folic acid consists of a pteridine ring linked to *p*-aminobenzoic acid joined at the other end to a molecule of glutamic acid. Food folates exist in various forms, containing different numbers of additional glutamate residues joined to the first glutamate. The folate or folic acid structure can vary by reduction of the pteridine moiety to form dihydrofolic acid and tetrahydrofolic acid (THF), elongation of the glutamate chain, and substitution of one carbon units to the polyglutamated form of the THF molecule.

carbon units that can be added at either or both of the N-5 or N-10 positions of the polyglutamyl form of the THF molecule include methyl (CH_3), methylene (—CH_2—), methenyl (—CH=), formyl (—CH=), or formimino (—CH=NH) groups.

Chemical Properties

The molecular weight of folic acid is 441.4, and although it is described as "water soluble," the acid form is only slightly soluble in water in contrast to the salt form, which is quite soluble. The THF molecule is labile in solution due to sensitivity to oxygen, light, and extremes in pH. In oxygenated solutions, THF breaks down to form pterin-6-carboxaldehyde, H_2 pterin, pterin, and xanthopterin. The molecule is rapidly cleaved at the C-9–N-10 bond forming *p*ABG.[1] In contrast to THF and N-10-substituted THF, which are unstable in the presence of oxygen, folic acid and THF substituted at N-5 (or N-5, N-10) are relatively stable when exposed to oxygen. Instability to light is a consistent feature of all forms of folate.

FOOD SOURCES

Naturally Occurring Food Folate

Folate that occurs naturally in the diet, referred to in this chapter as food folate, is concentrated in select foods including orange juice, strawberries, dark green leafy vegetables, peanuts, and dried beans such as black beans and kidney beans.[2] Meat in general is not a good source of folate, with the exception of liver.

Folic Acid in Fortified and Enriched Food Products

In addition to food folate, ready-to-eat breakfast cereals contribute significantly to folate intake in the United States since the majority of breakfast cereals in the United States marketplace contain ~100 μg per serving of folic acid and a smaller number contain 400 μg per serving.[3] Folic acid is an added ingredient in a large number of other food products including meal replacement and infant formulas, and an increasing number of ready-to-eat breakfast cereals, nutritional bars, and snack foods. In the United States, all "enriched" cereal grain products (e.g., bread, pasta, flour, breakfast cereal, and rice) and mixed food items containing these grains are required by the Food and Drug Administration to be fortified with folic acid for the purpose of reducing the risk of NTDs.[4] Although the effective date was January 1, 1998, the majority of food manufacturers had implemented folic acid fortification by mid-1997. Mandatory fortification has also been implemented in select countries in addition to the United States including Canada,[5] Chile,[6] and some Latin American countries.[7]

Effect of Folic Acid Fortification on Folate Intake and Status in the United States and Canada

Folic acid fortification has had a significant impact on folate status in the United States and Canada.[8,9] In the United States, recently reported nationally representative data from the National Health and Nutrition Examination Survey (NHANES) (1999–2000) were compared with that from the prefortification period (NHANES III 1988–1994).[8] The median serum folate concentration increased more than twofold (from 12.5 to 32.2 nmol/L) and the median red blood cell (RBC) folate concentration increased from 392 to 625 nmol/L from NHANES III (1988–1994) to NHANES (1999–2000). In Canada, the mean RBC folate concentration rose from 527 nmol/L during the prefortification period to 741 nmol/L postfortification in women of reproductive age.[9]

BIOAVAILABILITY

The bioavailability of folate may be defined as the portion of the nutrient that is physiologically available, which is influenced by numerous factors including but not limited to the following: (a) chemical form of folate; (b) food matrix; (c) the chemical environment in the intestinal tract; and (d) factors affecting the metabolic fate postabsorption.[10,11] Reported estimates of folate bioavailability are quite variable due in part to differences between experimental approaches and analytical methodologies used.[11–14]

The blood folate response to folic acid is greater than that observed in response to food folate.[10,11] The average bioavailability of food folate has been estimated to be no more than 50% relative to folic acid consumed alone in a fasting condition.[15] When folic acid is consumed with a light meal, the bioavailability is ~85% that of supplemental folic acid taken alone when fasting.[16]

METHODS

Food Folate

Food folate has historically been measured by a wide range of methods including microbiological assay, radiobinding or radiometric assay, and fluorometric, electrochemical, or spectrophotometric methods, with some methods in combination with high-performance liquid chromatography (HPLC).[17] A review of the interlaboratory variation using many of these different methods has been published.[18]

The microbiological assay has been considered to be one of the best and most versatile methods for the determination of food folate for the past half century. *Lactobacillus casei* subspecies *rhamnosus* (ATCC 7469) has been the most widely used microorganism since it responds almost equally to the widest variety of folate derivatives.[19] Folate values using the microbiological assay are currently obtained after heat extraction to release folate from folate-binding protein or the food matrix in the presence of a reducing agent such as ascorbic acid, followed by trienzymatic extraction and deconjugation.[20,21] This trienzyme procedure involves a combination of protease and α-amylase treatments to release folate bound to matrices of proteins and polysaccharides, respectively, in addition to pteroyl-γ-glutamyl carboxypeptidase (folate conjugase, EC 3.4.19.9), which hydrolyzes folate polyglutamates to folate with shorter glutamyl residues that can be used by the microorganisms.[19] Key studies have confirmed that the trienzyme assay results in significantly higher folate values compared with conjugase treatment alone and that the higher values are not an artifact of the assay procedure.[22,23] Based on the results of a recent collaborative study, the microbiological assay with trienzyme extraction has been recommended for adoption as the official AOAC method.[24]

Food folate can also be measured by HPLC methods[25,26] and procedures are also available to either allow the identification of specific one carbon derivatives of folate[27] or characterize the length of the polypeptide chain.[28,29] To identify the one carbon entities, folates are treated with folate conjugase to convert the polyglutamyl folates to monoglutamates and then separated by reverse phase HPLC.[27] To identify polyglutamate distributions, folates can be cleaved at the C-9–N-10 bond to yield (*p*ABPG) derivatives, which can be separated and identified by HPLC analysis.[28,29] The analysis of one carbon derivatives and polyglutamate chain length is complicated by the large number of folate derivatives present in food. To address this challenge, Selhub and coworkers[30] developed an affinity method using immobilized milk folate–binding protein to purify the extracted folates before reverse phase HPLC analysis. This method allows quantitation of individual folates in foods and can also be applied to tissues.

Biological Samples

Quantitation of folate in biological specimens includes microbiological growth procedures, protein–ligand-binding methods, chromatographic and mass spectrometric methods.[17,31] Several liquid chromatography–tandem mass spectrometry methods have been developed for the analysis of clinical specimens.[32,33] The classical *L. casei* method for measurement of both serum and RBC folate concentrations has been used in research laboratories for more than 50 years. When the microbiological assay is used, the standard cutoff to define inadequate folate status for serum folate is <7 nmol/L (<3 ng/mL) and for RBC folate is 305 nmol/L (<140 ng/mL).[34] The basis of this cutoff is the observation that in response to a folate-deficient diet (~5 μg/day), the appearance of hypersegmented neutrophils in the peripheral blood coincided with the approximate time when the RBC folate concentration was <305 nmol/L.[34] In a clinical setting, radioassay procedures are most commonly used with variable cutoffs depending on the specific kit used. Improvement and standardization of methods for quantitation of folate in biological samples remains the focus of ongoing research efforts due to substantial differences between commonly used methods in different laboratories.[35,36]

DIETARY REFERENCE INTAKES

The dietary reference intakes (DRIs) established by the Institute of Medicine (IOM) are a set of reference values including the estimated average requirement (EAR), recommended dietary allowance (RDA), adequate intake (AI), and tolerable upper intake level (UL).[37] The RDA for all males and nonpregnant females $\geq$14 years is 400 μg DFE/day. For pregnant and lactating women, the RDA increases to 600 and 500 μg DFE/day, respectively.[38] Dietary folate equivalent (DFE) is a unit of expression for the folate DRIs (except the upper level), and derived by the IOM as a means to account for differences in bioavailability of food folate and synthetic folic acid provided by fortified foods.[39] When expressed as DFEs, all forms of dietary folate, including folic acid in fortified products, are converted to an amount that is equivalent to food folate. The quantity of synthetic folic acid in the diet is first multiplied 1.7 times and this quantity is added to the microgram of food folate. The conversion factor (1.7) was based on the observation that when folic acid is consumed with a meal, which is the usual case for a fortified product, then the added folic acid is ~85% available[16] and food folate is ~50% available[15]; thus, the ratio 85:50 yielded the multiplier of 1.7 in the DFE calculation. A recent study provides confirming evidence for the validity of the use of the 1.7 multiplier to correct for the higher bioavailability of folic acid than the naturally occurring food folate.[40] Yang et al.[40] conducted a long-term-controlled human metabolic study in which the metabolic response to multiple combinations of food folate and folic acid (microgram of food folate or microgram of food folate plus microgram of folic acid $\times$ 1.7) was compared. The fact that the folate status responses to the different combinations within 400 and 800 μg DFE/day groups were not different supports the basis of the 1.7 equivalency conversion factor.

A tolerable UL was estimated (IOM 1998) for folic acid (1000 μg/day). In contrast, there is no UL for naturally occurring food folate. The UL for folic acid is not based on evidence of a toxic reaction to folic acid, since there are no substantiated side effects and no dose response associated with high doses of folic acid.[37] The basis of the UL is the reported correction of hematological abnormalities associated with a vitamin B_{12} deficiency, which may delay (mask) the detection of the B_{12} deficiency if the diagnosis is solely dependent on the presence of anemia.[41]

In addition to the DRIs for folate and folic acid, the IOM also established a separate recommendation specifically targeted to women capable of becoming pregnant to reduce the risk of NTDs. This recommendation is different from the RDA since the recommendation specifies that the supplemental form of the vitamin, folic acid (400 μg/day), be taken (or consumed as a fortified food) in addition to folate in a varied diet.

METABOLISM

ABSORPTION AND TRANSPORT

Dietary folate predominately occurs in a polyglutamate form, which must be first hydrolyzed to the monoglutamate form before intestinal epithelial cell uptake, which takes place primarily in the jejunum.[10] The enzyme responsible for the deconjugation of polyglutamyl folate is folylpoly-γ-glutamate carboxypeptidase (EC 3.4.12.10) (also referred to as folate conjugase or pteroylpolyglutamate hydrolase), which is located primarily in the jejunal brush-border membrane. Folylpoly-γ-glutamate carboxypeptidase functions as an exopeptidase that releases terminal glutamates sequentially with optimal activity at pH 6.5 to 7.0.[42] The next stage in the two-step process of dietary folate absorption is transport of monoglutamyl folate across the intestinal muscoa, which is maximum at a pH of 5–6.

The transport process for internalizing folate is not completely understood, however in general there appears to be two types of carrier-mediated mechanisms involved, a folate transporter and a folate receptor. These folate membrane transport systems are essential for normal folate absorption into the epithelial cells of the small intestine, for reabsorption by a similar epithelial layer in the proximal renal tubes, and for internalization through the plasma membranes of both the developing embryo and the adult organism.[43] In the intestine, the folate transporter is encoded by the reduced folate carrier (*RFC*) gene, which is also expressed in most tissues.[44,45] The RFC is mobile and therefore capable of mediating bidirectional flux.[43] The second type is the receptor-mediated processes in which folates are bound with high affinity at the membrane surface to a folate receptor-like protein, which mediates unidirectional flux following internalization of the receptor–folate complex.[43] The folate receptor is encoded by at least three genes with most tissues expressing the α-form. When high doses of folic acid are given (>10 μM), intestinal uptake takes place by a nonsaturable mechanism involving a diffusion-like process.[46]

Once internalized, folate is metabolized to 5-methyl THF, although the degree of metabolism depends on the folate dose, with unmetabolized folic acid appearing in the portal circulation when pharmacological doses are given.[47] With passage through the liver, folic acid is converted to 5-methyl THF,[48] however, large oral doses of folic acid result in a significant increase in urinary excretion of unmetabolized folic acid.[49]

Plasma folate, primarily 5-methyl THF, is largely bound to albumin, a low-affinity folate-binding protein (K_d folate ~1 mM), which accounts for ~50% of circulating bound folate.[50] A smaller proportion of plasma folate is bound to a high-affinity folate binder (K_d folate ~1 nM), which is a soluble form of a membrane-associated folate transporter.[51]

Cellular folate uptake is mediated by both RFCs and folate receptors.[51] Reversible internalization of folate is facilitated by RFC proteins in contrast to folate receptors, which mediate only unidirectional transport of cellular folate. The pathways for entry of folates are likely to be distinct in different cells depending on the relative efficiency of the RFC and the folate receptor-mediated mechanisms, as well as the intra- and extracellular concentration of folate.[51] The expression of folate transport proteins may adapt to extracellular folate concentrations. Folate in portal circulation is taken up by hepatic tissues by the RFC, which is a low-affinity, high-capacity system. In hepatic tissues, the RFC has a similar affinity for folic acid as it does for reduced folates; however in many other tissues, the affinity is much lower for folic acid relative to reduced folates.[44,45] In humans, the folate receptor is usually attached to the plasma membrane of cells via a glycosylphosphatidylinositol anchor. Tissues with the highest levels include the choroid plexus, kidney proximal tubes, placenta, and a number of human tumors. In the kidney, the folate receptor has a well-established role in receptor-mediated reabsorption of folate.[52] In the embryo and fetus, the folate receptor shows localized patterns of expression in that it is highly expressed in the neural folds before closure of the neural tube, and in the yolk sac. Folate is transported into RBCs exclusively during erythropoiesis and retained throughout the RBC life span since mature RBCs do not transport folate.

Intracellular Storage

To be retained intracellularly, folate polyglutamation by folylpolyglutamate synthetase (EC 6.3.2.17) is required.[53] To be released back into circulation, the polyglutamate form of folate must be reconverted to the monoglutamate form, a process that requires γ-glutamyl hydrolase (EC 3.4.19.9).[54,55] Tissue storage of folate in general is limited to the amounts required for metabolic function, which is estimated to be on average ~15–30 mg.[56,57]

Cellular folate accumulation displays saturation kinetics with the upper limit approximating the folate-binding capacity of the cell.[58] Within the cells, folate is bound by enzymes that catalyze folate-dependent reactions and by other folate proteins that sequester folate.[59]

Catabolism and Turnover

Folate is excreted in the urine primarily as breakdown products, with only a very small percentage as intact folate.[60,61] The percentage of ingested food folate that is excreted as intact urinary folate is estimated to be only 1%–2%, which indicates that folate is catabolized before urinary excretion.[62] The major fate of folates undergoing catabolism is cleavage of the C-9–N-10 bond producing pteridines and *p*ABG with the majority of *p*ABG N-acetylated to acetamidobenzolyglutamate (a*p*ABG) before excretion.[63,64] Studies conducted by Stover and coworkers have demonstrated that the iron-storage protein, ferritin, can catabolize folate in vitro and in vivo, and increased heavy-chain ferritin synthesis decreases intracellular folate concentrations independent of exogenous folate levels in cell culture models.[65]

The rates of whole-body folate turnover are very slow in humans with slow-turnover folate pools exhibiting mean residency times of >100 days.[66] Folate-binding proteins are not expressed in all tissues or are expressed to different degrees, which may explain the variability in different rates of tissue folate turnover since unbound folate is susceptible to catabolism.[67]

Excretion

The majority of plasma folate not associated with protein is freely filtered in the glomerulus and reabsorped in the proximal renal tubules.[68] A large quantity of folate is secreted daily into bile but is reutilized via enterohepatic recirculation.[68] The origins of folate excreted in feces include unabsorbed dietary folate, folate synthesized by colonic microbes, and folate contributed by endogenous secretions. It is estimated that the quantity of fecal folate excretion is comparable to that of urinary folate excretion.[63]

BIOCHEMICAL FUNCTIONS

Overview of Biochemical Functions

One carbon metabolism is synonymous with folate-requiring reactions and includes those involved with different phases of amino acid metabolism, pyrimidine and purine synthesis, and methylation reactions following the formation of the body's primary methylating agent, *S*-adenosylmethionine (SAM) (Figure 12.2). In each of these folate-dependent pathways, a specific form of the folate coenzyme donates a one carbon unit to the reaction, resulting in regeneration of THF, which is then free to accept other one carbon units from the folate pool and thus continue the cycle. A detailed description of the enzymatic conversions involved in the subcellular compartmentalization of folate-dependent reactions is reviewed elsewhere.[69]

Key Folate-Dependent Enzymatic Reactions Involved in One Carbon Metabolism

Serine–Glycine Interconversion

Serine hydroxymethyltransferase (SHMT) (EC 2.1.2.1) (Figure 12.2, Reaction 2) catalyzes the transfer of formaldehyde from serine to THF to form 5,10-methylene THF and glycine, a reversible reaction. Both serine and glycine are nonessential amino acids. Serine can be derived through glycolysis from 3-phosphoglycerate and much of the glycine requirement is provided by serine by the action of SHMT. The enzyme that contains pyridoxal 5′-phosphate is present in two different isoforms that carry out the interconversion of serine and glycine either in the mitochondria (mSHMT) or in the cytoplasm (cSHMT). The conversion of serine to glycine via SHMT generates a 1-C unit (5,10-methylene THF), which is the primary source of methyl groups for methionine, dTMP, and purine synthesis or it may be oxidized to CO_2 via 10-formyl THF.[69–71]

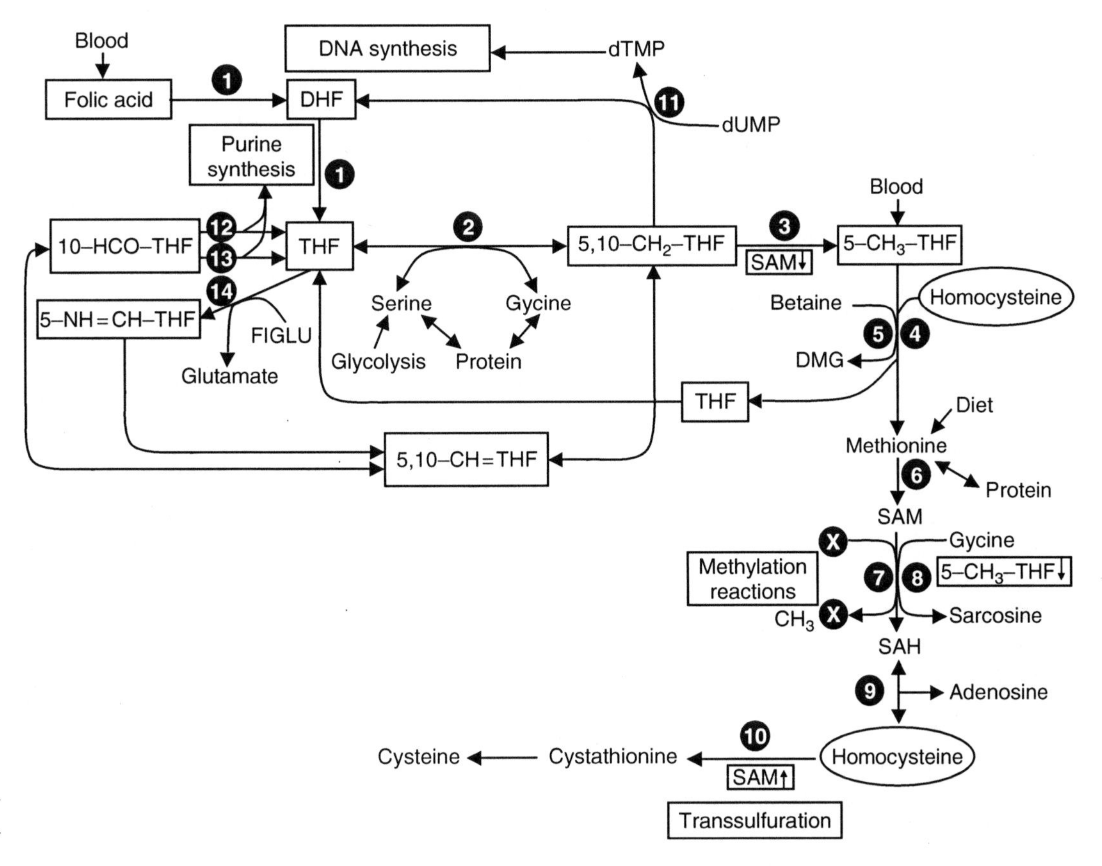

FIGURE 12.2 The diagram represents the major metabolic reactions and interconversions of folate coenzymes (polyglutamates). DHF, dihydrofolate; THF, tetrahydrofolate; DMG, dimethylglycine; SAM, *S*-adenosylmethionine; SAH, *S*-adenosylhomocysteine; FIGLU, formiminoglutamic acid. The enzymes and reaction numbers are noted in Table 12.1.

TABLE 12.1
Select Enzymes Involved in One Carbon Metabolism Depicted in Figure 12.2

Reaction	Enzyme	EC Number
1	Dihydrofolate reductase	1.5.1.3
2	Serine hydroxymethyltransferase	2.1.2.1
3	5,10-Methylene THF reductase	1.1.99.5
4	Methionine synthase	2.1.1.13
5	Betaine:homocysteine methyltransferase	2.1.1.5
6	Methionine adenosyltransferase	2.5.1.6
7	Variety methyltransferase reactions	Various
8	Glycine *N*-methyltransferase	2.1.1.20
9	*S*-Adenosylhomocysteine hydrolase	3.3.1.1
10	Cystathionine β-synthase	4.2.1.22
11	Thymidylate synthase	2.1.1.45
12	Glycinamide ribonucleotide transformylase	2.1.2.2
13	Aminocarboxamide ribotide transformylase	2.1.2.3
14	Formiminotransferase	2.1.2.5

Formation of 5-Methyltetrahydrofolate

A major cytosolic cycle of one carbon metabolism involves the reduction of 5,10–methylene THF to 5-methyl THF by 5,10-methylenetetrahydrofolate reductase (MTHFR) (EC 1.7.99.5) (Figure 12.2, Reaction 3). This reaction is dependent on FAD as a transfer agent for reducing equivalents from NADPH to the 5,10-methylene THF substrate to form 5-methyl THF. The binding of SAM to a specific regulatory domain of MTHFR results in allosteric inhibition, which can be reversed by adenosylhomocysteine (SAH).[72]

Homocysteine Remethylation

A key enzyme required for the remethylation process is methionine synthase (5-methyltetrahydrofolate:homocysteine methyltransferase; EC 2.1.1.13), which sequentially transfers a methyl group from 5-methyl THF to the cobalamin coenzyme and to homocysteine thus forming methionine and regenerating THF (Figure 12.2, Reaction 4). The methionine synthase reaction is the only reaction in which the methyl group of 5-methyl THF can be metabolized in mammalian tissues. The role of this enzyme is vitally important for both the folate cycle and for the production of methionine required for SAM-dependent transmethylation reactions. The methionine synthase reaction allows the reutilization of homocysteine as a carrier of methyl groups derived primarily from serine.

5-Methyl THF is the primary folate form supplied by the diet to the liver where it enters the folate pool by conversion to THF catalyzed by methionine synthase. This enzymatic step appears to be the obligatory step for assimilation of exogenous folate because 5-methyl THF is a very poor substrate for folate polyglutamate synthesis required for cellular folate retention.[69] For the methionine synthase enzyme to be active, the cobalamin cofactor must be reduced, which is accomplished enzymatically by methionine synthase reductase (MTRR) (EC 1.6.1.8).

The methyl-trap hypothesis was proposed[73] to explain why a cobalamin deficiency results in a secondary folate deficiency. The basis of this hypothesis is that a cobalamin deficiency inactivates methionine synthase trapping folate as 5-methyl THF since the MTHFR reaction is irreversible. The methyl-trap hypothesis provides the rationale for why either a cobalamin or folate deficiency may result in megaloblastic anemia due to insufficient THF to form 5,10-methylene THF required for normal DNA synthesis and cell division.

An alternative homocysteine remethylation cycle is the betaine-dependent remethylation catalyzed by betaine:homocysteine methyltransferase (BHMT) (EC 2.1.1.5) (Figure 12.2, Reaction 5).[74] The BHMT remethylation of homocysteine is an irreversible reaction in which choline is first oxidized to betaine (trimethylglycine) and then demethylated to glycine.[74] BMHT catalyzes the first demethylation step in which a methyl group of betaine is transferred to homocysteine, producing dimethylglycine and methionine, respectively.[74] Unlike the cobalamin-dependent remethylation of homocysteine catalyzed by methionine synthase, which is widely distributed in tissues throughout the body, BHMT tissue distribution in humans is limited to the liver and kidney.

Formation of *S*-Adenosylmethionine

Methionine is an essential amino acid that must be provided in the diet. Since methionine is usually one of the limiting amino acids in dietary protein, it has to be efficiently assimilated and recycled. In addition to protein synthesis, the other major function of methionine is the synthesis of SAM, the major methyl donor in mammalian systems. The transfer of the adenosyl component of ATP to methionine is dependent on methionine *S*-adenosyltransferase (EC 2.5.1.6) to form SAM (Figure 12.2, Reaction 6). When dietary methionine intake is adequate, SAM reduces the production of 5-methyl THF by allosteric inhibition of

TABLE 12.2
Examples of Transmethylation Reactions

Group	Methyl Group Acceptor/Function
DNA	DNA-cytosine/gene expression, regulation, inactivation, imprinting
RNA	mRNA-guanine/capping of mRNA
	tRNA-cytosine, -guanine, -adenine/alteration of tRNA flexibility
Histones	Lysine amino acid
Proteins—amino acids	Basic myelin protein; actin and myosin
Lipids	Phosphatidylethanolamine/synthesis of phosphatidylcholine
N-methyltransferases	Guanidinoacetic acid/creatine synthesis
	Nicotinamide/pyridine metabolism
	Histamine/inactivation
O-methyltransferases	Catechols (e.g., norepinephrine, epinephrine, dopamine)/inactivation

Source: Modified from Fowler, B., *Semin. Vasc. Med.*, 5 (2), 78, 2005. With permission.

MTHFR and hence the supply of methionine.[69] In contrast when dietary methionine is limited, SAM concentration decreases resulting in decreased inhibition of MTHFR, which allows for an increased production of 5-methyl THF. This leads to an increase in homocysteine remethylation to produce methionine for protein synthesis and methylation.[69]

Hepatic SAM concentration is regulated by glycine *N*-methyltransferase (EC 2.1.1.20), which catalyzes the SAM-dependent methylation of glycine to sarcosine and SAH (Figure 12.2, Reaction 8).[75] The glycine *N*-methyltransferase enzyme provides an alternate mechanism for maintaining the constant ratio of SAM to SAH, which is important to regulate methylation reactions, since SAH is a strong inhibitor of methyltransferases. Glycine *N*-methyltransferase is inhibited by 5-methyl THF, illustrating how folate controls SAM disposition and methyl group turnover.[76]

SAM is the methyl donor in >100 transmethylation reactions, including methylation of DNA, RNA, and membrane phospholipids (Figure 12.2, Reaction 7). A large variety of methyltransferase enzymes transfer the methyl groups from SAM, which in the process is converted to SAH. Examples of the >100 different SAM-dependent methylation reactions are listed in Table 12.2.[77]

Conversion of *S*-Adenosylmethionine to *S*-Adenosylhomocysteine

The conversion of SAM to SAH is a one-way process, which is subjected to competitive inhibition by SAH.[78] SAH has a higher affinity than SAM for the active site of the methyltransferases, therefore a build up of SAH and decreased SAM/SAH ratio is associated with methyltransferase inhibition.[78] SAH is hydrolyzed to homocysteine and adenosine by SAH hydrolase (EC 3.3.1.1) (Figure 12.2, Reaction 9) via a reversible reaction in which the thermodynamics of the SAH hydrolase reaction strongly favor SAH synthesis.[78] The utilization of adenosine by adenosine kinase and the remethylation of homocysteine provide the kinetic impetus that pulls this reaction in the direction of SAH hydrolysis.

Transsulfuration Pathway

The hydrolysis of SAH leads to the formation of homocysteine, which can then be metabolized to cysteine in the transsulfuration pathway or remethylated back to methionine by the methionine synthase reaction. Approximately half the homocysteine formed is converted by remethylation to methionine and the other half is irreversibly converted to cysteine.[79] It has been proposed that the real importance of transsulfuration in humans may be a catabolic pathway of homocysteine destruction, rather than a cysteine synthesis pathway.[80] In the transsulfuration pathway, homocysteine is first coupled with serine to form cystathionine in a pyridoxine-dependent reaction by cystathionine β-synthase (CBS) (EC 4.2.1.22) (Figure 12.2, Reaction 10). SAM functions as a switch between the methionine cycle and the transsulfuration pathway.[81] When SAM concentrations are low, homocysteine remethylation is unimpaired. In contrast, high concentrations of SAM inhibit 5,10-methylene THF[82] and BHMT.[81] Transsulfuration, in contrast is enhanced by SAM, which stimulates CBS activity and accelerates the elimination of homocysteine through the transsulfuration pathway.[83]

Nucleotide Biosynthesis

The rate-limiting step in DNA synthesis is the conversion of the pyrimidine deoxyuridylate (dUMP) to deoxythymidylate (dTMP), which is dependent on thymidylate synthase (EC 2.1.1.45) and 5,10-methylene THF as a source of one carbon groups (Figure 12.2, Reaction 11). The one carbon unit is initially at the formaldehyde oxidation level and is reduced to the methanol level during the reaction by the reducing power of the tetrahydropyrazine ring. The product of this reaction is dihydrofolate, which is inactive as a coenzyme and must be reduced back to the active THF coenzyme form by dihydrofolate reductase (EC 1.5.1.3) (Figure 12.2, Reaction 1). Both thymidylate synthase and dihydrofolate reductase act in a coordinated manner for efficient folate metabolism. The level of thymidylate synthase is much higher in rapidly growing or regenerating tissues than in adult liver.[84]

During the synthesis of the purine ring, 10-formyl THF is used in two reactions in which glycinamide ribonucleotide transformylase (EC 2.1.2.2) and aminocarboxamide ribotide transformylase (EC 2.1.2.3) add formyl groups at positions C-8 and C-2, respectively (Figure 12.2, Reactions 12 and 13).

Histidine Catabolism

In the final steps of histidine catabolism, the transfer of the formimino group of formiminoglutamate to THF is catalyzed by formiminotransferase (EC 2.1.2.5) (Figure 12.2, Reaction 14). The formimino moiety is converted to 5,10-methenyl THF in a formimidoyl THF cyclodeaminase (EC 4.3.1.4) reaction.

FACTORS AFFECTING FOLATE METABOLISM

Single Nucleotide Polymorphisms

The term polymorphism refers to a genetic mutation that occurs in a population at a frequency ≥1.0% of alleles that may or may not be detrimental.[85] There have been a large number of reports of single nucleotide polymorphisms affecting the enzymes and transport proteins required for normal folate metabolism that, in some cases, are linked to elevations in plasma homocysteine and clinical abnormalities.[85–88]

A polymorphism of particular importance to folate metabolism is the 677C→T base substitution in the gene encoding the enzyme MTHFR that catalyzes the reduction of 5,10-methylene THF to 5-methyl THF, the methyl donor for homocysteine remethylation to methionine.[85] Homozygosity for the 677C→T polymorphism (TT genotype) is associated with a 70% lower MTHFR enzyme activity.[85] The prevalence of the MTHFR 677C→T polymorphism in the overall population is ~12% for the homozygous variant (TT genotype) and ~50% for the heterozygous (CT genotype) variant.[89] When folate status is low, the MTHFR 677C→T polymorphism has been associated with significantly increased plasma homocysteine concentrations and reduced global DNA methylation.[90] Clinical abnormalities linked to the combined presence of low folate status and the homozygous variant for the MTHFR 677C→T polymorphism include increased risk for NTDs and vascular disease.[85,91] The influence of inadequate folate intake coupled with the 677C→T MTHFR polymorphism on folate metabolism has been determined in controlled feeding studies.[92,93] When low-folate diets (115–135 μg DFE/day) were consumed, both serum and RBC folate concentrations were lower and homocysteine concentrations were higher in women with the TT genotype versus CC genotype.[92,93] A larger percentage of women with the TT genotype had low folate status (serum folate <13.6 nmol/L) (59%) compared with women with the CC genotype (15%) in response to low-folate diets.[92]

The MTHFR 677C→T polymorphism in conjunction with low folate status has also been found to reduce global DNA methylation in epidemiological studies[90,94] and one controlled feeding study.[95] In a cross-sectional study conducted in a European population group, significantly less DNA methylation was observed in subjects with the TT genotype than those with the CC genotype.[90] In the United States, no differences could be detected in DNA methylation in women whose folate status was considerably higher than that observed in European countries due to consumption of fortified foods.[95] There was however a difference between genotype groups in the DNA methylation response to folate repletion following consumption (7 weeks) of a moderately low-folate diet. In individuals with the TT genotype, DNA methylation significantly increased in contrast to no observed change in the CC genotype group. These data provide additional evidence that the DNA methylation response to folate intake may be modified by the MTHFR 677C→T polymorphism and that an individual's MTHFR 677C→T genotype should be taken into account when evaluating the DNA methylation response to changes in folate intake.

Methionine synthase catalyzes homocysteine remethylation to methionine in a reaction in which the methyl group is donated by 5-methyl THF. A polymorphism of the methionine synthase enzyme 2756A→G results in the substitution of an aspartic acid with a glycine amino acid. Homozygous variants occur less frequently (<5%) than the MTHFR 677C→T variant (~12%).[85] Since human methionine synthase has not been expressed in vitro, functional studies of this polymorphism have not been performed. However, the corresponding amino acid (glutamine) in the bacterial enzyme (Q893) lies in a linker region connecting the activation domain to the cobalamin-binding domain.[85] The functional consequence of converting the bacterial Q893 residue into glycine was a slight decrease in activity with impaired reductive activation.[85] The polymorphism does not appear to be associated with hyperhomocysteinemia or with an increased risk of NTDs or vascular disease.[96–100]

The MTRR enzyme is required for maintaining methionine synthase in an active state by facilitating the reductive methylation of cobalamin.[101] A common polymorphism affecting this enzyme is the MTRR 66A→G variant, which is considered a genetic determinant of plasma homocysteine concentrations.[101,102] The coexistence of the MTRR 66A→G and the MTHFR 677C→T polymorphisms has been shown to exacerbate the homocysteine-elevating effect of the MTHFR TT genotype.[101]

The enzyme folylpoly-γ-glutamyl carboxypeptidase, which is encoded by the glutamate carboxypeptidase II gene (*GCPII*), is present in the intestinal brush border and responsible for the deconjugation of polyglutamate folate (predominant dietary form). A polymorphism (1561C→T) in the *GCPII* gene was first reported by Devlin et al. in a study in which the presence of this polymorphism was associated with lower folate status suggesting that the polymorphism may impair folate absorption.[103] In contrast to these initial findings, other reports indicate that the T allele did not affect the bioavailability of polyglutamyl folate[104] and was for unknown reasons associated with higher folate status.[104–106]

A common polymorphism affecting the *RFC1* gene (80G→A) may affect folate carrier function. A trend for higher homocysteine concentration was observed in individuals with the

80GG genotype, which increased and inversely affected RBC folate when the MTHFR 677 TT genotype was taken into account.[107]

Alcohol and Drugs

Alcohol interferes with folate absorption, hepatic uptake, and renal reabsorption and when consumed chronically in large amounts may contribute to folate deficiency.[108] The ability of alcohol to interfere with folate absorption has been linked to the negative effect of alcohol on the function of two proteins that regulate folate absorption, folylpoly-γ-glutamyl carboxypeptidase, and RFC.[108–111] Hepatic folate metabolism is impaired when chronic alcohol consumption is coupled with a low-folate diet.[108] A decreased hepatic uptake or retention of folic acid and reduced renal tubular reabsorption were observed in studies involving alcohol-fed monkeys.[112] Other studies have demonstrated increased urinary folate excretion in chronic alcoholic patients and alcohol-fed rats.[113,114] In addition to abnormalities in folate metabolism, the development of alcoholic liver injury is a frequent culmination of chronic high doses of alcohol coupled with a low-folate diet.[108]

Drugs (methotrexate, 5-fluorouracil, aminopterin, trimethoprim, trimetrexate, and triamterene) that interfere with folate metabolism are key components of chemotherapy for both neoplastic and nonneoplastic diseases. A major chemotherapeutic agent with antifolate activity, methotrexate (amethopterin) has been used in low doses to treat a large variety of both neoplastic and nonneoplastic diseases and has been especially effective in rheumatoid arthritis.[115] The molecular structure of methotrexate differs slightly from folate, however, these minor structural modifications result in a higher affinity for the drug's enzyme target, dihydrofolate reductase.[116] Treatment of rapidly growing malignant cells with methotrexate traps folate as dihydrofolate, which is nonfunctional as a coenzyme. Tissues that are growing slowly do not convert reduced folate to the dihydrofolate form rapidly; therefore, they are less affected by methotrexate than malignant cells. Patients receiving methotrexate may show significant increases in plasma homocysteine concentrations associated with the chronic use of this drug.[117]

Another major chemotherapeutic antifolate drug, 5-fluorouracil, inhibits the activity of thymidylate synthase. The mechanism of drug action involves the initial formation of a complex between the thymidylate synthase enzyme and folate in which the drug acts as a substrate.[116] Since the fluorine atom cannot be abstracted and the reaction completed, the drug functions as a covalent inhibitor of thymidylate synthase, which blocks DNA synthesis and reduces cell proliferation.[116]

Chronic use of the anticonvulsants diphenylhydantoin (phenytoin, Dilantin) and phenobarbital has been associated with impaired folate status; however, the mechanism of the folate–anticonvulsant interaction is not known.[118] An anti-inflammatory drug commonly used for the treatment of ulcerative colitis, salicylazosulfapyridine (Azulfidine, sulfasalazine) is known to inhibit folate absorption and metabolism.[115] Chronic use of drugs used for glycemic control in diabetes and some other conditions has been associated with impaired folate status and hyperhomocysteinemia.[119]

DEFICIENCY

Biomarkers and Status Assessment

Serum and Red Blood Cell Folate Concentration

Serum folate concentration is considered the earliest and most sensitive indicator of folate status but requires repeated measures over time to reflect long-term status.[120] In controlled metabolic studies in which folate intake is limited, serum folate concentration decreases rapidly within 1 to 3 weeks preceding changes in RBC folate concentration.[34,92,121] Cutoffs for serum folate concentrations used to define deficiency are variable depending on the method of analysis; however, when using the *L. casei* microbiological method of analysis a cutoff of <7 nmol/L (<3 ng/mL) is commonly used.[37]

Folate uptake into the RBC only occurs during the early stages of reticulocyte development in the bone marrow. Since the mature RBC membrane is not permeable to folate during the 120 day life span of the RBC, this indicator is considered a reflection of long-term status.[120] An early study involving liver biopsies provides evidence that RBC folate concentration parallels liver folate concentration and may be considered representative of tissue folate stores since ~50% of the body's folate is in the liver.[122] In response to controlled folate depletion, RBC concentration responds very slowly relative to serum folate and continues to decline initially when a folate repletion diet is consumed.[92,121] A cutoff value of <305 nmol/L (<140 ng/mL) is the criterion commonly used to define inadequate folate status when a microbiological assay is used.[37] Methodology for blood folate analysis is addressed later.

Homocysteine Concentration

Since changes in blood folate concentrations may or may not reflect metabolic abnormalities, it is essential to measure "functional" indictors of status. Elevated homocysteine concentration is considered a functional indicator of folate status in that it reflects a metabolic abnormality (insufficient 5-methyl THF to convert homocysteine to methionine) and not just a reduction in blood folate concentration associated with folate inadequacy.[37] It is difficult to define universally acceptable cutoff points for plasma homocysteine concentration because definitive evidence does not exist that values above a specific cutoff are associated with clinical abnormalities or increased disease risk. Homocysteine values are not considered specific for folate deficiency since other nutrient deficiencies, renal insufficiency, genetic polymorphisms, and lifestyle factors may lead to elevations in homocysteine concentrations.[85,123] A commonly used cutoff before fortification in the United States that was based on the upper percentile in the population was >14 μmol/L.[124] Multiple issues involved in defining a desirable homocysteine level have been addressed by Ubbink.[125] The methodologies available for the measurement of homocysteine have been reviewed.[126] The links between elevated homocysteine concentrations and vascular disease are discussed in the section Vascular Disease.

DNA Methylation

Genomic DNA methylation, an epigenetic modification of DNA (discussed in greater detail in Chapter 16), is evolving as a sensitive biomarker of dietary folate intake.[127,128] The primary methylating agent of the body, SAM, is dependent on an adequate supply of 5-methyl THF (Figure 12.2). Consumption of a low-folate diet in controlled human-feeding studies resulted in global DNA methylation that was responsive to folate repletion.[129,130] In individuals with the TT genotype for the MTHFR 677C→T polymorphism, the negative effect of low folate status on DNA methylation is accentuated[90] and the response to folate repletion may differ by MTHFR genotype.[95] McCabe and Caudill recently reviewed DNA methylation and its functions, examined the relationship between dietary methyl insufficiency and DNA methylation, and evaluated the associations between DNA methylation and cancer.[127] DNA methylation significantly decreases as a function of dietary folate depletion in human metabolic studies[129,130] as reviewed by McCabe and Caudill.[127] DNA methylation has been determined on the basis of the ability of genomic DNA to incorporate [^{3}H]methyl groups from labeled SAM in an in vitro assay.[129] New HPLC and mass spectrometry methods to measure genomic DNA methylation are now available.[90,95]

Hematological Indices

A folate deficiency leads to early hematological abnormalities in the bone marrow, which precede hypersegmentation of neutrophils in peripheral blood.[131] Macrocytic cells are produced in the bone marrow when folate supply to the bone marrow becomes rate limiting for erythropoiesis. Since the life span of the RBC is 120 days, megaloblastic anemia characterized by an increase in mean cell volume and a reduction in RBC number develops slowly after the earlier stages of folate-deficient megaloblastosis.[131] Impaired cell division is also evident in reduced leukocyte number and impaired regeneration of rapidly dividing gastrointestinal epithelial cells, both of which may have clinical consequences.[131]

Abnormal Pregnancy Outcomes

Folate requirements are increased in pregnant women to meet the demands for DNA synthesis and one carbon transfer reactions in rapidly dividing fetal and maternal cells.[132] When folate intake is restricted during pregnancy, impaired folate status has been associated with poor pregnancy outcomes including preterm delivery, low infant birth weight, and fetal growth retardation as previously reviewed.[132] Maternal hyperhomocysteinemia has been linked to increased habitual spontaneous abortion and pregnancy complications (e.g., abruptio placentae or placental infarction with fetal growth retardation and pre-eclampsia), which increase the risk of low birth weight and preterm delivery.[133,134] Although there is a reported link between hyperhomocysteinemia and low folate status with adverse pregnancy outcomes, it is not possible to determine whether low folate status and high homocysteine play a causative role or whether they are simply markers for abnormal pregnancy outcomes.[133,134] Randomized controlled trials with folic acid supplementation in women at high risk of these pregnancy complications are required to determine a cause and effect relationship.

Increased Risk of Birth Defects

Neural Tube Defects

The neural tube forms in the developing embryo from the neural plate during the first 28 days postconception and develops into the spinal cord and its protrusion that encases the brain.[135] Incomplete closure of the neural tube results in a group of birth defects collectively referred to as NTDs, which vary in severity depending on the location and size of the defect. There are marked geographical variations in the prevalence of NTDs. For example, during the 1980s, the prevalence at birth was 0.8 per 1000 births in the United States, 3.6 per 1000 in the Republic of Ireland, and 10.6 per 1000 in a Chinese province.[136]

Folic acid supplements taken periconceptionally significantly reduce the risk of NTDs, a major public health discovery based on findings from randomized controlled intervention trials supported by a large body of observational data.[37,137,138] Estimates of the effect of folic acid fortification on NTD prevalence are based on reports from the United States, Canada, and Chile, which indicate that fortification was associated with a significant reduction in NTDs, although the estimated reductions are quite variable (19%–50%) depending on the type of data evaluated.[139–143] The basis of folic acid–responsive NTDs is likely to be multifactorial involving both metabolic and genetic defects that may impair normal maternal folate metabolism, restricting delivery of adequate folate to the developing embryonic neural tube. Folate metabolic abnormalities proposed to increase NTD risk include elevations in homocysteine concentration,[144] increased SAH/SAM ratio, and impaired dTMP production, which interfere with DNA synthesis and cell division.[145] Other proposed mechanisms that may be involved in the etiology of NTDs include impaired maternal folate absorption[146] and maternal autoantibodies, which bind folate receptors and may block the cellular uptake of folate.[147]

The search for the genetic bases for the folic acid–responsive NTDs has focused on genes that encode for folate-related enzymes, receptors, and binding proteins.[87,148] A large number of polymorphisms in folate-related candidate genes (e.g., MTHFR, folate receptor alpha (FRα), RFC, CBS, MTR, MTRR, MTHFD, and SHMT) have been evaluated to determine if there is a link with NTDs. Only a few folate-related polymorphisms appear to be significant NTD risk factors[86,148,149] with the magnitude of the risk inversely associated with folate status[149–151] and the strongest evidence related to the MTHFR 677C→T polymorphism and NTD risk. Based on findings from a recent meta-analysis, the TT genotype (homozygosity for the 677C→T polymorphism) compared with the CC genotype was associated with a significant increase in risk for NTDs (odds ratio of 1.76 (95% confidence interval 1.45–2.14)).[91]

Congenital Heart Defects

In the United States, heart defects affect 1 in 110 newborns and account for a third or more of infant deaths due to birth defects, more than that for any other congenital anomaly including NTDs.[152] Periconceptional folic acid supplement use has also been associated with risk reduction for congenital heart defects in some[153–155] but not all studies.[156,157] Data from a randomized–controlled trial conducted in Hungary[158,159] and two population-based case–control studies in the United States[154,155] provide support for the link between periconceptional folic acid supplement use and reduced risk for congenital heart defects. Data from the Hungarian study indicate that prenatal multivitamins are associated with an overall 50% reduction in heart defects in general. The specific types of heart defects that appear to be most likely associated with periconceptional folic acid use include ventricular septal defects and some conotruncal defects, tetralogy of Fallot, and D-transposition of the great arteries.[160]

Increased Risk Chronic Disease

Vascular Disease

Elevated plasma homocysteine concentration is a significant risk factor for vascular disease, a conclusion based on a large body of epidemiological evidence as previously reviewed.[161] It is estimated that a 25% reduction in plasma homocysteine concentration is associated with an 11%–16% decrease in risk for ischemic heart disease[162] and a 19%–22% decrease in risk for stroke.[163]

Folic acid supplementation lowers plasma homocysteine concentration with the greatest homocysteine-lowering effect observed in individuals with the highest pretreatment homocysteine concentration.[164] After standardizing pretreatment homocysteine concentration to 12 μmol/L and serum folate to 12 nmol/L, the magnitude of the reduction in homocysteine achieved with different folic acid doses has been estimated in a series of meta-analyses conducted by the Homocysteine Lowering Trialist collaboration.[164,165] The magnitude of the reduction in homocysteine was ~25% for doses $\geq$0.8 mg with 90% and 60% of this effect associated with lower doses (0.4 and 0.2 mg/day, respectively).[164,165]

The improved folate status resulting from folic acid fortification in North America[166] would be expected to significantly attenuate the observed homocysteine-lowering response to folic acid (~25%) observed in studies primarily conducted in Europe where there is no mandatory fortification. The prevalence of elevated homocysteine was reduced by 50% when pre- and postfortification homocysteine concentrations were compared with the Framingham population.[167] Data from NHANES (1999–2000) indicate that ~80% of the entire US population currently have homocysteine concentrations $\leq$9 μmol/L and only 5% (~14% in elderly) have elevated ($\geq$13 μmol/L) concentrations.[166]

Whether the reductions in plasma homocysteine concentrations in response to supplemental folic acid are sufficient to be associated with a reduced incidence of vascular disease is the focus of controlled intervention trials currently underway in the United States, Canada, Europe, and Australia.[168] The North American trials may not have the statistical power necessary to detect a significant effect on vascular disease outcome due to the lower baseline homocysteine concentration resulting from fortification, as the recent Vitamin Intervention for Stroke Prevention (VISP) trial illustrates.[169] Ongoing randomized trials in European countries and Australia, which do not have mandatory folic acid fortification, are likely to provide a sustained homocysteine-lowering effect of folic acid thus increasing the probability of detecting vascular benefits.[170]

The presence of the MTHFR 677C→T polymorphism has been shown to significantly influence vascular disease risk based on a series of large meta-analyses.[162,171,172] Individuals with the TT genotype for the MTHFR 677C→T polymorphism have a significantly greater risk of stroke,[172] ischemic heart disease, and deep vein thrombosis[162] than individuals with the CC genotype. Individuals with the MTHFR 677 TT genotype were reported to have a 16% higher odds of coronary heart disease than individuals with the CC genotype based on a meta-analysis involving 11,162 coronary heart disease cases and 12,758 controls from 40 studies.[171] The data indicated that the TT genotype for the 677C→T polymorphism was only associated with increased coronary heart disease risk when folate status was low, illustrating the modulating effect of folate status on vascular disease risk associated with the MTHFR 677C→T polymorphism.

Cancer

Observational data provide population-based evidence for the conclusion that poor folate status is associated with an increase in cancer risk with the strongest support for colorectal cancer and its precancerous lesion, adenoma as previously reviewed.[173,174] In the Nurses' Health Study and the Health Professionals' Follow-Up Study, the risk for colorectal adenoma and cancer was 30%–40% lower in individuals with the highest folate intake (primarily supplement users) than those with the lowest folate intake.[173,174] In contrast to what might be predicted, the presence of the MTHFR 677C→T polymorphism has been associated with a significant reduction in colorectal cancer risk as previously reviewed.[175–177] In the Physician's Health Study for example, colorectal cancer risk was decreased threefold in individuals with the TT genotype for the MTHFR 677C→T polymorphism with normal folate status compared with the risk in the group with CC and CT genotypes combined.[175] When folate status was deficient, the protective effect of the MTHFR 677C→T polymorphism was absent. It is proposed that a reduction in MTHFR activity associated with the 677C→T polymorphism in the presence of adequate folate may lead to an increase in the 5,10-methylene THF required for DNA synthesis and normal cell division.[178]

In addition to colorectal cancer, accumulating evidence from large prospective epidemiological studies suggests that folate has a protective role against breast cancer, especially among alcohol users.[179–182] In the Nurses' Health Study,[179] there was a significant reduction in risk associated with total folate as well as folate from supplements among women who consume alcohol ($\geq$15 g/day). Similar findings were reported in the Canadian National Breast Screening Study[180] and the Iowa's Women's Health Study.[181] The evidence from these epidemiological investigations suggesting that the increased breast cancer risk associated with moderate alcohol consumption ($\geq$15 g/day; approximately one drink of any kind daily) can be significantly reduced by increased folate intake[179,180] indicates that both low folate intake and alcohol intake are potential modifiable cancer risk factors. The observation that alcohol consumption coupled with low folate intake increases cancer risk may be related to alcohol's ability to impair folate absorption, decrease hepatic folate uptake, and interfere with renal conservation of folate.[108]

Potential mechanisms by which folate status may modulate cancer risk include those that influence DNA stability or methylation.[178] When folate intake is limited, dTMP synthesis is impaired leading to a nucleotide imbalance and misincorporation of uracil into DNA, which has been associated with increased cancer risk. Excessive DNA uracil content as well as increased numbers of chromosomal breaks have been observed in folate-deficient humans and reversed with folic acid supplementation.[183] In addition to chromosomal instability due to uracil misincorporation, a folate deficiency may result in changes in DNA methylation, an "epigenetic" mechanism by which gene function is selectively activated or inactivated. It is hypothesized that a folate deficiency may alter the normal methylation patterns in neoplastic cells, which could potentially be associated with inactivation of tumor suppressor genes.[178]

SUMMARY AND CONCLUSIONS

This chapter presented highlights of folate's key role in one carbon metabolism and proposed links between metabolic abnormalities affecting folate-dependent pathways and health-related risks. Maintenance of normal folate status requires knowledge of food sources, stability and bioavailability, and physiological utilization of the vitamin in addition to recommended intakes and methods of status assessment, which are reviewed in this chapter. The potential for folate status or folate-related polymorphisms to influence the risk for developmental abnormalities and chronic disease is addressed in this chapter. Research challenges that evolve from our current understanding of folate metabolism and its relationship to health and disease will be best addressed in the future by a collaborative approach involving multiple disciplines including chemistry, biochemistry, physiology, genetics and molecular biology, clinical medicine, and epidemiology.

REFERENCES

1. Chippel, D. and Scrimgeour, K.G., Oxidative degradation of dihydrofolate and tetrahydrofolate, *Can. J. Biochem.*, 48 (9), 999–1009, 1970.
2. Suitor, C.W. and Bailey, L.B., Dietary folate equivalents: interpretation and application, *J. Am. Diet. Assoc.*, 100 (1), 88–94, 2000.
3. Bailey, L.B., Folate requirements and dietary recommendations, in *Folate in Health and Disease*, Bailey, L.B., ed., Marcel Dekker, New York, 1995, pp. 123–151.
4. Food standards: amendment of standards of identity for enriched grain products to require addition of folic acid, Final rule. 21 CFR Parts 136, 137, and 139, in *Fed. Regist.*, 1996, pp. 8781–8789.
5. Regulations amending the Food and Drug Regulations (1066), in *Canada Gazette*, Part I 1997, pp. 3702–3737.
6. Freire, W.B., Hertrampf, E., and Cortes, F., Effect of folic acid fortification in Chile: preliminary results, *Eur. J. Pediatr. Surg.*, 10 (Suppl 1), 42–43, 2000.
7. Freire, W.B., Howson, C.P., and Cordero, J.F., Recommended levels of folic acid and vitamin B_{12} fortification: a PAHO/MOD/CDC technical consultation, *Nutr. Rev.*, 62 (6 Pt 2), S1–S2, 2004.
8. Pfeiffer, C.M., Candill, S.P., Gunter, E.W., Osterloh, J., and Sampson, E.J., Biochemical indicators of B vitamin status in the U.S. population after folic acid fortification: results from the National Health and Nutrition Examination Survey 1999–2000, *Am. J. Clin. Nutr.*, 82 (2), 442–450, 2005.
9. Ray, J.G., Vermeulen, M.J., Boss, S.C., and Cole, D.E., Increased red cell folate concentrations in women of reproductive age after Canadian folic acid food fortification, *Epidemiology*, 13 (2), 238–240, 2002.

10. Gregory, J., The bioavailability of folate, in *Folate in Health and Disease*, Bailey, L., ed., Marcel Dekker, New York, 1995, pp. 195–235.
11. Gregory, J.F., III, Bioavailability of folate, *Eur. J. Clin. Nutr.*, 51 (Suppl 1), S54–S59, 1997.
12. Tamura, T. and Stokstad, E.L., The availability of food folate in man, *Br. J. Haematol.*, 25 (4), 513–532, 1973.
13. Babu, S. and Srikantia, S.G., Availability of folates from some foods, *Am. J. Clin. Nutr.*, 29 (4), 376–379, 1976.
14. Prinz-Langenohl, R., Bronstrup, A., Thorand, B., Hages, M., and Pietrzik, K., Availability of food folate in humans, *J. Nutr.*, 129 (4), 913–916, 1999.
15. Sauberlich, H.E., Kretsch, M.J., Skala, J.H., Johnson, H.L., and Taylor, P.C., Folate requirement and metabolism in nonpregnant women, *Am. J. Clin. Nutr.*, 46 (6), 1016–1028, 1987.
16. Pfeiffer, C.M., Rogers, L.M., Bailey, L.B., and Gregory, J.F., III, Absorption of folate from fortified cereal-grain products and of supplemental folate consumed with or without food determined by using a dual-label stable-isotope protocol, *Am. J. Clin. Nutr.*, 66 (6), 1388–1397, 1997.
17. Gregory, J.F., III, Chemical and nutritional aspects of folate research: analytical procedures, methods of folate synthesis, stability, and bioavailability of dietary folates, *Adv. Food Nutr. Res.*, 33, 1–101, 1989.
18. Finglas, P.M., Faure, U., and Southgate, D.A.T., First BCR-intercomparison on the determination of folates in food, *Food Chem.*, 46 (2), 199–213, 1993.
19. Tamura, T., Determination of food folate, *J. Nutr. Biochem.*, 9 (5), 285–293, 1998.
20. DeSouza, S. and Eitenmiller, R., Effects of different enzyme treatments on extraction of total folate from various foods prior to microbiological assay and radioassay, *J. Micronutrient Anal.*, 7 (1), 37–57, 1990.
21. Martin, J.I., Landen, W.O., Jr., Soliman, A.G., and Eitenmiller, R.R., Application of a tri-enzyme extraction for total folate determination in foods, *J. Assoc. Off. Anal. Chem.*, 73 (5), 805–808, 1990.
22. Tamura, T., Mizuno, Y., Johnston, K., and Jacob, R., Food folate assay with protease, a-amylase, and folate conjugase treatments, *J. Agric. Food Chem.*, 45 (1), 135–139, 1997.
23. Pfeiffer, C.M., Rogers, L.M., and Gregory, J.F., Determination of folate in cereal-grain food products using tri-enzyme extraction and combined affinity and reverse-phase liquid chromatography, *J. Agric. Food Chem.*, 45, 407–413, 1997.
24. Koontz, J., Phillips, K., Wunderlich, K., Exler, J., Holden, J., Gebhardt, S., and Haytowitz, D., Comparison of total folate concentrations in foods determined by microbiological assay at several experienced U.S. commercial laboratories, *J. AOAC Int.*, 88 (3), 805–813, 2005.
25. Finglas, P.M., Wigertz, K., Vahteristo, L., Witthoft, C., Southon, S., and de Froidmont-Gortz, I., Standardisation of HPLC techniques for the determination of naturally-occurring folates in food, *Food Chem.*, 64 (2), 245–255, 1999.
26. Konings, E.J., A validated liquid chromatographic method for determining folates in vegetables, milk powder, liver, and flour, *J. AOAC Int.*, 82 (1), 119–127, 1999.
27. Wilson, S.D. and Horne, D.W., Evaluation of ascorbic acid in protecting labile folic acid derivatives, *Proc. Natl. Acad. Sci., USA* 80 (21), 6500–6504, 1983.
28. Shane, B., High performance liquid chromatography of folates: identification of poly-gamma-glutamate chain lengths of labeled and unlabeled folates, *Am. J. Clin. Nutr.*, 35 (3), 599–608, 1982.
29. Brody, T., Shane, B., and Robert Stokstad, E.L., Separation and identification of pteroylpolyglutamates by polyacrylamide gel chromatography, *Anal. Biochem.*, 92 (2), 501–509, 1979.
30. Varela-Moreiras, G., Seyoum, E., and Selhub, J., Combined affinity and ion pair liquid chromatographies for the analysis of folate distribution in tissues, *J. Nutr. Biochem.*, 2 (1), 44–53, 1991.
31. Quinlivan, E.P., Hanson, A.D., and Gregory, J.F., The analysis of folate and its metabolic precursors in biological samples, *Anal. Biochem.*, 348 (2), 163–184, 2006.
32. Pawlosky, R.J., Flanagan, V.P., and Pfeiffer, C.M., Determination of 5-methyltetrahydrofolic acid in human serum by stable-isotope dilution high-performance liquid chromatography–mass spectrometry, *Anal. Biochem.*, 298 (2), 299–305, 2001.
33. Pfeiffer, C.M., Fazili, Z., McCoy, L., Zhang, M., and Gunter, E.W., Determination of folate vitamers in human serum by stable-isotope-dilution tandem mass spectrometry and comparison with radioassay and microbiologic assay, *Clin. Chem.*, 50 (2), 423–432, 2004.

34. Herbert, V., Experimental nutritional folate deficiency in man, *Trans. Assoc. Am. Physicians*, 75, 307–320, 1962.
35. Gunter, E.W., Bowman, B.A., Caudill, S.P., Twite, D.B., Adams, M.J., and Sampson, E.J., Results of an international round robin for serum and whole-blood folate, *Clin. Chem.*, 42 (10), 1689–1694, 1996.
36. van den Berg, H., Finglas, P.M., and Bates, C., FLAIR intercomparisons on serum and red cell folate, *Int. J. Vitam. Nutr. Res.*, 64 (4), 288–293, 1994.
37. Food and Nutrition Board, Institute of Medicine, Folate, in *Dietary Reference Intakes for Thiamin, Riboflavin, Niacin, Vitamin B_6, Folate, Vitamin B_{12}, Pantothenic Acid, Biotin, and Choline*, National Academy Press, Washington, DC, 1998, pp. 196–305.
38. Bailey, L.B., New standard for dietary folate intake in pregnant women, *Am. J. Clin. Nutr.*, 71 (5 Suppl), 1304S–1307S, 2000.
39. Bailey, L.B., Dietary reference intakes for folate: the debut of dietary folate equivalents, *Nutr. Rev.*, 56 (10), 294–299, 1998.
40. Yang, T.L., Hung, J., Caudill, M.A., Urrutia, T.F., Alamilla, A., Perry, C.A., Li, R., Hata, H., and Cogger, E.A., A long-term controlled folate feeding study in young women supports the validity of the 1.7 multiplier in the dietary folate equivalency equation, *J. Nutr.*, 135 (5), 1139–1145, 2005.
41. Savage, D.G. and Lindenbaum, J., Folate–cobalamin interactions, in *Folate in Health and Disease*, Bailey, L.B., ed., Marcel Dekker, New York, NY, 1995, pp. 237–285.
42. Chandler, C., Wang, T., and Halsted, C., Pteroylpolyglutamate hydrolase from human jejunal brush borders. Purification and characterization, *J. Biol. Chem.*, 261 (2), 928–933, 1986.
43. Sirotnak, F.M. and Tolner, B., Carrier-mediated transport of folates in mamalian cells, *Annu. Rev. Nutr.*, 19 (1), 91–122, 1999.
44. Moscow, J., Gong, M., He, R., Sgagias, M., Dixon, K., Anzick, S., Meltzer, P., and Cowan, K., Isolation of a gene encoding a human reduced folate carrier (*RFC1*) and analysis of its expression in transport-deficient, methotrexate-resistant human breast cancer cells, *Cancer Res.*, 55 (17), 3790–3794, 1995.
45. Said, H., Nguyen, T., Dyer, D., Cowan, K., and Rubin, S., Intestinal folate transport: identification of a cDNA involved in folate transport and the functional expression and distribution of its mRNA, *Biochim. Biophys. Acta*, 1281, 164–172, 1996.
46. Selhub, J., Dhar, G., and Rosenberg, I., Gastrointestinal absorption of folates and antifolates, *Pharmacol. Ther.*, 20 (3), 397–418, 1983.
47. Kelly, P., McPartlin, J., Goggins, M., Weir, D.G., and Scott, J.M., Unmetabolized folic acid in serum: acute studies in subjects consuming fortified food and supplements, *Am. J. Clin. Nutr.*, 65 (6), 1790–1795, 1997.
48. Kiil, J., Jagerstad, M., and Elsborg, L., The role of liver passage for conversion of pteroylmonoglutamate and pteroyltriglutamate to active folate coenzyme, *Int. J. Vitam. Nutr. Res.*, 49 (3), 296–306, 1979.
49. Caudill, M.A., Cruz, A.C., Gregory, J.F., III, Hutson, A.D., and Bailey, L.B., Folate status response to controlled folate intake in pregnant women, *J. Nutr.*, 127 (12), 2363–2370, 1997.
50. Ratnman, N. and Freisheim, J.H., Proteins involved in the transport of folates and antifolates by normal and neoplastic cells, in *Folic Acid Metabolism in Health and Disease*, Picciano, M.F., Stokstad, E.L.R., and Gregory, J.F., eds., Wiley-Liss, New York, 1990, pp. 93–120.
51. Antony, A.C., Folate receptors, *Annu. Rev. Nutr.*, 16, 501–521, 1996.
52. Hjelle, J.T., Christensen, E.I., Carone, F.A., and Selhub, J., Cell fractionation and electron microscope studies of kidney folate-binding protein, *Am. J. Physiol. Cell Physiol.*, 260 (2), C338–C346, 1991.
53. Shane, B., Folylpolyglutamate synthesis and role in the regulation of one-carbon metabolism, *Vitam. Horm.*, 45, 263–335, 1989.
54. Stokstad, E.L.R., Historical perspective on key advances in the biochemistry and physiology of folates, in *Folic Acid Metabolism in Health and Disease*, Picciano, M.F., Stokstad, E.L.R., and Gregory, J.F., eds., Wiley-Liss, New York, 1990, pp. 1–15.
55. McGuire, J.J. and Coward, J.K., Pteropolyglutamates: biosynthesis, degradation, and function, in *Folates and Pterins*, Blakley, R.L. and Benkovik, S.J., eds., John Wiley & Sons, New York, 1984, pp. 135–190.

56. Hoppner, K. and Lampi, B., Folate levels in human liver from autopsies in Canada, *Am. J. Clin. Nutr.*, 33 (4), 862–864, 1980.
57. Whitehead, V.M., Polygammaglutamyl metabolites of folic acid in human liver, *Lancet*, 1 (7806), 743–745, 1973.
58. Suh, J.R., Oppenheim, E.W., Girgis, S., and Stover, P.J., Purification and properties of a folate-catabolizing enzyme, *J. Biol. Chem.*, 275 (45), 35646–35655, 2000.
59. Shane, B., Folate chemistry and metabolism, in *Folate in Health and Disease*, Bailey, L.B., ed., Marcel Dekker, New York, 1995, pp. 1–22.
60. Scott, J.M., Catabolism of folates, in *Folates and Pterins*, Blakley, R.L. and Whitehead, V.M., eds., John Wiley & Sons, New York, 1986, pp. 307–327.
61. Caudill, M.A., Gregory, J.F., Hutson, A.D., and Bailey, L.B., Folate catabolism in pregnant and nonpregnant women with controlled folate intakes, *J. Nutr.*, 128 (2), 204–208, 1998.
62. Jukes, T., Franklin, A., Stokstad, E., and Boehne, J., The urinary excretion of pteroylglutamic acid and certain related compounds, *J. Lab. Clin. Med.*, 32, 1350–1355, 1947.
63. Krumdieck, C.L., Fukushima, K., Fukushima, T., Shiota, T., and Butterworth, C.E., Jr., A long-term study of the excretion of folate and pterins in a human subject after ingestion of ^{14}C folic acid, with observations on the effect of diphenylhydantoin administration, *Am. J. Clin. Nutr.*, 31 (1), 88–93, 1978.
64. Stea, B., Backlund, P.S., Jr., Berkey, P.B., Cho, A.K., Halpern, B.C., Halpern, R.M., and Smith, R.A., Folate and pterin metabolism by cancer cells in culture, *Cancer Res.*, 38 (8), 2378–2384, 1978.
65. Suh, J.R., Herbig, A.K., and Stover, P.J., New perspectives on folate metabolism, *Annu. Rev. Nutr.*, 21 (1), 255–282, 2001.
66. Stites, T.E., Bailey, L.B., Scott, K.C., Toth, J.P., Fisher, W.P., and Gregory, J.F., III, Kinetic modeling of folate metabolism through use of chronic administration of deuterium-labeled folic acid in men, *Am. J. Clin. Nutr.*, 65 (1), 53–60, 1997.
67. Stover, P.J., Physiology of folate and vitamin B_{12} in health and disease, *Nutr. Rev.*, 62 (6 Pt 2), S3–S13, 2004.
68. Whitehead, V.M., Pharmacokinetics and physiological disposition of folate and its derivatives, in *Folates and Pterins*, Blakley, R.L. and Whitehead, V.M., eds., John Wiley & Sons, New York, 1986, pp. 177–205.
69. Cook, R.J., Folate metabolism, in *Homocysteine in Health and Disease*, Carmel, R. and Jacobsen, D., eds., Cambridge University Press, Cambridge, UK, 2001, pp. 113–134.
70. Davis, S.R., Stacpoole, P.W., Williamson, J., Kick, L.S., Quinlivan, E.P., Coats, B.S., Shane, B., Bailey, L.B., and Gregory, J.F., III, Tracer-derived total and folate-dependent homocysteine remethylation and synthesis rates in humans indicate that serine is the main one-carbon donor, *Am. J. Physiol. Endocrinol. Metab.*, 286 (2), E272–E279, 2004.
71. Schalinske, K.L. and Steele, R.D., Quantitation of carbon flow through the hepatic folate-dependent one-carbon pool in rats, *Arch. Biochem. Biophys.*, 271 (1), 49–55, 1989.
72. Matthews, R., Ross, J., Baugh, C., Cook, J., and Davis, L., Interactions of pig liver serine hydroxymethyltransferase with methyl tetrahydropteroylpolyglutamate inhibitors and with tetrahydropteroylpolyglutamate substrates, *Biochemistry*, 21 (6), 1230–1238, 1982.
73. Herbert, V. and Zalusky, R., Interrelations of vitamin B_{12} and folic acid metabolism: folic acid clearance studies, *J. Clin. Invest.*, 41, 1263–1276, 1962.
74. Garrow, T., Betaine-dependent remethylation, in *Homocysteine in Health and Disease*, Carmel, R. and Jacobson, D., eds., Cambridge University Press, Cambridge, UK, 2001, pp. 145–152.
75. Ogawa, H., Gomi, T., Takusagawa, F., and Fujioka, M., Structure, function and physiological role of glycine *N*-methyltransferase, *Int. J. Biochem. Cell Biol.*, 30 (1), 13–26, 1998.
76. Konishi, K. and Fujioka, M., Rat liver glycine methyltransferase. Cooperative binding of *S*-adenosylmethionine and loss of cooperativity by removal of a short NH_2-terminal segment, *J. Biol. Chem.*, 263 (26), 13381–13385, 1988.
77. Fowler, B., Homocysteine: overview of biochemistry, molecular biology, and role in disease, *Semin. Vasc. Med.*, 5 (2), 76–86, 2005.
78. Melnyk, S., Pogribna, M., Pogribny, I.P., Yi, P., and James, S.J., Measurement of plasma and intracellular *S*-adenosylmethionine and *S*-adenosylhomocysteine utilizing coulometric electrochemical

detection: alterations with plasma homocysteine and pyridoxal 5′-phosphate concentrations, *Clin. Chem.*, 46 (2), 265–272, 2000.
79. Finkelstein, J. and Martin, J., Methionine metabolism in mammals. Distribution of homocysteine between competing pathways, *J. Biol. Chem.*, 259 (15), 9508–9513, 1984.
80. Kruger, W., The transsulfuration pathway, in *Homocysteine in Health and Disease*, Carmel, R. and Jacobson, D., eds., Cambridge University Press, Cambridge, UK, 2001, pp. 153–161.
81. Finkelstein, J. and Martin, J., Inactivation of betaine-homocysteine methyltransferase by adenosylmethionine and adenosylethionine, *Biochem. Biophys. Res. Commun.*, 118 (1), 14–19, 1984.
82. Daubner, S. and Matthews, R., Purification and properties of methylenetetrahydrofolate reductase from pig liver, *J. Biol. Chem.*, 257 (1), 140–145, 1982.
83. Finkelstein, J., Kyle, W., Martin, J., and Pick, A., Activation of cystathionine synthase by adenosylmethionine and adenosylethionine, *Biochem. Biophys. Res. Commun.*, 66 (1), 81–87, 1975.
84. Wakabayashi, M., Nakata, R., and Tsukamoto, I., Regulation of thymidylate synthase in regenerating rat liver after partial hepatectomy, *Biochem. Mol. Biol. Int.*, 34 (2), 345–350, 1994.
85. Rozen, R., Polymorphisms of folate and cobalamin metabolism, in *Homocysteine in Health and Disease*, Carmel, R. and Jacobsen, D., eds., Cambridge Press, Cambridge, UK, 2001, pp. 259–270.
86. Finnell, R.H., Gould, A., and Spiegelstein, O., Pathobiology and genetics of neural tube defects, *Epilepsia*, 44 (Suppl 3), 14–23, 2003.
87. Molloy, A.M., Folate and homocysteine interrelationships including genetics of the relevant enzymes, *Curr. Opin. Lipidol.*, 15 (1), 49–57, 2004.
88. Gellenkink, H., den Heijer, M., Heil, S., and Blom, H.J., Genetic determinants of plasma total homocysteine, *Semin. Vasc. Med.*, 5, 98–109, 2005.
89. Botto, L. and Yang, Q., 5,10-Methylenetetrahydrofolate reductase gene variants and congenital anomalies: a HuGE review, *Am. J. Epidemiol.*, 151 (9), 862–877, 2000.
90. Friso, S., Choi, S.W., Girelli, D., Mason, J.B., Dolnikowski, G.G., Bagley, P.J., Olivieri, O., Jacques, P.F., Rosenberg, I.H., Corrocher, R., and Selhub, J., A common mutation in the 5,10-methylenetetrahydrofolate reductase gene affects genomic DNA methylation through an interaction with folate status, *Proc. Natl. Acad. Sci., USA*. 99 (8), 5606–5611, 2002.
91. Vollset, E. and Botto, L.D., Neural tube defects, other congenital malformations and single nucleotide polymorphisms in the 5,10-methylenetetrahydrofolate reductase (MTHFR) gene, in *MTHFR Polymorphisms and Disease*, Ueland, P. and Rozen, R., eds., Landes Bioscience, Georgetown, TX, 2004, pp. 127–145.
92. Shelnutt, K.P., Kauwell, G.P.A., Chapman, C.M., Gregory, J.F., III, Maneval, D.R., Browdy, A.A., Theriaque, D.W., and Bailey, L.B., Folate status response to controlled folate intake is affected by the methylenetetrahydrofolate reductase 677C→T polymorphism in young women, *J. Nutr.*, 133 (12), 4107–4111, 2003.
93. Guinotte, C.L., Burns, M.G., Axume, J.A., Hata, H., Urrutia, T.F., Alamilla, A., McCabe, D., Singgih, A., Cogger, E.A., and Caudill, M.A., Methylenetetrahydrofolate reductase 677C→T variant modulates folate status response to controlled folate intakes in young women, *J. Nutr.*, 133 (5), 1272–1280, 2003.
94. Stern, L.L., Mason, J.B., Selhub, J., and Choi, S.-W., Genomic DNA hypomethylation, a characteristic of most cancers, is present in peripheral leukocytes of individuals who are homozygous for the C677T polymorphism in the methylenetetrahydrofolate reductase gene, *Cancer Epidemiol. Biomarkers Prev.*, 9 (8), 849–853, 2000.
95. Shelnutt, K.P., Kauwell, G.P.A., Gregory, I., Jesse, F., Maneval, D.R., Quinlivan, E.P., Theriaque, D.W., Henderson, G.N., and Bailey, L.B., Methylenetetrahydrofolate reductase 677C→T polymorphism affects DNA methylation in response to controlled folate intake in young women, *J. Nutr. Biochem.*, 15 (9), 554–560, 2004.
96. Morita, H., Kurihara, H., Sugiyama, T., Hamada, C., Kurihara, Y., Shindo, T., Oh-hashi, Y., and Yazaki, Y., Polymorphism of the methionine synthase gene: association with homocysteine metabolism and late-onset vascular diseases in the Japanese population, *Arterioscler. Thromb. Vasc. Biol.*, 19 (2), 298–302, 1999.
97. Tsai, M.Y., Welge, B.G., Hanson, N.Q., Bignell, M.K., Vessey, J., Schwichtenberg, K., Yang, F., Bullemer, F.E., Rasmussen, R., and Graham, K.J., Genetic causes of mild hyperhomocysteinemia in patients with premature occlusive coronary artery diseases, *Atherosclerosis*, 143 (1), 163–170, 1999.

98. Morrison, K., Edwards, Y.H., Lynch, S.A., Burn, J., Hol, F., and Mariman, E., Methionine synthase and neural tube defects, *J. Med. Genet.*, 34 (11), 958, 1997.
99. Shaw, G.M., Todoroff, K., Finnell, R.H., Lammer, E.J., Leclerc, D., Gravel, R.A., and Rozen, R., Infant methionine synthase variants and risk for spina bifida, *J. Med. Genet.*, 36 (1), 86–87, 1999.
100. van der Put, N.M., Eskes, T.K., and Blom, H.J., Is the common 677C→T mutation in the methylenetetrahydrofolate reductase gene a risk factor for neural tube defects? A meta-analysis, *Q. J. Med.*, 90 (2), 111–115, 1997.
101. Vaughn, J.D., Bailey, L.B., Shelnutt, K.P., Dunwoody, K.M., Maneval, D.R., Davis, S.R., Quinlivan, E.P., Gregory, J.F., III, Theriaque, D.W., and Kauwell, G.P., Methionine synthase reductase 66A→G polymorphism is associated with increased plasma homocysteine concentration when combined with the homozygous methylenetetrahydrofolate reductase 677C→T variant, *J. Nutr.*, 134 (11), 2985–2990, 2004.
102. Gaughan, D.J., Kluijtmans, L.A.J., Barbaux, S., McMaster, D., Young, I.S., Yarnell, J.W.G., Evans, A., and Whitehead, A.S., The methionine synthase reductase (MTRR) A66G polymorphism is a novel genetic determinant of plasma homocysteine concentrations, *Atherosclerosis*, 157 (2), 451–456, 2001.
103. Devlin, A.M., Ling, E.H., Peerson, J.M., Fernando, S., Clarke, R., Smith, A.D., and Halsted, C.H., Glutamate carboxypeptidase II: a polymorphism associated with lower levels of serum folate and hyperhomocysteinemia, *Hum. Mol. Genet.*, 9 (19), 2837–2844, 2000.
104. Melse-Boonstra, A., Lievers, K.J., Blom, H.J., and Verhoef, P., Bioavailability of polyglutamyl folic acid relative to that of monoglutamyl folic acid in subjects with different genotypes of the glutamate carboxypeptidase II gene, *Am. J. Clin. Nutr.*, 80 (3), 700–704, 2004.
105. Lievers, K.J.A., Kluijtmans, L.A.J., Boers, G.H.J., Verhoef, P., den Heijer, M., Trijbels, F.J.M., and Blom, H.J., Influence of a glutamate carboxypeptidase II (GCPII) polymorphism (1561C→T) on plasma homocysteine, folate and vitamin B_{12} levels and its relationship to cardiovascular disease risk, *Atherosclerosis*, 164 (2), 269–273, 2002.
106. Afman, L.A., Trijbels, F.J.M., and Blom, H.J., The H475Y polymorphism in the glutamate carboxypeptidase II gene increases plasma folate without affecting the risk for neural tube defects in humans, *J. Nutr.*, 133 (1), 75–77, 2003.
107. Chango, A., Emery-Fillon, N., de Courcy, G.P., Lambert, D., Pfister, M., Rosenblatt, D.S., and Nicolas, J.P., A polymorphism (80G→A) in the reduced folate carrier gene and its associations with folate status and homocysteinemia, *Mol. Genet. Metab.*, 70 (4), 310–315, 2000.
108. Halsted, C.H., Villanueva, J.A., Devlin, A.M., and Chandler, C.J., Metabolic interactions of alcohol and folate, *J. Nutr.*, 132 (8 Suppl), 2367S–2372S, 2002.
109. Naughton, C., Chandler, C., Duplantier, R., and Halsted, C., Folate absorption in alcoholic pigs: in vitro hydrolysis and transport at the intestinal brush border membrane, *Am. J. Clin. Nutr.*, 50 (6), 1436–1441, 1989.
110. Reisenauer, A., Buffington, C., Villanueva, J., and Halsted, C., Folate absorption in alcoholic pigs: in vivo intestinal perfusion studies, *Am. J. Clin. Nutr.*, 50 (6), 1429–1435, 1989.
111. Villanueva, J., Devlin, A., and Halsted, C., Reduced folate carrier: tissue distribution and effects of chronic ethanol intake in the micropig, *Alcohol. Clin. Exp. Res.*, 25 (3), 415–420, 2001.
112. Tamura, T. and Halsted, C., Folate turnover in chronically alcoholic monkeys, *J. Lab. Clin. Med.*, 101 (4), 623–628, 1983.
113. McMartin, K., Collins, T., Eisenga, B., Fortney, T., Bates, W., and Bairnsfather, L., Effects of chronic ethanol and diet treatment on urinary folate excretion and development of folate deficiency in the rat, *J. Nutr.*, 119 (10), 1490–1497, 1989.
114. Russell, R.M., Rosenberg, I.H., Wilson, P.D., Iber, F.L., Oaks, E.B., Giovetti, A.C., Otradovec, C.L., Karwoski, P.A., and Press, A.W., Increased urinary excretion and prolonged turnover time of folic acid during ethanol ingestion, *Am. J. Clin. Nutr.*, 38 (1), 64–70, 1983.
115. Morgan, S.L. and Baggot, J.E., Folate antagonists in nonneoplastic disease: proposed mechanism of efficacy and toxicity, in *Folate in Health and Disease*, Bailey, L.B., ed., Marcel Dekker, New York, 1995, pp. 435–462.
116. Priest, D.G. and Bunni, M.A., Folates and folate antagonists in cancer chemotherapy, in *Folate in Health and Disease*, Bailey, L.B., ed., Marcel Dekker, New York, 1995, pp. 379–404.

117. van Ede, A.E., Laan, R.F.J.M., Blom, H.J., Boers, G.H.J., Haagsma, C.J., Thomas, C.M.G., de Boo, T.M., and van de Putte, L.B.A., Homocysteine and folate status in methotrexate-treated patients with rheumatoid arthritis, *Rheumatology*, 41 (6), 658–665, 2002.
118. Young, S.N. and Ghadirian, A.M., Folic acid and psychopathology, *Prog. Neuropsychopharmacol. Biol. Psychiatry*, 13 (6), 841–863, 1989.
119. Carlsen, S.M., Folling, I., Grill, V., Bjerve, K.S., Schneede, J., and Refsum, H., Metformin increases total serum homocysteine levels in non-diabetic male patients with coronary heart disease, *Scand. J. Clin. Lab. Invest.*, 57 (6), 521–527, 1997.
120. Herbert, V., Making sense of laboratory tests of folate status: folate requirements to sustain normality, *Am. J. Hematol.*, 26 (2), 199–207, 1987.
121. Kauwell, G.P., Lippert, B.L., Wilsky, C.E., Herrlinger-Garcia, K., Hutson, A.D., Theriaque, D.W., Rampersaud, G.C., Cerda, J.J., and Bailey, L.B., Folate status of elderly women following moderate folate depletion responds only to a higher folate intake, *J. Nutr.*, 130 (6), 1584–1590, 2000.
122. Wu, A., Chanarin, I., Slavin, G., and Levi, A., Folate deficiency in the alcoholic—its relationship to clinical and haematological abnormalities, liver disease and folate stores, *Br. J. Haematol.*, 29 (3), 469–478, 1975.
123. Carmel, R., Cobalamin deficency, in *Homocysteine in Health and Disease*, Carmel, R. and Jacobson, D., eds., Cambridge University Press, Cambridge, UK, 2001, pp. 289–305.
124. Selhub, J., Jacques, P.F., Wilson, P.W., Rush, D., and Rosenberg, I.H., Vitamin status and intake as primary determinants of homocysteinemia in an elderly population, *JAMA* 270 (22), 2693–2698, 1993.
125. Ubbink, J., What is a desirable homocysteine level? in *Homocysteine in Health and Disease*, Carmel, R. and Jacobson, D., eds., Cambridge University Press, Cambridge, UK, 2001, pp. 485–490.
126. Rasmussen, K. and Moller, J., Methodologies of testing, in *Homocysteine in Health and Disease*, Carmel, R. and Jacobson, D., eds., Cambridge University Press, Cambridge, UK, 2001, pp. 199–211.
127. McCabe, D.C. and Caudill, M.A., DNA methylation, genomic silencing, and links to nutrition and cancer, *Nutr. Rev.*, 63 (6), 183–196, 2005.
128. Ulrey, C.L., Liu, L., Andrews, L.G., and Tollefsbol, T.O., The impact of metabolism on DNA methylation, *Hum. Mol. Genet.*, 14 (Suppl 1), R139–R147, 2005.
129. Rampersaud, G.C., Kauwell, G.P., Hutson, A.D., Cerda, J.J., and Bailey, L.B., Genomic DNA methylation decreases in response to moderate folate depletion in elderly women, *Am. J. Clin. Nutr.*, 72 (4), 998–1003, 2000.
130. Jacob, R.A., Gretz, D.M., Taylor, P.C., James, S.J., Pogribny, I.P., Miller, B.J., Henning, S.M., and Swendseid, M.E., Moderate folate depletion increases plasma homocysteine and decreases lymphocyte DNA methylation in postmenopausal women, *J. Nutr.*, 128 (7), 1204–1212, 1998.
131. Lindenbaum, J. and Allen, R., Clinical spectrum and diagnosis of folate deficiency, in *Folate in Health and Disease*, Bailey, L.B., ed., Marcel Decker, New York, NY, 1995, pp. 43–73.
132. Scholl, T.O. and Johnson, W.G., Folic acid: influence on the outcome of pregnancy, *Am. J. Clin. Nutr.*, 71 (5 Suppl), 1295S–1303S, 2000.
133. Vollset, S.E., Refsum, H., Irgens, L.M., Emblem, B.M., Tverdal, A., Gjessing, H.K., Monsen, A.L., and Ueland, P.M., Plasma total homocysteine, pregnancy complications, and adverse pregnancy outcomes: the Hordaland homocysteine study, *Am. J. Clin. Nutr.*, 71 (4), 962–968, 2000.
134. van der Molen, E.F., Arends, G.E., Nelen, W.L., van der Put, N.J., Heil, S.G., Eskes, T.K., and Blom, H.J., A common mutation in the 5,10-methylenetetrahydrofolate reductase gene as a new risk factor for placental vasculopathy, *Am. J. Obstet. Gynecol.*, 182 (5), 1258–1263, 2000.
135. O'Rahilly, R. and Muller, F., Neurulation in the normal human embryo, in *Neural Tube Defects. CIBA Foundation Symposium*, 181, Bock G.M.J., ed., John Wiley & Sons, West Sussex, England, 1994.
136. Elwood, J., Little, J., and Elwood, J., *Epidemiology and Control of Neural Tube Defects*, Oxford University Press, Oxford, 1992.
137. Institute of Medicine, Dietary reference intakes: energy, carbohydrate, fiber, fat, fatty acids, cholesterol, protein, and amino acids, in *Standing Committee on the Scientific Evaluation of Dietary Reference Intakes, Food and Nutrition Board*, National Academy of Sciences, Washington, DC, 2002.

138. Botto, L.D., Moore, C.A., Khoury, M.J., and Erickson, J.D., Neural-tube defects, *N. Engl. J. Med.*, 341 (20), 1509–1519, 1999.
139. Honein, M.A., Paulozzi, L.J., Mathews, T.J., Erickson, J.D., and Wong, L.Y., Impact of folic acid fortification of the US food supply on the occurrence of neural tube defects, *JAMA* 285 (23), 2981–2986, 2001.
140. Williams, L.J., Mai, C.T., Edmonds, L.D., Shaw, G.M., Kirby, R.S., Hobbs, C.A., Sever, L.E., Miller, L.A., Meaney, F.J., and Levitt, M., Prevalence of spina bifida and anencephaly during the transition to mandatory folic acid fortification in the United States, *Teratology*, 66 (1), 33–39, 2002.
141. Gucciardi, E., Pietrusiak, M.-A., Reynolds, D.L., and Rouleau, J., Incidence of neural tube defects in Ontario, 1986–1999, *Can. Med. Assoc. J.*, 167 (3), 237–240, 2002.
142. Persad, V.L., Van den Hof, M.C., Dube, J.M., and Zimmer, P., Incidence of open neural tube defects in Nova Scotia after folic acid fortification, *Can. Med. Assoc. J.*, 167 (3), 241–245, 2002.
143. Lopez-Camelo, J.S., Orioli, I.M., Dutra, M.D., Nazer-Herrera, J., Rivera, N., Ojeda, M.E., Canessa, A., Wettig, E., Fontannaz, A.M., Mellado, C., and Castilla, E.E., Reduction of birth prevalence rates of neural tube defects after folic acid fortification in Chile, *Am. J. Med. Genet. A.*, 135 (2), 120–125, 2005.
144. Daly, S., Cotter, A., Molloy, A., and Scott, J., Homocysteine and folic acid: implications for pregnancy, *Semin. Vasc. Med.*, 5, 190–200, 2005.
145. Scott, J.M., Evidence of folic acid and folate in the prevention of neural tube defects, *Bibl. Nutr. Dieta.*, 55, 192–195, 2001.
146. Boddie, A.M., Dedlow, E.R., Nackashi, J.A., Opalko, F.J., Kauwell, G.P., Gregory, J.F., III, and Bailey, L.B., Folate absorption in women with a history of neural tube defect-affected pregnancy, *Am. J. Clin. Nutr.*, 72 (1), 154–158, 2000.
147. Rothenberg, S.P., da Costa, M.P., Sequeira, J.M., Cracco, J., Roberts, J.L., Weedon, J., and Quadros, E.V., Autoantibodies against folate receptors in women with a pregnancy complicated by a neural-tube defect, *N. Engl. J. Med.*, 350 (2), 134–142, 2004.
148. Harris, M.J., Why are the genes that cause risk of human neural tube defects so hard to find? *Teratology*, 63 (5), 165–166, 2001.
149. Shaw, G.M., Lammer, E.J., Zhu, H., Baker, M.W., Neri, E., and Finnell, R.H., Maternal periconceptional vitamin use, genetic variation of infant reduced folate carrier (A80G), and risk of spina bifida, *Am. J. Med. Genet.*, 108 (1), 1–6, 2002.
150. Christensen, B., Arbour, L., Tran, P., Leclerc, D., Sabbaghian, N., Platt, R., Gilfix, B.M., Rosenblatt, D.S., Gravel, R.A., Forbes, P., and Rozen, R., Genetic polymorphisms in methylenetetrahydrofolate reductase and methionine synthase, folate levels in red blood cells, and risk of neural tube defects, *Am. J. Med. Genet.*, 84 (2), 151–157, 1999.
151. Molloy, A.M., Daly, S., Mills, J.L., Kirke, P.N., Whitehead, A.S., Ramsbottom, D., Conley, M.R., Weir, D.G., and Scott, J.M., Thermolabile variant of 5,10-methylenetetrahydrofolate reductase associated with low red-cell folates: implications for folate intake recommendations, *Lancet*, 349 (9065), 1591–1593, 1997.
152. Bailey, L.B. and Berry, R.J., Folic acid supplementation and the occurrence of congenital heart defects, orofacial clefts, multiple births, and miscarriage, *Am. J. Clin. Nutr.*, 81 (5), 1213S–1217S, 2005.
153. Czeizel, A.E., Periconceptional folic acid containing multivitamin supplementation, *Eur. J. Obstet. Gynecol. Reprod. Biol.*, 78, 151–161, 1998.
154. Botto, L.D., Mulinare, J., and Erickson, J.D., Occurrence of congenital heart defects in relation to maternal multivitamin use, *Am. J. Epidemiol.*, 151 (9), 878–884, 2000.
155. Shaw, G.M., Schaffer, D., Velie, E.M., Morland, K., and Harris, J.A., Periconceptional vitamin use, dietary folate, and the occurrence of neural tube defects, *Epidemiology*, 6 (3), 219–226, 1995.
156. Scanlon, K.S., Ferencz, C., Loffredo, C.A., Wilson, P.D., Correa-Villasenor, A., Khoury, M.J., and Willett, W.C., Preconceptional folate intake and malformations of the cardiac outflow tract. Baltimore–Washington Infant Study Group, *Epidemiology*, 9 (1), 95–98, 1998.
157. Werler, M.M., Hayes, C., Louik, C., Shapiro, S., and Mitchell, A.A., Multivitamin supplementation and risk of birth defects, *Am. J. Epidemiol.*, 150 (7), 675–682, 1999.
158. Czeizel, A.E., Reduction of urinary tract and cardiovascular defects by periconceptional multivitamin supplementation, *Am. J. Med. Genet.*, 62 (2), 179–183, 1996.

159. Czeizel, A.E., Periconceptional folic acid containing multivitamin supplementation, *Eur. J. Obstet. Gynecol. Reprod. Biol.*, 78 (2), 151–161, 1998.
160. Botto, L.D., Mulinare, J., and Erickson, J.D., Do multivitamin or folic acid supplements reduce the risk for congenital heart defects? Evidence and gaps, *Am. J. Med. Genet.*, 121A (2), 95–101, 2003.
161. Carmel, R. and Jacobson, D., *Homocysteine in Health and Disease*, Cambridge University Press, Cambridge, UK, 2001.
162. Wald, D.S., Law, M., and Morris, J.K., Homocysteine and cardiovascular disease: evidence on causality from a meta-analysis, *BMJ* 325 (7374), 1202–1206, 2002.
163. Homocysteine Studies Collaboration, Homocysteine and risk of ischemic heart disease and stroke: a meta-analysis, in *JAMA* 2015–2022, 2002.
164. Homocysteine Lowering Trialists Collaboration, Lowering blood homocysteine with folic acid based supplements: meta-analysis of randomised trials, *BMJ* 894–898, 1998.
165. Homocysteine Lowering Trialists Collaboration, Dose-dependent effects of folic acid on blood concentrations of homocysteine: a meta-analysis of the randomized trials, *Am. J. Clin. Nutr.*, 82 (4), 806–812, 2005.
166. Pfeiffer, C.M., Caudill, S.P., Gunter, E.W., Osterloh, J., and Sampson, E.J., Biochemical indicators of B vitamin status in the US population after folic acid fortification: results from the National Health and Nutrition Examination Survey 1999–2000, *Am. J. Clin. Nutr.*, 82 (2), 442–450, 2005.
167. Selhub, J., Jacques, P.F., Rosenberg, I.H., Rogers, G., Bowman, B.A., Gunter, E.W., Wright, J.D., and Johnson, C.L., Serum total homocysteine concentrations in the third National Health and Nutrition Examination Survey (1991–1994): population reference ranges and contribution of vitamin status to high serum concentrations, *Ann. Intern. Med.*, 131 (5), 331–339, 1999.
168. Clarke, S., Design of clinical trials to test the homocysteine hypothesis of vascular disease, in *Homocysteine in Health and Disease*, Carmel, R. and Jacobsen, D., eds., Cambridge University Press, Cambridge, UK, 2001, pp. 477–484.
169. Toole, J.F., Malinow, M.R., Chambless, L.E., Spence, J.D., Pettigrew, L.C., Howard, V.J., Sides, E.G., Wang, C.H., and Stampfer, M., Lowering homocysteine in patients with ischemic stroke to prevent recurrent stroke, myocardial infarction, and death: the Vitamin Intervention for Stroke Prevention (VISP) randomized controlled trial, *JAMA* 291 (5), 565–575, 2004.
170. Hankey, G.J., Eikelboom, J.W., Loh, K., Tang, M., Pizzi, J., Thom, J., and Yi, Q., Sustained homocysteine-lowering effect over time of folic acid-based multivitamin therapy in stroke patients despite increasing folate status in the population, *Cerebrovasc. Dis.*, 19 (2), 110–116, 2005.
171. Klerk, M., Verhoef, P., Clarke, R., Blom, H.J., Kok, F.J., Schouten, E.G., and the MTHFR Studies Collaboration Group, MTHFR 677C→T polymorphism and risk of coronary heart disease: a meta-analysis, *JAMA* 288 (16), 2023–2031, 2002.
172. Casas, J.P., Bautista, L.E., Smeeth, L., Sharma, P., and Hingorani, A.D., Homocysteine and stroke: evidence on a causal link from mendelian randomisation, *Lancet*, 365 (9455), 224–232, 2005.
173. Giovannucci, E., Stampfer, M.J., Colditz, G.A., Rimm, E.B., Trichopoulos, D., Rosner, B.A., Speizer, F.E., and Willett, W.C., Folate, methionine, and alcohol intake and risk of colorectal adenoma, *J. Natl. Cancer Inst.*, 85 (11), 875–884, 1993.
174. Giovannucci, E., Stampfer, M.J., Colditz, G.A., Hunter, D.J., Fuchs, C., Rosner, B.A., Speizer, F.E., and Willett, W.C., Multivitamin use, folate, and colon cancer in women in the Nurses' Health Study, *Ann. Intern. Med.*, 129 (7), 517–524, 1998.
175. Ma, J., Stampfer, M.J., Giovannucci, E., Artigas, C., Hunter, D.J., Fuchs, C., Willett, W.C., Selhub, J., Hennekens, C.H., and Rozen, R., Methylenetetrahydrofolate reductase polymorphism, dietary interactions, and risk of colorectal cancer, *Cancer Res.*, 57 (6), 1098–1102, 1997.
176. Giovannucci, E., Epidemiologic studies of folate and colorectal neoplasia: a review, *J. Nutr.*, 132 (8 Suppl), 2350S–2355S, 2002.
177. Robien, K. and Ulrich, C.M., 5,10-Methylenetetrahydrofolate reductase polymorphisms and leukemia risk: a HuGE minireview, *Am. J. Epidemiol.*, 157 (7), 571–582, 2003.
178. Kim, Y.I., Folate and DNA methylation: a mechanistic link between folate deficiency and colorectal cancer? *Cancer Epidemiol. Biomarkers Prev.*, 13 (4), 511–519, 2004.
179. Zhang, S., Hunter, D.J., Hankinson, S.E., Giovannucci, E.L., Rosner, B.A., Colditz, G.A., Speizer, F.E., and Willett, W.C., A prospective study of folate intake and the risk of breast cancer, *JAMA* 281 (17), 1632–1637, 1999.

180. Rohan, T.E., Jain, M.G., Howe, G.R., and Miller, A.B., Dietary folate consumption and breast cancer risk, *J. Natl. Cancer Inst.*, 92 (3), 266–269, 2000.
181. Sellers, T.A., Kushi, L.H., Cerhan, J.R., Vierkant, R.A., Gapstur, S.M., Vachon, C.M., Olson, J.E., Therneau, T.M., and Folsom, A.R., Dietary folate intake, alcohol, and risk of breast cancer in a prospective study of postmenopausal women, *Epidemiology*, 12 (4), 420–428, 2001.
182. Feigelson, H.S., Jonas, C.R., Robertson, A.S., McCullough, M.L., Thun, M.J., and Calle, E.E., Alcohol, folate, methionine, and risk of incident breast cancer in the American Cancer Society Cancer Prevention Study II Nutrition Cohort, *Cancer Epidemiol. Biomarkers Prev.*, 12 (2), 161–164, 2003.
183. Blount, B.C., Mack, M.M., Wehr, C.M., MacGregor, J.T., Hiatt, R.A., Wang, G., Wickramasinghe, S.N., Everson, R.B., and Ames, B.N., Folate deficiency causes uracil misincorporation into human DNA and chromosome breakage: implications for cancer and neuronal damage, *Proc. Natl. Acad. Sci., USA*. 94 (7), 3290–3295, 1997.

13 Vitamin B_{12}

Ralph Green and Joshua W. Miller

CONTENTS

HISTORY

The history of discovery of vitamin B_{12} is punctuated by a series of important contributions from diverse fields including human and animal nutrition, medicine, chemistry, microbiology, x-ray crystallography, and pharmaceutical science. Discoverers of some of the more important scientific milestones were awarded Nobel Prizes for their contributions. A full description of this rich tapestry of medical history intertwined with the leading edge of scientific discovery contains examples of the several threads drawn from the spools of scientific progress including insight, persistence, intuition, and serendipity, and lies beyond the scope of this chapter. However, several excellent monographs and articles have been written on the subject [1–3]. The original impetus that led ultimately to the discovery of B_{12} stemmed from the medical necessity to seek a cure for a mysterious and ultimately fatal disease first enigmatically described in 1855 by Thomas Addison, a physician at Guys Hospital in London, as "a very remarkable form of general anemia, occurring without any discoverable cause whatsoever" [1,4]. In tribute, this disease later acquired the eponym Addison's pernicious anemia. It was only some 20 years later that it was recognized that this type of anemia was often accompanied by a variety of neurological complications. After 70 years and many fatal outcomes following Addison's description, a group of physicians at the Thorndike Hospital in Boston made the epochal discovery that feeding a half-pound of lightly cooked liver to patients with pernicious anemia resulted in their cure. In point of fact, the intuition that prompted this group to try near-raw liver was far off the mark regarding the reason for its efficacy. To quote from their 1926 description: "Following the work of Whipple we made a few observations on patients concerning ... a diet ... [with] an abundance of liver ... on blood regeneration. The effect ... [was] quite similar to that which [Whipple] ... obtained in dogs. [This] ... led us to investigate the value of ... food rich in ... proteins and iron—particularly liver—[to treat] pernicious anemia" [5]. It is now well known that Whipple's earlier dog experiments worked because he was simply correcting iron deficiency in dogs that had been bled [6]. Moreover, since patients with pernicious anemia have lost the capacity to absorb vitamin B_{12} via the physiologic route, the efficacy of the liver fed to pernicious anemia patients was likely a function of two serendipitous circumstances. First, the large amount of B_{12} present in a half-pound of liver, permitting absorption of adequate B_{12} through a passive diffusion mechanism that allows for assimilation of 1%–2% of an oral dose, and second, the fact that liver is a rich source of folate, which would not be destroyed by the gentle heat used to prepare Minot and Murphy's unappetizing therapeutic dietary concoction. For reasons discussed later, folate can replace the need for B_{12} in its role in DNA synthesis.

For their seminal observations, Paul Minot, William Murphy, and George Whipple were awarded the Nobel Prize in Physiology and Medicine in 1934. By a simple, though unpalatable, nutritional intervention they had converted a disease with a median survival of 20 months and a 5 year survival of barely 10% and rendered it curable. Then began the intense and competitive search for the nutrient contained in liver in what became a veritable alchemist's dream of purifying the elusive precious elixir. This culminated some 20 years later when Karl Folkers and his group from Merck, and their transatlantic competitors at Glaxo led by E. Lester Smith, almost simultaneously announced successful purification and crystallization of reddish needle-like crystals of a new vitamin [7,8]. This vitamin showed clinical and biological activity by the gold standard assay of demonstrating efficacy in inducing and maintaining remission in patients with pernicious anemia. These teams undertook the gargantuan task that ultimately succeeded in scaling from the 60 g of dried liver that was required to induce remission in pernicious anemia to 1 μg of purified crystalline vitamin B_{12}, a 60 million-fold purification. Shortly thereafter, Smith gave some of his crystals to Dorothy Hodgkin, an x-ray crystallographer working at Oxford, to unravel the molecular structure of this compound that had an approximate molecular weight of 1300–1400 Da. She carefully and laboriously accomplished this task over 8 years, involving an estimated 10 million calculations [9]. Hodgkin was awarded the Nobel Prize in Chemistry in 1964 for her work on the elucidation of the structure of B_{12}, as well as the structures of penicillin and insulin. The next step, also a gigantic and ambitious undertaking, was the total chemical synthesis of B_{12}, which took 11 years to accomplish in 100 separate reactions and with almost as many coinvestigators [10]. This was led by Robert Woodward, who received the Nobel Prize for Chemistry in 1965.

Before all this took place, and during the years between the findings of Minot and his team and the crystallization of B_{12}, another investigator at the Thorndike Hospital, William Castle, in a series of brilliantly conceived experiments, set out to prove the hypothesis that there was a gastric factor that played a role in the normal absorption of the antianemic factor present in liver. His hypothesis was based on the earlier observations that in patients with pernicious anemia, the stomach lining appeared thin, without normal glandular structure, and gastric juice including acid production was reduced or absent [1]. He showed that gastric juice from normal individuals was capable of enhancing the ability of pernicious anemia patients to derive sufficient antianemic factor from a much smaller amount of liver than was the case without the gastric juice (10 g instead of >200 g). This led him to postulate a gastric intrinsic factor (IF) that was required to absorb the essential extrinsic factor in liver that later proved to be vitamin B_{12}.

These are the major milestones in the fascinating history of the pageant of B_{12} discovery, but it is by no means all. The identification of the biologically active forms of B_{12} (5′-deoxyadenosylcobalamin and methylcobalamin) and their roles in metabolic reactions; the development of sensitive assays to measure B_{12} at the concentrations found in the blood; methods to radioisotopically label B_{12} for tracer studies including measurement of B_{12} absorption; the discovery and characterization of B_{12}-binding proteins; the discovery of the autoimmune basis for pernicious anemia; and numerous other advances meld into our current state of knowledge about the unique and fascinating nutrient that is the topic of this chapter.

STRUCTURE AND CHEMISTRY

COBALAMINS

The ultimate source of vitamin B_{12} (B_{12})* for all living systems that require the vitamin is microbial biosynthesis. A detailed review of the complex, multistep biosynthesis of B_{12} by

*The term "vitamin B_{12}" should be restricted to cyanocobalamin. In this review, for purposes of simplicity, "B_{12}" will be used generically to refer to all forms of the vitamin. Specific forms of the vitamin will be referred to in the context of the narrative, when appropriate.

anaerobic (e.g., *Propionibacterium shermanii*, *Salmonella typhimurium*) and aerobic (e.g., *Pseudomonas dentrificans*) bacteria is beyond the scope of this chapter. The reader is referred to several excellent source references for specifics [11–13]. The structure and the chemistry of B_{12} are also complex and have been extensively reviewed [2,14–17,18]. In the context of this chapter, only a brief description of the chemistry is presented. B_{12} is an organometallic compound that has the highly unusual property among biological molecules of possessing a carbon–metal bond. The molecule consists of two halves: a planar group and nucleotide set at right angles to each other (Figure 13.1). The core planar group is a corrin ring with a single cobalt atom coordinated in the center of the ring. The nucleotide consists of the base, 5,6-dimethylbenzimidazole, and a phosphorylated sugar, ribose-3-phosphate. The corrin ring, like porphyrin, is comprised of four pyrroles, each of which is linked on either side to its two neighboring pyrroles by carbon–methyl or carbon–hydrogen methylene bridges, with one exception. In this exception, two neighboring pyrroles are joined directly to each other. The nitrogens of each of the four pyrroles are coordinated to the central cobalt atom. The fifth ligand of the cobalt, projecting above the plane of the molecule, is covalently bound to one of several groups, designated, R. In nature, the predominant form of B_{12} has 5′-deoxyadenosyl as the R-group (5′-deoxyadenosylcobalamin), which in eukaryotes is located primarily in

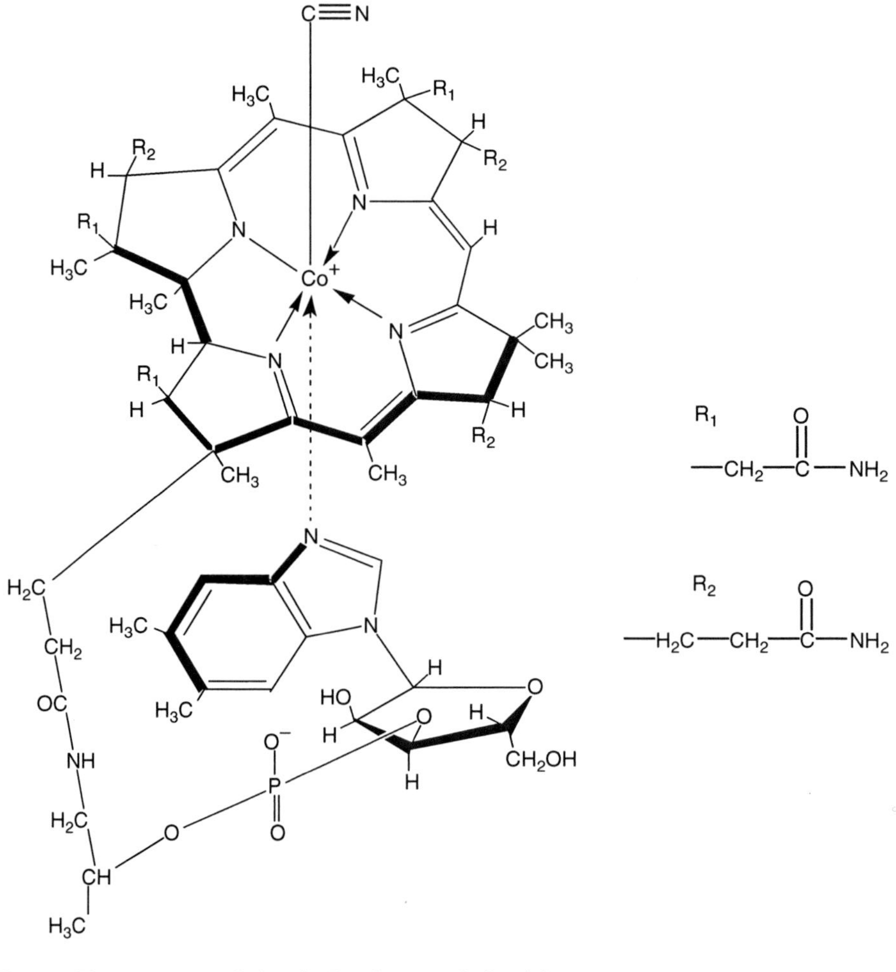

FIGURE 13.1 The structure of vitamin B_{12} (cyanocobalamin).

the mitochondria. It serves as the cofactor for the enzyme methylmalonyl CoA mutase. The other major natural form of B_{12} is methylcobalamin. This is the predominant form in human plasma and within the cytosol. It serves as the cofactor for the enzyme methionine synthase. There are also minor amounts of hydroxocobalamin, which is the form to which 5′-deoxyadenosylcobalamin and methylcobalamin are rapidly converted when the carbon–cobalt bond is disrupted by exposure to light. The cobalt atom in hydroxocobalamin is fully oxidized in the Co(III) state, whereas the cobalt exists as reduced Co(I) or Co(II) in the 5′-deoxyadenosylcobalamin and methylcobalamin forms.

The most stable pharmacological form of the vitamin is cyanocobalamin. In the presence of light and a source of cyanide, all forms of cobalamin are converted to cyanocobalamin. Cyanocobalamin is therefore the form used for pharmacological purposes, although hydroxocobalamin and methylcobalamin are also in use in some formularies. Several other forms of cobalamin have also been identified in cell and tissue extracts, including glutathionylcobalamin, sulfitocobalamin, and nitritocobalamin. Their physiological roles, if any, are not well understood, and with the exception of glutathionylcobalamin [19], may represent artifacts of the extraction process. Techniques to separate and identify the various forms of cobalamin include microbiological methods using thin layer chromatography and bioautography [20] and HPLC methods [21,22].

The sixth ligand of the central cobalt atom is occupied by one of the nitrogens of the 5,6-dimethylbenzimidazole base. The other nitrogen of the 5,6-dimethylbenzimidazole attaches to ribose, which connects to a phosphate, linking the lower axial ligand back to one of the seven amide groups of the corrin ring by an aminopropyl residue that serves as a molecular sling to attach it to the ring. It has been noted that compared with porphyrin rings, corrins are more flexible and less planar when viewed from the side. Putatively, this facilitates conformational changes required for cofactor activity.

Biologically active forms of B_{12} play many and varied roles in reactions involving different substrates. All of these may be classified into one of three categories: (1) mutases, involving exchanges of a hydrogen and some other group between two adjacent carbon atoms, which may or may not be followed by elimination of water or ammonia. There are several examples of such mutase reactions, including glutamate mutase, ornithine mutase, L-β-lysine mutase, α-methyleneglutarate mutase, and methylmalonyl CoA mutase. Examples of the elimination reactions are dioldehydrase, glycerol dehydrase, and ethanolamine ammonia lyase; (2) ribonucleotide reductase involving the reduction of the ribose in a ribonucleotide to deoxyribose; and (3) methyl group transfer reactions, such as methane synthase, acetate synthase, and methionine synthase. Of all these reactions, only methylmalonyl CoA mutase and methionine synthase are known to occur in eukaryotes, including mammals and humans.

The first two types of reactions (mutases and ribonucleotide reductase) involve a Co(II) intermediate oxidation state whereas the methyl group transfer reactions involve a Co(I) oxidation state. In all three types of reactions, the cobalt is Co(III) in the resting state. Key to the catalytic role of the cobalamin is the somewhat weak cobalt–carbon bond and the sensitivity of the active coenzymes to free radical damage by oxygen. Hence, the reactions are protected by anaerobic conditions.

B_{12} Analogs

Many analogs of B_{12}, collectively called corrinoids, are known to exist in nature [2,18]. These include two major subclassifications: (1) cobamides, which contain substitutions in the place of ribose, for example, adenoside; and (2) cobinamides, which lack a nucleotide. The analogs of B_{12} are distinguished microbiologically from the vitamin forms by organisms such as *Euglena gracilis* and *Lactobacillus leichmannii*, whose growth is sustained by the cobalamins, but not the cobamides or cobinamides. It is unclear whether B_{12} analogs are inert or inhibit B_{12}-dependent reactions. The sources of B_{12} analogs, whether from diet, gut bacteria, or endogenous breakdown of B_{12}, are unknown. B_{12} analogs have been found in fetal blood and tissues [23,24].

NUTRITIONAL ASPECTS

DIETARY SOURCES

Though required by eukaryotes, B_{12} is synthesized solely by prokaryotic microorganisms. Ruminants obtain B_{12} from the resident flora of their foregut. In some species, B_{12} is obtained through coprophagia or fecal contamination of the diet, but for humans and other omnivores, the only source of B_{12} (other than supplements) is foods of animal origin. The highest amounts of B_{12} are found in liver and kidney (>10 μg/100 g wet weight), but it is also present in shellfish, organ and muscle meats, fish, chicken, and dairy products—eggs, cheese, and milk—which contain smaller amounts (1–10 μg/100 g wet weight) [25]. Vegetables, fruits, and all other foods of nonanimal origin are free from B_{12} unless contaminated by bacteria. B_{12} in food is generally resistant to destruction by cooking.

REQUIREMENTS

The recommended dietary allowance (RDA) for males and females, age 14 years and older, is 2.4 μg/day. The RDA ranges from 0.9 to 1.8 μg/day for children age 1–13 years. Due to a lack of adequate data, no RDA has been established for infants <1 year of age. Instead, adequate intakes have been estimated of 0.4 μg/day for age 0–6 months and 0.5 μg/day for age 7–12 months. No upper limit of intake for B_{12} has been established as no discernible adverse effects have been observed even with several milligram daily doses of the vitamin [26].

ABSORPTION, TRANSPORT, AND METABOLISM

ABSORPTION AND INTESTINAL TRANSPORT

There are two distinct mechanisms for B_{12} absorption, one active and the other passive. The active physiological processes of B_{12} absorption are complex and involve discrete anatomical areas of the gastrointestinal tract, as well as specific B_{12}-binding and chaperone molecules (Figure 13.2). Dietary B_{12} is released from protein complexes primarily by enzymes in gastric juice, aided by the low pH of the stomach that is maintained by normal gastric output of hydrochloric acid from parietal cells. On release from proteins in food, B_{12} combines rapidly with a salivary R binder, part of a family of B_{12}-binding proteins known as haptocorrins. Subsequently, the salivary R binder is digested by pancreatic trypsin in the upper small intestine. The B_{12} is thus released and then transferred to the gastric glycoprotein, IF, produced by the same parietal cells responsible for gastric acid production. Binding of B_{12} to IF is favored by the less acidic milieu of the upper small intestine than the stomach.

All forms of B_{12} are absorbed by the same IF-dependent mechanism. The nucleotide portion of B_{12} fits into a pocket on the surface of the protein, while the –CN, –OH, $–CH_3$, or 5′-deoxyadenosyl group lies opposite to the site of attachment [27–30]. B_{12} analogs (cobamides and cobinamides, as described earlier) that attach to R binder do not attach to IF and therefore remain unabsorbed through the active physiological mechanism [31–35].

IF is a glycoprotein with a molecular weight of 45,000 Da (Table 13.1) [36]. It is produced in the microsomes or endoplasmic reticulum of the gastric parietal cells in the fundus and body of the stomach. The IF–B_{12} complex, in contrast to free IF, is resistant to enzyme digestion [37]. The formation of the complex is believed to protect not only the IF, but also the B_{12}, which is known to be susceptible to side-chain modification of the corrin ring, as well as perhaps removal of the alpha (lower-axial) ligand [2,38]. Because of protein folding, IF–B_{12} has a

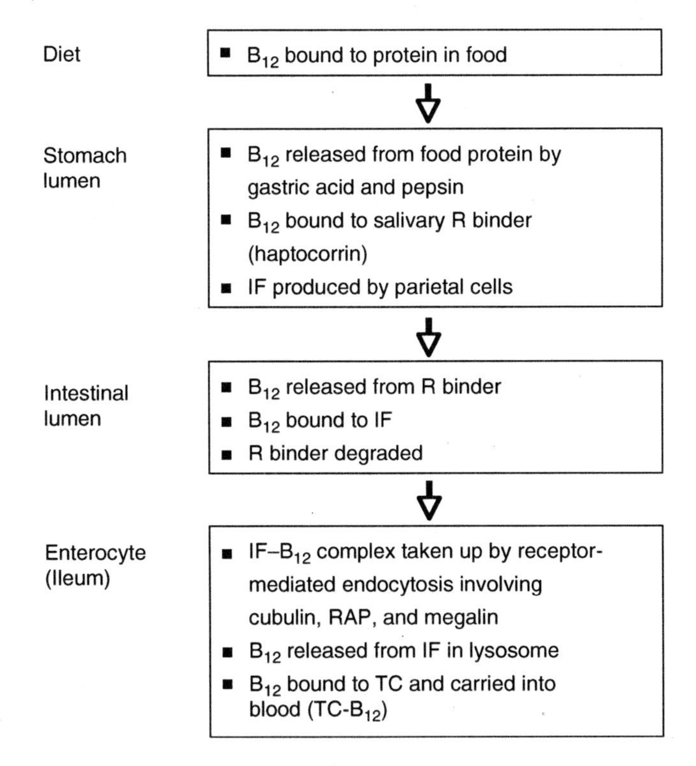

FIGURE 13.2 Normal physiology of B_{12} absorption.

smaller molecular radius than does free IF [39], and some peptide bonds that are accessible to proteolytic enzyme cleavage when IF is free are protected in the complex.

The IF–B_{12} complex traverses the entire length of the small intestine and binds to specific receptors located on the brush border of the terminal portion of the ileal mucosa. Several excellent reviews provide detailed summaries of the characteristics of IF–B_{12} receptors and the process of IF–B_{12} uptake [29,40–43]. The receptor consists of an α subunit facing outward, which binds IF, and a β subunit, which faces into the cell. These receptors consist of cubulin and a molecule designated as the receptor-associated protein (RAP). Cubilin (molecular weight 460,000 Da) is also present in yolk sac and in renal tubular epithelium. Internalization of the IF–B_{12} complex by the ileal receptor requires calcium ions and a

TABLE 13.1
Properties of Plasma B_{12} Transport Proteins

	Intrinsic Factor	Haptocorrin	Transcobalamin
Molecular weight	~45,000 Da	~150,000 Da	45,538 Da
Source	Gastric parietal cells	Granulocytes	Endothelial cells
Functions	Absorption	Storage, excretion of B_{12} analogs, antimicrobial	Cellular B_{12} uptake
Binding specificity	Very high for B_{12}	Low, binds B_{12} analogs	High for B_{12}
Membrane receptors	IF receptors on ileal enteroctyes (cubulin, RAP, megalin-mediated)	Nonspecific asialoglycoprotein receptors on hepatocytes	Transcobalamin receptors on all cell types
Saturation with B_{12}	—	80%–90%	10%–20%
Percentage of total plasma B_{12}	—	70%–80%	20%–30%
Plasma clearance	—	Slow ($t_{1/2}$ ~ 10 days)	Rapid ($t_{1/2}$ ~ 60–90 min)

near-neutral pH. Cubulin appears to traffic by means of megalin, a 600,000 Da endocytic receptor that mediates the uptake of a number of ligands. The role of RAP is to serve as a chaperone during receptor folding and internalization. Defects in the genes regulating this mechanism are implicated in autosomal recessive megaloblastic anemia (MGA1) characterized by intestinal malabsorption of B_{12} (Imerslund–Gräsbeck's disease) (see Genetics section). Following receptor-mediated endocytosis of the IF–B_{12} complex via clathryn-coated pits at the brush-border membrane of the ileal mucosa, B_{12} enters the enterocyte where it is processed to leave through the serosal surface into the portal circulation bound to the plasma transport protein, transcobalamin (see later). Following internalization of the IF–B_{12} complex, the exact fate of IF is unknown, but it is believed to undergo proteolytic degradation within the lysosome. Intact IF does not enter the bloodstream.

An important component of normal B_{12} absorption and body conservation of the vitamin is enterohepatic circulation. Between 0.5 and 5.0 μg of B_{12} enter the bile each day [44,45]. This B_{12} is available to bind to IF and thus a portion of biliary B_{12} is reabsorbed. B_{12} derived from sloughed intestinal cells also is reabsorbed in this process. There is evidence to suggest that bile may enhance B_{12} absorption [46]. Because of the appreciable amount of B_{12} undergoing enterohepatic recycling, B_{12} deficiency develops more rapidly in individuals who malabsorb the vitamin than is the case in vegans, who ingest none of the vitamin.

The ileum has a restricted capacity to absorb B_{12} because of a limited number of receptor sites. Although 50% or more of a single 1 μg oral dose of B_{12} may be absorbed, the proportion absorbed falls significantly with increasing amounts of B_{12} [18]. Moreover, after one dose of B_{12} has been presented, the ileal cells become refractory to further uptake of IF–B_{12} for ~6 h [18,47]. Nonetheless, the active mechanism for B_{12} absorption is extremely efficient for small (a few micrograms) oral doses of B_{12}. This is the mechanism by which the body acquires B_{12} from normal dietary sources. The other mechanism for B_{12} absorption is passive, occurring equally throughout the absorptive surface of the gastrointestinal tract. While rapid, it is extremely inefficient; ~1%–2% of an oral dose can be absorbed by this process [18]. Passive absorption of B_{12} can also occur through other mucous membranes, including the oral and the nasal mucosa.

Plasma Transport

Two main B_{12} transport proteins exist in human plasma, haptocorrin and transcobalamin. Both proteins bind B_{12} one molecule for one molecule. Plasma haptocorrin, previously known as transcobalamin I, is a glycoprotein (molecular weight ~150,000 Da) (Table 13.1). It is closely related to other haptocorrin B_{12}-binding proteins in milk, gastric juice, bile, saliva (R binder), and other fluids. These haptocorrins differ from each other only with respect to the carbohydrate moiety of the molecule. Transcobalamin III was a term used to describe a minor isoprotein of haptocorrin in plasma, which differs from the haptocorrin previously designated as transcobalamin I with respect to sugar composition and the level of saturation with B_{12}. Today, transcobalamins I and III are referred to collectively as haptocorrin. Plasma haptocorrins are derived primarily from neutrophil-specific granules.

Normally, plasma haptocorrin is ~80%–90% saturated with B_{12} and carries between 70% and 80% of the total circulating B_{12} [48,49]. However, haptocorrins do not facilitate B_{12} uptake or entry into extrahepatic tissues through a receptor-mediated mechanism. It is surmised that asialoglycoprotein receptors on liver cells are concerned in the removal of desialated haptocorrins from the plasma [50]. Because haptocorrins bind both B_{12} and B_{12} analogs asialoglycoprotein receptor-mediated uptake of haptocorrin into liver may represent a mechanism by which B_{12} analogs are removed from the circulation and subsequently excreted in the bile [50]. B_{12} analogs excreted in the bile are not reabsorbed through the IF-dependent mechanism, and thus are destined for excretion in the stool, though some reuptake by passive absorption may occur. Additionally, haptocorrin may have an antimicrobial function [51].

The other major B_{12} transport protein in plasma is transcobalamin (Table 13.1), previously known as transcobalamin II. Transcobalamin (molecular weight variously estimated to be between 38,000 and 43,000 Da by gel filtration and SDS-PAGE, and calculated to be 45,538 Da from the deduced amino acid sequence) [52–56] is a beta-globulin synthesized by liver and by other cells, including macrophages, endothelial cells, and ileal enterocytes. B_{12} absorbed in the ileal enterocyte by the IF-dependent mechanism enters the portal venous blood bound to transcobalamin. Indicative of this process is that B_{12} can be detected in serum bound to transcobalamin within 3–4 h after ingestion [57–59]. In contrast, newly absorbed B_{12} is not bound to haptocorrin. Consequentially, the potential increase in holotranscobalamin following absorption of orally administered B_{12} is far greater than that of holohaptocorrin. This may have important implications for evaluating B_{12} absorption through measurements of changes in holotranscobalamin and total B_{12} after an oral dose (see Absorption Tests section).

Transcobalamin is normally ~10%–20% saturated and carries only 20%–30% of the total circulating pool of B_{12} [48,60]. The large differences in percentage saturation and the proportion of the total circulating B_{12} bound between transcobalamin and haptocorrin are largely the function of their respective half-lives. Using intravenous injections of bound and unbound radiolabeled B_{12} ($^{57}Co–B_{12}$ or $^{58}Co–B_{12}$) the half-lives for the transcobalamin-B_{12} (holotranscobalamin) and haptocorrin-B_{12} (holohaptocorrin) complexes have been estimated to be <2 h and ~10 days, respectively [61,62]. Transcobalamin, but not haptocorrin, occurs in cerebrospinal fluid where it binds ~35 ng B_{12}/L [63]. Alterations may occur in transcobalamin and haptocorrin levels in plasma in a variety of disease states (Table 13.2). In general, an increase in haptocorrin causes an increase in total plasma B_{12}, whereas an increase in

TABLE 13.2
Effects of Disease States on Plasma B_{12} Transport Proteins

Haptocorrin

Increased (usually accompanied by elevated serum B_{12})

- Liver disease, including hepatitis, cirrhosis, and malignancy
- Renal disease[a]
- Myeloproliferative diseases, especially chronic myeloid leukemia, myelofibrosis, polycythemia vera
- Increased granulocyte production (e.g., inflammatory bowel disease, liver abscess)
- Eosinophilia due to hypereosinophilic syndrome

Decreased

- Congenital haptocorrin deficiency with decreased serum B_{12}, but no clear clinical abnormality

Transcobalamin

Increased (sometimes with no elevation in serum B_{12})

- Renal disease
- Gaucher's disease
- Autoimmune disease
- Pernicious anemia
- Long-term hydroxocobalamin therapy

Decreased

- Congenital transcobalamin deficiency with normal or decreased serum B_{12}, and megaloblastic anemia, pancytopenia, impaired B_{12} absorption, and defective cellular and humoral immunity
- Alcoholic liver disease

Source: Hoffbrand, A.V. and Green, R., Megaloblastic anaemia, in *Postgraduate Haematology, 5th edition*, Hoffbrand, A.V., Catovsky, D., and Tuddenham, E.G., eds., Blackwell Publishing, Oxford, 2005, chapter 5; Carmel, R. et al., *Clin. Lab. Haematol.*, 23, 365, 2001.

[a] In renal disease, transcobalamin levels are more elevated than haptocorrin.

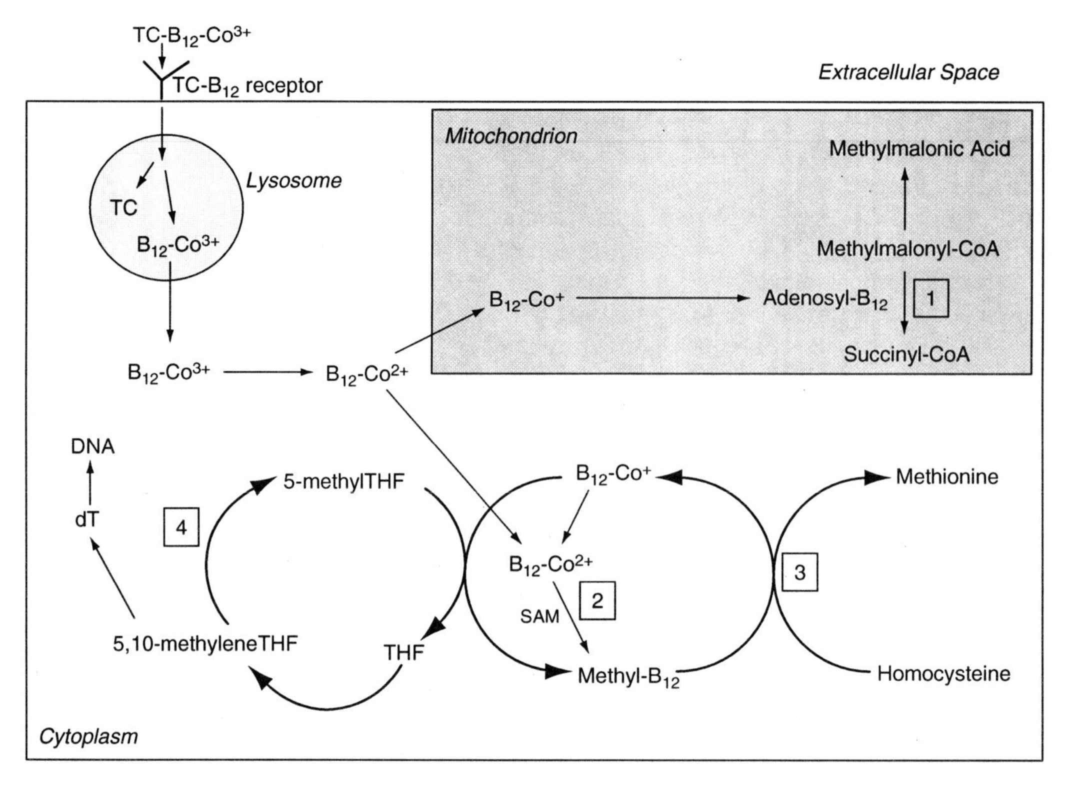

FIGURE 13.3 Cellular uptake and metabolism of B_{12}. Key enzymes: (1) methylmalonyl CoA mutase; (2) methionine synthase reductase; (3) methionine synthase; and (4) methylenetetrahydrofolate reductase. Abbreviations: Adenosyl-B_{12}, 5′-deoxyadenosylcobalamin; methyl-B_{12}, methylcobalamin; THF, tetrahydrofolate; SAM, *S*-adenosylmethionine; dT, deoxythymidine; TC, transcobalamin; Co, cobalt. (Modified from Rosenblatt, D.S., in Carmel, R., Green, R., Rosenblatt, D.S., and Watkins, D., *Hematology Am. Soc. Hematol. Educ. Program*, 62, 2003.)

transcobalamin does not [64]. One exception is in chronic renal disease, where the total plasma B_{12} is increased primarily because of raised levels of holotranscobalamin [65,66].

Receptors for holotranscobalamin are ubiquitously present in tissues, supporting the contention that transcobalamin is the primary B_{12} cellular delivery protein. After endocytosis, holotranscobalamin enters acidic lysosomes in which the transcobalamin protein is degraded, thus releasing B_{12} (Figure 13.3). The B_{12} is then available for metabolic processing to its cofactor forms.

Transcobalamin has a 20% amino acid homology and greater than 50% nucleotide homology with haptocorrin and IF. The regions of homology among the B_{12} binders are considered to be involved in B_{12} binding [56]. Properties of the plasma B_{12}-binding proteins are summarized in Table 13.1. Functionally important polymorphisms for transcobalamin exist and are discussed in the section Genetics.

Metabolism

Once within the cell, B_{12} participates as a cofactor in two important metabolic reactions, one mitochondrial and the other cytosolic (Figure 13.3). In the mitochondrial reaction, B_{12} in the form of 5′-deoxyadenosylcobalamin is required for the enzyme methylmalonyl CoA mutase. This enzyme catalyzes the conversion of methylmalonyl CoA to succinyl

CoA, an intermediate step in the conversion of propionate to succinate during the oxidation of odd-chain fatty acids and the catabolism of ketogenic amino acids. In the cytosolic reaction, B_{12} in the form of methylcobalamin is required in the folate-dependent methylation of the sulfur amino acid homocysteine to form methionine, which is catalyzed by methionine synthase. Methionine, apart from being necessary for adequate protein synthesis, is also a key precursor for the maintenance of methylation capacity through synthesis of the universal methyl donor *S*-adenosylmethionine. In addition, the methionine synthase reaction is ultimately necessary for normal DNA synthesis. The methyl group transferred to homocysteine during methionine synthesis is donated by the folate derivative methyltetrahydrofolate (methylTHF), forming tetrahydrofolate (THF). THF is subsequently converted to methylenetetrahydrofolate (methyleneTHF) by a one-carbon transfer from serine during its conversion to glycine. MethyleneTHF can be reduced to again form methylTHF, but it also serves as the critical one-carbon source for the de novo synthesis of thymidylate from deoxyuridylate required for DNA replication. B_{12} is thus an important cofactor in (1) the maintenance of normal DNA synthesis, as becomes evident under conditions of B_{12} deficiency, which lead to defective DNA synthesis and megaloblastic anemia; (2) the regeneration of methionine for the dual purposes of maintaining protein synthesis and methylation capacity; and (3) the avoidance of homocysteine accumulation, an amino acid metabolite implicated in vascular damage, thrombosis, and several associated degenerative diseases including coronary artery disease, stroke, Alzheimer disease, and osteoporosis [67].

GENETICS

Genetic causes of altered B_{12} metabolism have been identified that involve all of the various steps involved in B_{12} assimilation, transport, and metabolism. These may be considered in two broad categories: (1) severe but rare disorders involving gene deletion or mutation that generally result in serious complications during infancy and childhood, and which are associated with total absence or markedly compromised function of the encoded protein; and (2) milder and more subtle but considerably more common conditions that arise as a result of polymorphisms of genes involved in B_{12} pathways and those that are usually not associated with conspicuous clinical features. Polymorphisms are detected at any age, usually during population or epidemiological surveys. Inborn errors and polymorphisms are considered here separately, although there is an overlap between the two categories.

INBORN ERRORS OF METABOLISM

These conditions have been reviewed extensively elsewhere [68–70]. Affected individuals are usually identified because of hematological, neurological, or metabolic manifestations that may vary from mild to severe and even life-threatening. They may be considered in three categories as affecting ether intestinal absorption and assimilation, plasma transport, or intracellular metabolism.

Congenital Intrinsic Factor Deficiency or Functional Abnormality

Several mutations in the IF gene (gene locus 11q13) have been identified that result in either total absence of IF protein or an abnormal protein in which the IF can be detected immunologically, but is functionally inactive or is unstable [68–70]. In the latter case, IF is incapable of binding B_{12} or facilitating B_{12} uptake by the ileum. In all varieties of this disorder, and in contradistinction to pernicious anemia, affected individuals have a normal-appearing gastric mucosa and normal secretion of acid [71–73]. In addition, antibodies to parietal cells and IF are not present in the serum. Individuals with congenital IF deficiency usually come to medical attention when stores of B_{12}, maternally derived before birth, are exhausted. Affected infants and children between 1 and 3 years of age are found to have megaloblastic anemia, an unusual type of anemia at this age. Rarely, the disorder may be discovered in older children or even teenagers.

Imerslund–Gräsbeck Syndrome or Autosomal Recessive Megaloblastic Anemia

This disease, inherited as autosomal recessive, is the most common cause of megaloblastic anemia due to B_{12} deficiency encountered in infancy in western countries [68–70]. The patients, who usually present with megaloblastic anemia between the ages of 1 and 5 years, but who may present as early as 1 month or during teenage years, secrete normal amounts of IF and gastric acid, but are unable to absorb B_{12} because of a congenital defect in the ileum. Affected individuals have low levels of serum B_{12} despite normal IF production. B_{12} absorption tests like the Schilling test show malabsorption that is not corrected by exogenous IF. Several variants of the disorder have been identified that coincide with the geographical origin of the affected individual. Thus, in all Finnish families, the disease is caused by mutations in the CUBN gene that encodes for cubulin (gene locus 10p12.1) [74,75], the IF–B_{12} receptor described earlier. Interestingly, it appears that the frequency for the disease appears to be decreasing and it has been proposed that some environmental change, possibly diet, may influence expression of the disease [76]. Cubilin is also normally expressed on proximal renal tubules. In Norwegian MGA1 patients, CUBN mutations have not been found. Using linkage studies, a second candidate gene was identified in these patients [75]. Inactivation of this gene in the mouse is embryonic lethal, because the embryos lack an amnion, hence the gene designation AMN (human) or AMN (mouse) [77,78]. In humans, the AMN (gene locus 14q32) mutation results only in a mild MGA1 phenotype. It has been proposed that AMN may represent an example of a moonlighting protein [70,79]. This is a term used to describe proteins that possess two or more apparently unrelated functions depending on cell type, localization, cellular concentration of interacting molecules, developmental stage, and other variables. In the case of AMN, one proposed explanation is that the 5′-end of the gene product is required for B_{12} absorption, whereas the 3′-end is necessary for embryonic development [80]. In some cases of MGA1 ileal brush-border receptors for IF are nonfunctional, and impaired synthesis, processing, or ligand binding of cubilin have been implicated [81]. Apart from B_{12}, other tests of intestinal absorption are normal. Over 90% of patients with MGA1 show nonspecific proteinuria, but renal function is otherwise normal and renal biopsy has not shown any consistent defect. A few of these patients have shown aminoaciduria and congenital renal tract abnormalities.

Congenital Transcobalamin Deficiency

Transcobalamin (gene locus 22q11.2-qter) is functionally and clinically the most important of the plasma B_{12} carrier proteins. Consistent with this notion are observations of individuals with genetic transcobalamin deficiencies [68–70,82]. Infants with transcobalamin deficiency usually present with severe megaloblastic anemia within a few weeks of birth. Serum B_{12} levels are usually normal, because most of the B_{12} in plasma is bound to haptocorrin. Since haptocorrin-bound B_{12} is not available for cellular uptake, B_{12} needs to be given frequently by injection in large doses to cure and prevent anemia (e.g., 1 mg B_{12} three times weekly). This allows free B_{12} to enter marrow cells directly by passive diffusion in the absence of functional transcobalamin. Because these patients are young children, as in cases of Imerslund–Gräsbeck syndrome, the initially normal or near-normal total serum B_{12} levels are presumably attributable to maternally derived B_{12} acquired before birth. Though rare, the condition should be suspected in infants with unexplained anemia, particularly megaloblastic anemia, because it is easily treatable by B_{12} injections. Failure to institute adequate B_{12} therapy may lead to neurological damage. To make a diagnosis, it is necessary to measure transcobalamin directly, either immunologically or using an assay that specifically measures holotranscobalamin B_{12}. Less-severe cases are manifested later in childhood. In some cases, the protein is present in normal amounts, but is unable to bind B_{12} or to attach to the cell surface, and thus is functionally inert. It is not clear whether these types of transcobalamin deficiency display different phenotypes. Infants with transcobalamin deficiency do not show methylmalonic aciduria, but curiously display B_{12} malabsorption [70]. A proportion of patients have immune deficiency and reduced levels of serum immunoglobulins occur in some.

Congenital Haptocorrin Deficiency

In contrast to patients with transcobalamin deficiency, patients with congenital haptocorrin (gene locus 11q11-q12) deficiency display no apparent overt adverse clinical effects of their deficiency [83]. B_{12} absorption is normal in subjects with haptocorrin deficiency, but since the major fraction of serum B_{12} is normally associated with haptocorrin, these individuals have total serum B_{12} levels below normal. The low normal B_{12} levels in these individuals are not associated with biochemical sequelae or clinical symptoms of B_{12} deficiency. As a consequence of their low serum B_{12}, which may be found incidentally, these individuals may be erroneously suspected of B_{12} deficiency. Haptocorrin deficiency appears to be fairly common, and in one study was identified in as many as 15% of subjects found to have low serum B_{12} levels [83]. Many of these, with low but not totally absent haptocorrin, likely represent heterozygosity for haptocorrin deficiency. The gene frequency for haptocorrin deficiency thus appears to be quite high, but is benign in its effect. This suggests that whatever the function of haptocorrin, it is either not critical to maintenance of normal health, or there is a redundancy of function such that some other protein or mechanism compensates adequately for the role of haptocorrin.

Inborn Errors of Intracellular Cobalamin Metabolism

A number of underlying genetic abnormalities have been identified affecting proteins involved in the multistep pathway for cellular B_{12} uptake, intracellular transport and activation (Figure 13.4). These disorders have been classified as cobalamin mutations, generally designated either as *mut* or by sequential capital letters of the alphabet preceded by a *cbl* prefix (*cbl*A-*cbl*H), and identified by complementation analysis in cultured human fibroblasts [68,70]. In brief, the procedure of complementation analysis involves fusion of cultured fibroblasts from the individual who is being investigated with each of a panel of fibroblasts derived from individuals known to have the various cobalamin mutations. If the defects of the two fused cell lines involve different loci, then following fusion there is a correction to normal cobalamin metabolism compared with each unfused cell line. If the defects of the two cell lines involve the same gene locus, then there is no correction following fusion.

Individuals affected by one of the cobalamin mutations all share in common either or both hyperhomocysteinemia and methylmalonic acidemia, and this is usually discovered during investigation of infants or children (rarely young adults) with developmental delay, regression, a variety of other neurological and psychiatric manifestations, anemia, vomiting, failure to thrive, severe metabolic acidosis, ketosis, or thrombosis. Typically, these individuals are found to have normal serum B_{12} levels. Hyperhomocysteinemia, when present, is usually caused by abnormal functioning of the enzyme methionine synthase (*cbl*G) or a defect in the capacity to produce its cofactor, methylcobalamin (*cbl*E). Megaloblastic anemia is common in these patients, but frequently neurological and psychiatric symptoms are more prominent. Though usually discovered during early childhood, the disorder may on rare occasions first become apparent in adult life.

Methylmalonic acidemia may be the result of abnormal functioning of methylmalonyl coenzyme A mutase (*mut*) or caused by a defect in activation or production of its cofactor adenosylcobalamin (*cbl*A, *cbl*B, *cbl*H). In the case of the methylmalonyl coenzyme A mutase defects the enzyme may either be lacking (mut^{o}) or defective (mut^{-}). The *cbl*H variant appears to represent an interallelic variant of *cbl*A [84]. A proportion of infants with *cbl*A and *cbl*B respond to B_{12} in large doses, whereas those who are unresponsive include mut^{o} or mut^{-}.

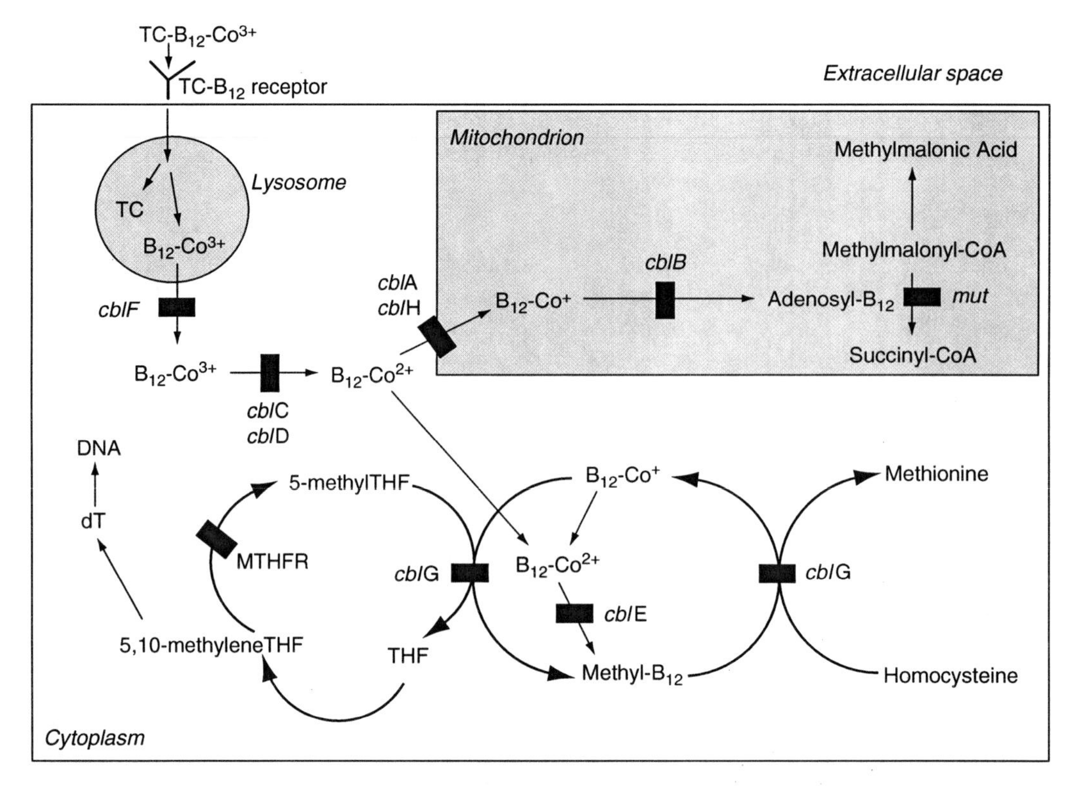

FIGURE 13.4 Inherited disorders of B_{12} metabolism showing known or putative sites of defects (black rectangles). Abbreviations: Adenosyl-B_{12}, 5′-deoxyadenosylcobalamin; methyl-B_{12}, methylcobalamin; THF, tetrahydrofolate; dT, deoxythymidine; TC, transcobalamin; Co, cobalt. (Modified from Rosenblatt, D.S., in Carmel, R., Green, R., Rosenblatt, D.S., and Watkins, D., *Hematology Am. Soc. Hematol. Educ. Program*, 62, 2003.)

Patients who are unable to produce either methylcobalamin or adenosylcobalamin have both hyperhomocysteinemia and methylmalonic acidemia (*cbl*C, *cbl*D, *cbl*F). Those with *cbl*C or *cbl*D have a defect in reduction of B_{12} from the cob(III)alamin to the cob(I)alamin state after transfer of B_{12} from the endocytic compartment to the cytoplasm. Over 100 cases of *cbl*C disease have been described. In *cbl*F, there is a defect in ability to release B_{12} from lysosomes [85].

The genes for some of the designated complementation mutations have been identified: *mut* (6p21, methylmalonyl coenzyme A mutase); *cbl*A (4q31.1-q31.2, a gene thought to encode for a mitochondrial cobalamin reductase) [86]; *cbl*B (12q24 caused by deficient activity of a cob(I)alamin adenosyltransferase) [87]; *cbl*E (5p15.2-15.3, methionine synthase reductase, a flavin-dependent enzyme) [88]; and *cbl*G caused either by greatly reduced levels of methionine synthase associated with diminished steady-state levels of mRNA or impairment of the reductive activation cycle of the enzyme [89,90].

Single Nucleotide Polymorphisms

Though inborn errors of metabolism or loss of function mutations in the various proteins involved in B_{12} absorption, transport, and metabolism can cause severe B_{12} deficiency syndromes, they are rare occurrences. Significantly more prevalent are single nucleotide polymorphisms (SNPs) that may have subtle, but potentially important effects on the handling of B_{12} and related functions.

Transcobalamin has received significant attention with respect to SNPs. In the 1970s and 1980s, distinct isopeptide forms of transcobalamin were identified by isoelectric focusing and polyacrylamide gel electrophoresis techniques [91–93]. Four relatively common transcobalamin isopeptides were identified, designated X, S, M, and F, according to their relative rates of electrophoretic mobility, that is, extra slow, slow, medium, and fast, respectively. Subsequently, molecular sequencing revealed several SNPs encoding for amino acid differences among transcobalamin isoforms [56,94–97]. The most prevalent polymorphism is a C-to-G substitution at base position 776 (776C > G) that results in an arginine in place of a proline in amino acid position 259. Comparison of the sequencing data with the isoelectric focusing and polyacrylamide gel electrophoresis data indicates that the M isoform of the protein generally corresponds to the 776C allele, while the X isoform generally corresponds to the 776G allele [95,96,98]. However, the correspondence between electrophoretic mobility and 776 allele (C or G) is not perfect [98] suggesting other base substitutions, separately or in combination with the 776 allele, influence the electrophoretic mobility of the protein. Which of the base substitutions among other SNPs known to exist for transcobalamin that correspond to the S and F isoforms is yet to be determined. The 776C > G polymorphism is highly prevalent in white populations with allele frequencies of ~55% and 45% for 776C and 776G, respectively [96,99–103]. The 776G allele is less prevalent in blacks, Hispanics, and native Americans, and more prevalent in Asians than in whites [102,103]. Blacks tend to have high frequencies of the F or S isoforms, depending on their ethnic origin, while these iosforms are rare in white, Asian, and native American populations [103].

The biochemical significance of the 776C > G polymorphism is indicated by studies comparing various indicators of B_{12} status among the genotypes, including total B_{12}, holotranscobalamin, methylmalonic acid, and homocysteine. The most consistent findings are that both apotranscobalamin and holotranscobalamin are lower in serum from individuals homozygous for the 776G allele than in those homozygous for the 776C allele [96,97,99,100,104–108]. Other observed differences include higher serum methylmalonic acid and a lower percentage of total B_{12} bound to transcobalamin (holotranscobalamin/total total B_{12} ratio) in 776G homozygotes [100]. Cerebrospinal fluid holotranscobalamin also is lower in 776G homozygotes [63]. Total B_{12} and homocysteine typically are not significantly different among the genotypes, though one study found a significant interaction between transcobalamin genotype and total B_{12} such that homocysteine was lower in individuals homozygous for the 776C wild-type allele who were also in the upper quartile of total B_{12} levels [109]. These observations suggest that the 776G allele encodes for a transcobalamin isoform with reduced affinity for B_{12} compared with that encoded by the 776C allele, though this remains to be proven empirically. Indeed, theoretical modeling predicts that the 776C > G polymorphism affects the secondary structure of the protein [97].

The clinical significance of the 776C > G polymorphism may be reflected by birth outcomes. Studies have found associations with spontaneous abortion and cleft lip or palate [110–112]. Another study found evidence that the 776C > G polymorphism influences the age of onset of Alzheimer's disease [107].

SNPs in other B_{12}-related proteins have been identified, including methionine synthase, methionine synthase reductase, and IF. The 2756A > G polymorphism in methionine synthase, which encodes for a glycine residue in place of aspartate, has been shown to affect the risk of various birth defects, including neural tube defects (NTDs), orofacial clefts, and Down syndrome [113–116]. Similarly, the 66A > G polymorphism in methionine synthase reductase, which encodes for methionine in place of isoleucine, is also associated with differential risk for NTDs and Down syndrome [114–118]. The effect of the 66A > G polymorphism on neural tube risk is mediated by B_{12} status such that the association is strongest for individuals with low B_{12} levels [117]. Recently, a polymorphism has been identified in IF, 68A > G, which encodes for arginine in place of glutamine. One study associated this polymorphism with congenital IF deficiency [71], but this finding was not confirmed in a separate study [73].

DEFICIENCY

Overview and Prevalence

B_{12} deficiency is a significant public health problem, particularly but not exclusively among the elderly. During the past decade, many investigators have reported a high prevalence of B_{12} deficiency in the elderly [119–127], primarily on the basis of raised serum or urine methylmalonic acid or homocysteine levels with or without low serum B_{12} concentrations. Some estimates suggest that the prevalence of B_{12} deficiency may be as high as 30%–40% among the elderly due to the condition of food B_{12} malabsorption caused by chronic gastritis, gastric atrophy, and perhaps other unknown causes [119]. As a result, there is a growing concern that the prevalence of B_{12} deficiency may have been underestimated [128]. The classic clinical manifestations of B_{12} deficiency, notably megaloblastic anemia, occur only in the most severely B_{12} depleted individuals [129], but neuropsychiatric manifestations [130] and metabolic abnormalities [131,132] often occur before serum B_{12} concentrations reach a level that would be considered deficient by standard criteria. Results of recent surveys of B_{12} status in the elderly indeed indicate that the prevalence of deficiency is much higher if based on serum or urine methylmalonic acid concentrations [120]. Lindenbaum et al. [120] have suggested that the usual cut-off values for serum B_{12} (i.e., <300 pg/mL or <221 pmol/L for mild deficiency and <200 pg/mL or <148 pmol/L for severe deficiency) are too low, and that <350 pg/mL (258 pmol/L) is the cut-off value below which serum methylmalonic acid and homocysteine concentrations may become elevated. Using the latter cut-off, the prevalence of serum B_{12} concentrations indicating deficiency in free-living elderly participating in the Framingham Heart Study was a staggering 40% [120]. Such observations underscore the need for more sensitive screening methods to identify B_{12} deficiency and malabsorption in the elderly.

In recent years, several studies have reported an apparently high prevalence of low B_{12} status and varying degrees of B_{12} deficiency in both children and young adults in diverse locations, such as Guatemala, Mexico, India, and Israel [133–137]. The causes of B_{12} deficiency in these populations are unclear, but may be related to a combination of low intake and unrecognized malabsorption. Infection with *Helicobacter pylori*, a widespread gastric pathogen, can be high in these populations [133,134], and there has been an increased attention to the protean effects of this organism on the gastrointestinal tract. *H. pylori* may cause gastritis leading to food B_{12} malabsorption. It has recently been suggested that *H. pylori* may also initiate autoimmune destruction of the gastric mucosa leading to pernicious anemia (Figure 13.5) [138,139].

Causes of B_{12} Deficiency

By far the most common cause of clinically evident B_{12} deficiency is malabsorption, although other causes, notably inadequate dietary intake, cause or contribute to B_{12} deficiency. Rarely, chemical inactivation by the anesthetic gas nitrous oxide (N_2O), as well a variety of inborn errors of metabolism affecting B_{12} absorption, transport and metabolism, result in conditions resembling B_{12} deficiency.

Dietary Deficiency

Dietary B_{12} deficiency arises in adult vegans who shun all meat, fish, eggs, cheese, and other animal products from their diet. The largest group of vegans in the world consists of Hindus and it is likely that many millions of individuals who are cultural or religious adherents of this or related creeds are at risk for deficiency of B_{12} on a nutritional basis. Not all vegans develop

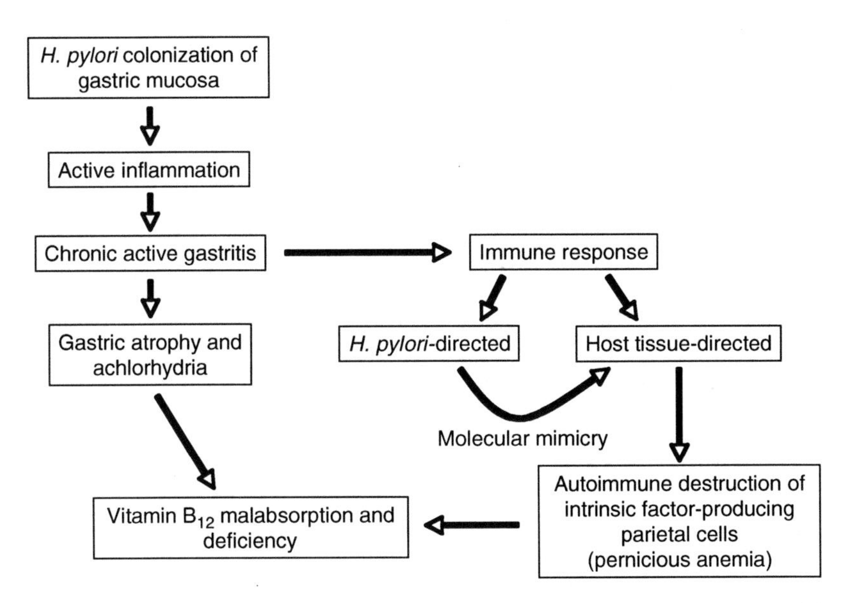

FIGURE 13.5 Putative role of *H. pylori* infection as an initiator of autoimmune gastritis. (Modified from Green, R., *Blood*, 107, 1247, 2006.)

B_{12} deficiency; dietary B_{12} deficiency may arise in nonvegetarian subjects who exist on grossly inadequate diets primarily because of poverty. Subnormal B_{12} levels have been found in up to 50% of randomly selected young adult Indian vegans [137]. Few, however, develop B_{12} deficiency of sufficient severity to cause anemia or neuropathy.

There are several possible explanations of why nutritional B_{12} deficiency may not progress to megaloblastic anemia, including the fact that the diet of most vegans is probably not totally lacking B_{12} because of dietary contamination. Furthermore, the serum B_{12} level may not be an accurate measure of body stores. Curiously, unlike serum B_{12}, red blood cell B_{12} levels in vegans have been found to be generally much closer to those of subjects on a normal diet [140]. The most likely explanation for the observation that vegans appear relatively protected from clinical B_{12} deficiency resides in the fact that the enterohepatic reabsorption of B_{12} excreted in the bile, discussed earlier [44,46], remains intact in vegans and thus biliary losses are less than those in conditions of malabsorption. Consequently, B_{12} deficiency, induced by dietary deficit alone, takes many years to develop in both humans and animals. Furthermore, it is possible that vegans may be protected against the hematological complications of B_{12} deficiency because of adequate folate intake.

In childhood, B_{12} deficiency has been described in infants born to severely B_{12}-deficient mothers [141–143]. These infants develop megaloblastic anemia at ~3–6 months of age, presumably because they are born with low stores of B_{12} and because they are fed breast milk of low B_{12} content. This occurs most commonly in Indian vegans, but a similar condition has also been described in unrecognized maternal pernicious anemia and in strict practitioners of veganism living in Western countries whose offspring have shown growth retardation, impaired psychomotor development, and other neurological sequelae [143]. B_{12} deficiency has also been observed in children fed macrobiotic diets [144,145].

Malabsorption—Gastric Causes

Pernicious anemia, the most well studied cause of B_{12} malabsorption, is usually caused by a lack of functional IF in the stomach resulting from autoimmune destruction of the gastric parietal cells. (For historical reviews of pernicious anemia, see Castle [1] and Chanarin [3].)

TABLE 13.3
Causes of B_{12} Malabsorption

Causes that often lead to megaloblastic anemia	
Autoimmune disorder	Pernicious anemia
Gastric	Congenital IF deficiency
	Total or partial gastrectomy
Intestinal	Intestinal stagnant loop syndrome: jejunal diverticulosis, ileocolic fistula, anatomical blind loop, intestinal structure, etc.
	Ileal resection and Crohn's disease
	Selective malabsorption with proteinuria (MGA1; Imerslund–Gräsbeck syndrome)
	Tropical sprue
	Congenital transcobalamin deficiency
	Fish tapeworm
Causes that usually do not lead to megaloblastic anemia	
Gastric	Simple atrophic gastritis (food B_{12} malabsorption)
	Zollinger-Ellison syndrome
	Gastric bypass surgery
	Use of proton pump inhibitors
Intestinal	Gluten-induced enteropathy
	Severe pancreatitis
	HIV infection
	Radiotherapy
	Graft versus host disease
Nutritional	Deficiencies of B_{12}, folate, protein, and possibly riboflavin and niacin
Drugs	Colchicine
	Para-aminosalicylate
	Neomycin
	Slow-release potassium chloride
	Anticonvulsant drugs
	Metformin
	Phenformin
	Cytotoxic drugs
	Alcohol

Source: Hoffbrand, A.V. and Green, R., Megaloblastic anemia, in *Postgraduate Haematology, 5th edition*, Hoffbrand, A.V., Catovsky, D., and Tuddenham, E.G., eds., Blackwell Publishing, Oxford, 2005, chapter 5.

Pernicious anemia may be defined as a severe lack of IF due to gastric atrophy following autoimmune gastritis (Table 13.3). It is a common disease in north Europeans but occurs in all countries and ethnic groups. In the United States, there are 37 million people over age 65 years (expected to rise to 70 million by the year 2030) and conservative estimates indicate that 2%–3% of this population has or develops pernicious anemia caused by progressive and ultimately complete abrogation of IF production and consequent B_{12} malabsorption [146,147]. The ratio of incidence in men and women is ~1:1.6. It is most commonly encountered in the elderly [146], but is not restricted to any age-group. The peak age of incidence is 60 years, with only 10% of cases presenting under 40 years of age. Among the African American and Latino populations, the age distribution of pernicious anemia is different, affecting a younger age-group, particularly women [148,149]. On rare occasions, a pernicious anemia-like condition can occur in children, arising from a genetic defect affecting the synthesis of IF (see Genetics section). Classical pernicious anemia or predisposition to its development has a genetic component, as it occurs more commonly than by chance in close relatives, in subjects with other organ-specific auto-immune diseases, particularly of the thyroid, and in those with premature graying, blue eyes, and vitiligo, as well as in persons of blood group A [146].

Apart from pernicious anemia, other causes of B_{12} deficiency involving the stomach are less common, not so well defined, and the malabsorption usually less complete. In part, this is because the area responsible for IF production within the stomach is extensive, and normally the amount of IF produced is in vast excess of what is required to accomplish physiologic B_{12} absorption. Surgical removal of all or most of the stomach in the operation of gastrectomy will have the same effect on the ability to absorb B_{12} as does autoimmune destruction of the IF-producing cell mass [146]. Following total gastrectomy, B_{12} deficiency is inevitable and prophylactic B_{12} therapy is routinely instituted following the operation. After partial gastrectomy, 10%–15% of patients may also develop B_{12} deficiency [146]. This usually manifests 4 years or more following the operation, but may occur sooner. The exact incidence and time of onset is most influenced by the size of the resection and the preexisting size of the body B_{12} store. The B_{12} deficiency following gastrectomy may cause uncomplicated megaloblastic anemia, but more frequently occurs in association with iron-deficiency anemia because gastric acidity favors iron absorption. This may render the identification of the nature of the anemia more obscure, since the typical macrocytosis of a megaloblastic anemia may be masked by the microcytic component of iron deficiency [150].

Following gastrectomy, the explanation of the B_{12} deficiency is usually lack of IF. Secretion of IF in postgastrectomy patients is stimulated by food; tests of absorption in the fasting state may therefore be misleading. In a few patients, the deficiency is due primarily to the creation of an intestinal stagnant loop that becomes bacterially contaminated or the development of abnormal flora in the jejunum. These conditions may contribute to B_{12} deficiency through microbial consumption of B_{12}. In addition to gastrectomy, B_{12} malabsorption leading to deficiency has been described following various procedures involving gastric reduction to treat morbid obesity [151].

In addition to the specific-disease pernicious anemia caused by autoimmune gastritis is the fairly common nonautoimmune chronic gastritis leading to gastric atrophy or the so-called simple atrophic gastritis [146,152]. This condition is characterized by a loss of stomach acid required for the extraction of B_{12} from food sources in the stomach. A substantial number of these patients show malabsorption of B_{12} from food with resulting borderline or low serum B_{12} levels, sometimes with raised serum levels of methylmalonic acid and homocysteine [153–155]. Typically, however, they do not develop clinically significant B_{12} deficiency, although some early literature reported in long-term follow-up of patients with gastritis that up to 25% developed anemia or neurological problems [146,156]. In malabsorption of food B_{12}, standard tests for free crystalline B_{12} absorption reveal no abnormality. A modified test using food-bound B_{12} must be used to demonstrate the malabsorption, as is described in the section on Absorption Tests. Another consequence of the failure of gastric acid production is that intestinal bacterial overgrowth can occur and further contribute to B_{12} malabsorption through competition for use of the vitamin [157]. In addition, there is growing evidence that infection with *H. pylori* is a major cause of nonspecific gastritis [158–160] and therefore potentially can result in B_{12} malabsorption [138–139,161,162]. It is not clear to what extent this may be responsible for B_{12} deficiency in developing countries where *H. pylori* infestation is endemic. Chronic gastritis and gastric atrophy also may affect >30% of elderly individuals globally [163], and may be responsible for the vast majority of lowered serum B_{12} levels seen in this age-group and the consequent deficiency that may develop.

Malabsorption—Intestinal Causes

Since the terminal portion of the ileum is the site for physiologic absorption of B_{12} via the IF-mediated mechanism, diseases, abnormalities, and removal of this portion of the intestine can result in B_{12} malabsorption and deficiency. Causes include inflammatory bowel disease (Crohn's disease); both tropical and nontropical sprue; HIV infection associated with AIDS; congenital B_{12} malabsorption (MGA1); as a sequel to radiation therapy for cancers of the abdominal or pelvic region; graft versus host disease; and ileal resection. The complete list of causes is shown in Table 13.3 [64,146,152]. In addition to diseases affecting the ileal lining, there are several causes of B_{12} malabsorption that arise in the lumen of the bowel and that compromise or abrogate absorption through disruption of the conditions of pH (excessive gastric hydrochloric acid production) or digestion (chronic pancreatic disease), as well as competition by abnormal bacterial flora or parasites such as *Giardia lamblia* and the fish tapeworm *Diphylobothrium latum* that consume B_{12}, making it unavailable to the host. Finally, a large number of drugs are known to interfere with B_{12} absorption. These are also listed in the Table 13.3. Of these drugs only a few, such as the proton pump inhibitors used to treat acid reflux and the biguanide oral antidiabetic agents, are likely to be used for a sufficiently long duration to cause significant B_{12} deficiency.

Miscellaneous Causes of B_{12} Deficiency

In addition to dietary deficiency and the various causes of malabsorption described earlier, chemical inactivation of B_{12} by inhalation of the anesthetic gas N_2O can also cause or substantially contribute to B_{12} deficiency [164–166]. N_2O irreversibly oxidizes methylcobalamin in the methionine synthase reaction during catalytic shunting of labile methyl groups from the active, fully reduced, Co(I) state in methylcobalamin to an inactive Co(III) state. This is of importance in the megaloblastic anemia that can occur in patients undergoing prolonged N_2O anesthesia, such as in intensive care units. In addition, a neuropathy resembling B_{12} neuropathy has been described in dentists and anesthetists who are repeatedly exposed to N_2O [165] and in monkeys that have been exposed experimentally to the gas for many months [167]. In patients with low B_{12} stores, megaloblastic anemia or B_{12} neuropathy may be precipitated after shorter exposure to N_2O [166]. The inactivation of methionine synthase results in accumulation of homocysteine in plasma. Though the effect of N_2O is at first restricted to methylcobalamin and methionine synthase, eventually due to irreversible oxidative damage there is generalized depletion of B_{12}, and methylmalonate levels rise in addition to the increase in homocysteine consequent on methionine inactivation. Recovery from N_2O exposure requires regeneration of methionine synthase, since this protein is damaged by active oxygen derived from the N_2O–B_{12} reaction [168].

Clinical and Biochemical Effects of B_{12} Deficiency

B_{12} deficiency has profound pathophysiological effects on the blood, nervous system, and possibly other organs. The most prominent effect is megaloblastic anemia, which is caused by the disruption of DNA synthesis. The reduction of methyleneTHF to methylTHF is an irreversible reaction under physiological conditions. Consequently, when B_{12} is deficient and THF synthesis is impaired, methylTHF has no metabolic outlet, forward or backward, and it becomes trapped. This methylfolate trap, first described by Herbert and Zalusky [169] in 1962, decreases the availability of folate for the synthesis of thymidylate and DNA. Unavailability of thymidine leads to misincorporation of dUTP in place of thymidine triphosphate (dTTP) during DNA polymerase-mediated base addition with stalling of the DNA replication mechanism [170]. Subsequent repeated futile cycles of DNA excision and repair continue while the state of thymidine starvation persists. This affects DNA synthesis throughout the body, but particularly in tissues undergoing rapid cellular turnover, including the hematopoietic system. This is the underlying cause of the megaloblastic anemia.

In bone marrow and other rapidly dividing cells, as a result of the defective nuclear DNA replication induced by B_{12} deficiency, there is unbalanced growth in dividing cell precursors resulting in delayed mitosis with normal cytoplasmic synthesis of RNA and protein. Dysynchrony between nuclear and cytoplasmic maturation occurs when a cell, undergoing programmed cytoplasmic development and growth (in the case of red cell precursors, this includes changes like hemoglobinization and involution of organelles), is not undergoing mitosis. This produces abnormally large cells with nuclear chromatin that has a fine, morphologically immature appearance. Although this condition mostly affects erythroid precursors in the bone marrow, giving rise to anemia with abnormally large erythrocytes (macrocytes), it can also affect the development of other hematopoietic cells, resulting in giant granulocyte precursors and mature neutrophils with abnormally large numbers of nuclear lobes (hypersegmented neutrophils) in the blood. In addition to anemia there may also be a net decrease in numbers of all the formed blood elements (pancytopenia). Disturbances in both cellular and humoral immune functions have also been reported in B_{12} deficiency-related disorders [146,171–173].

B_{12} deficiency, particularly if it progresses unrecognized for a protracted period, also affects the nervous system resulting in neuronal demyelination [174]. The primary manifestation is a demyelinating syndrome that affects both peripheral and central neurons. This is believed to be related to decreased synthesis of the universal methyl donor *S*-adenosylmethionine [175], which has a variety of functions in the nervous system. These include methylation reactions involving neurotransmitters and the membrane phospholipids contained in myelin. Particularly vulnerable to the demyelination that occurs in B_{12} deficiency are the long tracts of white matter in the posterior and lateral columns of the spinal cord containing sensory fibers that are responsible for conduction of vibration and position sense. Motor fiber myelination can also be affected. Although the hypothesis linking defective methylation with the myeloneuropathy of B_{12} deficiency is favored, there is some evidence that links disrupted odd-chain fatty acid metabolism related to the accumulation of methylmalonic acid and its precursors as a mechanism responsible for neurological damage due to B_{12} deficiency [176].

The neurological manifestations of B_{12} deficiency may precede the appearance of hematological changes and may, at times, occur in the absence of any hematological complications [130]. This renders the diagnosis more difficult, particularly since the neurological manifestations may be quite protean, running the gamut from peripheral neuropathy to depression, cognitive disturbances, dementia, and autonomic dysfunction [177,178]. The effect of deficiency on the nervous system is particularly catastrophic because the damage can be irreversible if allowed to continue without adequate B_{12} replacement.

The risk of irreversible neurological damage may be magnified in the context of folic acid supplementation. Impaired DNA synthesis due to B_{12} deficiency is essentially the result of a functional folic acid deficiency arising from sequestration of folate in the form of 5-methyltetrahydrofolate (the methylfolate trap), as discussed earlier. It is well recognized that folic acid supplementation reverses B_{12} deficiency-related megaloblastic anemia by providing folic acid for the synthesis of DNA, thus circumventing the methylfolate trap. The potentially deleterious effect of such treatment, however, is that by correcting the anemia, it masks the underlying B_{12} deficiency allowing neurological deterioration to continue undetected, often until irreversible damage has occurred. Since the U.S. Government has instituted the fortification of flour with folic acid to reduce the risk of NTDs in the general population [179–181], this raises the issue of whether such fortification may, in the long term, be detrimental to individuals with undetected and untreated B_{12} deficiency [26]. The elderly, who exhibit a high prevalence of B_{12} deficiency, may be particularly susceptible to this risk. Thus far, there has been no evidence that this is the case. In fact, one study of patients with low serum B_{12} found that there was no change in the proportion of these patients who presented with anemia after the initiation of folic acid fortification in the United States [182].

More recent evidence suggests that B_{12} deficiency may contribute to the risk of vascular disease (related to elevated levels of homocysteine in the blood) [131]. Other associations, discussed in the New Directions section, include cancer (particularly breast cancer), NTDs (spina bifida, anencephaly), and osteoporosis. B_{12} deficiency may also play a role in the rate of onset of clinical AIDS resulting from HIV infection.

The biochemical and metabolic hallmarks of B_{12} deficiency, other than a decrease in total serum B_{12} concentration, include an increase of methylmalonic acid in blood and urine due to the impairment of methylmalonyl CoA mutase (Figure 13.3) and an increase of homocysteine in blood and urine due to the impairment of methionine synthase (Figure 13.3). Accordingly, levels of serum and urinary methylmalonic acid and plasma homocysteine are important indicators of functional B_{12} status [131,183–185]. Additionally, serum holotranscobalamin decreases relatively early during negative B_{12} balance and therefore potentially provides the earliest indication of B_{12} deficiency [25,186]. The rationale and utility of using holotranscobalamin, methylmalonic acid, and homocysteine as indicators of B_{12} status, along with total B_{12}, are discussed in the Diagnosis and Treatment section.

DIAGNOSIS AND TREATMENT

DIAGNOSIS

The principal methods used for diagnosing B_{12} deficiency include clinical assessment, plasma, serum, and urine analyte assays, and tests of B_{12} absorptive capacity. Many of these tests are described later, and others, particularly those used to investigate possible causes of malabsorption (other than autoimmune pernicious anemia), lie beyond the scope of this chapter and are described in specialized texts of gastroenterology. B_{12} deficiency is usually suspected from the clinical picture, notably the presence of megaloblastic anemia and neurological symptoms, particularly in conjunction with a low serum B_{12}. Due to the potential seriousness of these clinical consequences, as well as recent recognition that low B_{12} status is highly prevalent not only in the elderly, but also in children and young adults throughout the world [187], an increasing emphasis is placed on other analyte assays, including holotranscobalamin, methylmalonic acid, and homocysteine, in the diagnosis of B_{12} deficiency.

Total Serum B_{12}

Measurement of total serum B_{12} remains the most widely used routine method of assessing B_{12} status. Measurement of serum B_{12} has evolved over the past 30 years beginning with microbiological assays using *Lactobacillus leichmanii* or other organisms [18]. More recent methods, which are still in use, include radioisotope dilution assays [188] and nonradioactive enzyme-linked and chemiluminescence assays [189]. These assays are frequently automated. Common to each of these assays is the initial release of all protein-bound B_{12} through destruction of the serum B_{12} carrier proteins or through change in pH. In addition, common to all competitive binding assays is the use of IF, added as a specific binding protein for cobalamin only, and not cobalamin analogs that may be present in some sera. Some early configurations of competitive binding assays for total serum B_{12} used or were contaminated with haptocorrin binders and gave spuriously high values for serum B_{12} because of interference by B_{12} analogs [190,191].

Both the microbiological and the competitive binding assays measure total serum B_{12}, the sum of both the haptocorrin and the transcobalamin protein-bound fractions. Serum B_{12} concentrations are typically expressed in pg/mL (or pmol/L), with values <200 pg/mL (<148 pmol/L) considered deficient (reference range $=$ 200–900 pg/mL or 148–664 pmol/L). While this range is diagnostically useful for the majority of cases of B_{12} deficiency, there are individuals with values that would be considered deficient, but who exhibit no clinical signs of deficiency [131]. Conversely, there are individuals who have serum B_{12} concentrations that would be considered normal, but who clearly exhibit B_{12}-related abnormalities (e.g., megaloblastic anemia, neurological deficits) that resolve on B_{12} supplementation [130–132]. Thus, the use of total serum B_{12} for detecting B_{12} deficiency has limitations. The less-than-adequate positive and negative predictive value of total serum B_{12} for detecting B_{12} deficiency is plausibly explained on the basis of the distribution of serum B_{12} among its plasma carrier proteins [131]. Holotranscobalamin exhibits a higher rate of turnover (<2 h) than holohaptocorrin (up to 10 days), and consequently only 20%–30% of B_{12} in serum at any given time is actually bound to transcobalamin, with the remainder bound to haptocorrin (Table 13.1) [48,49,60]. Because dietary and biliary B_{12} are absorbed across the enterocyte and appear in the serum initially bound to transcobalamin, a significant decrease in serum holotranscobalamin concentration may precede any significant decreases in holohaptocorrin concentration during a state of B_{12} negative balance. Because holotranscobalamin represents only a small fraction of the total serum B_{12}, a reduction in holotranscobalamin during the early stages of B_{12} negative balance may have little effect on total serum B_{12} concentration. An abnormally low total serum B_{12} concentration is frequently a late occurrence in the continuum from the onset of negative B_{12} balance to overt deficiency (i.e., the development of megaloblastic anemia and neurological deficits) [186].

In general, the more severe the deficiency, the lower the serum B_{12} level. In patients with spinal cord damage and megaloblastic anemia due to B_{12} deficiency, the level is usually <100 pg/mL (<74 pmol/L). Values between 100 pg/mL (74 pmol/L) and 200 pg/mL (148 pmol/L) are regarded as borderline and may be found in patients with mild B_{12} deficiency. Serum B_{12} levels above the normal reference range (if not due to recent therapy or supplement use) are usually due to a rise in holohaptocorrin, or to liver or renal disease with increased saturation of haptocorrin and transcobalamin (Table 13.2) [65,66]. Elevation of serum B_{12} through one of these mechanisms, unrelated to B_{12} status, may obscure an underlying condition of B_{12} deficiency.

Holotranscobalamin

Experimental evidence to support the hypothesis that serum holotranscobalamin concentrations reflect recent B_{12} malabsorption and negative balance includes the following: (1) Low concentrations of serum holotranscobalamin are found in patients with a failure of B_{12} absorption due to pernicious anemia [186] or due to gastric atrophy [192]. (2) There is a rapid fall (within 7 days) of serum holotranscobalamin concentrations after damage to the intestine caused by pelvic radiotherapy for the treatment of cancer, while total plasma B_{12} concentrations remain in the normal range (>200 pg/mL or >148 pmol/L) [193]. (3) Low serum holotranscobalamin concentrations (defined as <40 pg/mL or <30 pmol/L) were found in >50% of 100 sequentially studied AIDS patients who had generalized intestinal malabsorption [194], although most of these patients had serum B_{12} concentrations in the normal range (>200 pg/mL or >148 pmol/L). Intramuscular B_{12} treatment was reported to improve their cognitive function and hematopoiesis. (4) In long-term vegans, holotranscobalamin concentrations remain in the low-normal range (defined as 40–60 pg/mL or 30–44 pmol/L) for many years because absorption of some B_{12} through the enterohepatic recirculation is maintained despite low dietary B_{12} intake [195]. Thus, it should be anticipated that in contrast to B_{12} malabsorption, holotranscobalamin would remain in the normal range even when B_{12} stores become markedly depleted, as long as absorption of the vitamin remains intact. (5) In elderly individuals, in whom B_{12} malabsorption syndromes are prevalent, low holotranscobalamin concentrations have been observed: serum holotranscobalamin concentrations <40 pg/mL (<30 pmol/L) were reported in 35% of 150 Veterans Administration outpatients age 65–95 years [152]; in well- and poorly nourished nursing home residents with a mean age of 84 years, low holotranscobalamin (defined as <60 pg/mL or <44 pmol/L) was observed in 15% and 36% of individuals, respectively [196]; and the proportion of the total serum B_{12} carried by transcobalamin was found to be significantly lower in older adults (~4%) than young adults (~15%) [129].

Taken together, these observations offer compelling support that holotranscobalamin may be a sensitive indicator of B_{12} absorption and status. Measurement of holotranscobalamin has been confounded, however, by assay limitations. For many years, holotranscobalamin was measured almost exclusively using the method of Jacob and Herbert [197], or some minor modification thereof. This assay used microfine silica as an agent for removal of transcobalamin from serum. Total B_{12} was measured in serum before and after treatment with the microfine silica, with the calculated difference between the two measurements equal to the holotranscobalamin concentration. This method suffered from technical flaws, as well as conceptual limitations. A study examining the potential usefulness of holotranscobalamin measurement to identify B_{12} deficiency among a miscellaneous group of patients with macrocytosis concluded that the test was not useful [198]. Refinements and improvements to this assay were subsequently described, using Sepharose beads coated with antitranscobalamin antibody [100,199,200] or heparin-conjugated Sepharose [201]. Like the approach using microfine silica, all suffered from the drawback that holotranscobalamin levels, rather than being measured directly, were calculated by difference.

More recently, more precise and accurate methods to measure holotranscobalamin have been developed in which the concentration of this fraction of the total B_{12} is measured directly. These methods have been commercialized and are based on separating transcobalamin from haptocorrin using a monoclonal transcobalamin antibody followed by direct measurement by radioassay of the B_{12} bound to transcobalamin [202] or using a monoclonal antibody specific for holotranscobalamin in an automated chemiluminescence assay format [203]. Numerous studies have appeared in the literature recently assessing the clinical and epidemiological utility of holotranscobalamin measurement for detection of B_{12} deficiency or B_{12} status determination for population screening [204–210]. In general, these studies indicate that used singly, holotranscobalamin measurement is about equivalent to total serum B_{12} with respect to sensitivity and specificity.

Although holotranscobalamin levels may reflect total body B_{12}, apotranscobalamin (unsaturated transcobalamin) or the percentage saturation of total transcobalamin is not a reliable indicator of B_{12} status. This may be because apotranscobalamin levels, which normally are present in plasma in a fivefold to tenfold excess over holotranscobalamin levels, are reported to rise several fold as an acute phase protein in response to infection and inflammatory processes [211]. In contrast, holotranscobalamin levels are not affected by infection or inflammation.

Methylmalonic Acid and Homocysteine

Metabolite assays that provide an indication of B_{12} status are also available. These include serum and urinary methylmalonic acid and total plasma homocysteine [131]. The assays are sometimes termed functional or biochemical because they assess the metabolic pathways in which B_{12} participates directly. They are useful because metabolic disturbances generally precede overt clinical symptoms, thus allowing for the detection of deficiency before serious and potentially irreversible structural changes occur. In addition, B_{12}-responsive elevations of serum methylmalonic acid and plasma homocysteine concentrations may be observed despite a total serum B_{12} concentration in the normal range (i.e., >200 pg/mL) [130,131].

Several factors limit the usefulness of these measurements, however. The most reliable methods for determining methylmalonic acid use elaborate derivatization procedures followed by gas chromatography or mass spectrometry [212–214]. The methods are technically daunting, require specialized equipment and training, and are expensive. In addition, it is known that serum methylmalonic acid concentrations may become elevated in B_{12}-replete individuals with renal insufficiency, thus reducing specificity of the assay for identifying B_{12} deficiency. Methods for measuring homocysteine use simpler derivatization procedures or enzymatic conversion to *S*-adenosylhomocysteine, followed by high-pressure liquid chromatography [215,216]. They are somewhat less expensive than methylmalonic acid assays, but still require specialized equipment and training. More recently, assays that use a simpler format have been introduced that do not involve chromatographic separation [217]. Importantly, however, plasma homocysteine is not a specific indicator of B_{12} status. Several other common conditions, including folate and vitamin B_6 deficiencies, certain genetic enzyme defects, renal insufficiency, hypothyroidism, and particular drugs, can cause plasma homocysteine to become elevated [218]. Thus, although methylmalonic acid and homocysteine are certainly important and useful clinical assays, they nonetheless have significant limitations when used for determining B_{12} status [219].

Multiple Analyte Testing

As described earlier, the limitations of individual analyte assays indicate that no single assay is completely adequate for assessment of B_{12} status. In recent years, several novel or refined strategies have been proposed for the diagnosis or detection of B_{12} deficiency or for screening of populations. These promote the use of either sequential tests as described by an algorithmic approach [131] or panels of two or more measurements performed in sequence or simultaneously [204–207,220]. Preliminary evidence from our laboratory suggests that the ratio of holotranscobalamin to total B_{12} may also serve as a useful indicator of functional B_{12} status (unpublished observations). In addition to various combinations and permutations of total B_{12}, holotranscobalamin, methylmalonic acid, and homocysteine, these panels of tests may also include two other metabolites that rise in B_{12} deficiency, 2-methylcitric acid, and cystathionine [221].

Deoxyuridine Suppression Test

In cultured normal bone marrow, addition of deoxyuridine (dU) considerably suppresses the uptake of radioactive thymidine into DNA. This is due to conversion of dU to deoxythymidine (dT) by the enzyme thymidylate synthase in a reaction in which methyleneTHF serves as cosubstrate. The dT so formed through what is termed the de novo pathway is converted to dTMP through the action of thymidine kinase and ultimately to dTTP for incorporation into DNA. dTMP arising through the de novo pathway inhibits preformed thymidine uptake through the salvage pathway. dU suppresses radioactive thymidine incorporation less effectively in megaloblastic anemia due to either folate or B_{12} deficiency because of a block in dU monophosphate conversion to dTMP [222]. In B_{12} deficiency, the test can be corrected with B_{12} or 5-formyltetrahydrofolate (folinic acid), but not with 5-methyltetrahydrofolate. In contrast, in folate deficiency both the folate analogs, but not B_{12}, correct the test [223]. Performance of the dU suppression test is laborious and the test is rarely performed other than in specialized laboratories.

Immune Phenomena

Autoimmune mechanisms play an important role in the pathogenesis of pernicious anemia. Tests based on the demonstration of immune phenomena are available to assist in the diagnosis of the disease. Two types of IF antibody may be found in the sera of patients with pernicious anemia: both are IgG immunoglobulins. One, the blocking or Type I antibody, prevents the combination of IF and B_{12}; whereas the other, the binding, Type II, or precipitating antibody, attaches to IF whether bound to B_{12} or not and prevents attachment of IF to the ileal mucosa. The blocking antibody occurs in the serum of ~70% of patients with pernicious anemia and the binding antibody in 35%–40% of patients [224–226]. Binding antibodies are found only in those patients who also have blocking antibodies. IF antibodies cross the placenta and cause temporary IF deficiency in the new-born infant [227–229]. Pernicious anemia patients also show cell-mediated immunity to IF. An increased CD4/CD8 lymphocyte ratio in blood has been described in pernicious anemia patients with IF antibodies [230]. In addition, complement-dependent cytotoxicity has been observed in pernicious anemia patients [231].

IF antibodies are rarely found in conditions other than pernicious anemia. Type I antibody has been detected occasionally not only in the sera of patients without pernicious anemia, but with other autoimmune diseases such as thyrotoxicosis, myxoedema, Hashimoto's disease, or diabetes mellitus, or in relatives of pernicious anemia patients [18]. There is a clinical association between pernicious anemia and thyroid diseases, vitiligo, hypoparathyroidism, and Addison's disease of the adrenal, and a higher prevalence of these diseases is found in patients with pernicious anemia [18]. IF antibodies have also been detected in gastric juice in a proportion of pernicious anemia patients [232]. These antibodies may reduce absorption of dietary B_{12} by combining with small amounts of residual IF in the gastric juice, thus further reducing the already limited capacity to absorb B_{12} in pernicious anemia.

Antibodies directed against parietal cells may be detected immunohistochemically in microscopic sections of the gastric mucosa by immunoflourescence or by complement fixation techniques. These antibodies are present in the sera of nearly 90% of adult patients with pernicious anemia, but they are frequently present in other diseases as well [19]. Parietal cell antibodies have been detected in as many as 16% of randomly selected women over the age of 60 years and in a smaller proportion of younger control subjects [233]. They are found more frequently than in controls in relatives of pernicious anemia patients, and in patients with simple atrophic gastritis, autoimmune thyroid disorders, Addison's disease of the adrenal, rheumatoid arthritis, and other autoimmune conditions [18]. Parietal cell antibodies have also been found in the gastric juice in pernicious anemia. It is directed against the α and β subunits of the gastric proton pump (H^+-K^+-ATPase). The serum of pernicious anemia patients may also contain an autoantibody to the gastrin receptor [234].

Absorption Tests

The Schilling test [235] has been the gold standard method for detecting B_{12} malabsorption and is the only test of B_{12} absorption ever to be widely used in clinical practice. The test requires the oral administration of cobalt-57-labeled B_{12} (^{57}Co–B_{12}) to a fasting subject and complete collection of urine during the subsequent 24 h. A large dose of nonradioactive B_{12} (1000 μg) is administered by intramuscular injection up to 2 h after the oral radioactive dose. This temporarily saturates all available plasma B_{12}-binding proteins such that any of the ^{57}Co–B_{12} dose that is absorbed, which is of low molecular weight, is flushed into the urine. Low excretion of the radioactivity in urine indicates impairment of the ability to absorb the vitamin. Patients identified as having malabsorbtion are given a Stage II test in which an exogenous source of IF (usually porcine) is administered orally with ^{57}Co–B_{12} to check for gastric pernicious anemia. If the IF does not correct the malabsorption (evidenced by continued low excretion of ^{57}Co–B_{12} in the urine) then the patient does not have classical pernicious anemia or any other gastric defect resulting in failure of IF production. This points to an intestinal cause of the B_{12} malabsorption. The patient may then be treated with antibiotics and have an additional Stage III test to determine if malabsorption was due to bacterial overgrowth.

In clinical practice, the radioactivity is usually provided as crystalline B_{12}, which can be absorbed by elderly individuals even if they lack gastric acid and pepsin. The labeled vitamin must be mixed and equilibrated with food (e.g., egg protein), called the food-bound Schilling test or the egg-yolk B_{12} absorption test, to simulate dietary B_{12} absorption [236–242]. Only the food-bound Schilling test is abnormal in most individuals with chronic gastritis or gastric atrophy because they do not produce enough hydrochloric acid or pepsin to release B_{12} from its attachment to dietary protein.

Even with the high prevalence of B_{12} deficiency in the elderly and its clinical importance, absorption is now rarely tested. The reasons for the disinclination of physicians to prescribe the Schilling test for patients suspected of having B_{12} deficiency relate to several factors, including reduced availability of test components (i.e., ^{57}Co–B_{12} and IF), cost (several hundreds of dollars for each stage), the lengthy protocol (up to 1 week to carry out all three parts), and the requirement for oral consumption of a radioactive compound requiring management and disposal of radioactive waste, thus precluding its use in women of childbearing age as well as in children. In addition, the pharmacological dose of B_{12} injected intramuscularly as part of the test delays and sometimes obscures subsequent assessment of responses in B_{12} status to medical and nutritional therapy. Furthermore, the test requires normal renal function and complete collection of 24 h urine output and is invalidated by either incomplete urine collection or underlying chronic renal disease. Because of these limitations, physicians are reluctant to order the test for their B_{12}-deficient patients suspected of having pernicious anemia and other malabsorption disorders. Instead, patients found or suspected to have B_{12} deficiency are frequently prescribed lifelong monthly intramuscular injections of B_{12} without adequate diagnosis of the underlying cause of the deficiency. Because food-bound B_{12} is not usually used in the Schilling test, many patients referred with low serum B_{12} concentrations resulting from atrophic gastritis are incorrectly determined to have normal B_{12} absorption [241,242], adding to the perception that the test is of limited value.

Alternatives to the Schilling test are currently considered. One method [243,244] employs a strategy of giving three consecutive 9 μg oral doses of nonradioactive B_{12}, given 6 h apart. Change in serum holotranscobalamin level is then assessed 24 h after the initial B_{12} dose. Initial studies suggest that change in holotranscobalamin distinguishes between individuals with B_{12} malabsorption and those with intact B_{12} absorptive capacity with reasonable sensitivity and specificity. A second strategy considered exploits a newly developed method for the microbial synthesis of B_{12} labeled with carbon-14 (^{14}C–B_{12}) and accelerator mass spectrometry (AMS) [59]. AMS provides the capacity to detect levels of ^{14}C in biological samples at attomolar range, and thus is uniquely suited to detect the appearance in the blood of minimally radioactive substances. Initial studies have shown that ^{14}C–B_{12}, given as a physiological dose (1.5 μg) and containing one-twentieth of the level of radioactivity typically used in the Schilling test (0.05 μCi ^{14}C–B_{12} vs. 1.0 μCi ^{57}Co–B_{12}), can be detected in plasma after oral ingestion in a healthy adult, with peak label appearing between 6 and 8 h after ingestion. Future studies will determine if measurement of plasma ^{14}C–B_{12} after oral ingestion can distinguish B_{12} malabsorbers from those with intact absorptive capacity.

Therapeutic Trial

Response to treatment of subjects with suspected B_{12} deficiency (treatment strategies are described in detail later) can be employed as a means for definitive diagnosis [188], though nowadays it is rarely used. This works particularly well for the diagnosis of B_{12} deficiency as the cause of megaloblastic anemia. It involves treatment with a physiological dose of B_{12} (e.g., 1–2 μg intramuscularly daily) and monitoring of the hematological response. A therapeutic trial is less definitive in the diagnosis of neurological deficits caused by B_{12} deficiency. If the deficiency has been prolonged (over 1 year), then the neurological deficits may not respond to B_{12} supplementation [245,246]. Response to treatment is discussed in more detail in the next section.

TREATMENT

Response to Treatment

Following treatment of vitamin B_{12} deficiency, a series of observable changes occur, depending on the degree of deficiency. Classically, in B_{12} deficiency, the observable changes relate to hematological reversal of megaloblastic abnormalities and the accompanying macrocytic anemia. Typically, these changes begin to occur rapidly, with correction of megaloblastic abnormalities in the bone marrow beginning to occur after 8–12 h and complete disappearance of abnormal morphology within 2–3 days. It is known that megaloblasts are incapable of normal maturation and effective hematopoiesis, and they undergo apoptosis within the bone marrow [247]. It therefore requires time for newly committed progenitor cells to mature to reticulocytes within the marrow so that the number of reticulocytes begin to rise abruptly 3–5 days after treatment is instituted, reaching a zenith after 4–10 days. There is a more gradual rise in the red cell count and the hemoglobin concentration as the depleted circulating red cell mass is reconstituted. Parallel with the rise in red cell count, there is an increase in the platelet and white cell counts if these were also low at the time treatment was initiated. The intensity of the hematological response is, in general, proportional to the original degree of anemia. The pattern of response provides important information in that it confirms there was, indeed, a B_{12} deficiency, and also may indicate the presence of additional complicating factors such as associated deficiencies of other hematinic factors. In such situations, the reticulocyte response and rise in hemoglobin concentration or red cell count are suboptimal. This occurs typically when there is an associated iron deficiency that frequently coexists in conditions like gastric atrophy and pernicious anemia.

In the absence of hematological abnormalities, an objective response to treatment is more difficult to evaluate. Neurological changes attributable to B_{12} deficiency may show a variable response to B_{12} replacement therapy, depending on the severity and the duration of the abnormality [177]. With respect to the myeloneuropathy, symptoms of <3 months duration are generally completely reversible and improvement begins within weeks, particularly those of muscular weakness. So, too, do psychiatric manifestations such as irritability, confusion, and even hallucinations. Sensory abnormalities like paresthesias take longer to remit and may never completely disappear. Some studies have reported improvements in objective measurements of neurological function following B_{12} treatment, including visual and auditory-evoked potentials and nerve conduction velocity [248–252].

There are also objective biochemical changes that occur following effective treatment of B_{12} deficiency, some specific and others nonspecific. Specific biochemical changes include reduction in plasma methylmalonic acid and homocysteine. Typically, these metabolites fall significantly within days after initiation of B_{12} replacement therapy [132,253]. Methylmalonic acid and homocysteine may be elevated in subjects without hematological or neurological abnormalities, including a proportion with normal levels of serum B_{12}. These metabolites, nonetheless, may fall to normal with B_{12} therapy. The significance of these biochemical changes is controversial [119,131,254–256]. They may imply functional B_{12} deficiency not reflected by subnormal levels of the vitamin or by disturbed hematopoiesis. This suggests that the accepted normal serum level of B_{12} reflects body stores that are sufficiently high to prevent hematological changes, but in some subjects may not be optimal for prevention of other complications, including thrombosis, vascular disease (putatively associated with hyperhomocysteinemia), and fetal NTDs.

Among the nonspecific biochemical changes that occur in response to B_{12} treatment are an increase in previously low-serum alkaline phosphatase, an increase in serum uric acid (depressed to varying degrees in B_{12} deficiency), a fall in serum lactic dehydrogenase and unconjugated bilirubin (both raised during the B_{12}-deficient state), and a fall in the serum iron concentration caused by sudden increase in the rate of erythropoiesis with a resulting consumption of available iron. The erthyropoietic burst also rapidly consumes extracellular potassium that can result in a precipitous and life-threatening lowering of serum potassium [257].

In addition to the objective, measurable changes in blood count values, there are a number of dramatic subjective changes experienced by a B_{12}-deficient patient following treatment. This is variously described in superlatives by patients who experience a general sense of well-being and improved alertness. Mood may become elevated, as well.

Forms of Treatment

Treatment protocols for established B_{12} deficiency are fairly straightforward. The form of B_{12} is cyanocobalamin in the United States and hydroxocobalamin in the United Kingdom. In several countries both forms are used, and in Japan methylcobalamin is popular. The advantages claimed for hydroxocobalamin over cyanocobalamin are that the former shows better retention following a large intramuscular dose and that cyanocobalamin is metabolically inactive until the cyanide group is cleaved from the upper axial ligand position of cobalamin [64].

Regardless of the form of B_{12}, it is generally necessary to continue lifelong treatment with B_{12} once the decision has been made that a patient is B_{12}-deficient, particularly if the deficiency is due to conditions other than dietary deficiency. The traditional approach has been to administer the B_{12} by intramuscular injection. Initially, the B_{12} is given in doses of 1000 μg twice weekly for 2 weeks and then 1000 μg weekly for another 4 weeks. This generally replenishes the depleted B_{12} tissue stores. Thereafter, B_{12} may be given by monthly injection of 1000 μg. So large a dose of cyanocobalamin is not well retained and most of this dose is excreted in the urine. The use of hydroxocobalamin reduces the need to administer as many doses initially (six 1000 μg injections at 3–7 day intervals suffice initially with maintenance injections of 1000 μg required only every 3 months). Toxic reactions to vitamin B_{12} are extremely rare and there is no upper limit defined [26].

Because a small fraction (1%–2%) of any oral dose of B_{12} can be absorbed passively through diffusion, even in the total absence of the normal IF-mediated physiologic mechanism for B_{12} absorption, B_{12} replacement may be given orally to treat deficiency [258]. To ensure that an oral dose of B_{12} is adequate, it has been recommended that daily doses of 1000–2000 μg be given [259]. Sublingual and intranasal routes of B_{12} administration have also been proposed and marketed [260–263].

NEW DIRECTIONS

Gene Expression

As stated in the Chemistry section, the details of the microbial biosynthesis of B_{12} are complex. One aspect of B_{12} biosynthesis that warrants mention, recent advances in the understanding of how intracellular B_{12} appears to regulate its own biosynthesis in bacteria, as well as transport of available extracellular B_{12} into the bacterial cell. In the presence of 5′-deoxyadenosylcobalamin, expression of the *cob* operon of *S. typhimurium*, which encodes for the B_{12} biosynthetic pathway, is significantly decreased. Likewise, the expression of the btuB gene of *Escherichia coli* and *S. typhimurium*, which encodes for the membrane cobalamin transporter, is decreased in the presence of 5′-deoxyadenosylcobalamin [11,264–266]. Mutational analysis has revealed that the mechanism by which this occurs is at the level of translation initiation and involves two elements in the leader sequences of the *cob* and btuB genes, a so-called B_{12} box and an RNA hairpin structure [267–271]. Binding of 5′-deoxyadenosylcobalamin to the B_{12} box alters and stabilizes the tertiary structure of the RNA hairpin, thus inhibiting ribosomal binding and the initiation of translation. In this way, B_{12} acts as a riboswitch, a function beyond its well-known role as a cofactor in enzymatic reactions. B_{12} is not unique in this regard; several other small molecules are known to serve as riboswitches, including thiamine pyrophosphate, flavin mononucleotide, *S*-adenosylmethionine, lysine, guanine, and adenine [272,273]. It is important to note that riboswitches seem to be restricted to prokaryotic systems. To date, a eukaryotic riboswitch has not been identified. This notable evolutionary distinction suggests the possibility that riboswitches, including the B_{12} riboswitch, might be exploited as targets for novel antimicrobial drugs [272].

Though riboswitches have not been identified in eukaryotic cells, there is evidence that B_{12} acts to promote the translation of at least one mammalian gene. B_{12} has been known for many years to induce the activity of methionine synthase (but not methylmalonylCoA mutase) [274–276]. A series of investigations by Banerjee and coworkers [277–279] have established that the increased activity of methionine synthase in the presence of B_{12} is not solely the result of conversion of apo-enzyme to holo-enzyme, nor is it the result of increased transcription of the methionine synthase gene or stabilization of the protein. Instead, induction of enzyme activity seems to be initiated from an internal ribosomal entry site (IRES) that spans 71 bases immediately upstream of the translation start codon of the methionine synthase mRNA. B_{12} increases the efficiency of IRES-dependent translation of the protein. The effect is not due to direct binding of B_{12} to the mRNA sequence, but rather appears to be the result of interaction of B_{12} with an IRES transactivating factor (ITAF) [279]. The working model is that B_{12} binds to an as yet unidentified ITAF protein and induces a conformational change that promotes the interaction of the ITAF with the IRES. This in turn enhances recruitment of ribosomes and promotes translation. It is proposed that this may constitute a mechanism by which B_{12}, a rare commodity in the environment, may be rapidly sequestered within the cell [278]. Thus, methionine synthase may have, as additional purpose to its primary function of enzymatic conversion of homocysteine to methionine, the role of providing an intracellular storage silo for the vitamin. It will be of great interest in the future to see if this effect of B_{12} is unique to methionine synthase in mammalian cells or if B_{12} promotes IRES-dependent translation of other proteins, particularly those involved in B_{12} metabolism.

Inflammation

Vitamin B_{12} may be a modulator of the inflammatory response. Evidence for a relationship between B_{12} and inflammation comes from the totally gastrectomized (TGX) rat model of B_{12} deficiency [280]. Removal of the stomach eliminates the source of IF required for the physiologic absorption of B_{12}. Consequently, B_{12} deficiency occurs within several months, as demonstrated by Scalabrino and colleagues [281] who have described significantly elevated levels of homocysteine and methylmalonic acid in the blood as well as subacute combined degeneration of the spinal cord (SACD). Inhibition of methionine synthesis with resulting alterations of methylation and abnormal methylmalonate incorporation into odd-chain fatty acids have been implicated as pathogenetic mechanisms underlying SACD (see Deficiency section). An alternative proposition, however, is that B_{12} deficiency causes neurodegeneration through a mechanism mediated by the inflammatory cytokine, tumor necrosis factor alpha (TNF-α) [282]. Intracerebroventricular microinjection of TNF-α into nongastrectomized rats induces spinal cord pathology similar to that observed in the TGX rat. In addition, TNF-α is overexpressed in the spinal cords of TGX rats, and this overexpression can be reversed with intramuscular injections of B_{12}. Moreover, intracerebroventricular microinjections of TNF-α antibodies or cytokine inhibitors of TNF-α production, such as transforming growth factor ß1 and interleukin 6, prevent SACD lesions in the TGX rat. The relevance to humans of these findings is supported by the observation that serum and cerebrospinal fluid TNF-α levels are elevated in patients with B_{12} deficiency and are normalized by B_{12} replacement therapy [283,284]. It is unclear from these rat and human studies, however, if the increased expression of TNF-α is secondary to the primary biochemical impairments induced by B_{12} deficiency, or if B_{12} plays a more direct role in TNF-α expression at the transcriptional or translational level. This latter possibility, for which there is no experimental support, could represent a novel IRES-dependent type role for B_{12} in the regulation of gene expression that lies beyond the currently recognized B_{12}-related proteins, similar to that postulated in the previous section.

The observed association between B_{12} deficiency and increased TNF-α may underlie several clinical observations [285]. First, a connection between Alzheimer's disease and B_{12} deficiency has long been suspected. Alzheimer's disease, with its characteristic amyloid plaques and neurofibrillary tangles in the brain, is ultimately a disease with a strong inflammatory component. The potential for developing antiinflammatory drugs to prevent or slow the progression of Alzheimer's disease is currently an active line of investigation. If B_{12} deficiency promotes inflammation by inducing increased expression of TNF-α, this could exacerbate the damage caused by the disease. Second, in vitro studies have shown that methylcobalamin inhibits inflammatory cytokine production [286]. This observation has led to the use of methylcobalamin in the treatment of rheumatoid arthritis [286]. Last, B_{12} has been shown to inhibit HIV infection of lymphocytes and monocytes in vitro [287]. In contrast, TNF-α is known to promote HIV replication. Together, these observations suggest that B_{12} may inhibit HIV infectivity by suppressing TNF-α production. Of note is that low B_{12} status has been associated with an accelerated rate of onset of clinical AIDS after HIV infection [288].

Diagnostic Imaging and Drug Delivery

Cancer cells have the capacity to take up and sequester B_{12} at a higher rate and efficiency than that required for normal metabolism and cell replication [289]. This may be the result of a high density of transcobalamin receptor sites on cancer cells [290]. This implies an increased need for B_{12} to support rapid DNA replication and cell proliferation that are characteristic of cancer cells. The differential uptake of B_{12} between cancer cells and normal cells has been proposed as a phenomenon that can be exploited for both in vivo imaging and drug delivery. Common to these approaches is the attachment of the label or drug to the central cobalt atom of B_{12} in the upper axial ligand position.

Labeling of B_{12} or B_{12} analogs with gamma-emitting Indium-111 has been used to image high-grade primary and metastatic malignancies of the breast, lung, colon, thyroid, prostate, and central nervous system [291]. The use of nonradioactive fluorescently labeled B_{12} has also been explored [292]. Initial experiments have demonstrated that fluorescently labeled B_{12} can be used for lymphatic mapping in a porcine model, thus opening the possibility of a minimally invasive method to visualize malignant cells in the lymphatic system [293].

With respect to drug delivery, promising results have been obtained with a conjugate of B_{12} and colchicine. Colchicine is highly cytotoxic, primarily through inhibition of tubulin polymerization and the blocking of mitosis during metaphase [294]. Colchicine has not been useful in cancer treatment because of very high systemic toxicity. However, if colchicine can be preferentially targeted to cancer cells, then the drug may yet prove an effective anticarcinogen. A B_{12}–colchicine conjugate has been synthesized and uptake into breast, brain, and melanoma cancer cell lines has been demonstrated in vitro [294]. LC_{50} values for the conjugate are in the nanomolar range, suggesting this mode of drug delivery may ultimately prove clinically beneficial.

Emerging Epidemiological Associations

Because of the prominent role of B_{12} in both DNA synthesis and homocysteine metabolism, there is a biochemical basis for investigating associations between B_{12} and chronic degenerative diseases of aging. In addition to putative associations between B_{12} and vascular and neurodegenerative diseases discussed earlier, other associations that have some epidemiological support include cancer (in particular breast cancer), bone health, age-related hearing loss, and NTDs.

Breast Cancer

The association with breast cancer was first observed in 1999 in postmenopausal women [295,296]. In a prospective study, median serum B_{12} levels were lower in cases versus controls and the lowest quintile of serum B_{12} was associated with an elevated odds ratio for breast cancer. A subsequent prospective study found an inverse association between B_{12} and incident breast cancer, but only in premenopausal women [297]. Proposed mechanisms by which B_{12} may play a role in cancer are similar to those proposed for folate deficiency, that is, an increase in DNA strand breaks due to uracil misincorporation and a decrease in DNA methylation, which can affect gene expression patterns and genome stability [295,296].

Osteoporosis

In recent years, there has been growing interest in a possible relationship between osteoporosis and B_{12} status. In middle-age and older adults, associations have been observed between B_{12} and bone mineral content, bone mineral density, risk of osteoporosis and osteopenia, and risk of hip fracture [298–303]. Associations have also been observed between B_{12} and markers of bone turnover, including serum osteocalcin and urinary deoxypyridinoline excretion [302]. Notably, B_{12} supplements increase osteocalcin levels in individuals with B_{12} deficiency [304]. Relationships between B_{12} and bone are not limited to the elderly; low bone mineral density associated with low B_{12} status (including elevated methylmalonic acid) has been observed in adolescents formerly fed a macrobiotic diet low in B_{12} [300]. A mechanism by which B_{12} influences bone is suggested by in vitro and clinical studies linking B_{12} with osteoblastic activity [304,305]. Alternatively, the relationship between B_{12} and bone health may be mediated by homocysteine. Two prominent studies have linked hyperhomocysteinemia to increased risk of osteoporotic fractures in older adults, though the dependence of this relationship on B_{12} status was not assessed in these studies [306,307]. There is also evidence that lowering homocysteine with a combination of B_{12} and folate supplement reduces the risk of hip fracture [308].

Hearing Loss

Among the many and varied symptoms of B_{12} deficiency that have been reported are tinnitus and auditory hallucinations, suggesting a role for B_{12} in hearing. Limited epidemiological evidence provides some support for an association. In a small cohort of older women (age 60–71 years) serum B_{12} was significantly lower in subjects with impaired hearing defined as a hearing threshold >20 dB than in subjects with a threshold <20 dB [309]. In addition, pure-tone air conduction thresholds were inversely correlated with B_{12} levels. A study of military personnel exposed to excessive noise also suggests an association; subjects with a combination of tinnitus and noise-induced hearing loss had a higher prevalence of low serum B_{12} than those with noise-induced hearing loss without tinnitus or normal hearing [310]. Moreover, a lessening of the tinnitus was reported in the B_{12}-deficient subjects who received B_{12} supplements. Mechanisms by which B_{12} might affect hearing could be damage to the vascular system of the ear associated with hyperhomocysteinemia, alterations in bone conduction properties resulting from metabolic bone changes, or direct neurotoxic effects of homocysteine or methylmalonic acid on the neural components of the ear [309].

Neural Tube Defects

The success of folic acid fortification of the food supply in reducing the incidence of NTDs in the United States, Canada, and other countries is well documented [181,311]. Because of the interrelated biochemical functions of folate and B_{12} in the conversion of homocysteine to methionine, it was predicted that B_{12} status might also be an important factor in neural tube development. The strongest support for a role of B_{12} in neural tube development comes from case-control studies; mean total B_{12} level is consistently lower in the amniotic fluid from NTD pregnancies than normal pregnancies [312]. In contrast, the majority of studies find no difference in mean serum B_{12} between cases and controls [312]. These observations suggest that women susceptible to an NTD-affected birth have a higher requirement for B_{12} to support normal neural tube development, thus implicating genetic differences in delivery of B_{12} to the fetus, B_{12} metabolism, or cofactor function that may contribute to NTDs. In support of this contention are data indicating that a common polymorphic variant in methionine synthase reductase (A66G) influences the risk of NTDs, particularly when maternal B_{12} status is low [117]. Therefore, with folic acid fortification, it can be hypothesized that some of the residual NTD incidence is related to a combination of genetic factors and low B_{12} nutrition. The effect of polymorphisms in this situation may arise either as a result of maternal or fetal SNPs, or the coexistence of both.

REFERENCES

1. Castle, W.B., The conquest of pernicious anemia, in *Blood, Pure and Eloquent*, Wintrobe, M.M., ed., McGraw Hill, NY, 1980, 283.
2. Smith, L.E., *Vitamin B_{12}*, John Wiley, NY, 1965.
3. Chanarin, I., Historical review: a history of pernicious anemia, *Br. J. Haematol.*, 111, 407, 2000.
4. Addison, T., *On the Constitutional and Local Effects of Disease of the Suprarenal Capsules*, Samuel Highley, London, 1855, 43.
5. Minot, G.R. and Murphy, W.P., Observations on patients with pernicious anemia partaking a special diet: A. Clinical aspects, *Trans. Assoc. Am. Physicians*, 44, 72, 1926.
6. Whipple, G.H. and Robscheit-Robbins, F.S., Iron and its utilization in experimental anemia, *Am. J. Med. Sci.*, 191, 11, 1936.
7. Rickes, E.L. et al., Crystalline vitamin B_{12}, *Science*, 107, 396, 1948.
8. Smith, E.L. and Parker, L.F.J., Purification of antipernicious anaemia factor, *Biochem. J.*, 43, viii, 1948.
9. Hodgkin, D.C. et al., Structure of vitamin B_{12}, *Nature*, 178, 64, 1956.
10. Woodward, R.B., The total synthesis of vitamin B_{12}, *Pure Appl. Chem.*, 33, 145, 1973.
11. Roth, J.R., Lawrence, J.G., and Bobik, T.A., Cobalamin (coenzyme B_{12}): synthesis and biological significance, *Annu. Rev. Microbiol.*, 50, 137, 1996.
12. Scott, A.I., Discovering nature's diverse pathways to B_{12}: a 35-year odyssey, *J. Org. Chem.*, 68, 2529, 2003.
13. Martens, J.-H. et al., Microbial production of vitamin B_{12}, *Appl. Microbiol. Biotechnol.*, 58, 275, 2002.
14. Banerjee, R., *Chemistry and Biochemistry of B_{12}*, John Wiley, NY, 1999.
15. Dolphin, J.D., *B_{12}: Vol. 1: Chemistry; Vol. 2: Biochemistry and Medicine*, John Wiley, NY, 1982.

16. Pratt, J.M., *Inorganic Chemistry of Vitamin B_{12}*, Academic Press, NY, 1972.
17. Halpern, J. and Dolphin, D., *Chemistry and Significance of Vitamin B_{12} Model Systems*, John Wiley, NY, 1982.
18. Chanarin, I., *The Megaloblastic Anemias*, Blackwell Scientific Publications, Oxford, 1969.
19. Pezacka, E., Green, R., and Jacobsen, D.W., Glutathionylcobalamin as an intermediate in the formation of cobalamin coenzymes, *Biochem. Biophys. Res. Commun.*, 169, 443, 1990.
20. Linnell, J.C., Hussein, A.-A., and Matthews, D.M., A two-dimensional chromato-bioautographic method for complete separation of individual plasma cobalamins, *J. Clin. Pathol.*, 23, 820, 1970.
21. Frenkel, E.P., Kitchens, R.L., and Prough, R., High-performance liquid chromatographic separation of cobalamins, *J. Chromatogr.*, 174, 393, 1979.
22. Jacobsen, D.W., Green, R., and Brown, K.L., Analysis of cobalamin coenzymes and other corrinoids by high-performance liquid chromatography, *Meth. Enzymol.*, 123, 14, 1986.
23. Kondo, H., Kolhouse, J.F., and Allen, R.H., Presence of cobalamin analogues in animal tissue, *Proc. Natl. Acad. Sci.*, 77, 817, 1980.
24. Muir, M. and Landon, M., Endogenous origin of microbiologically-inactive cobalamins (cobalamin analogues) in the human fetus, *Br. J. Haematol.*, 61, 303, 1985.
25. Herbert, V.D. and Colman, N., Folic acid and vitamin B_{12}, in *Modern Nutrition in Health and Disease*, 7th edition, Shils, M.E. and Young, V.R., eds., Lea and Febiger, Philadelphia, 1988, 388.
26. Institute of Medicine, Vitamin B_{12}, *Dietary Reference Intakes for Thiamin, Riboflavin, Niacin, Vitamin B_6, Folate, Vitamin B_{12}, Pantothenic Acid, Biotin, and Choline*, The National Academies Press, Washington, DC, 2000, 306.
27. Fedosov, S.N. et al., Comparative analysis of cobalamin binding kinetics and ligand protection for intrinsic factor, transcobalamin, and haptocorrin, *J. Biol. Chem.*, 277, 9989, 2002.
28. Andrews, E.R., Pratt, J.M., and Brown, K.L., Molecular recognition in the binding of vitamin B_{12} by the cobalamin-specific intrinsic factor, *FEBS Lett.*, 281, 90, 1991.
29. Grasbeck, R., Intrinsic factor and the other vitamin B_{12} transport proteins, in *Progress in Hematology*, Brown, E.B. and Moore, C.V., eds., Grune and Stratton, NY, 1969, 233.
30. Seetharam, B., Receptor-mediated endocytosis of cobalamin (vitamin B_{12}), *Annu. Rev. Nutr.*, 19, 173, 1999.
31. Kolhouse, J.F. and Allen, R.H., Absorption, plasma transport, and cellular retention of cobalamin analogues in the rabbit, *J. Clin. Invest.*, 60, 1381, 1977.
32. Stupperich, E. and Nexo, E., Effect of the cobalt–N coordination on the cobamide recognition by the human vitamin B_{12} binding proteins intrinsic factor, transcobalamin and haptocorrin, *Eur. J. Biochem.*, 199, 299, 1991.
33. Gottlieb, C.W., Retief, F.P., and Herbert, V., Blockade of vitamin B_{12}-binding sites in gastric juice, serum and saliva by analogues and derivatives of vitamin B_{12} and by antibody to intrinsic factor, *Biochim. Biophys. Acta*, 141, 560, 1967.
34. Hippe, E., Haber, E., and Olesen, H., Nature of vitamin B_{12} binding. II. Steric orientation of vitamin B_{12} on binding and number of combining sites of human intrinsic factor and the transcobalamins, *Biochim. Biophys. Acta*, 243, 75, 1971.
35. Bunge, M.B., Schilling, R.F., and Schloesser, L.L., Intrinsic factor studies. IV. Selective absorption and binding of cyanocobalamin by gastric juice in the presence of excess pseudovitamin B_{12} or 5,6-dimethylbenzimidazole, *J. Lab. Clin. Med.*, 48, 735, 1956.
36. Fedosov, S.N. et al., Assembly of the intrinsic factor domains and oligomerization of the protein in the presence of cobalamin, *Biochemistry*, 43, 15095, 2004.
37. Abels, J. and Schilling, R.F., Protection of intrinsic factor by vitamin B_{12}, *J. Lab. Clin. Med.*, 64, 375, 1964.
38. Kondo, H. et al., Presence and formation of cobalamin analogues in multivitamin-mineral pills, *J. Clin. Invest.*, 70, 889, 1982.
39. Hippe, E., Changes in Stokes radius on binding of vitamin B_{12} to human intrinsic factor and transcobalamins, *Biochim. Biophys. Acta*, 208, 337, 1970.
40. Moestrup, S.K. and Verroust, P.J., Megalin- and cubulin-mediated endocytosis of protein-bound vitamins, lipids, and hormones in polarized epithelia, *Annu. Rev. Nutr.*, 21, 407, 2001.
41. Kozyraki, R., Cubulin, a multifunctional epithelial receptor: an overview, *J. Mol. Med.*, 79, 161, 2001.

42. Barth, J.L. and Argraves, W.S., Cubulin and megalin: partners in lipoprotein and vitamin metabolism, *Trends Cardiovasc. Med.*, 11, 26, 2001.
43. Birn, H., The kidney in vitamin B_{12} and folate homeostasis: characterization of receptors for tubular uptake of vitamins and carrier proteins, *Am. J. Physiol. Renal Physiol.*, 291, 22, 2006.
44. El Kholty, S. et al., Portal and biliary phases of enterohepatic circulation of corrinoids in humans, *Gastroenterology*, 101, 1399, 1991.
45. Green, R. et al., Enterohepatic circulation of cobalamin in the nonhuman primate, *Gastroenterology*, 81, 773, 1981.
46. Green, R. et al., Absorption of biliary cobalamin in baboons following total gastrectomy, *J. Lab. Clin. Med.*, 100, 771, 1982.
47. Heyssel, R.M. et al., Vitamin B_{12} turnover in man. The assimilation of vitamin B_{12} from natural foodstuff by man and estimates of minimal daily dietary requirements, *Am. J. Clin. Nutr.*, 18, 176, 1966.
48. Hall, C.A., The carriers of native vitamin B_{12} in normal human serum, *Clin. Sci. Mol. Med.*, 53, 453, 1977.
49. Morkbak, A.L. et al., Effect of vitamin B_{12} treatment on haptocorrin, *Clin. Chem.*, 52, 1104, 2006.
50. Burger, R.L. et al., Human plasma R-type vitamin B_{12}-binding proteins: II. The role of transcobalamin I, transcobalamin III, and the normal granulocyte vitamin B_{12}-binding protein in the plasma transport of vitamin B_{12}, *J. Biol. Chem.*, 250, 7707, 1975.
51. Adkins, Y. and Lonnerdal, B., Potential host-defense role of a human milk vitamin B_{12}-binding protein, haptocorrin, in the gastrointestinal tract of breastfed infants, as assessed with porcine haptocorrin in vitro, *Am. J. Clin. Nutr.*, 77, 1234, 2003.
52. Quadros, E.V. et al., Purification and molecular characterization of human transcobalamin II, *J. Biol. Chem.*, 261, 15455, 1986.
53. Allen, R.H. and Majerus, P.W., Isolation of vitamin B_{12}-binding proteins using affinity chromatography. 3. Purification and properties of human plasma transcobalamin II, *J. Biol. Chem.*, 247, 7709, 1972.
54. Lindemans, J., Van Kapel, J., and Abels, J., Purification of human transcobalamin II-cyanocobalamin by affinity chromatography using thermolabile immobilization of cyanocobalamin, *Biochim. Biophys. Acta*, 579, 40, 1979.
55. Van Kapel, J. et al., An improved method for large scale purification of human holo-transcobalamin II, *Biochim. Biophys. Acta*, 676, 307, 1981.
56. Platica, O. et al., The cDNA sequence and the deduced amino acid sequence of human transcobalamin II show homology with rat intrinsic factor and human transcobalamin I, *J. Biol. Chem.*, 266, 7860, 1991.
57. Booth, C.C. and Mollin, D.L., Plasma, tissue, and urinary radioactivity after oral administration of 56Co-labelled vitamin B_{12}, *Br. J. Haematol.*, 2, 223, 1956.
58. Doscherholmen, A. and Hagen, P.S., Radioactive vitamin B_{12} absorption studies: results of direct measurement of radioactivity in the blood, *J. Clin. Invest.*, 35, 699, 1956.
59. Carkeet, C. et al., Human Vitamin B_{12} absorption measurement by accelerator mass spectrometry using specifically labeled 14C-cobalamin, *Proc. Natl. Acad. Sci.*, 103, 5649, 2006.
60. Refsum, H. et al., Holotranscobalamin and total transcobalamin in human plasma: determination, determinants, and reference values in healthy adults, *Clin. Chem.*, 52, 129, 2006.
61. Hom, B.L., Plasma turnover of 57Cobalt-vitamin B_{12} bound to transcobalamin I and II, *Scand. J. Haematol.*, 4, 32, 1967.
62. Finkler, A.E. and Hall C.A., Nature of the relationship between vitamin B_{12} binding and cell uptake, *Arch. Biochem. Biophys.*, 120, 79, 1967.
63. Zetterberg, H. et al., The transcobalamin (TC) codon 259 genetic polymorphism influences holo-TC concentration in cerebrospinal fluid from patients with Alzheimer disease, *Clin. Chem.*, 49, 1195, 2003.
64. Hoffbrand, A.V. and Green R., Megaloblastic anaemia, in *Postgraduate Haematology, 5th edition*, Hoffbrand, A.V., Catovsky, D., and Tuddenham, E.G., eds., Blackwell Publishing, Oxford, 2005, Chapter 5.
65. Carmel, R. et al., High serum cobalamin levels in the clinical setting—clinical associations and holo-transcobalamin changes, *Clin. Lab. Haematol.*, 23, 365, 2001.

66. Garrod, M.G. et al., Renal insufficiency is associated with elevated holotranscobalamin II in the elderly, *FASEB J.*, 18, 138.16, 2004.
67. Refsum, H. et al., Homocysteine and cardiovascular disease, *Annu. Rev. Med.*, 49, 31, 1998.
68. Rosenblatt, D.S. and Fenton, W.A., Inherited disorders of folate and cobalamin transport and metabolism, in *The Metabolic and Molecular Bases of Inherited Metabolic Disease*, 8th edition, Scriver, C.R. et al., eds., McGraw-Hill, NY, 2001, 3897.
69. Whitehead, V.M., Acquired and inherited disorders of cobalamin and folate in children, *Br. J. Haematol.*, 134, 125, 2006.
70. Carmel, R., Green, R., Rosenblatt, D.S., and Watkins, D., Update on cobalamin, folate, and homocysteine, *Hematology Am. Soc. Hematol. Educ. Program*, 62, 2003.
71. Gordon, M.M. et al., A genetic polymorphism in the coding region of the gastric intrinsic factor gene (GIF) is associated with congenital intrinsic factor deficiency, *Hum. Mutat.*, 23, 85, 2004.
72. Yassin, F. et al., Identification of a 4-base deletion in the gene in inherited intrinsic factor deficiency, *Blood*, 103, 1515, 2004.
73. Tanner, S.M. et al., Hereditary juvenile cobalamin deficiency caused by mutations in the intrinsic factor gene, *Proc. Natl. Acad. Sci.*, 102, 4130, 2005.
74. Kristiansen, M. et al., Cubulin P1297L mutation associated with hereditary megaloblastic anemia 1 causes impaired recognition of intrinsic factor-vitamin B_{12} by cubulin, *Blood*, 96, 405, 2000.
75. Tanner, S.M. et al., Genetically heterogeneous selective malabsorption of vitamin B_{12}: founder effects, consanguinity, and high clinical awareness explain aggregations in Scandinavia and the Middle East, *Hum. Mutat.*, 23, 327, 2004.
76. Aminoff, M. et al., Selective intestinal malabsorption of vitamin B_{12} displays recessive Mendelian inheritance: assignment of a locus to chromosome 10 by linkage, *Am. J. Hum. Genet.*, 57, 824, 1995.
77. Wang, X. et al., A candidate gene for the amnionless gastrulation stage mouse mutation encodes a TRAF-related protein, *Dev. Biol.*, 177, 274, 1996.
78. Tomihara-Newberger, C. et al., The amn gene product is required in extraembryonic tissues for the generation of middle primitive streak derivatives, *Dev. Biol.*, 204, 34, 1998.
79. Jeffery, C.J., Moonlighting proteins, *TIBS*, 24, 8, 1999.
80. Tanner, S.M. et al., Amnionless, essential for mouse gastrulation, is mutated in recessive hereditary megaloblastic anemia, *Nat. Genet.*, 33, 426, 2003.
81. Kozyraki, R. et al., The human intrinsic factor-vitamin B_{12} receptor, cubulin: molecular characterization and chromosomal mapping of the gene to 10p within the autosomal recessive megaloblastic anemia (MGA1) region, *Blood*, 91, 3593, 1998.
82. Frater-Schroder, M., Genetic patterns of transcobalamin II and the relationships with congenital defects, *Mol. Cell. Biochem.*, 56, 5, 1983.
83. Carmel, R., Mild transcobalamin I (haptocorrin) deficiency and low serum cobalamin concentrations, *Clin. Chem.*, 49, 1367, 2003.
84. Watkins, D., Matiaszuk, N., and Rosenblatt, D.S., Complementation studies in the cblA class of inborn errors of cobalamin metabolism: evidence for interallelic complementation and for a new complementation class (*cbl*H), *J. Med. Genet.*, 37, 510, 2000.
85. Watkins, D. and Rosenblatt, D.S., Failure of lysosomal release of vitamin B_{12}: a new complementation group causing methylmalonic aciduria (*cbl*F), *Am. J. Hum. Genet.*, 39, 404, 1986.
86. Dobson, C.M. et al., Identification of the gene responsible for the *cbl*A complementation group of vitamin B_{12}-responsive methylmalonic acidemia based on analysis of prokaryotic gene arrangements, *Proc. Natl. Acad. Sci.*, 99, 15554, 2002.
87. Dobson, C.M. et al., Identification of the gene responsible for the *cbl*B complementation group of vitamin B_{12}-dependent methylmalonic aciduria, *Hum. Mol. Genet.*, 11, 3361, 2002.
88. Leclerc, D. et al., Cloning and mapping of a cDNA for methionine synthase reductase, a flavoprotein defective in patients with homocystinuria, *Proc. Natl. Acad. Sci.*, 95, 3059, 1998.
89. Gulati, S. et al., Defects in human methionine synthase in *cbl*G patients, *Hum. Mol. Genet.*, 5, 1859, 1996.
90. Leclerc, D. et al., Human methionine synthase: cDNA cloning and identification of mutations in patients of the *cbl*G complementation group of folate/cobalamin disorders, *Hum. Mol. Genet.*, 5, 1867, 1996.
91. Daiger, S.P. et al., Detection of genetic variation with radioactive ligands: III. Genetic polymorphism of transcobalamin II in human plasma, *Am. J. Hum. Genet.*, 30, 202, 1978.

92. Frater-Schroder, M., Hitzig, W.H., and Butler, R., Studies on transcobalamin (TC): 1. Detection of TC II isoproteins in human serum, *Blood*, 53, 193, 1979.
93. Hansen, M. and Frater-Schroder, M., Human transcobalamin isopeptides: separation by isoelectric focusing and by polyacrylamide gel electrophoresis, *Electrophoresis*, 8, 221, 1987.
94. Li, N. et al., Isolation and sequence analysis of variant forms of human transcobalamin II, *Biochim. Biophys. Acta*, 1172, 21, 1993.
95. Li, N. et al., Polymorphism of human transcobalamin II: substitution of proline and/or glutamine residues by arginine, *Biochim. Biophys. Acta*, 1219, 515, 1994.
96. Namour, F. et al., Isoelectric phenotype and relative concentration of transcobalamin II isoproteins related to the codon 259 Arg/Pro polymorphism, *Biochem. Biophys. Res. Commun.*, 251, 769, 1998.
97. Afman, L.A. et al., Single nucleotide polymorphisms in the transcobalamin gene: relationship with transcobalamin concentrations and risk for neural tube defects, *Eur. J. Hum. Genet.*, 10, 433, 2002.
98. McCaddon, A. et al., Transcobalamin polymorphism and homocysteine, *Blood*, 98, 3497, 2001.
99. Namour, F. et al., Transcobalamin codon 259 polymorphism in HT-29 and Caco-2 cells and in Caucasians: relation to transcobalamin and homocysteine concentration in blood, *Blood*, 97, 1092, 2001.
100. Miller, J.W. et al., Transcobalamin II 775G > C polymorphism and indices of vitamin B_{12} status in healthy older adults, *Blood*, 100, 718, 2002.
101. Zetterberg, H. et al., The transcobalamin codon 259 polymorphism should be designated 776C > G, not 775G > C, *Blood*, 101, 3749, 2003.
102. Bowen, R.A., Wong, B.Y., and Cole, D.E., Population-based differences in frequency of the transcobalamin II Pro259Arg polymorphism, *Clin. Biochem.*, 37, 128, 2004.
103. Roychoudhury, A.K. and Nei, M., *Human Polymorphic Genes: World Distribution*, Oxford University Press, NY, 1988, 175.
104. Afman, L.A. et al., Reduced vitamin B_{12} binding by transcobalamin II increases risk of neural tube defects, *QJM*, 94, 159, 2001.
105. Geisel, J. et al., The role of genetic factors in the development of hyperhomocysteinemia, *Clin. Chem. Lab. Med.*, 41, 1427, 2003.
106. Wans, S. et al., Analysis of the transcobalamin II 776C > G (259P > R) single nucleotide polymorphism by denaturing HPLC in healthy elderly: associations with cobalamin, homocysteine and holo-transcobalamin II. *Clin. Chem. Lab. Med.*, 41, 1532, 2003.
107. McCaddon, A. et al., Transcobalamin polymorphism and serum holo-transcobalamin in relation to Alzheimer's disease, *Dement. Geriatr. Cogn. Disorders*, 17, 215, 2004.
108. von Castel-Dunwoody, K.M. et al., Transcobalamin 776C > G polymorphism negatively affects vitamin B_{12} metabolism, *Am. J. Clin. Nutr.*, 81, 1436, 2005.
109. Lievers, K.J. et al., Polymorphisms in the transcobalamin gene: association with plasma homocysteine in healthy individuals and vascular disease patients, *Clin. Chem.*, 48, 1383, 2002.
110. Zetterberg, H. et al., The transcobalamin codon 259 polymorphism influences the risk of human spontaneous abortion, *Hum. Reprod.*, 17, 3033, 2002.
111. Zetterberg, H. et al., Gene-gene interaction between fetal MTHFR 677C > T and transcobalamin 776C > G polymorphisms in human spontaneous abortion, *Hum. Reprod.*, 18, 1948, 2003.
112. Martinelli, M. et al., Study of four genes belonging to the folate pathway: transcobalamin 2 is involved in the onset of non-syndromic cleft lip with or without cleft palate, *Hum. Mutat.*, 27, 294, 2006.
113. Christensen, B. et al., Genetic polymorphisms in methylenetetrahydrofolate reductase and methionine synthase, folate levels in red blood cells, and risk of neural tube defects, *Am. J. Med. Genet.*, 84, 151, 1999.
114. Doolin, M.-T. et al., Maternal genetic effects, exerted by genes involved in homocysteine remethylation, influence the risk of spina bifida, *Am. J. Hum. Genet.*, 71, 1222, 2002.
115. Bosco, P. et al., Methionine synthase (MTR) 2756 (A-G) polymorphism, double heterozygosity methionine synthase 2756 AG/methionine synthase reductase (MTRR) 66 AG, and elevated homocysteinemia are 3 risk factors for having a child with Down syndrome, *Am. J. Med. Genet.*, 121A, 219, 2003.

116. Motowska, A., Hozyasz, K.K., and Jagodzinski, P.P., Maternal MTR genotype contributes to the risk of non-syndromic cleft lip and palate in the Polish population, *Clin. Genet.*, 69, 512, 2006.
117. Wilson, A. et al., A common variant in methionine synthase reductase combined with low cobalamin (vitamin B_{12}) increases risk for spina bifida, *Mol. Genet. Metab.*, 67, 317, 1999.
118. Hobbs, C.A. et al., Polymorphisms in genes involved in folate metabolism as maternal risk factors for Down syndrome, *Am. J. Hum. Genet.*, 67, 623, 2000.
119. Pennypacker, L. et al., High prevalence of cobalamin deficiency in elderly outpatients, *J. Am. Geriatr. Soc.*, 39, 1155, 1991.
120. Lindenbaum, J. et al., Prevalence of cobalamin deficiency in the Framingham elderly population, *Am. J. Clin. Nutr.*, 60, 2, 1994.
121. Groene, L.A. et al., Serum homocysteine and methylmalonic acid levels in elderly outpatients with borderline serum cobalamin, *J. Am. Geriatr. Soc.*, 43, SA22, 1995.
122. Nilsson-Ehle, H. et al., Low serum cobalamin levels in a population study of 70- and 75-year-old subjects: gastrointestinal causes and hematological effects, *Dig. Dis. Sci.*, 34, 716, 1989.
123. Hanger, H.C. et al., A community study of vitamin B_{12} and folate levels in the elderly, *J. Am. Geriatr. Soc.*, 39, 1155, 1991.
124. Russell, R.M., Vitamin B_{12}, in *Nutrition in the Elderly: The Boston Nutritional Status Survey*, Hartz, S.C., Rosenberg, I.H., and Russell, R.M., eds., Smith-Gordon & Co Ltd., London, 1992.
125. Norman, E.J. and Morrison, J.A., Screening elderly populations for cobalamin (vitamin B_{12}) deficiency using the urinary methylmalonic acid assay by gas chromatography mass spectrometry, *Am. J. Med.*, 94, 589, 1993.
126. Joosten, E. et al., Metabolic evidence that deficiencies of vitamin B_{12} (cobalamin), folate, and vitamin B_6 occur commonly in elderly people, *Am. J. Clin. Nutr.*, 58, 468, 1993.
127. Crystal, H.A. et al., Serum vitamin B_{12} levels and incidence of dementia in a healthy elderly population: a report from the Bronx longitudinal aging study, *J. Am. Geriatr. Soc.*, 42, 933, 1994.
128. Allen, L.H. and Casterline, J., Vitamin B_{12} deficiency in elderly individuals: diagnosis and requirements, *Am. J. Clin. Nutr.*, 60, 12, 1994.
129. Marcus, D.L. et al., Low serum B_{12} levels in a hematologically normal elderly subpopulation, *J. Am. Geriatr. Soc.*, 35, 635, 1987.
130. Lindenbaum, J. et al., Neuropsychiatric disorders caused by cobalamin deficiency in the absence of anemia or macrocytosis, *N. Engl. J. Med.*, 318, 1720, 1988.
131. Green, R., Metabolite assays in cobalamin and folate deficiency, *Baillières Clin. Haematol.*, 8, 533, 1995.
132. Allen, R.H. et al., Metabolic abnormalities in cobalamin (vitamin B_{12}) and folate deficiency, *FASEB J.*, 7, 1344, 1993.
133. Rogers, L.M. et al., High prevalence of cobalamin deficiency in Guatemalan school children: association with elevated serum methylmalonic acid and plasma homocysteine, and low plasma holotranscobalamin II concentrations, *Am. J. Clin. Nutr.*, 77, 433, 2003.
134. Rogers, L.M. et al., Predictors of cobalamin deficiency in Guatemalan school children: diet, *Helicobacter pylori*, or bacterial overgrowth? *J. Pediatr. Gastroenterol. Nutr.*, 36, 27, 2003.
135. Allen, L.H. et al., Vitamin B_{12} deficiency and malabsorption are highly prevalent in rural Mexican communities, *Am. J. Clin. Nutr.*, 62, 1013, 1995.
136. Gielchinsky, Y. et al., High prevalence of low serum vitamin B_{12} in a multi-ethnic Israeli population, *Br. J. Haematol.*, 115, 707, 2001.
137. Refsum, H. et al., Hyperhomocysteinemia and elevated methylmalonic acid indicate a high prevalence of cobalamin deficiency in Asian Indians, *Am. J. Clin. Nutr.*, 74, 233, 2001.
138. Hershko, C. et al., Variable hematological presentation of autoimmune gastritis: age-related progression from iron deficiency to cobalamin depletion, *Blood*, 107, 1673, 2006.
139. Green, R., Protean *H. pylori*: perhaps "pernicious" too? *Blood*, 107, 1247, 2006.
140. Inamdor-Deshmurkh, A.B. et al., Erythrocyte vitamin B_{12} activity in healthy Indian lactovegetarians, *Br. J. Haematol.*, 32, 395, 1976.
141. Jadhav, M. et al., Vitamin B_{12} deficiency in Indian infants: a clinical syndrome, *Lancet*, 2, 903, 1962.
142. Graham, S.M., Arvela, O.M., and Wise, G.A., Long-term neurologic consequences of nutritional vitamin B_{12} deficiency in infants, *J. Pediatr.*, 121, 710, 1992.

143. Higginbottom, M.C., Sweetman, L., and Nyhan, W.L., A syndrome of methylmalonic aciduria, homocystinuria, megaloblastic anemia and neurologic abnormalities in a vitamin B_{12}-deficient breast-fed infant of a strict vegetarian, *N. Engl. J. Med.*, 299, 317, 1978.
144. Schneede, J. et al., Methylmalonic acid and homocysteine in plasma as indicators of functional cobalamin deficiency in infants on macrobiotic diets, *Pediatr. Res.*, 36, 194, 1994.
145. van Dusseldorp, M. et al., Risk of persistent cobalamin deficiency in adolescents fed a macrobiotic diet in early life, *Am. J. Clin. Nutr.*, 69, 664, 1999.
146. Chanarin, I., *The Megaloblastic Anemias*, 2nd edition, Blackwell Scientific Publications, Oxford, 1979.
147. Carmel, R., Prevalence of undiagnosed pernicious anemia in the elderly, *Arch. Intern. Med.*, 156, 1097, 1996.
148. Carmel, R. et al., Profiles of black and Latin-American patients having pernicious anemia: HLA antigens, lymphocytotoxic antibody, anti-parietal cell antibody serum gastrin levels, and ABO blood groups, *Am. J. Clin. Pathol.*, 75, 291, 1981.
149. Solanki, D.L. et al., Pernicious anemia in blacks: a study of 64 patients from Washington, DC and Johannesburg, South Africa, *Am. J. Clin. Pathol.*, 75, 96, 1991.
150. Spivak, J.L., Masked megaloblastic anemia, *Arch. Intern. Med.*, 142, 2111, 1982.
151. MacLean, L.D., Rhode, B.M., and Shizgal, H.M., Nutrition following gastric operations for morbid obesity, *Ann. Surg.*, 198, 347, 1983.
152. Baik, H.W. and Russell, R.M., Vitamin B_{12} deficiency in the elderly, *Annu. Rev. Nutr.*, 19, 357, 1999.
153. Sipponen, et al., Prevalence of low vitamin B_{12} and high homocysteine in serum in an elderly male population: association with atrophic gastritis and *Helicobacter pylori* infection, *Scand. J. Gastroenterol.*, 38, 1209, 2003.
154. Santarelli, L. et al., Atrophic gastritis as a cause of hyperhomocysteinaemia, *Aliment. Pharmacol. Ther.*, 19,107, 2004.
155. Aimone-Gastin, I. et al., Prospective evaluation of protein bound vitamin B_{12} (cobalamin) malabsorption in the elderly using trout flesh labelled in vivo with 57Co-cobalamin, *Gut*, 41, 475, 1997.
156. Wood, I.J. et al., Vitamin B_{12} deficiency in chronic gastritis, *Gut*, 5, 27, 1964.
157. King, C.E. and Toskes, P.P., Small intestinal bacterial overgrowth, *Gastroenterology*, 76, 1035, 1979.
158. Blaser, M.J. and Brown, W.R., Campylobacters and gastroduodenal inflammation, *Adv. Intern. Med.*, 34, 21, 1989.
159. Dooley, C.P. et al., Prevalence of *Helicobacter pylori* infection and histologic gastritis in asymptomatic persons, *N. Engl. J. Med.*, 321, 1562, 1989.
160. Rauws, E.A.J. et al., Campylobacter pyloridis-associated chronic active antral gastritis, *Gastroenterology*, 94, 33, 1988.
161. Carmel, R., Perez-Perez, G.I., and Blaser, M.J., *Helicobacter pylori* and food-cobalamin malabsorption, *Dig. Dis. Sci.*, 39, 309, 1994.
162. Fong, T.-L. et al., *Helicobacter pylori* infection in pernicious anemia: a prospective controlled study, *Gastroenterology*, 100, 328, 1991.
163. Krasinski, S.D. et al., Fundic atrophic gastritis in an elderly population: effect on hemoglobin and several serum nutritional indicators, *J. Am. Geriatr. Soc.*, 34, 800, 1986.
164. Amess, J.A. et al., Megaloblastic haemopoiesis in patients receiving nitrous oxide, *Lancet*, 2, 339, 1978.
165. Layzer, R.B., Myeloneuropathy after prolonged exposure to nitrous oxide, *Lancet*, 2, 1227, 1978.
166. O'Leary, P.W., Combs, M.J., and Schilling, R.F., Synergistic deleterious effects of nitrous oxide exposure and vitamin B_{12} deficiency, *J. Lab. Clin. Med.*, 105, 428, 1985.
167. Scott, J.M. et al., Pathogenesis of subacute combined degeneration: a result of methyl group deficiency, *Lancet*, 2, 334, 1981.
168. Drummond, J.T. and Matthews, R.G., Nitrous oxide degradation by cobalamin-dependent methionine synthase: characterization of the reactants and products in the inactivation reaction, *Biochemistry*, 33, 3732, 1994.
169. Herbert, V. and Zalusky, R., Interrelations of vitamin B_{12} and folic acid metabolism: folic acid clearance studies, *J. Clin. Invest.*, 41, 1263, 1962.

170. Goulian, M., Bleile, B., and Tseng, B.Y. Methotrexate-induced misincorporation of uracil into DNA, *Proc. Natl. Acad. Sci.*, 77, 1956, 1980.
171. Wright, P.E. and Sears, D.A., Hypogammaglobulinemia and pernicious anemia, *South. Med. J.*, 80, 243, 1987.
172. Kätkä, K., Immune functions in pernicious anemia before and after treatment with vitamin B_{12}, *Scand. J. Haematol.*, 32, 76, 1984.
173. Hitzig, W.H. et al., Hereditary transcobalamin II deficiency: clinical findings in a new family, *J. Pediatr.*, 85, 622, 1974.
174. Green, R. and Kinsella, L.J., Current concepts in the diagnosis of cobalamin deficiency, *Neurology*, 45, 1435, 1995.
175. Dinn, J.J. et al., Methyl group deficiency in nerve tissue: a hypothesis to explain the lesion of subacute combined degeneration, *Ir. Med. J.*, 149, 1, 1980.
176. Frenkel, E.P., Abnormal fatty acid metabolism in peripheral nerves of patients with pernicious anemia, *J. Clin. Invest.*, 52, 1237, 1973.
177. Savage, D.G. and Lindenbaum, J., Neurological complications of acquired cobalamin deficiency: clinical aspects, *Baillières Clin. Haematol.*, 8, 657, 1995.
178. Karnaze, D.S. and Carmel, R., Low serum cobalamin levels in primary degenerative dementia: do some patients harbor atypical cobalamin deficiency states? *Arch. Intern. Med.*, 147, 429, 1987.
179. Jacques, P.F. et al., The effect of folic acid fortification on plasma folate and total homocysteine concentrations, *N. Engl. J. Med.*, 340, 1449, 1999.
180. Choumenkovitch, S.F. et al., Folic acid fortification increases red blood cell folate concentrations in the Framingham study, *J. Nutr.*, 131, 3277, 2001.
181. Honein, M.A. et al., Impact of folic acid fortification of the US food supply on the occurrence of neural tube defects, *JAMA*, 285, 2981, 2001.
182. Mills, J.L. et al., Low vitamin B_{12} concentrations in patients without anemia: the effect of folic acid fortification of grain, *Am. J. Clin. Nutr.*, 77, 1474, 2003.
183. Allen, R.H. et al., Diagnosis of cobalamin deficiency: I. Usefulness of serum methylmalonic acid and total homocysteine concentrations, *Am. J. Hematol.*, 34, 90, 1990.
184. Lindenbaum, J. et al., Diagnosis of cobalamin deficiency: II. Relative sensitivities of serum cobalamin, methylmalonic acid, and total homocysteine concentrations, *Am. J. Hematol.*, 34, 99, 1990.
185. Norman, E.J., Urinary methylmalonic acid/creatinine ratio: a gold standard test for tissue vitamin B_{12} deficiency, *J. Am. Geriatr. Soc.*, 47, 1158, 1999.
186. Herzlich, B. and Herbert, V., Depletion of serum holotranscobalamin II: an early sign of negative vitamin B_{12} balance, *Lab. Invest.*, 58, 332, 1988.
187. Stabler, S.P. and Allen, R.H., Vitamin B_{12} deficiency as a worldwide problem, *Annu. Rev. Nutr.*, 24, 299, 2004.
188. Dawson, D.W., Hoffbrand, A.V., and Worwood, M., Investigation of megaloblastic anemia and iron-deficiency anaemias, in *Practical Hematology*, 7th edition, Dacie, J.V. and Lewis, S.M., eds., Churchill Livingstone, NY, 397, 1991.
189. Wilson, D.H. et al., Development and multisite evaluation of an automated assay for B_{12} on the Abbott AxSYM analyzer, *Clin. Chem.*, 45, 428, 1999.
190. Raven, J.L. et al., Comparison of three methods for measuring vitamin B_{12} in serum: radioisotopic, *Euglena gracilis* and *Lactobacillus leichmannii*, *Br. J. Haematol.*, 22, 21, 1972.
191. Green, R. et al., The use of chicken serum for measurement of serum vitamin B_{12} concentration by radioisotope dilution: description of method and comparison with microbiological assay results, *Br. J. Haematol.*, 27, 507, 1974.
192. Lindgren et al., Holotranscobalamin—a sensitive marker of cobalamin malabsorption, *Eur. J. Clin. Invest.*, 29, 321, 1999.
193. Vu, T. et al., New assay for the rapid determination of plasma holotranscobalamin II levels: preliminary evaluation in cancer patients, *Am. J. Haematol.*, 42, 202, 1993.
194. Herbert, V. et al., Low holotranscobalamin II is the earliest serum marker for subnormal vitamin B_{12} (cobalamin) absorption in patients with AIDS, *Am. J. Haematol.*, 34, 132, 1990.
195. Herbert, V., Recommended dietary intakes (RDI) of vitamin B_{12} in humans, *Am. J. Clin. Nutr.*, 45, 671, 1987.

196. Guzik, H.J. et al., Prevalence of negative vitamin B_{12} balance in well and malnourished frail elderly, *J. Am. Geriatr. Assoc.*, 41, A412, 1993.
197. Jacob, E. and Herbert, V., Measurement of unsaturated "granulocyte-related" (TC I and TC III) and "liver-related" (TC II) B_{12} binders by instant batch separation using microfine precipitate of silica (QUSO G-32), *J. Lab. Clin. Med.*, 86, 505, 1975.
198. Wickramasinghe, S.N. and Ratnayaka, I.D., Limited value of serum holo-transcobalamin II measurements in the differential diagnosis of macrocytosis, *J. Clin. Pathol.*, 49, 755, 1996.
199. Goh, Y.T., Jacobsen, D.W., and Green, R., Diagnosis of functional cobalamin deficiency: utility of transcobalamin-bound vitamin B_{12} determination in conjunction with total serum homocysteine and methylmalonic acid, *Blood*, 78, 100a, 1991.
200. Lindemans, J., Schoester, M., and van Kapel, J., Application of a simple immunoadsorption assay for the measurement of saturated and unsaturated transcobalamin II and R-binders, *Clin. Chim. Acta*, 132, 53, 1983.
201. Van Kapel, J., Wouters, N.M.H., and Lindemans, J., Application of heparin-conjugated Sepharose for the measurement of cobalamin-saturated and unsaturated transcobalamin II and R-binders, *Clin. Chim. Acta*, 172, 297, 1988.
202. Ulleland, M. et al., Direct assay for cobalamin bound to transcobalamin (holo-transcobalamin) in serum, *Clin. Chem.*, 48, 526, 2002.
203. Orning, L. et al., Characterization of a monoclonal antibody with specificity for holo-transcobalamin, *Nutr. Metab. (Lond.)*, 3, 3, 2006.
204. Miller, J.W. et al., Measurement of total vitamin B_{12} and holotranscobalamin, singly and in combination, in screening for metabolic vitamin B_{12} deficiency, *Clin. Chem.*, 52, 278, 2006.
205. Herrmann, W. et al., Functional vitamin B_{12} deficiency and determination of holotranscobalamin in populations at risk, *Clin. Chem. Lab. Med.*, 41, 1478, 2003.
206. Obeid, R. et al., Vitamin B_{12} status in the elderly as judged by available biochemical markers, *Clin. Chem.*, 50, 238, 2004.
207. Lloyd-Wright, Z. et al., Holotranscobalamin as an indicator of dietary vitamin B_{12} deficiency, *Clin. Chem.*, 49, 2076, 2003.
208. Hvas, A.M. and Nexo E., Holotranscobalamin as a predictor of vitamin B_{12} status, *Clin. Chem. Lab. Med.*, 41, 1489, 2003.
209. Nexo, E. et al., Holo-transcobalamin is an early marker of changes in cobalamin homeostasis: a randomized placebo-controlled study, *Clin. Chem.*, 48, 1768, 2002.
210. Hvas, A.M. and Nexo, E., Holotranscobalamin–a first choice assay for diagnosing early vitamin B deficiency? *J. Intern. Med.*, 257, 289, 2005.
211. Remacha, A.F. et al., Vitamin B_{12} transport proteins in patients with HIV-1 infection and AIDS, *Haematologica*, 78, 84, 1993.
212. Marcell, P.D. et al., Quantitation of methylmalonic acid and other dicarboxylic acids in normal serum and urine using capillary gas chromatography-mass spectrometry, *Anal. Biochem.*, 150, 58, 1985.
213. Rasmussen, K., Solid-phase sample extraction for rapid determination of methylmalonic acid in serum and urine by a stable-isotope-dilution method, *Clin. Chem.*, 35, 260, 1989.
214. Kushnir, M.M. et al., Analysis of dicarboxylic acids by tandem mass spectrometry: high-throughput quantitative measurement of methylmalonic acid in serum, plasma, and urine, *Clin. Chem.*, 47, 1993, 2001.
215. Araki, A. and Sako, Y., Determination of free and total homocysteine in human plasma by high-performance liquid chromatography with fluorescence detection, *J. Chromatogr.*, 422, 43, 1987.
216. Jacobsen, D.W., Gatautis, V.J., and Green, R., Determination of plasma homocysteine by high-performance liquid chromatography with fluorescence detection, *Anal. Biochem.*, 178, 208, 1989.
217. Donnelly, J.G. and Pronovost, C., Evaluation of the Abbott IMx fluorescence polarization immunoassay and the bio-rad enzyme immunoassay for homocysteine: comparison with high-performance liquid chromatography, *Ann. Clin. Biochem.*, 37, 194, 2000.
218. Green, R. and Jacobsen, D.W., Clinical implications of hyperhomocysteinemia, in *Folate in Health and Disease*, Bailey, L.B., ed., Marcel Dekker, NY, 75, 1995.

219. Green, R., Screening for vitamin B_{12} deficiency: caveat emptor, *Ann. Intern. Med.*, 124, 509, 1996.
220. Clarke, R. et al., Screening for vitamin B_{12} and folate deficiency in older persons, *Am. J. Clin. Nutr.*, 77, 1241, 2003.
221. Stabler, S.P., Lindenbaum, J., and Allen, R.H., The use of homocysteine and other metabolites in the specific diagnosis of vitamin B_{12} deficiency, *J. Nutr.*, 126, 1266S, 1996.
222. Metz, J., The deoxyuridine suppression test, *Crit. Rev. Clin. Lab. Sci.*, 20, 205, 1984.
223. Taheri, M.R. et al., The effect of folate analogues and vitamin B_{12} on provision of thymine nucleotides for DNA synthesis in megaloblastic anemia, *Blood*, 59, 634, 1982.
224. Rose, M.S. and Chanarin, I., Studies on intrinsic factor antibodies, *Br. J. Haematol.*, 15, 325, 1968.
225. Bardhan, K.D. et al., Blocking and binding autoantibody to intrinsic factor, *Lancet*, I, 62, 1968.
226. Toh, B.H., van Driel, I.R., and Gleeson, P.A., Pernicious anemia, *N. Engl. J. Med.*, 337, 1441, 1997.
227. Bar-Shany, S. and Herbert, V., Transplacentally acquired antibody to intrinsic factor with vitamin B_{12} deficiency, *Blood*, 30, 777, 1967.
228. Goldberg, L.S., Barnett, E.V., and Desai, R., Effect of transplacental transfer of antibody to intrinsic factor, *Pediatrics*, 40, 851, 1967.
229. Fisher, J.M. and Taylor, K.B., Placental transfer of gastric antibodies, *Lancet*, I, 695, 1967.
230. Wodzinski, M.A. et al., Lymphocyte subpopulations in patients with hydroxycobalamin responsive megaloblastic anaemia, *J. Clin. Pathol.*, 38, 582, 1985.
231. De Aizpurua, H.J. et al., Autoantibodies cytotoxic to gastric parietal cells in serum of patients with pernicious anemia, *N. Engl. J. Med.*, 309, 625, 1983.
232. Rose, M.S. and Chanarin, I., Dissociation of intrinsic factor from its antibody: application to study of pernicious anemia gastric juice specimens, *Br. Med. J.*, i, 468, 1969.
233. Doniach, D. and Roitt, I.M., An evaluation of gastric and thyroid auto-immunity in relation to hematological disorders, *Semin. Hematol.*, I, 313, 1964.
234. De Aizpurua, H.J., Ungar, B., and Toh, B.H., Autoantibody to gastrin receptor in pernicious anemia, *N. Engl. J. Med.*, 313, 479, 1985.
235. Schilling, R., Intrinsic factor studies: II. The effect of gastric juice on the urinary excretion of radioactivity after the oral administration of radioactive B_{12}, *J. Lab. Clin. Med.*, 42, 860, 1953.
236. Carmel, R., Sinow, R.M., and Karnaze, D.S., Atypical cobalamin deficiency: subtle biochemical evidence of deficiency is commonly demonstrable in patients without megaloblastic anemia and is often associated with protein-bound cobalamin malabsorption, *J. Lab. Clin. Med.*, 109, 454, 1987.
237. Gozzard, D.I., Dawson, D.W., and Lewis, M.J., Experiences with dual protein bound aqueous vitamin B_{12} absorption test in subjects with low serum vitamin B_{12} concentrations, *J. Clin. Pathol.*, 40, 633, 1987.
238. Dawson, D.W., Sawers, A.H., and Sharma, R.K., Malabsorption of protein-bound vitamin B_{12}, *Br. Med. J. [Clin. Res.]*, 228, 675, 1984.
239. Jones, B.P. et al., Incidence and clinical significance of protein-bound vitamin B_{12} malabsorption, *Eur. J. Haematol.*, 38, 131, 1987.
240. Doscherholmen, A. and Swaim, W., Impaired assimilation of egg 57Co vitamin B_{12} in patients with hypochlorhydria and after gastric resection, *Gastroenterology*, 64, 913, 1973.
241. Carmel, R., Subtle and atypical cobalamin deficiency states, *Am. J. Hematol.*, 34, 108, 1990.
242. Scarlett, J.D., Read, H., and O'Dea, K., Protein-bound cobalamin absorption declines in the elderly, *Am. J. Hematol.*, 39, 79, 1992.
243. Bor, M.V., Nexo, E., and Hvas, A.M., Holo-transcobalamin concentration and transcobalamin saturation reflect recent vitamin B_{12} absorption better than does serum vitamin B_{12}, *Clin. Chem.*, 50, 1043, 2005.
244. Bor, M.V. et al., Nonradioactive vitamin B_{12} absorption test evaluated in controls and in patients with inherited malabsorption of vitamin B_{12}, *Clin. Chem.*, 51, 2151, 2005.
245. Martin, D.C. et al., Time dependency of cognitive recovery with cobalamin replacement: a report of a pilot study, *J. Am. Geriatr. Soc.*, 40, 168, 1992.
246. Abyad, A., Prevalence of vitamin B_{12} deficiency among demented patients and cognitive recovery with cobalamin replacement, *J. Nutr. Health Aging*, 6, 254, 2002.
247. Koury, M.J. et al., Apoptosis of late-stage erythroblasts in megaloblastic anemia: association with DNA damage and macrocyte production, *Blood*, 89, 4617, 1997.

248. Carmel, R. et al., The frequently low cobalamin levels in dementia usually signify treatable metabolic, neurologic and electrophysiologic abnormalities, *Eur. J. Haematol.*, 54, 245, 1995.
249. Karnaze, D.S. and Carmel, R., Neurologic and evoked potential abnormalities in subtle cobalamin deficiency states, including deficiency without anemia and with normal absorption of free cobalamin, *Arch. Neurol.*, 47, 1008, 1990.
250. Puri, V. et al., Vitamin B_{12} deficiency: a clinical and electrophysiological profile, *Electromyogr. Clin. Neurophysiol.*, 45, 273, 2005.
251. Misra, U.K., Kalita, J., and Das, A., Vitamin B_{12} deficiency neurological syndromes: a clinical, MRI and electrodiagnostic study, *Electromyogr. Clin. Neurophysiol.*, 43, 57, 2003.
252. Hemmer, B. et al., Subacute combined degeneration: clinical, electrophysiological, and magnetic resonance imaging findings, *J. Neurol. Neurosurg. Psychiatr.*, 65, 822, 1998.
253. Stabler, S.P. et al., Clinical spectrum and diagnosis of cobalamin deficiency, *Blood*, 76, 871, 1990.
254. Carmel, R., Subtle cobalamin deficiency, *Ann. Intern. Med.*, 124, 338, 1996.
255. Schilling, R.F. and Williams, W.J., Vitamin B_{12} deficiency: underdiagnosed, overtreated? *Hosp. Pract. (Minneap.)*, 30, 47, 1995.
256. Hvas, A.M., Ellegaard, J., and Nexo, E., Vitamin B_{12} treatment normalizes metabolic markers but has limited clinical effect: a randomized placebo-controlled study, *Clin. Chem.*, 47, 1396, 2001.
257. Lawson, D.H. et al., Hypokalemia in megaloblastic anemia, *Lancet*, 2, 588, 1970.
258. Crosby, W.H., Improvisation revisited: oral cyanocobalamin without intrinsic factor for pernicious anemia, *Arch. Intern. Med.*, 140, 1582, 1980.
259. Kuzminski, A.M. et al., Effective treatment of cobalamin deficiency with oral cobalamin, *Blood*, 92, 1191, 1998.
260. Sharabi, A. et al., Replacement therapy for vitamin B_{12} deficiency: comparison between the sublingual and oral route, *Br. J. Clin. Pharmacol.*, 56, 635, 2003.
261. Delpre, G., Stark, P., and Niv, Y., Sublingual therapy for cobalamin deficiency as an alternative to oral and parenteral cobalamin supplementation, *Lancet*, 354, 740, 1999.
262. Monto, R.W. and Rebuck, J.W., Observations on the mechanism of intranasal absorption of vitamin B_{12} in pernicious anemia, *Blood*, 10, 1151, 1955.
263. Slot, W.B. et al., Normalization of plasma vitamin B_{12} concentration by intranasal hydroxycobalamin in vitamin B_{12}-deficient patients, *Gastroenterology*, 113, 430, 1997.
264. Kadner, R.J., Repression of synthesis of the vitamin B_{12} receptor in *Escherichia coli*, *J. Bacteriol.*, 136, 1050, 1978.
265. Wei, B.Y., Bradbeer, C., and Kadner, R.J., Conserved structural and regulatory regions in the Salmonella typhimurium btuB gene for the outer membrane vitamin B_{12} transport protein, *Res. Microbiol.*, 143, 459, 1992.
266. Escalente-Semerena, J.C. and Roth, J.R., Regulation of cobalamin biosynthetic operons in *Salmonella typhimurium*, *J. Bacteriol.*, 169, 2251, 1987.
267. Franklund, C.V. and Kadner, R.J., Multiple transcribed elements control expression of the *Escherichia coli* btuB gene, *J. Bacteriol.*, 179, 4039, 1997.
268. Nou, X. and Kadner, R.J., Coupled changes in translation and transcription during cobalamin-dependent regulation of btuB expression in *Escherichia coli*, *J. Bacteriol.*, 180, 6719, 1998.
269. Nou, X. and Kadner, R.J., Adenosylcobalamin inhibits ribosome binding to btuB RNA, *Proc. Natl. Acad. Sci.*, 97, 7190, 2000.
270. Ravnum, S. and Andersson, D.L., An adenosyl-cobalamin (coenzyme-B_{12})-repressed translational enhancer in the cob mRNA of Salmonella typhimurium, *Mol. Microbiol.*, 39, 1585, 2001.
271. Nahvi, A. et al., Genetic control by a metabolite binding mRNA, *Chem. Biol.*, 9, 1043, 2002.
272. Hasselberth, J.R. and Ellington, A.D., A (ribo) switch in the paradigms of genetic regulation, *Nature Struct. Biol.*, 9, 891, 2002.
273. Mandel, M. et al., Riboswitches control fundamental biochemical pathways in Bacillus subtilis and other bacteria, *Cell*, 113, 577, 2003.
274. Mangum, J.H. and North, J.A., Vitamin B_{12}-dependent methionine biosynthesis in HEp-2 cells, *Biochem. Biophys. Res. Commun.*, 32, 105, 1968.
275. Mangum, J.H., Murray, B.K., and North, J.A., Vitamin B_{12} dependent methionine biosynthesis in cultured mammalian cells, *Biochemistry*, 8, 3496, 1969.

276. Kerwar, S.S. et al., Studies on vitamin B_{12} metabolism in HeLa cells, *Arch. Biochem. Biophys.*, 142, 231, 1971.
277. Gulati, S., Brody, L.C., and Banerjee, R., Posttranscriptional regulation of mammalian methionine synthase by B_{12}, *Biochem. Biophys. Res. Commun.*, 259, 436, 1999.
278. Oltean, S. and Banerjee, R., Nutritional modulation of gene expression and homocysteine utilization by vitamin B_{12}, *J. Biol. Chem.*, 278, 20778, 2003.
279. Oltean, S. and Banerjee, R., A B_{12}-responsive internal ribosome entry site (IRES) element in human methionine synthase, *J. Biol. Chem.*, 280, 32662, 2005.
280. Scalabrino, G. et al., Subacute combined degeneration and induction of ornithine decarboxylase in spinal cord of totally gastrectomized rats, *Lab. Invest.*, 62,297, 1990.
281. Scalabrino, G. et al., Enhanced levels of biochemical markers for cobalamin deficiency in totally gastrectomized rats: uncoupling of the enhancement from the severity of spongy vacuolation in spinal cord, *Exp. Neurol.*, 144, 258, 1997.
282. Buccellato, F.R. et al., Myelinolytic lesions in the spinal cord of cobalamin-deficient rats are TNF-α-mediated, *FASEB J.*, 13, 297, 1999.
283. Peracchi, M. et al., Human cobalamin deficiency: alterations in serum tumour necrosis factor-α and epidermal growth factor, *Eur. J. Haematol.*, 67, 123, 2001.
284. Scalabrino, G. et al., High tumor necrosis factor-alpha levels in cerebrospinal fluid of cobalamin-deficient patients, *Ann. Neurol.*, 56, 886, 2004.
285. Miller, J.W., Vitamin B_{12} deficiency, tumor necrosis factor-alpha, and epidermal growth factor: a novel function for vitamin B_{12}? *Nutr. Rev.*, 60, 142, 2002.
286. Yamashiki, M., Nishimura, A., and Kosaka, Y., Effects of methylcobalamin (vitamin B_{12}) on in vitro cytokine production of peripheral blood mononuclear cells, *J. Clin. Lab. Immunol.*, 37, 173, 1992.
287. Weinberg, J.B. et al., Inhibition of productive human immunodeficiency virus-1 infection by cobalamins, *Blood*, 86, 1281, 1995.
288. Tang, A.M. et al., Low serum vitamin B_{12} concentrations are associated with faster human immunodeficiency virus type 1 (HIV-1) disease progression, *J. Nutr.*, 127, 345, 1997.
289. Schneider, Z. and Stroinski, A., *Comprehensive B_{12}*, De Gruyter, Berlin, 1987.
290. Amagasaki, T., Green, R., and Jacobsen, D.W., Expression of transcobalamin II receptors by human leukemia K562 and HL-60 cells, *Blood*, 76, 1380, 1990.
291. Collins, D.A. et al., Biodistribution of radiolabeled adenosylcobalamin in patients diagnosed with various malignancies, *Mayo Clin. Proc.*, 75, 568, 2000.
292. Smeltzer, C.C. et al., Synthesis and characterization of fluorescent cobalamin (CobalaFluor) derivatives for imaging, *Org. Lett.*, 3, 799, 2001.
293. McGreevy, J.M., Cannon, M.J., and Grissom, C.B., Minimally invasive lymphatic mapping using fluorescently labeled vitamin B_{12}, *J. Surg. Res.*, 111, 38, 2003.
294. Bagnato, J.D. et al., Synthesis and characterization of a cobalamin-colchicine conjugate as a novel tumor-targeted cytotoxin, *J. Org. Chem.*, 69, 8987, 2004.
295. Choi, S.W., Vitamin B_{12} deficiency: a new risk factor for breast cancer? *Nutr. Rev.*, 57, 250, 1999.
296. Wu, K. et al., A prospective study on folate, B_{12}, and pyridoxal 5′-phosphate (B_6) and breast cancer, *Cancer Epidemiol. Biomarkers Prev.*, 8, 209, 1999.
297. Zhang, S.M. et al., Plasma folate, vitamin B_6, vitamin B_{12}, homocysteine, and risk of breast cancer, *J. Natl. Cancer Inst.*, 95, 373, 2003.
298. Dhonukshe-Rutten, R.A. et al., Vitamin B_{12} status is associated with bone mineral content and bone mineral density in frail elderly women but not in men, *J. Nutr.*, 133, 801, 2003.
299. Stone, K.L. et al., Low serum vitamin B_{12} levels are associated with increased hip bone loss in older women: a prospective study, *J. Clin. Endocrinol. Metab.*, 89, 1217, 2004.
300. Dhonukshe-Rutten, R.A. et al., Low bone mineral density and bone mineral content are associated with low cobalamin status in adolescents, *Eur. J. Nutr.*, 44, 341, 2005.
301. Tucker, K.L. et al., Low plasma vitamin B_{12} is associated with lower BMD: the Framingham osteoporosis study, *J. Bone Miner. Res.*, 20, 152, 2005.
302. Dhonukshe-Rutten, R.A. et al., Homocysteine and vitamin B_{12} status relate to bone turnover markers, broadband ultrasound attenuation, and fractures in healthy elderly people, *J. Bone Miner. Res.*, 20, 921, 2005.

303. Morris, M.S., Jacques, P.F., and Selhub, J., Relation between homocysteine and B-vitamin status indicators and bone mineral density in older Americans, *Bone*, 37, 234, 2005.
304. Carmel, R. et al., Cobalamin and osteoblast-specific proteins, *N. Engl. J. Med.*, 319, 70, 1988.
305. Kim, G.S. et al., Effects of vitamin B_{12} on cell proliferation and cellular alkaline phosphatase activity in human bone marrow stromal osteoprogenitor cells and UMR106 osteoblastic cells, *Metabolism*, 45, 1443, 1996.
306. van Meurs, J.B. et al., Homocysteine levels and the risk of osteoporotic fracture, *N. Engl. J. Med.*, 350, 2033, 2004.
307. McLean, R.R. et al., Homocysteine as a predictive factor for hip fracture in older persons, *N. Engl. J. Med.*, 350, 2042, 2004.
308. Sato, Y. et al., Effect of folate and mecobalamin on hip fractures in patients with stroke: a randomized controlled trial, *JAMA*, 293, 1082, 2005.
309. Houston, D.K. et al., Age-related hearing loss, vitamin B_{12}, and folate in elderly women, *Am. J. Clin. Nutr.*, 69, 564, 1999.
310. Shemesh, Z. et al., Vitamin B_{12} deficiency in patients with chronic-tinnitus and noise-induced hearing loss, *Am. J. Otolaryngol.*, 2, 94, 1993.
311. Ray, J.G., Folic acid food fortification in Canada, *Nutr. Rev.*, 62, S35, 2004.
312. Ray, J.G. and Blom, H.J., Vitamin B_{12} insufficiency and the risk of fetal neural tube defects, *QJM*, 96, 289, 2003.

14 Choline

Timothy A. Garrow

CONTENTS

INTRODUCTION

Optimal nutrition requires dietary choline but this nutrient is not a vitamin. The functions of choline in animals have no resemblance to the B vitamins, vitamin C, or the fat-soluble vitamins. The relatively large daily requirement humans have for choline (~0.5 g/day) and its metabolism are more akin to the amino acids than any other class of nutrients. Choline is made from serine and methionine, and its oxidation in the mitochondria is an energy-yielding process. Biochemically, choline is required for phospholipid and acetylcholine biosynthesis, and its oxidation to betaine and ultimately glycine is important for osmolyte homeostasis and one-carbon metabolism, respectively.

This chapter focuses on the role of choline in mammalian biology. There have been many reviews on different aspects of choline chemistry and biology and the reader is referred to several excellent sources of additional information [1–10], including earlier editions of this handbook.

HISTORY

Choline was discovered by Adolph Strecker in 1862 [11]. He isolated the platinum salt of a substance from pig and oxen gall with the chemical formula of $C_5H_{13}NO$, $HCl + PtCl_2$, which he termed cholin and correctly surmised it to be an ammonium base. In 1868, he later went on to show that choline is an integral part of egg yolk lecithin and cites Wurtz as the first to chemically synthesize choline by heating ethylene oxide with trimethylamine under acidic conditions [12]. Later, choline was shown to be a component of sphingomyelin [13,14]. Other key discoveries include the elucidation of the pathway for the biosynthesis of choline by du Vigneaud et al. in 1941 [15], its incorporation into phosphatidylcholine (lecithin) by Kennedy and Weiss in 1956 [16], and the potent pharmacological actions of acetylcholine by Hunt and Taveau in 1906 [17].

The nutritional importance of choline was first recognized by its lipotrope action. Lipotrope is a term that was coined for compounds that prevent the accumulation of neutral lipid in the liver. Best and Huntsman showed in depancreatized dogs maintained on insulin that phosphatidylcholine conferred lipotrope activity [18,19]. Fatty liver is the most well-known outcome of choline deficiency, a symptom that occurs rapidly in every animal species tested, including monkeys [20]. Long-term choline deficiency has been shown to lead to the development of liver cancer in rodents, a pathology that occurs in part because of the complications associated with prolonged fatty infiltration as well as other independent mechanisms caused by the deficiency [21–24]. The importance of choline for liver function represents the basis for its relatively recent designation by the National Academy of Sciences (United States) as an essential nutrient for humans. Removing choline from the diet of adult men resulted in a decrease in plasma choline and an elevation of serum alanine aminotransferase levels, despite adequate levels of dietary methionine, folic acid, and vitamin B_{12} [25]. Before its designation as an essential nutrient, choline was excluded from this status because of its well-characterized pathway of biosynthesis and the lack of a human deficiency syndrome, the latter due to its abundance in many commonly consumed foods. Although supplemental methionine reportedly oblates the need for dietary choline as a growth stimulant in all animals tested except chicks [26], such a diet cannot be recommended for humans because the combination of high dietary methionine coupled with low choline will likely result in elevated levels of plasma total homocysteine ([27] and references therein), a proposed risk factor for vascular diseases and thrombosis [28–30].

CHEMISTRY

STRUCTURE, NOMENCLATURE, AND CHEMICAL PROPERTIES

The structure of choline and choline-containing biomolecules can be seen in Figure 14.1 and Figure 14.2. Free choline [2-hydroxy-*N,N,N*-trimethylethanaminium or (b-hydroxyethyl) trimethylammonium], $(CH_3)_3N^+CH_2CH_2CH_2OH$, is an organic base that is very hydroscopic. It is soluble in water and alcohol but not in chloroform or ether. The most common salts used in diet formulations are choline chloride (trade names: Biocolinea, Hepacholine, and Lipotil)

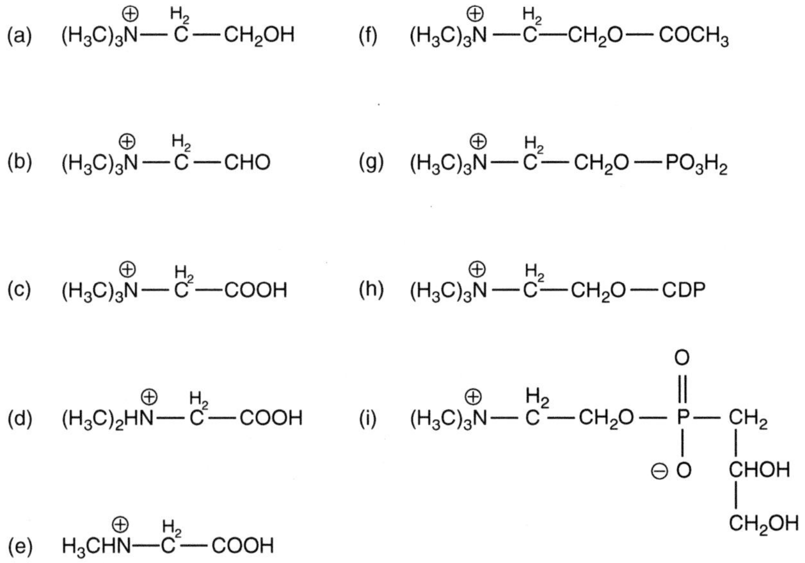

(a) $(H_3C)_3N^{\oplus}{-}CH_2{-}CH_2OH$ (f) $(H_3C)_3N^{\oplus}{-}CH_2{-}CH_2O{-}COCH_3$

(b) $(H_3C)_3N^{\oplus}{-}CH_2{-}CHO$ (g) $(H_3C)_3N^{\oplus}{-}CH_2{-}CH_2O{-}PO_3H_2$

(c) $(H_3C)_3N^{\oplus}{-}CH_2{-}COOH$ (h) $(H_3C)_3N^{\oplus}{-}CH_2{-}CH_2O{-}CDP$

(d) $(H_3C)_2HN^{\oplus}{-}CH_2{-}COOH$ (i) $(H_3C)_3N^{\oplus}{-}CH_2{-}CH_2O{-}P(=O)(O^{\ominus}){-}CH_2{-}CHOH{-}CH_2OH$

(e) $H_3CHN^{\oplus}{-}CH_2{-}COOH$

FIGURE 14.1 The structure of choline and derived water-soluble metabolites. The structures of (a) choline, (b) betaine aldehyde, (c) betaine, (d) dimethylglycine, (e) sarcosine, (f) acetylcholine, (g) phosphocholine, (h) CDP-choline, and (i) glycerophosphocholine are shown.

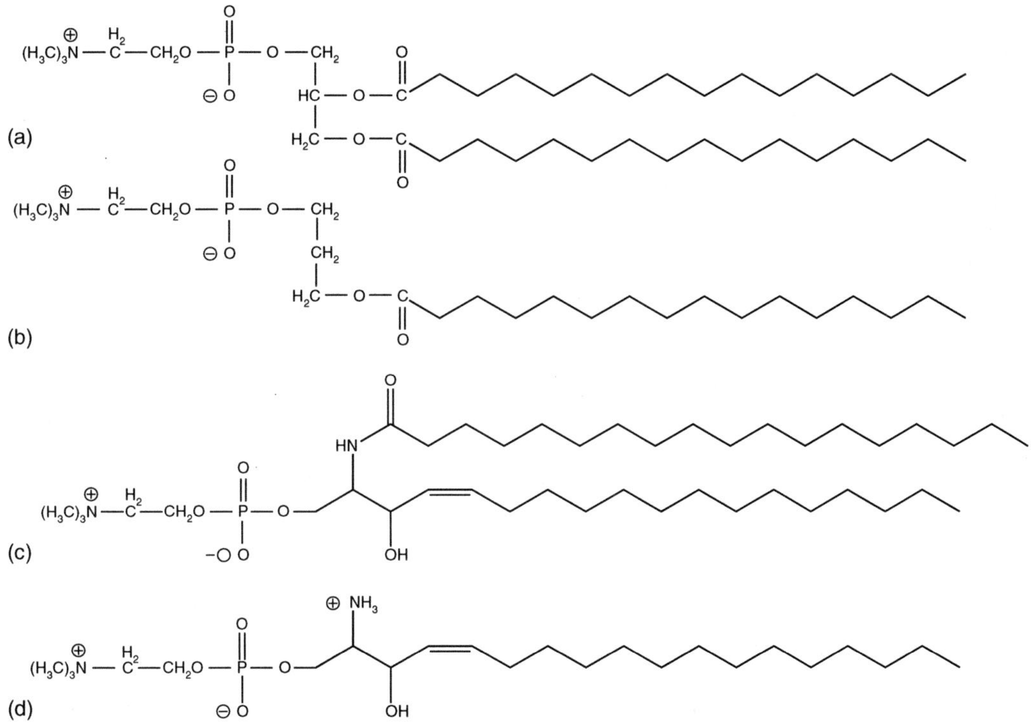

(a) $(H_3C)_3N^{\oplus}{-}CH_2{-}CH_2O{-}P(=O)(O^{\ominus}){-}O{-}CH_2{-}HC(O{-}C(=O){-}R){-}H_2C{-}O{-}C(=O){-}R$

(b) $(H_3C)_3N^{\oplus}{-}CH_2{-}CH_2O{-}P(=O)(O^{\ominus}){-}O{-}CH_2{-}CH_2{-}H_2C{-}O{-}C(=O){-}R$

(c) $(H_3C)_3N^{\oplus}{-}CH_2{-}CH_2O{-}P(=O)(-O){-}O{-}$ ... HN, OH

(d) $(H_3C)_3N^{\oplus}{-}CH_2{-}CH_2O{-}P(=O)(O^{\ominus}){-}O{-}$ ... $^{\oplus}NH_3$, OH

FIGURE 14.2 The structure of lipid-soluble choline-containing metabolites. The structures of (a) phosphatidylcholine, (b) lysophosphatidylcholine, (c) sphingomyelin, and (d) lysosphingomyelin are shown. Note that the fatty acid composition, both aliphatic chain length and degree of saturation, can vary in these metabolites.

and choline bitartrate, the latter of which has largely supplanted the use of the former because it is less hydroscopic. Choline is commonly made from trimethylamine and ethylene chlorohydrin or ethylene oxide (U.S. Patent 2,774,759 to American Cyanamid). It decomposes in alkaline solutions releasing trimethylamine.

Choline Antagonists

There have been hundreds of compounds made to probe the biochemistry and metabolism choline and its derived metabolites. One of the first choline antagonists used in animals was 2-amino-2-methyl-1-propanol. This compound slows choline synthesis and oxidation and causes many of the symptoms associated with choline deficiency [31–34]. Diethanolamine is an environmental contaminant that is a choline antagonist. It has been shown to cause hepatic choline deficiency and liver cancer in rodents [4,35,36]. Choline-specific transporters are inhibited to varying degrees by hemicholinium-3. This compound has been particularly useful in the classification of choline transporters [37]. Hemicholinium-3 is also a weak inhibitor of choline kinase (CK) [38]. Triethylcholine and homocholine have also been used to characterize choline transport mechanisms [39,40], and these and other *N*-ethyl analogs of choline have been studied as false neurotransmitters [41–43]. A new inhibitor, *N*-cyclohexylcholine, has been shown to be a high-affinity ligand for the blood–brain barrier choline transporter [44]. Ever since the development of the cholinergic hypothesis of decline in dementia, inhibitors of acetylcholine degradation have been developed. There are four acetycholine esterase (AChE) inhibitors currently used to treat dementia, namely, tacrine, donepezil, riastigmine, and galantamine [45]. Analogs of *trans*-1-methyl-4-(1-naphthylvinyl)-pyridinium are potent inhibitors of choline acetyltransferase (ChAT) [46]. Because phosphocholine is now known to be a signaling molecule that has a role in cell proliferation there is renewed interest in the development of CK inhibitors. The structure of new inhibitors [47,48] as well as the more classical CK inhibitors have been recently reviewed [38]. Finally, specific- and high-affinity inhibitors have been made for betaine-homocysteine S-methyltransferase (BHMT) [49], an enzyme in the pathway of choline oxidation. Treating mice with one of these inhibitors, carboxybutylhomocysteine, blocks the enzyme in vivo [27].

ASSAY PROCEDURES

Many procedures have been developed to quantify the various metabolites of choline in different matrixes. Most methods are restricted to choline and one or two other choline-containing metabolites. However, after choline was classified as an essential nutrient for humans [20] and the U.S. FDA allowed health claims for choline [50] quantifying choline and all the choline-containing compounds in foods has attracted greater attention. In brief, choline and acetylcholine can be measured using a classic radioisotope method [51] or one of several newer methods that employ liquid chromatography with electrochemical or fluorescent detection [52–54], continuous-flow fast atom bombardment mass spectrometry [55], or biosensor technology [56]. The combination of liquid or gas chromatography with various mass spectrometer techniques [57,58] or proton nuclear magnetic resonance [59] has greatly expanded the number of metabolites of choline that can be accurately measured from a single sample. A recent procedure using liquid chromatography with electrospray ionization–isotope dilution mass spectrometry enables researchers to measure all of the major choline metabolites in foods or tissues [60]. This method was recently employed to generate the most comprehensive database of total choline in foods to date [61]. In addition, there is an AOAC method (*Official Method 999.14*) for the determination of choline in milk and infant formulas [62,63]. This method is simple and does not require expensive equipment, although it only measures total choline content and not the distribution of the choline moiety in various molecules. The AOAC method is based on the principle that choline-containing compounds can by hydrolyzed by acid or base to generate free choline, and, following neutralization, the sample can be treated with bacterial choline oxidase to convert choline to betaine while generating two equivalents of hydrogen peroxide. The hydrogen peroxide generated is then used for the peroxidase-dependent oxidation of phenol, which in turn reacts with 4-aminoantipyrine to generate a quinoneimine chromophore. This method was recently adapted to measure the total choline content of dietary supplements [64].

CONTENT IN FOOD

Zeisel et al. [61] recently published a comprehensive evaluation of the choline content of 145 commonly consumed foods. Measurements included choline, phosphocholine, glycerophosphocholine, phosphatidylcholine, and sphingomyelin. The amount of acetylcholine and cytidinediphosphocholine (CDP-choline) in foods is negligible. The sum of all of these forms was added to give a total choline value since all of the choline derivatives mentioned earlier can be metabolically converted to free choline (Figure 14.3).

All whole and unprocessed foods contain some choline. In terms of total choline, the richest sources (mg/100 g) are beef liver (418), chicken liver (290), eggs (251), wheat germ (152), bacon (125), soybeans (116), and pork (103) [61]. Of these rich sources, the predominant form is phosphatidylcholine, which is 95% of the choline in eggs and about 55%–70% of the choline in meats and soybeans. In wheat germ the predominant form is free choline (45%), while phosphatidylcholine is the second most abundant form (30%). In general, whole fruits and vegetables contain about 5–40 mg total choline/100 g [61].

An important metabolite derived from choline, betaine (Figure 14.4), has also been quantified in foods [60,65,66]. The level of betaine in foods varies, particularly in plants, because its concentration increases in tissues during periods of water or salt stress [67]. In general, wheat products are good sources of betaine, with the germ and the bran being very rich sources (>1000 mg/100 g product). Other rich sources include shellfish, such as shrimp, mussel, oyster, and scallops (100–1000 mg/100 g product). In general, fruits and vegetables contain much less betaine (<10 mg/100 g product), except beets and spinach, which are good sources (~100–600 mg/100 g product). Choline and betaine are stable during different cooking procedures, although betaine [65] and presumably the water-soluble forms of choline can leach from boiled foods. The free choline content of foods can increase following mechanical disruption (dicing, grinding) because of the release of phospholipase activity [60].

METABOLISM

ABSORPTION, TRANSPORT, AND PLASMA CONCENTRATIONS

Choline bioavailability is linked to fat absorption since phosphatidylcholine is the predominant source of dietary choline. Most dietary fat is triglyceride (>95%), with the remainder containing some phosphatidylcholine and lesser amounts of sphingomyelin and other choline metabolites. Phosphatidylcholine is hydrolyzed by pancreatic and intestinal phospholipase A_2 to form lysophosphatidylcholine, which is absorbed into the mucosal cell by passive diffusion [68]. Much of the absorbed lysophosphatidylcholine is reacylated back to phosphatidylcholine and secreted into the lymph with the chylomicron particle. Significant amounts of absorbed lysophosphatidylcholine can also be deacylated by intestinal phospholipase B to form glycerophosphocholine and a fatty acid [6]. Dietary sphingomyelin is hydrolyzed by an intestinal alkaline sphingomyelinase to form ceramide and phosphocholine [69]. Phosphocholine is hydrolyzed by intestinal phosphatase to form free choline. Little is known about the digestion

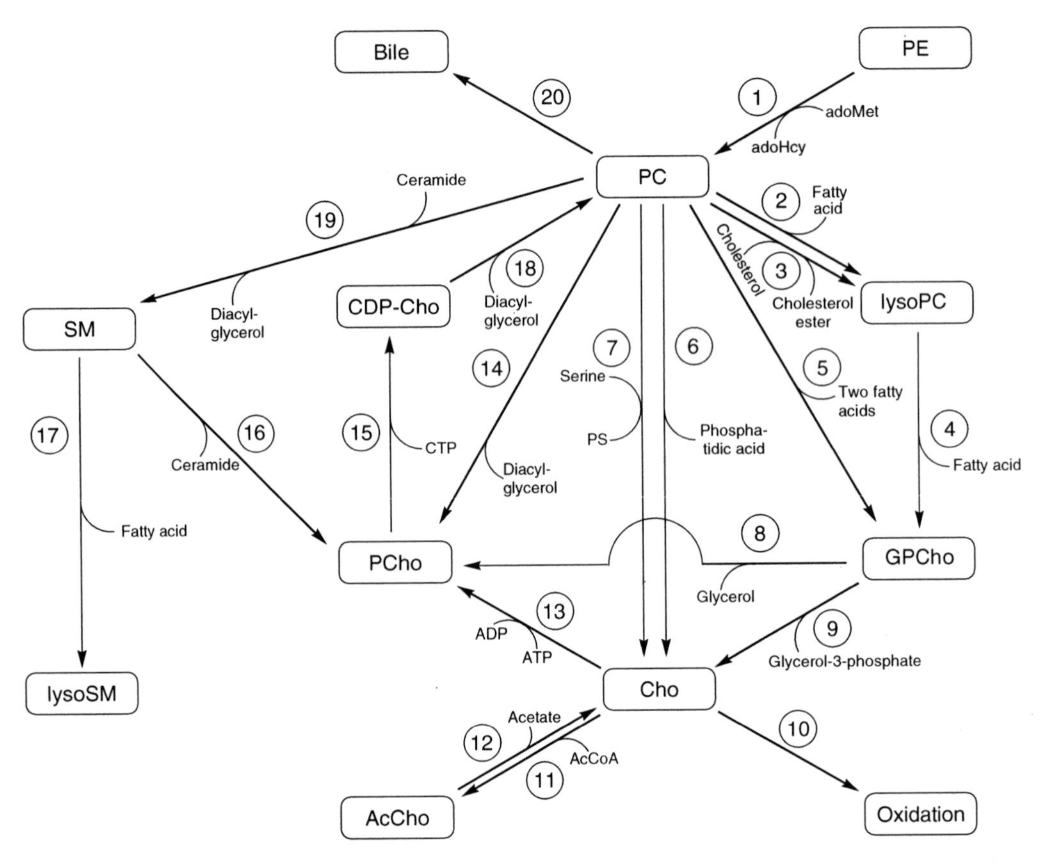

FIGURE 14.3 Choline metabolism. The enzyme reactions of choline metabolism are (1) phoshatidylethanolamine methyltransferase (PEMT); (2) phospholipase A_2; (3) lecithin–cholesterol acyltransferase (LCAT); (4) lysophospholipase; (5) phospholipase B; (6) phospholipase D; (7) phosphatidylserine synthase-1; (8) and (9) glycerophosphodiester phosphodiesterases; (10) choline oxidations enzymes (see Figure 14.4); (11) choline acetyltransferase (ChAT); (12) acetylcholine esterase (AChE); (13) choline kinase (CK); (14) phospholipase C; (15) CTP:phosphocholine cytidylyltransferase (CT); (16) sphingomyelinases; (17) sphingomyeline deacylase; (18) cholinephophotransferase (CPT); (19) sphingomyelin synthase; and (20) multidrug-resistance protein-3 (human MDR-3). Diagram abbreviations: AcCho, acetylcholine; adoHcy, S-adenosylhomocysteine; adoMet, S-adenosylmethionine; CDP, cytosine diphosphate; CDP-Cho, cytosine diphosphate Cho; CDP-choline, cytosine diphosphate choline; CTP, cytosine triphosphate; GPCho, glycerophosphocholine; lysoPC, lysophosphatidylcholine; lysoSM, lysosphingomyelin; PCho, phosphocholine; PC, phosphatidylcholine; PE, phosphatidylethanolamine; PS, phosphatidylserine; and SM, sphingomyelin.

and the absorption of the other choline metabolites. The choline released from sphingomyelin degradation and that found in the diet are absorbed through a sodium-independent choline transporter that is moderately sensitive to hemicholinium-3 inhibition. The properties of this uptake mechanism are consistent with the intermediate-affinity choline transporter-like (CTL) family of transporters described later. The concentration of free choline in plasma ranges from 10 to 50 μM [37], the variation reflecting recent intake [6,70]. Betaine, an oxidation product of choline, is also found in the diet and is absorbed by the IMINO proline transporter [71]. The concentration of betaine in plasma ranges from 25 to 50 μM [72,73], and its uptake by tissues is discussed in conjunction with osmolyte regulation (section Osmotic Regulation).

Choline is a positively charged quaternary amine and its entrance into cells requires protein-mediated transfer. Biochemically, choline transport has been classified into three

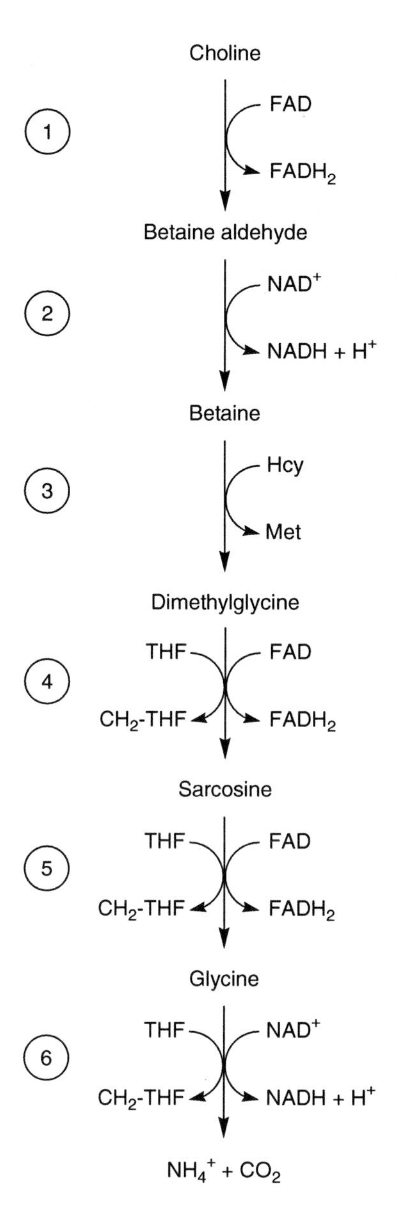

FIGURE 14.4 Choline oxidation. The enzymes of choline oxidation are (1) choline dehydrogenase (CHDH); (2) betaine-aldehyde dehydrogenase (BADH); (3) betaine-homocysteine S-methyltransferase (BHMT); (4) dimethylglycine dehydrogenase; and (5) sarcosine dehydrogenase. Reaction 6 is catalyzed by the glycine cleavage system. All of the reactions shown are mitochondrial, except BHMT, which is cytosolic.

general phenomena based on kinetic studies with radiolabeled choline: (i) low-affinity ($K_m > 30$–$100\ \mu M$) facilitative diffusion that is insensitive to hemicholinium-3, (ii) intermediate-affinity sodium-independent transport that is moderately sensitive to hemicholinium-3 inhibition, and (iii) high-affinity ($K_m < 10\ \mu M$) sodium-dependent transport that is very sensitive to hemicholinium-3 inhibition [37]. A given cell may express more than one of these general classes of transporters. In general, the low- and intermediate-affinity systems are used to transport choline through the plasma membrane and for some other unique choline transport needs, for example, the blood–brain barrier, mitochondrial and intestinal transporters. The high-affinity system is unique to the cholinergic neurons. Choline transport has been reported to be rate-limiting for acetylcholine synthesis [74] and for the oxidation of choline to betaine in the mitochondria [75]. In recent years there has been significant progress elucidating the molecular biology of choline transporters and assigning their genes to the biochemical classes of choline transporters mentioned earlier [37,74,76–78].

The high-affinity choline transport system is specific to the cholinergic neurons of the brain, brain stem, and spinal cord. This system is now believed to be the product of one gene, which has been cloned from several mammalian species [37,74]. The gene has been designated *CHT1* and it encodes a 63 kDa protein whose function is sodium-dependent. Its primary sequence has consensus motifs for several kinases and there is emerging evidence that the transport of choline through CHT1 is inhibited by protein kinase C-dependent phosphorylation [74]. Because this transporter can be rate-limiting for acetylcholine synthesis, a neurotransmitter required for normal central and peripheral nervous system function, further study of the structure and function of CHT1 promises to yield results with therapeutic potential. For example, abnormal cholinergic function is associated with some neurodegenerative diseases, including Alzheimer's, Parkinson's, and amyotrophic lateral sclerosis [37,74].

The intermediate-affinity transporters are encoded by a family of five genes, CTL1–5 (choline-specific transporter-like proteins), some of which produce complex alternative splice variants [37,79]. Many tissues express one or more CTL genes, but the CTL1 gene has been the most thoroughly characterized. The deduced protein sequences of the two known splice variants (hCTL1a and hCTL1b) of human CTL1 are composed of 657 and 654 residues [37] and each contains five putative protein kinase C phosphorylation sites. Expression of both isoforms in cultured cells indicates little-to-no sodium dependence for choline transport [37]. The CHT1 and CTL families of transporters are specific for choline.

Three organic cation transporters, OTC1, OTC2, and OTC3, are members of the solute carrier superfamily (SLC) of transporters and are low-affinity transporters of choline. These transporters have broad specificity and further work is required to clarify their precise role in choline transport in vivo [37,80]. These transporters are expressed in many tissues, are about 60–65 kDa, and *OTC1* and *OTC2* are known to produce at least one splice variant [80].

Tissue Deposition and Storage

There have been very few studies that have investigated the quantities and the distribution of all the choline metabolites in the major organs of mammals. Most of the choline in the body is found in the form of phosphatidylcholine [57,60]. For example, in rodent liver phosphatidylcholine accounts for 90% of the total choline. Lysophosphatidylcholine and phosphocholine generally account for an additional 7%–9%, whereas free choline is only 0.5%–1% of the total tissue choline. Liver and brain contain about 25 μmol total choline/g tissue [57,60], whereas muscle, heart, and kidney contain about 20%–30% of that found in liver and brain. Each organ has a similar distribution of choline metabolites except kidney, which contains significantly more glycerophosphocholine, presumably for osmotic control (section Osmotic Regulation). There are no known mechanisms to store choline in tissues. All of the molecules that contain the choline moiety are either intermediates in pathways, signaling molecules, or reside in lipid bilayers providing structural and functional properties to membranes. Although pathway intermediates, particularly phosphocholine, can fluctuate because of recent intake, there is no evidence indicating that these metabolite changes are nothing other than a transient mass–action effect. Rather, excess choline is catabolized via the choline oxidation pathway (section Choline Oxidation).

Cellular Metabolism

Biosynthesis and Turnover of Phosphatidylcholine

Phosphatidylcholine can be synthesized in animals by the S-adenosylmethionine-dependent methylation of phosphatidylethanolamine, which is catalyzed by phosphatidylethanolamine methyltransferase (PEMT). This enzyme is liver-specific and accounts for about 30% of the phosphatidylcholine made in hepatocytes [81]. PEMT knockout mice have an absolute requirement for dietary choline. Lack of dietary choline results in a dramatic reduction of phosphatidylcholine and the accumulation of triglycerides in the liver, and the mice live only 3–5 days [82]. The liver damage in these mice can be reversed by supplemental choline [83], but levels of liver phosphocholine remain lower than normal [84]. These mice also have lower levels of plasma total homocysteine and their hepatocytes secrete less homocysteine [85,86], indicating that PEMT-dependent biosynthesis of phosphatidylcholine is a major draw on the S-adenosylmethionine pool.

Other nucleated cells of the body rely solely on the CDP-choline pathway for phosphatidylcholine biosynthesis (Figure 14.3), whereas the liver synthesizes about 70% of its phosphatidylcholine via this pathway [81]. The CDP-choline pathway requires free choline and is composed of three enzymes: CK, CTP:phosphocholine cytidylyltransferase (CT), and CDP-choline:1,2-diacylglycerol choline phosphotransferase (or cholinephosphotransferase, CPT). These reactions are also referred to as the Kennedy pathway because of the significant work of Eugene Kennedy and Weiss in this area during the 1950s [16]. Each reaction of this pathway is briefly discussed below.

CK is a cytosolic enzyme that catalyzes the ATP-dependent phosphorylation of choline. It also displays kinase activity toward ethanolamine, but there are also ethanolamine-specific kinases in the human and mouse genomes [87]. There are two CK genes in mice: *Chok/Etnk-α* and *Chok/Etnk-β*, which encode CK-α and CK-β proteins, respectively. CK-β (45 kDa) seems to be ubiquitously expressed but is most abundant in the heart and the liver. Two isoforms of CK-α, CK-α1 (50 kDa) and CK-α2 (52 kDa) have been shown to result from alternative splicing of the *Chok/Entk-α* mouse gene. Although their mRNAs can be detected in all tissues tested, the alpha proteins are only strongly immunodetectable in the liver and the testes. CK enzymes are dimers, with homodimers (a/a and b/b) and heterodimers (a/b) found in tissues. The first crystal structure of a CK (*Caenorhabditis elegans*) was recently solved and shown to have structural similarities to protein kinases and aminoglycoside phosphotransferases [88]. There are no known allosteric effectors of CK, nor is the enzyme's activity known to be modulated by any posttranslational modification. CK may be the rate-limiting step of the Kennedy pathway under some metabolic scenarios, for example, mitogen-stimulated phosphatidylcholine synthesis, although the key regulatory enzyme of this pathway is generally believed to be CT [89–91].

CT is encoded by two genes in mice, *Pcyt1a* and *Pcyt1b*. Both genes produce multiple transcripts that encode the CTα and CTβ isoforms, respectively. The CTα mRNAs are more ubiquitously expressed, and are highest in the heart, the liver, and the kidney. CTβ mRNAs are most abundant in brain. A key difference between these genes is that the *Pcyt1a* gene products contain a nuclear import motif, whereas the *Pcyt1b* gene products do not. Both proteins contain a membrane-binding and phosphorylation domain. These gene characteristics explain why CT activity has been detected in the nuclear envelope, as well as in the cytosolic-assessable membranes of various tissues. Both CTα and CTβ are regulated by lipids in a similar manner. Phosphatidylcholine is believed to feed back and inhibit CT activity since there is an inverse relationship between membrane phosphatidylcholine and CT content. Diacylglycerol stimulates activity by mass action (a substrate) and by enhancing the translocation of the soluble, inactive forms of CT to their active, membrane-bound forms.

Fatty acids, phosphatidylethanolamine, and anionic phospholipids also enhance the translocation of CT to the membranes. The membrane-associated form of CT is less phosphorylated that the soluble form of the enzyme. Although the C-terminal region encodes a so-called phosphorylation domain with many putative phosphorylation sites and some kinases have been shown to phosphorylate the enzyme in vitro, whether phosphorylation has a key role in intracellular location or in the regulation of its activity remains unknown. It is also unknown which enzymes phosphorylate and dephosphorylate the enzyme in vivo. It is clear that CT activity is also regulated by changes in the steady-state levels of CT mRNA, as affected by changes in transcription and mRNA turnover, but aside from an increased mRNA abundance in various cells stimulated to proliferate, much needs to be learned regarding the molecular signals that mediate these changes. There have been several recent reviews covering the biochemistry and molecular biology of CT [89–92].

The last enzyme of the Kennedy pathway, CPT, is an integral membrane protein that is most abundant in the endoplasmic reticulum and whose specific activity is highest in liver, small intestine, adipose, and brain. This condensation reaction converts CDP-choline and diacylglycerol to phosphatidylcholine. There are two genes in humans that encode CPT, one is a specific CPT and the other also has ethanolaminephosphotransferase activity [87,93]. The latter is ubiquitously expressed whereas the phosphocholine-specific enzyme has a more limited tissue distribution, with highest levels expressed in the small intestine and the testis.

Phosphatidylcholine can be catabolized by at least five different lipases (Figure 14.3) generating diacylglycerol (phospholipase C), phosphatidic acid (phospholipase D), arachadonic acid (phospholipases B and A_2), and lysophosphatidylcholine [phospholipase A_2 and lecithin–cholesterol acyltransferase (LCAT)], all of which have roles in signal transduction. The major pathway for phosphatidylcholine degradation is via lysophosphatidylcholine, which is then converted to glycerophosphocholine and then choline (or phosphocholine) by the action of lysophospholipases and glycerophosphodiester phosphodiesterases, respectively [94]. The last known way to the formation of choline from phosphatidylcholine is by the base exchange reaction catalyzed by PS synthase 1, which catalyzes the conversion of phosphatidylcholine and serine to PS and choline [91,95].

Biosynthesis and Turnover of Sphingomyelin

The pathways of sphingomyelin synthesis and degradation have been recently reviewed [96,97]. This choline-containing phospholipid is synthesized by sphingomyelin synthases localized in the Golgi apparatus, which catalyze the conversion of phosphatidylcholine and ceramide to sphingomyelin and DAG. Sphingomyelin is then transported to the plasma membrane by an exocytic pathway. Sphingomyelin is degraded to ceramide and phosphocholine by sphingomyelinases (Figure 14.3), of which seven have been described that have differing cellular locations and enzymatic properties [98–100]. Sphingomyelin can also be converted to lysosphingomyelin (also known as sphingosylphosphorylcholine) by a sphingomyelin deacylase activity that remains uncharacterized. The routes of degradation of lysosphingomyelin remain unknown but may involve hydrolysis resulting in the generation of sphingosine-1-phosphate and choline. The synthesis and degradation of sphingomyelin generates signaling molecules (section Choline-Containing Signaling Molecules), and its structural role in membranes as a component of lipid rafts help form centers of signal transduction activity (section Membrane Structure and Function).

Choline Oxidation

There is no storage system for choline and so homeostasis can only be achieved by changing rates of synthesis and degradation. Choline oxidation is a process that requires enzymes found in the cytosol and the mitochondria (Figure 14.4). Many tissues express some of the enzymes of choline oxidation, but the liver is the primary organ where the whole complement of enzymes is abundantly expressed [101,102]. The oxidation of choline is an energy-yielding process that is anapleurotic to the one-carbon pool. Since the majority of one-carbon metabolism, on a whole body basis, occurs in liver, the localization of choline oxidation in this organ and the amount of choline in the diet are consistent with choline being a major one-carbon donor [103,104].

The oxidation of choline begins with its transport into the mitochondria, a process that has been proposed to be rate-limiting for its oxidation [75]. The K_m for choline transport into rat liver mitochondria is about 220 μM [105], which is considerably higher than the K_m value obtained for rat liver CK (13 μM) [106]. Since the concentration of free choline in rodent liver is reportedly 50–250 μM [60,107,108], and probably increases when choline is supplemented in the diet, together these data indicate that the oxidation of choline fluctuates relative to liver choline concentrations while phosphorylation is almost always proceeding at maximum capacity and is probably only limited by the expression of CK. However, at least in rodents, the capacity of the choline oxidation pathway is robust. Experiments indicate that choline oxidation accounts for most of its metabolism (60%–90%) shortly after administration of a radiolabeled tracer dose [109–111]. After transport into the mitochondria, choline is oxidized to betaine aldehyde by choline dehydrogenase (CHDH), the first enzyme of the choline oxidation pathway. Rodent and human genes for CHDH share a surprising homology to *Escherichia coli* CHDH [112], and recently the rat cDNA has been overexpressed in cultured cells [113]. CHDH is a member of the glucose–methanol–choline family of oxidoreductases, with each member containing a consensus FAD-binding domain [114]. Many members of this oxidoreductase family are soluble proteins but mammalian CHDH is associated with the inner mitochondrial membrane [115]. Preparations from liver mitochondria have shown that its activity can be measured by oxygen uptake, indicating that the electrons produced from this reaction enter the electron transport system and coenzyme Q has been identified as the electron acceptor [116,117]. The rat liver enzyme has been purified to homogeneity [116,118]. It has a molecular mass of 66 kDa, which is consistent with the coding sequence of its gene [113,115,117], and it has been shown to contain FAD [118]. There are no known regulatory features of this enzyme.

The second enzyme in the oxidation of choline is betaine-aldehyde dehydrogenase (BADH), which catalyzes the NAD-dependent conversion of betaine aldehyde to betaine. BADH activity is detected in the cytosol (93%–95%) and mitochondria (5%–7%) of rat liver [115,119,120]. Since there are many aldehyde dehydrogenase genes and isozymes, the identification of the enzymes that are responsible for BADH activities has been sought for a considerable period of time. Recent work has shown that the E3 aldehyde dehydrogenase isozyme (product of the *ALDH9* gene) displays high specificity toward betaine aldehyde [121]. However, this enzyme also has considerable activity toward aminobutyraldehyde and γ-trimethylamino-butyraldehyde [119], the latter being an intermediate of carnitine biosynthesis. The E3 isozyme is abundant in liver cytosol, and recent works suggest that it is present in the mitochondria as well [119,122], consistent with earlier studies on the subcellular fractionation of BADH activity [115,119,120]. Although it has not been confirmed, it seems likely that the cytosolic and mitochondrial isoforms of BADH are both products of the *ALDH9* nuclear gene [122]. Whether any betaine aldehyde is metabolized to betaine in the cytosol is not known for certain but seems doubtful. Studies with isolated mitochondria fail to detect any betaine aldehyde leaving the mitochondria following incubation with ^{14}C-choline, and yet betaine rapidly appears in the extramitochondrial space [115,123,124]. This observation, in addition to the knowledge that CHDH can also oxidize betaine aldehyde as well as choline [116], suggests that choline is rapidly converted to betaine in mitochondria by the combined actions of CHDH and the mitochondrial isoform of E3 aldehyde dehydrogenase. The crystal structure of a class 9 BADH from cod liver has recently been reported [125].

The third enzyme of the choline oxidation pathway is catalyzed by BHMT. This enzyme catalyzes a methyl transfer from betaine to homocysteine to form dimethylglycine and methionine. This is one of the most abundant enzymes found in liver, typically measured at 0.5%–2% of the total soluble protein in this organ [126]. Lesser amounts are found in the kidney proximal tubules of guinea pigs, pigs, and primates, including humans [101,102,127]. The expression of this enzyme is influenced by methionine and choline intake [108,128,129]. The levels of hepatic BHMT mRNA increase fivefold or more when dietary methionine is restricted and choline (or betaine) is supplemented [129]. The level of enzyme activity and immunodetectable protein mirrors the diet-induced changes in mRNA; however, kidney BHMT expression is refractory to these dietary changes [130]. The diet-induced changes in BHMT expression are most likely driven by the effect these nutrients have on liver S-adenosylmethionine concentrations. S-adenosylmethionine has been shown to inhibit BHMT transcription in human hepatoma cells [131]. Dimethylglycine is a potent inhibitor of BHMT due to the formation of an abortive ternary complex with enzyme and homocysteine [132], but it remains unclear whether this inhibition is physiologically significant when animals are consuming diets that are not supplemented with excessive amounts of choline or betaine. The human BHMT gene has been cloned and sequenced [129], and a highly related gene called BHMT2 has also been found in mouse and human genomes [133]. However, the BHMT2 protein does not catalyze a betaine-dependent methyl transfer to homocysteine, but rather uses S-methylmethionine as a methyl donor [134], a compound only known to be produced by plants and fungi. Crystal structures of human and rat BHMT have been solved [135,136].

The last two reactions of the choline oxidation pathway convert dimethylglycine to glycine and are catalyzed by genetically related folate- and flavin-dependent enzymes, dimethylglycine and sarcosine dehydrogenases, respectively [137–148]. Like the other enzymes of choline oxidation, these enzymes are abundant in the liver and the kidney; however, they are also expressed at significant levels in many other organs [149,150]. These enzymes are found in the matrix of the mitochondria and catalyze the oxidative demethylation of dimethylglycine and sarcosine-producing $FADH_2$ and methylenetetrahydrofolate. The methylene group of methylenetetrahydrofolate can be oxidized to formate in the mitochondria, generating ATP and reduced nicotinamide dinucleotides. Formate then leaves the mitochondria and can be incorporated into the cytosolic folate pool and used for the biosynthesis of purines, pyrimidines, serine, and methionine (section One-Carbon Metabolism), the latter via the methyltetrahydrofolate- and vitamin B_{12}-dependent methionine synthase [151].

BIOCHEMICAL FUNCTION

Membrane Structure and Function

Phosphatidylcholine is the predominant phospholipid in mammalian membranes and lipoproteins. In the cell membrane most of the phosphatidylcholine is located in the outer leaflet (extracellular), an asymmetry that is maintained by the action of membrane-associated translocases, floppases, and scramblases [96,152,153] that act on the various membrane phospholipids. In the liver, about 90% of the choline moiety is found in phosphatidylcholine [91,95]. Sphingomyelin is also found in all membranes within the cell, but at much lower levels than phosphatidylcholine. The plasma, Golgi, and lysosomal membranes are particularly rich in sphingomyelin. Like phosphatidylcholine, the sphingomyelin content in the outer leaflet of the plasma membrane is greater than that in the inner leaflet. The concentration of sphingomyelin in the outer leaflet has recently been shown to be an important structural component of specialized membrane domains called lipid rafts. Lipid rafts are rich in cholesterol and are referred to as rafts because they are resistant to disruption by nonionic detergents. Lipid rafts are centers for signal transduction enzymes and receptors [96].

In addition to the fact that phosphatidylcholine is an integral part of membranes and lipoproteins, the liver secretes large amounts of phosphatidylcholine into bile [91,95] where it acts as a surfactant to facilitate lipid digestion (Figure 14.3). It has been estimated that mouse liver secretes as much phosphatidylcholine into bile each day as is present in the entire organ. This process takes place at the cannicular membranes via a phosphatidylcholine-specific flippase known as multiple drug-resistant protein 3 in humans, or multidrug-resistant protein 2 in mice [95]. Mice devoid of PEMT activity die with only half of the liver phosphatidylcholine content of their wild-type littermates. However, mice devoid of both MDR2 and PEMT activities (*mdr2 −/−*, *pemt −/−*) survive more than 90 days without dietary choline because the draw of phosphatidylcholine into bile via MDR2 is ablated and the oxidation of choline is dramatically reduced [95]. Combined, these changes increase the recycling of any choline released from phospholipid catabolism back into the CDP-choline pathway to regenerate phosphatidylcholine, thus allowing the liver to retain function.

Choline in Neurotransmission and Brain Development

Acetylcholine is a neurotransmitter. Although the amount of choline used for acetylcholine synthesis is very small relative to that funneled into the CDP-choline and choline oxidation pathways, this molecule is indispensable for central and peripheral nervous function. Cholinergic neurons are involved in a diverse array of cognitive and neuromuscular functions and are affected by neurodegenerative diseases such as Alzheimer's and Parkinson's.

Acetylcholine is synthesized from choline and acetyl-coenzyme A by ChAT. It is made in the cytosol of nerve terminals and is concentrated in synaptic vesicles with the aid of a unique choline transporter, VAChT (vesicular acetylcholine transporter). The VAChT gene is located within intron 1 of the ChAT gene, and hence ChAT and VAChT expressions are coordinated. It has been shown that ChAT is normally phosphorylated and many putative phosphorylation sites for many kinases exist in the deduced amino acid sequence of the enzyme. Phosphorylation sites for calcium- or calmodulin-dependent kinase II and protein kinase C have been identified, yet at present it is unclear how changes in phosphorylation at each site affect ChAT activity, subcellular localization, and interaction with other cellular proteins [154]. At nerve depolarization, acetylcholine is released from the vesicles by exocytosis and elicits its neurotransmitter action by binding to nicotinic and muscarinic receptors. Free choline is then rapidly hydrolyzed to choline and acetate by AChE. Recently it has been appreciated that the once orphan esterase, butyrylcholine esterase, also has AChE activity but this activity only accounts for 5% of acetylcholine hydrolysis in humans [45]. Choline in the synaptic cleft is then efficiently reused for acetylcholine synthesis following uptake by the high-affinity, CHT1 choline-specific transporter. Acetylcholine synthesis and release may be affected by choline nutritional status [155] and can be augmented by supplemental choline [6].

Choline is important for brain development. Rodent pups receiving choline supplements (in utero or early after birth) experience a lifelong memory and attention span improvement. Exactly how choline supplementation elicits these effects is not understood but is known to involve increased sensitivity of the hippocampal neurons to stimulate of long-term potentiation and increased working spatial memory. In rodents, choline has been shown to influence nerve cell division, differentiation, migration, apoptosis, and other processes that affect development of the hippocampus and neural tube closure. More in-depth coverage of the role of choline in neurotransmission and brain function can be obtained from recent articles [9,156].

Choline-Containing Signaling Molecules

The metabolism of phosphatidylcholine and sphingomyelin can generate the following signaling molecules: diacylglycerol, phosphatidic acid, arachidonic acid, ceramide, sphingosine-1-phosphate, lysophosphatidylcholine, and lysosphingomyelin (Figure 14.3). Of these, lysophosphatidylcholine and lysosphingomyelin contain the choline moiety and both are signaling lipids that are involved in a complex array of biological functions. Besides its production intracellularly by phospholipase A_2, lysophosphatidylcholine is produced in plasma by the action of LCAT, which transfers a fatty acid from phosphatidylcholine to cholesterol. Lysophosphatidylcholine is known to be proinflammatory and stimulates atherogenesis, at least in part by upregulating proinflammatory molecules (e.g., vascular cell adhesion molecule-1 and intracellular adhesion molecule-1), cytokines, and matrix metalloproteinase-2. Lysosphingomyelin has been shown to affect cell growth and is probably involved in angiogenesis, wound healing, and muscle contraction. Both lysophosphatidylcholine and lysosphingomyelin exert their bioactivity through families of lipid-specific G protein-coupled receptors that function, at least in part, to increase intracellular calcium concentrations.

In addition to lysophosphatidylcholine and lysosphingomyelin, platelet-activating factor (PAF) is a choline-containing phospholipid (not shown). This signaling phospholipid is involved in a diverse set of physiological events including wound healing, angiogenesis, apoptosis, and reproduction. Traditionally, PAF referred to as 1-*O*-alkyl-2-acetyl-*sn*-glycero-3-phosphocholine, but it has now been recognized that this molecule is one of a larger family of 1-alkyl or 1-acyl derivatives containing a short *sn*-2 group that may or may not be oxidized. Although many derivatives have been described, only the analogs with an *sn*-2 acetyl group are known to be bioactive. The most characterized pathway for the synthesis of PAFs involves the action of phospholipase A_2 on 1-*O*-alkyl- or 1-*O*-acyl-2-arachidonoyl-glycerophosphcholine, which releases arachidonate to generate 1-*O*-alkyl- or 1-*O*-acyl-2-lysoglycerophosphocholine. These molecules can then be acted on by an acetyltransferase (acetyl-CoA:1-*O*-alkyl-2-lyso-glycerophosphcholine acetyltransferase) to generate alkyl-PAF and acyl-PAF, respectively. Like lysophosphatidylcholine and lysosphingomyelin, the action of PAF molecules is mediated by G protein-coupled receptors that are expressed in a wide variety of tissues and cells. The deduced amino acid sequences of the lysophosphatidylcholine, lysosphingomyelin, and PAF receptors have considerable homology (~35%–50%) and may have overlapping ligand specificities, perhaps explaining some of their overlapping physiological effects.

Recent work has indicated that phosphocholine is also a signaling molecule important for cell division, including malignant transformation [38,87]. A detailed review of the choline-containing signaling molecules is beyond the scope of this work but the interested reader is referred to many recent reviews for a more advanced introduction to this exciting and rapidly evolving area of research [38,87,157–167].

One-Carbon Metabolism

One-carbon metabolism refers generically to the reactions that use tetrahydrofolate coenzymes and those reactions that transfer a methyl group, the latter being primarily S-adenosylmethionine-dependent methyltransferases. Folate-dependent reactions transfer one-carbon units at different oxidation states. 10-formyltetrahydrofolate is required for purine and formylmethionine biosynthesis; 5,10-methylenetetrahydofolate is used for the interconversion of serine and glycine and thymidylate biosynthesis; and 5-methyltetrahydrofolate is required for the methylation of homocysteine to regenerate methionine (i.e., remethylation). The folate-dependent remethylation of homocysteine is catalyzed by methionine synthase, which is also a cobalamin (vitamin B_{12})-dependent enzyme. It is known that serine (via mitochondrial serine hydroxymethyltransferase), glycine (via the mitochondrial glycine cleavage system), and choline are the major sources of one-carbon units that support folate metabolism, but much more research is required to understand their relative contributions and how their contributions change because of changes in nutritional and physiological states.

When oxidized, four of the five carbon atoms that make up choline enter the one-carbon pool (Figure 14.4). This process is mediated by the enzymes that metabolize betaine to glycine and the mitochondrial glycine cleavage system, the latter of which oxidizes glycine to ammonium ion, carbon dioxide, and methylenetetrahydrofolate. All of the major enzymes that generate one-carbon units for folate-dependent reactions are mitochondrial, except BHMT, yet the predominant need for these one-carbon units is extramitochondrial. The transfer of one-carbon units generated in the mitochondria to the cystosol is mediated by two sets of folate-interconverting enzymes that operate in opposite directions in the cytosol (reductive direction) and mitochondria (oxidative direction), with formate being the one-carbon intermediate linking these compartments [151].

Since there is no storage form of choline, animals in maintenance must oxidize each day an amount that equals what is taken in by the diet plus that which is synthesized de novo via PEMT (minus any incomplete choline oxidation products that might be excreted), which can total to be a gram or more. In humans, classic studies showed that choline intake and the need to synthesize methyl groups de novo are inversely related [103,104]. Simple choline deficiency results in reduced hepatic methionine, S-adenosylmethionine [168–170], and DNA hypomethylation [171,172], and in vivo inhibition of BHMT causes fasting hyperhomocysteinemia and increases postmethionine load hyperhomocysteinemia [27]. These outcomes of choline deficiency emphasize the importance of choline oxidation to one-carbon metabolism.

Osmotic Regulation

Cells regulate their volume by finely adjusting the levels of intracellular osmolytes. Osmolytes can be inorganic, for example, sodium, potassium, and chloride ions, or organic, for example, betaine, glycerophosphocholine, *myo*-inositol, sorbitol, and amino acids such as taurine, glutamate, and others [173]. The organic osmolytes have been the focus of much study over the last two decades. Changes in the intracellular concentration of osmolytes result in changes in cell volume by affecting the water content of the cell by osmosis. Two important osmolytes are derived from choline: betaine and glycerophosphocholine. The tissue of the body with the greatest need for osmotic regulation is the kidney inner medulla since these cells are exposed to very high extracellular osmolarity during the normal process of concentrating urine for excretion. It is not surprising, therefore, that most research on the biology of osmolytes in mammals have focused on the kidney inner medulla [174–177].

Betaine is an intermediate of choline oxidation (Figure 14.4), and several processes can facilitate the ability of the inner medulla to modulate betaine concentrations, including changes in synthesis from choline, changes in betaine import and export, and changes in betaine degradation. The renal cortex and the medulla have been shown to express CHDH and BADH, indicating that both regions of the kidney have some capacity to synthesize betaine. Hypertonicity due to hypernatremia caused a 50% increase in betaine synthesis in rat kidney cortex, but had no effect on medullary betaine synthesis [178]. This study suggested that enhanced betaine synthesis in the kidney cortex and perhaps efflux out of this tissue could be a mechanism to increase the availability of betaine for transport into the medulla. Another mechanism to enhance the availability of betaine for medullary cells includes decreased degradation by BHMT. It has been shown that guinea pig liver and kidney cortex dramatically downregulate BHMT expression during hypernatremia [127]. BHMT is not expressed in the kidney medulla [101,127], precluding the catabolism of betaine in these cells. Aside from these few studies that imply changes in betaine synthesis and degradation might be mechanisms to facilitate betaine accumulation by the renal medulla, there has been much more research on the ability of the medulla to transport betaine into the cell, and to a lesser extent, on betaine efflux mechanisms [173,175,179]. Betaine is transported into the renal medullary epithelial cells by the betaine/γ-aminobutyric acid transporter (BGT1). BGT1 is expressed in the basolateral membrane and is a sodium- and chloride-coupled cotransporter. Its levels have been shown to increase or decrease under hypertonic or hypotonic conditions, respectively, with a corresponding effect on intracellular betaine concentrations. Betaine has also been shown to rapidly efflux out of medullary cells when they are exposed to hyper-osmotic conditions. The molecular mechanisms responsible for changes in betaine synthesis and degradation due to changes in osmolarity have not been described, but changes in BGT1 mRNA expression have been shown to be driven by the tonicity element binding protein (tonEBP) interacting with the tonicity elements (tonE) of the *BGT1* gene [180].

The biosynthesis of glycerophosphocholine from phosphatidylcholine is shown in Figure 14.3. To date, there is no evidence that glycerophosphocholine can be directly produced from choline. The rate-limiting step in glycerophosphocholine biosynthesis is reportedly the production of lysophosphatidylcholine from phosphatidylcholine [181]. Work to date suggests that changes in glycerophosphocholine synthesis rate is not the primary mechanism responsible for the increase in medullary glycerophosphocholine content observed during hypertonic stress. This conclusion is supported by the finding that phospholipase activities required for glycerophosphocholine synthesis from phosphatidylcholine are refractory or change very little in response to changes in osmolarity [182,183]. Rather, work to date suggests that the rate of glycerophosphocholine degradation is the primary mechanism influencing medullary glycerophosphocholine concentrations, a conclusion based on the observation that medullary glycerophosphocholine:choline phosphodiesterase, which converts glycerophosphocholine into choline and phosphoglycerol, and alkaline phosphatase activity decrease under conditions of high osmolarity [182,184,185].

DEFICIENCY SIGNS AND METHODS OF NUTRITIONAL ASSESSMENT

There are many publications that detail the symptoms and the assessment of choline deficiency in animals and cells [5–7,21–23,83,95,168,170,172,186–210]. In animals the most frequently measured metabolite changes associated with choline deficiency include reductions in liver choline metabolites (including betaine), methionine and S-adenosylmethionine. Liver triglyceride levels increase dramatically, and as discussed earlier, fatty liver has historically been the hallmark of choline (or lipotrope) deficiency. Another common occurrence of experimental choline deficiency in weanling animals is renal hemorrhage [198], which appears to be due to a lack of betaine, an organic osmolyte critical for normal renal function. Choline deficiency in experimental animals results in liver cell proliferation, apoptosis, and eventual transformation. Indeed, choline is the only nutrient deficiency that results in the spontaneous development of cancer (hepatocarcinoma). Choline deficiency in rodents has been shown to affect learning and attentional processes throughout the lifespan [3,9].

Far less is known about choline deficiency in humans. Most assessment tools are limited to what can be obtained from a blood sample, although fatty liver can now be confirmed by nuclear magnetic resonance imaging [211]. Due to its wide distribution in foods [61], and the fact that the average total choline intake of adult humans meets or exceeds the dietary reference intakes for choline [20,212], a primary deficiency of choline has not been observed. However, suboptimal choline status has been observed in humans undergoing total parental nutrition [20,213]. Healthy humans fed diets low or devoid in choline have reduced plasma choline and increased serum alanine amino transferase [25], increased plasma creatine phosphokinase [214], increased lymphocyte DNA damage and apoptosis [215], and increased plasma total homocysteine following a methionine load [196]. It has recently been reported that women who had lower choline intakes during pregnancy had significantly increased risk of giving birth to a child with a neural tube defect [216].

NUTRITIONAL REQUIREMENT

ANIMALS

The recommended intakes of choline for rat, mouse, guinea pig, and hamster range from 7.1 to 7.9 mmol/kg diet [217]. This is equivalent to 1.8–2.0 g of choline bitartrate/kg diet. These recommendations assume that the diets of these laboratory animals contain adequate methionine (but nonsupplemental levels), folate, and vitamin B_{12}. The primary basis for these recommendations is the level of choline required to prevent fatty liver, a phenomena that happens quickly (one to several days) after the consumption of a diet devoid of choline ensues.

HUMANS

In 1998, the Food and Nutrition Board of the Institute of Medicine set the first recommended intakes of choline for humans [20]. Adequate intakes were set at 125 mg/day for infants 0–6 months, 150 mg/day for infants 7–12 months, 200 mg/day for children 1–3 years, 250 mg/day for children 4–8 years, 375 mg/day for boys and girls 9–13 years, 400 mg/day for girls 14–18 years, 550 mg/day for boys 14–18 and men greater than 19 years, and 425 mg/day for women 19 years or older. The requirement was set at 450 mg/day and 550 mg/day for pregnancy and lactation, respectively. An intake of 500 mg/day was the level required to prevent an increase in plasma alanine aminotransferase activity [25] in humans consuming adequate methionine, folate, and vitamin B_{12}, and this one report was the only data set used to extrapolate this set of current recommended values. Hence, these values may change in the future as more knowledge of the level of choline intake required to maintain optimal health is gained.

FACTORS INFLUENCING CHOLINE STATUS

NUTRITIONAL FACTORS

There are several nutritional factors that affect choline status. The best documented is the interrelationship between methionine intake and the requirement for choline. Most early studies focused on quantifying the ability of methionine to replace choline in the diet using growth and liver lipid content as indicators of choline status. Using these indicators most studies concluded that choline was not an essential nutrient because supplemental methionine could compensate for the lack choline by rescuing growth rate and reducing liver lipids. The only exception to this was the growing chick, which no amount of dietary methionine (below toxic levels) could rescue the growth depression observed when they were fed a diet devoid of choline [26]. The general interpretation of these data was that in most animals the supplemental methionine enhanced the availability of S-adenosylmethionine for the synthesis of phosphatidylcholine from phosphatidylethanolamine, thereby abolishing the need for dietary choline. However, as indicated earlier (section History), the combination of high dietary methionine coupled with low choline likely results in elevated levels of plasma total homocysteine [27], a proposed risk factor for vascular diseases and thrombosis [28–30]. In addition, recent studies indicate that reducing dietary methionine reduces mitochondrial oxidative damage and increases longevity [218–222]. These data suggest that replacing any of the choline requirement with supplemental methionine does not result in optimal, long-term health.

Dietary betaine can replace part of the choline requirement, as indicated by its ability to promote growth and prevent liver lipid accumulation in animals fed choline-deficient diets [223,224]. These effects are likely due to betaine's ability to offset the role choline normally provides one-carbon units for methionine biosynthesis and folate-dependent reactions, which requires oxidation to betaine and beyond (Figure 14.4). In addition, betaine can prevent the renal hemorrhage associated with choline deficiency in weanling animals [198], indicating that this phenomena must be due primarily to the lack of the osmolyte rather than any other metabolic role for choline.

Severe folate deficiency has been shown to significantly reduce liver choline and phosphocholine concentrations [225] in rats consuming diets that contain what is normally an adequate level of choline. These changes are probably due to reduced methionine synthesis from homocysteine via the folate- and vitamin B_{12}-dependent methionine synthase reaction, which in turn decreases the availability of S-adenosylmethionine for choline (phosphatidylcholine) biosynthesis via PEMT. In addition, there may be enhanced choline oxidation to bolster methionine biosynthesis through the BHMT-catalyzed reaction, a process that would be expected to deplete liver choline levels.

Pharmaceuticals

Any drug that interferes with folate, vitamin B_{12}, or sulfur amino acid metabolism should be tested for, and probably disrupts choline metabolism because the function of these nutrients intersect at the level of one-carbon metabolism (section Osmotic Regulation). For example, methotrexate, one of the most widely recognized antifolates, is currently in clinical use for the treatment of childhood lymphoblastic leukemias, rheumatoid arthritis, and psoriasis. In experimental animals this drug causes a reduction in tissue folate [171,172,206], phosphocholine and glycerophosphocholine [168], and in the S-adenosylmethionine-to-S-adenosylhomocysteine ratio [168,226]. Tissue homocysteine levels become elevated [169,172]. These metabolite changes are likely due to the reduced conversion of homocysteine to methionine by the folate- and vitamin B_{12}-dependent methionine synthase, and these metabolite changes are also observed when animals are fed a choline-deficient diet [168,169,172]. Methotrexate also causes a reduction in liver betaine levels [227], which is consistent with enhanced flux through the choline oxidation pathway as a mechanism to bolster methionine production via BHMT (Figure 14.4). An outcome of the methotrexate-induced disturbances in sulfur amino acid metabolism is a general reduction in S-adenosylmethionine-dependent methylation reactions, including phosphatidylcholine biosynthesis (causing fatty liver) [228,229] and DNA methylation [172]. Supplementing choline to methotrexate-treated animals greatly attenuates or abolishes the reduction in the S-adenosylmethionine-to-S-adenosylhomocysteine ratio and downstream events including the development of fatty liver [229], whereas restricting dietary choline exacerbates these pathological changes [206].

Genetics

The possibility that genetic variation can affect the dietary requirement for choline is an area that requires more research. It has been noted that some humans are more susceptible to developing clinical signs of choline deficiency (increased liver lipid and plasma alanine amino transferase and creatine phosphokinase activities) than others when placed on diets very low in choline. To date there have been two reports investigating whether single nucleotide polymorphisms in the genes involved in choline and one-carbon metabolism have a role in this phenomena. These studies indicate that individuals with the *MTHFD1* +1958 G→A (rs 2236225) polymorphism [230] or the *PEMT* promoter −744 G→C (rs 12325817) or CHDH +432 G→T (rs 12676) polymorphism [211] are more susceptible to choline deficiency symptoms, and that women harboring these polymorphisms are more affected than men. It is proposed that all of these polymorphisms may result in a functional reduction of phosphatidylcholine biosynthesis by either reducing PEMT expression or reducing the flux of one-carbon units entering the S-adenosylmethionine pool, the latter of which is required for optimal PEMT activity. The observation that these polymorphisms made women more susceptible to signs of choline deficiency than men could be very important because it was shown recently that deficient maternal dietary choline intake was associated with a fourfold increased risk of giving birth to a child with a neural tube defect [216], a condition most notably associated with disturbed folate metabolism or folate deficiency. Due to the relatively small number of subjects in the two studies mentioned earlier, additional studies using a larger numbers of subjects are required to confirm these observations.

EFFICACY AND HAZARDS OF PHARMACOLOGICAL DOSES OF CHOLINE

Animals and humans can tolerate high intakes of choline with no adverse side effects. For humans the tolerable upper limit has been set at 3.5 g/day for adults 19 years and older [20]. Very high levels of choline intake (>5 g/day) in humans have been associated with a fishy body odor, excessive sweating and salivation, vomiting, and gastrointestinal distress. The fishy body odor is known to be due to the excretion of high amounts of trimethylamine, a bacterial degradation product of choline [231]. Individuals with trimethylaminuria, renal or liver disease, depression, and Parkinson's disease may have increased sensitivity to pharmacological doses of choline. These hazards and others associated with pharmacological intakes of choline were outlined by the Institute of Medicine [20].

REFERENCES

1. Sarter, M. and Parikh, V.: Choline transporters, cholinergic transmission and cognition. *Nat. Rev. Neurosci.*, 2005, 6(1):48–56.
2. Ackerstaff, E., Glunde, K., and Bhujwalla, Z.M.: Choline phospholipid metabolism: a target in cancer cells? *J. Cell Biochem.*, 2003, 90(3):525–533.
3. Meck, W.H. and Williams, C.L.: Metabolic imprinting of choline by its availability during gestation: implications for memory and attentional processing across the lifespan. *Neurosci. Biobehav. Rev.*, 2003, 27(4):385–399.
4. Newberne, P.M.: Choline deficiency associated with diethanolamine carcinogenicity. *Toxicol. Sci.*, 2002, 67(1):1–3.
5. Garrow, T.A.: Choline and carnitine. In: *Present Knowledge in Nutrition.* Edited by Bowman B.A., Russel., R.M., eighth edn. Washington, DC: ILSI Press; 2001: 261–272.
6. Zeisel, S.H.: Dietary choline: biochemistry, physiology, and pharmacology. *Annu. Rev. Nutr.*, 1981, 1:95–121.
7. Zeisel, S.H.: Choline deficiency. *J. Nutr. Biochem.*, 1990, 1(7):332–349.
8. Zeisel, S.H.: Choline: an essential nutrient for humans. *Nutrition*, 2000, 16(7–8):669–671.
9. Zeisel, S.H.: Nutritional importance of choline for brain development. *J. Am. Coll. Nutr.*, 2004, 23(6 Suppl):621S–626S.
10. Zeisel, S.H.: Choline, homocysteine, and pregnancy. *Am. J. Clin. Nutr.*, 2005, 82(4):719–720.
11. Strecker, A.: Ueber einige neue Bestandtheile der Schweinegalle. *Annal der Chemie u Parmacie*, 1862, 123:353–360.
12. Strecker, A.: Ueber das lecithin. *Annal der Chemie u Parmacie*, 1868, 148:77–90.
13. Levene, P.A.: On sphingomyelin II. *J. Biol. Chem.*, 1914, 18:453–463.
14. Levene, P.A.: Spingomyelin III. *J. Biol. Chem.*, 1916, 24:68–69.

15. du Vigneaud, V., Cohn, M., Chandler, J.P., Schenck, J.R., and Simmonds, S.: The utilization of the methyl group of methioinine in the biological synthesis of choline and creatine. *J. Biol. Chem.*, 1941, 140:625–641.
16. Kennedy, E.P. and Weiss, S.B.: The function of cytidine coenzymes in the biosynthesis of phospholipides. *J. Biol. Chem.*, 1956, 222(1):193–214.
17. Hunt, R. and Taveau, R.M.: The pharmacological action of certain choline derivatives and new methodology for detecting choline. *Br. Med. J.*, 1906, 2:1788–1791.
18. Best C.H. and Huntsman, M.E.: The effects of the components of lecithin upon deposition of fat in the liver. *J. Physiol.*, 1932, 75:405–412.
19. Best C.H. and Huntsman, M.E.: The effect of choline on the liver fat of rats in various states of nutrition. *J. Physiol.*, 1935, 83:255–274.
20. Choline. In: *Dietary Reference Intakes for Thiamin, Riboflavin, Niacin, Vitamin* B_6, *Folate, Vitamin* B_{12}, *Biotin and Choline*. Washington, DC: National Academy Press; 1998:390–422.
21. Ghoshal, A.K.: New insight into the biochemical pathology of liver in choline deficiency. *Crit. Rev. Biochem. Mol. Biol.*, 1995, 30(4):263–273.
22. Ghoshal, A.K. and Farber, E.: Choline deficiency, lipotrope deficiency and the development of liver disease including liver cancer: a new perspective. *Lab. Invest.*, 1993, 68(3):255–260.
23. Ghoshal, A.K. and Farber, E.: Liver biochemical pathology of choline deficiency and of methyl group deficiency: a new orientation and assessment. *Histol. Histopathol.*, 1995, 10(2):457–462.
24. Zeisel, S.H., da Costa, K.A., Albright, C.D., and Shin, O.H.: Choline and hepatocarcinogenesis in the rat. *Adv. Exp. Med. Biol.*, 1995, 375:65–74.
25. Zeisel, S.H., Da Costa, K.A., Franklin, P.D., Alexander, E.A., Lamont, J.T., Sheard, N.F., and Beiser, A.: Choline, an essential nutrient for humans. *FASEB J.*, 1991, 5(7):2093–2098.
26. Baker, D.H., Halpin, K.M., Czarnecki, G.L., and Parsons, C.M.: The choline-methionine interrelationship for growth of the chick. *Poult. Sci.*, 1983, 62(1):133–137.
27. Collinsova, M., Strakova, J., Jiracek, J., and Garrow, TA.: Inhibition of betaine-homocysteine s-methyltransferase causes hyperhomocysteinemia in mice. *J. Nutr.*, 2006, 136(6):1493–1497.
28. Guthikonda, S. and Haynes, W.G.: Homocysteine: role and implications in atherosclerosis. *Curr. Atheroscler. Rep.*, 2006, 8(2):100–106.
29. Homocysteine-lowering trials for prevention of cardiovascular events: a review of the design and power of the large randomized trials. *Am. Heart. J.*, 2006, 151(2):282–287.
30. Undas, A., Brozek, J., and Szczeklik, A.: Homocysteine and thrombosis: from basic science to clinical evidence. *Thromb. Haemost.*, 2005, 94(5):907–915.
31. Mulford, D.J. and Outland, C.E.: The effect of 2-amino-2-methyl-1-propanol on the incidence of kidney lesions in male rats of different ages fed diets low in choline. *J. Nutr.*, 1957, 61(3):381–388.
32. Outland, C.E., Mealey, E.H., Longmore, W.J., and Mulford, D.J.: The effect of ethanolamine and its *N*-methyl derivatives on kidney hemorrhagic degeneration in rats due to 2-amino-2-methyl-1-propanol. *J. Nutr.*, 1959, 67(4):655–663.
33. Wells, I.C. and Remy, C.N.: Inhibition of de novo choline biosynthesis by 2-amino-2-methyl-1-propanol. *Arch. Biochem. Biophys.*, 1961, 95:389–399.
34. Haubrich, D.R. and Gerber, N.H.: Choline dehydrogenase. Assay, properties and inhibitors. *Biochem. Pharmacol.*, 1981, 30(21):2993–3000.
35. Lehman-McKeeman, L.D., Gamsky, E.A., Hicks, S.M., Vassallo, J.D., Mar, M.H., and Zeisel S.H.: Diethanolamine induces hepatic choline deficiency in mice. *Toxicol. Sci.*, 2002, 67(1):38–45.
36. Stott, W.T., Bartels, M.J., Brzak, K.A., Mar, M., Markham, D.A., Thornton, C.M., and Zeisel, S.H.: Potential mechanisms of tumorigenic action of diethanolamine in mice. *Toxicol. Lett.*, 2000, 114(1–3):67–75.
37. Michel, V., Yuan, Z., Ramsubir, S., and Bakovic, M.: Choline transport for phospholipid synthesis. *Exp. Biol. Med. (Maywood)*, 2006, 231(5):490–504.
38. Janardhan, S., Srivani, P. and Sastry, G.N.: Choline kinase: an important target for cancer. *Curr. Med. Chem.*, 2006, 13(10):1169–1186.
39. Collier, B.: The structural specificity of choline transport into cholinergic nerve terminals. *J. Neurochem.*, 1981, 36(3):1292–1294.
40. Deves, R. and Krupka, R.M.: The binding and translocation steps in transport as related to substrate structure. A study of the choline carrier of erythrocytes. *Biochim. Biophys. Acta*, 1979, 557(2):469–485.

41. Boksa, P. and Collier, B.: *N*-ethyl analogues of choline as precursors to cholinergic false transmitters. *J. Neurochem.*, 1980, 35(5):1099–1104.
42. Bowman, W.C. and Rand, M.J.: Actions of triethylcholine on neuromuscular transmission. 1961. *Br. J. Pharmacol.*, 1997, 120(4 Suppl):228–247; discussion 226–227.
43. Buccafusco, J.J. and Aronstam, R.S.: Precursors of cholinergic false transmitters: central effects on blood pressure and direct interactions with cholinergic receptors. *Neuropharmacology*, 1988, 27(3):227–233.
44. Geldenhuys, W.J., Lockman, P.R., Philip, A.E., McAfee, J.H., Miller, B.L., McCurdy, C.R., and Allen, D.D.: Inhibition of choline uptake by *N*-cyclohexylcholine, a high affinity ligand for the choline transporter at the blood–brain barrier. *J. Drug. Target.*, 2005, 13(4):259–266.
45. Ballard, C.G., Greig, N.H., Guillozet-Bongaarts, A.L., Enz, A., and Darvesh, S.: Cholinesterases: roles in the brain during health and disease. *Curr. Alzheimer. Res.*, 2005, 2(3):307–318.
46. Chandrasekaran, V., McGaughey, G.B., Cavallito, C.J., and Bowen, J.P.: Three-dimensional quantitative structure-activity relationship (3D-QSAR) analyses of choline acetyltransferase inhibitors. *J. Mol. Graph. Model.*, 2004, 23(1):69–76.
47. Campos, J.M., Sanchez-Martin, R.M., Conejo-Garcia, A., Entrena, A., Gallo, M.A., and Espinosa, A.: (Q)SAR studies to design new human choline kinase inhibitors as antiproliferative drugs. *Curr. Med. Chem.*, 2006, 13(11):1231–1248.
48. Conejo-Garcia, A., Entrena, A., Campos, J.M., Sanchez-Martin, R.M., Gallo, M.A., and Espinosa, A.: Towards a model for the inhibition of choline kinase by a new type of inhibitor. *Eur. J. Med. Chem.*, 2005, 40(3):315–319.
49. Jiracek, J., Collinsova, M., Rosenberg, I., Budesinsky, M., Protivinska, E., Netusilova, H., and Garrow, T.A.: S-alkylated homocysteine derivatives: new inhibitors of human betaine-homocysteine S-methyltransferase. *J. Med. Chem.*, 2006, 49(13):3982–3989.
50. Nutrient Content Claims Notification for Choline Containing Foods: http://www.cfsan.fda.gov/~dms/flcholin.html.
51. Goldberg, A.M. and McCaman, R.E.: The determination of picomole amounts of acetylcholine in mammalian brain. *J. Neurochem.*, 1973, 20(1):1–8.
52. Ikarashi, Y., Sasahara, T., and Maruyama, Y.: Determination of choline and acetylcholine levels in rat brain regions by liquid chromatography with electrochemical detection. *J. Chromatogr.*, 1985, 322(1):191–199.
53. Damsma, G. and Flentge, F.: Liquid chromatography with electrochemical detection for the determination of choline and acetylcholine in plasma and red blood cells. Failure to detect acetylcholine in blood of humans and mice. *J. Chromatogr.*, 1988, 428(1):1–8.
54. Ricny, J., Tucek, S., and Vins, I.: Sensitive method for HPLC determination of acetylcholine, choline and their analogues using fluorometric detection. *J. Neurosci. Methods*, 1992, 41(1):11–17.
55. Ishimaru, H., Ikarashi, Y., and Maruyama, Y.: Use of high-performance liquid chromatography continuous-flow fast atom bombardment mass spectrometry for simultaneous determination of choline and acetylcholine in rodent brain regions. *Biol. Mass Spectrom.*, 1993, 22(12):681–686.
56. Panfili, G., Manzi, P., Compagnone, D., Scarciglia, L., and Palleschi, G.: Rapid assay of choline in foods using microwave hydrolysis and a choline biosensor. *J. Agric. Food Chem.*, 2000, 48(8):3403–3407.
57. Pomfret, E.A., daCosta, K.A., Schurman, L.L., and Zeisel, S.H.: Measurement of choline and choline metabolite concentrations using high-pressure liquid chromatography and gas chromatography–mass spectrometry. *Anal. Biochem.*, 1989, 180(1):85–90.
58. Acevedo, L.D., Xu, Y., Zhang, X., Pearce, R.J., and Yergey, A.: Quantification of acetylcholine in cell culture systems by semi-micro high-performance liquid chromatography and electrospray ionization mass spectrometry. *J. Mass Spectrom.*, 1996, 31(12):1399–1402.
59. Holmes, H.C., Snodgrass, G.J., and Iles, R.A.: Changes in the choline content of human breast milk in the first 3 weeks after birth. *Eur. J. Pediatr.*, 2000, 159(3):198–204.
60. Koc, H., Mar, M.H., Ranasinghe, A., Swenberg, J.A., and Zeisel, S.H.: Quantitation of choline and its metabolites in tissues and foods by liquid chromatography/electrospray ionization-isotope dilution mass spectrometry. *Anal. Chem.*, 2002, 74(18):4734–4740.
61. Zeisel, S.H., Mar, M.H., Howe, J.C., and Holden, J.M.: Concentrations of choline-containing compounds and betaine in common foods. *J. Nutr.*, 2003, 133(5):1302–1307.

62. Woollard, D.C. and Indyk, H.E.: Determination of choline in milk and infant formulas by enzymatic analysis: collaborative study. *J. AOAC Int.*, 2000, 83(1):131–138.
63. *Official Method 999.14*, 17th edn. Gaithersburg, M.D.: AOAC International; 2000.
64. Rader, J.I., Weaver, C.M., and Trucksess, M.W.: Extension of AOAC official method 999.14 (choline in infant formula and milk) to the determination of choline in dietary supplements. *J. AOAC Int.*, 2004, 87(6):1297–1304.
65. de Zwart, F.J., Slow, S., Payne, R.J., Lever, M., George, P.M., Gerrard, J.A., and Chambers, S.T.: Glycine betaine and glycine betaine analogues in common foods. *Food Chem.*, 2003, 83:197–204.
66. Slow, S., Donaggio, M., Cressey, P.J., Lever, M., George, P.M., and Chambers, S.T.: The betaine content of New Zealand foods and estimated intake in the New Zealand diet. *J. Food Composit. Anal.*, 2005, 18:473–485.
67. Rontein, D., Basset, G., and Hanson, A.D.: Metabolic engineering of osmoprotectant accumulation in plants. *Metab. Eng.*, 2002, 4(1):49–56.
68. Tso, P. and Balint, J.A.: Formation and transport of chylomicrons by enterocytes to the lymphatics. *Am. J. Physiol.*, 1986, 250(6 Pt 1):G715–G726.
69. Nilsson, A. and Duan, R.D.: Absorption and lipoprotein transport of sphingomyelin. *J. Lipid. Res.*, 2006, 47(1):154–171.
70. Savendahl, L., Mar, M.H., Underwood, L.E., and Zeisel, S.H.: Prolonged fasting in humans results in diminished plasma choline concentrations but does not cause liver dysfunction. *Am. J. Clin. Nutr.*, 1997, 66(3):622–625.
71. Kowalczuk, S., Broer, A., Munzinger, M., Tietze, N., Klingel, K., and Broer, S.: Molecular cloning of the mouse IMINO system: an Na^+- and Cl^--dependent proline transporter. *Biochem. J.*, 2005, 386(Pt 3):417–422.
72. Schwab, U., Torronen, A., Meririnne, E., Saarinen, M., Alfthan, G., Aro, A., and Uusitupa, M.: Orally administered betaine has an acute and dose-dependent effect on serum betaine and plasma homocysteine concentrations in healthy humans. *J. Nutr.*, 2006, 136(1):34–38.
73. Melse-Boonstra, A., Holm, PI., Ueland, P.M., Olthof, M., Clarke, R., and Verhoef, P.: Betaine concentration as a determinant of fasting total homocysteine concentrations and the effect of folic acid supplementation on betaine concentrations. *Am. J. Clin. Nutr.*, 2005, 81(6):1378–1382.
74. Ribeiro, F.M., Black, S.A., Prado, V.F., Rylett, R.J., Ferguson, S.S., and Prado, M.A.: The "ins" and "outs" of the high-affinity choline transporter CHT1. *J. Neurochem.*, 2006, 97(1):1–12.
75. Kaplan, C.P., Porter, R.K., and Brand, M.D.: The choline transporter is the major site of control of choline oxidation in isolated rat liver mitochondria. *FEBS Lett.*, 1993, 321(1):24–26.
76. Nouri-Sorkhabi, M.H., Chapman, B.E., Kuchel, P.W., Gruca, M.A., and Gaskin, K.J.: Parallel secretion of pancreatic phospholipase A(2), phospholipase A(1), lipase, and colipase in children with exocrine pancreatic dysfunction. *Pediatr. Res.*, 2000, 48(6):735–740.
77. Lockman, P.R. and Allen, D.D.: The transport of choline. *Drug. Dev. Ind. Pharm.*, 2002, 28(7):749–771.
78. Allen, D.D. and Lockman, P.R.: The blood–brain barrier choline transporter as a brain drug delivery vector. *Life Sci.*, 2003, 73(13):1609–1615.
79. Traiffort, E., Ruat, M., O'Regan, S., and Meunier, F.M.: Molecular characterization of the family of choline transporter-like proteins and their splice variants. *J. Neurochem.*, 2005, 92(5):1116–1125.
80. Jonker, J.W. and Schinkel, A.H.: Pharmacological and physiological functions of the polyspecific organic cation transporters: OCT1, 2, and 3 (SLC22A1-3). *J. Pharmacol. Exp. Ther.*, 2004, 308(1):2–9.
81. Reo, N.V., Adinehzadeh, M., and Foy, B.D.: Kinetic analyses of liver phosphatidylcholine and phosphatidylethanolamine biosynthesis using (13)C NMR spectroscopy. *Biochim. Biophys. Acta*, 2002, 1580(2–3):171–188.
82. Walkey, C.J., Donohue, L.R., Bronson, R., Agellon, L.B., and Vance, D.E.: Disruption of the murine gene encoding phosphatidylethanolamine *N*-methyltransferase. *Proc. Natl. Acad. Sci., USA*. 1997, 94(24):12880–12885.
83. Waite, K.A., Cabilio, N.R., and Vance, D.E.: Choline deficiency-induced liver damage is reversible in Pemt(−/−) mice. *J. Nutr.*, 2002, 132(1):68–71.
84. Zhu, X., Song, J., Mar, M.H., Edwards, L.J., and Zeisel, S.H.: Phosphatidylethanolamine *N*-methyltransferase (PEMT) knockout mice have hepatic steatosis and abnormal hepatic choline metabolite concentrations despite ingesting a recommended dietary intake of choline. *Biochem. J.*, 2003, 370(Pt 3):987–993.

85. Noga, A.A., Stead, L.M., Zhao, Y., Brosnan, M.E., Brosnan, J.T., and Vance, D.E.: Plasma homocysteine is regulated by phospholipid methylation. *J. Biol. Chem.*, 2003, 278(8):5952–5955.
86. Jacobs, R.L., Stead, L.M., Devlin, C., Tabas, I., Brosnan, M.E., Brosnan, J.T., and Vance, D.E.: Physiological regulation of phospholipid methylation alters plasma homocysteine in mice. *J. Biol. Chem.*, 2005, 280(31):28299–28305.
87. Aoyama, C., Liao, H., and Ishidate, K.: Structure and function of choline kinase isoforms in mammalian cells. *Prog. Lipid. Res.*, 2004, 43(3):266–281.
88. Peisach, D., Gee, P., Kent, C., and Xu, Z.: The crystal structure of choline kinase reveals a eukaryotic protein kinase fold. *Structure*, 2003, 11(6):703–713.
89. Clement, J.M. and Kent, C.: CTP:phosphocholine cytidylyltransferase: insights into regulatory mechanisms and novel functions. *Biochem. Biophys. Res. Commun.*, 1999, 257(3):643–650.
90. Kent, C.: Regulatory enzymes of phosphatidylcholine biosynthesis: a personal perspective. *Biochim. Biophys. Acta*, 2005, 1733(1):53–66.
91. Vance, J.E. and Vance, D.E.: Phospholipid biosynthesis in mammalian cells. *Biochem. Cell Biol.*, 2004, 82(1):113–128.
92. Cornell, R.B. and Northwood, I.C.: Regulation of CTP:phosphocholine cytidylyltransferase by amphitropism and relocalization. *Trends. Biochem. Sci.*, 2000, 25(9):441–447.
93. Lykidis, A. and Jackowski, S.: Regulation of mammalian cell membrane biosynthesis. *Prog. Nucleic. Acid. Res. Mol. Biol.*, 2001, 65:361–393.
94. Hatch, G.M., Oskin, A., and Vance, D.E.: Involvement of the lysosome in the catabolism of intracellular lysophosphatidylcholine and evidence for distinct pools of lysophosphatidylcholine. *J. Lipid. Res.*, 1993, 34(11):1873–1881.
95. Li, Z., Agellon, L.B., and Vance, D.E.: Phosphatidylcholine homeostasis and liver failure. *J. Biol. Chem.*, 2005, 280(45):37798–37802.
96. Ohanian, J. and Ohanian, V.: Sphingolipids in mammalian cell signalling. *Cell Mol. Life Sci.*, 2001, 58(14):2053–2068.
97. Padron, J.M.: Sphingolipids in anticancer therapy. *Curr. Med. Chem.*, 2006, 13(7):755–770.
98. Liu, B., Obeid, L.M., and Hannun, Y.A.: Sphingomyelinases in cell regulation. *Semin. Cell Dev. Biol.*, 1997, 8(3):311–322.
99. Levade, T., Andrieu-Abadie, N., Segui, B., Auge, N., Chatelut, M., Jaffrezou, J.P., and Salvayre. R.: Sphingomyelin-degrading pathways in human cells role in cell signalling. *Chem. Phys. Lipids.*, 1999, 102(1–2):167–178.
100. Levade, T. and Jaffrezou, J.P.: Signalling sphingomyelinases: which, where, how and why? *Biochim. Biophys. Acta*, 1999, 1438(1):1–17.
101. Delgado-Reyes, C.V., Wallig, M.A., and Garrow, T.A.: Immunohistochemical detection of betaine-homocysteine S-methyltransferase in human, pig, and rat liver and kidney. *Arch. Biochem. Biophys.*, 2001, 393(1):184–186.
102. Sunden, S.L., Renduchintala, M.S., Park, E.I., Miklasz, S.D., and Garrow, T.A.: Betaine-homocysteine methyltransferase expression in porcine and human tissues and chromosomal localization of the human gene. *Arch. Biochem. Biophys.*, 1997, 345(1):171–174.
103. Mudd, S.H., Ebert, M.H., and Scriver, C.R.: Labile methyl group balances in the human: the role of sarcosine. *Metabolism*, 1980, 29(8):707–720.
104. Mudd, S.H. and Poole, J.R.: Labile methyl balances for normal humans on various dietary regimens. *Metabolism*, 1975, 24(6):721–735.
105. Porter, R.K., Scott, J.M., and Brand, M.D.: Choline transport into rat liver mitochondria. Characterization and kinetics of a specific transporter. *J. Biol. Chem.*, 1992, 267(21):14637–14646.
106. Porter, T.J. and Kent, C.: Purification and characterization of choline/ethanolamine kinase from rat liver. *J. Biol. Chem.*, 1990, 265(1):414–422.
107. Haubrich, D.R., Wang, P.F., Chippendale, T., and Proctor, E.: Choline and acetylcholine in rats: effect of dietary choline. *J. Neurochem.*, 1976, 27(6):1305–1313.
108. Finkelstein, J.D., Martin, J.J., Harris, B.J., and Kyle, W.E.: Regulation of the betaine content of rat liver. *Arch. Biochem. Biophys.*, 1982, 218(1):169–173.
109. Haubrich, D.R., Wang, P.F., and Wedeking, P.W.: Distribution and metabolism of intravenously administered choline[methyl-3-H] and synthesis in vivo of acetylcholine in various tissues of guinea pigs. *J. Pharmacol. Exp. Ther.*, 1975, 193(1):246–255.

110. Galletti, P., De Rosa, M., Nappi, M.A., Pontoni, G., del Piano, L., Salluzzo, A., and Zappia, V.: Transport and metabolism of double-labelled CDPcholine in mammalian tissues. *Biochem. Pharmacol.*, 1985, 34(23):4121–4130.
111. Weinhold, P.A. and Sanders, R.: The oxidation of choline by liver slices and mitochondria during liver development in the rat. *Life Sci.*, 1973, 13(5):621–629.
112. Andresen, P.A., Kaasen, I., Styrvold, O.B., Boulnois, G., and Strom, A.R.: Molecular cloning, physical mapping and expression of the bet genes governing the osmoregulatory choline–glycine betaine pathway of *Escherichia coli. J. Gen. Microbiol.*, 1988, 134(6):1737–1746.
113. Huang, S. and Lin, Q.: Functional expression and processing of rat choline dehydrogenase precursor. *Biochem. Biophys. Res. Commun.*, 2003, 309(2):344–350.
114. Cavener, D.R.: GMC oxidoreductases. A newly defined family of homologous proteins with diverse catalytic activities. *J. Mol. Biol.*, 1992, 223(3):811–814.
115. de Ridder, J.J. and van Dam, K.: Control of choline oxidation by rat-liver mitochondria. *Biochim. Biophys. Acta*, 1975, 408(2):112–122.
116. Tsuge, H., Nakano, Y., Onishi, H., Futamura, Y., and Ohashi, K.: A novel purification and some properties of rat liver mitochondrial choline dehydrogenase. *Biochim. Biophys. Acta*, 1980, 614(2):274–284.
117. Barrett, M.C. and Dawson, A.P.: The reaction of choline dehydrogenase with some electron acceptors. *Biochem. J.*, 1975, 151(3):677–683.
118. Qiu, Z.H. and Lin, Q.S.: Spectra properties of rat liver mitochondrial choline dehydrogenase. *Sci. China. B.*, 1990, 33(8):955–963.
119. Pietruszko, R. and Chern, M.: Betaine aldehyde dehydrogenase from rat liver mitochondrial matrix. *Chem. Biol. Interact.*, 2001, 130–132(1–3):193–199.
120. Wilken, D.R., McMacken, M.L., and Rodriquez, A.: Choline and betaine aldehyde oxidation by rat liver mitochondria. *Biochim. Biophys. Acta*, 1970, 216(2):305–317.
121. Chern, M.K. and Pietruszko, R.: Human aldehyde dehydrogenase E3 isozyme is a betaine aldehyde dehydrogenase. *Biochem. Biophys. Res. Commun.*, 1995, 213(2):561–568.
122. Chern, M.K. and Pietruszko, R.: Evidence for mitochondrial localization of betaine aldehyde dehydrogenase in rat liver: purification, characterization, and comparison with human cytoplasmic E3 isozyme. *Biochem. Cell Biol.*, 1999, 77(3):179–187.
123. Porter, R.K., Scott, J.M., and Brand, M.D.: The nature of betaine efflux from rat liver mitochondria. *Biochem. Soc. Trans.*, 1992, 20(3):247S.
124. Porter, R.K., Scott, J.M., and Brand, M.D.: Characterization of betaine efflux from rat liver mitochondria. *Biochim. Biophys. Acta*, 1993, 1141(2–3):269–274.
125. Johansson, K., El-Ahmad, M., Ramaswamy, S., Hjelmqvist, L., Jornvall, H., and Eklund, H.: Structure of betaine aldehyde dehydrogenase at 2.1 A resolution. *Protein. Sci.*, 1998, 7(10):2106–2117.
126. Garrow, T.A.: Purification, kinetic properties, and cDNA cloning of mammalian betaine-homocysteine methyltransferase. *J. Biol. Chem.*, 1996, 271(37):22831–22838.
127. Delgado-Reyes, C.V. and Garrow, T.A.: High sodium chloride intake decreases betaine-homocysteine S-methyltransferase expression in guinea pig liver and kidney. *Am. J. Physiol. Regul. Integr. Comp. Physiol.*, 2005, 288(1):R182–R187.
128. Finkelstein, J.D., Martin, J.J., Harris, B.J., and Kyle, W.E.: Regulation of hepatic betaine-homocysteine methyltransferase by dietary betaine. *J. Nutr.*, 1983, 113(3):519–521.
129. Park, E.I. and Garrow, T.A.: Interaction between dietary methionine and methyl donor intake on rat liver betaine-homocysteine methyltransferase gene expression and organization of the human gene. *J. Biol. Chem.*, 1999, 274(12):7816–7824.
130. Slow, S. and Garrow, T.A.: Liver choline dehydrogenase and kidney betaine-homocysteine S-methyltransferase expression are not affected by methionine or choline intake in growing rats. *J. Nutr.*, 2006, 136:2279–2283.
131. Castro, C., Breksa, A.P., Salisbury, E.M., and Garrow, T.A.: Betaine-homocysteine S-methyltransferase transcription is inhibited by S-adenosylmethionine. In: 12th International Symposium on Pteridines and Folates: 2001. Washington, DC: Kluwer Academic Publishers; 2001.
132. Castro, C., Gratson, A.A., Evans, J.C., Jiracek, J., Collinsova, M., Ludwig, M.L., and Garrow, T.A.: Dissecting the catalytic mechanism of betaine-homocysteine S-methyltransferase by use of intrinsic tryptophan fluorescence and site-directed mutagenesis. *Biochemistry*, 2004, 43(18):5341–5351.

133. Chadwick, L.H., McCandless, S.E., Silverman, G.L., Schwartz, S., Westaway, D., and Nadeau, J.H.: Betaine-homocysteine methyltransferase-2: cDNA cloning, gene sequence, physical mapping, and expression of the human and mouse genes. *Genomics*, 2000, 70(1):66–73.
134. Garrow, T.A., Szegedi, S.S., and Castro, C.: Assigning enzymatic function to betaine-homocysteine methyltransfease-2 as an S-methylmethionine-specific homocysteine methyltransfease. *FASEB J.*, 2006, 20:A606.
135. Evans, J.C., Huddler, D.P., Jiracek, J., Castro, C., Millian, N.S., Garrow, T.A., and Ludwig, M.L.: Betaine-homocysteine methyltransferase: zinc in a distorted barrel. *Structure*, 2002, 10(9):1159–1171.
136. Gonzalez, B., Pajares, M.A., Martinez-Ripoll, M., Blundell, T.L., and Sanz-Aparicio, J.: Crystal structure of rat liver betaine homocysteine s-methyltransferase reveals new oligomerization features and conformational changes upon substrate binding. *J. Mol. Biol.*, 2004, 338(4):771–782.
137. Cook, R.J. and Wagner, C.: Dimethylglycine dehydrogenase and sarcosine dehydrogenase: mitochondrial folate-binding proteins from rat liver. *Methods Enzymol.*, 1986, 122:255–260.
138. Porter, D.H., Cook, R.J., and Wagner, C.: Enzymatic properties of dimethylglycine dehydrogenase and sarcosine dehydrogenase from rat liver. *Arch. Biochem. Biophys.*, 1985, 243(2):396–407.
139. Wittwer, A.J. and Wagner, C.: Identification of the folate-binding proteins of rat liver mitochondria as dimethylglycine dehydrogenase and sarcosine dehydrogenase. Flavoprotein nature and enzymatic properties of the purified proteins. *J. Biol. Chem.*, 1981, 256(8):4109–4115.
140. Wittwer, A.J. and Wagner, C.: Identification of the folate-binding proteins of rat liver mitochondria as dimethylglycine dehydrogenase and sarcosine dehydrogenase. Purification and folate-binding characteristics. *J. Biol. Chem.*, 1981, 256(8):4102–4108.
141. Frisell, W.R. and Mackenzie, C.G.: Separation and purification of sarcosine dehydrogenase and dimethylglycine dehydrogenase. *J. Biol. Chem.*, 1962, 237:94–98.
142. Hoskins, D.D. and Mackenzie, C.G.: Solubilization and electron transfer flavoprotein requirement of mitochondrial sarcosine dehydrogenase and dimethylglycine dehydrogenase. *J. Biol. Chem.*, 1961, 236:177–183.
143. Steenkamp, D.J. and Husain, M.: The effect of tetrahydrofolate on the reduction of electron transfer flavoprotein by sarcosine and dimethylglycine dehydrogenases. *Biochem. J.*, 1982, 203(3):707–715.
144. Brizio, C., Barile, M., and Brandsch, R.: Flavinylation of the precursor of mitochondrial dimethylglycine dehydrogenase by intact and solubilised mitochondria. *FEBS Lett.*, 2002, 522(1–3):141–146.
145. Otto, A., Stoltz, M., Sailer, H.P., and Brandsch, R.: Biogenesis of the covalently flavinylated mitochondrial enzyme dimethylglycine dehydrogenase. *J. Biol. Chem.*, 1996, 271(16):9823–9829.
146. Lang, H., Polster, M., and Brandsch, R.: Rat liver dimethylglycine dehydrogenase. Flavinylation of the enzyme in hepatocytes in primary culture and characterization of a cDNA clone. *Eur. J. Biochem.*, 1991, 198(3):793–799.
147. Cook, R.J., Misono, K.S., and Wagner, C.: The amino acid sequences of the flavin-peptides of dimethylglycine dehydrogenase and sarcosine dehydrogenase from rat liver mitochondria. *J. Biol. Chem.*, 1985, 260(24):12998–13002.
148. Cook, R.J., Misono, K.S., and Wagner, C.: Identification of the covalently bound flavin of dimethylglycine dehydrogenase and sarcosine dehydrogenase from rat liver mitochondria. *J. Biol. Chem.*, 1984, 259(20):12475–12480.
149. Bergeron, F., Otto, A., Blache, P., Day, R., Denoroy, L., Brandsch, R., and Bataille, D.: Molecular cloning and tissue distribution of rat sarcosine dehydrogenase. *Eur. J. Biochem.*, 1998, 257(3):556–561.
150. Lang, H., Minaian, K., Freudenberg, N., Hoffmann, R., and Brandsch, R.: Tissue specificity of rat mitochondrial dimethylglycine dehydrogenase expression. *Biochem. J.*, 1994, 299(Pt 2):393–398.
151. Appling, D.R.: Compartmentation of folate-mediated one-carbon metabolism in eukaryotes. *FASEB J.*, 1991, 5(12):2645–2651.
152. Devaux, P.F.: Static and dynamic lipid asymmetry in cell membranes. *Biochemistry*, 1991, 30(5):1163–1173.
153. Zwaal, R.F. and Schroit, A.J.: Pathophysiologic implications of membrane phospholipid asymmetry in blood cells. *Blood*, 1997, 89(4):1121–1132.
154. Dobransky, T. and Rylett, R.J.: A model for dynamic regulation of choline acetyltransferase by phosphorylation. *J. Neurochem.*, 2005, 95(2):305–313.

155. Zeisel, S.H.: Dietary influences on neurotransmission. *Adv. Pediatr.*, 1986, 33:23–47.
156. Zeisel, S.H. and Niculescu, M.D.: Perinatal choline influences brain structure and function. *Nutr. Rev.*, 2006, 64(4):197–203.
157. Roudebush, W.E., Massey, J.B., Elsner, C.W., Shapiro, D.B., Mitchell-Leef, D., and Kort, H.I.: The significance of platelet-activating factor and fertility in the male primate: a review. *J. Med. Primatol.*, 2005, 34(1):20–24.
158. Alfaro, V.: Role of histamine and platelet-activating factor in allergic rhinitis. *J. Physiol. Biochem.*, 2004, 60(2):101–111.
159. Chen, C.H.: Platelet-activating factor acetylhydrolase: is it good or bad for you? *Curr. Opin. Lipidol.*, 2004, 15(3):337–341.
160. Stafforini, D.M., McIntyre, T.M., Zimmerman, G.A., and Prescott, S.M.: Platelet-activating factor, a pleiotrophic mediator of physiological and pathological processes. *Crit. Rev. Clin. Lab. Sci.*, 2003, 40(6):643–672.
161. Bazan, N.G.: Synaptic lipid signaling: significance of polyunsaturated fatty acids and platelet-activating factor. *J. Lipid. Res.*, 2003, 44(12):2221–2233.
162. Kostenis, E.: Novel clusters of receptors for sphingosine-1-phosphate, sphingosylphosphorylcholine, and (lyso)-phosphatidic acid: new receptors for "old" ligands. *J. Cell Biochem.*, 2004, 92(5):923–936.
163. Meyer zu Heringdorf, D., Himmel, H.M., and Jakobs, K.H.: Sphingosylphosphorylcholine-biological functions and mechanisms of action. *Biochim. Biophys. Acta*, 2002, 1582(1–3):178–189.
164. Xu, Y.: Sphingosylphosphorylcholine and lysophosphatidylcholine: G protein-coupled receptors and receptor-mediated signal transduction. *Biochim. Biophys. Acta*, 2002, 1582(1–3):81–88.
165. Kougias, P., Chai, H., Lin, P.H., Lumsden, A.B., Yao, Q., and Chen, C.: Lysophosphatidylcholine and secretory phospholipase A2 in vascular disease: mediators of endothelial dysfunction and atherosclerosis. *Med. Sci. Monit.*, 2006, 12(1):RA5–16.
166. Lagarde, M., Bernoud, N., Brossard, N., Lemaitre-Delaunay, D., Thies, F., Croset, M., and Lecerf, J.: Lysophosphatidylcholine as a preferred carrier form of docosahexaenoic acid to the brain. *J. Mol. Neurosci.*, 2001, 16(2–3):201–204; discussion 215–221.
167. Prokazova, N.V., Zvezdina, N.D., and Korotaeva, A.A.: Effect of lysophosphatidylcholine on transmembrane signal transduction. *Biochemistry (Mosc)*, 1998, 63(1):31–37.
168. Pomfret, E.A., daCosta, K.A., and Zeisel, S.H.: Effects of choline deficiency and methotrexate treatment upon rat liver. *J. Nutr. Biochem.*, 1990, 1(10):533–541.
169. Svardal, A.M., Ueland, P.M., Berge, R.K., Aarsland, A., Aarsaether, N., Lonning, P.E., and Refsum, H.: Effect of methotrexate on homocysteine and other sulfur compounds in tissues of rats fed a normal or a defined, choline-deficient diet. *Cancer. Chemother. Pharmacol.*, 1988, 21(4):313–318.
170. Zeisel, S.H., Zola, T., daCosta, K.A., and Pomfret, E.A.: Effect of choline deficiency on S-adenosylmethionine and methionine concentrations in rat liver. *Biochem. J.*, 1989, 259(3):725–729.
171. Alonso-Aperte, E. and Varela-Moreiras, G.: Brain folates and DNA methylation in rats fed a choline deficient diet or treated with low doses of methotrexate. *Int. J. Vitam. Nutr. Res.*, 1996, 66(3):232–236.
172. Varela-Moreiras, G., Ragel, C., and Perez de Miguelsanz, J.: Choline deficiency and methotrexate treatment induces marked but reversible changes in hepatic folate concentrations, serum homocysteine and DNA methylation rates in rats. *J. Am. Coll. Nutr.*, 1995, 14(5):480–485.
173. Wehner, F., Olsen, H., Tinel, H., Kinne-Saffran, E., and Kinne, R.K.: Cell volume regulation: osmolytes, osmolyte transport, and signal transduction. *Rev. Physiol. Biochem. Pharmacol.*, 2003, 148:1–80.
174. Beck, F.X. and Neuhofer, W.: Response of renal medullary cells to osmotic stress. *Contrib. Nephrol.*, 2005, 148:21–34.
175. Kempson, S.A. and Montrose, M.H.: Osmotic regulation of renal betaine transport: transcription and beyond. *Pflugers Arch.*, 2004, 449(3):227–234.
176. Ferraris, J.D. and Burg, M.B.: Drying and salting send different messages. *J. Physiol.*, 2004, 558(Pt 1):3.
177. Burg, M.B.: Response of renal inner medullary epithelial cells to osmotic stress. *Comp. Biochem. Physiol. A. Mol. Integr. Physiol.*, 2002, 133(3):661–666.

178. Grossman, E.B., and Hebert, S.C.: Renal inner medullary choline dehydrogenase activity: characterization and modulation. *Am. J. Physiol.*, 1989, 256(1 Pt 2):F107–F112.
179. Beck, F.X., Burger-Kentischer, A., and Muller, E.: Cellular response to osmotic stress in the renal medulla. *Pflugers Arch.*, 1998, 436(6):814–827.
180. Kwon, H.M.: Transcriptional regulation of the betaine/gamma-aminobutyric acid transporter by hypertonicity. *Biochem. Soc. Trans.*, 1996, 24(3):853–856.
181. Bauernschmitt, H.G. and Kinne, R.K.: Metabolism of the 'organic osmolyte' glycerophosphorylcholine in isolated rat inner medullary collecting duct cells. I., Pathways for synthesis and degradation. *Biochim. Biophys. Acta*, 1993, 1148(2):331–341.
182. Bauernschmitt, H.G. and Kinne, R.K.: Metabolism of the 'organic osmolyte' glycerophosphorylcholine in isolated rat inner medullary collecting duct cells. II. Regulation by extracellular osmolality. *Biochim. Biophys. Acta*, 1993, 1150(1):25–34.
183. Kwon, E.D., Jung, K.Y., Edsall, L.C., Kim, H.Y., Garcia-Perez, A., and Burg, M.B.: Osmotic regulation of synthesis of glycerophosphocholine from phosphatidylcholine in MDCK cells. *Am. J. Physiol.*, 1995, 268(2 Pt 1):C402–C412.
184. Kanfer, J.N. and McCartney, D.G.: GPC phosphodiesterase and phosphomonoesterase activities of renal cortex and medulla of control, antidiuresis and diuresis rats. *FEBS Lett.*, 1989, 257(2):348–350.
185. Kwon, E.D., Zablocki, K., Jung, K.Y., Peters, E.M., Garcia-Perez, A., and Burg, M.B.: Osmoregulation of GPC:choline phosphodiesterase in MDCK cells: different effects of urea and NaCl. *Am. J. Physiol.*, 1995, 269(1 Pt 1):C35–C41.
186. Albright, C.D., da Costa, K.A., Craciunescu, C.N., Klem, E., Mar, M.H., and Zeisel, S.H.: Regulation of choline deficiency apoptosis by epidermal growth factor in CWSV-1 rat hepatocytes. *Cell Physiol. Biochem.*, 2005, 15(1–4):59–68.
187. Albright, C.D., Liu, R., Bethea, T.C., Da Costa, K.A., Salganik, R.I., and Zeisel, S.H.: Choline deficiency induces apoptosis in SV40-immortalized CWSV-1 rat hepatocytes in culture. *FASEB J.*, 1996, 10(4):510–516.
188. Albright, C.D., Mar, M.H., Craciunescu, C.N., Song, J., and Zeisel, S.H.: Maternal dietary choline availability alters the balance of netrin-1 and DCC neuronal migration proteins in fetal mouse brain hippocampus. *Brain Res. Dev. Brain Res.*, 2005, 159(2):149–154.
189. Albright, C.D., Mar, M.H., Friedrich, C.B., Brown, E.C., and Zeisel, S.H.: Maternal choline availability alters the localization of p15Ink4B and p27Kip1 cyclin-dependent kinase inhibitors in the developing fetal rat brain hippocampus. *Dev. Neurosci.*, 2001, 23(2):100–106.
190. Albright, C.D., Siwek, D.F., Craciunescu, C.N., Mar, M.H., Kowall, N.W., Williams, C.L., and Zeisel, S.H.: Choline availability during embryonic development alters the localization of calretinin in developing and aging mouse hippocampus. *Nutr. Neurosci.*, 2003, 6(2):129–134.
191. Albright, C.D., Tsai, A.Y., Friedrich, C.B., Mar, M.H., and Zeisel, S.H.: Choline availability alters embryonic development of the hippocampus and septum in the rat. *Brain Res. Dev. Brain Res.*, 1999, 113(1–2):13–20.
192. Albright, C.D. and Zeisel, S.H.: Choline deficiency causes increased localization of transforming growth factor-beta1 signaling proteins and apoptosis in the rat liver. *Pathobiology*, 1997, 65(5):264–270.
193. Albright, C.D., Zeisel, S.H., and Salganik, R.I.: Choline deficiency induces apoptosis and decreases the number of eosinophilic preneoplastic foci in the liver of OXYS rats. *Pathobiology*, 1998, 66(2):71–76.
194. Craciunescu, C.N., Albright, C.D., Mar, M.H., Song, J., and Zeisel, S.H.: Choline availability during embryonic development alters progenitor cell mitosis in developing mouse hippocampus. *J. Nutr.*, 2003, 133(11):3614–3618.
195. da Costa, K.A., Cochary, E.F., Blusztajn, J.K., Garner, S.C., and Zeisel, S.H.: Accumulation of 1,2-sn-diradylglycerol with increased membrane-associated protein kinase C may be the mechanism for spontaneous hepatocarcinogenesis in choline-deficient rats. *J. Biol. Chem.*, 1993, 268(3):2100–2105.
196. da Costa, K.A., Gaffney, C.E., Fischer, L.M., and Zeisel, S.H.: Choline deficiency in mice and humans is associated with increased plasma homocysteine concentration after a methionine load. *Am. J. Clin. Nutr.*, 2005, 81(2):440–444.

197. da Costa, K.A., Garner, S.C., Chang, J., and Zeisel, S.H.: Effects of prolonged (1 year) choline deficiency and subsequent re-feeding of choline on 1,2-sn-diradylglycerol, fatty acids and protein kinase C in rat liver. *Carcinogenesis*, 1995, 16(2):327–334.
198. Griffith, W.H.: The renal lesions in choline deficiency. *Am. J. Clin. Nutr.*, 1958, 6(3):263–273.
199. Holmes-McNary, M.Q., Baldwin, A.S. Jr., and Zeisel, S.H.: Opposing regulation of choline deficiency-induced apoptosis by p53 and nuclear factor kappaB. *J. Biol. Chem.*, 2001, 276(44):41197–41204.
200. Holmes-McNary, M.Q., Loy, R., Mar, M.H., Albright, C.D., and Zeisel, S.H.: Apoptosis is induced by choline deficiency in fetal brain and in PC12 cells. *Brain Res. Dev. Brain Res.*, 1997, 101(1–2):9–16.
201. Kulinski, A., Vance, D.E., and Vance, J.E.: A choline-deficient diet in mice inhibits neither the CDP-choline pathway for phosphatidylcholine synthesis in hepatocytes nor apolipoprotein B secretion. *J. Biol. Chem.*, 2004, 279(23):23916–23924.
202. Niculescu, M.D., Craciunescu, C.N., and Zeisel, S.H.: Dietary choline deficiency alters global and gene-specific DNA methylation in the developing hippocampus of mouse fetal brains. *FASEB J.*, 2006, 20(1):43–49.
203. Niculescu, M.D., Yamamuro, Y., and Zeisel, S.H.: Choline availability modulates human neuroblastoma cell proliferation and alters the methylation of the promoter region of the cyclin-dependent kinase inhibitor 3 gene. *J. Neurochem.*, 2004, 89(5):1252–1259.
204. Niculescu, M.D. and Zeisel, S.H.: Diet, methyl donors and DNA methylation: interactions between dietary folate, methionine and choline. *J. Nutr.*, 2002, 132(8 Suppl):2333S–2335S.
205. Rogers, A.E., Zeisel, S.H., and Groopman, J.: Diet and carcinogenesis. *Carcinogenesis*, 1993, 14(11):2205–2217.
206. Selhub, J., Seyoum, E., Pomfret, E.A., and Zeisel, S.H.: Effects of choline deficiency and methotrexate treatment upon liver folate content and distribution. *Cancer Res.*, 1991, 51(1):16–21.
207. Shin, O.H., Mar, M.H., Albright, C.D., Citarella, M.T., da Costa, K.A., and Zeisel, S.H.: Methyl-group donors cannot prevent apoptotic death of rat hepatocytes induced by choline-deficiency. *J. Cell Biochem.*, 1997, 64(2):196–208.
208. Yen, C.L., Mar, M.H., Meeker, R.B., Fernandes, A., and Zeisel, S.H.: Choline deficiency induces apoptosis in primary cultures of fetal neurons. *FASEB J.*, 2001, 15(10):1704–1710.
209. Yen, C.L., Mar, M.H., and Zeisel, S.H.: Choline deficiency-induced apoptosis in PC12 cells is associated with diminished membrane phosphatidylcholine and sphingomyelin, accumulation of ceramide and diacylglycerol, and activation of a caspase. *FASEB J.*, 1999, 13(1):135–142.
210. Zeisel, S.H.: Choline: an important nutrient in brain development, liver function and carcinogenesis. *J. Am. Coll. Nutr.*, 1992, 11(5):473–481.
211. da Costa, K.A., Kozyreva, O.G., Song, J., Galanko, J.A., Fischer, L.M., and Zeisel, S.H.: Common genetic polymorphisms affect the human requirement for the nutrient choline. *FASEB J.*, 2006, 20(9):1336–1344.
212. Fischer, L.M., Scearce, J.A., Mar, M.H., Patel, J.R., Blanchard, R.T., Macintosh, B.A., Busby, M.G., and Zeisel, S.H.: Ad libitum choline intake in healthy individuals meets or exceeds the proposed adequate intake level. *J. Nutr.*, 2005, 135(4):826–829.
213. Buchman, A.L.: Choline deficiency during parenteral nutrition in humans. *Nutr. Clin. Pract.*, 2003, 18(5):353–358.
214. da Costa, K.A., Badea, M., Fischer, L.M., and Zeisel, S.H.: Elevated serum creatine phosphokinase in choline-deficient humans: mechanistic studies in C2C12 mouse myoblasts. *Am. J. Clin. Nutr.*, 2004, 80(1):163–170.
215. da Costa, K.A., Niculescu, M.D., Craciunescu, C.N., Fischer, L.M., and Zeisel, S.H.: Choline deficiency increases lymphocyte apoptosis and DNA damage in humans. *Am. J. Clin. Nutr.*, 2006, 84(1):88–94.
216. Shaw, G.M., Carmichael, S.L., Yang, W., Selvin, S., and Schaffer, D.M.: Periconceptional dietary intake of choline and betaine and neural tube defects in offspring. *Am. J. Epidemiol.*, 2004, 160(2):102–109.
217. Subcommittee on Laboratory Animal Nutrition CoAN, Board on Agriculture, National Research Council: *Nutrient Requirements of Laboratory Animals*, fourth edn. Washington, DC: National Academy Press; 1995.

218. Sanz, A., Caro, P., Ayala, V., Portero-Otin, M., Pamplona, R., and Barja, G.: Methionine restriction decreases mitochondrial oxygen radical generation and leak as well as oxidative damage to mitochondrial DNA and proteins. *FASEB J.*, 2006, 20(8):1064–1073.
219. Pamplona, R. and Barja, G.: Mitochondrial oxidative stress, aging and caloric restriction: the protein and methionine connection. *Biochim. Biophys. Acta*, 2006, 1757(5–6):496–508.
220. Uthus, E.O. and Brown-Borg, H.M.: Methionine flux to transsulfuration is enhanced in the long living Ames dwarf mouse. *Mech. Ageing Dev.*, 2006, 127(5):444–450.
221. Linnebank, M., Fliessbach, K., Kolsch, H., Rietschel, M., and Wullner, U.: The methionine synthase polymorphism c.2756Aright curved arrow G (D919G) is relevant for disease-free longevity. *Int. J. Mol. Med.*, 2005, 16(4):759–761.
222. Miller, R.A., Buehner, G., Chang, Y., Harper, J.M., Sigler, R., and Smith-Wheelock, M.: Methionine-deficient diet extends mouse lifespan, slows immune and lens aging, alters glucose, T4, IGF-I and insulin levels, and increases hepatocyte MIF levels and stress resistance. *Aging Cell*, 2005, 4(3):119–125.
223. Young, R.J., Lucas, C.C., Patterson, J.M., and Best, C.H.: Lipotropic dose–response studies in rats; comparisons of choline, betaine, and methionine. *Can. J. Biochem. Physiol.*, 1956, 34(4):713–720.
224. Best, C.H., Lucas, C.C., Ridout, J.H., and Patterson, J.M.: Dose-response curves in the estimation of potency of lipotropic agents. *J. Biol. Chem.*, 1950, 186(1):317–329.
225. Kim, Y.I., Miller, J.W., da Costa, K.A., Nadeau, M., Smith, D., Selhub, J., Zeisel, S.H., and Mason, J.B.: Severe folate deficiency causes secondary depletion of choline and phosphocholine in rat liver. *J. Nutr.*, 1994, 124(11):2197–2203.
226. Rhee, M.S., Johnson, T.B., Priest, D.G., and Galivan, J.: The effect of methionine on methotrexate metabolism in rat hepatocytes in monolayer culture. *Biochim. Biophys. Acta*, 1989, 1011(2–3):122–128.
227. Barak, A.J. and Kemmy, R.J.: Methotrexate effects on hepatic betaine levels in choline-supplemented and choline-deficient rats. *Drug Nutr. Interact.*, 1982, 1(4):275–278.
228. Freeman-Narrod, M.: Choline antagonism of methotrexate liver toxicity in the rat. *Med. Pediatr. Oncol.*, 1977, 3(1):9–14.
229. Freeman-Narrod, M., Narrod, S.A., and Custer, R.P.: Chronic toxicity of methotrexate in rats: partial to complete projection of the liver by choline: brief communication. *J. Natl. Cancer Inst.*, 1977, 59(3):1013–1017.
230. Kohlmeier, M., da Costa, K.A., Fischer, L.M., and Zeisel, S.H.: Genetic variation of folate-mediated one-carbon transfer pathway predicts susceptibility to choline deficiency in humans. *Proc. Natl. Acad. Sci., USA*. 2005, 102(44):16025–16030.
231. Zeisel, S.H., Wishnok, J.S., and Blusztajn, J.K.: Formation of methylamines from ingested choline and lecithin. *J. Pharmacol. Exp. Ther.*, 1983, 225(2):320–324.

15 Ascorbic Acid

Carol S. Johnston, Francene M. Steinberg, and Robert B. Rucker

CONTENTS

INTRODUCTION AND HISTORY

Ascorbic acid (vitamin C) plays a role as a redox cofactor and catalyst in a broad array of biochemical reactions and processes. Vitamin C is designated as ascorbic acid because of its ability to cure and prevent scurvy [1–6]. Ascorbic acid comes from the Scandinavian terms, skjoerberg or skorbjugg, and from the English, scarfy or scorby. From a historical perspective, it is instructive to visit the original treatise on scurvy by James Lind, *Treatise on the Scurvy*, published in 1753 [7], although it was over 100 years later that a connection between scurvy and diet was established and an additional 100 years before the first biological and chemical descriptions of ascorbic acid began to appear [1].

Scurvy has had a direct influence on all of our lives. Scurvy was endemic in many areas throughout seventeenth to nineteenth centuries. The military diets of the seventeenth and eighteenth centuries adhered to protocols that promoted scurvy, that is, lack of fruits and vegetables. For example, Britain's general lack of success in earliest explorations of the New World compared with the Spanish and French is an example of how scurvy influenced the historical face of "New World" development. Over 2 million sailors are reported to have died of scurvy during the era, often called the "Age of Sail" [8]. Indeed, it was not until 1804, that the British Navy adopted the use of lime juice as a part of rations, which resulted in the nickname "limeys" for British sailors [8–10]. In the United States, thousands of settlers died from scurvy, particularly in route to the west [11]. During the Civil War, poor nutrition, resulting in scurvy (and also pellagra), also took its toll and debatably influenced the outcome of a number of key battles [8–12].

An important breakthrough in the understanding of scurvy was the observation that guinea pigs were susceptible to scurvy. This observation, reported in 1907 by Holst and Frohlich, was one of the first examples of use of an animal model to study a nutritional disease [13]. Eventually, it was demonstrated that primates were also susceptible to scurvy [1]. Next, Zilva and his associates isolated antiscorbutic activity from a crude fraction of lemon [4,9,10]. Zilva showed that the activity was destroyed by oxidation and protected by reducing agents. Important to the evolving nomenclature for vitamins, it was suggested that the new antiscorbutic factor be designated "factor or vitamin C" since "A" and "B" had been previously designated as potential health and growth factors [9].

Throughout the 1930s, work progressed rapidly with validation and identification of vitamin C in a number of foods. Early papers by Szent-Gyorgyi, Haworth, King, and coworkers document in part this effort as well as chemical identification and elucidation of ascorbic acid's structure [10]. In 1937, both Szent-Gyorgyi and Haworth received Nobel Prizes in medicine and chemistry, respectively, for work related to vitamin C.

CHEMISTRY AND FOOD SOURCES

NOMENCLATURE AND STRUCTURE

The IUPAC–IUB Commission on Biochemical Nomenclature changed vitamin C (2-oxo-L-theo-hexono-4-lactone-2,3-enediol) to ascorbic acid or L-ascorbic acid in 1965. The chemical structures of ascorbic acid are given in Figure 15.1. The molecule has a near planar five-member ring. Ascorbic acid has two chiral centers, which contain four stereoisomers. Dehydroascorbic acid, the oxidized form of ascorbic acid retains vitamin C activity and can exist as a hydrated hemiketal. Crystalline dehydro-L-ascorbic acid can exist as a dimer [14–16].

PHYSICAL AND CHEMICAL PROPERTIES

Physical and chemical features of ascorbic acid are summarized in Table 15.1. Data are also available regarding X-ray crystallographic, [^{1}H] and [^{13}C]NMR spectroscopic, IR- and

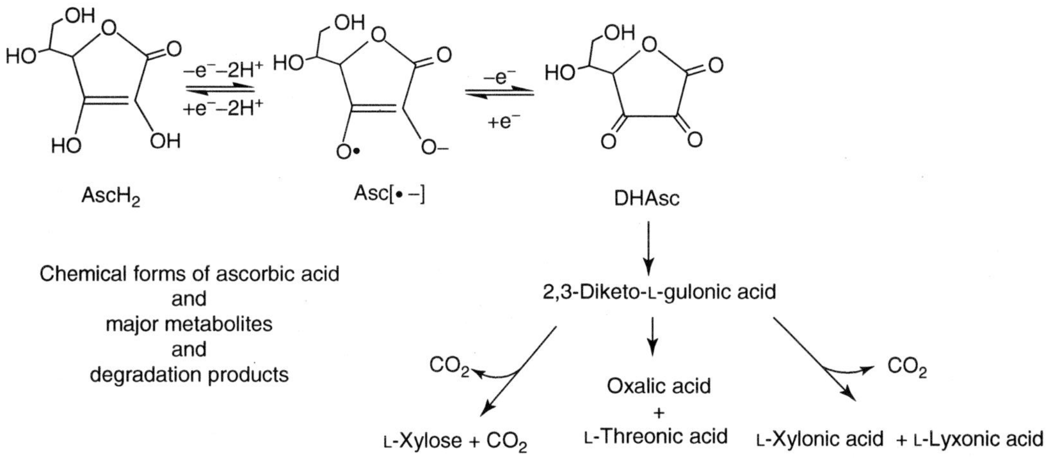

$AscH_2$ ⇌ Asc[• −] ⇌ DHAsc

−e⁻−2H⁺ / +e⁻−2H⁺ ; −e⁻ / +e⁻

Chemical forms of ascorbic acid and major metabolites and degradation products

DHAsc → 2,3-Diketo-L-gulonic acid → Oxalic acid + L-Threonic acid; → L-Xylose + CO_2 (CO_2); → L-Xylonic acid + L-Lyxonic acid (CO_2)

FIGURE 15.1 Ascorbic acid and various oxidation products. Ascorbic acid can exist in several different forms. The two predominant forms and some of their associated oxidation products are shown. In solution, ascorbic acid probably exists as the hydrated semiketal. $AscH_2$ (reduced ascorbic acid) ↔ Asc[−] (ascorbate radical) ↔ DHASC (dehydroascorbic acid). Under basic conditions, cleavage occurs rapidly at carbon-1 or carbon-2.

UV-spectroscopic, and mass spectroscopic characteristics [12,17]. The most important chemical property of ascorbic acid is the reversible oxidation to semidehydro-L-ascorbic acid and oxidation further to dehydro-L-ascorbic acid [12,14,16]. This property is the basis for its known physiological activities. In addition, the proton on oxygen-3 is acidic ($pK_1 = 4.17$), which contributes to the acidic nature of ascorbic acid.

Degradation reactions of L-ascorbic acid in aqueous solutions depend on a number of factors such as pH, temperature, the presence of oxygen, or metals. In general, ascorbic acid is

TABLE 15.1
Selected Physical Properties of Ascorbic Acid

Empirical formula	$C_6H_8O_6$
Molar mass	176.13
Crystalline form	Monoclinic, mix of platelets and needles
Melting point	190°C–192°C
Optical rotation	$[\alpha]25/D + 20.5°$ to 21.51° (cm = 1 in water)
pH, at 5 mg/mL	~3
at 50 mg/mL	~2
pK_1	4.17
pK_2	11.57
Redox potential (dehydroascorbic acid/ascorbate)	−174 mV
(ascorbate • −, H^+/ascorbate$^-$)	+282 mV
Solubility, g/mL	
Water	0.33
Ethanol, abs.	0.02
Ether, chloroform, benzene	Insoluble
Absorption spectra	
at pH 2	E_{max} (1%, 10 mm) 695 at 245 nm
at pH 6.4	E_{max} (1%, 10 mm) 940 at 265 nm

not very stable in aqueous media at room temperature. Above pH 7.0, alkali-catalyzed degradation results in over 50 compounds, mainly mono-, di-, and tricarboxylic acids [15,18,19]. The vitamin can be stabilized in biological samples with trichloroacetic acid or metaphosphoric acid. Ascorbic acid is reasonably stable in blood or enteral or intravenous solutions when stored at or below 20°C [20–22].

As noted, in addition to redox and acid–base properties, ascorbic acid can exist as a free radical [14,16,18,19,23]. The ascorbate radical is an important intermediate in reactions involving oxidants and ascorbic acid's antioxidant activity. The physiologically dominate ascorbic acid monoanions and dianions have p*K*s of 4.1 (pK_1) and 11.79 (pK_2), respectively.

Rate constants for the generation of ascorbate radicals vary considerably, for example, $10^4-10^8\ s^{-1}$. When ascorbate radicals are generated by oxyanions, the rate constants are on the order of $10^4-10^7\ s^{-1}$, when generated by halide radicals, $10^6-10^8\ s^{-1}$, and when generated by tocopherol and flavonoids radicals, $10^6-10^8\ s^{-1}$ [14,15]. Once formed, the ascorbate radical decays slowly, usually by disproportionation [15,16]. Changing ionic strength or pH can influence the rate of dismutation of ascorbic acid (i.e., either increase or decrease). Certain oxyanions, for example, phosphate, accelerate dismutation [16]. The acceleration is attributed to the ability of various protonated forms of phosphate to donate a proton efficiently to the ascorbate radical, particularly dimer forms of ascorbate.

In biological systems, the unusual stability of the ascorbate radical dictates that accessory enzymatic systems be made available to reduce the potential transient accumulation of the ascorbate radical. Excess ascorbate radicals may initiate free-radical cascade reactions or nonspecific oxidations. In plants, NADH:monodehydroascorbate reductase (EC 1.6.5.4) has evolved to maintain ascorbic acid in its reduced form. NADH:monodehydroascorbate reductase plays a major role in stress-related responses in plants. In animal tissues, glutathione dehydroascorbate reductase (EC 1.8.5.1) serves this purpose. Such enzymes keep vitamin C operating at maximum efficiency, so that other enzyme systems may take advantage of the univalent redox-cycling capacity of ascorbate [12]. As an example, without an interaction between dopamine hydroxylase (EC 1.14.17.1) and cytochrome b_5 reductase (EC 1.10.2.1), increasing the concentration of ascorbate will scavenge the dopamine radical and replace it with an ascorbate radical. Similarly, dopamine can reduce the radical intensity of ascorbate [24,25]. Enzymatically coupled reactions reduce the potential of radical accumulation.

Isolation

Ascorbic acid is stable in many organic and inorganic acids. *m*-Phosphoric acid–containing ethylenediamine tetraacetic acid (0.5%–2%), oxalic acid, dilute trichloroacetic acid, dilute perchloric acid, or 2,3-dimercaptopropanol are often used as solvents or solutions for tissue extraction [20,26]. Extraction of ascorbic acid should be carried out under subdued light and an inert atmosphere to avoid the potential for degradation [26].

Chemical and Biological Synthesis

The approach used for ascorbic acid synthesis often depends on the eventual use of the final product [27]. For example, strategies for radiochemical labeling of ascorbic acid involve coupling either a C-1 fragment to a C-5 fragment or a C-2 fragment to a C-4 fragment. Alternatively, the approach may involve the conversion of the six-carbon form of ascorbic acid or an analog to a suitable radiolabeled derivative. Although procedural details are beyond the scope of this chapter, most approaches in making or modifying ascorbic acid involve first derivatizing ascorbic acid [28,29]. In this regard, selective derivatization of ascorbic acid can be difficult because of delocation of the negative charge of ascorbate in its anionic form. For example, by protecting the C-2 and C-3 hydroxyl groups, alkylation or

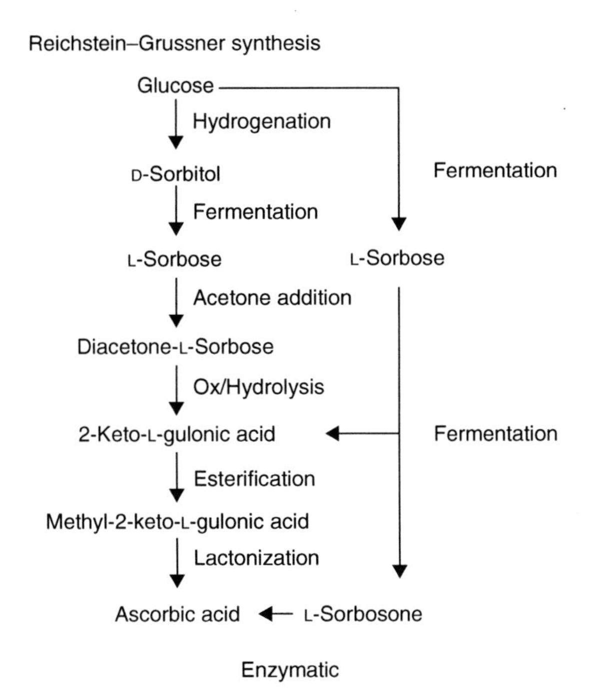

FIGURE 15.2 Basic steps in the commercial synthesis of ascorbic acid from D-glucose via the Reichstein–Grussner synthesis pathway or fermentation starting with D-glucose or L-sorbitol. If ample quantities of sorbosone are produced, ascorbic acid can be generated by the action of sorbosone dehydrogenase.

acylation can take place at the more sterically accessible primary hydroxyl group on C-6. Reactions at the C-5 position occur only after derivatizations of the C-2, C-3, and C-6 are completed [30]. The formation of acetates or ketals of ascorbic acid is useful for protection of the molecule while reactions at the other carbons are carried out [30]. The chemical pathway for industrial synthesis of ascorbic acid from glucose is given in Figure 15.2. This process was first developed in the 1930s and is still in use. More biological approaches involve the use of a novel enzyme, for example, L-sorbosone dehydrogenase, which directly converts polyalcohols, such as L-sorbosone to L-ascorbic acid and 2-keto-L-gulonic acid [31,32].

Analysis

Ascorbic acid has strong UV absorption, which is the basis of spectrophotometric methods for the measurement of ascorbic acid (see Table 15.1). Treatment of material to be analyzed with ascorbic acid oxidase is often used as a blank to correct for interfering substances in biological samples. A number of high-performance liquid chromatographic methods have now been developed for isolation of ascorbic acid [33–43].

Electrochemical detection is also used for measuring ascorbic acid and derivatives in eluates [36]. Electrochemical detection allows for the simultaneous measurement of ascorbic and dehydroascorbic acid, isomers, and derivatives. Chromatographic approaches include ion exchange, gas, reversed phase, and ion-pairing HPLC chromatographic protocols.

In direct assays of ascorbic acid in crude mixtures, the 2,2′-dipyridyl calorimetric method is often used, which is based on the reduction of Fe(III) to Fe(II) by ascorbic acid [39]. Fe(II) reacts with 2,2′-dipyridyl to form a complex that can be quantified calorimetrically. In addition to 2,2′-dipyridyl, ferozine and Folin phenol reagent have also been used. Further, methods based on fluorometric and chemiluminescence detection provide highly sensitive approaches for the determination of ascorbic acid [38,40].

Enzymatic methods using ascorbate oxidase have the advantage of selectively measuring the biological activity of ascorbic acid [44]. Conventional and isotope ratio mass spectrometry techniques have also been used to analyze ascorbic acid. Isotope ratio mass spectrometry is particularly useful and sensitive, when ^{13}C ascorbic acid is available for use as a reference or standard in the analysis of complex matrices [40,43].

As a final point, in addition to the problems associated with accurately measuring ascorbic acid, the presence of ascorbic acid may also interfere with many urine and blood chemical tests. Examples include the analysis of glucose, uric acid, creatinine, bilirubin, glycohemoglobin, hemoglobin A, cholesterol, triglycerides, leukocytes, and inorganic phosphate [45,46], because as a reductant, ascorbic acid can cause nonspecific color formation.

Sources of Ascorbic Acid

Ascorbic acid occurs in significant amounts in vegetables, fruits, and animal organs such as liver, kidney, and brain. Potatoes and cabbage are also among the important sources of vitamin C. Typical values are given in Table 15.2.

BIOCHEMICAL FUNCTIONS

Plants

Ascorbic acid is detected in yeast and prokaryotes, except cyanobacteria [12]. Ascorbic acid is synthesized in plants from D-glucose and other sugars. Ascorbic acid functions in many mono- and dioxygenases to maintain metals in a reduced state. For example, mono- and dioxygenases usually contain copper or iron as redox cofactors, respectively. As an additional characteristic, dioxygenases require α-ketoglutarate and O_2 as cosubstrates in reactions whereas monooxygenases require only O_2. The pathway for ascorbic acid synthesis in plants and animals is shown in Figure 15.3.

Animals and Animal Models

In the kidney of fish, reptiles, and birds, and the liver of mammals, the key enzyme in the synthesis of ascorbic acid is L-gulonolactone oxidase (EC 1.1.3.8; cf. Figure 15.3). During the course of evolution, the ability to express L-gulonolactone oxidase functional activity disappeared in the guinea pig, some fruit-eating bats, and most primates, including man [47].

Regarding specific steps in the pathway in animals, L-gulonolactone is generated by the direct oxidation of glucose [48,49]. In this regard, it may be asked whether the amounts of ascorbic acid synthesized per day in animals with gulonolactone oxidase correspond to the amounts needed in the diets of the guinea pig or primate. Grollman and Lehninger [48] used liver homogenates and gulonic acid as substrates for ascorbic acid synthesis. They found that the amounts varied from ~0.01 g of L-ascorbic acid synthesized per day per kilogram body weight for the pig to 0.2 g/kg body weight for the rat. Linus Pauling in his monograph, *Vitamin C and the Common Cold* [50], used such data to infer that the ascorbic acid needs in humans were in grams per day range. What is ignored is that ascorbic acid production can be no more than the amount of glucose or galactose shunted through the gulonate oxidative pathway. In a 70 kg person, this value ranges from 5 to 15 g/day. Only ~1% of the gulonate flux is in the direction of ascorbate synthesis [48,51,52]. Therefore, given that 5–15 g of glucose and galactose are shunted through the glucuronate and gulonate pathway in humans,

TABLE 15.2
Vitamin C in Selected Food

Sources	Edible Portion (mg/100 g)	Sources	Edible Portion (mg/100 g)
Animal products		*Vegetables*	
Cows milk	0.5–2	*Asparagus*	15–30
Human milk	3–6	Avocado	10
Beef	1–2	Broccoli	80–90
Pork	1–2	Beet	6–8
Veal	1–1.5	Beans, various	10–15
Ham	20–25	Brussels sprout	100–120
Liver, chicken	15–20	Cabbage	30–70
Beef	10	Carrot	5–10
Kidney, chicken	6–8	Cucumber	6–8
Heart, chicken	5	Cauliflower	50–70
Gizzard, chicken	5–7	Eggplant	15–20
Crab muscle	1–4	Chive	40–50
Lobster	3	Kale	70–100
Scrimp muscle	2–4	Onion	10–15
Fruits		Pea	8–12
Apple	3–30	Potato	4–30
Banana	8–16	Pumpkin	15
Blackberry	8–10	Radish	25
Cherry	15–30	Spinach	35–40
Currant, red	20–50	*Spices and condiments*	
Currant, black	150–200	Chicory	33
Grape	2–5	Coriander (spice)	90
Grapefruit	30–70	Garlic	16
Kiwi fruit	80–90	Horseradish	45
Lemon	40–50	Lettuce, various	10–30
Melons	9–60	Leek	5
Mango	10–15	Parsley	200–300
Orange	30–50	Papaya	39
Pear	2–5	Pepper, various	150–200
Pineapple	15–25		
Plums	2–3		
Rose hips	250–800		
Strawberry	40–70		
Tomato	10–201		

this would amount to ~50–150 mg of ascorbate per day, if humans were capable of making ascorbate. This is the same order of magnitude, as the reported need for ascorbic acid in humans [51,53–55].

Interestingly, examination of two animal genetic models (1) the gulonolactone oxidase null mouse [56] and (2) the osteogenic disorder Shionogi (ODS) rat [57], in which a missense mutation of L-gulono-γ-lactone oxidase causes scurvy-prone disorders, leads to the same conclusion. The L-ascorbic acid requirement for normal growth and metabolism for these two animal models is in the order of 300–400 mg L-ascorbic acid/kg of diet [58], that is, about the same as that for the guinea pig, ~200 mg L-ascorbic acid/kg diet for optimal growth. Expressed per unit of food energy intake, this amounts to 80–160 mg L-ascorbic acid/1000 kcal (4187 kJ), that is, 150–300 mg/day in "human terms." Moreover, human milk contains 50 mg L-ascorbic acid/L or 150–250 mg/kg of milk solids. The point is that a strong case may be made that for vitamins, ascorbate as a specific example, requirements in

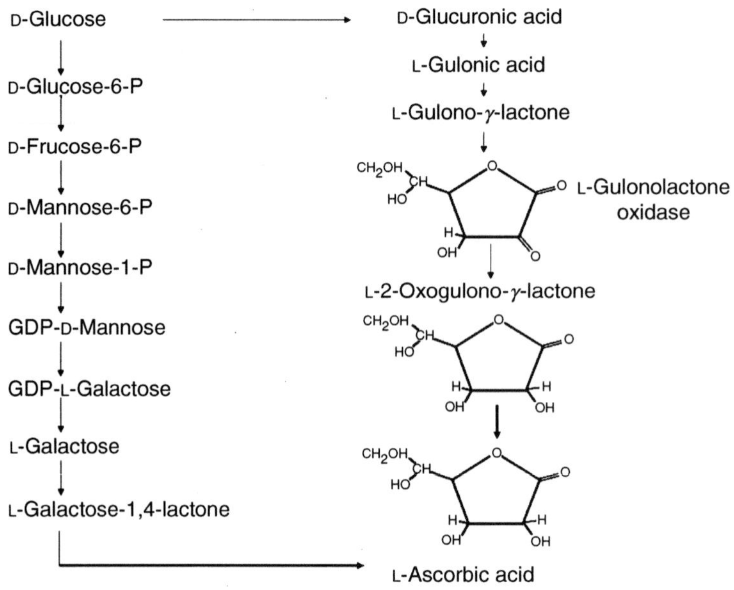

FIGURE 15.3 Cellular pathways for the synthesis of ascorbic acid. The direct oxidative pathway for glucose is utilized in animals that make ascorbic acid. Gulonolactone oxidase is compromised or absent in animals that cannot make ascorbic acid. In plants and bacteria that make L-ascorbic acid (pathway to the left), galactose and mannose, in addition to D-glucose can contribute to ascorbic acid production.

homeothermic (warm-blooded) animals are similar or are of the same magnitude when expressed relative to units of energy intake.

Selected Enzymes and Biochemical Processes

Ascorbic acid deprivation and scurvy include a range of signs and symptoms that involve defects in specific enzymatic steps and processes (cf. Table 15.3). Other examples are summarized in Selected Clinical Features Important to Ascorbic Acid Status.

Ascorbic Acid and Glutathione Interrelationships

Cells deal with excessive oxidants by a number of mechanisms. The most important is the utilization of L-γ-glutamyl-L-cysteine-glycine (GSH) as a reductant [59–67]. GSH is synthesized by a two-step reaction involving γ-L-glutamyl cysteine synthetase and GSH synthetase. When GSH synthesis is blocked, for example, by use of inhibitors, such as L-buthionine-(*SR*)-sulfoximine, newborn animals die within a few days due to oxidative stress, which can result in proximal renal tubular damage, liver damage, and disruption of lamella bodies in lung [65]. The cellular damage involves mostly mitochondrial changes. A role for ascorbic acid is depicted in Figure 15.4.

Meister and his associates reported that administration of ascorbic acid ameliorates most of the signs of chemically induced GSH deficiency [65]. The effect is very pronounced in newborn rats, which do not efficiently synthesize ascorbic acid in contrast to adult rats, and guinea pigs. When L-buthionine-(*SR*)-sulfoximine is administered, in addition to the loss in GSH, there is a marked increase in dehydroascorbic acid. This has led to the hypothesis that GSH is very important to dehydroascorbic acid reduction and, as a consequence, ascorbic acid recycling. Moreover, in studies using guinea pigs, treatment with GSH ester significantly delays the onset of scurvy. The sparing effect is probably due to the need for both ascorbic

TABLE 15.3
Functions of Ascorbic Acid Associated with Specific Enzymes

Function	Associated Enzymes	Associated Mechanism and Features
Extracellular matrix maturation (collagen biosynthesis)	Prolyl-3-hydroxylase Prolyl-4-hydroxylase Lysyl hydroxylase	Dioxygenase; Fe^{2+}
Cq1 Complement synthesis	Prolyl-4-hydroxylase	Dioxygenase; Fe^{2+}
Carnitine biosynthesis	6-*N*-Trimethyl-L-lysine hydroxylase γ-Butyrobetaine hydroxylase	Dioxygenase; Fe^{2+}
Pyridine metabolism	Pyrimidine deoxyribonucleoside Hydroxylase (fungi)	Dioxygenase; Fe^{2+}
Cephalosporin synthesis	Deacetoxycephalosporin C synthetase	Dioxygenase; Fe^{2+}
Tyrosine metabolism	Tyrosine-4-hydroxyphenylpyruvate hydrolase	Dioxygenase; Fe^{2+}
Norepinephrine biosynthesis	Dopamine-β-monooxygenase or hydrolase	Monooxygenase; Cu^{1+}
Peptidylglycine α-amidation in the activation of hormones	Peptidylglycine α-amidating monooxygenase	Monooxygenase; Cu^{1+}

acid and GSH in counteracting the deleterious effects of reactive oxidant species. Keys to understanding the steps in the ascorbate–GSH relationships are the enzymes thioredoxin and thioredoxin reductase [68,69]. The mammalian thioredoxin reductases are found within a family of selenium-containing pyridine nucleotide–disulfide oxidoreductases. They are catalyzed by the NADPH-dependent reduction of thioredoxin, as well as of other endogenous and

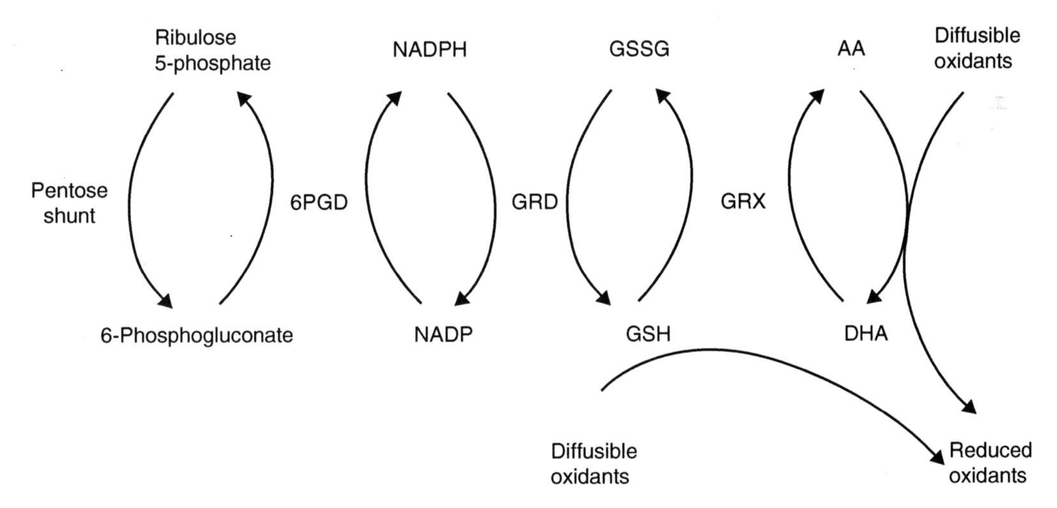

FIGURE 15.4 Interaction between ascorbic acid and glutathione. Excess oxidants can be reduced directly and indirectly by ascorbic acid and glutathione by complex processes that are depicted conceptually although in a very simplified fashion. The most important reductant in the cell is glutathione (L-γ-glutamyl-L-cysteine-glycine, GSH), which is synthesized by a two-step reaction involving L-glutamyl cysteine synthetase and GSH synthetase. In addition to reducing equivalents derived from the pentose shunt or hexose monophosphate shunt pathway via NADPH (catalyzed by 6-phosphogluconate dehydrogenase [6-PGD] and transferred by glutathione reductase [GD]), reduced ascorbic acid can transfer reducing equivalents to oxidized glutathione (GSSG) catalyzed by thioredoxin (TRX) and perhaps to some species of diffusible oxidants.

exogenous compounds. The importance of thioredoxin to many aspects of cell function appears in part related to the recycling of ascorbate from its oxidized form [66,67].

Although ascorbic acid also has pro-oxidant properties and may cause apoptosis of lymphoid and myeloid cells, Puskas and associates [70–74] have shown that dehydroascorbate, the oxidized form of vitamin C, also stimulates the antioxidant defenses in some cells by preferentially importing dehydroascorbate over ascorbate. While 200–800 μM vitamin C caused apoptosis of Jurkat and H9 human T lymphocytes, pretreatment with 200–1000 μM dehydroascorbate stimulates the activity of the pentose phosphate pathway enzymes glucose 6-phosphate dehydrogenase (G6PD), 6-phosphogluconate dehydrogenase, and transaldolase, and elevates intracellular glutathione levels. A 3.3-fold elevation in glutathione was observed after 48 h stimulation with 800 μM dehydroascorbate [73].

Norepinephrine and Adrenal Hormone Synthesis

Synthesis of norepinephrine (Figure 15.5) depends on ascorbic acid and explains in part the need for a high concentration of ascorbic acid in brain tissue and the adrenal glands. Ascorbic acid is a cofactor required both in catecholamine biosynthesis and in adrenal steroidogenesis. In studies using animal models with a deletion in the ascorbic acid transporter *SVCT2* gene, reduced tissue levels of ascorbic acid occur. Animals die soon after birth and there is a significant decrease in tissue catecholamine levels in the adrenals. The drop in ascorbic acid is accompanied by decreased plasma levels of corticosterone and altered morphology of mitochondrial membranes, that is, a clear validation of the importance of ascorbic acid on adrenal cortical function [75,76]. At the enzymatic level, a primary effect is on dopamine-β-hydroxylase (EC 1.14.17.1), which is present in catecholamine storage granules in nervous tissues and in chromaffin cells of the adrenal medulla. This is the site of the final and rate-limiting step in the synthesis of norepinephrine. Dopamine-β-hydroxylase is a tetramer containing two Cu(I) ions per monomer, which consumes ascorbate stoichiometrically with O_2 during its catalytic cycle. At a steady state, the predominant enzyme form is an enzyme–product complex.

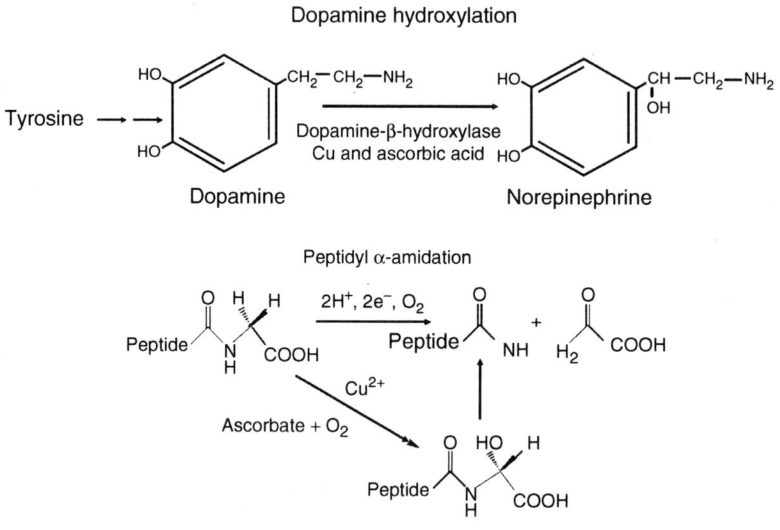

FIGURE 15.5 Steps in norepinephrine synthesis catalyzed by dopamine-β-hydroxylase (dopamine hydroxylation) and C-terminal amide formation via peptidyl α-amidations (peptidyl α-amidation). Mechanistically, these reactions occur in two steps. The enzyme receives single e^- sequentially from two ascorbic acid molecules resulting in ascorbate free radical as intermediate. This intermediate is later reduced back to ascorbate by transmembrane electron transfers via cytochrome b_{561}.

The primary function of ascorbate is to maintain copper in a reduced state in this complex. Only the reduced enzyme seems to be catalytically competent, with bound cuprous ions as the only reservoir of reducing equivalents. Under acute stress, ascorbic acid levels in neural tissue are also rapidly depleted [12,77,78].

Hormone Activation (α-Amidations)

Many hormones and hormone-releasing factors are activated by posttranslational steps involving α-amidations [12]. Examples of hormone activation include melanotropins, calcitonin, releasing factors for growth hormone, corticotrophin and thyrotropin, pro-ACTH, vasopressin, oxytocin, cholecystokinin, and gastrin [79,80]. Peptidylglycine α-amidating monooxygenase (EC 1.14.17.3), the enzyme that carries out α-amidation, is found in secretory granules of neuroendocrine cells in the brain, pituitary, thyroid, and submaxillary glands [81–83]. For peptides that undergo amidation, a glycine must be at the C terminus. The process involves C-terminal amidation with the release of glyoxylate (Figure 15.5). Similar to dopamine-β-hydroxylase, in the ascorbate-dependent α-amidases, ascorbic acid serves as a reductant to maintain copper in a reduced state at the active site of the enzyme.

Ascorbic Acid as an Antioxidant

The Food and Nutrition Board's panel on Dietary Antioxidant and Related Compounds of the NAS has defined an antioxidant as "any substance that, when present at low concentrations compared to those of an oxidizable substrate (e.g. proteins, lipids, carbohydrates and nucleic acids), significantly delays or prevents oxidation of that substrate" [84]. Ascorbic acid readily scavenges reactive oxygen and nitrogen species, such as superoxide and hydroperoxyl radicals, aqueous peroxyl radicals, singlet oxygen, ozone, peroxynitrite, nitrogen dioxide, nitroxide radicals, and hypochlorous acid. Excesses of such products have been associated with lipid, DNA, and protein oxidation.

Lipids

Although mostly inferential, numerous in vitro and in vivo studies have focused on the ability of ascorbic acid to reverse lipid peroxidation [85,86]. When the peroxyl radicals are generated in plasma, vitamin C is consumed faster than other antioxidants, for example, uric acid, bilirubins, and vitamin E [86]. Ascorbic acid is 10^3 more reactive than a polyunsaturated fatty acid in reacting with peroxyl radicals. In contrast, ascorbic acid is not as effective in scavenging hydroxyl or alkoxyl radicals [86].

In assays for lipid peroxidation, low-density lipoprotein (LDL) particles are often used as the lipid source [85,87,88]. LDL oxidation susceptibility is estimated by the lag time and propagation rate of lipid peroxidation in LDL exposed to copper ions or catalyst to initiate oxidation. Many studies in humans and animals support the observation that ascorbic acid generally retards peroxyl radical formation in LDL. Studies have been carried out with smokers, nonsmokers, and hypercholesterolemic subjects [89]. In all cases, with the combination of ascorbic acid and vitamin E, a significant reduction in oxidized LDL has been reported [88]. In studies using only vitamin C, however, the effect on LDL oxidation is more varied.

DNA

Oxidative damage to DNA is of particular importance in somatic cells, because of the risk of mutations, which can lead to cancer or birth defects. In addition to protection against lipid peroxidative damage, ascorbic acid has also been shown to provide a degree of protection with respect to DNA oxidation. In DNA, 8-oxoguanosine and its respective nucleoside 8-oxo-deoxyguanosine are the products [90–92]. These modified nucleic acid bases are found in all cells, and are excreted in urine. Estimation of 8-oxo-deoxyguanosine derivatives and other modified bases has led to the view that cells must repair 10^4 to 10^5 oxidative lesions per cell per day [93]. Fraga et al. [90,91] were among the first to demonstrate a significant decrease in human sperm 8-oxo-deoxyguanosine levels following vitamin C supplementation. However, since the nucleus of many cells contains relatively low concentrations of ascorbic acid, it remains unclear as to the relative importance of ascorbic acid to DNA protection.

Protein

Examples of protein oxidation include the lifelong oxidation of long-lived proteins, such as the crystallin in the lens of the eye, the oxidation of α-proteinase inhibitor, and the advanced glycation end products associated with diabetes. Tyrosine, N-terminal amino acids, and cysteine are often targets of such reactions [94–96]. Although data are limited, ascorbic acid supplementation appears to have a protective effect and certain categories of protein oxidation. Protein carbonyl formation, a precursor for glycation products, is increased in scorbutic guinea pigs and reduced on ascorbic acid repletion [97]. Vitamin C supplementation has also been shown to reduce the formation of nitrotyrosine levels in patients with *Helicobacter pylori* gastritis [98].

In summary, ascorbate is an electron donor, which may account for many of its known functions. However, much remains to be resolved. In spite of the ability of ascorbic acid to influence the production of hydroxyl and alkoxyl radicals, whether this is the principle effect or mechanism that occurs in vivo remains uncertain. There seems to be good evidence for the antioxidant protection of lipids by vitamin C in biological fluids (both with and without iron cosupplementation, e.g., Ref. [88]) with the data on protein oxidation and DNA oxidation somewhat inconsistent.

Carnitine Biosynthesis

Researchers have suggested that early features of scurvy (fatigue and weakness) may be attributed to carnitine deficiency [99–101]. Ascorbate is a cofactor of two-enzyme hydroxylation in the pathway of carnitine biosynthesis (Figure 15.6), γ-butyrobetaine hydroxylase, and ε-*N*-trimethyllysine hydroxylase [98–100]. High doses of ascorbic acid in guinea pigs fed high-fat diets contribute to enhanced carnitine synthesis. Ascorbate deficiency results in as much as a 50% decrease in carnitine in heart and skeletal muscle compared with guinea pig fed ascorbic acid [49,100,102].

Extracellular Matrix and Ascorbic Acid

Ascorbic acid is an essential cofactor in extracellular matrix (ECM) metabolism. Vitamin C deficiency differentially affects the expression of collagen, laminin, various cell surface integrins, as well as elastin [103]. The effects of ascorbic acid may be observed at both the functional and regulatory gene levels. Ascorbic acid is a cofactor for enzymes important to the posttranslational modification of matrix proteins and perhaps the transcriptional regulation of specific proteins. As examples, the role of ascorbic acid in prolyl and lysyl hydroxylase will be highlighted.

Collagen is the predominant structural protein in animals. To date, 25 (possibly more) distinct types of collagen polypeptide chains have been identified. Each of these forms assembles into distinct fibrillar or laminar structures [104]. The fibrillar types are typically formed by triple helical arrangements of glycine- and proline-enriched polypeptide chains. For such chains to form stable structures, specific prolyl residues in each chain must be hydroxylated. The hydroxylation is catalyzed by prolyl hydroxylase.

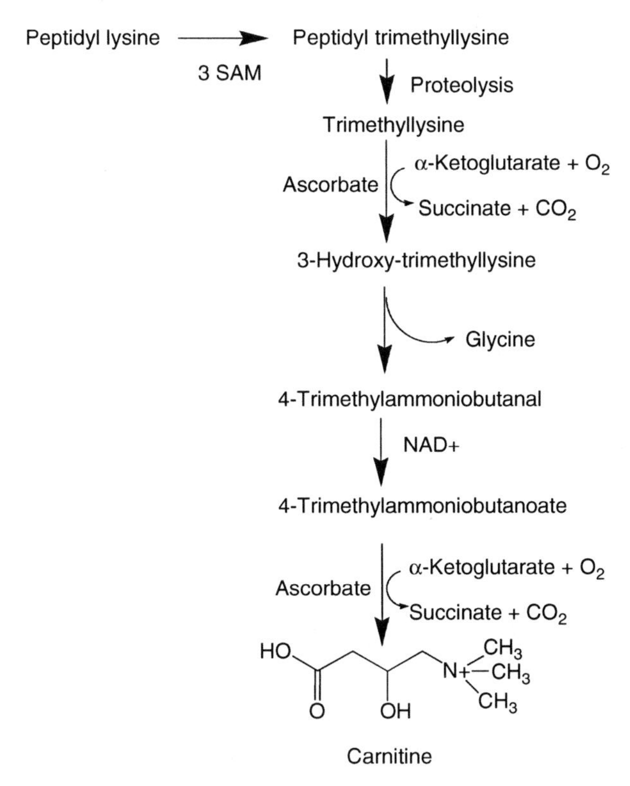

FIGURE 15.6 Steps in carnitine biosynthesis. In order to form L-carnitine from lysine, three consecutive methylation reactions are required utilizing *S*-adenosylmethionine (SAM) as the methyl donor. This step occurs as a posttranslational protein modification. Next, trimethyllysine is obtained (after protein hydrolysis). Trimethyllysine is enzymatically transformed into 3-hydroxy-trimethyllysine in a reaction requiring α-ketoglutarate, O_2, and ascorbic acid. Following the loss of glycine and oxidation to trimethylammoniobutyrate, a second hydroxylation involving an ascorbic acid-assisted step results in carnitine.

Moreover, lysyl groups in collagen are also hydroxylated. Some of the resulting residues of hydroxyl lysine becomes a part of the complex network of cross-links, which aid in stabilizing the helical forms of collagen into stable fibers [79,80,105].

When collagen fibers are under-hydroxylated, intracellular cellular assembly of collagen fibers is compromised, with possible alterations in the distribution and types of cross-links. The result is excessive degradation and turnover of collagen. Physiologic consequences range from impaired wound healing to capillary fragility, the hallmarks of scurvy. An important perspective is that some collagens have very long half-lives and are developmentally regulated [105]. Consequently, if scurvy occurs at critical times in development there may be very profound and long-lasting consequences affecting the deposition of bone, the modeling of the vascular, and pulmonary alveolar matrix [79,80,105–108].

Elastin is another protein that is hydroxylated, although it is the over-hydroxylation, in contrast to the under-hydroxylation, that causes decreased production of the ultimate product, an insoluble elastin fiber [105–108]. When elastin producing cells are subjected to medium containing high concentrations of ascorbic acid (e.g., near millimolar concentrations), there is a decrease in expression of elastin. The short-term response is abnormal assembly, which causes a shift in the partitioning of elastin into insoluble matrix to more "soluble" and easily degraded forms of elastin. The net result is less insoluble elastin [106,107].

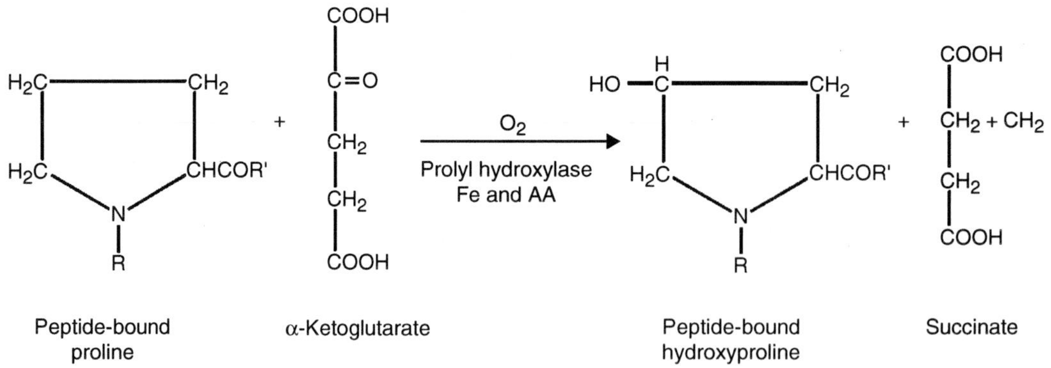

FIGURE 15.7 Hydroxylation of peptidyl proline. The reaction sequence for prolyl hydroxylase (prolyl-glycyl-peptide-2-oxoglutarate:oxygen oxidoreductase, EC 1.14.11.2) is shown. Lysyl hydroxylase carries out a similar sequence of steps. In contrast to the mechanism or sequence of steps described in the previous figures, iron is utilized instead of copper as the redox metal. Ascorbate role is to maintain iron in a reduced state.

As noted, the effects of ascorbate on collagen and elastin are both posttranslational and possibly transcriptional. Collagen fibers begin to assemble in the endoplasmic reticulum (ER) and Golgi complexes. Specific proline residues are hydroxylated by two hydroxylases, prolyl 4-hydroxylase and prolyl 3-hydroxylase. Vitamin C is necessary to maintain the enzyme prolyl hydroxylase in an active form by keeping iron, an essential cofactor for prolyl hydroxylase, reduced. Note that for the mono- and dioxygenases that utilize ascorbic acid as a reductant, copper and iron are often the targets for reduction. Reduced iron and copper are required for coordination with oxygen, the principal cosubstrate for the mono- and dioxygenases [79,80].

Another cosubstrate is α-ketoglutarate. Oxidative decomposition of α-ketoglutarate forms CO_2 plus succinate and leads to the generation of Fe(IV)-oxo or activated oxygen species, which next interacts with and hydroxylates the primary substrate. Ascorbate's role is to return the metal to its reduced state for another catalytic cycle. In this regard, ascorbic acid persists for 6–12 catalytic cycles (Figure 15.7).

Regarding ECM expression and ascorbate status, there is the need to resolve a number of factors. In cell culture, high concentrations of ascorbate can act as a pro-oxidant. Inverse correlations exist between antioxidants (e.g., vitamin E added to cultures) and ascorbic acid in fibroblast and smooth muscle cultures when collagen mRNA or collagen production is used as the dependent variable [109]. Ascorbic acid promotes collagen production, which may be countered by the addition of α-tocopherol to cultures. The phenomenon appears most related to the pro-oxidant effects of ascorbic acid and malonaldehyde formation as a product of lipid peroxidation. Malonaldehyde has been shown to promote collagen expression, possibly by upregulation of c-*jun* nuclear kinase [110].

In summary, the response to ascorbic acid with respect to ECM is complex. The role of ascorbate as a cosubstrate or cofactor for prolyl and lysyl hydroxylase (dioxygenases) is clear and mechanistically understood. Many facets of ascorbate role in gene expression, however, remain unresolved, given that changes in redox potential, oxidation productions, and the stability of ECM can all impact changes in gene expression.

Ascorbic Acid and Gene Expression

The influence of ascorbic acid on the mRNA transcription of specific genes remains unclear [12,99,111–113]. As illustrated by the ECM and ascorbic acid interactions, it is clear that controlling for changes in oxidative potential is essential to truly determine the specific effects of ascorbic acid on the expression of given genes. For example, disruption of the ECM has profound effects on cell differentiation and gene expression. Further, an interesting phenomenon is the formation of the complex of ascorbate and RNA (at GC and AU base pairs). This can apparently occur with little change in RNA secondary structure [114], which may influence the stabilization or destabilization of given transcripts. With regard to hydroxylated proteins, particularly collagen, transcription may be influenced by the amounts of intracellular under-hydroxylated products or peptides [109,115–117]. If there is a redox-controlled mechanism that involves ascorbic acid, additional detail is often needed to determine the influence of products of lipid peroxidation, which may also influence gene expression [109,116–118]. The opening and closing of certain ion channels (e.g., the cystic fibrosis transmembrane chloride channel) is also sensitive to ascorbic acid, which may in turn influence gene expression [119].

Regarding genes that are known to be influenced by ascorbic acid, the transcription of the 72 kDa type IV collagenase (matrix metalloproteinase-2) is downregulated by ascorbic acid in cultured human amnion-derived cells [113]. Tyrosine hydroxylase transcription [120] and the mRNA encoding of various forms of cytochrome P450 in liver microsomes are enhanced by ascorbic acid. Other mRNAs whose transcription appears to be regulated by ascorbic acid are the ubiquitins, the collagen-related integrins, and the *fra-1* gene, which encodes a transcription factor of the *Fos* family and downregulates the activator protein-1 (AP-1) target gene [74,121]. In plants, the maize *Hrgp* gene is induced by ascorbic acid [113].

ASCORBIC ACID METABOLISM AND REGULATION

Ascorbic acid is transported into all types of cells. Simple diffusion accounts for some of this movement. The major transport, however, is carrier mediated [75]. For ascorbate, there are Na^+ cotransporters that actively transport ascorbate into cells [75]. In contrast, dehydroascorbate is taken into cells by the facilitative glucose transporters.

Cell accumulation of ascorbic acid occurs as dehydroascorbate is converted to ascorbic acid. This also serves to keep the intracellular concentration of dehydroascorbate low, favoring uptake into the cell along a concentration gradient. As examples, the erythrocyte and neutrophil dehydroascorbate reduction system are capable of rapidly generating ascorbic acid [75]. Neutrophils utilize ascorbate as a reductant to generate H_2O_2 for "killer activity." Inside the neutrophil, dehydroascorbate is converted to ascorbate by a dehydroascorbic acid reductase that utilizes glutathione as a reductant. Activated neutrophils accumulate ascorbate to levels that range from 2 mM to as much as 10 mM and can effectively recycle ascorbic acid. The increase in the intracellular ascorbic acid concentration occurs at a time when the cell needs maximum antioxidant protection against the products of its own oxidative burst reactions.

Of clinical significance, diabetes can influence ascorbate cellular transport. High glucose can compete for ascorbic acid, presumably by interfering with ascorbic acid uptake via the glucose transporter isoforms, GLUT1 and GLUT2, which transport the oxidized form of vitamin C, dehydroascorbic acid [122–125]. Dehydroascorbic acid also enters mitochondria via the facilitative glucose transporter 1 (Glut1) and accumulates in the mitochondria as ascorbic acid.

Specific active transporters for ascorbic acid have also been identified and are found in tissues that accumulate ascorbic acid [124–127]. The activity of the transporters has been observed to vary inversely with intracellular ascorbate, with the net result of maintaining a relatively constant intracellular concentration. Two different isoforms of specific sodium–vitamin C cotransporters (SVCT1/SLC23A1 and SVCT2/SLC23A2) have been cloned. The tissue distributions of the transporters differ, with SVCT1 occurring primarily in epithelial tissues such as intestine, liver, and kidney. Whereas SVCT2 is widely distributed and detected in choroid plexus cells and neurons, cardiac muscle, placenta, and most other tissues [128–130].

With regard to intestinal absorption, in guinea pigs and in humans, the ileum and jejunum are major sites of absorption. The process is efficient. Ascorbic acid is easily absorbed (cf. Requirements and Allowances). Similar to the cellular uptake of ascorbic acid by red cells and neutrophils, enterocyte uptake is Na^+ dependent [122].

Ascorbic acid circulates in plasma at micromolar concentrations, whereas it is found in some tissues, often at millimolar concentrations. Ascorbic acid oxidation to CO_2 and C-4 and C-5 derivatives and excretion are major paths by which ascorbic acid is lost from the body [131].

SELECTED CLINICAL FEATURES IMPORTANT TO ASCORBIC ACID STATUS

Defining Ascorbic Acid Status

Although leukocyte concentrations are generally considered to be the best indicator of vitamin C status, the measurement of leukocyte vitamin C is technically complex [131,132]. The varying amounts of ascorbic acid in differing leukocyte fractions and the lack of standardized reporting procedures [131–134] also complicate interpretation of data. Hence, the measurement of plasma vitamin C concentration is currently the most widely applied test for vitamin C status. Plasma concentrations between 11 and 28 μmol/L represent marginal vitamin C status. At this level, there is a moderate risk for developing clinical signs of vitamin C deficiency due to inadequate tissue stores of vitamin C.

Data from the Second National Health and Nutrition Examination Survey, 1976–1980 (NHANES II) [135], indicated that the prevalence of vitamin C deficiency (plasma vitamin C concentrations <11 μmol/L) ranged from 0.1% in children (3–5 years of age) to 3% in females (25–44 years of age) and 7% in males (45–64 years of age). A decade later, the more sensitive measures utilized by NHANES III indicated that the prevalence of vitamin C deficiency was 12% for adult females and 17% for adult males [136]. Marginal vitamin C status (plasma vitamin C concentrations from 11 to 28 μmol/L) was noted in 20%–23% of adults [136]. Smokers are more likely to have marginal vitamin C status compared with nonsmoking adults. Several studies suggest that smokers require >200 mg ascorbate daily to maintain plasma concentrations at a level equivalent to nonsmokers consuming 60 mg vitamin daily (cf. Ref. [137] and references cited therein). The current vitamin C recommendation for smokers is ~40% greater than that for nonsmokers, 110 and 125 mg daily for females and males, respectively [138].

In its most extreme form, scurvy is characterized by subcutaneous and intramuscular hemorrhages, leg edema, neuropathy, and cerebral hemorrhage, and, if untreated, the condition is ultimately fatal. Presently, even in affluent countries, scurvy should be considered when signs and symptoms such as cutaneous and oral lesions are observed, particularly in alcoholics, the institutionalized elderly, or persons who live alone and consume restrictive diets containing little or no fruits and vegetables. Patients may also complain of lassitude, weakness, and vague myalgias, and seek medical attention following the appearance of a skin rash or lower extremity edema. Discussion of the functional roles of ascorbic acid in body systems and prevention of chronic disease is provided later.

Clinical Features

Immune Function

Since the publication of *Vitamin C and the Common Cold* by Pauling [50], the role of vitamin C in immune function has been a topic of lively debate. The high concentration of vitamin C in leukocytes, and the rapid decline in plasma and leukocyte vitamin C concentrations during stress and infection, has been used as evidence that vitamin C plays a role in immune function [139–143]. Dozens of basic research studies and clinical trials have been conducted in attempts to resolve the role of vitamin C in common cold and other viral and bacterial infections [140–153]; most reviewers of the literature concur that there is little justification for routine vitamin C mega-dose prophylaxis [148–153]. However, in certain high-risk populations, vitamin C supplementation may provide some benefit. Ultra–marathon runners are likely to suffer upper-respiratory-tract infections in the immediate postrace period [154–157]. In a double-blind, placebo-controlled trial, vitamin C supplementation (600 mg/day), beginning 21 days before the start of the race, reduced by 50% the incidence of postrace upper-respiratory-tract infections in runners [148]. In the same study, the incidence of upper-respiratory-tract infections in sedentary controls was not affected by vitamin C supplementation, although the duration of symptoms was significantly less (−1.4 days) in control subjects receiving vitamin C supplements. Three of four randomized, double-blind, placebo-controlled trials utilizing 1–2 g vitamin C daily have reported a significant reduction in the incidence of respiratory-tract infections among military personnel [150]. A lesser dosage, 300 mg/day, was not associated with reduction in common cold infections among military recruits; but a 50% reduction in the most severe respiratory infection was noted [149]. Elderly patients hospitalized with acute respiratory infections and receiving 200 mg vitamin C daily were also reported to fare better than patients receiving placebo [153]. Although the difference was not statistically significant, the elderly patients receiving placebo were five times more likely to die from complications of respiratory-tract infection than patients receiving the ascorbate supplement.

The mechanism by which vitamin C reduces the incidence or severity of respiratory-tract infections is not known. Studies show that a low salivary IgA secretion rate midrace predicted the occurrence of upper-respiratory-tract infections in ultra–marathon runners [148–151]. Vitamin C supplementation (1500 mg/day for the 7 days before race day) did not affect the reductions in salivary IgA noted at midrace and postrace [151]. Other trials investigating alterations in immune responses after high-intensity running have been unable to demonstrate a countering effect of vitamin C supplementation on changes in interleukin-6, natural killer cell activity, lymphocyte proliferation, and granulocyte phagocytosis [153,158]. However, a more consistent finding is that vitamin C can also accelerate the destruction of histamine, a mediator of allergy and cold symptoms [159–162]. Vitamin C supplementation reduces blood histamine concentrations from 30% to 40% in adult subjects [161,162], and an acute dosages of vitamin C (e.g., 2 g) reduces bronchial responsiveness to inhaled histamine in patients with allergy [163]. In addition, supplementation with 250 mg vitamin C/day for 6 weeks significantly reduces monocyte ICAM-1 mRNA expression (−50%) in healthy male subjects [164], an important observation because the expression of this adhesion molecule by inflammatory and endothelial cell types is associated with airway hyperresponsiveness characteristic of the common cold, allergic asthma, and seasonal allergic rhinitis.

Ascorbic acid can also influence neutrophil chemotaxis [165–170]; however, enhancement is most often obtained at nonphysiological concentrations of vitamin C. For example, neutrophil chemotaxis is enhanced following an intravenous injection of 1 g ascorbic acid [168] and following high doses of ascorbic acid (2 or 3 g/day for one or more weeks) [169–171]. Ascorbic acid supplementation (1 g/day) has also been shown to significantly improve leukocyte chemotaxis in patients with Chediak–Higashi syndrome, a disease characterized by impaired neutrophil microtubule assembly [172,173] and in patients with chronic granulomatous disease, a condition characterized by depressed neutrophil activation [174]. In guinea pigs, vitamin C deficiency does not affect neutrophil activity, but it does decrease neutrophil killing of internalized pathogens [175].

Data regarding the effect of vitamin C status on lymphocyte proliferation are somewhat equivocal. Vitamin C depletion for a 9 week period in human subjects did not appear to alter

T-cell number or T-cell proliferation in assays in vitro [175]; and the decline in lymphocyte proliferation noted in aged populations is not restored by vitamin C in vitro [176]. In another metabolic depletion–repletion study, vitamin C ingested daily in amounts ranging from 5 to 251 mg for 92 days also did not affect mitogen-induced lymphocyte proliferation [177]. Indeed, it may be that it is the restoration of function after a deficiency rather than response to supplementation that will prove to be the most important factor. Moreover, the mechanism is complex and appears to involve mitogen-induced proliferative processes [169,178–180], as well as reduction in or in combination with a reduction in the rate of apoptosis in T cells maintained in culture.

Vitamin C may also influence other immune system parameters. Vitamin C status in guinea pigs is directly related to serum concentrations of the complement component C1q, a protein that, in association with the other complement proteins, mediates nonspecific humoral immunity [181,182]. Vitamin C dose-dependently inhibits intracytoplasmic production of the proinflammatory cytokines IL-10 and TNF-α in whole blood cultures [183], possibly by inhibiting NFκB activation [184]. Finally, several investigators have suggested that the antihistamine effect of vitamin C may indirectly enhance immune responsiveness, that is, ascorbic acid enhances mitogen-dependent lymphocyte blastogenesis by inhibiting histamine production in spleen cell cultures [185].

Progression of Selected Chronic Diseases

Atherosclerosis

Epidemiologic studies have shown that death due to cardiovascular disease is inversely related to regular use of vitamin C supplements [186–190]. Individuals participating in the NHANES II Mortality Study with tissue-saturating concentrations of serum ascorbic acid ($\geq$62 μmol/L) were 34% less likely to die from cardiovascular disease [186–190]. Males with vitamin C deficiency (plasma vitamin C <11 μmol/L) were at significantly increased risk of myocardial infarction after controlling for potentially confounding variables [189,190,191]. The mean plasma vitamin C concentration in male patients admitted within the first 12 h of onset of an acute myocardial infarction was significantly lower than that of control subjects (19.5 and 37.0 μmol/L, respectively).

The oxidation of LDL has been implicated in the etiology of atherosclerosis in addition to endothelial dysfunction and inflammatory processes. Vitamin C may be involved in the recycling of vitamin E, which in turn may donate electrons to prevent LDL oxidation [192,193], or improve vascular health by promoting endothelial nitric oxide synthesis [192,194] or by reducing blood pressure in hypertensive patients [196]. However, as described earlier, clinical trials of ascorbate supplementation, either alone or with other antioxidant vitamins, have yet to yield significant reductions in cardiovascular disease risk or clinical events that indicate ascorbic acid is a truly independent factor in cardiovascular risk protection [195–200]. Much is still needed to clarify mechanisms that may eventually lead to understanding why the results of certain studies suggest some level of efficacy.

Stroke

Risk of stroke, both cerebral infarction and hemorrhagic stroke, is inversely related to vitamin C status. In two large prospective studies in Finland and Japan, serum vitamin C (>45 μmol/L) was associated with a 30%–50% lower risk of stroke [196,201,202]. However, the regular use of vitamin C supplements was not associated with reduced risk for stroke [203] suggesting that other factors in fruits and vegetables may be responsible for the beneficial effects of diets rich in vitamin C.

Cancer

In epidemiologic studies, all-cause cancer incidence and deaths appear inversely related to serum vitamin C concentrations in men but not women [185–187]. Risk of fatal lung cancer was inversely related to serum vitamin C in both men and women [204]. The regular use of vitamin C supplements is related to a reduced risk of gastric and intestinal cancers in large US cohorts [205]; yet, a short-term, intervention trial in a Chinese population at high risk for stomach cancer did not demonstrate a benefit of vitamin C supplementation (120 mg/day) on the incidence of gastric cancer [206–208]. The chemopreventive properties of vitamin C may be linked to antioxidant effects that protect against oxidative DNA damage, or to protective effects against carcinogenic mechanisms that disrupt the cell cycle [209,210]. Although the pro-oxidant effects of ascorbic acid in vitro suggest a possible role for vitamin C in mutagenesis, investigations utilizing physiologically relevant cell culture systems demonstrate that vitamin C is most often associated with decreased frequency of DNA mutations.

Cataracts

Epidemiologic studies have also shown that the risk of cataract is significantly higher in individuals with moderate to low blood concentrations of vitamin C [211–213]. After controlling for potentially confounding variables, including diabetes, smoking, sunlight exposure, and regular aspirin use, taking vitamin C supplements for ~10 years was associated with reduced risk for early (odds ratio, 0.23; 95% CI, 0.09–0.60) and moderate (odds ratio, 0.17; 95% CI, 0.03–0.87) age-related lens opacities in women. In a separate study, high dietary vitamin C (>200 mg/day) was associated with a 30% reduction in cataract risk, and serum ascorbic acid concentrations >49 μmol/L were associated with a 60%–70% reduction in all types of cataract [211]. Interestingly, a high-quality diet rich in fruits, vegetables, and whole grains is associated with a reduced prevalence of cataract in nonusers of vitamin C supplements but not in users of vitamin C supplements, suggesting an important role for vitamin C in cataract prevention [211–214].

Pulmonary Function

In large population-based studies, vitamin C is associated with forced expiratory volume (FEV_1) and forced vital capacity, the common functional markers for pulmonary function [215,216]. Vitamin C appears to decrease oxidant damage to the lung [210,217] and may modulate the development of chronic lung diseases and declines in lung function. A prospective study of diet and lung function demonstrated that an additional 100 mg higher than average intake of vitamin C was related to a significantly smaller reduction in FEV_1 after a 9 year follow-up [218]. Dietary vitamin C is inversely related to self-reported respiratory symptoms (morning cough, chronic cough, and wheezing) in adults, a relationship that tends to be related to smoking status [219,220]. Hence, smokers, as well as populations with chronic exposure to air pollutants [217,219,221], benefit from optimizing intakes of vitamin C.

Bone Density

Ascorbic acid increases collagen accumulation and alkaline phosphatase activity in osteogenic cells thereby affecting bone formation. Abnormal bone development and fractures are noted in scurvy, yet the role of vitamin C in protecting against age-related bone loss is less clear. Vitamin C from the diet is not consistently associated with bone mineral density in postmenopausal women [222,223], but dietary vitamin C, as well as fruit and vegetable consumption, is protective against bone loss in young and early menopausal women [222,223]. Long-term vitamin C supplementation (400–750 mg/day for >10 year), however, is positively associated with bone mineral density in postmenopausal women [222–226]. In a population at risk for hip fracture (female smokers aged 40–76 years), low dietary vitamin C was associated with a threefold increased risk for hip fracture as compared with nonsmoking women; smokers consuming adequate dietary vitamin C (>67 mg daily) were not at an increased risk of hip fracture [226].

Wound Healing and Connective Tissue Metabolism

As discussed, the mechanisms that link ascorbic acid intake to connective regulation and deposition are related to its role as an enzymatic cofactor (and stabilizing factor) for prolyl and lysyl hydroxylases.

REQUIREMENTS, ALLOWANCES, AND UPPER LIMITS

The 2000 RDA for vitamin C, 75 mg daily for adult females and 90 mg daily for adult males, represents a 25%–50% increase over the 1989 RDA, 60 mg [227]. Plasma vitamin C concentrations range from 45 to 50 μmol/L in well-nourished individuals with a typical vitamin C intake of 90–100 mg dietary vitamin C daily [227]. Plasma vitamin C concentrations in people who regularly consume vitamin C supplements are 30%–70% higher, ranging from 50 to 60 μmol/L to 75–80 μmol/L in individuals who regularly supplement 100 mg to 500–1000 mg vitamin C [227–229], respectively. Plasma vitamin C concentrations in newborn infants are much higher, ~150 μmol/L [230–234].

In humans, vitamin C bioavailability is nearly 100% for single oral doses ≤200 mg but falls to ~75% at an oral dose of 500 mg and to ~50% at an oral dose of 1250 mg [57]. At the higher oral doses, 500 and 1250 mg, nearly 100% of the absorbed dose is excreted nonmetabolized in urine; thus, effective homeostatic mechanisms operate to control plasma vitamin C concentrations over wide ranges of intake.

REBOUND SCURVY

There is some evidence that accelerated metabolism or disposal of ascorbic acid may occur after prolonged supplementation of high doses. Presumably, when vitamin C supplementation ceases abruptly, the accelerated disposal of vitamin C creates a vitamin C-deficient state, that is, "rebound scurvy." The phenomenon seems to have some support from animal studies [12] and historical records [10]. However, there are concerns regarding rebound scurvy that come largely from work by Cochrane [233]. Of 42 cases of infantile scurvy at Children's Hospital in Halifax, Nova Scotia (from October 1959 to January 1961), only two could not be attributed to inadequate dietary vitamin C. The possibility of rebound scurvy was considered, because the mothers of both of the infants reported taking vitamin C supplements during pregnancy (400 mg daily). However, the regression plots of plasma ascorbic acid depletion during withdraw from low-dose vitamin C (60 mg/day for 2 weeks) and from high-dose vitamin C (600 mg/day for 3 weeks) display similar slopes, indicating similar rates of vitamin C metabolism and disposal independent of initial vitamin C status. In guinea pigs, high intakes of vitamin C upregulate enzymes important to ascorbic acid degradation [12]. Whether this is truly the case in humans and in the appropriate setting lead to as suggested by the observations of Cochrane [233] needs further clarification and validation.

OXALIC ACID AND URIC ACID

About 75% of kidney stones contain calcium oxalate; another 5%–10% is composed of uric acid. High doses of vitamin C have been shown to increase urinary excretion of both oxalic acid and uric acid; and thus, theoretically promote the formation of kidney stones [235–238].

Case reports have described the development of hyperoxaluria with associated pathologies (tubular necrosis and hematuria) in previously healthy individuals consuming 5–8 g vitamin C daily [235–237]. These individuals appeared to possess abnormally high capacities to absorb dietary ascorbic acid and to convert ascorbic acid to oxalate. Yet clinical investigations indicate that calcium oxalate stone-formers and normal subjects respond similarly to megadoses of vitamin C [238,239]. The crystallization of calcium oxalate in urine was increased ~60% in both stone-forming patients and healthy subjects consuming 1 g vitamin C for 3 days [239]. A prospective cohort study of 45,600 men without a history of nephrolithiasis demonstrated a significant association between incident kidney stones and vitamin C ingestion after a 14 year follow-up [240,241]. The multivariate risk ratio in men who consumed $\geq$1000 mg daily as compared with $<$90 mg daily was 1.41 (95% CI: 1.11–1.80). Consequently, it would seem prudent for calcium oxalate stone-formers to abstain from consuming supplemental vitamin C. For others, daily intakes of vitamin C more than the tolerable upper intake level set by the Food and Nutrition Board, 2000 mg, are not recommended.

Iron-Related Disorders

Red cell hemolysis, related to G6PD deficiency, has been reported as a toxic effect of ascorbic acid [242]. Although the mechanism is not clear, it is possible that ascorbic acid in excess can act as a pro-oxidant catalyst in the presence of available iron and the absence of an important source of reducing equivalents in red cells, that is, the NADPH that is generated by G6PD.

Since dietary vitamin C may enhance mealtime iron absorption, some have speculated that high-dose vitamin C regimens may aggravate conditions associated with increased iron absorption and storage, notably hemochromatosis. About 0.5% and 10% of the US population are homozygous and heterozygous, respectively, for the hemochromatosis *HFE* gene mutation. Ascorbic acid fortification of foods did increase nonheme iron absorption in homozygous patients compared with wild-type controls, but increased iron absorption was not observed in heterozygous patients [243]. Vitamin C supplementation may also have adverse effects in thalassemia major, an iron-overload disease characterized by impaired globin chain synthesis, ineffective erythroporesis, and anemia. Supplemental vitamin C may mobilize iron stores creating iron-overloaded plasma and risk for increased oxidative stress.

Vitamin B_{12}

Herbert et al. [244] reported that patients who received ascorbic acid in high doses had low serum vitamin B_{12}. These data have not been replicated by others, and this concern has never been confirmed. The long-term use of supplemental vitamin C is not likely to adversely affect serum vitamin B_{12} concentrations [245,246].

SUMMARY

Ascorbic acid is the cell's universal reducing agent. It performs redox reactions by free-radical mechanisms to activate the mono- and dioxygenases vital for many aspects of normal cellular metabolism. Ascorbic acid is required for the growth and repair of all tissues owing in part to its role as a cofactor for prolyl and lysyl hydroxylase activity, which is essential for collagen formation and wounds healing. Ascorbic acid also directly moderates oxidative stress by neutralizing free radicals, and indirectly by affecting the metabolism of glutathione and vitamin E. In animals that lack the gene for L-gulonolactone oxidase, or possess a mutated gene, ascorbic acid cannot be synthesized and becomes a dietary essential. Poor ascorbic acid status has been related to risk for chronic disease (e.g., atherosclerosis and cataracts) and the worsening of respiratory function in high-risk populations, such as the elderly and smokers. Although ascorbic acid is considered relatively nontoxic, supplementation by some populations (e.g., oxalate stone-formers and individuals suffering from iron-overload diseases) is not recommended. Clearly in past centuries and up to the first decades of the twentieth century, vitamin C deficiencies were common, especially during the winter months and during long ocean voyages. In its most severe form, for example, scurvy, vitamin C deficiency has altered human history. Studies of its chemistry and functions were the underpinning of two Nobel Prizes: to Albert von Szent-Gyorgyi Nagyrapolt in Medicine (1937) for his discoveries in connection with biological combustion processes, with special reference to vitamin C; and to Sir Walter N. Haworth in Chemistry (1937) for his studies on carbohydrates and vitamin C.

REFERENCES

1. Lorenz, A.J. (1954) The conquest of scurvy. *J. Am. Diet. Assoc.*, 30, 665–670.
2. Szent-Gyorgyi, A. (1928) Observations on the function of peroxidase systems and the chemistry of the adrenal cortex. Description of a new carbohydrate derivative. *Biochem. J.*, 22, 1387–1409.
3. Drummond, J.C. (1920) The nomenclature of the so-called accessory food factors (vitamins). *Biochem. J.*, 14, 660.
4. Zilva, S.S. (1932) The non-specificity of the phenolindophenol reducing capacity of lemon juice and its fractions as a measure of their antiscorbutic activity. *Biochem. J.*, 26, 1624–1627.
5. Hirst, E.L. and Zilva, S.S. (1933) Ascorbic acid as the anti-scorbutic factor. *Biochem. J.*, 27, 1271–1278.
6. Waugh, W.A. and King, C.G. (1932) Isolation and identification of vitamin C. *J. Biol. Chem.*, 97, 325–331.
7. Lind, J. (1753) *A Treatise of the Scurvy in Three Parts. Containing an inquiry into the Nature, Causes and Cure of that Disease, together with a Critical and Chronological View of what has been published on the subject.* A. Millar, London.
8. Bown, S.R. (2005) *Scurvy.* Thomas Dunne Books, St. Martin's Griffen, NY, pp. 1–254.
9. Goldblith, S.A. and Joslyn, M.A. (1964) *Milestones in Nutrition.* Avi Publishing Company, Westport, CT, pp. 331–446.
10. Carpenter, K. (1986) *The History of Scurvy and Vitamin C.* Cambridge University Press, Cambridge, pp. 1–346.
11. Lorenz, A.J. (1957) Scurvy in the gold rush. *J. Hist. Med. Allied. Sci.*, 7, 501–510.
12. Asard, H., May, J., and Smirnoff, N. (eds.) (2004) *Vitamin C: Function and Biochemistry in Animals and Plants.* BIOS Scientific Publishers, New York City, New York, pp. 1–323.
13. Holst, A. and Frohlich, T. (1907) Experimental studies relating to ship beriberi and scurvy II, on the etiology of scurvy. *J. Hygiene.*, 7, 634–671.
14. Bielski, B.H.J. (1982) Chemistry of ascorbic acid radicals. In: Seib, P.A., Tolbert, B.M., eds., *Ascorbic Acid: Chemistry, Metabolism, and Uses. Advances in Chemistry Series.* American Chemical Society, Washington DC, 81–100.
15. Halliwell, B. and Whiteman, M. (1997) Antioxidant and prooxidant properties of vitamin C. In: *Vitamin C in Health and Disease.* Marcel Dekker, New York, pp. 25–94.
16. Bielski, B.H.J., Allen, A.O., and Schwarz, H.A. (1981) Mechanism of disproportionation of ascorbate radicals. *J. Am. Chem. Soc.*, 103, 3516–3518.
17. Seib, P.A. and Tolbert, B.M. (1982) *Ascorbic Acid: Chemistry Metabolism, and Uses. Advances in Chemistry Series 200.* American Chemical Society, Washington DC, pp. 1–605.
18. Carr, A. and Frei, B. (1999) Does vitamin C act as a pro-oxidant under physiological conditions? *FASEB J.*, 13, 1007–1024.
19. Bors, W. and Buettner, G.R. (1997) The vitamin C radical and its reactions. In: *Vitamin C in Health and Disease.* Marcel Dekker, New York.
20. Smith, J.L., Canham, J.E., Kirkland, W.D., and Wells, P.A. (1988) Effect of intralipid, amino acids, container, temperature, and duration of storage on vitamin stability in total parenteral nutrition admixtures. *J. Parenter. Enteral. Nutr.*, 12, 478–483.
21. Dahl, G.B., Jeppsson, R.I., and Tengborn, H.J. (1986) Vitamin stability in a TPN mixture stored in an EVAP plastic bag. *J. Clin. Hospital. Pharm.*, 11, 271–279.
22. Wang, S., Eide, T.C., Sogn, E.M., Berg, K.J., and Sund, R.B. (1999) Plasma ascorbic acid in patients undergoing chronic haemodialysis. *Eur. J. Clin. Pharmacol.*, 55, 527–532.

23. Halliwell, B. (1996) Vitamin C: antioxidant or pro-oxidant in vivo. *Free Radic. Res.*, 25, 439–454.
24. Soto-Otero, R., Mendez-Alvarez, E., Hermida-Ameijeiras, A., Munoz-Patino, A.M., and Labandeira-Garcia, J.L. (2000) Autoxidation and neurotoxicity of 6-hydroxydopamine in the presence of some antioxidants: potential implication in relation to the pathogenesis of Parkinson's disease. *J. Neurochem.*, 74, 1605–1612.
25. Sakagami, H., Satoh, K., Ida, Y., Hosaka, M., Arakawa, H., and Maeda, M. (1998) Interaction between sodium ascorbate and dopamine. *Free. Radic. Biol. Med.*, 25, 1013–1020.
26. Behrens, W.A. and Madère, R. (1994) A procedure for the separation and quantitative analysis of ascorbic acid. Dehydroascorbic acid, isoascorbic acid, and dehydroisoascorbic acid in food and animal tissue. *J. Liquid Chromatogr.*, 17, 2445–2455.
27. Crawford, T.C. (1982) Synthesis of L-ascorbic acid. In: Seib, F.A. and Tolbert, B.M., eds., *Ascorbic Acid: Chemistry, Metabolism, and Uses. Advances in Chemistry Series*, American Chemical Society, Washington, DC, pp. 1–36.
28. Andrews, G.C. and Crawford, T. (1982) Recent advances in the derivatization of L-ascorbic acid. In: Seib, P.A. and Tolbert, B.M., eds., *Ascorbic Acid: Chemistry, Metabolism, and Uses. Advances in Chemistry Series*, American Chemical Society, Washington, DC, pp. 59–80.
29. Lee, C.H., Seib, P.A., and Liang, Y.T. (1978) Chemical synthesis of several phosphoric esters of L-ascorbic acid. *Carbohydrate Res.*, 67, 127–138.
30. Weber, P.F. (1999) The role of vitamins in the prevention of osteoporosis a brief status report. *Int. J. Vitam. Nutr. Res.*, 69, 194–197.
31. Miyazaki, T., Saginaw, T., and Hoshino, T. (2006) Pyrroloquinoline quinone-dependent dehydrogenases from *Ketogulonicigenium vulgare* catalyze the direct conversion of L-sorbosone to L-ascorbic acid. *Appl. Environ. Microbiol.*, 72, 1487–1495.
32. Chotani, G., Dodge, T., Hsu, A., Kumar, M., LaDuca, R., Trimbur, D., Weyler, W., and Sanford, K. (2000) The commercial production of chemicals using pathway engineering. *Biochim. Biophys. Acta*, 1543, 434–455.
33. Kimoto, E., Terada, S., and Yamaguchi, T. (1997) Analysis of ascorbic acid, dehydroascorbic acid, and transformation products by ion-pairing high-performance liquid chromatography with multiwavelength ultraviolet and electrochemical detection. *Methods Enzymol.*, 279, 3–12.
34. Terada, M., Watanabe, Y., Kunitomo, M., and Hayashi, E. (1978) Differential rapid analysis of ascorbic acid and ascorbic acid 2-sulfate by dinitrophenylhydrazine method. *Anal. Biochem.*, 84, 604–608.
35. Tsao, C.S. and Young, M. (1985) Analysis of ascorbic acid derivatives by high performance liquid chromatography with electrochemical detection. *J. Chromatogr.*, 13, 855–856.
36. Thomson, C.O. and Trenerry, V.C. (1995) A rapid method for the determination of total L-ascorbic acid in fruits and vegetables by micellar electrokinetic capillary chromatography. *Food Chem.*, 53, 43–50.
37. McGown, E.L., Rusnak, M.G., Lewis, C.M., and Tillotson, J.A. (1982) Tissue ascorbic acid analysis using ferrozine compared with the dinitrophenylhydrazine method. *Anal. Biochem.*, 119, 55–61.
38. Kampfenkel, K., Van Montagu, M., and Inze, D. (1995) Extraction and determination of ascorbate and dehydroascorbate from plant tissue. *Anal. Biochem.*, 225, 165–167.
39. Margolis, S.A. and Duewer, D.L. (1996) Measurement of ascorbic acid in human plasma and serum: stability, intralaboratory repeatability, and interlaboratory reproducibility. *Clin. Chem.*, 42, 1257–1262.
40. Gensler, M., Rossmann, A., and Schmidt, H.-L. (1995) Detection of added L-ascorbic acid in fruit juices by isotope ratio mass spectrometry. *J. Agric. Food Chem.*, 43, 2662–2666.
41. Moeslinger, T., Brunner, M., Volf, I., and Spieckermann, P.G. (1995) Spectrophotometric determination of ascorbic acid and dehydroascorbic acid. *Clin. Chem.*, 41, 1177–1181.
42. Tangney, C.C. (1988) Analyses of vitamin C in biological samples with an emphasis on recent chromatographic techniques. *Prog. Clin. Biol. Res.*, 259, 331–362.
43. Frenich, A.G., Torres, M.E., Vega, A.B., Vidal, J.L., and Bolanos, P.P. (2005) Determination of ascorbic acid and carotenoids in food commodities by liquid chromatography with mass spectrometry detection. *J. Agric. Food Chem.*, 53, 7371–7376.
44. Liu, T.Z., Chin, N., Kiser, M.D., and Bigler, W.N. (1982) Specific spectrophotometry of ascorbic acid in serum or plasma by use of ascorbate oxidase. *Clin. Chem.*, 28, 2225–2228.

45. Benzie, I.F.F. and Strain, J.J. (1995) The effect of ascorbic acid on the measurement of total cholesterol and triglycerides: possible artefactual lowering in individuals with high plasma concentration of ascorbic acid. *Clin. Chim. Acta*, 239, 185–190.
46. Freemantle, J., Freemantle, M.J., and Badrick, T. (1994) Ascorbate interferences in common clinical assays performed on three analyzers. *Clin. Chem.*, 40, 950–951.
47. Chatergee, I.B. (1973) Evolution and the biosynthesis of ascorbic acid. *Science*, 182, 1271–1273.
48. Grollman, A.P. and Lehninger, A. (1957) Enzymatic synthesis of L-ascorbic acid in different animal species. *Arch. Biochem. Biophys.*, 69, 458–467.
49. Englard, S. and Seifter, S. (1986) The biochemical functions of ascorbic acid. *Annu. Rev. Nutr.*, 6, 365–406.
50. Pauling, L. (1970) *Vitamin C and the Common Cold.* WH Freeman & Co, San Francisco.
51. Rucker, R.B. and Steinberg, F.M. (2002) Vitamin requirements. *Biochem. Mol. Biol. Educ.*, 30, 86–89.
52. Rucker, R.B., Dubick, M.A., and Mouritsen, J. (1980) Hypothetical calculations of ascorbic acid synthesis based on estimates in vitro. *Am. J. Clin. Nutr.*, 33, 961–964.
53. Levine, M., Conry-Cantilena, C., Wang, Y., Welch, R.W., Washko, P.W., Dhariwal, K.R., Park, J.B., Lazarev, A., Graumlich, J., King, J., and Cantilena, L.R. (1996) Vitamin C pharmacokinetics in health volunteers: evidence for a recommended dietary allowance. *Proc. Natl. Acad. Sci., USA* 93, 3704–3709.
54. Carr, A.C. and Frei, B. (1999) Toward a new recommended dietary allowance for vitamin C based on antioxidant and health effects in humans. *Am. J. Clin. Nutr.*, 69, 1086–1107.
55. Chen, H., Karne, R.J., Hall, G., Campia, U., Panza, J.A., Cannon, R.O., 3rd, Wang, Y., Katz, A., Levine, M., and Quon, M.J. (2006) High-dose oral vitamin C partially replenishes vitamin C levels in patients with Type 2 diabetes and low vitamin C levels but does not improve endothelial dysfunction or insulin resistance. *Am. J. Physiol. Heart Circ. Physiol.*, 290, H137–H145.
56. Maeda, N., Hagihara, H., Nakata, Y., Hiller, S., Wilder, J., and Reddick, R. (2000) Aortic wall damage in mice unable to synthesize ascorbic acid. *Proc. Natl. Acad. Sci., USA* 97, 841–846.
57. Kawai, T., Nishikimi, M., Ozawa, T., and Yagi, K. (1992) A missense mutation of L-gulono-gamma-lactone oxidase causes the inability of scurvy-prone osteogenic disorder rats to synthesize L-ascorbic acid. *J. Biol. Chem.*, 267, 21973–21976.
58. Horio, F., Ozaki, K., Kohmura, M., Yoshida, A., Makino, S., and Hayashi, Y. (1986) Ascorbic acid requirement for the induction of microsomal drug-metabolizing enzymes in a rat mutant unable to synthesize ascorbic acid. *J. Nutr.*, 116, 2278–2289.
59. Meister, A. (1992) On the antioxidant effects of ascorbic acid and glutathione. *Biochem. Pharmacol.*, 44, 1905–1915.
60. Martensson, J., Han, J., Griffith, O.W., and Meister, A. (1993) Glutathione ester delays the onset of scurvy in ascorbate-deficient guinea pigs. *Proc. Natl. Acad. Sci., USA* 90, 317–321.
61. Martensson, J. and Meister, A. (1991) Glutathione deficiency decreases tissue ascorbate levels in newborn rats: ascorbate spares glutathione and protects. *Proc. Natl. Acad. Sci., USA* 88, 4656–4660.
62. Martensson, J. and Meister, A. (1992) Glutathione deficiency increases hepatic ascorbic acid synthesis in adult mice. *Proc. Natl. Acad. Sci., USA* 89, 11566–11568.
63. Meister, A. (1992) Biosynthesis and functions of glutathione, an essential biofactor. *J. Nutr. Sci., Vitaminol (Tokyo)* Spec No, 1–6.
64. Meister, A. (1992) Depletion of glutathione in normal and malignant human cells in vivo by L-buthionine sulfoximine: possible interaction with ascorbate. *J. Natl. Cancer Inst.*, 84, 1601–1602.
65. Meister, A. (1994) Glutathione, ascorbate, and cellular protection. *Cancer Res.*, 54, 1969s–1975s.
66. Meister, A. (1994) Glutathione–ascorbic acid antioxidant system in animals. *J. Biol. Chem.*, 269, 9397–9400.
67. Meister, A. (1995) Mitochondrial changes associated with glutathione deficiency. *Biochim. Biophys. Acta*, 1271, 35–42.
68. Mustacich, D. and Powis, G. (2000) Thioredoxin reductase. *Biochem. J.*, 346 (Pt 1), 1–8.
69. Powis, G., Mustacich, D., and Coon, A. (2000) The role of the redox protein thioredoxin in cell growth and cancer. *Free Radic. Biol. Med.*, 29, 312–322.
70. Banhegyi, G., Marcolongo, P., Puskas, F., Fulceri, R., Mandl, J., and Benedetti, A. (1998) Dehydroascorbate and ascorbate transport in rat liver microsomal vesicles. *J. Biol. Chem.*, 273, 2758–2762.
71. Braun, L., Puskas, F., Csala, M., Gyorffy, E., Garzo, T., Mandl, J., and Banhegyi, G. (1996) Gluconeogenesis from ascorbic acid: ascorbate recycling in isolated murine hepatocytes. *FEBS Lett.*, 390, 183–186.

72. Braun, L., Puskas, F., Csala, M., Meszaros, G., Mandl, J., and Banhegyi, G. (1997) Ascorbate as a substrate for glycolysis or gluconeogenesis: evidence for an interorgan ascorbate cycle. *Free Radic. Biol. Med.*, 23, 804–808.
73. Puskas, F., Gergely, P., Jr, Banki, K., and Perl, A. (2000) Stimulation of the pentose phosphate pathway and glutathione levels by dehydroascorbate, the oxidized form of vitamin C. *FASEB J.*, 14, 1352–1361.
74. Puskas, F., Gergely, P., Niland, B., Banki, K., and Perl, A. (2002) Differential regulation of hydrogen peroxide and Fas-dependent apoptosis pathways by dehydroascorbate, the oxidized form of vitamin C. *Antioxid. Redox. Signal*, 4, 357–369.
75. Wilson, J.X. (2005) Regulation of vitamin C transport. *Annu. Rev. Nutr.*, 25, 105–125.
76. Patak, P., Willenberg, H.S., and Bornstein, S.R. (2004) Vitamin C is an important cofactor for both adrenal cortex and adrenal medulla. *Endocrine. Res.*, 30, 871–875.
77. Roscetti, G., del Carmine, R., Trabucchi, M., Massotti, M., Purdy, R.H., and Barbaccia, M.L. (1998) Modulation of neurosteroid synthesis/accumulation by L-ascorbic acid. *J. Neurochem.*, 71, 1108–1117.
78. Karanth, S., Yu, W.H., Walczewska, A., Mastronardi, C., and McCann, S.M. (2000) Ascorbic acid acts as an inhibitory transmitter in the hypothalamus to inhibit stimulated luteinizing hormone-releasing hormone release by scavenging nitric oxide. *Proc. Natl. Acad. Sci., USA* 97, 1891–1896.
79. Rucker, R.B. and McGee, C. (1993) Chemical modifications of proteins in vivo: selected examples important to cellular regulation. *J. Nutr.*, 123, 977–990.
80. Rucker, R.B. and Wold, F. (1988) Cofactors in and as posttranslational protein modifications. *FASEB J.*, 2, 2252–2261.
81. Prigge, S.T., Mains, R.E., Eipper, B.A., and Amzel, L.M. (2000) New insights into copper monooxygenases and peptide amidation: structure, mechanism and function. *Cell Mol. Life Sci.*, 57, 1236–1259.
82. Prigge, S.T., Kolhekar, A.S., Eipper, B.A., Mains, R.E., and Amzel, L.M. (1999) Substrate-mediated electron transfer in peptidylglycine alpha-hydroxylating monooxygenase. *Nat. Struct. Biol.*, 6, 976–983.
83. Prigge, S.T., Kolhekar, A.S., Eipper, B.A., Mains, R.E., and Amzel, L.M. (1997) Amidation of bioactive peptides: the structure of peptidylglycine alpha-hydroxylating monooxygenase. *Science*, 278, 1300–1305.
84. Food and Nutrition Board (1998) *Dietary Reference Intakes*. National Academy Press, Washington, DC.
85. Niki, E. and Noguchi, N. (1997) Protection of human low-density lipoprotein from oxidative modification by vitamin C. In: Packer, L., Fuchs, J., eds., *Vitamin C in Health and Disease*. Marcel Dekker, New York, pp. 183–192.
86. Buettner, G.R. (1993) The pecking order of free radicals and antioxidants: lipid peroxidation, A-tocopherol, and ascorbate. *Arch. Biochem. Biophys.*, 300, 535–543.
87. Urso, M.L. and Clarkson, P.M. (2003) Oxidative stress, exercise, and antioxidant supplementation. *Toxicology*, 189, 41–54.
88. Carr, A.C., Zhu, B.Z., and Frei, B. (2000) Potential antiatherogenic mechanisms of ascorbate (vitamin C) and alpha-tocopherol (vitamin E). *Circ. Res.*, 87, 349–354.
89. Steinberg, F.M. and Chait, A. (1998) Antioxidant vitamin supplementation and lipid peroxidation smokers. *Am. J. Clin. Nutr.*, 68, 319–327.
90. Fraga, C.G., Motchnik, P.A., Shigenaga, M.K., Helbock, H.J., Jacob, R.A., and Ames, B.N. (1991) Ascorbic acid protects against endogenous oxidative DNA damage in human sperm. *Proc. Natl. Acad. Sci., USA*. 88, 11003–11006.
91. Fraga, C.G., Motchink, P.A., Wyrobek, A.J., Rempel, D.M., and Ames, B.N. (1996) Smoking and low antioxidant levels increase oxidative damage to sperm DNA. *Mutat. Res.*, 351, 199–203.
92. Lindahl, T. (1993) Instability and decay of the primary structure of DNA. *Nature*, 362, 709–715.
93. Ames, B.N., Shigenaga, M.K., and Gold, L.S. (1993) DNA lesions, inducible DNA repair, and cell division: three key factors in mutagenesis and carcinogenesis. *Environ. Health Perspect*, 101 (Suppl 5), 35–44.
94. Stadtman, E.R. (1991) Ascorbic acid and oxidative inactivation of proteins. *Am. J. Clin. Nutr.*, 54, 125S–1128S.

95. Berlett, B.S. and Stadtman, E.R. (1997) Protein oxidation in aging, disease, and oxidative stress. *J. Biol. Chem.*, 272, 20313–20316.
96. Dean, R.T., Fu, S., Stocker, R., and Davies, M.J. (1997) Biochemistry and pathology of radical-mediated protein oxidation. *Biochem. J.*, 324, 1–18.
97. Ortwerth, B.J. and Monnier, V.M. (1997) Protein glycation by the oxidation products of ascorbic acid. In: Packer, L., Fuchs, J., eds., *Vitamin C in Health and Disease*. Marcel Dekker, New York, pp. 123–142.
98. Mannick, E.E., Bravo, L.E., Zarama, G., Realpe, J.L., Zhang, X.-J., Ruiz, B., Fontham, E.T.H., Mera, R., Miller, M.J.S., and Correa, P. (1996) Inducible nitric oxide synthase, nitrotyrosine, and apoptosis in *Helicobacter pylori* gastritis: effect of antibiotics and antioxidants. *Cancer Res.*, 56, 3238–3243.
99. Naidu, K.A. (2003) Vitamin C in human health and disease is still a mystery? An overview. *Nutr. J.*, 2, 7.
100. Rebouche, C.J. (1991) Ascorbic acid and carnitine biosynthesis. *Am. J. Clin. Nutr.*, 54, 1147S–1152S.
101. Johnston, C.S., Solomon, R.E., and Corte, C. (1996) Vitamin C depletion is associated with alterations in blood histamine and plasma free carnitine in adults. *J. Am. Coll. Nutr.*, 15, 586–591.
102. Englard, S. and Seiffer, S. (1986) The biochemical functions of ascorbic acid, and transmembrane electron transfer. *Am. J. Clin. Nutr.*, 54, 1173S–1178S.
103. Tinker, D. and Rucker, R.B. (1985) Role of selected nutrients in synthesis, accumulation, and chemical modification of connective tissue proteins. *Physiol. Rev.*, 65, 607–657.
104. Wess, T.J. (2005) Collagen fibril form and function. *Adv. Protein Chem.*, 70, 341–374.
105. Reiser, K., McCormick, R.J., and Rucker, R.B. (1992) Enzymatic and nonenzymatic cross-linking of collagen and elastin. *FASEB J.*, 6, 2439–2449.
106. Critchfield, J.W., Dubick, M., Last, J., Cross, C.E., and Rucker, R.B. (1985) Changes in response to ascorbic acid administered orally to rat pups: lung collagen, elastin and protein synthesis. *J. Nutr.*, 115, 70–77.
107. Davidson, J.M., LuValle, P.A., Zoia, O., Quaglino, D. Jr., and Giro, M. (1997) Ascorbate differentially regulates elastin and collagen biosynthesis in vascular smooth muscle cells and skin fibroblasts by pretranslational mechanisms. *J. Biol. Chem.*, 272, 345–352.
108. Quaglino, D., Fornieri, C., Botti, B., Davidson, J.M., and Pasquali-Ronchetti, I. (1991) Opposing effects of ascorbate on collagen and elastin deposition in the neonatal rat aorta. *Eur. J. Cell Biol.*, 54, 18–26.
109. Chojkier, M., Houglum, K., Solis-Herruzo, J., and Brenner, D.A. (1989) Stimulation of collagen gene expression by ascorbic acid in cultured human fibroblasts. A role for lipid peroxidation? *J. Biol. Chem.*, 264, 16957–16962.
110. Aleffi, S., Petrai, I., Bertolani, C., Parola, M., Colombatto, S., Novo, E., Vizzutti, F., Anania, F.A., Milani, S., Rombouts, K., Laffi, G., Pinzani, M., and Marra, F. (2005) Upregulation of proinflammatory and proangiogenic cytokines by leptin in human hepatic stellate cells. *Hepatology*, 42, 1339–1348.
111. Shiga, M., Kapila, Y.L., Zhang, Q., Hayami, T., and Kapila, S. (2003) Ascorbic acid induces collagenase-1 in human periodontal ligament cells but not in MC3T3-E1 osteoblast-like cells: potential association between collagenase expression and changes in alkaline phosphatase phenotype. *J. Bone Miner. Res.*, 18, 67–77.
112. Shin, D.M., Ahn, J.I., Lee, K.H., Lee, Y.S., and Lee, Y.S. (2004) Ascorbic acid responsive genes during neuronal differentiation of embryonic stem cells. *Neuroreport*, 15, 1959–1963.
113. Arrigoni, O. and De Tullio, M.C. (2002) Ascorbic acid: much more than just an antioxidant. *Biochim. Biophys. Acta*, 1569, 1–9.
114. Djoman, M.C., Neault, J.F., Hashemi-Fesharaky, S., and Tajmir-Riahi, H.A. (1998) RNA-ascorbate interaction. *J. Biomol. Struct. Dyn.*, 15, 1115–1120.
115. Houglum, K.P., Brenner, D.A., and Chojkier, M. (1991) Ascorbic acid stimulation of collagen biosynthesis independent of hydroxylation. *Am. J. Clin. Nutr.*, 54, 1141S–1143S.
116. Geesin, J.C., Hendricks, L.J., Falkenstein, P.A., Gordon, J.S., and Berg, R.A. (1991) Regulation of collagen synthesis by ascorbic acid: characterization of the role of ascorbate-stimulated lipid peroxidation. *Arch. Biochem. Biophys.*, 290, 127–132.

117. Houglum, K., Brenner, D.A., and Chojkier, M. (1991) D-alpha-tocopherol inhibits collagen alpha 1(I) gene expression in cultured human fibroblasts. Modulation of constitutive collagen gene expression by lipid peroxidation. *J. Clin. Invest.*, 87, 2230–2235.
118. Parola, M., Pinzani, M., Casini, A., Albano, E., Poli, G., Gentilini, A., Gentilini, P., and Dianzani, M.U. (1993) Stimulation of lipid peroxidation or 4-hydroxynonenal treatment increases procollagen alpha 1(I) gene expression in human liver fat-storing cells. *Biochem. Biophys. Res. Commun.*, 194, 1044–1050.
119. Fischer, H., Schwarzer, C., and Illek, B. (2004) Vitamin C controls the cystic fibrosis transmembrane conductance regulator chloride channel. *Proc. Natl. Acad. Sci., USA* 101, 3691–3696.
120. Seitz, G., Gebhardt, S., Beck, J.F., Bohm, W., Lode, H.N., Niethammer, D., and Bruchelt, G. (1998) Ascorbic acid stimulates DOPA synthesis and tyrosine hydroxylase gene expression in the human neuroblastoma cell line SK-N-SH. *Neurosci. Lett.*, 244, 33–36.
121. Carinci, F., Pezzetti, F., Spina, A.M., Palmieri, A., Laino, G., De Rosa, A., Farina, E., Illiano, F., Stabellini, G., Perrotti, V., and Piattelli, A. (2005) Effect of vitamin C on pre-osteoblast gene expression. *Arch. Oral Biol.*, 50, 481–496.
122. MacDonald, L., Thumser, A.E., and Sharp, P. (2002) Decreased expression of the vitamin C transporter SVCT1 by ascorbic acid in a human intestinal epithelial cell line. *Br. J. Nutr.*, 87, 97–100.
123. Takanaga, H., Mackenzie, B., and Hediger, M.A. (2004) Sodium-dependent ascorbic acid transporter family SLC23. *Pflugers Arch.*, 447, 677–682.
124. Liang, W.J., Johnson, D., Ma, L.S., Jarvis, S.M., and Wei-Jun, L. (2002) Regulation of the human vitamin C transporters expressed in COS-1 cells by protein kinase C [corrected]. *Am. J. Physiol. Cell Physiol.*, 283, C1696–C1704.
125. Kashiba, M., Oka, J., Ichikawa, R., Kasahara, E., Inayama, T., Kageyama, A., Kageyama, H., Osaka, T., Umegaki, K., Matsumoto, A., Ishikawa, T., Nishikimi, M., Inoue, M., and Inoue, S. (2002) Impaired ascorbic acid metabolism in streptozotocin-induced diabetic rats. *Free Radic. Biol. Med.*, 33, 1221–1230.
126. Sotiriou, S., Gispert, S., Cheng, J., Wang, Y., Chen, A., Hoogstraten-Miller, S., Miller, G.F., Kwon, O., Levine, M., Guttentag, S.H., and Nussbaum, R.L. (2002) Ascorbic-acid transporter Slc23a1 is essential for vitamin C transport into the brain and for perinatal survival. *Nat. Med.*, 8, 514–517.
127. Erichsen, H.C., Eck, P., Levine, M., and Chanock, S. (2001) Characterization of the genomic structure of the human vitamin C transporter SVCT1 (SLC23A2). *J. Nutr.*, 131, 2623–2627.
128. Garcia Mde, L., Salazar, K., Millan, C., Rodriguez, F., Montecinos, H., Caprile, T., Silva, C., Cortes, C., Reinicke, K., Vera, J.C., Aguayo, L.G., Olate, J., Molina, B., and Nualart, F. (2005) Sodium vitamin C cotransporter SVCT2 is expressed in hypothalamic glial cells. *Glia.*, 50, 32–47.
129. Gispert, S., Dutra, A., Lieberman, A., Friedlich, D., and Nussbaum, R.L. (2000) Cloning and genomic organization of the mouse gene *slc23a1* encoding a vitamin C transporter. *DNA Res.*, 7, 339–345.
130. Goldenberg, H. and Schweinzer, E. (1994) Transport of vitamin C in animal and human cells. *J. Bioenerg. Biomembr.*, 26, 359–367.
131. Wilson, J.X. (2005) Regulation of vitamin C transport. *Annu. Rev. Nutr.*, 25, 105–125.
132. Rumey, S.C. and Levine, M. (1998) Absorption, transport, and disposition of ascorbic acid in humans. *J. Nutr. Biochem.*, 9, 116–130.
133. Jacob, R.A., Skala, J.H., and Omaye, S.T. (1987) Biochemical indices of human vitamin C status. *Am. J. Clin. Nutr.*, 46, 818–826.
134. Blanchard, J., Conrad, K.A., Watson, R.R., Garry, P.J., and Crawley, J.D. (1989) Comparison of plasma, mononuclear, and polymorphonuclear leukocyte vitamin C levels in young and elderly women during depletion and supplementation. *Eur. J. Clin. Nutr.*, 43, 97–106.
135. Omaye, S.T., Schaus, E.E., Kutnink, M.A., and Hawkes, W.C. (1987) Measurement of vitamin C in blood components by high-performance liquid chromatography. Implication in assisting vitamin C status. *Ann. NY Acad. Sci.*, 498, 389–401.
136. Hematological and nutritional biochemistry reference data for persons 6 months–74 years of age: United States, 1976–80 (1984) US Department of Health and Human Services; Public Health Service; National Center for Health Statistics. Hyattsville, MD, DHHS Publication No. (PHS) 83, 138–143.
137. Hampl, J.S., Taylor, C.A., and Johnston, C.S. (2004) Vitamin C deficiency and depletion in the United States: the Third National Health and Nutrition Examination Survey, 1988 to 1994. *Am. J. Public Health*, 94, 870–875.

138. Schectman, G., Byrd, J.C., and Hoffmann, R. (1991) Ascorbic acid requirements for smokers: analysis of a population survey. *Am. J. Clin. Nutr.*, 53, 1466–1470.
139. Standing Committee on the Scientific Evaluation of dietary reference intakes, Food and Nutrition Board (2000) *Dietary Reference Intakes for Vitamin C, Vitamin E, Selenium, and Beta Carotene, and Other Carotenoids*. National Academy Press, Washington, DC.
140. Schwerdt, P.R. and Schwerdt, C.E. (1975) Effect of ascorbic acid on rhinovirus replication in WI-38 cells (38724). *Proc. Soc. Exp. Biol. Med.*, 148, 1237–1245.
141. Betanzos-Cabrera, G., Ramirez, F.J., Munoz, J.L., Barron, B.L., and Maldonado, R. (2004) Inactivation of HSV-2 by ascorbate-Cu(III) and its protecting evaluation in CF-1 mice against encephalitis. *J. Virol. Methods*, 120, 161–165.
142. Harakeh, S. and Jariwalla, R.J. (1991) Comparative study of the anti-HIV activities of ascorbate and thiol-containing reducing agents in chronically HIV infected cells. *Am. J. Clin. Nutr.*, 54, 1231S–1235S.
143. Muller, F., Svardal, A.M., Norday, I., Berge, R.K., Aukrust, P., and Froland, S.S. (2000) Virological and immunological effects of antioxidant treatment in patients with HIV infection. *Eur. J. Clin. Invest.*, 30, 905–914.
144. Zhang, H.M., Wakisaka, N., Naeda, O., and Yamamoto, T. (1997) Vitamin C inhibits the growth of a bacterial risk factor for gastric carcinoma: *Helicobacter pylori*. *Cancer*, 80, 1897–1903.
145. Simon, J.A., Hudes, E.S., and Perez-Perez, G.I. (2003) Relation of serum ascorbic acid to *Helicobacter pylori* serology in US adults: the Third National Health and Nutrition Examination Survey. *J. Am. Coll. Nutr.*, 22, 283–289.
146. Douglas, R., Hemila, H., D'Souza, R., Chalker, E., and Treacy, B. (2004) Vitamin C for preventing and treating the common cold. *Cochrane Database Syst. Rev.*, 18, CD000980.
147. Hemila, H. (1997) Vitamin C intake and susceptibility to the common cold. *Br. J. Nutr.*, 77, 59–72.
148. Hemila, H. (1996) Vitamin C and common cold incidence: a review of studies with subjects under heavy physical stress. *Int. J. Sports Med.*, 17, 379–383.
149. Nieman, D.C., Dumke, C.I., Henson, D.A., McAnulty, S.R., McAnulty, L.S., Lind, R.H., and Morrow, J.D. (2003) Immune and oxidative changes during and following the Western States Endurance Run. *Int. J. Sports Med.*, 24, 541–547.
150. Peters, E.M., Goetzsche, J.M., Grobbelaar, B., and Noakes, T.D. (1993) Vitamin C supplementation reduces the incidence of postrace symptoms of upper-respiratory-tract infection in ultra marathon runners. *Am. J. Clin. Nutr.*, 57, 170–174.
151. Hemila, H. (2004) Vitamin C supplementation and respiratory infections: a systematic review. *Military Med.*, 169, 920–925.
152. Hunt, C., Chakravorty, N.K., Annan, G., Habibzadeh, N., and Schorah, C.J. (1994) The clinical effects of vitamin C supplementation in elderly hospitalized patients with acute respiratory infections. *Int. J. Vitam. Nutr. Res.*, 64, 212–219.
153. Nieman, D.C. (2000) Is infection risk linked to exercise workload? *Med. Sci. Sports Exerc.*, 32 (Suppl), S406–S411.
154. Palmer, F.M., Nieman, D.C., Henson, D.A., McAnulty, S.R., McAnulty, L., Swick, N.S., Utter, A.C., Vinci, D.M., and Morrow, J.D. (2003) Influence of vitamin C supplementation on oxidative and salivary IgA changes following an ultra marathon. *Eur. J. Appl. Physiol.*, 89, 100–107.
155. Krause, R., Patruta, S., Daxbock, F., Fladerer, P., Biegelmayer, C., and Wenisch, C. (2001) Effect of vitamin C on neutrophil function after high-intensity exercise. *Eur. J. Clin. Invest.*, 31, 258–263.
156. Nieman, D.C., Henson, D.A., Butterworth, D.E., Warren, B.J., Davis, J.M., Fagoaga, O.R., and Nehlsen-Cannarella, S.L. (1997) Vitamin C supplementation does not alter the immune response to 2.5 h of running. *Int. J. Sport Nutr.*, 7, 173–184.
157. Tauler, P., Aguilo, A., Gimeno, I., Noguera, A., Agusti, A., Tur, J.A., and Pons, A. (2003) Differential response of lymphocytes and neutrophils to high intensity physical activity and to vitamin C diet supplementation. *Free Radic. Res.*, 37, 931–938.
158. Sharma, P., Raghavan, S.A., Saini, R., and Dikshit, M. (2004) Ascorbate-mediated enhancement of reactive oxygen species generation from polymorphonuclear leukocytes: modulatory effect of nitric oxide. *J. Leukoc. Biol.*, 75, 1070–1078.
159. Chatterjee, I.B., Majumder, A.K., Nandi, B.K., and Subramanian, N. (1975) Synthesis and some major functions of vitamin C in animals. *Ann. NY Acad. Sci.*, 258, 24–45.

160. Uchida, K., Mitsui, M., and Kawakishi, S. (1989) Monooxygenation of *N*-acetylhistamine mediated by L-ascorbate. *Biochim. Biophys. Acta*, 991, 377–379.
161. Johnston, C.S., Solomon, R.E., and Corte, C. (1996) Vitamin C depletion is associated with alterations in blood histamine and plasma free carnitine in adults. *J. Am. Coll. Nutr.*, 15, 586–591.
162. Johnston, C.S., Retrum, K.R., and Srilakshmi, J.C. (1992) Antihistamine effects and complications of supplemental vitamin C. *J. Am. Diet. Assoc.*, 92, 988–989.
163. Bucca, C., Rolla, G., Oliva, A., and Farina, J.C. (1990) Effect of vitamin C on histamine bronchial responsiveness of patients with allergic rhinitis. *Ann. Allergy*, 65, 311–314.
164. Rayment, S.J., Shaw, J., Woollard, K.J., Lunee, J., and Griffiths, H.R. (2003) Vitamin C supplementation in normal subjects reduces constitutive ICAM-1 expression. *Biochem. Biophys. Res. Commun.*, 308, 339–345.
165. Goetzl, E.J. (1976) Defective responsiveness to ascorbic acid of neutrophil random and chemotactic migration in Felty's syndrome and systemic lupus erythematosus. *Ann. Rheum. Dis.*, 35, 510–515.
166. Sandler, J.A., Gallin, J.I., and Vaughan, M. (1975) Effects of serotonin, carbamylcholine, and ascorbic acid on leukocyte cyclic GMP and chemotaxis. *J. Cell Biol.*, 67, 480–484.
167. Goetzl, E.J., Waserman, S.I., Gigli, I., and Austen, K.F. (1974) Enhancement of random migration and chemotactic response of human leukocytes by ascorbic acid. *J. Clin. Invest.*, 53, 813–818.
168. Anderson, R. and Theron, A. (1979) Effects of ascorbate on leucocytes. *S. Afr. Med. J.*, 56, 394–400.
169. Anderson, R. (1981) Ascorbate-mediated stimulation of neutrophil motility and lymphocyte transformation by inhibition of the peroxidase/H_2O_2/halide system in vitro and in vivo. *Am. J. Clin. Nutr.*, 34, 1906–1911.
170. Johnston, C.S., Martin, L.J., and Cai, X. (1992) Antihistamine effect of supplemental ascorbic acid and neutrophil chemotaxis. *J. Am. Coll. Nutr.*, 11, 172–176.
171. Anderson, R., Oosthuizen, R., Maritz, R., Theron, A., and Van Rensburg, A.J. (1890) The effects of increasing weekly doses of ascorbate on certain cellular and humoral immune functions in normal volunteers. *Am. J. Clin. Nutr.*, 33, 71–76.
172. Weening, R.S., Schoorel, E.P., Roos, D., van Schaik, M.L.J., Voetman, A.A., Bot, A.A.M., Batenburg-Plenter, A.M., Willems, C., Zeijlemaker, W.P., and Astaldi, A. (1980) Effect of ascorbate on abnormal neutrophil, platelet, and lymphocyte function in a patient with the Chediak–Hagashi syndrome. *Blood*, 57, 856–865.
173. Boxer, L.A., Watanabe, A.M., Rister, M., Besch, H.R., Allen, J., and Baehner, R.L. (1976) Correction of leukocyte function in Chediak–Higashi syndrome by ascorbate. *N. Engl. J. Med.*, 295, 1041–1045.
174. Anderson, R. (1981) Assessment of oral ascorbate in three children with chronic granulomatous disease and defective neutrophil motility over a 2-year period. *Clin. Exp. Immunol.*, 43, 180–188.
175. Goldschmidt, M.C. (1991) Reduced bactericidal activity in neutrophils from scorbutic animals and the effect of ascorbic acid on these target bacteria in vivo and in vitro. *Am. J. Clin. Nutr.*, 54, 1214S–1220S.
176. Kay, N.E., Holloway, D.E., Hutton, S.W., Bone, N.D., and Duane, W.C. (1982) Human T-cell function in experimental ascorbic acid deficiency and spontaneous scurvy. *Am. J. Clin. Nutr.*, 36, 127–130.
177. Douziech, N., Seres, I., Larbi, A., Szikszay, E., Roy, P.M., Arcand, M., Dupuis, G., and Fulop, T. (2002) Modulation of human lymphocyte proliferative response with aging. *Exp. Gerontol.*, 37, 369–387.
178. Jacob, R.A., Kelley, D.S., Pianalto, F.S., Swendseid, M.E., Henning, S.M., Zhang, J.Z., Ames, B.N., Fraga, C.G., and Peters, J.H. (1991) Immunocompetence and oxidant defense during ascorbate depletion of healthy men. *Am. J. Clin. Nutr.*, 54, 1302S–1309S.
179. Panush, R.S., Delafuente, J.C., Katz, P., and Johnson, J. (1982) Modulation of certain immunologic responses by vitamin C. III. Potentiation of in vitro and in vivo lymphocyte responses. *Int. J. Vit. Nutr. Res.*, 23 (Suppl), 35–47.
180. Campbell, J.D., Cole, M., Bunditrutavorn, B., and Vella, A.T. (1999) Ascorbic acid is a potent inhibitor of various forms of T cell apoptosis. *Cell Immunol.*, 194, 1–5.
181. Johnston, C.S., Kolb, W.P., and Haskell, B.E. (1987) The effect of vitamin C nutriture on complement component C1q concentrations in guinea pig plasma. *J. Nutr.*, 117, 764–768.
182. Johnston, C.S. (1991) Complement component C1q levels unaltered by ascorbate nutriture. *J. Nutr. Biochem.*, 2, 499–501.

183. Hartel, C., Strunk, T., Bucsky, P., and Schultz, C. (2004) Effects of vitamin C on intracytoplasmic cytokine production in human whole blood monocytes and lymphocytes. *Cytokine*, 27, 101–106.
184. Carcamo, J.M., Pedraza, A., Borquez-Ojeda, O., and Golde, D.W. (2002) Vitamin C suppresses TNFα-induced NFκB activation by inhibiting IκBα phosphorylation. *Biochemistry*, 41, 12995–13002.
185. Oh, C. and Nakano, K. (1988) Reversal by ascorbic acid of suppression by endogenous histamine of rat lymphocyte blastogenesis. *J. Nutr.*, 118, 639–644.
186. Enstrom, J.E., Kanim, L.E., and Klein, M.A. (1992) Vitamin C intake and mortality among a sample of the United States population. *Epidemiology*, 3, 194–202.
187. Knekt, P., Ritz, J., Pereira, M.A., O'Reilly, E.J., Augustsson, K., Fraser, G.E., Goldbourt, U., Heitmann, B.L., Hallmans, G., Liu, S., Pietinen, P., Spiegelman, D., Stevens, J., Virtamo, J., Willett, W.C., Rimm, E.B., and Ascherio, A. (2004) Antioxidant vitamins and coronary heart disease risk: a pooled analysis of 9 cohorts. *Am. J. Clin. Nutr.*, 80, 1508–1520.
188. Simon, J.A., Hudes, E.S., and Tice, J.A. (2001) Relation of serum ascorbic acid to mortality among US adults. *J. Am. Coll. Nutr.*, 20, 255–263.
189. Nyyssonen, K., Parvianinen, M.T., Salonen, R., Tuomilehto, J., and Salonen, J.T. (1997) Vitamin C deficiency and risk of myocardial infarction: prospective population study of men from Eastern Finland. *Br. Med. J.*, 314, 634–638.
190. Riemersma, R.A., Carruthers, K.F., Elton, R.A., and Fox, K.A.A. (2000) Vitamin C and the risk of acute myocardial infarction. *Am. J. Clin. Nutr.*, 71, 1181–1186.
191. Gale, C.R., Martyn, C.N., Winter, P.D., and Cooper, C. (1995) Vitamin C and risk of death from stroke and coronary heart disease in a cohort of elderly people. *Br. Med. J.*, 310, 1563–1566.
192. May, J.M. and Mendiratta, S. (1998) Protection and recycling of alpha-tocopherol in human erythrocytes by intracellular ascorbic acid. *Arch. Biochem. Biophys.*, 349, 281–289.
193. Hodis, H.N., Mack, W.J., LaBree, L., Mahrer, P.R., Sevanian, A., Liu, C.R., Liu, C.H., Hwang, J., Selzer, R.H., and Azen, S.P. (2002) Alpha-tocopherol supplementation in healthy individuals reduces low-density lipoprotein oxidation but not atherosclerosis: the Vitamin E Atherosclerosis Prevention Study (VEAPS). *Circulation*, 106, 1453–1459.
194. Heller, R., Unbehaun, A., Schellenberg, B., Mayer, B., Werner-Felmayer, G., and Werner, E.R. (2001) L-Ascorbic acid potentates endothelial nitric oxide synthesis via a chemical stabilization of tetrahydrobiopterin. *J. Biol. Chem.*, 276, 40–47.
195. Mullan, B.A., Young, I.S., Fee, H., and McCance, D.R. (2002) Ascorbic acid reduces blood pressure and arterial stiffness in type 2 diabetes. *Hypertension*, 40, 804–809.
196. Duffy, S.J., Gokce, N., Holbrook, M., Huang, A., Frei, B., Keaney, J.F., and Vita, J.A. (1999) Treatment of hypertension with ascorbic acid. *Lancet*, 354, 2048–2049.
197. Salonen, R.M., Nyyssonen, K., Kaikkonen, J., Porkkala-Sarataho, E., Voutilainen, S., Rissanen, T.H., Tuomainen, T.P., Valkonen, V.P., Ristonmaa, U., Lakka, H.M., Vanharanta, M., Salonen, J.T., and Poulsen, H.E. (2003) Antioxidant Supplementation in Atherosclerosis Prevention Study. Six-year effect of combined vitamin C and E supplementation on atherosclerotic progression: the Antioxidant Supplementation in Atherosclerosis Prevention (ASAP) Study. *Circulation*, 107, 947–953.
198. Heart Protection Study Collaborative Group (2002) Heart Protection Study Collaborative Group MRC/BHF Heart Protection Study of antioxidant vitamin supplementation in 20,536 high-risk individuals: a randomized placebo-controlled trial. *Lancet*, 360, 23–33.
199. Brown, B.G., Cheung, M.C., Lee, A.C., Zhao, X.Q., and Chait, A. (2002) Antioxidant vitamins and lipid therapy, End of a long romance? *Arterioscler. Thromb. Vasc.*, 22, 1535–1546.
200. Jialal, I. and Singh, U. (2006) Is vitamin C an anti-inflammatory agent? *Am. J. Clin. Nutr.*, 83, 525–526.
201. Kurl, S., Tuomainen, T.P., Laukkanen, J.A., Nyyssonen, K., Lakka, T., Sivenius, J., and Salonen, J.T. (2002) Plasma vitamin C modifies the association between hypertension and risk of stroke. *Stroke*, 33, 1568–1573.
202. Yokoyama, T., Date, C., Kokubo, Y., Yoshiike, N., Matsumura, Y., and Tanaka, H. (2000) Serum vitamin C concentration was inversely associated with subsequent 20-year incidence of stroke in a Japanese rural community. *Stroke*, 31, 2287–2294.
203. Khaw, K.T., Bingham, S., Welch, A., Luben, R., Wareham, N., Oakes, S., and Day, N. (2001) Relation between plasma ascorbic acid and mortality in men and women in EPIC-Norfolk prospective study: a prospective population study. European Prospective Investigation into Cancer and Nutrition. *Lancet*, 35, 657–663.

204. Jacobs, E.J., Connell, C.J., Patel, A.V., Chao, A., Rodriguez, C., Seymour, J., McCullough, M.L., Calle, E.E., and Thun, M.J. (2001) Vitamin C and vitamin E supplement use and colorectal cancer mortality in a large American Cancer Society cohort. *Cancer Epidemiol. Biomarkers Prev.*, 10, 17–23.
205. Jacobs, E.J., Connell, C.J., McCullough, M.L., Chao, A., Jonas, C.R, Rodriguez, C., Calle, E.E., and Thun, M.J. (2002) Vitamin C, vitamin E, and multivitamin supplement use and stomach cancer mortality in the Cancer Prevention Study II cohort. *Cancer Epidemiol. Biomarkers Prev.*, 11, 35–41.
206. Mayne, S.T., Risch, H.A., Dubrow, R., Chow, W.H., Gammon, M.D., Vaughan, T.L., Farrow, D.C., Schoenberg, J.B., Stanford, J.L., Ahsan, H., West, A.B., Rotterdam, H., Blot, W.J., and Fraumeni, J.F. (2001) Nutrient intake and risk of subtypes of esophageal and gastric cancer. *Cancer Epidemiol. Biomarkers Prev.*, 10, 1055–1062.
207. Blot, W.J., Ki, J.Y., Taylor, P.R., Guo, W., Dawsey, S., Wang, G.Q., Yang, C.S., Zheng, S.F., Gail, M., Li, G.Y. et al. (1993) Nutrition intervention trials in Linxian, China: supplementation with specific vitamin/mineral combinations, cancer incidence, and disease-specific mortality in the general population. *J. Natl. Cancer Inst.*, 85, 148–1492.
208. Lee, K.W., Lee, H.J., Surh, Y.J., and Lee, C.Y. (2003) Vitamin C and cancer chemoprevention: reappraisal. *Am. J. Clin. Nutr.*, 78, 1074–1078.
209. Lutsenko, E.A., Carcamo, J.M., and Golde, D.W. (2002) Vitamin C prevents DNA mutation induced by oxidative stress. *J. Biol. Chem.*, 277, 16895–16899.
210. Jacques, P.F. and Chylack, L.T. (1991) Epidemiologic evidence of a role for the antioxidant vitamins and carotenoids in cataract prevention. *Am. J. Clin. Nutr.*, 53, 325S–355S.
211. Jacques, P.F., Taylor, A., Hankinson, S.E., Willet, W.C., Mahnken, B., Lee, Y., Vaid, K., and Lahav, M. (1997) Long-term vitamin C supplement use and prevalence of early age-related lens opacities. *Am. J. Clin. Nutr.*, 66, 911–916.
212. Valero, M.P., Fletcher, A.E., DeStavola, B.L., Vioque, J., and Alepuz, V.C. (2002) Vitamin C is associated with reduced risk of cataract in a Mediterranean population. *J. Nutr.*, 132, 1299–1306.
213. Moeller, S.M., Taylor, A., Tucker, K.L., McCullough, M.L., Chylack, L.T., Hankinson, S.E., Willett, W.C., and Jacques, P.F. (2004) Overall adherence to the dietary guidelines for Americans is associated with reduced prevalence of early age-related nuclear lens opacities in women. *J. Nutr.*, 134, 1812–1819.
214. Schunemann, H.J., McCann, S., Grant, B.J.B., Trevisan, M., Muti, P., and Freudenheim, J.L. (2002) Lung function in relation to intake of carotenoids and other antioxidant vitamins in a population-based study. *Am. J. Epidemiol.*, 155, 463–471.
215. Hu, G. and Cassano, P.A. (2000) Antioxidant nutrients and pulmonary function: the Third National Health and Nutrition Examination Survey (NHANES III). *Am. J. Epidemiol.*, 151, 975–981.
216. Hatch, G.E. (2002) Asthma, inhaled oxidants, and dietary antioxidants. *Am. J. Clin. Nutr.*, 61 (Suppl), 625S–630S.
217. McKeever, T.M., Scrivener, S., Broadfield, E., Jones, Z., Britton, J., and Lewis, S.A. (2002) Prospective study of diet and decline in lung function in a general population. *Am. J. Respir. Crit. Care Med.*, 165, 1299–1303.
218. Omenaas, E., Fluge, O., Buist, A.S., Vollmer, W.M., and Gulsvik, A. (2003) Dietary vitamin C intake is inversely related to cough and wheeze in young smokers. *Respir. Med.*, 97, 134–142.
219. Bodner, C., Godden, D., Brown, K., Little, J., Ross, S., and Seaton, A. (1999) Antioxidant intake and adult-onset wheeze: a case–control study. *Eur. Respir. J.*, 13, 22–30, 1999.
220. Mudway, I.S., Krishna, M.T., Frew, A.J., MacLeod, D., Sandstrom, T., Holgate, S.T., and Kelly, F.J. (1999) Compromised concentrations of ascorbate in fluid lining the respiratory tract in human subjects after exposure to ozone. *Occup. Environ. Med.*, 56, 473–481.
221. Leveille, S.G., LaCroix, A.Z., Doepsell, T.D., Beresford, S.A., VanBelle, G., and Buchner, D.M. (1999) Dietary vitamin C and bone mineral density in postmenopausal women in Washington State, USA. *J. Epidemiol. Commun. Health*, 51, 479–485.
222. Simon, J.A. and Hudes, E.S. (2001) Relation of ascorbic acid to bone mineral density and self-reported fractures among US adults. *Am. J. Epidemiol.*, 154, 427–433.
223. Macdonald, H.M., New, S.A., Golden, M.H., Campbell, M.K., and Reid, D.M. (2004) Nutritional associations with bone loss during the menopausal transition: evidence of a beneficial effect of calcium, alcohol, and fruit and vegetable nutrients and of a detrimental effect of fatty acids. *Am. J. Clin. Nutr.*, 79, 155–165.

224. Morton, D.J., Barrett-Connor, E.L., and Schneider, D.L. (2001) Vitamin C supplement use and bone mineral density in postmenopausal women. *J. Bone Miner. Res.*, 16, 135–140.
225. Melhus, H., Michaelsson, K., Holberg, L., Wolk, A., and Ljunghall, S. (1999) Smoking, antioxidant vitamins, and the risk of hip fracture. *J. Bone Miner. Res.*, 14, 129–135.
226. Ervin, R.B., Wright, J.D., Wang, C.Y., and Kennedy-Stephenson, J. (2004) Dietary intake of selected vitamins for the United States population: 1999–2000. Advance Data; Vital and Health Statistics, US Department of Health and Human Services, No. 339.
227. Block, G., Mangels, A.R., Patterson, B.H., Levander, O.A., Norkus, E.P., and Taylor, P.R. (1999) Body weight and prior depletion affect plasma ascorbate levels attained on identical vitamin C intake: a controlled-diet study. *J. Am. Coll. Nutr.*, 18, 628–637.
228. Dickinson, V.A., Block, G., and Russek-Cohen, E. (1994) Supplement use, other dietary and demographic variables, and serum vitamin C in NHANES II. *J. Am. Coll. Nutr.*, 13, 22–32.
229. vanZoeren-Grobben, D., Lindeman, J.H.N., Houdkamp, E., Brand, R., Schrijver, J., and Berger, H.M. (1994) Postnatal changes in plasma chain-breaking antioxidants in healthy preterm infants fed formula and/or human milk. *Am. J. Clin. Nutr.*, 60, 900–906.
230. Padayatt, S.J., Sun, H., Wang, Y., Riordan, H.D., Hewitt, S.M., Katz, A., Wesley, R.A., and Levine, M. (2004) Vitamin C pharmacokinetics: implications for oral and intravenous use. *Ann. Intern. Med.*, 140, 533–537.
231. Hamabe, A., Takase, B., Uehata, A., Kurita, A., Ohsuzu, F., and Tamai, S. (2001) Impaired endothelium-dependent vasodilatation in the brachial artery in variant angina pectoris and the effect of intravenous administration of vitamin C. *Am. J. Cardiol.*, 87, 1154–1159.
232. Ellis, G.R., Anderson, R.A., Chirkov, Y.Y., Morris-Thurgood, J., Jackson, S.K., Lewis, M.J., Horowitz, J.D., and Frenneaux, M.P. (2001) Acute effects of vitamin C on platelet responsiveness to nitric oxide donors and endothelial function in patients with chronic heart failure. *J. Cardiovasc. Pharmacol.*, 37, 564–570.
233. Cochrane, W.A. (1965) Over nutrition in prenatal and neonatal life: a problem? *Can. Med. Assoc. J.*, 93, 893–899.
234. Omaye, S.T., Skala, J.H., and Jacob, R.A. (1989) Plasma ascorbic acid in adult males: effects of depletion and supplementation. *Am. J. Clin. Nutr.*, 44, 257–264.
235. Kallner, A. (1988) Plasma ascorbic acid in adult males. *Am. J. Clin. Nutr.*, 47, 340–341.
236. Auer, B.L., Auer, D., and Rodgers, A.L. (1998) Relative hyperoxaluria, crystalluria and haematuria after megadose ingestion of vitamin C. *Eur. J. Clin. Invest.*, 28, 695–700.
237. Mashour, S., Turner, J.F., and Merrell, B. (2000) Acute renal failure, oxalosis, and vitamin C supplementation. *Chest*, 118, 561–563.
238. Traxer, O., Huet, B., Poindexter, J., Pak, C.Y., and Pearle, M.S. (2003) Effect of ascorbic acid consumption on urinary stone risk factors. *J. Urol.*, 170, 397–401.
239. Baxmann, A.C., Mendonca, C.O.G., and Heilberg, I.P. (2003) Effect of vitamin C supplements on urinary oxalate and pH in calcium stone-forming patients. *Kidney Int.*, 63, 1066–1071.
240. Taylor, E.N., Stampfer, M.J., and Curhan, G.C. (2004) Dietary factors and the risk of incident kidney stones in men: new insights after 14 years of follow-up. *J. Am. Soc. Nephrol.*, 15, 3225–3232.
241. Campbell, G.D., Steinberg, M.H., and Bower, J.D. (1975) Ascorbic acid-induced hemolysis in G6PD deficiency. *Ann. Intern. Med.*, 82, 810.
242. Hunt, J.R. and Zeng, H. (2004) Iron absorption by heterozygous carriers of the HFE C282Y mutation associated with hemochromatosis. *Am. J. Clin. Nutr.*, 80, 924–931.
243. Reller, K., Dresow, B., Collell, M., Fischer, R., Engelhardt, R., Nielsen, P., Durken, M., Politis, C., and Piga, A. (1998) Iron overload and antioxidant status in patients with β-thalassemia major. *Ann. NY Acad. Sci.*, 850, 463–465.
244. Herbert, V., Jacob, E., Wong, K.T., Scott, J., and Pfeffer, R.D. (1978) Low serum vitamin B_{12} levels in patients receiving ascorbic acid in megadoses: studies concerning the effect of ascorbate on radioisotope vitamin B_{12} assay. *Am. J. Clin. Nutr.*, 31, 253–258.
245. Jacob, R.A., Otradovec, C.L., Russell, R.M., Munro, H.N., Hartz, S.C., McGandy, R.B., Morrow, F.D., and Sadowski, J.A. (1988) Vitamin C status and nutrient interactions in a healthy elderly population. *Am. J. Clin. Nutr.*, 48, 1436–1442.
246. Simon, J.A. and Hudes, E.S. (1999) Relation of serum ascorbic acid to serum vitamin B_{12}, serum ferritin, and kidney stones in US adults. *Arch. Intern. Med.*, 159, 619–624.

16 Vitamin-Dependent Modifications of Chromatin: Epigenetic Events and Genomic Stability

James B. Kirkland, Janos Zempleni, Linda K. Buckles, and Judith K. Christman

CONTENTS

INTRODUCTION

DNA and DNA-binding proteins make up the bulk of chromatin. DNA-binding proteins comprise a diverse group of compounds, including histones, high-mobility group proteins, transcription factors, and enzymes that mediate covalent modifications of DNA and histones.

For many years, the nucleotide sequence of DNA has been considered the sole driver of heredity. Consistent with this notion, heritable changes in phenotypic traits were thought to be determined by genetic mutations and recombinations. More recently, however, the discovery of epigenetic mechanisms for gene regulation has dramatically expanded our understanding of mechanisms used by eukaryotes to regulate gene expression through remodeling in chromatin structure and chemical modifications of both DNA and DNA-binding proteins. It is now well established that enzymatic methylation of cytosine residues in DNA and methylation, acetylation, and phosphorylation of amino acids in histones can establish changes in gene expression and chromatin conformation that are maintained through many generations of cell division in mammalian cells. More recently, these covalent modifications of DNA and its binding proteins have been found to play essential roles in maintaining genomic stability and DNA repair. However, the role of vitamins such as folate, biotin, vitamin B, and short-chain fatty acids is less appreciated. This chapter focuses on two unique modifications of histones by biotinylation and poly(ADP-ribosyl)ation and the role of folate and other dietary sources of methyl groups on modification of DNA and histones.

ROLES FOR VITAMINS IN EPIGENETIC EVENTS

Introduction to Chromatin Structure and Modifications of Histones

Vitamin-dependent modifications of chromatin may target both DNA and its binding proteins. In this section, we review the following examples for nutrient-dependent modifications of chromatin, which play roles in epigenetic events and genomic stability: biotinylation, acetylation and poly(ADP-ribosyl)ation of histones, and methylation of DNA.

Chromatin in the mammalian cell nucleus is composed primarily of DNA and DNA-binding proteins, that is, histones and nonhistone proteins (Figure 16.1). Histones play a

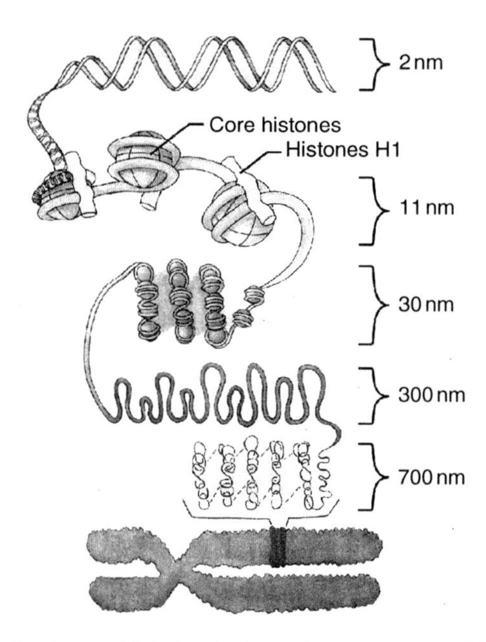

FIGURE 16.1 DNA is organized at multiple levels through interactions with specific proteins and other cellular molecules, eventually increasing in diameter from 2 nm for double-stranded DNA up to 700 nm for a fully condensed chromosome. This complex structure is highly regulated and is responsive to the supply of several micronutrients, including biotin, folate, and niacin.

predominant role in the folding of DNA into chromatin (1). Five major classes of histones have been identified in mammals: H1, H2A, H2B, H3, and H4. Histones consist of a globular domain and a more flexible amino terminus (histone tail). Lysine and arginine residues account for a combined >20% of all amino acid residues in histones, leading to a positive net charge of these proteins at physiological pH (1).

DNA and histones form repetitive nucleoprotein units, the nucleosomes (1). Each nucleosome (nucleosomal core particle) consists of 146 base pairs of DNA wrapped around an octamer of core histones (one H3–H3–H4–H4 tetramer and two H2A–H2B dimers). The binding of DNA to histones is of electrostatic nature, and is mediated by the association of negatively charged phosphate groups of DNA with positively charged ε-amino groups (lysine moieties) and guanidino groups (arginine moieties) of histones. The DNA located between nucleosomal core particles is associated with histone H1.

The amino-terminal tail of histones protrudes from the nucleosomal surface; covalent modifications of this tail affect the structure of chromatin and form the basis for gene regulation (2–7), mitotic and meiotic chromosome condensation (8,9), and DNA repair (10–15). Histone tails are modified by covalent acetylation (16–18), methylation (1), phosphorylation (1), ubiquitination (1), poly(ADP-ribosyl)ation (12,19,20), and biotinylation (see later) of ε-amino groups (lysine), guanidino groups (arginine), carboxyl groups (glutamate), and hydroxyl groups (serine). Multiple signaling pathways converge on histones to mediate covalent modifications of specific amino acid residues (8,21). Site-specific modifications of histones have distinct functions; for example, dimethylation of lysine-4 in histone H3 is associated with transcriptional activation of surrounding DNA (6,22). Modifications of histone tails (histone code) considerably extend the information potential of the DNA code and gene regulation (6,23,24). Modifications of histone tails may affect binding of chromatin-associated proteins, triggering cascades of downstream histone modifications. For example, methylation of arginine-3 in histone H4 recruits the histone acetyltransferase Esa1 to yeast chromatin, leading to acetylation of lysine-5 in histone H4 (6). Histone modifications can influence each other in synergistic or antagonistic ways, mediating gene regulation. For example, phosphorylation of serine-10 inhibits methylation of lysine-9 in histone H3, but is coupled with acetylation of lysine-9 and lysine-14 during mitogenic stimulation in mammalian cells (6). Covalent modifications of histones can be reversed by a large variety of enzymatic processes (6).

Acetylation of histones itself represents a vitamin-dependent form of chromatin structure regulation. It does not receive much attention from a nutrition perspective as pantothenic acid deficiency is never a practical issue. However, as stated earlier, methylation of histones can alter acetylation patterns, and deacetylation is dependent on NAD pools and dietary niacin status, so there are many opportunities for nutrient interactions. Deacetylation plays a key role in chromatin silencing and is discussed further in the section on niacin.

Biotinylation of Histones

Histone Biotinyl Transferases and Hydrolases

Histones are modified by covalent attachment of the vitamin biotin. Hymes et al. have proposed a reaction mechanism by which cleavage of biocytin (biotin-ε-lysine) by biotinidase leads to the formation of a biotinyl–thioester intermediate (cysteine-bound biotin) at or near the active site of biotinidase (25–27). In the next step, the biotinyl moiety is transferred from the thioester to the ε-amino group of lysine in histones. Biocytin is generated in the breakdown of biotin-dependent carboxylases, which contain biotin linked to the ε-amino group of a lysine moiety (28,29).

Biotinidase belongs to the nitrilase superfamily of enzymes, which consists of 12 families of amidases, *N*-acyltransferases, and nitrilases (30). Some members of the nitrilase superfamily (vanins-1, -2, and -3) share significant sequence similarities with biotinidase (31); it is unknown whether vanins use histones as acceptor molecules in transferase reactions. Biotinidase is ubiquitous in mammalian cells and 26% of the cellular biotinidase activity is located in the nuclear fraction (28). Human biotinidase has been characterized at the gene level (32,33). The 5′-flanking region of exon 1 contains a CCAAT element, three initiator sequences, an octamer sequence, three methylation consensus sites, two GC boxes, and one HNF-5 site, but has no TATA element (33). The 62 amino acid region that harbors the active site of biotinidase is highly conserved among various mammals and *Drosophila* (34).

Subsequent to the elucidation of the biotinidase-mediated mechanism of histone biotinylation in vitro (25,26), biotinylated histones H1, H2A, H2B, H3, and H4 were detected in human peripheral blood mononuclear cells in vivo (35). Biotinylated histones were also detected in human lymphoma cells (36), small cell lung cancer cells (37), choriocarcinoma cells (38), and chicken erythrocytes (39). These studies also suggested that biotinidase may not be the only enzyme mediating histone biotinylation. For example, evidence was provided that biotinylation of histones increases in response to cell proliferation, whereas biotinidase activity was similar in nuclei from proliferating cells and quiescent controls (35). Finally, Narang et al. identified holocarboxylase synthetase (HCS) as another enzyme that may catalyze biotinylation of histones (40).

Mechanisms mediating debiotinylation of histones are largely unknown. Recent studies suggested that biotinidase may catalyze both biotinylation and debiotinylation of histones (41). Variables such as the microenvironment in chromatin and posttranslational modifications and alternate splicing of biotinidase might determine whether biotinidase acts as biotinyl histone transferase or histone debiotinylase. This assumption is based on the following lines of reasoning. First, the availability of substrate might favor either biotinylation or debiotinylation of histones. For example, locally high concentrations of biocytin might increase the rate of histone biotinylation in confined regions of chromatin. Note that the pH is unlikely to affect the biotinylation equilibrium, given that the pH optimum is similar (pH 8) for both the biotinylating activity (25) and the debiotinylating activity of biotinidase (41). Second, proteins may interact with biotinidase at the chromatin level, favoring either biotinylation or debiotinylation of histones. Third, three alternatively spliced variants of biotinidase have been identified (42). Theoretically, these variants may have unique functions in histone metabolism. Fourth, some variants of biotinidase are modified posttranslationally by glycosylation (32,42), potentially affecting enzymatic activity. An assay for analysis of histone debiotinylases is available (41).

Identification of Biotinylation Sites

Biotinylation sites in human histones were identified by using synthetic peptides (43,44). Briefly, this approach is based on the following analytical sequence: (i) short peptides (<20 amino acids in length) are synthesized chemically; the amino acid sequences in these peptides are based on the sequence in a given region of a given histone; (ii) peptides are incubated with biotinidase or HCS to conduct enzymatic biotinylation; (iii) peptides are resolved by electrophoresis; and (iv) biotin in peptides is probed using streptavidin peroxidase. Amino acid substitutions (e.g., lysine-to-alanine substitutions) and modifications (e.g., acetylation of lysines) in synthetic peptides can be used to corroborate identification of biotinylation sites and to investigate the cross talk between biotinylation and other known modifications of histones, respectively (43). Using this approach the following biotinylation sites have been identified in human histones: K9, K13, K125, K127, and K127 in histone H2A (45), K4, K9, and K18 in histone H3 (46), and K8 and K12 in histone H4 (43). Acetylation and phosphorylation of lysine and serine residues, respectively, decrease biotinylation of adjacent lysine residues (43,45,46). In contrast, dimethylation of arginine residues enhances biotinylation of adjacent lysine residues (45,46). This is consistent with studies suggesting that histones in livers from biotin-deficient rats showed unusual patterns of phosphorylation, methylation, and acetylation compared with biotin-sufficient controls (47).

Biological Functions of Histone Biotinylation

Biotinylation of histones is a relatively new field of research; evidence of biological roles for biotinylation of histones is scarce. However, biotinylation of histones appears to participate in the following biological processes.

First, evidence was provided that biotinylation of histones increases in response to cell proliferation in human peripheral blood mononuclear cells (35). Biotinylation of histones increases early in the cell cycle (G1 phase) and remains increased during later phases (S, G2, and M phases) compared with quiescent controls; the increase is greater than fourfold. Fibroblasts from patients with HCS deficiency are severely deficient in histone biotinylation (40). It remains to be determined whether this is associated with decreased proliferation rates. Note that these early studies were conducted before specific biotinylation sites in histones were identified and before biotinylation site-specific antibodies became available. Subsequent studies used site-specific antibodies to demonstrate that biotinylation of K8 and K12 in histone H4 increases in M phase of the cell cycle compared with G1 phase in human small cell lung cancer cells (48).

Second, studies in chicken erythrocytes have provided circumstantial evidence that biotinylated histones are enriched in transcriptionally silent chromatin (39). These studies have recently been expanded by using chromatin immunoprecipitation (ChIP) assays (49) in combination with antibodies to K8-biotinylated and K12-biotinylated histone H4. These studies provided evidence that biotinylated histone H4 is associated with heterochromatin in pericentromeric regions and inactive euchromatin (49a).

Third, biotinylation of histones might play a role in the cellular response to DNA damage (39,50). If formation of thymine dimers is caused by exposure of lymphoid cells to UV light, the global biotinylation of histones increases (39). If double-stranded DNA breaks are caused by exposure of lymphoid and choriocarcinoma cells to etoposide, biotinylation of K12 in histone H4 shows a rapid and transient decrease (50). This is consistent with a role for histone biotinylation in signaling DNA damage. These studies suggest that distinct kinds of DNA damage cause unique changes in histone biotinylation. Currently, it is unknown whether biotinylation of histones is a mechanism leading to DNA repair or apoptosis.

Biotin Supply

Effects of biotin supply on biotinylation of histones have been investigated in various human-derived cell lines (36–38). In these studies cell lines were cultured in media containing deficient, physiological, and pharmacological concentrations of biotin for several weeks. Biotin concentrations in culture media had only a moderate impact on biotinylation of histones; in contrast, biotinylation of carboxylases correlated strongly with biotin concentrations in culture media (36–38). The reader should note that even small changes in biotinylation of histones might be physiologically meaningful, given that these changes might affect other modifications of histones such as acetylation and methylation. Consistent with this hypothesis, evidence has been provided that biotin deficiency is associated with decreased rates of DNA repair by nonhomologous endjoining (49b).

Niacin and Chromatin Structure

Dietary niacin can be consumed in the form of tryptophan (converted at low efficiency), niacin (nicotinic acid), and nicotinamide (see Figure 6.3). Niacin exerts its impact on cellular functions through the formation of the pyridine nucleotides, NAD and NADP, which exist in oxidized and reduced forms. Although these molecules are critical to the redox reactions present in essentially all metabolic pathways, there are a large number of nonredox roles for niacin. Most of these make use of NAD^+ as a substrate, and belong to the ADP-ribosylation class of reactions. These include mono- and poly(ADP-ribosyl)ation, cyclic ADP-ribose formation, and NAD-dependent deacetylation reactions.

Mono(ADP-ribosyl)ation reactions are posttranslational modifications of proteins, in many cases GTP-binding proteins, with a wide variety of poorly understood metabolic roles. Cyclic ADP-ribose regulates intracellular calcium signaling. Although these two may impact on chromatin structure through cell-signaling events, little is known in this area at present, and this chapter concentrates on the effects of poly(ADP-ribosyl)ation and deacetylase activities.

Poly(ADP-ribosyl)ation and PARP-1

The human disease of niacin deficiency, pellagra, is characterized by sun sensitivity, which is suggestive of problems in DNA repair and genomic stability. The connection between niacin and sun sensitivity was illuminated by the discovery that NAD is required for the synthesis of poly(ADP-ribose) by the enzyme poly(ADP-ribose) polymerase-1 (PARP-1) (see Figure 6.5). Poly(ADP-ribose) is a anionic chain of ADP-ribose units synthesized on protein acceptors using NAD^+ as a substrate. PARP-1 is a zinc-finger protein that binds to strand breaks in DNA. This binding causes catalytic activation, leading to the synthesis of poly(ADP-ribose) on a variety of nuclear proteins. The predominant acceptor is PARP-1 itself, in a reaction referred to as automodification (51). Many other proteins are covalently modified by PARP-1, including histone H1, core histones, high-mobility group proteins, and protamines (52). Poly(ADP-ribose) is highly negatively charged, and modified proteins tend to lose affinity for DNA. Due to charge repulsion, automodified PARP-1 eventually dissociates from DNA strand breaks, allowing repair to proceed (53). Similarly, histones modified with poly(ADP-ribose) dissociate from DNA and the local chromatin structure becomes more relaxed (52). Catalytically active PARP-1 can cause complete dissociation of the nucleosome structure through covalent modification of histones H1, H2A and HB, H3 and H3d, H4, and H5 (52). In vivo experiments show that H1 and H2B are the predominant substrates. In vivo, active turnover of poly(ADP-ribose) by a specific glycohydrolase generates shorter chains on acceptor proteins and causes a proportionate shift toward histone modification. Thus, the early understanding of the role of PARP-1 in chromatin structure followed this picture; DNA damage leads to strand breaks through the action of base excision repair; strand breaks lead to PARP-1 binding and catalytic activation, causing poly(ADP-ribosyl) ation of PARP-1, histones, and high-mobility group proteins. The relaxation of chromatin occurs in a localized fashion around strand breaks, and this relaxation allows for proper access by DNA polymerase and other repair proteins. Automodified PARP-1 then dissociates from strand breaks, allowing completion of repair and the removal of poly(ADP-ribose) from substrates via glycohydrolase activity (52). Although some simplified in vitro systems have questioned aspects of this process, they have not always represented the appropriate level of chromatin structure to be valid models for eukaryotic nuclear processes (53).

This early model remains valid, but appears to represent the tip of the iceberg with respect to ADP-ribosylation reactions in chromatin. In addition to acting as acceptor proteins for covalent addition of poly(ADP-ribose), histones also have noncovalent poly(ADP-ribose)-binding sites.

These sites have very high-affinity binding, resisting dissociation by salts, detergents, and acids. The C-terminus of H1 and the N-termini of H3 and H4 were found to be the sites of noncovalent poly(ADP-ribose)-binding, and these are also the tail regions involved in DNA condensation (54). Thus, PARP-1 enzymes, automodified with long chains of poly(ADP-ribose), draw nearby histones out of the chromatin structure by noncovalent binding, leading to local chromatin relaxation. The histones return when the polymer is degraded by glycohydrolase activity, generating a process referred to as histone shuttling (54). Covalent and noncovalent effects of poly(ADP-ribosyl)ation on histones are thought to be important in the accurate repair of DNA damage and prevention of recombination events at sites of injury. Although the removal of histones and relaxation of the chromatin should allow the access of repair enzymes to the site of damage, this relaxed state associated with strand breaks also encourages nonhomologous recombination events, potentially leading to chromosomal translocations that are known to play an important role in carcinogenesis. The cloud of negatively charged poly(ADP-ribose) at these sites is thought to fulfill a second purpose of repelling other strands of DNA, thereby discouraging recombination events.

DNA strand breaks and chromatin remodeling may also take place as an intentional process in the absence of exogenous DNA damaging agents. One example of this occurs in the development of mammalian sperm. During spermatogenesis, an extremely compact form of chromatin develops because of the progressive replacement of histones by transitional proteins, and eventually protamines. Just before this exchange of chromatin-binding proteins, there is an appearance of DNA strand breaks and active synthesis of poly(ADP-ribose), presumably by both PARP-1 and PARP-2, which are both activated by DNA ends (55).

Another example of PARP-1 controlling chromatin structure in the absence of obvious DNA damage is seen in the puffing of polytene chromosomes in fruit flies. Following stresses such as heat shock, there are rapid increases in the expression of certain mRNA species, like certain heat shock proteins. The transcription of these genes requires local decondensation of the giant polytene chromosomes, and these areas are seen as distinct puffs by microscopy. It was recently shown that PARP-1 accumulates rapidly at these puff loci and is required for the decondensation of chromatin and subsequent changes in gene expression (56). It is not known if this is organized by strand breaks or if this mechanism acts in other types and species of chromosomes.

In a similar finding, Cohen-Armon et al. showed that PARP-1 is required in *Aplysia* for the formation of long-term memory. These nematodes undergo well-established learning patterns related to feeding and stress avoidance. PARP-1 was activated during these learning processes, and long-term memory was blocked by PARP inhibition (57). The mechanism may be similar to the puff loci, in that PARP-1 appears to facilitate the formation of new mRNA and proteins, enabling shifts in gene expression. Strand breaks did not appear to be a key component of the response.

The previous two examples suggest that PARP-1 activity modifies chromatin structure in the absence of strand breaks, and this has now been demonstrated. In addition to the zinc-finger structures that bind DNA strand breaks, PARP-1 contains further DNA-binding domains, which bind to non-B structures like hairpins, cruciforms, and stably unpaired regions. This type of binding, in the absence of strand breaks, causes catalytic activation of PARP-1, leading to PARP-1 automodification and histone poly(ADP-ribosyl)ation (58). This opens the potential role of PARP-1 in chromatin structure regulation to all cellular processes, not just those following DNA damage.

PARP-1 also participates directly in chromatin structure by a mechanism that is actually disrupted by poly(ADP-ribose) formation. Nonmodified PARP-1 competes with histone H1 binding to linker DNA. The binding of PARP-1 between nucleosomes increases the repeat length and sedimentation constant, generating a compact form of chromatin that is likely to be transcriptionally repressed (59). Increasing NAD^+ leads to automodification of PARP-1 and its release from chromatin, providing a mechanism for integration of energy metabolism, chromatin structure, and gene expression.

PARP-1 also communicates laterally with other epigenetic pathways. DNA methyltransferase 1 (DNMT1) adds methyl groups to cytosine residues in promoter regions of DNA, regulating gene expression (see later section of this chapter). DNMT1 has a high-affinity binding site for poly(ADP-ribosyl)ated PARP-1. This binding inactivates DNMT1 in vitro, and PARP-1 activity was shown to be a negative regulator of DNA methylation in cultured cells (60).

Additional PARP Enzymes

Reports that PARP-null mice still synthesize small amounts of poly(ADP-ribose) (61) have been validated by the discovery of five other poly(ADP-ribose)-synthesizing enzymes, including two other nuclear enzymes involved in excision repair (PARP-2, PARP-3) (62,63), a vault-associated protein (VPARP) (64), and two telomere-associated proteins (tankyrase-1 and tankyrase-2) (65). Analysis of genome sequences reveals 12 additional genes with the consensus sequence for PARP activity (66). PARP-2 has been found to be similar to PARP-1 in function; both are catalytically activated by DNA damage, heterodimerize, and interact with other DNA repair proteins like XRCC1 (67). Disruption of *PARP-1* or *PARP-2* genes causes genomic instability, whereas a double knockout causes embryonic lethality (68). PARP-1 and PARP-2 may have similar roles in the regulation of chromatin structure.

Tankyrase-1 binds TRF1, which is a negative regulator of telomerase. Tankyrase-1 synthesizes poly(ADP-ribose) on TRF1, and the electrostatic repulsion forces it to be released from its binding at the telomere, which allows telomerase to access and elongate the end of the chromosome (69). Tankyrase-2 shares 85% amino acid identity with tankyrase-1, has a similar subcellular distribution, and also interacts with TRF1 (70). Thus, the tankyrases have a similar action on TRF1 to that of PARP-1 and histones, and appear important in the regulation of chromatin structure within the telomeric regions. This is an emerging field, and the impact of poly(ADP-ribose) synthesis by tankyrases on telomeric stability will likely be a focus of future research. There is also evidence from yeast studies that Sir2 localizes to the telomere, and may interact with tankyrases in the regulation of telomeric chromatin structure (see later).

The function of VPARP, and vault particles in general, is poorly understood. Vault particles are cytosolic barrel-like structures that appear to have a storage function. Although VPARP is found mainly in the cytosol, associated with vault particles, PARP-1, tankyrase-1, and VPARP have also been found to localize to centromeres or spindle apparatus during mitosis (64,71,72), and there may be a coordinated role for poly(ADP-ribose) synthesis in the regulation of the cell cycle and segregation of chromosomes. The remaining 12 gene products containing the consensus sequence for PARP activity may add several additional components to the already complex model of poly(ADP-ribose) and chromatin structure.

To summarize the interrelationship between poly(ADP-ribose) metabolism and chromatin structure, it is obvious that the dominant physical characteristic of this polymer is its similarity to DNA. The majority of polymer synthesis takes place in the nucleus, and it is a highly anionic structure that competes with many DNA-binding sites on proteins, or forces acceptor proteins away from DNA by electrostatic repulsion. By using NAD as a substrate, these reactions also represent a connection between nuclear regulation and the energy status of the cell. With the potential for 18 different poly(ADP-ribosyl)ating enzymes in human cells, it is apparent that many regulatory processes are using this mechanism, and we anticipate a variety of new research findings in this area.

Sirtuin Family of Deacetylases

An additional role for NAD in the regulation of chromatin structure is through the action of the sirtuins, which act as NAD-dependent protein deacetylases (73). Acetyl groups are added to lysine residues in histones, neutralizing charge and decreasing DNA histone interaction. This leads to a more open chromatin structure and increased gene expression. Deacetylation leads to a more compact chromatin structure and gene silencing. It also appears to protect sensitive areas of chromatin, like telomeres (74), against translocation events and to play a role in extended life span associated with caloric restriction (75). Inhibitors of the deacetylation enzymes are being developed for cancer therapy and are presumably active against cancer cells by the derepression of gene expression favoring cell differentiation and apoptosis (76).

The activity of sirtuins, like Sir2 in yeast or SIRT1 in mammalian cells (family of seven members), is actually an ADP-ribosylation reaction. The acetyl group is transferred from the lysine residue of a histone, to the ADP-ribose portion of NAD^+, forming *O*-acetyl-ADP-ribose, in a reaction driven by the release of energy associated with nicotinamide cleavage. In fact, many sirtuins mono(ADP-ribosyl)ate themselves or related proteins as an alternate reaction. Interest in this area expanded with the recent finding that Sir2 activity was the critical factor in the life span induction caused by calorie restriction in budding yeast. The end result of enhanced Sir2 activity was an improvement in genomic stability, which limited the age-related accumulation of extrachromosomal rDNA circles (75). Although mammalian cells do not suffer from rDNA accumulation, similar forces are involved in genomic instability at both levels of nuclear organization, and it appears that the mammalian sirtuins play similar roles. A major focus of the yeast longevity work has been to define the mechanisms by which caloric restriction is coupled to Sir2 activity and longevity. Sir2 activity is closely tied to the energy status of the cell; it uses NAD^+ as a substrate, and is inhibited by nicotinamide and NADH. Lin et al. provide evidence that decreased NADH levels are the physiological triggers connecting caloric restriction to enhanced Sir2 activity and longevity (77). This is a critical concept to explore in higher models, as caloric restriction has extended life span in all animal models in which it has been tested. A pharmacological approach to the same pathway could have a large impact on chronic diseases related to genomic instability. Along this line of thought, chemical activators of sirtuins, such as resveratrol, have been identified. Resveratrol is a polyphenol found in red grape juice and wine, which extends life span in *Caenorhabditis elegans* and *Drosophila melanogaster* (78). The effect of resveratrol is dependent on Sir2 activity and is not additive with caloric restriction, providing a strong proof of principle for sirtuins and aging. Increased sirtuin activity has also been shown to protect neurons from the type of degeneration seen in Alzheimer's and Parkinson's diseases (79), but it must be remembered that sirtuins are involved in the deacetylation of a variety of proteins other than histones, including p53, a major regulator of cell survival and apoptosis (80).

Dietary Niacin Status and Chromatin Structure

There has not been any direct work on niacin status and chromatin structure in whole animal models. However, niacin deficiency and pharmacological supplementation have been shown to dramatically alter poly(ADP-ribose) levels in rat bone marrow cells, and to have a significant impact on genomic stability (81–83). DNA damage-induced poly(ADP-ribose) levels in rat bone marrow vary from 10 to 600 pmol/million cells, depending on dietary niacin status (81,82). Although chromatin structure has not been directly measured under these conditions, it seems likely that the local relaxation around strand breaks will differ. The end result of chromosomal instability during niacin deficiency is evidenced by increased levels of sister chromatid exchanges, chromosomal aberrations, DNA strand breaks, and enhanced leukemogenesis (discussed in more detail in Chapter 6).

PARP has a relatively high K_m for NAD^+ (84), and a loss of PARP activity appears to occur at stages of NAD depletion (e.g., 50% of control NAD^+ in cultured cells) (85), which do not affect basic redox reactions and energy metabolism, as judged by cell division (11). In vitro, tankyrase-1 is responsive to NAD concentrations through the physiological range, producing larger-sized poly(ADP-ribose) as the NAD concentration is increased (65). The K_m for NAD^+ of SIRT1 is reported to be over 500 μM (86), putting this enzyme in an affinity range that would be sensitive to dietary niacin status. Conversely, mitochondria are very efficient in sequestering NAD, and enzymes in redox metabolism may have higher affinities for NAD than do ADP-ribosylation enzymes. In this fashion, cells could maintain critical energy metabolism during niacin deficiency, while allowing the ADP-ribosylation reactions (which consume NAD) to fail.

In summary, niacin-dependent cofactors play a major role in the regulation of chromatin structure and genomic stability through a wide variety of ADP-ribosylation reactions, with many more appearing to be on the verge of discovery. In addition to acting as the substrate for these reactions, NAD cofactors reflect the energy status of the cell and provide a link between DNA damage events and chromatin structure. Deregulation of these mechanisms will have an impact on carcinogenesis and aging, as discussed in more detail in Chapter 6.

Modification of Chromatin by Methylation

In 1948, Rollin Hotchkiss was the first to detect 5-methylcytosine (5mC) in mammalian DNA (87). By 1954, it was already known that 5mC was not randomly distributed in DNA and that the only dinucleotide with significant 5mC content was 5mC,G (88,89). Once it was shown that cytosine residues were enzymatically methylated after incorporation into DNA, the basis for the field of epigenetics was established (90,91). Epigenetic determinants can be defined as meiotically and mitotically heritable modulators of gene regulation that are not encoded in the primary DNA sequence. Postreplicative methylation of cytosine residues in DNA fits this definition. More recently, methylation of histones has also been shown to play a major role in epigenetic regulation of gene expression, but is yet to be established as meiotically heritable.

DNA methylation and histone methylation are inextricably associated with diet since several vitamins function as cofactors and substrates in the synthesis of *S*-adenosylmethionine (AdoMet or SAM), the predominant methyl donor used by cellular methyltransferases (MTases) (92). AdoMet is generated when methionine is adenylated by methionine adenosyltransferase (MAT, EC 2.5.1.6, Figure 16.2). Methionine required for AdoMet formation can be generated through two interrelated pathways. In one, homocysteine:methionine synthase (MTR, also known as methionine synthase (MS), EC 2.1.1.13) uses the methyl group from 5-methyltetrahydrofolate (methyl-THF) to produce AdoMet. In the other, homocytseine is methylated by betaine–homocysteine *S*-methyltransferase (BHMT, EC 2.1.1.5) to generate AdoMet (Figure 16.2). The charged sulfur atom in AdoMet reduces the thermodynamic barrier for transfer of the methyl group to RNA, DNA, proteins, and phospholipids, subsequently regulating a wide range of cellular functions (93–95). AdoMet can also serve as a donor of its decarboxylated aminopropyl moiety for polyamine synthesis (96). Thus, it is important to recognize that although disruptions in AdoMet metabolism may play a critical role in altering epigenetic marks, a decrease in AdoMet availability could profoundly impact a variety of cellular functions through nonepigenetic pathways.

Specific nutrients that function to regulate the supply of cellular AdoMet include folic acid, cobalamin (vitamin B_{12}), pyridoxine (vitamin B_6), methionine, and choline (also referred to as lipotropes) (97). Dietary betaine also serves as an important source of methyl groups for humans (98). Riboflavin (vitamin B_2) and zinc (Zn^{2+}) are additional key dietary factors involved in one-carbon metabolism. The steps at which these nutrients function in one-carbon metabolism through the folate cycle are indicated in Figure 16.2.

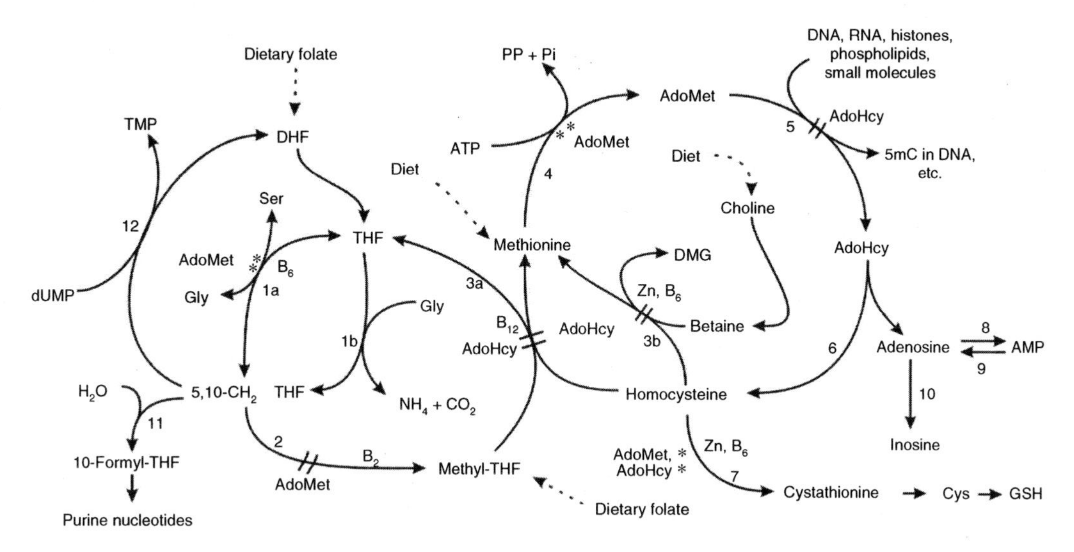

FIGURE 16.2 Methyl metabolism. Dietary factors, enzymes, and substrates involved in methyl metabolism. Enzymes in methyl metabolism identified by number: 1a, glycine hydroxymethyltransferase (GHMT); 1b, serine transhydroxymethylase; 2, methylenetetrahydrofolate reductase (MTHFR); 3a, 5-methyltetrahydrofolate:homocysteine *S*-methyltransferase (methionine synthase or MS); 3b, betaine–homocysteine *S*-methyltransferase (BHMT); 4, methionine adenosyltransferase (MAT); 5, various methyltransferases, including DNA methyltransferase (DNMT); 6, *S*-adenosylhomocysteine hydrolase (SAHH); 7, cystathionine-β-synthase (CBS); 8, adenosine kinase (AK); 9, 5-nucleotidase (5-NT); 10, adenosine deaminase (ADA); 11, methylenetetrahydrofolate cyclohydrolase; 12, thymidylate synthetase (TS). Abbreviations: DHF = dihydrofolate; Ser = serine; Gly = glycine; Cys = cysteine; THF = tetrahydrofolate; B_6 = vitamin B_6; B_{12} = vitamin B_{12} or cobalamin; B_2 = vitamin B_2 or riboflavin; 5,10-CH_2 THF = 5,10-methylenetetrahydrofolate; methyl-THF = 5-methyltetrahydrofolate; Zn = zinc; DMG = dimethylglycine; AdoMet = *S*-adenosylmethionine; AdoHcy = *S*-adenosylhomocysteine; GSH = glutathione (reduced); ATP = adenosine triphosphate; Pi = inorganic phosphate; PP = pyropyrophosphate; TMP = thymidine monophosphate; dUMP = deoxyuridylate monophosphate; AMP = adenosine monophosphate; // = inhibits; * * = activates.

Since acute deficiencies of these nutrients are no longer prevalent in populations residing in modernized countries, interest has shifted to defining the health consequences of suboptimal intakes of nutrients that influence epigenetic events associated with aging or relevant to development of cancer or other diseases. However, the contribution of suboptimal intakes of specific vitamins to altered cellular DNA or histone methylation status is not completely understood at the present time.

DNA methylation of cytosine residues contributes to chromatin structure, but the sequence of events and the specific mechanisms by which DNA methylation status controls chromatin structure also remain to be clarified. For example, it has been shown that methyl-CpG-binding proteins, such as the MeCP1 complex and the MeCP2 protein, bind specifically to methylated CpG sequences and promote transcription repression (99–101). Transcription factors, including AP-2, c-Myc, CREB, E2F, and NF-κB, which recognize and bind to GC-rich regulatory sequences exhibit impaired binding to methylated DNA elements within their corresponding recognition sequences (102,103). Increased DNA methylation has also been shown to follow transcriptional silencing (104), and a loss of DNA methylation can follow transcriptional activation (105). Additionally, DNA methylation has been shown to trigger methylation of lysine 9 (K9) in the N terminus of histone H3 (H3) (106). The H3-K9 epigenetic mark is associated with transcriptionally silent chromatin (107). An extensive literature based on findings from multiple independent observations has led to the recognition that methylation of cytosine residues in DNA plays a role in regulating the association of a variety of proteins with a localized region of DNA and serves as a regulatory component in the complex process of gene expression. However, it has been noted that DNA methylation does not appear to be involved in gene silencing in insects and other invertebrates whereas histone methylation "has an evolutionarily conserved role in gene silencing" (108). Thus, it would not be surprising to find that in some cases posttranslational modification of histones determines whether DNA methylation occurs, whereas in others DNA methylation is a leading event that stimulates chromatin remodeling or is even sufficient to maintain gene silencing in the absence of histone methylation.

Overview of Mammalian DNA Methylation

Epigenetic modifications associated with DNA methylation tend to be stable and heritable in somatic cells, but exhibit plasticity associated with temporal growth stages. The most dramatic epigenetic changes occur during gametogenesis proceeding through conception into early embryonic development where an initial genome-wide loss of methylation is followed by reestablishment of DNA methylation patterns (97,109,110). Aging is also marked by a gradual, genome-wide decrease in DNA methylation, yet is accompanied by an increase in de novo methylation that can silence expression of specific genes (111,112).

Alterations in DNA methylation are observed in numerous pathological conditions ranging from cancer (113) to atherosclerosis (114) and are investigated as possible contributors to human behavioral disorders such as schizophrenia and autism (115). Chronic inflammation has also been associated with alterations in DNA methylation patterns (116,117). Both loss of methylation and gain of methylation play a role. Loss of methylation is one of the earliest events in the linear progression model of familial adenomatous polyposis coli and appears to be linked with loss of imprinting of IGF2 (118). However, there is also ample evidence of silencing of tumor suppressor genes due to hypermethylation as the disease progresses (119). Although more investigation is needed to discern whether changes in DNA methylation in some of these diseases are the result of the pathological process and play a causal role in their development, it is clear that DNA methylation is essential in mammals and that alterations in DNA methylation patterns, promoting alterations in chromatin structure, accompany disease progression (95).

The addition of a methyl group at the 5-carbon position of cytosine ($C \rightarrow 5$ mC) is the only enzymatically mediated covalent modification of genomic DNA in mammalian cells (103). Methylation of cytosine occurs predominantly at C residues $5'$ to guanosine (G) in the DNA sequence ($5'$-CG-$3'$) in the CpG dinucleotide site, which is recognized as a methylation target by all known catalytically active mammalian DNA methyltransferases (DNMTs). Approximately 70% of C residues within the CpG dinucleotide context are methylated in mammalian cells (120–122). Since CpG dinucleotides are observed at ~20%–25% of the expected frequency in bulk DNA (123–125), it has been postulated that deamination of 5mC→T has resulted in a high frequency of mutation at these sites. C residues within genomic regions exhibiting a relative paucity of CpGs are normally heavily methylated, and are primarily localized within repetitive DNA elements, parasitic DNA, and pericentromeric regions (126–128). On the other hand, CpG islands (CGIs), currently defined as discrete regions within bulk DNA that exhibit a $C+G$ content of $>55\%$ and have a length >200 base pairs, remain relatively unmethylated (125,129–131). Many CGIs are localized in the promoter region of transcribed genes where they function to regulate gene expression (129,132). In summary, CpG methylation influences critical cellular events inclusive of transcription regulation, genomic stability, differential maintenance of the density of chromatin structure, X chromosome inactivation, and the silencing of parasite DNA elements (122).

DNA Methyltransferases

DNMTs catalyze the transfer of a methyl group from the universal donor, AdoMet, to carbon 5 of the cytosine moiety within DNA. In the process of methyl group transfer, the target C residue is flipped out of the DNA double-helix structure for the covalent modification (133). Mammalian DNMTs include DNMT1, DNMT2, DNMT3a, DNMT3b, and DNMT3L. However, only DNMT1, DNMT3a, and DNMT3b have been shown to exhibit significant catalytic activity (DNMT, EC 2.1.1.37). Reviews of the structures and functions of DNMTs provide more detailed information than that presented herein (97,122,134,135). DNMT1 is considered a maintenance MTase, because it exhibits 5- to >100-fold preference for hemi-methylated DNA substrates over unmethylated DNA (97,136). Hemi-methylated DNA is generated during cell division, where the original template DNA strand retains the 5mC epigenetic mark, but the newly synthesized daughter strand does not bear this epigenetic modification until methylated by DNMT1 to maintain the preexisting methylation patterns. DNMT1 is a component of the multiprotein DNA replication complex and appears to complete the task concurrently with DNA synthesis (137). In general, in vitro studies show that DNMT3a and DNMT3b exhibit little or no preference for hemi-methylated versus fully unmethylated sites; in vitro they exhibit catalytic efficiencies at least one log lower than that of DNMT1 toward hemi-methylated sites. DNMT3a and DNMT3b are de novo MTases in vivo. They play a key role in establishing new DNA methylation patterns (138,139), although with different specificity. DNMT3a, in concert with the catalytically inactive DNMT3L, is critical in establishing imprinting (140). Although both DNMT3a and DNMT3b can methylate C residues that are in CpA and CpT sites, a recent study presented convincing data that 15%–20% of cytosine methylation in embryonal stem cells occurs in non-CpG sites. In contrast, non-CpG methylation was negligible in somatic tissues (141).

Both DNMT3a and DNMT3b can methylate pericentric major satellite repeats and DNMT3b appears to be a major regulator of genomic stability. There is also evidence that DNMT3b is involved in maintenance methylation (142,143). Although the mechanisms regulating the specificity of the DNMTs are still under active investigation, it has been shown that, unlike DNMT1, flanking sequences of up to ± 4 base pairs surrounding the CpG target influence the catalytic activity of DNMT3a and DNMT3b (144) (Farrell and Christman, unpublished data). In addition, short, double-stranded RNA can induce DNA methylation (145).

Mammalian DNMTs function as components within large multiprotein complexes associated with chromatin. For example, DNMT1, DNMT3a, and DNMT3b have been observed to bind directly to histone deacetylases (HDACs) and repress gene expression (122). DNMTs, histone methytransferases (SUV39H1), HDAC1, HDAC2, individual 5mC-binding proteins (MBD1, MBD2, MBD3, MBD4, MeCP2, KAISO) or 5mC-binding protein complexes (MeCP1), and heterochromatin-binding protein (HP1) interact with methylated DNA. Many of these proteins are observed to colocalize in chromatin regions within the cell and to directly interact with each other by yeast two-hybrid assays and coimmunoprecipitation (101,146–148). Thus, a complex network of connections between DNMTs and a wide range of chromatin-associated proteins contribute to epigenetic signaling through DNA methylation.

Role of Folate in Regulation of Nucleic Acid Stability

Dietary folate is a critical component in maintaining chromatin stability, because it is essential for both AdoMet synthesis and de novo synthesis of purines required for synthesis of DNA and RNA (97,149,150). However, folate, choline, and methionine can compensate for each other in the event of a deficiency of one of these nutrients (151). During the course of one-carbon metabolism, a carbon unit from either serine or glycine is transferred to tetrahydrofolate (THF) to generate 5,10-methylenetetrahydrofolate (5,10-CH_2 THF).

The latter compound is used in the synthesis of thymidine, the rate-limiting step in DNA synthesis (152). Insufficient thymidine pools that can result from vitamin deficiencies promote incorporation of uracil into DNA contributing to a futile cycle of removal of the misincorporated base followed by reintroduction of uracil back into DNA (153). This futile cycle contributes to DNA strand breaks that can lead to irreparable DNA damage and hypomethylation of DNA (154). 5,10-CH_2 THF can be converted to 10-formyl-THF for de novo synthesis of purines used in the synthesis of DNA and RNA. Finally, 5,10-CH_2 THF can be reduced to methyl-THF, by methylenetetrahydrofolate reductase (MTHFR, EC 1.5.1.20), to serve as the methyl donor for the reaction that methylates homocysteine to form methionine in the cyclic pathway that synthesizes AdoMet.

Methyl transfer from AdoMet releases *S*-adenosylhomocysteine (AdoHyc), which acts as a competitive inhibitor of most MTases (97,155). Therefore, cellular homocysteine and AdoHyc levels are tightly regulated through multiple cellular processes. *S*-adenosylhomocysteine hydrolase (SAHH, EC 3.3.1.1) catalyzes a reversible reaction that converts AdoHyc to adenosine and homocysteine. Although the formation of AdoHyc is favored, four additional metabolic pathways limit AdoHyc formation. One of these pathways converts adenosine to inosine. Another pathway, catalyzed by the cystathionine-β-synthase enzyme (CBS, EC 4.2.1.22), condenses serine with homocysteine to form cystathionine. Two additional pathways regenerate methionine either by adding a methyl group to homocysteine by MTR or by using the BHMT enzyme pathway. Limiting levels of folate and vitamin B_{12} can interfere with methionine synthesis via the MTR enzyme. Vitamin B_6 serves as a cofactor for both the CBS and BHMT enzymes that function to reduce cellular homocysteine levels.

Nutrient Intake, DNA Methylation Status, and Disease Risk

For humans, the primary dietary sources of methyl groups include methionine (~10 mmol of methyl/day), folate (~5–10 mmol of methyl/day), and choline (~30 mmol of methyl/day) (151). The tight association of these three sources of methyl-donor groups within the one-carbon metabolic pathway necessitates that all three be assessed when studying dietary influence of DNA methylation status. Unfortunately, no published human studies that correlate the combined intake of all three with DNA methylation status are available. However, some human studies showing that folate status does influence DNA methylation have been completed. Serum folate levels have been reported to be inversely associated with plasma homocysteine levels and DNA hypomethylation status of colonic mucosa, although disease outcome was not reported (156). It has also been found that an experimentally induced, low-folate diet promoted a global decrease in DNA methylation in leukocytes from 20 to 30 year old women (157). Thus, it is reasonable to conclude that deficiencies of other vitamins known to function in the one-carbon metabolic pathway could influence the status of DNA.

Human epidemiological studies also offer indirect evidence that vitamin intakes may influence DNA methylation status changes associated with chronic disease. The association between dietary insufficiency of nutrients that regulate one-carbon metabolism and disorders such as colon cancer, cardiovascular disease, depression and other psychiatric disorders, birth defects, and diabetes has been reviewed (97,158–165). However, direct studies linking the intake of nutrients that are sources of methyl groups with DNA methylation status and disease risk are needed to clarify the role of dietary effects on DNA methylation as a factor determining disease risk.

For example, despite the need for adequate folate consumption, recent animal studies have led to recommendations for caution in recommending population-wide folic acid fortification (166). A study conducted by Song et al. (167) showed that folate supplementation inhibited ileal adenoma formation in mice harboring the $Apc^{Min/+}$ mutation during a 3 month time frame. However, in the mice treated with supplemental folate for 6 months, this protective effect was no longer observed. In fact, at 6 months the $Apc^{Min/+}$ mice receiving the folate-deficient diet exhibited the lowest number of ileal adenomas. These studies suggest that folate deficiency inhibits tumor progression in individuals harboring premalignant lesions, whereas folate supplementation promotes tumor progression. However, there are several caveats regarding comparison of the effects of lowering the level of DNMT1 by knockout and lowering it by feeding folate- or folate- and choline-deficient diets. Simple lowering the level of DNMT1 does not have a direct effect on the availability of AdoMet for methylation of other proteins or RNA or synthesis of polyamines. This may account for the fact that reviews of human epidemiological data only support an inverse association or no significant difference between folate intake and risk of colorectal and other cancers.

Another emerging concern among epidemiologists is that nutrient consumption during midlife, the age of most epidemiological study populations, may not have the same health protective effects that would be conferred from this intake behavior if it occurred during critical growth periods of the in utero stages through childhood (168–170). It has been proposed that nutritional deprivation during the formative growth stages of human life may preset metabolic processes that will persist through adulthood even if nutritional intakes are adequate during the adult stage of life. This concern has been strengthened by the results from investigations using animal models to demonstrate the influence of nutritional exposure on patterns of DNA methylation and subsequent, life-long gene expression. A review of both human epidemiological data and animal model data suggest the relative risk of adult-onset chronic disease can be increased by prenatal and early life growth responses to nutrition (166). Waterland and Jirtle have demonstrated that the methylation status of an intracisternal A particle (IAP) retrotransposon within the promoter of the *agouti* (*A*) allele of mice renders expression of the gene (A^{vy}) responsive to the effects of maternal nutrition during fetal growth. CpG methylation in the IAP varies greatly among A^{vy} mice. Hypomethylation of the IAP in A^{vy} animals allows maximal production of yellow phaelomelanin in hair follicles leading to a yellow coat, whereas hypermethylation leads to A^{vy} gene silencing and a psuedoagouti (brown) coat. Variation in the extent of methylation generally results in a wide variety of individual coat color, adiposity, glucose tolerance, and tumor susceptibility in A^{vy}/a(nonagouti-loss of function) mice. However, supplementation of a/a dams with the dietary methyl donors of folic acid, vitamin B_{12}, choline, and betaine promotes an increase of genomic methylation within the A^{vy} gene promoter of their pups, contributing to shift in coat color of the pups from yellow to brown. Previously, it had been shown that yellow-phenotype dams, possessing an A^{vy} allele, produced yellow-coated and mottled pups but no pseudoagouti offspring (171). The phenotype of the sires possessing an A^{vy} allele exhibited no influence on progeny coat color. Although these studies may not have direct implications for human health, they do demonstrate that (i) DNA methylation on maternal chromosomes is not completely erased during oogenesis and can be passed to progeny and (ii) that nutritional exposure early in life can establish stable epigenetic modifications that regulate gene expression during adulthood.

It has long been recognized that single-carbon metabolism is adversely affected by alcohol consumption (172). Chronic overconsumption of alcohol is frequently associated with poor food intake, and additionally, can cause malabsorption of nutrients leading to deficiencies. Therefore, it is not surprising that the combination of a low-folate intake coupled with high alcohol consumption has been linked with an increased risk of chronic disease, particularly cancer (173–177). It was also observed that an inverse relationship between folate intake and colon cancer risk was most pronounced in smokers, whereas, caffeine intake had no effect on the relative risk of colon cancer (178). More recent data continue to identify individuals who smoke or consume higher amounts of alcohol to be at risk for chronic disease formation, which is believed to be partially due to a depletion of lipotropes (179).

Germ-line polymorphisms within genes, which generate proteins functioning within the one-carbon metabolic pathways, add another complicating layer to the influence of vitamin intake on DNA methylation status. For instance, a 677C→T polymorphism in the MTHFR enzyme has been shown to impair DNA methylation in women subjected to inadequate folate intakes (157). It is uncertain how this 677C→T polymorphism may impact the long-term health status of the U.S. population following mandated folic acid fortification of grain products since 1998 (180). Quite possibly, the observation of frank folate deficiencies may be confined predominantly to smokers and to individuals who abuse alcohol.

Rodents have been used to study the effects of dietary lipotrope deficiencies on DNA methylation status. However, a complicating factor is that these nutrients are synthesized by the intestinal flora (181). Antibiotics can be administered to ablate the intestinal flora, but it is uncertain if the study results are entirely due to the target nutrient deficiency or to an interaction of the nutrient deficiency in combination with health consequences associated with altered intestinal physiology created by antibiotic therapy. As reviewed in Dizik et al. (182), lipotrope-deficient diets synergize with chemical carcinogens to promote tumors in rats and mice. Furthermore, prolonged intake of diets lacking methionine, choline, vitamin B_{12}, and folic acid is sufficient to induce hepatocellular carcinoma in rats, and rats subjected to methyl-deficient diets exhibit hypomethylation of DNA as early as 7 days (183). Thus, hypomethylation of hepatic tissue DNA precedes hepatocellular carcinoma in these rats. In addition, it was observed that mRNA levels of protooncogenes were elevated within rats subjected to methyl-deficient diets (184). On refeeding of an adequate diet for 1–3 weeks, hemi-methylated sites resulting from replication of DNA in the absence of sufficient AdoMet were remethylated and the levels of mRNA of selected genes were restored to levels exhibited by rats fed a normal diet. However, hypomethylated sites within the *c-myc*, *c-fos*, and *c-Ha-ras* genes were observed to persist for at least 1 year of refeeding with adequate dietary sources of methyl groups. These studies open the possibility that intermittent or long-term exposure to inadequate dietary sources of methyl-donor groups may result in heritable epigenetic changes within growth regulatory genes, which renders cells more permissive of hyperplasia and tumorigenesis.

Methylation of Histones

The role of AdoMet depletion or AdoHcy accumulation in inhibition of histone methylation was recognized over 30 years ago, but is now receiving greater attention because of the demonstrated importance of this modification in regulating chromatin structure (97,185). Although the effects of dietary folate deprivation remain to be investigated, it has been found that 36 weeks of feeding a low-methionine diet lacking choline, vitamin B_{12}, and folic acid not only induced loss of DNA methylation but led to a decrease in H4-K20 trimethylation, H3-K9 trimethylation, and a gradual decrease in expression of both Suv4–20h2 and Suv39h1 histone methyltransferase (HMT) accompanying preneoplastic changes. Widespread reduction in DNA methylation coupled with reduced histone methylation would be predicted to lead to aberrant activation of genes normally silenced in hepatocytes as well as protooncogenes and endogenous retroposons. Interestingly, with a longer course of methyl deprivation expression of Suv39h1 HMT and histone H3-K9 methylation increased in neoplastic nodules and tumors (186). Since H3-K9 is predominantly localized to centromeric and telomeric regions of the chromosomes, these changes could contribute to chromosomal instability and activation of telomerase leading to tumor progression.

CONCLUSION

It is now well established that chemical modifications of DNA and DNA-binding proteins alter the structure of chromatin without altering the nucleotide sequence of DNA. Some of these modifications are associated with heritable changes in gene function, genomic stability, and DNA repair. There is growing evidence that a number of vitamins and other dietary components play an essential role in establishing and maintaining epigenetic regulation of chromatin structure and gene expression. First, biotinylation of histones has the potential to regulate gene silencing, cell proliferation, and cellular response to DNA damage. Second, poly(ADP-ribosyl)ation of histones plays several roles in DNA repair and apoptotic events in response to DNA damage. Third, folate-dependent production of AdoMet is required for both DNA- and histone-mediated gene silencing. In addition, although not a focus of this chapter, vitamin B_{12}, B_6, and riboflavin all contribute to the synthesis of AdoMet and regulation of AdoHcy levels. These findings are consistent with roles for vitamins that go far beyond their classical roles as coenzymes or antioxidants. We are just beginning to understand how vitamin metabolism interfaces with epigenetics. Future studies are likely to find many new roles for vitamins and are likely to unravel the true magnitude of vitamin-driven events regulating chromatin structure and DNA repair.

ACKNOWLEDGMENTS

This work was supported by NIH grants DK063945, 1U54CA100926, NSF EPSCoR grant EPS-0346476, USDA grant 2006-35200-01540, the Leukemia Research Foundation, and DAMD 17-02-10505. Previous funding from the American Institute for Cancer Research for studies on diet and DNA methylation are gratefully acknowledged. The work of J. Kirkland on niacin has been supported by NSERC, NCIC, and CRS. Thanks to Megan Kirkland for the drawing of Figure 16.1.

REFERENCES

1. A. Wolffe. *Chromatin*, 3rd edn. San Diego, CA: Academic Press, 1998.
2. M.A. Gorovsky. Macro- and micronuclei of *Tetrahymena pyriformis*: a model system for studying the structure of eukaryotic nuclei. *J. Protozool.*, 20:19–25, 1973.
3. D.J. Mathis, P. Oudet, B. Waslyk, and P. Chambon. Effect of histone acetylation on structure and in vitro transcription of chromatin. *Nucleic Acids Res.*, 5:3523–3547, 1978.
4. J.E. Brownell, J. Zhou, T. Ranalli, R. Kobayashi, D.G. Edmondson, S.Y. Roth, and C.D. Allis. *Tetrahymena* histone acetyltransferase A: a homolog to yeast Gcn5p linking histone acetylation to gene activation. *Cell*, 84:843–851, 1996.
5. J. Taunton, C.A. Hassig, and S.L. Schreiber. A mammalian histone deacetylase related to a yeast transcriptional regulator Rpd3. *Science*, 272:408–411, 1996.
6. T. Jenuwein and C.D. Allis. Translating the histone code. *Science*, 293:1074–1080, 2001.
7. A.-D. Pham and F. Sauer. Ubiquitin-activating/conjugating activity of TAFII250, a mediator of activation of gene expression in *Drosophila*. *Science*, 289:2357–2360, 2000.
8. P. Cheung, C.D. Allis, and P. Sassone-Corsi. Signaling to chromatin through histone modifications. *Cell*, 103:263–271, 2000.
9. A.L. Clayton and L.C. Mahadevan. MAP kinase-mediated phosphoacetylation of histone H3 and inducible gene regulation. *FEBS Lett.*, 546:51–58, 2003.
10. H. Juarez-Salinas, J.L. Sims, and M.K. Jacobson. Poly(ADP-ribose) levels in carcinogen-treated cells. *Nature*, 282:740–741, 1979.
11. B.W. Durkacz, O. Omidiji, D.A. Gray, and S. Shall. (ADP-ribose)$_n$ participates in DNA excision repair. *Nature*, 283:593–596, 1980.
12. T. Boulikas, B. Bastin, P. Boulikas, and G. Dupuis. Increase in histone poly(ADP-ribosylation) in mitogen-activated lymphoid cells. *Exp. Cell Res.*, 187:77–84, 1990.
13. F. Althaus. Poly ADP-ribosylation: a histone shuttle mechanism in DNA excision repair. *J. Cell Sci.*, 102:663–670, 1992.

14. Y.S. Yoon, J.W. Kim, K.W. Kang, Y.S. Kim, K.H. Choi, and C.O. Joe. Poly(ADP-ribosyl)ation of histone H1 correlates with internucleosomal DNA fragmentation during apoptosis. *J. Biol. Chem.*, 271:9129–9134, 1996.
15. A.W. Bird, D.Y. Yu, M.G. Pray-Grant, Q. Qiu, K.E. Harmon, P.C. Megee, P.A. Grant, M.M. Smith, and M.F. Christman. Acetylation of histone H4 by Esa1 is required for DNA double-strand break repair. *Nature*, 419:411–415, 2002.
16. J. Ausio, and K.E. van Holde. Histone hyperacetylation: its effect on nucleosome conformation and stability. *Biochemistry*, 25:1421–1428, 1986.
17. T.R. Hebbes, A.W. Thorne, and C. Crane-Robinson. A direct link between core histone acetylation and transcriptionally active chromatin. *EMBO J.*, 7:1395–1402, 1988.
18. D.Y. Lee, J.J. Hayes, D. Pruss, and A.P. Wolffe. A positive role for histone acetylation in transcription factor access to nucleosomal DNA. *Cell*, 72:73–84, 1993.
19. P. Chambon, J.D. Weill, J. Doly, M.T. Strosser, and P. Mandel. On the formation of a novel adenylic compound by enzymatic extracts of liver nuclei. *Biochem. Biophys. Res. Commun.*, 25:638–643, 1966.
20. T. Boulikas. At least 60 ADP-ribosylated variant histones are present in nuclei from dimethylsulfate-treated and untreated cells. *EMBO J.*, 7:57–67, 1988.
21. V. Laudet and H. Gronemeyer. *The Nuclear Receptor Facts Book*. San Diego, CA: Academic Press, 2002.
22. W. Fischle, Y. Wang, and C.D. Allis. Histone and chromatin cross-talk. *Curr. Opin. Cell Biol.*, 15:172–183, 2003.
23. B.D. Strahl and C.D. Allis. The language of covalent histone modifications. *Nature*, 403:41–45, 2000.
24. B.M. Turner. Histone acetylation and epigenetic code. *Bioessays*, 22:836–845, 2000.
25. J. Hymes, K. Fleischhauer, and B. Wolf. Biotinylation of histones by human serum biotinidase: assessment of biotinyl-transferase activity in sera from normal individuals and children with biotinidase deficiency. *Biochem. Mol. Med.*, 56:76–83, 1995.
26. J. Hymes and B. Wolf. Human biotinidase isn't just for recycling biotin. *J. Nutr.*, 129:485S–489S, 1999.
27. R. Rodriguez-Melendez, and J. Zempleni. Regulation of gene expression by biotin. *J. Nutr. Biochem.*, 14:680–690, 2003.
28. J. Pispa. Animal biotinidase. *Ann. Med. Exp. Biol. Fenn.*, 43:4–39, 1965.
29. B. Wolf and G.S. Heard. Biotinidase deficiency. In: L. Barness and F. Oski, eds. *Advances in Pediatrics*. Chicago, I.L.: Medical Book Publishers, 1991:1–21.
30. C. Brenner. Catalysis in the nitrilase superfamily. *Curr. Opin. Struct. Biol.*, 12:775–782, 2002.
31. B. Maras, D. Barra, S. Dupre, and G. Pitari. Is pantetheinase the actual identity of mouse and human vanin-1 proteins. *FEBS Lett.*, 461:149–152, 1999.
32. H. Cole, T.R. Reynolds, J.M. Lockyer, G.A. Buck, T. Denson, J.E. Spence, J. Hymes, and B. Wolf. Human serum biotinidase cDNA cloning, sequence, and characterization. *J. Biol. Chem.*, 269:6566–6570, 1994.
33. H. Cole Knight, T.R. Reynolds, G.A. Meyers, R.J. Pomponio, G.A. Buck, and B. Wolf. Structure of the human biotinidase gene. *Mamm. Genome*, 9:327–330, 1998.
34. K.L. Swango and B. Wolf. Conservation of biotinidase in mammals and identification of the putative biotinidase gene in *Drosophila melanogaster*. *Mol. Genet. Metab.*, 74:492–499, 2001.
35. J.S. Stanley, J.B. Griffin, and J. Zempleni. Biotinylation of histones in human cells: effects of cell proliferation. *Eur. J. Biochem.*, 268:5424–5429, 2001.
36. K.C. Manthey, J.B. Griffin, and J. Zempleni. Biotin supply affects expression of biotin transporters, biotinylation of carboxylases, and metabolism of interleukin-2 in Jurkat cells. *J. Nutr.*, 132:887–892, 2002.
37. S.B. Scheerger and J. Zempleni. Expression of oncogenes depends on biotin in human small cell lung cancer cells NCI-H69. *Int. J. Vitam. Nutr. Res.*, 73:461–467, 2003.
38. S.E.R.H. Crisp, G. Camporeale, B.R. White, C.F. Toombs, J.B. Griffin, H.M. Said, and J. Zempleni. Biotin supply affects rates of cell proliferation, biotinylation of carboxylases and histones, and expression of the gene encoding the sodium-dependent multivitamin transporter in JAr choriocarcinoma cells. *Eur. J. Nutr.*, 43:23–31, 2004.
39. D.M. Peters, J.B. Griffin, J.S. Stanley, M.M. Beck, and J. Zempleni. Exposure to U.V. light causes increased biotinylation of histones in Jurkat cells. *Am. J. Physiol. Cell Physiol.*, 283:C878–C884, 2002.

40. M.A. Narang, R. Dumas, L.M. Ayer, and R.A. Gravel. Reduced histone biotinylation in multiple carboxylase deficiency patients: a nuclear role for holocarboxylase synthetase. *Hum. Mol. Genet.*, 13:15–23, 2004.
41. T.D. Ballard, J. Wolff, J.B. Griffin, J.S. Stanley, Sv. Calcar, and J. Zempleni. Biotinidase catalyzes debiotinylation of histones. *Eur. J. Nutr.*, 41:78–84, 2002.
42. C.M. Stanley, J. Hymes, and B. Wolf. Identification of alternatively spliced human biotinidase mRNAs and putative localization of endogenous biotinidase. *Mol. Genet. Metab.*, 81:300–312, 2004.
43. G. Camporeale, E.E. Shubert, G. Sarath, R. Cerny, and J. Zempleni. K8 and K12 are biotinylated in human histone H4. *Eur. J. Biochem.*, 271:2257–2263, 2004.
44. G. Camporeale, Y.C. Chew, A. Kueh, G. Sarath, and J. Zempleni. Use of synthetic peptides for identifying biotinylation sites in human histones. In: R.J. McMahon, ed. *Avidin-Biotin Technology in the Life Sciences*. Totowa, NJ: Humana Press, 2005.
45. Y.C. Chew, G. Camporeale, N. Kothapalli, G. Sarath, and J. Zempleni. Lysine residues in N- and C-terminal regions of human histone H2A are targets for biotinylation by biotinidase. *J. Nutr. Biochem.*, 17:225–233, 2006.
46. K. Kobza, G. Camporeale, B. Rueckert, A. Kueh, J.B. Griffin, G. Sarath, and J. Zempleni. K4, K9, and K18 in human histone H3 are targets for biotinylation by biotinidase. *FEBS J.*, 272:4249–4259, 2005.
47. F. Petrelli, S. Coderoni, P. Moretti, and M. Paparelli. Effect of biotin on phosphorylation, acetylation, methylation of rat liver histones. *Mol. Biol. Rep.*, 4:87–92, 1978.
48. N. Kothapalli and J. Zempleni. Biotinylation of histones depends on the cell cycle in NCI-H69 small cell lung cancer cells. *FASEB J.*, 19:A55, 2005.
49. A.M. Oommen, J.B. Griffin, G. Sarath, and J. Zempleni. Roles for nutrients in epigenetic events. *J. Nutr. Biochem.*, 16:74–77, 2005.
49a. G. Camporeale, A.M. Oommen, J.B. Griffin, G. Sarath, and J. Zempleni. K12-biotinylated histone H4 marks heterochromatin in human lymphoblastoma Cells. *J. Nutr. Biochem.*, (in press).
49b. N. Kothapalli, G. Sarath, and J. Zempleni. Biotinylation of K12 in histone H4 decreases in response to DNA double strand breaks in human JAr choriocarcinoma cells. *J. Nutr.*, 135:2337–2342, 2005.
50. N. Kothapalli and J. Zempleni. Double strand breaks of DNA decrease biotinylation of lysine-12 in histone H4 in JAr cells. *FASEB J.*, 18:A103–A104, 2004.
51. D. Lautier, J. Lagueux, J. Thibodeau, L. Menard, and G.G. Poirier. Molecular and biochemical features of poly (ADP-ribose) metabolism. *Mol. Cell. Biochem.*, 122:171–193, 1993.
52. D. D'Amours, S. Desnoyers, I. D'Silva, and G.G. Poirier. Poly(ADP-ribosyl)ation reactions in the regulation of nuclear functions. *Biochem. J.*, 342 (Pt 2):249–268, 1999.
53. M.S. Satoh, G.G. Poirier, and T. Lindahl. NAD(+)-dependent repair of damaged DNA by human cell extracts. *J. Biol. Chem.*, 268:5480–5487, 1993.
54. F.R. Althaus, S. Bachmann, L. Hofferer, H.E. Kleczkowska, M. Malanga, P.L. Panzeter, C. Realini, and B. Zweifel. Interactions of poly(ADP-ribose) with nuclear proteins. *Biochimie*, 77:423–432, 1995.
55. M.L. Meyer-Ficca, H. Scherthan, A. Burkle, and R.G. Meyer. Poly(ADP-ribosyl)ation during chromatin remodeling steps in rat spermiogenesis. *Chromosoma*, 114:67–74, 2005.
56. A. Tulin and A. Spradling. Chromatin loosening by poly(ADP)-ribose polymerase (PARP) at Drosophila puff loci. *Science*, 299:560–562, 2003.
57. M. Cohen-Armon, L. Visochek, A. Katzoff, D. Levitan, A.J. Susswein, R. Klein, M. Valbrun, and J.H. Schwartz. Long-term memory requires polyADP-ribosylation. *Science*, 304:1820–1822, 2004.
58. I. Lonskaya, V.N. Potaman, L.S. Shlyakhtenko, E.A. Oussatcheva, Y.L. Lyubchenko, and V.A. Soldatenkov. Regulation of poly(ADP-ribose) polymerase-1 by DNA structure-specific binding. *J. Biol. Chem.*, 280:17076–17083, 2005.
59. M.Y. Kim, S. Mauro, N. Gevry, J.T. Lis, and W.L. Kraus. NAD+-dependent modulation of chromatin structure and transcription by nucleosome binding properties of PARP-1. *Cell*, 119:803–814, 2004.
60. A. Reale, G.D. Matteis, G. Galleazzi, M. Zampieri, and P. Caiafa. Modulation of DNMT1 activity by ADP-ribose polymers. *Oncogene*, 24:13–19, 2005.
61. W.M. Shieh, J.C. Ame, M.V. Wilson, Z.Q. Wang, D.W. Koh, M.K. Jacobson, and E.L. Jacobson. Poly(ADP-ribose) polymerase null mouse cells synthesize ADP-ribose polymers. *J. Biol. Chem.*, 273:30069–30072, 1998.

62. J.C. Ame, V. Rolli, V. Schreiber, C. Niedergang, F. Apiou, P. Decker, S. Muller, T. Hoger, J. Menissier-de Murcia, and G. de Murcia. PARP-2, a novel mammalian DNA damage-dependent poly(ADP-ribose) polymerase. *J. Biol. Chem.*, 274:17860–17868, 1999.
63. M. Johansson. A human poly(ADP-ribose) polymerase gene family (ADPRTL): cDNA cloning of two novel poly(ADP-ribose) polymerase homologues. *Genomics*, 57:442–445, 1999.
64. V.A. Kickhoefer, A.C. Siva, N.L. Kedersha, E.M. Inman, C. Ruland, M. Streuli, and L.H. Rome. The 193-kD vault protein, VPARP, is a novel poly(ADP-ribose) polymerase. *J. Cell Biol.*, 146:917–928, 1999.
65. S. Smith, I. Giriat, A. Schmitt, and T. de Lange. Tankyrase, a poly(ADP-ribose) polymerase at human telomeres. *Science*, 282:1484–1487, 1998.
66. J. Diefenbach and A. Burkle. Introduction to poly(ADP-ribose) metabolism. *Cell. Mol. Life Sci.*, 62:721–730, 2005.
67. V. Schreiber, J.C. Ame, P. Dolle, I. Schultz, B. Rinaldi, V. Fraulob, J. Menissier-de Murcia, and G. de Murcia. Poly(ADP-ribose) polymerase-2 (PARP-2) is required for efficient base excision DNA repair in association with PARP-1 and XRCC1. *J. Biol. Chem.*, 277:23028–23036, 2002.
68. J. Menissier-de Murcia, M. Ricoul, L. Tartier, C. Niedergang, A. Huber, F. Dantzer, V. Schreiber, J.C. Ame, A. Dierich, M. LeMeur, L. Sabatier, P. Chambon, and G. de Murcia. Functional interaction between PARP-1 and PARP-2 in chromosome stability and embryonic development in mouse. *EMBO J.*, 22:2255–2263, 2003.
69. S. Smith and T. de Lange. Tankyrase promotes telomere elongation in human cells. *Curr. Biol.*, 10:1299–1302, 2000.
70. P.G. Kaminker, S.H. Kim, R.D. Taylor, Y. Zebarjadian, W.D. Funk, G.B. Morin, P. Yaswen, and J. Campisi. TANK2, a new TRF1-associated poly(ADP-ribose) polymerase, causes rapid induction of cell death upon overexpression. *J. Biol. Chem.*, 276:35891–35899, 2001.
71. M. Kanai, M. Uchida, S. Hanai, N. Uematsu, K. Uchida, and M. Miwa. Poly(ADP-ribose) polymerase localizes to the centrosomes and chromosomes. *Biochem. Biophys. Res. Commun.*, 278:385–389, 2000.
72. S. Smith and T. de Lange. Cell cycle dependent localization of the telomeric PARP, tankyrase, to nuclear pore complexes and centrosomes. *J. Cell Sci.*, 112 (Pt 21):3649–3656, 1999.
73. J. Landry, A. Sutton, S.T. Tafrov, R.C. Heller, J. Stebbins, L. Pillus, and R. Sternglanz. The silencing protein SIR2 and its homologs are NAD-dependent protein deacetylases. *Proc. Natl. Acad. Sci., USA* 97:5807–5811, 2000.
74. N.C. Emre, K. Ingvarsdottir, A. Wyce, A. Wood, N.J. Krogan, K.W. Henry, K. Li, R. Marmorstein, J.F. Greenblatt, A. Shilatifard, and S.L. Berger. Maintenance of low histone ubiquitylation by Ubp10 correlates with telomere-proximal Sir2 association and gene silencing. *Mol. Cell*, 17:585–594, 2005.
75. J.M. Denu. Linking chromatin function with metabolic networks: Sir2 family of NAD(+)-dependent deacetylases. *Trends Biochem. Sci.*, 28:41–48, 2003.
76. S.Y. Roth, J.M. Denu, and C.D. Allis. Histone acetyltransferases. *Annu. Rev. Biochem.*, 70:81–120, 2001.
77. S.J. Lin, E. Ford, M. Haigis, G. Liszt, and L. Guarente. Calorie restriction extends yeast life span by lowering the level of NADH. *Genes Dev.*, 18:12–16, 2004.
78. J.G. Wood, B. Rogina, S. Lavu, K. Howitz, S.L. Helfand, M. Tatar, and D. Sinclair. Sirtuin activators mimic caloric restriction and delay ageing in metazoans. *Nature*, 430:686–689, 2004.
79. A. Bedalov and J.A. Simon. Neuroscience. NAD to the rescue. *Science*, 305:954–955, 2004.
80. H. Vaziri, S.K. Dessain, E. Ng Eaton, S.I. Imai, R.A. Frye, T.K. Pandita, L. Guarente, and R.A. Weinberg. hSIR2(SIRT1) functions as an NAD-dependent p53 deacetylase. *Cell*, 107:149–159, 2001.
81. A.C. Boyonoski, J.C. Spronck, L.M. Gallacher, R.M. Jacobs, G.M. Shah, G.G. Poirier, and J.B. Kirkland. Niacin deficiency decreases bone marrow poly(ADP-ribose) and the latency of ethylnitrosourea-induced carcinogenesis in rats. *J. Nutr.*, 132:108–114, 2002.
82. A.C. Boyonoski, J.C. Spronck, R.M. Jacobs, G.M. Shah, G.G. Poirier, and J.B. Kirkland. Pharmacological intakes of niacin increase bone marrow poly(ADP-ribose) and the latency of ethylnitrosourea-induced carcinogenesis in rats. *J. Nutr.*, 132:115–120, 2002.
83. J.C. Spronck and J.B. Kirkland. Niacin deficiency increases spontaneous and etoposide-induced chromosomal instability in rat bone marrow cells in vivo. *Mutat. Res.*, 508:83–97, 2002.
84. J.B. Kirkland and J.M. Rawling. Niacin. In: R.B. Rucker, W Suttie, D.B. McCormick, L.J. Machlin, eds. *Handbook of Vitamins*, 3rd edn. New York, NY: Marcel Dekker, Inc., 2001:211–252.

85. E.L. Jacobson, V. Nunbhakdi-Craig, D.G. Smith, H.Y. Chen, B.L. Wasson, and M.K. Jacobson. ADP-ribose polymer metabolism: implications for human nutrition. In: G.G. Poirier, P Moreau, eds. *ADP-Ribosylation Reactions*. New York, NY: Springer Verlag, Inc., 1992:153–162.
86. K.T. Howitz, K.J. Bitterman, H.Y. Cohen, D.W. Lamming, S. Lavu, J.G. Wood, R.E. Zipkin, P. Chung, A. Kisielewski, L.L. Zhang, B. Scherer, and D.A. Sinclair. Small molecule activators of sirtuins extend Saccharomyces cerevisiae lifespan. *Nature*, 425:191–196, 2003.
87. R.D. Hotchkiss. The quantitative separation of purines, pyrimidines, and nucleosides by paper chromatography. *J. Biol. Chem.*, 168:315–332, 1948.
88. E. Chargaff and C.F. Crampton. Separation of calf thymus deoxyribonucleic acid into fractions of different composition. *Nature*, 172:289–292, 1953.
89. R.L. Sinsheimer. The action of pancreatic desoxyribonuclease. I. Isolation of mono- and dinucleotides. *J. Biol. Chem.*, 208:445–459, 1954.
90. M. Gold and J. Hurwitz. The enzymatic methylation of the nucleic acids. *Cold Spring Harb. Symp. Quant. Biol.*, 28:149–156, 1963.
91. P.R. Srinivasan and E. Borek. Enzymatic alteration of nucleic acid structure. *Science*, 145:548–553, 1964.
92. E.B. Fauman and R.M. Blumenthal. Structure and evolution of AdoMet-dependent methyltransferases. In: X Cheng, R.M. Blumenthal, eds. *S-Adenosylmethionine-Dependent Methyltransferases: Structure and Function*. World Scientific Publishing, Hackensack, NJ, 1999.
93. E. Wainfan, M. Dizik, M. Hluboky, and M.E. Balis. Altered tRNA methylation in rats and mice fed lipotrope-deficient diets. *Carcinogenesis*, 7:473–476, 1986.
94. D. Tollervey. Small nucleolar RNAs guide ribosomal RNA methylation. *Science*, 273:1056–1057, 1996.
95. G. Egger, G. Liang, A. Aparicio, and P.A. Jones. Epigenetics in human disease and prospects for epigenetic therapy. *Nature*, 429:457–463, 2004.
96. A.E. Pegg, D.B. Jones, and J.A. Secrist, III. Effect of inhibitors of *S*-adenosylmethionine decarboxylase on polyamine content and growth of L1210 cells. *Biochemistry*, 27:1408–1415, 1988.
97. J.K. Christman. Diet, DNA methylation and cancer. In: J Zempleni, H Daniel, eds. *Molecular Nutrition*. Wallingford: CAB International, 2003:237–265.
98. S.A. Craig. Betaine in human nutrition. *Am. J. Clin. Nutr.*, 80:539–549, 2004.
99. P.L. Jones, G.J. Veenstra, P.A. Wade, D. Vermaak, S.U. Kass, N. Landsberger, J. Strouboulis, and A.P. Wolffe. Methylated DNA and MeCP2 recruit histone deacetylase to repress transcription. *Nat. Genet.*, 19:187–191, 1998.
100. X. Nan, H.H. Ng, C.A. Johnson, C.D. Laherty, B.M. Turner, R.N. Eisenman, and A. Bird. Transcriptional repression by the methyl-CpG-binding protein MeCP2 involves a histone deacetylase complex. *Nature*, 393:386–389, 1998.
101. S.G. Jin, C.L. Jiang, T. Rauch, H. Li, and G.P. Pfeifer. MBD3L2 interacts with MBD3 and components of the NuRD complex and can oppose MBD2-MeCP1-mediated methylation silencing. *J. Biol. Chem.*, 280:12700–12709, 2005.
102. P.H. Tate and A.P. Bird. Effects of DNA methylation on DNA-binding proteins and gene expression. *Curr. Opin. Genet. Dev.*, 3:226–231, 1993.
103. R. Singal and G.D. Ginder. DNA methylation. *Blood*, 93:4059–4070, 1999.
104. T. Enver, J.W. Zhang, T. Papayannopoulou, and G. Stamatoyannopoulos. DNA methylation: a secondary event in globin gene switching? *Genes Dev.*, 2:698–706, 1988.
105. C.H. Sullivan, J.T. Norman, T. Borras, and R.M. Grainger. Developmental regulation of hypomethylation of delta-crystallin genes in chicken embryo lens cells. *Mol. Cell. Biol.*, 9:3132–3135, 1989.
106. K.E. Bachman, B.H. Park, I. Rhee, H. Rajagopalan, J.G. Herman, S.B. Baylin, K.W. Kinzler, and B. Vogelstein. Histone modifications and silencing prior to DNA methylation of a tumor suppressor gene. *Cancer Cell*, 3:89–95, 2003.
107. S. Kubicek and T. Jenuwein. A crack in histone lysine methylation. *Cell*, 119:903–906, 2004.
108. M. Mandrioli and F. Borsatti. Histone methylation and DNA methylation: a missed pas de deux in invertebrates. *Invert. Surv. J.*, 2:159–161, 2005.
109. W. Mayer, A. Niveleau, J. Walter, R. Fundele, and T. Haaf. Demethylation of the zygotic paternal genome. *Nature*, 403:501–502, 2000.
110. H.D. Morgan, F. Santos, K. Green, W. Dean, and W. Reik. Epigenetic reprogramming in mammals. *Hum. Mol. Genet.*, 14 Spec No 1:R47–58, 2005.

111. J.P. Issa. Aging, DNA methylation and cancer. *Crit. Rev. Oncol. Hematol.*, 32:31–43, 1999.
112. L. Liu, R.C. Wylie, L.G. Andrews, and T.O. Tollefsbol. Aging, cancer and nutrition: the DNA methylation connection. *Mech. Ageing Dev.*, 124:989–998, 2003.
113. J.P. Issa. CpG island methylator phenotype in cancer. *Nat. Rev. Cancer*, 4:988–993, 2004.
114. S. Zaina, M.W. Lindholm, and G. Lund. Nutrition and aberrant DNA methylation patterns in atherosclerosis: more than just hyperhomocysteinemia? *J. Nutr.*, 135:5–8, 2005.
115. I.I. Gottesman, and D.R. Hanson. Human development: biological and genetic processes. *Annu. Rev. Psychol.*, 56:263–286, 2005.
116. J.P. Issa, N. Ahuja, M. Toyota, M.P. Bronner, and T.A. Brentnall. Accelerated age-related CpG island methylation in ulcerative colitis. *Cancer Res.*, 61:3573–3577, 2001.
117. T. Ushijima and E. Okochi-Takada. Aberrant methylations in cancer cells: where do they come from? *Cancer Sci.*, 96:206–211, 2005.
118. A.P. Feinberg, R. Ohlsson, and S. Henikoff. The epigenetic progenitor origin of human cancer. *Nat. Rev. Genet.*, 7:21–33, 2006.
119. E.R. Fearon and B. Vogelstein. A genetic model for colorectal tumorigenesis. *Cell*, 61:759–767, 1990.
120. A. Razin and A.D. Riggs. DNA methylation and gene function. *Science*, 210:604–610, 1980.
121. M. Ehrlich and R.Y. Wang. 5-Methylcytosine in eukaryotic DNA. *Science*, 212:1350–1357, 1981.
122. K.D. Robertson. DNA methylation and chromatin—unraveling the tangled web. *Oncogene*, 21:5361–5379, 2002.
123. M.N. Swartz, T.A. Trautner, and A. Kornberg. Enzymatic synthesis of deoxyribonucleic acid. XI. Further studies o.n. nearest neighbor base sequences in deoxyribonucleic acids. *J. Biol. Chem.*, 237:1961–1967, 1962.
124. G.J. Russell, P.M. Walker, R.A. Elton, and J.H. Subak-Sharpe. Doublet frequency analysis of fractionated vertebrate nuclear DNA. *J. Mol. Biol.*, 108:1–23, 1976.
125. A.P. Bird. CpG-rich islands and the function of DNA methylation. *Nature*, 321:209–213, 1986.
126. J.A. Yoder, C.P. Walsh, and T.H. Bestor. Cytosine methylation and the ecology of intragenomic parasites. *Trends Genet.*, 13:335–340, 1997.
127. A. Eden, F. Gaudet, A. Waghmare, and R. Jaenisch. Chromosomal instability and tumors promoted by DNA hypomethylation. *Science*, 300:455, 2003.
128. F. Gaudet, J.G. Hodgson, A. Eden, L. Jackson-Grusby, J. Dausman, J.W. Gray, H. Leonhardt, and R. Jaenisch. Induction of tumors in mice by genomic hypomethylation. *Science*, 300:489–492, 2003.
129. F. Antequera and A. Bird. Number of CpG islands and genes in human and mouse. *Proc. Natl. Acad. Sci., USA* 90:11995–11999, 1993.
130. S.H. Cross and A.P. Bird. CpG islands and genes. *Curr. Opin. Genet. Dev.*, 5:309–314, 1995.
131. D. Takai and P.A. Jones. Comprehensive analysis of CpG islands in human chromosomes 21 and 22. *Proc. Natl. Acad. Sci., USA* 99:3740–3745, 2002.
132. P.W. Laird. The power and the promise of DNA methylation markers. *Nat. Rev. Cancer*, 3:253–266, 2003.
133. S. Klimasauskas, S. Kumar, R.J. Roberts, and X. Cheng. HhaI methyltransferase flips its target base out of the DNA helix. *Cell*, 76:357–369, 1994.
134. A. Jeltsch. Beyond Watson and Crick: DNA methylation and molecular enzymology of DNA methyltransferases. *Chembiochem.*, 3:274–293, 2002.
135. A. Hermann, H. Gowher, and A. Jeltsch. Biochemistry and biology of mammalian DNA methyltransferases. *Cell. Mol. Life Sci.*, 61:2571–2587, 2004.
136. M. Okano, S. Xie, and E. Li. Cloning and characterization of a family of novel mammalian DNA (cytosine-5) methyltransferases. *Nat. Genet.*, 19:219–220, 1998.
137. P.M. Vertino, J.A. Sekowski, J.M. Coll, N. Applegren, S. Han, R.J. Hickey, and L.H. Malkas. DNMT1 is a component of a multiprotein DNA replication complex. *Cell Cycle*, 1:416–423, 2002.
138. C.L. Hsieh. In vivo activity of murine de novo methyltransferases, Dnmt3a and Dnmt3b. *Mol. Cell. Biol.*, 19:8211–8218, 1999.
139. I. Suetake, F. Shinozaki, J. Miyagawa, H. Takeshima, and S. Tajima. DNMT3L stimulates the DNA methylation activity of Dnmt3a and Dnmt3b through a direct interaction. *J. Biol. Chem.*, 279:27816–27823, 2004.
140. M. Kaneda, M. Okano, K. Hata, T. Sado, N. Tsujimoto, E. Li, and H. Sasaki. Essential role for de novo DNA methyltransferase Dnmt3a in paternal and maternal imprinting. *Nature*, 429:900–903, 2004.

141. B.H. Ramsahoye, D. Biniszkiewicz, F. Lyko, V. Clark, A.P. Bird, and R. Jaenisch. Non-CpG methylation is prevalent in embryonic stem cells and may be mediated by DNA methyltransferase 3a. *Proc. Natl. Acad. Sci., USA* 97:5237–5242, 2000.
142. J.E. Dodge, M. Okano, F. Dick, N. Tsujimoto, T. Chen, S. Wang, Y. Ueda, N. Dyson, and E. Li. Inactivation of Dnmt3b in mouse embryonic fibroblasts results in DNA hypomethylation, chromosomal instability, and spontaneous immortalization. *J. Biol. Chem.*, 280:17986–17991, 2005.
143. T. Chen, N. Tsujimoto, and E. Li. The PWWP domain of Dnmt3a and Dnmt3b is required for directing DNA methylation to the major satellite repeats at pericentric heterochromatin. *Mol. Cell. Biol.*, 24:9048–9058, 2004.
144. V. Handa and A. Jeltsch. Profound flanking sequence preference of Dnmt3a and Dnmt3b mammalian DNA methyltransferases shape the human epigenome. *J. Mol. Biol.*, 348:1103–1112, 2005.
145. H. Kawasaki and K. Taira. Transcriptional gene silencing by short interfering RNAs. *Curr. Opin. Mol. Ther.*, 7:125–131, 2005.
146. H.G. Yoon, D.W. Chan, A.B. Reynolds, J. Qin, and J. Wong. N-CoR mediates DNA methylation-dependent repression through a methyl CpG binding protein Kaiso. *Mol. Cell.*, 12:723–734, 2003.
147. A.P. Feinberg and B. Tycko. The history of cancer epigenetics. *Nat. Rev. Cancer*, 4:143–153, 2004.
148. J.M. Craig. Heterochromatin–many flavours, common themes. *Bioessays*, 27:17–28, 2005.
149. C.D. Davis and E.O. Uthus. DNA methylation, cancer susceptibility, and nutrient interactions. *Exp. Biol. Med.* (Maywood), 229:988–995, 2004.
150. Y.I. Kim. Folate and DNA methylation: a mechanistic link between folate deficiency and colorectal cancer? *Cancer Epidemiol. Biomarkers Prev.*, 13:511–519, 2004.
151. M.D. Niculescu and S.H. Zeisel. Diet, methyl donors and DNA methylation: interactions between dietary folate, methionine and choline. *J. Nutr.*, 132:2333S–2335S, 2002.
152. B.C. Blount, M.M. Mack, C.M. Wehr, J.T. MacGregor, R.A. Hiatt, G. Wang, S.N. Wickramasinghe, R.B. Everson, and B.N. Ames. Folate deficiency causes uracil misincorporation into human DNA and chromosome breakage: implications for cancer and neuronal damage. *Proc. Natl. Acad. Sci., USA* 94:3290–3295, 1997.
153. B.N. Ames and P. Wakimoto. Are vitamin and mineral deficiencies a major cancer risk? *Nat. Rev. Cancer*, 2:694–704, 2002.
154. B.M. Ryan and D.G. Weir. Relevance of folate metabolism in the pathogenesis of colorectal cancer. *J. Lab. Clin. Med.*, 138:164–176, 2001.
155. S.F. De Cabo, J. Santos, and J. Fernandez-Piqueras. Molecular and cytological evidence of *S*-adenosyl-L-homocysteine as an innocuous undermethylating agent in vivo. *Cytogenet. Cell Genet.*, 71:187–192, 1995.
156. M. Pufulete, R. Al-Ghnaniem, J.A. Rennie, P. Appleby, N. Harris, S. Gout, P.W. Emery, and T.A. Sanders. Influence of folate status on genomic DNA methylation in colonic mucosa of subjects without colorectal adenoma or cancer. *Br. J. Cancer*, 92:838–842, 2005.
157. K.P. Shelnutt, G.P. Kauwell, J.F. Gregory, III, D.R. Maneval, E.P. Quinlivan, D.W. Theriaque, G.N. Henderson, and L.B. Bailey. Methylenetetrahydrofolate reductase 677C→T polymorphism affects DNA methylation in response to controlled folate intake in young women. *J. Nutr. Biochem.*, 15:554–560, 2004.
158. E. Giovannucci and W.C. Willett. Dietary factors and risk of colon cancer. *Ann. Med.*, 26:443–452, 1994.
159. C.A. Garay and P.F. Engstrom. Chemoprevention of colorectal cancer: dietary and pharmacologic approaches. *Oncology* (Williston Park) 13:89–97; discussion 97–100, 105, 1999.
160. J.D. Potter. Colorectal cancer: molecules and populations. *J. Natl. Cancer Inst.*, 91:916–932, 1999.
161. C.A. Tomeo, G.A. Colditz, W.C. Willett, E. Giovannucci, E. Platz, B. Rockhill, H. Dart, and D.J. Hunter. Harvard Report on Cancer Prevention. Volume 3: prevention of colon cancer in the United States. *Cancer Causes Control*, 10:167–180, 1999.
162. C.S. Fuchs, W.C. Willett, G.A. Colditz, D.J. Hunter, M.J. Stampfer, F.E. Speizer, and E.L. Giovannucci. The influence of folate and multivitamin use on the familial risk of colon cancer in women. *Cancer Epidemiol. Biomarkers Prev.*, 11:227–234, 2002.
163. S. Maier and A. Olek. Diabetes: a candidate disease for efficient DNA methylation profiling. *J. Nutr.*, 132:2440S–2443S, 2002.

164. I.B. Van den Veyver. Genetic effects of methylation diets. *Annu. Rev. Nutr.*, 22:255–282, 2002.
165. M.A. Sanjoaquin, N. Allen, E. Couto, A.W. Roddam, and T.J. Key. Folate intake and colorectal cancer risk: a meta-analytical approach. *Int. J. Cancer*, 113:825–828, 2005.
166. R.A. Waterland and R.L. Jirtle. Transposable elements: targets for early nutritional effects on epigenetic gene regulation. *Mol. Cell. Biol.*, 23:5293–5300, 2003.
167. J. Song, A. Medline, J.B. Mason, S. Gallinger, and Y.I. Kim. Effects of dietary folate on intestinal tumorigenesis in the apcMin mouse. *Cancer Res.*, 60:5434–5440, 2000.
168. J.A. McKay, E.A. Williams, and J.C. Mathers. Folate and DNA methylation during in utero development and aging. *Biochem. Soc. Trans.*, 32:1006–1007, 2004.
169. K.B. Michels and W.C. Willett. Breast cancer—early life matters. *N. Engl. J. Med.*, 351:1679–1681, 2004.
170. W.C. Willett. Diet and cancer: an evolving picture. *JAMA*, 293:233–234, 2005.
171. H.D. Morgan, H.G. Sutherland, D.I. Martin, and E. Whitelaw. Epigenetic inheritance at the agouti locus in the mouse. *Nat. Genet.*, 23:314–318, 1999.
172. J.D. Finkelstein, J.P. Cello, and W.E. Kyle. Ethanol-induced changes in methionine metabolism in rat liver. *Biochem. Biophys. Res. Commun.*, 61:525–531, 1974.
173. R. Jiang, F.B. Hu, E.L. Giovannucci, E.B. Rimm, M.J. Stampfer, D. Spiegelman, B.A. Rosner, and W.C. Willett. Joint association of alcohol and folate intake with risk of major chronic disease in women. *Am. J. Epidemiol.*, 158:760–771, 2003.
174. E. Giovannucci. Alcohol, one-carbon metabolism, and colorectal cancer: recent insights from molecular studies. *J. Nutr.*, 134:2475S–2481S, 2004.
175. L.E. Kelemen, T.A. Sellers, R.A. Vierkant, L. Harnack, and J.R. Cerhan. Association of folate and alcohol with risk of ovarian cancer in a prospective study of postmenopausal women. *Cancer Causes Control*, 15:1085–1093, 2004.
176. S.C. Larsson, E. Giovannucci, and A. Wolk. Dietary folate intake and incidence of ovarian cancer: the Swedish Mammography Cohort. *J. Natl. Cancer Inst.*, 96:396–402, 2004.
177. T.A. Sellers, D.M. Grabrick, R.A. Vierkant, L. Harnack, J.E. Olson, C.M. Vachon, and J.R. Cerhan. Does folate intake decrease risk of postmenopausal breast cancer among women with a family history? *Cancer Causes Control*, 15:113–120, 2004.
178. S.C. Larsson, E. Giovannucci, and A. Wolk. A prospective study of dietary folate intake and risk of colorectal cancer: modification by caffeine intake and cigarette smoking. *Cancer Epidemiol. Biomarkers Prev.*, 14:740–743, 2005.
179. G. Poschl, F. Stickel, X.D. Wang, and H.K. Seitz. Alcohol and cancer: genetic and nutritional aspects. *Proc. Nutr. Soc.*, 63:65–71, 2004.
180. D.A. Kessler and D.E. Shalala. Food standards: amendment of standards of identity for enriched grain products to require addition of folic acid. *Fed. Regist.*, 61:8781–8797, 1996.
181. L.V. Hooper, T. Midtvedt, and J.I. Gordon. How host–microbial interactions shape the nutrient environment of the mammalian intestine. *Annu. Rev. Nutr.*, 22:283–307, 2002.
182. M. Dizik, J.K. Christman, and E. Wainfan. Alterations in expression and methylation of specific genes in livers of rats fed a cancer promoting methyl-deficient diet. *Carcinogenesis*, 12:1307–1312, 1991.
183. E. Wainfan, M. Dizik, M. Stender, and J.K. Christman. Rapid appearance of hypomethylated DNA in livers of rats fed cancer-promoting, methyl-deficient diets. *Cancer Res.*, 49:4094–4097, 1989.
184. J.K. Christman, G. Sheikhnejad, M. Dizik, S. Abileah, and E. Wainfan. Reversibility of changes in nucleic acid methylation and gene expression induced in rat liver by severe dietary methyl deficiency. *Carcinogenesis*, 14:551–557, 1993.
185. S. Huang. Histone methyltransferases, diet nutrients and tumour suppressors. *Nat. Rev. Cancer*, 2:469–476, 2002.
186. I.P. Pogribny, S.A. Ross, V.P. Tryndyak, M. Pogribna, L.A. Poirier, and T.V. Karpinets. Histone H3 lysine 9 and H4 lysine 20 trimethylation and the expression of Suv4-20h2 and Suv-39h1 histone methyltransferases in hepatocarcinogenesis induced by methyl deficiency in rats. *Carcinogenesis*, 27:1180–1186, 2006.

17 Accelerator Mass Spectrometry in the Study of Vitamins and Mineral Metabolism in Humans

Fabiana Fonseca de Moura, Betty Jane Burri, and Andrew J. Clifford

CONTENTS

HISTORICAL BACKGROUND

Accelerator mass spectrometry (AMS) harnesses the power of advanced nuclear instruments to solve important and heretofore unsolvable problems in human nutrition and metabolism. AMS methods are based on standard nuclear physics concepts. Isotopes of a given element differ from one another by the number of neutrons in their nucleus. Generally, the isotope with the lowest number of neutrons in its nucleus is the natural isotope (e.g., ^{1}H,^{12}C). Adding one neutron typically creates a stable isotope (e.g., ^{2}H,^{13}C), which is similar in most properties to the natural isotope, but differs in mass and can thus be separated and detected by mass spectrometry. Isotopes with even greater numbers of neutrons (e.g., ^{3}H,^{14}C) become unstable. An unstable nucleus such as ^{14}C has excess energy, which is released in the form of particles of radiation. These radioisotopes can also be detected by mass spectrometry, while more common and familiar instruments such as liquid scintillation and Geiger counters can detect their radioactive decay products.

The antecedents of AMS date back to the beginning of the nuclear era. In 1903, Marie Curie and her husband Pierre Curie established quantitative standards for measuring the rate of radioactive emission, and it was Marie Curie who found that there was a decrease in the rate of radioactive emissions over time (radioactive decay), which could be calculated and predicted.[1] In 1911, Ernest Rutherford bombarded atoms with α-rays and defined the structure of the atom.[2] By 1912, more than 30 radioactive species were known and current isotope terminology was introduced. The α-particle is a nucleus of the element helium, β-particles are electrons whereas γ-radiation is composed of electromagnetic rays (their names were intended to be temporary until better identification could be obtained). By 1921, several instruments had been constructed to determine the masses of isotopes and their relative proportions. These instruments evolved into what we now call mass spectrometers.

In the 1930s, J.D. Cockroft and E.T.S. Walton were the first to construct a true accelerator at the Cavendish Laboratory, at Cambridge, UK.[3] The Cockroft–Walton accelerator accelerated protons by driving off electrons from atoms. In this accelerator, hydrogen protons were generated by an electric discharge in hydrogen gas. The proton ions traveled inside an evacuated tube containing electrodes. Each time the ions oscillated from one electrode to the other, they accelerated; by the time the ions passed through the tube they were accelerated into a narrow bundle or beam of particles that could be separated and measured. This first accelerator generated a little over a million volts. Shortly thereafter, Robert J. Van de Graaff developed the eponymous generator, which uses static electricity to generate very high voltages. In this accelerator, a pulley-driven rubber belt moves at high speed to generate electricity. As the pulley rotates, the inside of the belt becomes negatively charged and the outside positive. The positive charges are then collected in an outer metal sphere. The Van de Graaff generators produced as much as 10 million volts.

In 1932, the most famous of all accelerators, the Ernest O. Lawrence cyclotron, was built at the Radiation Laboratory of the University of California at Berkeley.[4] In this accelerator the particle beams circled, allowing the particles to pass through the same electrodes many times. Between 1934 and 1939, a large number of radionuclides were produced, identified, and characterized by bombarding elements with every available particle in accelerating machines.

Cyclotrons could also in principle be used as extremely sensitive mass spectrometers, but it was not until 1977 that a cyclotron was used in this way for radiocarbon dating.[5] The cyclotron increased the sensitivity of radiocarbon dating dramatically because it allowed direct measurement of the actual mass of radioactive ^{14}C, instead of the typical methods, which only count radioactive decays. Mass spectrometry methods had also been suggested for the measurement of $^{14}C/^{12}C$ ratios for carbon dating, but had difficulties distinguishing between the ^{14}N and ^{14}C. To solve that problem, two research groups in 1977 proposed using a tandem Van de Graaff accelerator instead of a cyclotron for radiocarbon dating.[6,7] The Van de Graaff accelerator can discriminate between ^{14}N and ^{14}C and it is also capable of accelerating and separating all three carbon isotopes (^{12}C,^{13}C, and ^{14}C) simultaneously.[8] Nowadays, the Van de Graaff accelerator is the most commonly used accelerator for ^{14}C measurements.

In the early 1960s, before the advancement of AMS, there were ^{14}C measurements of human blood and tissues from individuals who were exposed to elevated atmospheric ^{14}C from nuclear weapons testing,[9,10] as well as ^{14}C studies of the metabolism of nutrients in hospitalized patients.[11,12] However, these studies had to use large amounts of ^{14}C capable of being detected by a liquid scintillation counter. The possibility of using AMS in biomedical research has been reported since 1978[13] and was reenforced in a review published in 1987.[14] However, it was not until the early 1990s that AMS began to be used regularly for biomedical and clinical applications.[15–19]

DESCRIPTION OF ACCELERATOR MASS SPECTROMETRY

A photo of the accelerator mass spectrometer at Lawrence Livermore National Laboratory (Livermore, CA, USA) used in our studies is shown in Figure 17.1. An accelerator mass spectrometer is a form of an isotope ratio spectrometer, ideal for measuring long-lived radioisotopes because it measures the actual mass rather than the radioactive decay. AMS separates and measures the individual atoms of isotopic species. AMS is an extremely sensitive technique, able to detect isotope concentrations to parts per quadrillion and quantify labeled elements to attomole levels in milligram-sized samples.[20]

Since AMS measures individual isotopomers, it is millions of times more sensitive than the more familiar methods of Geiger counting and liquid scintillation counting, which only measure radioactive decays. However, data from liquid scintillation counting and AMS can be linearly extrapolated and compared.[8,21] Radioisotope methods have inherent superiorities to stable and natural isotope methods. Specifically, the total radioisotope activity can be collected and measured, regardless of whether the compounds measured have been identified. This allows for the collection and measurement of all the metabolites, before they are identified. Stable isotope methods, in contrast, are difficult to use to identify metabolites, and in general can only be used to measure metabolites that have already been identified by other methods. A second advantage is that AMS is more sensitive than almost all stable isotope methods currently available; by using such small dosages, it allows researchers to conduct true-tracer studies. This is especially advantageous in nutrient metabolism research, where the observed behaviors in nutrient metabolism may depend on the size of the administered labeled dose.

The most common use of AMS in nutrition is to measure carbon or hydrogen isotopes, although calcium and aluminum have also been measured.[22–24] In this chapter, we illustrate the use of AMS for human metabolism research, using folic acid, vitamin A, β-carotene, and calcium as examples.

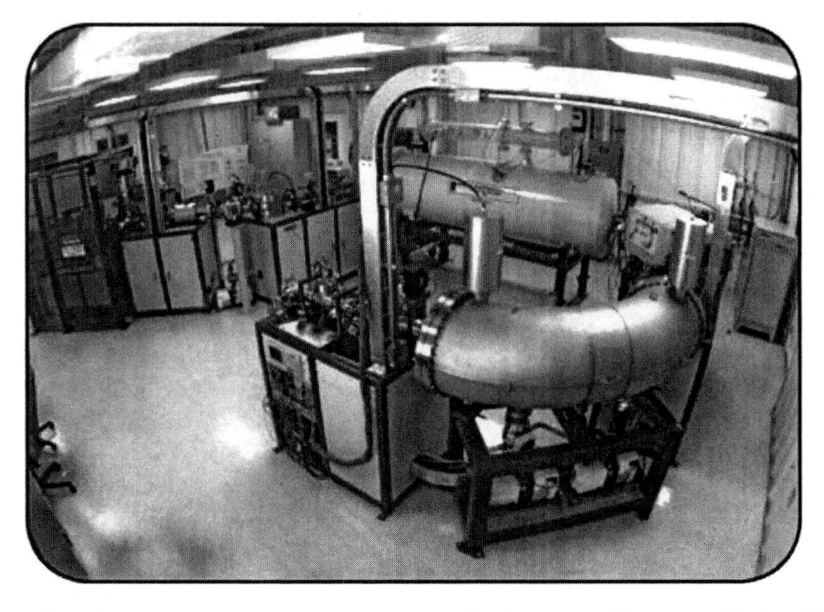

FIGURE 17.1 1 MV accelerator mass spectrometer at the Lawrence Livermore National Laboratory (LLNL). (From http://bioams.llnl.gov/equipment.php.)

ACCELERATOR MASS SPECTROMETRY METHOD

AMS methods require careful sample preparation. Before AMS measurement, the carbon of biological samples must be converted to graphite. The first method for rapid production of graphite from biological samples was developed in 1992.[25] A description of a high-throughput method for measuring ^{14}C is given below.[26] In the first step, dried biological samples are placed in combustion tubes containing cupric oxide and heated to 650°C for 2.5 h. All of the carbon present in the sample is oxidized to carbon dioxide. In the second step, carbon dioxide is reduced to graphite in the presence of titanium hydride and zinc powder at 500°C for 3 h then 550°C for 2 h, using cobalt as catalyst.[26] The graphitized samples are then loaded into the AMS instrument and 1 mg (or more) of carbon is added to each sample in the form of 50 μL 33.3 mg/mL of tributyrin in methanol. It is important that the biological material to be analyzed does not get contaminated with ^{14}C during sample preparation. To avoid sample cross contamination, disposable materials are used throughout the entire process of graphitization.

Most AMS instruments use cesium as an ion source.[20,27] Samples are bombarded with cesium vapor, which causes the graphitized samples to form negative ions that are extracted by a series of plates held thousands of volts more positive than the ion source. The negative ion beam enters an injection magnet where the ions are separated and selected by their mass-to-charge ratio, so that ^{12}C, ^{13}C, and ^{14}C ions pass through separately as a series of pulses in sequence.[28] The pulsed ion beams pass into a tandem electrostatic Van de Graaff particle accelerator where the negative ions flow toward a positive terminal held at 1 to 5 million volts. As the ions travel, they attain very high energies, and these high-energy ion beams are focused to collide with argon gas molecules (on a 0.02 μmol thin carbon foil) in a collision cell. This collision strips the outer valence electrons from the atoms, so that the charge on the atoms changes from negative to positive and all molecular species are converted to atoms. These positive atomic ion beams are now repelled by the positive high terminal voltage used and exit the accelerator. The beams then pass into a high-energy analyzing magnet where the ^{12}C, ^{13}C, and ^{14}C atoms are separated by their mass moment charge state ratio. ^{12}C and ^{13}C are measured with Faraday cups whereas the less abundant ^{14}C beam is focused by a quadropole and electrostatic cylindrical analyzer and counted in a gas ionization detector. The rare isotope (^{14}C) count is compared to the abundant (^{12}C) isotope count to determine the relative abundance of the ^{14}C atoms in the original sample.[28] Measurements are normalized to improve precision, by comparing the $^{14}C/^{12}C$ ratio in the sample with the same ratio obtained from a known standard, graphitized sucrose with an accepted $^{14}C/^{12}C$ ratio of 1.5081 modern (Australian National University [ANU], Canberra, Australia).[26,27] ^{14}C determinations are made at the Center for Accelerator Mass Spectrometry at Lawrence Livermore Laboratory (Livermore, CA, USA).

AMS can also be used to detect ^{3}H tracers in milligram-sized samples.[29,30] Sample preparation for analysis by tritium AMS is a multistep process in which the organic samples are converted to titanium hydride.[29] First, the organic sample is oxidized to carbon dioxide and water. Then the water is reduced to hydrogen gas, which reacts with titanium to produce titanium hydride. The ratio of $^{3}H/^{1}H$ is measured by AMS. This technique is currently under development, but once established it can be a very powerful tool because ^{3}H is the most widely and least expensive radioisotope used in biomedical research. In addition, ^{3}H AMS could be used with ^{14}C AMS for double-labeled experiments to study the interaction of two compounds or the metabolites of a single compound labeled in two separate locations.[31,32]

CONSIDERATIONS FOR HUMAN SUBJECTS

Several studies conducted in the 1960s used relatively large doses of radioisotopes to study the metabolism of vitamins in hospitalized subjects. Classic studies of vitamins A, C, E, and other nutrients were all conducted this way.[11,12,33,34] The information from these studies formed the basis of our current understanding of nutrient metabolism and requirement. Those experimental protocols would not meet current Institutional Review Boards' requirements since the amount of radiation used ranged from 10 to 194 μCi. AMS, an extremely sensitive technique, allows the use of radiation dosages that are several 1000 fold lower, on average, a radiation exposure of 100 nCi,[35–39] which corresponds to 11 μSv or 1.1 mrem. This amount of radiation exposure is equivalent to that received during a 3 h flight in an airplane or from 1 day of cosmic radiation at sea level. The U.S. Food and Drug Administration defines a safe radiation dose as <3 rem to the whole body, blood-forming organs, lens of the eye, and gonads or 5 rem for the remaining organs.[40] Additionally, tissues and fluids with a specific activity >2 nCi/g must be declared as radioactive material. The blood, urine, and fecal specimens from the low doses of ^{14}C used in current AMS studies (≤ 200 nCi) are below the 2 nCi/g cutoff; therefore, the specimens are not considered radioactive material by the U.S. Federal Regulation.[40]

MATHEMATICAL MODELING

Our understanding of nutrient metabolism is hindered because metabolism occurs over time, often in inaccessible tissues. It is very difficult, even impossible, to collect experimental data for some critical steps in nutrient metabolism *in vivo*. Kinetic modeling is a systems analysis approach that constructs a quantitative overview of the dynamic and kinetic behavior of metabolism of a nutrient as it might occur *in vivo*. A mathematical model is built to realize as complete a description as possible of the metabolic system under investigation. The advance of computer hardware and modeling software makes it possible to solve (and manipulate) differential equations meant to predict kinetic behavior efficiently and accurately. Therefore, mathematical modeling has become an attractive tool for collecting and processing research data and information needed to understand the dynamics of nutrient metabolism *in vivo*. Kinetic models are built to mimic the metabolism of a nutrient as it might occur *in vivo* and to estimate values for critical parameters, so that unobserved portions of the dynamic and kinetic behavior of the nutrient under investigation can be predicted. Specific information obtained about the nutrient under investigation includes the number of storage sites (pools) for the nutrient and their sizes, how they are connected, and how their masses change over time.

Modeling begins with a thorough review existing knowledge of the metabolism of the nutrient under investigation to formulate an initial structure for the model. Then initial constants (for transfer of nutrient to recipient compartments from donor compartments) are estimated and adjusted in physiologically relevant ways until the model structure and rate constants predict best fits for the experimental data. Final parameter values are generated using iterative nonlinear least squares routines. The following references describe a series of conferences on mathematical modeling in nutrition and health sciences.[41–47]

HUMAN FOLATE METABOLISM

Folate is necessary for purine and pyrimidine synthesis and for the metabolism of homocysteine to methionine. There have been extensive studies of folate metabolism in humans using pharmacological dosages of radiolabeled folate measured with liquid scintillation counting.[48–52] These studies yield useful information about folate absorption, metabolism, and excretion. However, all but one were of short duration and thus gave no information about long-term storage and metabolism of folate.[52]

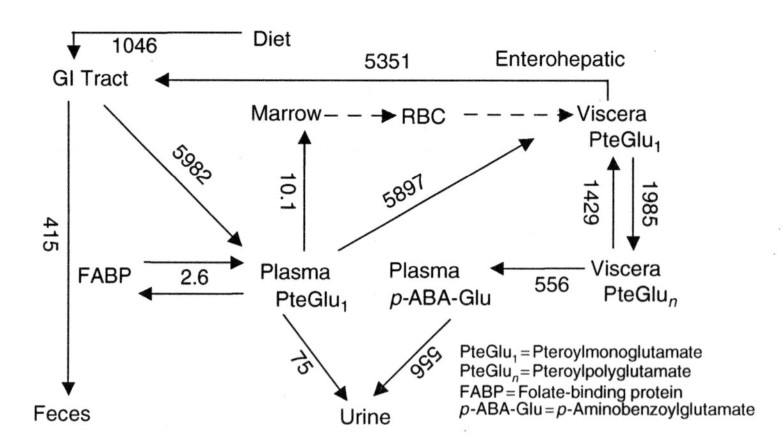

FIGURE 17.2 Kinetic model of folate metabolism. The numbers represent steady-state folate fluxes (nanomoles per day).

We investigated short- and long-range human folate metabolism with AMS following an oral dose of ^{14}C-pteroylmonoglutamate in healthy adults.[38] Thirteen free-living adults received 0.5 nmol ^{14}C-pteroylmonoglutamate (100 nCi) plus 79.5 nmol nonlabeled pterolylmonoglutamate orally in water. The subjects were typical American adults with no known disease and had a mean dietary folate intake of 1046 nmol/day. ^{14}C was followed in plasma, erythrocytes, urine, and feces for 40 days. Kinetic models were used to analyze and interpret the data. Model parameters were optimized using the SAAM II kinetic analysis software such that hypotheses that were inconsistent with the datasets observed for each of the 13 subjects could be rejected. A diagram of the final model is shown in Figure 17.2. Our model consisted of four pools of folate: gastrointestinal tract (lumen), plasma, erythrocyte, and viscera (all other tissues).

Apparent absorption of ^{14}C-pteroylmonoglutamate was 79%. Mean total body folate was 225 μmol. Pteroylpolyglutamate synthesis, recycling, and catabolism were 1985, 1429, and 556 nmol/day, respectively. Mean residence times were 0.525 day as visceral pteroylmonoglutamate, 119 days as visceral pteroylpolyglutamate, 0.0086 day as plasma folate, and 0.1 day as gastrointestinal folate.

The kinetic model predicted that only 0.25% of plasma folate was destined for bone marrow, even though folate metabolism is important for healthy bones. It also predicted an important role for bile in folate metabolism. Most folate was recycled in tissues through bile. Visceral pteroylmonoglutamate, which is transported to the gastrointestinal tract via bile, provided a large pool of extracellular pteroylmonoglutamate (5351 nmol/day) that could blunt between-meal fluctuations in folate supply to the cells to sustain folate concentrations during periods of folate deprivation. Therefore, the digestibility of the dietary folate plus the folate recovered in the bile (1046 + 5351 nmol/day, respectively) was 92%. We accounted for the gastric transit time of 1 day to the absorption site. The 6.15 days erythron transit time was a new observation that fit well with the week-long maturation of hematopoietic progenitor cells.[53]

Intact pteroylmonoglutamate that was eliminated in the urine represented ~6% of ingested folate, a value that compared well with already published values.[54–56] However, the novel and testable hypothesis represented by our model is that fully one-half of excreted folate was derived from visceral pteroylpolyglutamate and appeared in the urine as *p*-aminobenzoylglutamate (and its metabolic successors).

The model makes several important predictions. First, the fractional absorption of folate was high and independent of the gastrointestinal folate load. Second, ~33% of visceral pteroylmonoglutamate was converted to the polyglutamate form. Third, most of the body folate was visceral (>99%), and most of the visceral folate was pteroylpolyglutamate (>98%). Fourth, the model predicted that bile folate was 25 times greater than prior estimates and that steady-state folate distributions were approximately fivefold larger than prior estimates.[57]

In addition, the model predicted two distinct chemical forms of folate in plasma: pteroylmonoglutamate and *p*-aminobenzoylglutamate. For visceral pteroylglutamate to be recycled by conversion to visceral pteroylmonoglutamate was no surprise, but for visceral pteroylpolyglutamate to also be converted directly to *p*-aminobenzoylglutamate is a new pathway that fits nicely with other recent discoveries in pteroylpolyglutamate catabolism.[58]

HUMAN VITAMIN A AND β-CAROTENE METABOLISM

Vitamin A (retinol and its metabolites) plays an important role in vision, growth, cell division, and differentiation.[59] Retinol status has been difficult to assess using nonisotopic methods, because its serum concentrations are tightly regulated and 90% or more of its body stores are in inaccessible tissues such as liver and kidney.[60–64] Therefore, much of what is known about the human absorption and metabolism of retinoids is based on one small radioisotope study.[65]

Recently we fed deuterated retinyl acetate to adult men and women. Our results show that a single large peak appears in the blood at ~4–8 h postdose, reaching its maximum at 12–24 h postdose.[66] The vitamin A half-lives ranged from 75 to 241 days for men fed a vitamin A-deficient diet[65] and 56 to 243 days for men and women fed a vitamin A-adequate diet.[36,67,68]

The reasons for the large variations in metabolic half-life are unknown, but the main factors that appear to influence vitamin A metabolism are the individual's vitamin A nutritional status and dietary intake. People with higher retinol status appear to absorb retinol more efficiently than people with lower retinol status.[36,65,66] Very low intakes of retinol appear to reduce (rather than increase) retinol utilization, even when retinol stores are still adequate.[65] Other factors, such as, gender, race, and body composition, did not have a strong influence on vitamin A metabolism in our studies, but might well have an impact in more heterogeneous groups.[66]

Although retinoids are key essential nutrients, they are not widely dispersed among foods. In developing countries, β-carotene, found in yellow-orange fruits and vegetables, is the major source of vitamin A.[69] β-carotene has also been reported to have various biological effects; among them are enhancement of the immunological system, to stimulate gap junction communication between cells *in vitro*, and a possible antioxidant activity.[70–72] We conducted a long-term kinetic study of β-carotene[30] using ^{14}C-β-carotene derived by growing spinach in an atmospherically sealed chamber pulsed with $^{14}CO_2$. A healthy 35 year old male received a single oral dose of ^{14}C-β-carotene (306 μg; 200 nCi) and the tracer was followed for 209 days in plasma, 17 days in urine, and 10 days in feces. Aliquots of plasma (30 μL), urine (100 μL), and stool (150 μL) samples were analyzed. Plasma ^{14}C-β-carotene, ^{14}C-retinyl esters, ^{14}C-retinol, and several ^{14}C-retinoic acids were separated by reversed phase HPLC.

The results showed that 57.4% of the administered dose was recovered in the stool within 48 h postdose; therefore, 42.6% of β-carotene was bioavailable. Urine was not a major excrete route for intact β-carotene. There was a 5.5 h delay between dosing and the

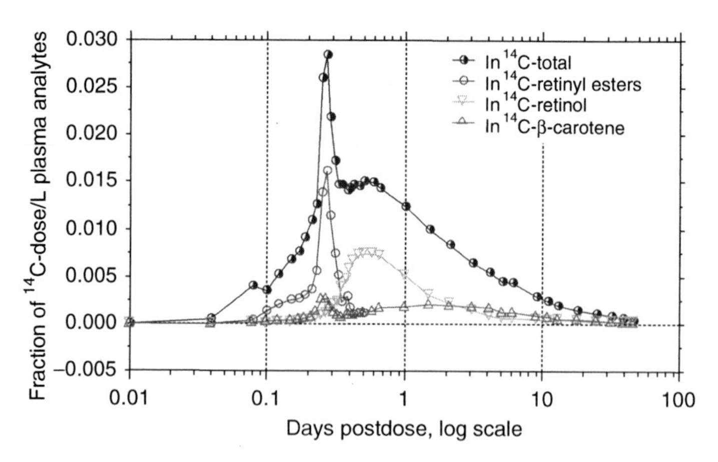

FIGURE 17.3 Patterns of ^{14}C in plasma following an oral dose of ^{14}C-β-carotene to a normal adult. (From Burri, B.J. and Clifford, A.J., *Arch. Biochem. Biophys.*, 430 (1), 110, 2004.) The ^{14}C in plasma, which is associated with the labeled retinyl esters, retinol, and β-carotene fractions, accounts for about one-half of the total radioactivity. The remainder is associated with yet-unidentified carotenoid and retinoid metabolites, possibly epoxides, apo-carotenals, and retinoic acids.

appearance of ^{14}C in plasma. The losses of ^{14}C-β-carotene and its metabolites after an oral dose of ^{14}C-β-carotene are shown in Figure 17.3. ^{14}C-β-carotene and ^{14}C-retinyl esters presented similar kinetic profiles for the first 24 h. Both ^{14}C-β-carotene and ^{14}C-retinyl esters rose to a plateau spanning between 14 and 21.3 h. The concentration of ^{14}C-retinol rose linearly for 28 h postdose before declining. Therefore, the substantial disappearance of retinyl esters from plasma between 21 and 25 h closely preceded the transition from increasing retinol concentrations. This observation suggests that retinyl ester was handed off to retinol into circulation. The area under the curve suggested a molar vitamin A value of 0.53 for β-carotene, with a minimum of 62% of the absorbed β-carotene cleaving to vitamin A. The pattern of total ^{14}C,^{14}C-β-carotene, ^{14}C-retinyl esters, and ^{14}C-retinol in plasma is shown in Figure 17.4.

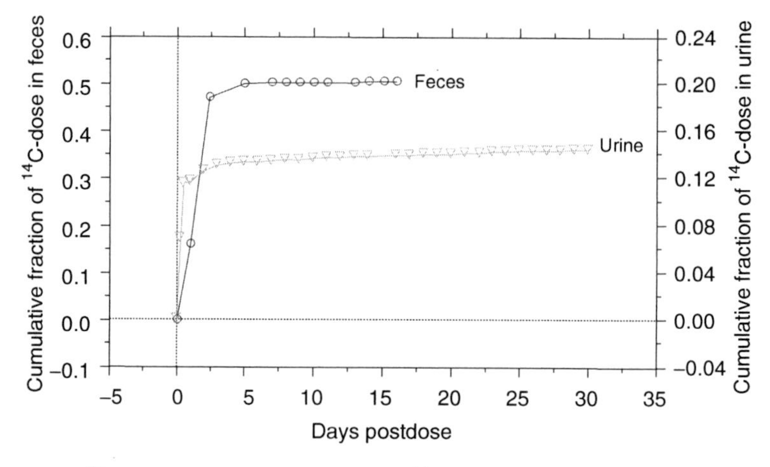

FIGURE 17.4 Loss of ^{14}C in feces and urine from oral ^{14}C-β-carotene in a healthy adult. (From Lemke, S.L., Dueker, S.R., Follett, J.R., Lin, Y., Carkeet, C., Buchholz, B.A., Vogel, J.S., and Clifford, A.J., *J. Lipid Res.*, 44 (8), 1591, 2003.)

In addition, the effect of vitamin A nutritional status on β-carotene metabolism was elucidated.[36] Two healthy adult women received an oral dose of ^{14}C-β-carotene (0.5–1.0 nmol with specific activity of 98.8 mCi/mmol) in a banana "milk shake." Seven weeks after this first dose, both women began taking a vitamin A supplement, 3000 RE (10,000 IU) retinyl palmitate per day. They consumed the supplement for 21 days and then received a second dose of ^{14}C-β-carotene. The women continued taking the 3000 RE supplements for 14 days after the second dose was given, then the amount of vitamin A supplement was decreased to 1500 RE (5000 IU) per day for the remainder of the study. Concentrations of ^{14}C-β-carotene, ^{14}C-retinyl esters, and ^{14}C-retinol in plasma were measured for 46 days after the first dose and 56 days after the second dose.

Using AUCs and irreversible losses of ^{14}C in feces and urine, a yield of 0.54 mol ^{14}C-vitamin A from 1 mol of ^{14}C-β-carotene before supplementation and 0.74 mol ^{14}C-vitamin A after supplementation was calculated. These data indicate that more vitamin A was formed from β-carotene when subjects were taking vitamin A supplementation. This suggests that retinoid status can influence carotenoid status and vice versa.

CALCIUM

Calcium is the most abundant divalent cation of the human body and is important for the maintenance of bone mineral density, blood clotting, nerve conduction, muscle contraction, enzyme regulation, and membrane permeability.[73] Calcium has three radioisotopes, ^{47}Ca, ^{45}Ca, and ^{41}Ca. ^{47}Ca and ^{45}Ca have relatively short half-lives (4.5 and 165 days, respectively) but ^{41}Ca is a very long-lived radioisotope ($t_{1/2} \sim$ 116,000 years). Osteoporosis, the decrease in bone mass and density due in part to loss of calcium, is a growing problem as people age; therefore, long-term studies on bone calcium turnover and bone resorption are extremely important.[74,75] Short-term studies of calcium metabolism can be done by a variety of stable and radioisotope techniques, using ^{47}Ca and ^{45}Ca, but these cannot resolve long-term small but significant differences in bone resorption. The advent of AMS has made possible the use of the long-lived radioisotope ^{41}Ca, which potentially could be traced for decades.[76] In 1990, Elmore et al. assessed the potential for using ^{41}Ca for bone resorption study by measuring ^{41}Ca by AMS in dogs.[77] The authors demonstrated that ^{41}Ca behaves identically to ^{45}Ca *in vivo*. Freeman et al. developed an improved protocol,[78] then administered 5 nCi of ^{41}Ca dissolved in orange juice to 25 subjects and measured the tracer in urine by AMS.[24] Fink et al. described the protocols for measuring ^{41}Ca/^{40}Ca ratios to a sensitivity of 6×10^{-16}.[79] These studies have clearly demonstrated the feasibility of the AMS approach. Freeman et al. have also shown that the osteoporosis drug, alendronate, markedly suppressed bone resorption by effecting ^{41}Ca loss in urine.[24] The use of ^{41}Ca and AMS to better understand long-term calcium metabolism in humans, and to trace the impact on osteoporosis of minute differences in calcium metabolism, occurring over many years, offers many exciting possibilities.

SUMMARY

AMS is an isotope ratio method ideal for measuring the ratios of long-lived radioisotopes such as ^{14}C/^{12}C for biological and chemical research. It is capable of measuring nutrients and their metabolites in attomol (10^{-18}) concentrations in milligram-sized samples. The detection sensitivity and small sample size requirements of AMS satisfies both the analytical and ethical requirements for tracer applications in human subjects.

ACKNOWLEDGMENTS

The literature on the AMS method has been published mostly by the researchers at the Center for Accelerator Mass Spectrometry at Lawrence National Laboratory (LLNL) in the United States, the Center for Biomedical Accelerator Mass Spectrometry in York, UK, and the Radiocarbon Laboratory of the GeoBiosphere Center in Lund, Sweden. All of the work reported by our laboratory was performed in collaboration with the researchers at the Center for AMS at LLNL. The best current description of the method for preparing AMS samples is given in: Getachew, G., Kim, S.H., Burri, B.J., Kelly, P.B., Haack, K.W., Ognibene, T.J., Buchholz, B.A., Vogel, J.S., Modrow, J., and Clifford, A.J. How to convert biological carbon into graphite for AMS. Radiocarbon, 48, 325–336, 2006.

REFERENCES

1. Glasstone, S., *Source Book on Atomic Energy*, 3rd ed. D. Van Nostrand Company, Inc., New York, 1967, chap. 2.
2. Faires, R.A. and Parks, B.H., *Radioisotope Laboratory Techniques*, 1st ed. George Newnes, Ltd., London, 1958, chap. 1.
3. Wilson, R.R. and Littauer, R., *Accelerators: Machines of Nuclear Physics*, 1st ed. Anchor Books, New York, 1960, chap. 3.
4. Heilbron, J.L. and Seidel, R.W., *Lawrence and his Laboratory: A History of the Lawrence Berkley Laboratory*, 1st ed. University of California Press, Berkley and Los Angeles, 1989, chap. 1.
5. Muller, R.A., Radioisotope dating with a cyclotron, *Science*, 196, 489–494, 1977.
6. Nelson, D.E., Korteling, R.G., and Stott, W.R., Carbon-14: direct detection at natural concentrations, *Science*, 198, 507–508, 1977.
7. Bennett, C.L. et al., Radiocarbon dating using electrostatic accelerators: negative ions provide the key, *Science*, 198, 508–510, 1977.
8. Garner, R.C., Barker, J., Flavell, C., Garner, J.V., Whattam, M., Young, G.C., Cussans, N., Jezequel, S., and Leong, D., A validation study comparing accelerator MS and liquid scintillation counting for analysis of ^{14}C-labelled drugs in plasma, urine and faecal extracts, *J. Pharm. Biomed. Anal.*, 24 (2), 197–209, 2000.
9. Broecker, W.S., Schulert, A., and Olson, E.A., Bomb carbon-14 in human beings, *Science*, 130 (3371), 331–332, 1959.
10. Libby, W.F., Berger, R., Mead, J.F., Alexander, G.V., and Ross, J.F., Replacement rates for human tissue from atmospheric radiocarbon, *Science*, 146, 1170–1172, 1964.
11. Goodman, D.S., Blomstrand, R., Werner, B., Huang, H.S., and Shiratori, T., The intestinal absorption and metabolism of vitamin A and beta-carotene in man, *J. Clin. Invest.*, 45 (10), 1615–1623, 1966.
12. Blomstrand, R. and Werner, B., Studies on the intestinal absorption of radioactive beta-carotene and vitamin A in man. Conversion of beta-carotene into vitamin A, *Scand. J. Clin. Lab. Invest.*, 19 (4), 339–345, 1967.
13. Keilson, J. and Waterhouse, C., *First Conference on Radiocarbon Dating with Accelerators*. H.E. Gove University of Rochester, Rochester, 1978.
14. Elmore, D. and Phillips, F.M., Accelerator mass spectrometry for measurement of long-lived radioisotopes, *Science*, 236, 543–550, 1987.
15. Turteltaub, K.W., Felton, J.S., Gledhill, B.L., Vogel, J.S., Southon, J.R., Caffee, M.W., Finkel, R.C., Nelson, D.E., Proctor, I.D., and Davis, J.C., Accelerator mass spectrometry in biomedical dosimetry: relationship between low-level exposure and covalent binding of heterocyclic amine carcinogens to DNA, *Proc. Natl. Acad. Sci., USA* 87 (14), 5288–5292, 1990.
16. Shapiro, S.D., Endicott, S.K., Province, M.A., Pierce, J.A., and Campbell, E.J., Marked longevity of human lung parenchymal elastic fibers deduced from prevalence of D-aspartate and nuclear weapons-related radiocarbon, *J. Clin. Invest.*, 87 (5), 1828–1834, 1991.
17. Turteltaub, K.W., Frantz, C.E., Creek, M.R., Vogel, J.S., Shen, N., and Fultz, E., DNA adducts in model systems and humans, *J. Cell Biochem. Suppl.*, 17F, 138–148, 1993.

18. Felton, J.S. and Turteltaub, K.W., Accelerator mass spectrometry for measuring low-dose carcinogen binding to DNA, *Environ. Health Perspect.*, 102 (5), 450–452, 1994.
19. Turteltaub, K.W., Mauthe, R.J., Dingley, K.H., Vogel, J.S., Frantz, C.E., Garner, R.C., and Shen, N., MeIQx–DNA adduct formation in rodent and human tissues at low doses, *Mutat. Res.*, 376 (1–2), 243–252, 1997.
20. Vogel, J.S. and Turteltaub, K.W., Accelerator mass spectrometry as a bioanalytical tool for nutritional research, *Adv. Exp. Med. Biol.*, 445, 397–410, 1998.
21. Vogel, J.S., Turteltaub, K.W., Finkel, R., and Nelson, D.E., Accelerator mass spectrometry–isotope quantification at attomole sensitivity, *Anal. Chem.*, 67 (11), 353A–359A, 1995.
22. Hotchkis, M., Fink, D., Tuniz, C., and Vogt, S., Accelerator mass spectrometry analyses of environmental radionuclides: sensitivity, precision and standardisation, *Appl. Radiat. Isot.*, 53 (1–2), 31–37, 2000.
23. Priest, N.D., The biological behaviour and bioavailability of aluminium in man, with special reference to studies employing aluminium-26 as a tracer: review and study update, *J. Environ. Monit.*, 6 (5), 375–403, 2004.
24. Freeman, S.P.T.H. et al., The study of skeletal calcium metabolism with ^{41}Ca and ^{45}Ca, *Nucl. Instr. Meth. Phys. Res. B*, 172, 930–933, 2000.
25. Vogel, J.S., Rapid production of graphite without contamination for biomedical AMS, *Radiocarbon*, 34, 344–350, 1992.
26. Ognibene, T.J., Bench, G., Vogel, J.S., Peaslee, G.F., and Murov, S., A high-throughput method for the conversion of CO_2 obtained from biochemical samples to graphite in septa-sealed vials for quantification of ^{14}C via accelerator mass spectrometry, *Anal. Chem.*, 75 (9), 2192–2196, 2003.
27. Barker, J. and Garner, R.C., Biomedical applications of accelerator mass spectrometry–isotope measurements at the level of the atom, *Rapid. Commun. Mass Spectrom.*, 13 (4), 285–293, 1999.
28. Lappin, G. and Garner, R.C., Current perspectives of ^{14}C-isotope measurement in biomedical accelerator mass spectrometry, *Anal. Bioanal. Chem.*, 378 (2), 356–364, 2004.
29. Roberts, M.L., Velsko, C., and Turteltaub, K.W., Tritium AMS for biomedical applications, *Nucl. Instr. Meth. Phys. Res. B*, 92, 459–462, 1994.
30. Hamm, R.W. et al., *A Compact Tritium Analysis System*. John Wiley & Sons, Boston, 2001.
31. Dingley, K.H., Roberts, M.L., Velsko, C.A., and Turteltaub, K.W., Attomole detection of ^{3}H in biological samples using accelerator mass spectrometry: application in low-dose, dual-isotope tracer studies in conjunction with ^{14}C accelerator mass spectrometry, *Chem. Res. Toxicol.*, 11 (10), 1217–1222, 1998.
32. Ognibene, T.J. and Vogel, J.S., *Highly Sensitive ^{14}C and ^{3}H Quantification of Biochemical Samples using Accelerator Mass Spectrometry*. John Wiley & Sons, Boston, 2003.
33. MacMahon, M.T. and Neale, G., The absorption of alpha-tocopherol in control subjects and in patients with intestinal malabsorption, *Clin. Sci.*, 38 (2), 197–210, 1970.
34. Kelleher, J. and Losowsky, M.S., The absorption of alpha-tocopherol in man, *Br. J. Nutr.*, 24 (4), 1033–1047, 1970.
35. Buchholz, B.A., Arjomand, A., Dueker, S.R., Schneider, P.D., Clifford, A.J., and Vogel, J.S., Intrinsic erythrocyte labeling and attomole pharmacokinetic tracing of ^{14}C-labeled folic acid with accelerator mass spectrometry, *Anal. Biochem.*, 269 (2), 348–352, 1999.
36. Dueker, S.R., Lin, Y., Buchholz, B.A., Schneider, P.D., Lame, M.W., Segall, H.J., Vogel, J.S., and Clifford, A.J., Long-term kinetic study of beta-carotene, using accelerator mass spectrometry in an adult volunteer, *J. Lipid Res.*, 41 (11), 1790–1800, 2000.
37. Lemke, S.L., Dueker, S.R., Follett, J.R., Lin, Y., Carkeet, C., Buchholz, B.A., Vogel, J.S., and Clifford, A.J., Absorption and retinol equivalence of beta-carotene in humans is influenced by dietary vitamin A intake, *J. Lipid Res.*, 44 (8), 1591–1600, 2003.
38. Lin, Y., Dueker, S.R., Follett, J.R., Fadel, J.G., Arjomand, A., Schneider, P.D., Miller, J.W., Green, R., Buchholz, B.A., Vogel, J.S., Phair, R.D., and Clifford, A.J., Quantitation of in vivo human folate metabolism, *Am. J. Clin. Nutr.*, 80 (3), 680–691, 2004.
39. Burri, B.J. and Clifford, A.J., Carotenoid and retinoid metabolism: insights from isotope studies, *Arch. Biochem. Biophys.*, 430 (1), 110–119, 2004.
40. U.S. Code Fed. Reg., Prescription drugs for human use generally recognized as safe and effective and not misbranded: drugs used in research. U.S. Code Title 21, chapter 1 (4-1-03 ed.), Part 361, pp. 300–305.

41. Abumrad, N., Mathematical models in experimental nutrition, *J. Parenter. Enteral Nutr.*, 15, 44–98, 1991.
42. Canolty, N. and Cain, T., *Mathematical Models in Experimental Nutrition*. University of Georgia, Athens, GA, 1985.
43. Coburn, S. and Townsend, D., Mathematical modeling in experimental nutrition, *Adv. Food Nutr. Res.*, 40, 1, 1996.
44. Hoover-Plow, J. and Chandra, R., Mathematical modeling in experimental nutrition, *Prog. Food Nutr. Sci.*, 12, 211, 1988.
45. Siva Subramanian, K. and Wastney, M., *Kinetics Model of Trace Element and Mineral Metabolism during Development*. CRC Press, New York, 1955.
46. Clifford, A. and Mueller, H., Mathematical modeling in nutrition research, *Adv. Exp. Med. Biol.*, 445, 1–423, 1998.
47. Novotny, J., Green, M., and Boston, R., Mathematical modeling in nutrition research and the health sciences, *Adv. Exp. Med. Biol.*, 537, 1–420, 2003.
48. Anderson, B., Belcher, E.H., Chanarin, I., and Mollin, D.L., The urinary and faecal excretion of radioactivity after oral doses of H3-folic acid, *Br. J. Haematol.*, 6, 439–455, 1960.
49. Baker, S.J., Kumar, S., and Swaminathan, S.P., Excretion of folic acid in bile, *Lancet*, 10, 685, 1965.
50. Butterworth, C.E., Jr., Baugh, C.M., and Krumdieck, C., A study of folate absorption and metabolism in man utilizing carbon-14-labeled polyglutamates synthesized by the solid phase method, *J. Clin. Invest.*, 48 (6), 1131–1142, 1969.
51. Perry, J. and Chanarin, I., Intestinal absorption of reduced folate compounds in man, *Br. J. Haematol.*, 18 (3), 329–339, 1970.
52. Krumdieck, C.L., Fukushima, K., Fukushima, T., Shiota, T., and Butterworth, C.E., Jr., A long-term study of the excretion of folate and pterins in a human subject after ingestion of ^{14}C folic acid, with observations on the effect of diphenylhydantoin administration, *Am. J. Clin. Nutr.*, 31 (1), 88–93, 1978.
53. Steinberg, S.E., Campbell, C.L., and Hillman, R.S., Kinetics of the normal folate enterohepatic cycle, *J. Clin. Invest.*, 64 (1), 83–88, 1979.
54. Cooperman, J.M., Pesci-Bourel, A., and Luhby, A.L., Urinary excretion of folic acid activity in man, *Clin. Chem.*, 16 (5), 375–381, 1970.
55. Sauberlich, H.E., Kretsch, M.J., Skala, J.H., Johnson, H.L., and Taylor, P.C., Folate requirement and metabolism in nonpregnant women, *Am. J. Clin. Nutr.*, 46 (6), 1016–1028, 1987.
56. Kownacki-Brown, P.A., Wang, C., Bailey, L.B., Toth, J.P., and Gregory, J.F., III, Urinary excretion of deuterium-labeled folate and the metabolite *p*-aminobenzoylglutamate in humans, *J. Nutr.*, 123 (6), 1101–1108, 1993.
57. Institute of Medicine, *Dietary reference intakes for Thiamin, Riboflavin, Niacin, Vitamin B6, Folate, Vitamin B12, Pantothenic acid, Biotin, and Choline*. National Academy of Sciences Press, Washington, DC, 1998.
58. Suh, J.R., Oppenheim, E.W., Girgis, S., and Stover, P.J., Purification and properties of a folate-catabolizing enzyme, *J. Biol. Chem.*, 275 (45), 35646–35655, 2000.
59. Institute of Medicine, *Dietary reference intakes for Vitamin A, Vitamin K, Arsenic, Boron, Chromium, Copper, Iodine, Iron, Manganese, Molybdenum, Nickel, Silicon, Vanadium, and Zinc*. National Academy of Sciences Press, Washington, DC, 2000.
60. Azais-Braesco, V. and Pascal, G., Vitamin A in pregnancy: requirements and safety limits, *Am. J. Clin. Nutr.*, 71 (5 Suppl), 1325S–1333S, 2000.
61. Berdanier, C.D., Everts, H.B., Hermoyian, C., and Mathews, C.E., Role of vitamin A in mitochondrial gene expression, *Diabetes Res. Clin. Pract.*, 54 (Suppl 2), S11–S27, 2001.
62. Clagett-Dame, M. and DeLuca, H.F., The role of vitamin A in mammalian reproduction and embryonic development, *Annu. Rev. Nutr.*, 22, 347–381, 2002.
63. Harrison, E.H. and Hussain, M.M., Mechanisms involved in the intestinal digestion and absorption of dietary vitamin A, *J. Nutr.*, 131 (5), 1405–1408, 2001.
64. Olson, J.A., Serum levels of vitamin A and carotenoids as reflectors of nutritional status, *J. Natl. Cancer Inst.*, 73 (6), 1439–1444, 1984.
65. Sauberlich, H.E., Hodges, R.E., Wallace, D.L., Kolder, H., Canham, J.E., Hood, J., Raica, N., Jr., and Lowry, L.K., Vitamin A metabolism and requirements in the human studied with the use of labeled retinol, *Vitam. Horm.*, 32, 251–275, 1974.

66. Burri, B.J. and Park, J.Y., Compartmental models of vitamin A and beta-carotene metabolism in women, *Adv. Exp. Med. Biol.*, 445, 225–237, 1998.
67. Novotny, J.A., Dueker, S.R., Zech, L.A., and Clifford, A.J., Compartmental analysis of the dynamics of beta-carotene metabolism in an adult volunteer, *J. Lipid Res.*, 36 (8), 1825–1838, 1995.
68. Novotny, J.A., Zech, L.A., Furr, H.C., Dueker, S.R., and Clifford, A.J., Mathematical modeling in nutrition: constructing a physiologic compartmental model of the dynamics of beta-carotene metabolism, *Adv. Food Nutr. Res.*, 40, 25–54, 1996.
69. Bender, D.A., *Nutritional Biochemistry of Vitamins*, 2nd ed. Cambridge University Press, Cambridge, 2003.
70. Santos, M.S., Meydani, S.N., Leka, L., Wu, D., Fotouhi, N., Meydani, M., Hennekens, C.H., and Gaziano, J.M., Natural killer cell activity in elderly men is enhanced by beta-carotene supplementation, *Am. J. Clin. Nutr.*, 64 (5), 772–777, 1996.
71. Sies, H. and Stahl, W., Carotenoids and intercellular communication via gap junctions, *Int. J. Vitam. Nutr. Res.*, 67 (5), 364–367, 1997.
72. Mosca, L., Rubenfire, M., Mandel, C., Rock, C., Tarshis, T., Tsai, A., and Pearson, T., Antioxidant nutrient supplementation reduces the susceptibility of low density lipoprotein to oxidation in patients with coronary artery disease, *J. Am. Coll. Cardiol.*, 30 (2), 392–399, 1997.
73. Groff, J.L. and Gropper, S.S., *Advanced Nutrition and Human Metabolism*, 3rd ed. Wadsworth, Belmont, 2000.
74. Heaney, R.P., Factors influencing the measurement of bioavailability; taking calcium as a model, *J. Nutr.*, 131, 1344S–1348S, 2001.
75. Heaney, R.P., Long-lasting deficiency diseases: insights from calcium and vitamin D, *Am. J. Clin. Nutr.*, 78, 912–919, 2003.
76. Weaver, C.M. and Liebman, M., Biomarkers of bone health appropriate for evaluating functional foods designed to reduce risk of osteoporosis, *Br. J. Nutr.*, 88 (Suppl 2), S225–S232, 2002.
77. Elmore, D. et al., Calcium-41 as a long-term biological tracer for bone resorption, *Nucl. Instr. Meth. Phys. Res. B*, 52, 531–535, 1990.
78. Freeman, S.P.H.T. et al., Biological sample preparation and ^{41}Ca AMS measurement at LLNL, *Nucl. Instr. Meth. Phys. Res. B*, 99, 557–561, 1995.
79. Fink, D., Middleton, R., Klein, J., and Sharma, P., ^{41}Ca: measurement by accelerator mass spectrometry and applications, *Nucl. Instr. Meth. Phys. Res. B*, 47, 79–96, 1990.

18 Dietary Reference Intakes for Vitamins

Suzanne P. Murphy and Susan I. Barr

CONTENTS

INTRODUCTION

Dietary reference intakes (DRIs) are nutrient reference standards to be used for planning and assessing diets of apparently healthy individuals and groups. DRIs were developed by the United States and Canada to update, expand on, and replace the former recommended nutrient intakes for Canadians and recommended dietary allowances (RDA) for Americans. The process was overseen by the Standing Committee on the Scientific Evaluation of Dietary Reference Intakes of the Food and Nutrition Board, Institute of Medicine, The National Academies, in collaboration with Health Canada. Instead of releasing a report that covered all nutrients in a single volume, as was done previously, a series of reports on groups of related nutrients was released, reflecting the work of nutrient panels composed of Canadian and American scientists (1–6). The first nutrient report was released in 1997 and covered calcium, phosphorus, magnesium, vitamin D, and fluoride (1); the final nutrient report was released in 2004 and covered electrolytes and water (6). Reports were also published on using a risk assessment model to establish upper levels (ULs) (7) and on the use of DRIs in dietary assessment and planning (8,9).

There are several types of DRIs and each has a specific definition. Figure 18.1 shows how these DRIs relate to one another.

ESTIMATED AVERAGE REQUIREMENT

The estimated average requirement (EAR) is defined as "the daily intake value that is estimated to meet the requirement, as defined by the specified indicator of adequacy, in half the apparently healthy individuals in a life stage or gender group" (6). Several aspects of this definition warrant further elaboration:

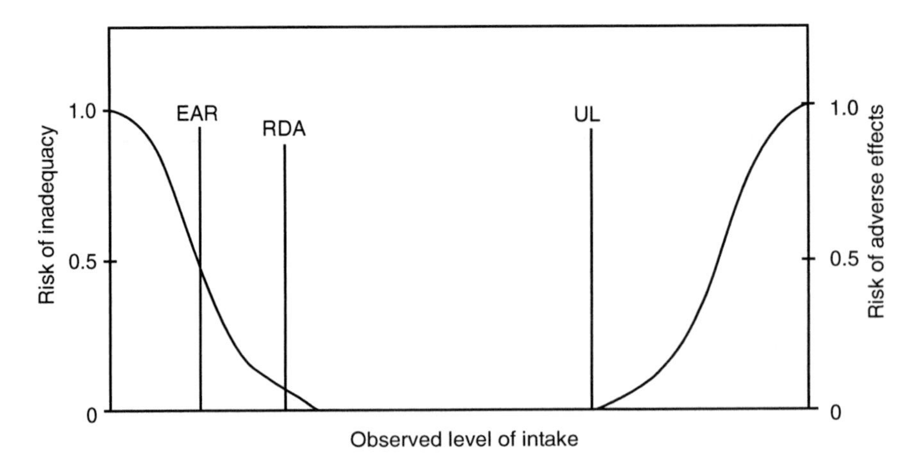

FIGURE 18.1 Dietary reference intakes. This figure shows that the estimated average requirement (EAR) is the intake at which the risk of inadequacy is 0.5 (50%) to an individual. The recommended dietary allowance (RDA) is the intake at which the risk of inadequacy is very small—only 2%–3%. The adequate intake (AI) does not bear a consistent relationship to the EAR or the RDA because it is set without the ability to estimate the requirement (however, it is thought to meet the needs of most individuals). At intakes between the RDA (or AI) and the tolerable upper intake level (UL), the risks of inadequacy and of excess are both close to zero. At intakes above the UL, the risk of adverse effects may increase (although the intake level at which this may occur is not known with precision). (Adapted from Food and Nutrition Board, Institute of Medicine, *Dietary Reference Intakes: Applications in Dietary Assessment*, National Academies Press, Washington, DC, 2000. With permission.)

Daily intake value: All DRIs are expressed as amounts per day; however, they are more appropriately considered as average intakes over a longer period of time (e.g., weeks or months).

Requirement: A requirement is defined as "the lowest continuing value of a nutrient that, for a specified indicator of adequacy, will maintain a defined level of nutriture in an individual" (6). The specified indicator of adequacy is identified for each nutrient, although in some cases it may differ among different age groups. The indicators of adequacy used for the vitamins are described in the next section (Dietary Reference Intakes for Vitamins).

Half the apparently healthy individuals: Although the word "average" is used in the EAR, its definition implies a median value rather than an average. The EAR is expected to meet or exceed the requirements of 50% of healthy individuals in a life stage or gender group, and to fall below the requirements of the other 50%. The median and the average remain the same when the requirement distribution is symmetrical, which is assumed to be the case for all of the vitamins.

Recommended Dietary Allowance

The RDA is defined as "the average daily intake level that is sufficient to meet the nutrient requirement of nearly all (97%–98%) apparently healthy individuals in a particular life stage and gender group" (6). The primary use of the RDA is as a daily intake goal for individuals: at this level of intake, there is a very high probability (97%–98%) that the given individuals will meet or exceed their requirements. This is in contrast to the EAR, which would be expected to fall below the requirements of 50% of individuals.

The RDA for vitamin intakes is set based on the EAR plus twice the standard deviation (SD) of the EAR: RDA = EAR + 2SD. As the requirements are thought to be normally distributed, intake at the RDA will be sufficient for 97%–98% of individuals. If sufficient data are not available to calculate the SD, a coefficient of variation (CV; SD/EAR) of 10% is frequently used in place of the SD. This is based on the variability of other biological variables. In this case, the RDA is set as the EAR and twice the CV of 10%: $RDA = EAR + 2(0.1 \times EAR) = 1.2 \times EAR$. In some cases, when there is evidence of greater variability (but still insufficient data to accurately identify the SD), a larger CV was assumed. For example, for vitamin A the CV was assumed to be 20%; thus, the $RDA = 1.4 \times EAR$. For niacin, the CV was 15%, so that the RDA is $1.3 \times EAR$.

Adequate Intake

For some nutrients, sufficient scientific evidence was not available to establish an EAR, and in these situations, adequate intakes (AIs) were set instead. The AI is defined as "the recommended average daily intake value based on observed or experimentally determined approximations or estimates of nutrient intake by a group (or groups) of apparently healthy people who are assumed to be adequate—used when an RDA cannot be determined" (6). In the case of vitamins, AIs were established for vitamin D, vitamin K, pantothenic acid, biotin, and choline. As a recommended intake, the AI is expected to meet or exceed the amount needed to maintain a defined nutritional state or criterion of adequacy in almost all members of an apparently healthy population. In other words, it is likely that the AI would be at or above the RDA if it had been possible to determine the requirement distribution and set a value for the RDA. This is particularly likely to be the case if an AI was based on average intakes of free-living individuals. For example, AIs for infants aged 0–6 months were set for all nutrients (except vitamin D) as the average intake by full-term infants born to presumably healthy, well-nourished mothers and exclusively fed human milk. Under these conditions, infants grow well and it is therefore assumed that their intake from human milk meets or exceeds their requirements.

The AI is similar to the RDA in that both are recommended intake levels for individuals, expected to meet or exceed amounts needed to maintain a specified indicator of adequacy in almost all individuals. However, there is much less certainty about AIs than RDAs, and the presence of an AI is an indication that additional research is required. Eventually, it is hoped that additional knowledge of nutrient requirements will allow AIs to be replaced by EARs and RDAs.

Tolerable Upper Intake Level

The UL is the "highest level of daily nutrient intake that is likely to pose no risk of adverse health effects in almost all apparently healthy individuals in the specified life stage group. As intake increases above the UL, the potential risk of adverse effects increases" (6). Although the UL is thought to represent an intake that the body can biologically tolerate, it is not a recommended intake. There are no established benefits to healthy individuals of intakes that exceed the RDA or AI. It is important to note that the UL is intended to apply to chronic consumption rather than to intakes on any given day, and that it does not apply to individuals who are treated while under medical supervision. For example, the UL for niacin for adults is 35 mg/day, an amount which may be exceeded by individuals who are treated for hypercholesterolemia (2). However, in this situation the individual can be monitored by their physician for adverse effects.

The ULs for nutrients are based on evaluations conducted using a risk assessment framework. An important feature of this process is the concept that adverse effects of nutrients are not expected until intake exceeds a threshold. Just as requirements for nutrients vary among individuals, it appears that the thresholds for adverse effects also vary. An intake that might be tolerated by one individual could result in adverse effects in another. The intent is to set the UL so that it is below the threshold of even the most sensitive members of a group.

At present, ULs have not been set for all vitamins: specifically, vitamin K, thiamin, riboflavin, vitamin B_{12}, biotin, and pantothenic acid do not have ULs. This does not mean that these vitamins are safe in unlimited quantities. In most cases, the data are not sufficient to identify the potential risk of adverse effects.

DIETARY REFERENCE INTAKES FOR VITAMINS

The first DRIs were released in 1997 (1), and included those for vitamin D. Additional vitamin DRIs were published through 2001 (2–4). Table 18.1 shows the DRIs that apply to vitamins, and gives the values for nonpregnant, nonlactating adults. The complete sets of DRI values, including those for infants, children, and adolescents, may be found at http://www.iom.

TABLE 18.1
Vitamin DRIs for Males and Females 19 Years of Age and Older

	EAR	RDA	AI	UL
Vitamin A (μg RAE/day)[a]	500/625[b]	700/900[b]		3000[c]
Vitamin D (μg/day)			5/10/15[d]	50
Vitamin K (μg/day)			90/120[b]	—
Vitamin E (mg/day)	12	15		1000[e]
Vitamin C (mg/day)	60/75[b]	75/90[b]		2000
Thiamin (mg/day)	0.9/1.0[b]	1.1/1.2[b]		—
Riboflavin (mg/day)	0.9/1.1[b]	1.1/1.3[b]		—
Niacin (mg NE/day)[f]	11/12[b]	14/16[b]		35[e]
Vitamin B_6 (mg/day)	1.1/1.3/1.4[g]	1.3/1.5/1.7[g]		100
Vitamin B_{12} (μg/day)	2.0	2.4[h]		—
Folate (μg DFE/day)[i]	320	400		1000[e]
Pantothenic acid (mg/day)			5	—
Biotin (μg/day)			30	—
Choline (mg/day)[j]			425/550[b]	3500

Sources: Food and Nutrition Board, Institute of Medicine, *Dietary Reference Intakes for Calcium, Phosphorus, Magnesium, Vitamin D and Fluoride*, National Academies Press, Washington, DC, 1997; Food and Nutrition Board, Institute of Medicine, *Dietary Reference Intakes for Thiamin, Riboflavin, Niacin, Vitamin B_6, Folate, Vitamin B_{12}, Pantothenic Acid, Biotin, and Choline*, National Academies Press, Washington, DC, 1998; Food and Nutrition Board, Institute of Medicine, *Dietary Reference Intakes for Vitamin C, Vitamin E, Selenium and Carotenoids*, National Academies Press, Washington, DC, 2000; Food and Nutrition Board, Institute of Medicine, *Dietary Reference Intakes for Vitamin A, Vitamin K, Arsenic, Boron, Chromium, Copper, Iodine, Iron, Manganese, Molybdenum, Nickel, Silicon, Vanadium, and Zinc*, National Academies Press, Washington, DC, 2001.

[a] RAE = Retinol activity equivalent.
[b] For women/men.
[c] Applies to intake of preformed vitamin A (retinol) only.
[d] For ages 19–50/51–70/>70 years; amount needed in the absence of adequate exposure to sunlight.
[e] Applies to synthetic forms in supplements and fortified foods.
[f] NE = Niacin equivalent.
[g] For ages 19–50/women >50/men >50.
[h] Adults over 50 are advised to meet the RDA mainly by consuming foods fortified with B_{12} or a supplement containing B_{12}.
[i] DFE = Dietary folate equivalent.
[j] Although AIs have been set for choline, there are few data to assess whether a dietary supply of choline is needed at all stages of the life cycle, and it may be that the choline requirement can be met by endogenous synthesis at some of these stages.

edu/file.asp?id = 21372. Note that most nutrients have several DRIs (e.g., vitamin C has an EAR, an RDA, and a UL); thus it is inappropriate to refer to "the DRI" for a nutrient.

For many of the vitamins, values for children and adolescents are extrapolated from those for adults. For infants <1 year of age, an AI is set based on the vitamin content of breast milk (age 0–6 months) and the combination of breast milk and solid food (age 7–12 months). The requirements for pregnant and lactating women are based on those for nonpregnant, nonlactating females, plus an allowance for daily accumulations by the fetus (during pregnancy) or the average amount secreted in breast milk (during lactation). Following is a brief discussion of the functional criteria used for DRIs for each of the vitamins, as well as any special considerations when using the DRIs. More details on the functions of each vitamin are given in the respective chapters earlier in this book. As discussed later, for some vitamins (vitamin A, vitamin E, and folate), the units for the DRIs differ from those used for the former RDAs and thus may not match the units traditionally used to measure intakes (10,11).

- *Vitamin A* (μg RAE/day): An EAR and RDA, as well as a UL, have been set for vitamin A (4). The primary functional criterion for the EAR is adequate liver vitamin A stores; however, an additional (lower) EAR was also identified for the correction of abnormal dark adaptation in adults. The DRIs for vitamin A are given in microgram of Retinol Activity Equivalents (RAEs), rather than in microgram of retinol equivalents (REs). The new unit reflects current bioavailability studies showing a lower conversion of provitamin A carotenoids to vitamin A. The conversion factors are now one-half of those used previously, so that intake of vitamin A in RAE is lower than intake in RE if any provitamin A carotenoids are in the diet. Thus, intakes in RE should not be used to evaluate vitamin A intakes relative to the DRIs. No DRIs were set for specific carotenoids, although provitamin A carotenoids in the diet contribute to meeting the recommended intakes for vitamin A. The UL for vitamin A applies only to preformed vitamin A (retinol). The UL is based on a risk of liver abnormalities as the critical adverse effect for adults, the risk of teratogenicity for women of child-bearing age, and the risk of a bulging fontanel in infants. The UL for children and adolescents is extrapolated from the UL for adults on the basis of relative body weights.
- *Vitamin D* (μg/day): An AI and a UL were set for vitamin D (as cholecalciferol) for all age groups. One microgram of cholecalciferol is equal to 40 IU of vitamin D. The primary functional criterion for the AI is the maintenance of serum 25(OH) vitamin D concentrations at 27.5 nmol/L. The AI is intended to apply to individuals who do not obtain adequate exposure to sunlight. The requirements are higher for older adults (over 50 years of age) because a variety of factors may reduce cutaneous production of this vitamin. The UL is based on a risk of hypercalcemia at higher intakes of vitamin D.
- *Vitamin K* (μg/day): An AI is set for vitamin K for all age groups. The AI for all age groups except infants is based on the median intake of vitamin K from a national nutrition survey. No UL was set for this vitamin.
- *Vitamin E* (mg/day): Vitamin E has an EAR, RDA, and UL. The functional criterion for the requirement for most age groups is the prevention of hydrogen peroxide–induced hemolysis of red blood cells. The units for the EAR and RDA are milligrams of α-tocopherol (α-T), and not for milligrams of α-tocopherol equivalents (α-TE), as have been used in the past. Other tocopherols and tocotrienols no longer are thought to have vitamin E activity. Furthermore, the requirements apply only to RRR-α-tocopherol (the form of α-tocopherol that occurs naturally in foods), and the 2R-stereoisomeric forms which contribute about half of the α-tocopherol used in most fortified foods and supplements. Thus, vitamin E intakes in α-TE will be higher than intakes in α-T and should not be used to evaluate intakes relative to the DRIs. An approximate conversion factor is milligram α-T = 0.8 × milligram α-TE.

Conversion factors for supplemental and fortification vitamin E in international units (IUs) are 0.45 mg/IU for synthetic vitamin E and 0.67 mg/IU for natural vitamin E. The UL for vitamin E is based on hemorrhagic effects at high intakes. ULs for children and adolescents were extrapolated from those for adults. No UL was set for infants. The UL applies only to forms of the vitamin used for fortification and dietary supplements. Furthermore, the UL applies to all forms of synthetic vitamin E (both the 2R and 2S stereoisomers).

- *Vitamin C* (mg/day): An EAR, RDA, and UL were set for vitamin C. The criterion for the requirement is near-maximal neutrophil concentration of vitamin C. The EAR for most age groups is extrapolated from the EAR for adults 19 through 30 years old. The EAR and RDA are 35 mg/day higher for smokers due to increased oxidative stress and metabolic turnover of vitamin C. A UL was set for all age groups except infants, based on an increased risk of osmotic diarrhea and gastrointestinal disturbances. The ULs for children and adolescents were extrapolated from the UL for adults.
- *Thiamin* (mg/day): The EAR and RDA for thiamin are based on the amount of thiamin needed to achieve and maintain normal erythrocyte transketolase activity while avoiding excessive thiamin excretion. Although body size and energy intake were considered in setting the requirements, the EAR and RDA are not expressed per 1000 kcal, as has been done in the past. No UL was set for this vitamin.
- *Riboflavin* (mg/day): Riboflavin has an EAR and RDA that are based on a combination of indicators, including the excretion of riboflavin and its metabolites, blood values for riboflavin, and the erythrocyte glutathione reductase activity coefficient. As with thiamin, the EAR and RDA for riboflavin are daily intake values and are not expressed relative to energy intake. No UL was set for this vitamin.
- *Niacin* (mg NE/day): For niacin, the EAR and RDA are based on urinary excretion of niacin metabolites. They are expressed in niacin equivalents (NE) to allow for some conversion of tryptophan to niacin. As with thiamin and riboflavin, the EAR and RDA are not expressed relative to energy intake. The UL is based on a risk of flushing at higher niacin intakes in adults, and was extrapolated to children and adolescents. No UL was set for infants. The UL applies only to synthetic forms of the nutrient used for fortification and dietary supplements.
- *Vitamin* B_6 (mg/day): The EAR and RDA for vitamin B_6 are based on the maintenance of an adequate plasma pyridoxal phosphate concentration. Although typical protein intakes were considered when setting the requirements, the requirements are not expressed relative to protein intake. The UL is based on a risk of sensory neuropathy at high intakes. No UL was set for infants.
- *Vitamin* B_{12} (μg/day): For vitamin B_{12}, the EAR and RDA are based on the amount needed for the maintenance of hematological status and serum B_{12} values. No UL was set for this vitamin.
- *Folate* (μg DFE/day): The EAR and RDA for folate are based on the amount needed to maintain erythrocyte folate. The folate requirement applies to naturally occurring folate in food, as well as the monoglutamate form (folic acid) used in fortified foods and supplements. The DRIs for folate are given as micrograms of dietary folate equivalents (DFEs), not in micrograms of folate as has been used in the past. A microgram of food folate is equal to a microgram of DFE, but a microgram of folic acid (from fortification or supplements) is equal to 1.67 DFE. Thus, folate intakes in micrograms will be lower than folate intakes in micrograms DFE, and should not be used to evaluate intakes relative to the DRIs. The UL for folate applies only to synthetic forms of the nutrient used for fortification and dietary supplements. It is based on an examination of case studies of the progression of neurological effects in vitamin B_{12}-deficient individuals taking folate supplements. No UL was set for infants.

- *Pantothenic acid* (mg/day): The AI for pantothenic acid is based on data on pantothenic acid intake that is sufficient to replace urinary excretion. No UL was set for this vitamin.
- *Biotin* (μg/day): The AI for biotin for infants is based on the content of breast milk. For children and adults, the AI is based primarily on an extrapolation from the AI for infants, as well as on limited data on current intakes. No UL was set for this vitamin.
- *Choline* (mg/day): The AI for choline is based on the intake required to maintain liver function as assessed by serum alanine aminotransferase levels. Although an AI was set for all of the age groups, the data for determining the necessity of choline are sparse for some stages of the life cycle. The UL for choline is based primarily on a risk of hypotension. No UL was set for infants.

When this volume was published, all the vitamin DRIs were at least 7 years old, and the DRI for vitamin D was set 10 years ago. Given the availability of new knowledge about the functions and requirements for the vitamins, a periodic review and revision of the vitamin DRIs should be considered.

APPROPRIATE USES OF VITAMIN DIETARY REFERENCE INTAKES

The many uses of the DRIs fall into two broad categories: intake assessment and intake planning (8,12) (Figure 18.2). A further subdivision within each category separates applications for individuals and applications for population groups. Each is briefly discussed here, and in more detail in two reports from the Subcommittee on Interpretation and Uses of the DRIs (8,9). A new paradigm is utilized for many of these applications because the distribution of requirements is specified for most nutrients. This distribution is defined by the EAR, which is the mean of the distribution, and the standard deviation of the EAR. For all vitamins, the distribution is assumed to be normal.

Assessment of individuals: Many uses of the DRIs involve assessing the diets of individuals. Examples include dietary counseling and nutrition education. As the distribution of requirements is given for most nutrients, it is possible to estimate the probability of adequacy (or the probability of inadequacy) for a given intake, assuming that the intake represents an individual's "usual" intake (i.e., what is usually consumed over a long period of time). For example, usual intake at the EAR would have a 50% probability of inadequacy, since by definition, half of the people in the age–sex category have requirements below the EAR and

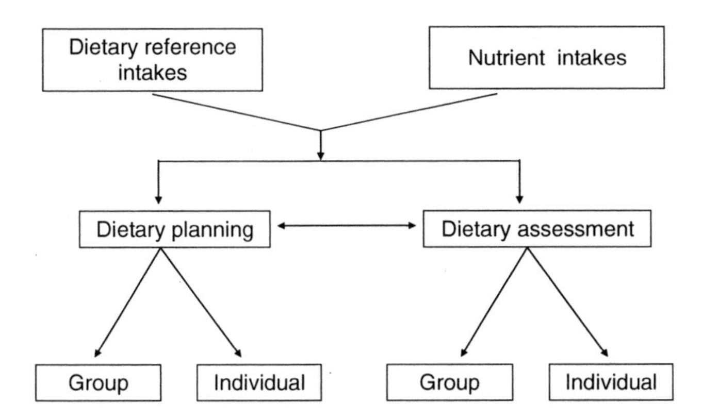

FIGURE 18.2 Conceptual framework for uses of dietary reference intakes. (Adapted from Beaton, G.H. Criteria of an adequate diet. In: Shils, M.E., Olson, J.A., and Shike, M., Eds. *Modern Nutrition in Health and Disease*, 8th Edition. Philadelphia: Lea & Febiger. pp. 1491–1505, 1994; Food and Nutrition Board, Institute of Medicine, *Dietary Reference Intakes: Applications in Dietary Assessment*, National Academies Press, Washington, DC, 2000.)

half have requirements above it. Usual intake at the RDA would have a 97%–98% probability of adequacy, because the RDA is set at a level that meets the needs of 97%–98% of the individuals in the category. Using a simple statistical algorithm, it is possible to calculate the probability of adequacy for any usual intake level. As intakes that are reported or observed are not usually long-term intakes, because of the effect of day-to-day variations in intake, the confidence that these probability estimates are correct is reduced if only a few days of intake are available. An adjustment for this reduced confidence can be made, which allows an evaluation of the *confidence* of adequacy, as well as the *probability* of adequacy. In the past, individual assessment was based on the percent of the RDA in a usual diet because the distribution of requirements was not stated. However, unlike the probability and confidence of adequacy, the percent of the RDA cannot be meaningfully interpreted.

For nutrients with an AI, rather than an EAR/RDA, usual intakes of individuals may be evaluated by comparing the intake to the AI. If intake is above the AI, it is likely to be adequate. However, if the intake is below the AI, the probability of adequacy is unknown. Because an AI is usually higher than an RDA (if one were known), intakes below the AI may still have a high probability of adequacy. An individual's usual intake also may be compared to the UL for a nutrient. Usual intakes above the UL are not desirable because they are at risk of being excessive.

In summary, several DRIs may be used to assess an individual's usual intake: the EAR to estimate the probability of adequacy; the AI, if an EAR is not available, to determine if the probability of adequacy is high; and the UL to estimate whether the intake is at risk of being excessive.

Planning for individuals: The DRIs are frequently used to plan diets for individuals. For example, food guides and dietary guidelines help consumers choose nutritionally adequate diets because they are based on the DRIs. The Nutrition Facts and Supplement Facts labels on consumer products use nutrient standards, although these have not yet been updated to reflect the current DRIs. In addition, both consumers and health professionals may use the DRIs to plan diets with a high probability of nutrient adequacy and a low probability of being excessive. For all of these uses, the RDA is the appropriate target for an individual's intake, and when an RDA is not available, the AI may be used for the same purpose. The EAR is not meant to be a target for individuals. If an individual's usual intake is at or above the RDA or AI, the probability of adequacy is high. Likewise, if the usual intake is below the UL, the risk of adverse effects is low.

Assessment of population groups: The DRIs may be used to assess the intakes of groups of people. This type of assessment is used for national nutrition surveys (such as the National Health and Nutrition Examination Survey, NHANES), and to evaluate food assistance programs (such as the National School Lunch Program). Several statistical assumptions are involved in both assessing and planning intakes of population groups, and these assumptions require that the group contains a minimum number of people. Although the minimum varies across nutrients and applications, a group with 100 people is likely to be sufficient for appropriate statistical calculations.

Assessing the intakes of groups is conceptually more complex than assessing the intakes of individuals, although computer algorithms can greatly simplify this process. For group assessment, the goal is to estimate the *prevalence* of inadequacy within the group, as well as the prevalence of intakes at risk of being excessive. The prevalence of inadequacy may be calculated as the average of the probabilities of inadequacy for each individual in the group. However, for many nutrients, an even easier estimate of the prevalence of inadequacy is possible—the proportion of the group with usual intakes below the EAR is approximately equal to the proportion of the group with inadequate intakes. This EAR "cut-point" approach may be used for nutrients with a normal distribution of requirements, which is thought to be the case for all vitamins. The cut-point approach also assumes that the variation of usual intakes is greater than the variation of requirements within the group, which is true for most intake distributions among free-living populations. Finally, it assumes that intakes and requirements are essentially uncorrelated, which is thought to be true for vitamins. The cut-point method is a useful statistical method of estimating the prevalence of inadequacy in a group. However, it does not mean that the EAR should be used to identify specific individuals in the group with adequate or inadequate intakes. As noted earlier, individuals with usual intakes at the EAR still have a 50% probability of inadequacy.

For nutrients with an AI, the prevalence of inadequate intakes cannot be determined. However, if the median intake of a group is at or above the AI, a low prevalence of inadequacy within the group is likely. This is particularly likely to be true if the AI was based on the intakes of a healthy group. If the median intake is below the AI, it is still possible that the prevalence of inadequacy is low. Thus, no statement about the prevalence of inadequacy can be made for groups with median intakes below the AI.

The prevalence of excessive intakes may be estimated by determining the proportion of usual intakes that is above the UL. It should be noted that this will *not* correspond to the prevalence of the adverse effect used to set the UL. For example, the UL for vitamin C for adults is set at 2000 mg/day, based on the adverse effect of osmotic diarrhea. If a survey indicated that 10% of a group had intakes above the UL, these individuals would be at *potential risk* of the adverse effect. There would not be a 10% prevalence of diarrhea; the actual prevalence would likely be considerably lower because the UL is intended to protect even the most sensitive individuals in the group.

It is important to ensure that the effect of day-to-day variation in intakes has been removed from the intake distribution before calculating either the prevalence of inadequacy or the prevalence of excess. This type of adjustment to the distribution of intakes can be made using computer algorithms. One algorithm is described in Appendix E of the IOM report on planning diets (9). Software to make the adjustment is also available (13). Figure 18.3 shows

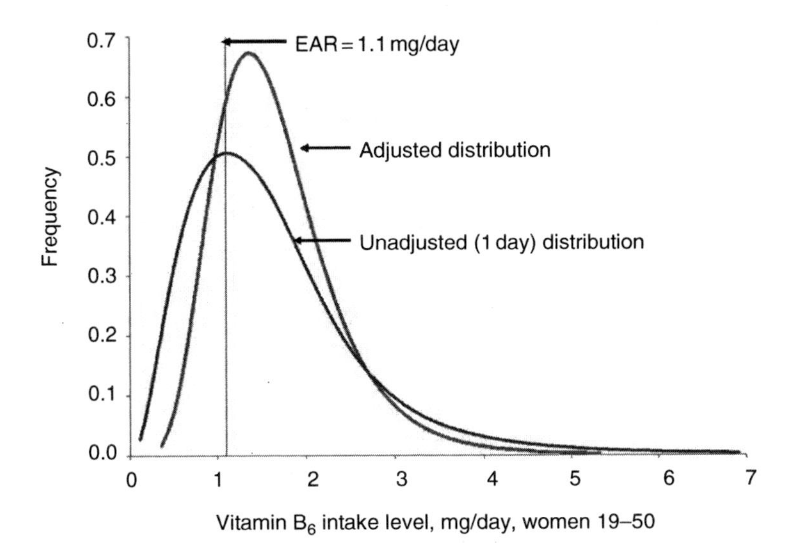

FIGURE 18.3 Vitamin B_6 intake distributions for women 19–50 years. A distribution of 1 day intakes is compared to a distribution that has been adjusted to represent usual intakes. Note that the proportion of the distribution that falls below the EAR is considerably less with the adjusted usual intake distribution than with 1 day of intake. (Adapted from Food and Nutrition Board, Institute of Medicine, *Dietary Reference Intakes: Applications in Dietary Assessment*, National Academies Press, Washington, DC, 2000.)

the effect of removing day-to-day variation from a distribution of vitamin B_6 intakes, and the difference in estimates of the prevalence of inadequacy before and after the adjustment.

In summary, several of the DRIs are used to assess the intakes of groups: the EAR is used to estimate the prevalence of inadequate intakes, and the UL is used to estimate the prevalence of excessive intakes. It is important to adjust intake distributions to reflect usual intakes before using these procedures. For nutrients with an AI, but not an EAR, it is only possible to determine if the prevalence of inadequacy is likely to be low. The RDA is not used to assess the intake of groups.

Planning for groups: There are numerous uses of the DRIs for planning intakes of population groups. Examples include planning for institutional feeding, food assistance programs, and military rations. Planning intakes for population groups relies on the same concepts as assessing intakes of groups. The goal of the planning activity is to minimize the prevalence of inadequate intakes and also the prevalence of excessive intakes within the group of interest. Planning and assessment are closely linked, as it is not usually possible to predict the actual outcome of the planning activity.

Planning intakes for groups involves several steps. The first is to identify the nutrients of interest, as well as the acceptable prevalences of inadequacy and excess. Although 2%–3% has often been used as an acceptable prevalence for both of these indicators, such targets may not always be feasible or even desirable. The next step is to examine the current usual intake distribution for a nutrient and decide if the distribution needs to be shifted up (or down) to improve the prevalences of adequacy and excess. As with any assessment using the DRIs, it is important that intake distribution be adjusted to reflect usual intakes. The third step is to determine the amount of the shift that is needed. The magnitude of the shift can be approximated using the EAR and the UL as cut-points. For example, if 30% of the group has usual intakes of vitamin C below the EAR, then intakes need to be increased by an amount that shifts the distribution so that only 2%–3% have vitamin C intakes below the EAR (if that is the target that was chosen). Such a shift would require that all intakes increase by a specific amount (e.g., 10 mg of vitamin C) if the shape of the distribution is unchanged. It is also important to determine if the shift would cause an undesirable increase in the prevalence of intakes above the UL, again assuming that the shape of the intake distribution does not change. Because assuming that the distribution shape will not change is likely to be unrealistic, it is crucial that an assessment activity takes place after the new feeding plan is implemented.

In some cases, it may be desirable to try to change the shape of the distribution as part of the planning activity. This might be accomplished, for example, by trying to target those individuals whose usual intake has the highest probability of inadequacy. For these individuals, nutrition education programs could be provided, or specific foods or supplements could be made available to them. Once the group is subdivided so that particular individuals are targeted, their diets would be planned using the methodology described earlier for planning intakes for individuals. The group planning activity would now apply to the remainder of the group, with these individuals removed.

The AI may be used as the target for the median intake of the group, if an EAR is not available. For nutrients with an AI, the goal is to increase the median intake to at least the level of the AI, without increasing the prevalence of excessive intakes.

Planning intakes for groups is not a simple task. The steps described earlier need to be undertaken for each nutrient of interest, and then the results must be translated into foods to be provided and menus for actual meals. This activity also requires assumptions about the amount of food that will be chosen and consumed by individuals in the group. Again, given the many assumptions involved, it is crucial that an assessment activity follows the implementation of the feeding plan.

For some groups, the individuals within the group are not homogeneous. For example, there may be a mix of gender categories within the group, such as boys and girls

TABLE 18.2
Uses of Dietary Reference Intakes (DRIs) for Planning and Assessing Nutrient Intakes of Apparently Healthy Individuals and Groups

DRI	Individual	Group
Assessment		
EAR	Use (with information on variability of requirement and intake) to examine the probability that usual intake is inadequate	The proportion of the group with usual intake below the EAR estimates the group prevalence of inadequacy
RDA	Usual intake at or above the RDA has a low probability of inadequacy	Do not use to assess intakes of groups
AI	Intake at or above the AI can be assumed adequate. No assessment can be made if intake is below the AI	Median usual intake at or above the AI implies a low prevalence of inadequate intakes.[a] No assessment can be made if median intake is below the AI
UL	Usual intake above the UL may place an individual at risk of adverse effects from excessive intake	The proportion of a group with usual intake above the UL is at potential risk of adverse effects of excessive intake
Planning		
EAR	Do not use the EAR as an intake goal; usual intake at this level has a 50% probability of inadequacy	Plan for an acceptably low proportion of a group with intakes below the EAR. Note that mean intake is likely to be above the RDA
RDA	Aim for this intake; usual intake at or above the RDA has a low probability of inadequacy	Do not use the RDA to plan mean intakes for groups. In almost all cases, mean intake at the RDA will lead to an unacceptably high prevalence of inadequate intakes
AI	Aim for this intake; usual intake at or above the AI has a low probability of inadequacy	Plan for median intake at this level; median usual intake at or above the AI implies a low prevalence of inadequate intakes[a]
UL	Plan for usual intake to remain below the UL to avoid potential risk of adverse effect from excessive intake	Plan to minimize the proportion of a group with intakes above the UL to minimize potential risk of adverse effects of excessive intake

Sources: Food and Nutrition Board, Institute of Medicine, *Dietary Reference Intakes: Applications in Dietary Assessment*, National Academies Press, Washington, DC, 2000; Food and Nutrition Board, Institute of Medicine, *Dietary Reference Intakes: Applications in Dietary Planning*, National Academies Press, Washington, DC, 2003.

[a] The AI should be used with less confidence if it has not been established as a median intake of a healthy group.

in a school feeding program. If the EAR and UL for boys are used for the planning activity, then the prevalences of inadequacy and excess may not be acceptable for the girls. Often, an iterative process is necessary to set appropriate planning goals for such heterogeneous groups.

The appropriate uses of the DRIs are summarized in Table 18.2. These issues are discussed in more detail in the IOM reports on uses of the DRIs (8,9) and also in several published journal articles (14–19).

CONCLUSIONS

DRIs are available for 14 vitamins. All the DRIs are based on a specific functional indicator of adequacy (for the EAR, RDA, and AI) or indicator of risk of adverse effects (for the UL). Furthermore, a distribution of requirements is given for most of the vitamins, which allows many new uses of these nutrient standards. In addition to new applications related to assessing and planning intakes for individuals, there are expanded opportunities to assess and plan intakes for population groups. The first vitamin DRIs (for vitamin D) were released in 1997 and thus are now over 10 years old. A periodic review and revision of the vitamin DRIs should be considered.

REFERENCES

1. Food and Nutrition Board, Institute of Medicine. *Dietary Reference Intakes for Calcium, Phosphorus, Magnesium, Vitamin D and Fluoride.* Washington, DC: National Academies Press, 1997.
2. Food and Nutrition Board, Institute of Medicine. *Dietary Reference Intakes for Thiamin, Riboflavin, Niacin, Vitamin B_6, Folate, Vitamin B_{12}, Pantothenic Acid, Biotin, and Choline.* Washington, DC: National Academies Press, 1998.
3. Food and Nutrition Board, Institute of Medicine. *Dietary Reference Intakes for Vitamin C, Vitamin E, Selenium and Carotenoids.* Washington, DC: National Academies Press, 2000.
4. Food and Nutrition Board, Institute of Medicine. *Dietary Reference Intakes for Vitamin A, Vitamin K, Arsenic, Boron, Chromium, Copper, Iodine, Iron, Manganese, Molybdenum, Nickel, Silicon, Vanadium, and Zinc.* Washington, DC: National Academies Press, 2001.
5. Food and Nutrition Board, Institute of Medicine. *Dietary Reference Intakes for Energy, Carbohydrate, Fiber, Fat, Fatty Acids, Cholesterol, Protein, and Amino Acids (Macronutrients).* Washington, DC: National Academies Press, 2002.
6. Food and Nutrition Board, Institute of Medicine. *Dietary Reference Intakes for Water, Potassium, Sodium, Chloride, and Sulfate.* Washington, DC: National Academies Press, 2004.
7. Food and Nutrition Board, Institute of Medicine. *Dietary Reference Intakes: A Risk Assessment Model for Establishing Upper Intake Levels for Nutrients.* Washington, DC: National Academies Press, 1998.
8. Food and Nutrition Board, Institute of Medicine. *Dietary Reference Intakes: Applications in Dietary Assessment.* Washington, DC: National Academies Press, 2000.
9. Food and Nutrition Board, Institute of Medicine. *Dietary Reference Intakes: Applications in Dietary Planning.* Washington, DC: National Academies Press, 2003.
10. Murphy, S.P. Dietary reference intakes for the US and Canada: Update on implications for nutrient databases. *J. Food Comp. Anal.*, 2002;15:411–417.
11. Murphy, S.P. Changes in dietary guidance: Implications for food and nutrient databases. *J. Food Comp. Anal.*, 2001;14:269–278.
12. Beaton, G.H. Criteria of an adequate diet. In: Shils, M.E., Olson, J.A., and Shike, M., Eds. *Modern Nutrition in Health and Disease*, 8th Edition. Philadelphia: Lea & Febiger. pp. 1491–1505, 1994.
13. Carriquiry, A. Assessing the prevalence of nutrient adequacy. *Public Health Nutr.*, 1999;2:23–33.
14. Murphy, S.P., Barr, S.I., and Poos, M.I. Using the new dietary reference intakes to assess diets: A map to the maze. *Nutr. Rev.*, 2002;60:267–275.
15. Murphy, S.P. Impact of the new Dietary Reference Intakes on nutrient calculation programs. *J. Food Comp. Anal.*, 2003;16:365–372.
16. Stumbo, P.J. and Murphy, S.P. Simple plots tell a complex story: Using the EAR, RDA, AI and UL to evaluate nutrient intakes. *J. Food Comp. Anal.*, 2004;17:485–492.
17. Barr, S.I., Murphy, S.P., Agurs-Collins, T., and Poos, M.I. Planning diets for individuals using the Dietary Reference Intakes. *Nutr. Rev.*, 2003;61:352–360.
18. Murphy, S.P. and Barr, S.I. Challenges in using the DRIs to plan diets for groups. *Nutr. Rev.*, 2005; 105:1275–1279.
19. Barr, S.I., Murphy, S., and Poos, M.I. Interpreting and using the dietary reference intakes in assessment of individuals and groups. *J. Am. Diet Assoc.*, 2002;102:780–788.

Index

B

C

D

E

F

G

I

J

K

L

M

N

O

P

Q

R

S

U

V

W

X

Y

Z